Advanced Practice Nursing *of* Adults *in* Acute Care

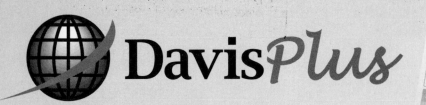
 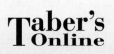

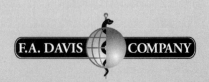

Advanced Practice Nursing *of* Adults *in* Acute Care

Janet G. Whetstone Foster, PhD, APRN, CNS, CCRN
Associate Professor
Texas Woman's University College of Nursing
Houston, Texas

Suzanne S. Prevost, RN, PhD, COI
Associate Dean, Practice and Community Engagement
President, Sigma Theta Tau International
Robert Wood Johnson Executive Nurse Fellow
University of Kentucky College of Nursing
Lexington, Kentucky

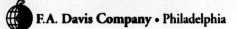 **F.A. Davis Company** • Philadelphia

F. A. Davis Company
1915 Arch Street
Philadelphia, PA19103
www.fadavis.com

Printed in the United States of America

Last digit indicates print number: 10 9 8 7 6 5 4 3 2 1

Publisher, Nursing: Joanne Patzek DaCunha, RN, MSN
Director of Content Development: Darlene D. Pedersen
Project Editor: Jamie M. Elfrank
Design and Illustration Manager: Carolyn O'Brien

As new scientific information becomes available through basic and clinical research, recommended treatments and drug therapies undergo changes. The author(s) and publisher have done everything possible to make this book accurate, up to date, and in accord with accepted standards at the time of publication. The author(s), editors, and publisher are not responsible for errors or omissions or for consequences from application of the book, and make no warranty, expressed or implied, in regard to the contents of the book. Any practice described in this book should be applied by the reader in accordance with professional standards of care used in regard to the unique circumstances that may apply in each situation. The reader is advised always to check product information (package inserts) for changes and new information regarding dose and contraindications before administering any drug. Caution is especially urged when using new or infrequently ordered drugs.

Library of Congress Cataloging-in-Publication Data

Foster, Janet G. Whetstone.
  Advanced practice nursing of adults in acute care / Janet G. Whetstone Foster, Suzanne S. Prevost.
    p. ; cm.
  Includes bibliographical references and index.
  ISBN 978-0-8036-2162-6 (alk. paper)
  I. Prevost, Suzanne S. II. Title.
  [DNLM: 1. Acute Disease—nursing. 2. Advanced Practice Nursing—methods. WB 105]

  616.20231—dc23

                                                    2011036226

To my husband, Bob, who has provided inspiration and support for this and all my projects throughout the years. Love and kisses . . .

To my parents, who taught me to value hard work and appreciate the good that could come of it.

To my siblings, Ellen, Rich, Rob, and Dave, who have always expressed their pride in my accomplishments (without "rivalry").

To niece Cathy and sister Marge, who were always on my mind as I edited the hematology/oncology chapter.

To my dog Rockstar, who was snuggled at my feet at the beginning of the project, and Lemon, who is here for the conclusion.

Janet G. Whetstone Foster

To my husband, Frank—for 28 years of support, encouragement, and friendship. Thanks for tolerating my workaholic tendencies and for occasionally forcing me to break away for fun.

To my daughter Liz—my most important contribution to the nursing profession. Thanks for allowing me to vicariously relive my professional youth through your clinical encounters and for the constant reminder of the challenges experienced by acute care nurses.

To my daughter Emily—the spiritual and creative one. Thanks for keeping the faith, for challenging me to make use of new technology, and for reminding me to also use the right side of my brain.

To my dean, Jane Kirschling—for being an inspirational leader, mentor, and friend. Thank you for giving all of us the support and flexibility to do work such as this.

Suzanne S. Prevost

The idea for this book arose from our experience teaching clinical nurse specialist (CNS) students over the years, when we were forced to "piecemeal" required readings from numerous sources because no one textbook provided content appropriate to CNS practice. A majority of CNSs practice in hospitals (versus outpatient or primary care settings). They manage patients who suffer from disease and nondisease causes of illness, with acuity levels falling below that of critical illness, and who are cared for outside of the intensive care unit. We mention this because the textbooks we have historically used were written for either primary care or critical care practitioners. Additionally, CNSs are charged with not only influencing care for individual patients but also enhancing quality outcomes for populations of patients and improving systems of care for hospitalized patients. Our visions for this text were to integrate the CNS competencies and spheres of influence with advanced clinical management and to focus on health problems for hospitalized adult patients, with an acuity level that falls between primary care and critical care.

The book is organized around a "body systems" approach to enable advanced practice nurses to safely care for hospitalized adults in the acute care setting. In addition, nursing sensitive indicators, nondisease etiologic causes of illness, and assessment and management at the advanced level are addressed, including nursing and medical management, differential diagnosis, and pharmacologic and nonpharmacologic aspects of prescriptive authority. The three spheres of influence and seven core competencies of the CNS provide the conceptual framework for the role components addressed in the text and are incorporated into each chapter.

Chapters 1 and 2 focus on *Influencing Practice*. Chapter 1 provides a historical perspective of advanced practice and the four roles, with an emphasis on the CNS. The spheres of influence are explained, along with core competencies. Chapter 2 addresses nondisease causes of illness that are problematic for patients, cost outliers for hospitals, and challenges for nurses that often necessitate the expertise of the CNS.

Chapters 3 through 7 concentrates on *Clinical Issues of Concern*. Chapter 3 includes a detailed account of the pathophysiology of pain and a comprehensive approach to management. Chapter 4 focuses on health problems associated with aging and incorporates newly released competencies for CNSs working with older adults. Chapter 5 covers palliative and end-of-life care for patients and families, a common source of expertise often provided by CNSs. Chapter 6 concerns psychosocial health problems that sometimes serve as a primary reason for hospitalization (injuries associated with violence and abuse) or are comorbid conditions that the CNS must address in the plan of care (substance abuse and withdrawal syndromes, anxiety, and depression). Chapter 7 addresses management of challenging wounds associated with a variety of conditions such as diabetes, peripheral vascular disease, and compartment syndrome.

Chapters 8 through 17 addresses *System-Based Health Problems* and incorporates every major body system. Each chapter includes numerous diseases that CNSs are most likely to encounter in hospitalized patients. A comprehensive account of background such as incidence/prevalence, risk factors, etiology, and associated costs; pathophysiology; diagnostic procedures; and management is included. In addition, each chapter provides examples of ways CNSs influence the care of patients, practice of nurses and other professionals, and health care systems through operationalizing the relevant CNS core competencies.

Although the text will provide many links to electronic resources, we hope that this text is comprehensive enough to meet the educational needs of CNS students so that faculty no longer find it necessary to "piecemeal" resources for students. We hope that students are spared the need to purchase multiple texts in an attempt to meet the educational requirements of their specialty and still fall short of the depth and breadth required of expert clinicians. Finally and most importantly, we hope that patients and families, nurses and other professionals, and health care organizations can benefit from having CNSs prepared with a comprehensive approach: integration of patient management problems with CNS core competencies.

Paul Arnstein, PhD, APRN-BC, FAAN
Clinical Nurse Specialist for Pain Relief
Massachusetts General Hospital
Boston, Massachusetts

Paul Bernstein, MD
Clinical Associate Professor of Medicine
Department of Internal Medicine
Division of Nephrology
Rochester General Hospital
University of Rochester
Program Director
Rochester General Hospital Internal Medicine
Residency Program
Rochester, New York

Amy Brin, MSN, MA, APRN, ACHPN, CNL
Advanced Practice Nurse
Hospice of the Bluegrass/Palliative Care Center of the
  Bluegrass
Adjunct Faculty
University of Kentucky College of Nursing
Lexington, Kentucky

**Damon B. Cottrell, MS, RN, CCNS, CCRN,
  ACNS-BC, CEN**
Assistant Professor
University of New England
Portland, Maine

Margaret M. Ecklund, MS, RN, CCRN, ACNP-BC
Nurse Practitioner
Pulmonary Medicine
Rochester General Health System
Rochester, New York

**Janet G. Whetstone Foster, PhD, APRN, CNS,
  CCRN**
Associate Professor
Texas Woman's University College of Nursing
Houston, Texas

Tari Gilbert, MSN, FNP-BC
Nurse Practitioner
Study Coordinator
Principal Investigator
University of California, San Diego
San Diego, California

Marvin Grieff, MD
Clinical Associate Professor of Medicine
Department of Internal Medicine
Division of Nephrology
Rochester General Hospital and University of
  Rochester School of Medicine
Rochester, New York

Diana Jones, MSN, RN, ACNS-BC
St. Vincent Hospital
Indianapolis, Indiana

Yassaman Khalili, MSc, RN, CNS
Adult Clinical Nurse Specialist—Surgical Unit
Massachusetts General Hospital
Boston, Massachusetts

Stephen D. Krau, PhD, RN, CNE
Associate Professor
Vanderbilt University School of Nursing
Nashville, Tennessee

**Laura G. Leahy, MSN, APN, CRNP,
  PMH-CNS/FNP, BC**
Psychiatric Advanced Practice Nurse
Associate Clinical Professor
University of Pennsylvania, School of Nursing
Philadelphia, Pennsylvania

**Cheryl A. Lehman, PhD, RN, CNS-BC, RN-BC,
  CRRN**
Associate Professor/Clinical
The University of Texas Health Science Center
  at San Antonio
School of Nursing
San Antonio, Texas

**Celia Levesque, RN, MSN, CNS-BC, CDE,
  BC-ADM**
Advanced Practice Nurse, Division of Internal Medicine
Department of Endocrine Neoplasia and Hormonal
  Disorders
MD Anderson Cancer Center
Houston, Texas

Sarah L. Livesay, MSN, APRN, CNS
Manager of Neuroscience Clinical Programs
St. Luke's Episcopal Hospital
Houston, Texas

Sharon E. Lock, PhD, APRN, FNP-BC
Associate Professor
Coordinator of Primary Care Nurse Practitioner Track
University of Kentucky College of Nursing
Lexington, Kentucky

Rebecca Long, MS, RN, CMSRN, ACNS-BC
Clinical Nurse Specialist
Academic Educator
VA Healthcare System/San Diego University
VA Health Care San Diego
San Diego, California

Karen C. Lyon, PhD, APRN, ACNS, NEA
Associate Dean and Professor
Nelda C. Stark College of Nursing
Texas Woman's University
Houston, Texas

Hannah Felton Lyons, MSN, RN, AOCN
Oncology Clinical Nurse Specialist
Massachusetts General Hospital
Boston, Massachusetts

Kate Moore, DNP, RN, CCRN, CEN, ACNP-BC, ANP-BC, GNP-BC
Acute Care Nurse Practitioner
Trauma and Critical Care Surgery
Assistant Professor
College of Nursing
University of Kentucky
Lexington, Kentucky

Paul Netzel, MSN, RN, ACNP
Acute Care Nurse Practitioner
University of Kentucky
Lexington, Kentucky

Jan Powers, PhD, RN, CCNS, CCRN, CNRN, FCCM
Director of Clinical Nurse Specialist and Nursing Research
Critical Care Clinical Nurse Specialist
St. Vincent Hospital
Indianapolis, Indiana

Suzanne S. Prevost, RN, PhD, COI
Associate Dean, Practice and Community Engagement
President, Sigma Theta Tau International
Robert Wood Johnson Executive Nurse Fellow
University of Kentucky College of Nursing
Lexington, Kentucky

Julie E. Rosof-Williams, MSN, APRN, FNP-BC, SANE-P, SANE-A
Assistant in the Department of Pediatrics
Vanderbilt University, School of Medicine
Instructor in Nursing
Vanderbilt University, School of Nursing
Nashville, Tennessee

Brenda K. Shelton, MS, RN, CCRN, AOCN, CNS
Clinical Nurse Specialist
The Sidney Kimmel Comprehensive Cancer Center at Johns Hopkins
Baltimore, Maryland

Cathy J. Thompson, PhD, RN, CCNS
Associate Professor, CNS Option Coordinator
University of Colorado, Denver
College of Nursing
Aurora, Colorado

Christopher A. Weatherspoon, RN, MS, FNP-BC
Tennessee Valley Healthcare System
Nashville Campus
Veterans Affairs
Nashville, Tennessee

Deborah L. Weatherspoon, RNH, CRNA, MSN
Assistant Professor
Middle Tennessee State University
Murfreesboro, Tennessee

Tricia Bernecker, MSN, PhDc, RN, ACNS-BC
Assistant Professor
DeSales University
Center Valley, Pennsylvania

Linda Callahan, PhD, RN, CRNA, NP
Professor
School of Nursing
California State University, Long Beach
Long Beach, California

Stephanie Chalupka, EdD, RN, PHCNS-BC,
   FAAOHN
Professor and Director
Master of Science in Nursing Programs
Worcester State College
Worcester, Massachusetts

Julie Ann Davey, MSN, RN, ANP, ACNP, NP
Clinical Faculty
Emory University
Atlanta, Georgia

Tracy K. Fasolino, PhD, FNP-BC
Assistant Professor
Clemson University
Salem, South Carolina

Jane Flanagan, PhD, ANP-BC
Assistant Professor
Boston College
Chesnut Hill, Massachusetts

Debra Hain, DNS, APRN, GNP-BC
Assistant Professor
Florida Atlantic University
Christine E. Lynn College of Nursing
Boca Raton, Florida

Mary Jane S. Hanson, PhD, CRNP, CNS, RN,
   FNP-BC, ACNS-BC, ANP-BC
Professor and Director
Graduate Nursing Program
The University of Scranton
Scranton, Pennsylvania

Valerie Hart, EdD, APRN, BC, CNS
Associate Professor of Nursing
University of Southern Maine
Portland, Maine

Heidi He, MSN, FNP
Nursing Faculty, Lecture
California State University, Bakersfield
Bakersfield, California

Mary Alice Hodge, PhD, TN
Assistant Professor/BSN Director
Gardner-Webb University
Boiling Springs, North Carolina

Joyce Young Johnson, MN, PhD, RN
Dean, College of Sciences and Health Professions
Albany State University
Albany, Georgia

Katharine A. Kelly, DNP, RN, FNP-C, CEN
Assistant Professor, Nursing
California State University, Sacramento
Sacramento, California

Ramona Browder Lazenby, EdD, RN, FNP-BC, CNE
Professor and Associate Dean of Nursing
Auburn University at Montgomery School of Nursing
Montgomery, Alabama

Christine E. Lynn
College of Nursing
Florida Atlantic University
Boca Raton, Florida

Mary Sue Marz, PhD, RN
Professor
School of Nursing
Eastern Michigan University
Ypsilanti, Michigan

Susan E. Steele, PhDm, RN, CWOCN
Assistant Professor
Georgia College and State University
Milledgeville, Georgia

Nancy Stephenson, PhD, APRN, BC
Associate Professor
East Carolina University
Beaufort, North Carolina

Laura B. Sutton, PhD, CNS-BC
Clinical Assistant Professor
University of Florida College of Nursing
Gainesville, Florida

Sharon J. Thompson, PhD, RN, MPH
Associate Professor of Nursing
Advisor, Nurse Anesthesia Option
Gannon University
Villa Maria School of Nursing
Erie, Pennsylvania

Vickie Walker, DNP, RN
Assistant Professor
Gardner-Webb University
Boiling Springs, North Carolina

Barbara Wilder, DSN, CRNP
Associate Professor
Auburn University School of Nursing
Auburn, Alabama

ACKNOWLEDGMENTS

There are many people who have helped bring this project to fruition. We would like to acknowledge Joanne DaCunha, who sold our idea to the decision-makers at F. A. Davis in the beginning and has been with us throughout the development to offer her thoughtful feedback, possible only from a seasoned veteran in the business. Numerous other individuals at F. A. Davis deserve recognition: Tyler Baber guided us early on; Maureen Grealish has been steadfast in keeping us on schedule; and Jamie Elfrank has an attention for detail required of any leading publisher of textbooks. Many others in the art and production departments warrant recognition; some of the chapters required extraordinary artwork and creativity to enhance the quality of the book, for which we are grateful.

We would like to express a special thank you to our contributors. These are very busy people who enthusiastically took on the work of writing a chapter, in addition to their usual workload. Many are former students of ours. They are all respected experts in their field, and we are humbled to have them participate in this project.

CONTENTS

CHAPTER 1

Advanced Practice Nursing: Clinical Nurse Specialist (CNS) Practice

Damon B. Cottrell, MS, RN, CCNS, CCRN, ACNS-BC, CEN

INTRODUCTION

A number of forces are present in the current health care environment that beget a myriad of opportunities for application of advanced nursing practice. The aging population, current and worsening nursing shortage, steadily increasing patient acuity, escalating complexity of patient care, rapid evolution of medical technology, and expansion of nursing and medical knowledge all lend great need for nurses engaged in advanced practice roles. In addition to these environmental forces, there has been significant movement within the advancement of the nursing profession, specifically, within advanced practice nursing.

There has been a great emphasis on care quality and patient safety since the landmark Institute of Medicine (IOM) report "To Err Is Human: Building a Safer Healthcare System" published in 1999 that indicated between 44,000 and 98,000 deaths occur each in year hospitals due to medical error (1). Following this report, the IOM published "Crossing the Quality Chasm: A New Health System for the 21st Century" in 2001 (2). This report called for monumental change in the U.S. health care delivery system, reporting that the system falls short of integrating knowledge gained through medical science and technology into practice (2). Due to this "chasm," in many cases patients do not receive optimal care and some are even harmed (2). A multitude of regulatory agencies and health care–related organizations have taken note. Regulatory agencies such as The Joint Commission (TJC) and the Centers for Medicare and Medicaid Services (CMS) have built quality initiatives into their standards, with the expectation that organizations will comply and

improve the quality of care they provide to their clients. As of October 1, 2008, CMS has implemented a pay-for-performance initiative that bases reimbursement on quality standard achievement of individual organizations. This initiative is one of many that led to the impetus for great change in the way care delivery occurs, and it is likely to be followed by private insurers. Other organizations, such as the Institute for Healthcare Improvement (IHI), have initiated campaigns in which specific initiatives and "bundles" of evidence-based care have been provided to assist health care facilities in achieving the goal of quality patient care.

Health care redesign, restructuring, and reform have increased the demand for advanced practice registered nurses (APRNs). This turbulent, difficult time in health care sets the stage for advanced practice nurses to contribute their significant knowledge, skill, and passion for optimal patient and family outcomes. Even more than before, the time is right for demonstrating the benefits of the breadth and depth of advanced training, education, and practice. The four roles—nurse practitioners, nurse midwives, nurse anesthetists, and clinical nurse specialists (CNSs)—each have distinct and vital contributions. The first three primarily make significant contributions to direct care. The CNS is uniquely prepared for addressing quality via direct care, indirect care working through and with others, and from a systems perspective.

A FOCUS ON QUALITY

Since the landmark IOM report and subsequent reports of breaks in quality of care, there has been a significant emphasis put forward by quality-driven organizations to oversee and drive the changes required to address these troublesome issues.

The National Quality Forum (NQF) is a nonprofit organization driven to implement a national strategy for health care quality measurement and reporting (3). The NQF has developed a list of 28 medical errors called *never events*. The meaning is exactly what it infers—that these particular events should never occur. Facilities must enact processes to ensure that these events do not occur. As noted, the list is expansive and includes 28 specific situations. Some examples include surgery performed on the wrong patient or body part, patient death or injury related to medication error, patient death or injury associated with hypoglycemia, pressure ulcers, and more.

Over 1100 health care facilities contribute to the National Database of Nursing Quality Indicators (NDNQI), which is the only database with data collected at the nursing unit level (4). The database began in 1994 and has secured an ongoing focus on nursing sensitive indicators. The data are submitted by participating facilities and then benchmarked against like groupings of units. These indicators include rate of falls, pressure ulcer prevalence, and others.

The CMS has sets of core measures that are evidence-based practices (EBPs) known to improve the care for patients with specific problems or diagnoses. These measures are selected due to high patient volumes combined with a myriad of opportunities for improvement within clinical care. The broad categories include heart failure, acute myocardial infarction, pneumonia, and surgical care, with more on the horizon. Institutions are required to report outcomes on these specific measures and outcomes drive reimbursement; the better the institutional outcomes and the greater the reimbursement.

TJC continues to be a source driving quality within health care institutions. Each year, a new set of national patient safety goals (NPSGs) are developed and intended to be implemented. Again, the focus is on quality and preventing adverse events. There are many other organizations with the focus on quality-driven outcomes. The IHI has implemented a 100,000 Lives Campaign and the subsequent Five Million Lives campaign. These initiatives led to the implementations of other quality processes, including rapid response teams, heart failure care, pressure ulcer prevention, preventing central line infections, and more.

Other related designations have come into the health care arena that have a significant focus on quality, but perhaps from a larger perspective. The Magnet designation is awarded by the credentialing arm of the American Nurses Association (ANA), or the American Nurses Credentialing Center (ANCC). This designation focuses on nursing as a whole within a particular organization. It uses forces of magnetism to guide organizations through distinctive and exceptional processes, leading to an environment that is a "magnet" for nurses to work and want to work. Magnet facilities are known for a high degree of autonomy and quality outcomes.

On a similar note, the American Association of Critical Care Nurses provides a Beacon award for adult and pediatric critical care and progressive care units. This particular award looks at individual units and evaluates more than 30 criteria that are indicative of overall quality and exceptional care environments.

WHAT IS ADVANCED PRACTICE NURSING?

There are many definitions of *advanced practice nursing*. It is important to reiterate that this term is an umbrella term for the four specific APRN roles. Most of these definitions are quite similar. An APRN is a nurse who is prepared through a master's or doctoral program and has acquired advanced clinical knowledge and skills that are built on a foundation of nursing practice. It is the advanced clinical knowledge and skill in the provision of direct care that form the linchpin of advanced practice. The APRN is prepared for and responsible for the use of prescription of pharmacologic and nonpharmacologic interventions. The comprehensive definition of an APRN as delineated in the APRN Consensus Model document is included in Table 1–1.

Within the four APRN roles, the nurse midwife and nurse anesthetist roles have traditionally been well defined in practice. The nurse practitioner role has also been fairly well defined; however, there has been some lack of clarity between the roles of the nurse practitioner and the CNS. The nurse practitioner typically devotes the majority of time in direct care to patients. Direct care is confined to a patient population, according to education and demonstrated knowledge and skill in preparation for the role. These populations have traditionally included family, adult, geriatric, pediatric, and acute care. Nurse practitioners manage problems, promote health, and provide patient education.

The CNS also provides direct care. This provision of care is often only a part or even perhaps only represents a percentage of the responsibilities of the role. This role also has other significant subroles. The CNS also spends a significant amount of time acting within these educator, leader, researcher and consultant subroles. The subroles allow the CNS to navigate highly complex systems in order to achieve quality outcomes.

The Clinical Nurse Specialist (CNS)

The National Association of Clinical Nurse Specialists (NACNS) defines a CNS as a licensed registered nurse with graduate preparation in a CNS program who is an expert clinician in a specialized area of nursing that may include a population, setting, disease, medical subspecialty,

TABLE 1–1 Definition of the APRN

Graduate level education preparing for one of the four APRN roles (CNS, NP, NM, CRNA)

Passed a national certification examination that measures the APRN role and population-focused competencies (includes maintenance of certification indicating continued competence)

Acquired advanced clinical knowledge and skill in preparing for direct care to patients (includes indirect care activities, yet the "defining factor" is that a significant component of the educational program is focused on direct care)

Practice built on registered nurse foundation, yet greater depth and breadth of knowledge, synthesis of data, complexity of skills/interventions, and increased role autonomy

Educationally prepared, accountable, and responsible for health promotion/maintenance, assessment, diagnosis, and management of patient problems (includes preparation for prescription of pharmacologic and nonpharmacologic interventions)

Clinical experience reflecting the intended license

Licensed to practice as an APRN in one of the four roles (CRNA, CNS, NP, CNM)

type of care, or patient problem (5). It is the highly focused training within a specialty that sets the CNS apart. The CNS is uniquely trained to provide expert practice. They consult and participate in quality improvement initiatives in order to reduce medical errors. The CNS also ensures the use and implementation of EBP by nursing staff through education and contributes to nursing and medical knowledge through research. Within an even larger scope, the CNS implements and evaluates systems and processes within the matrix of highly complex health delivery systems.

History and Milestones in CNS Practice

There are references crediting the first thought of nursing specialization back to 1900 as portrayed in an article in the *American Journal of Nursing* (6, 7). In her article and in the context of the time period, Katherine DeWitt wrote about the earlier times when the physician practiced within all specialties, including gynecology, surgery, apothecary, and more, and later within her text indicated that nurses will follow suit (8). She skillfully asks the question regarding why these "generalist"-type physicians are no longer seen and then answers with a profoundly forward-thinking statement, "Because present civilization and modern science demand a perfection along each line of work formerly unknown" (8, p. 14)

After specialization, however, within the 1930s and 1940s, there is some debate about the advent of the concept of the CNS, although there is agreement that the term *nurse clinician* began with Frances Reiter in 1943 (6, 9). It is noted that Reiter did not believe a master's degree was pivotal to be a nurse clinician; however, it was the belief that it was an efficient method to achieve such preparation (9). Ultimately, it was Hildegard Peplau who developed the first master's program focused on advanced training psychiatric

CNSs in 1954 (6, 10). Expansion of nursing training began to include CNS preparation in a graduate program by 1963 and a growth in CNS programs continued into the 1980s (6).

Psychiatric CNSs continued to move forward. Then, during the 1970s, critical care and oncology specialties began to form, leading to a period of significant growth for CNSs (10). Unfortunately, a lack of organizational understanding of the role began. It is interesting to note that some of the confusion about the role and required education existing today is not necessarily new. Individuals were employed who called themselves CNSs; however, they did not have the required background or education (7). Today, statutes exist ensuring title protection for the CNS in many states and jurisdictions. Although this prevents the use of the title, it has only brought some change, as confusion continues with implementation of the role under a different title. Beginning in 1980, the ANA published, *Nursing: A Social Policy Statement*, which defined CNS preparation as a graduate degree from a program focused on scientific knowledge, including supervised advanced practice, and as having met eligibility requirements for national certification in a specialty (7, 10, 11). The 1980s marked growth in CNS programs and utilization within organizations. This expansion was also marked by the beginning of articulation of research supporting CNS practice outcomes and publication supporting the role (10).

During the 1990s, the health care industry underwent great financial challenges due to changes in Medicare reimbursement. This decade proved problematic for the CNS because due to budget constraints, there were significant reductions in CNS positions (10). In 1995, the NACNS was established. Through its leadership, this organization has led to great developments in opportunities for CNSs (10). Many specialty organizations have also been significant advocates of CNS practice. Despite this, the 1990s continued with decreasing numbers of CNS programs, positions, and organizational support for the role. This was rather unfortunate due to the added value that the CNS lends to practice and outcomes. It is suggested that CNSs had not quantified their role sufficiently in terms of outcomes or financial impact and that today's critical shortage of CNSs is directly attributable to these factors (12). Although these times are keenly remembered by some practicing CNSs, today's focus on quality presents a different picture given the current state of the nation's economy. The 2000s began with the significant focus on quality after the landmark reports outlining the health care challenges ahead. It seemed that the value of CNS practice had been rekindled, and in 2002, the NACNS was receiving increased numbers of recruiter requests for CNS positions (12). As we move forward through difficult financial times in which health care quality and outcomes are in the forefront, it will be more important for CNSs to document their contribution to patient and financial outcomes.

Spheres of Influence

In 1998, the NACNS Research and Practice Committee published the *Statement on Clinical Nurse Specialist Practice and Education* that spoke to the three spheres of influence in which a CNS practices (16, 18): the patient or client, nurse or nursing, and organization or system. There is a critical interplay of themes within these spheres. The social context, organizational structure, process, financial resources, and public policy all apply within a continuum of the navigation between these spheres. For example, a CNS may be consulted by a bedside nurse to assist in the solving of a patient problem. Once this immediate issue is completed, the CNS may find that the implications of this situation extend beyond the borders of the patient, unit, patient population, and perhaps through the organization. The CNS by virtue of the three spheres is committed to solving the larger, system or process issue. By using leadership, collaboration, and consultation skills, the CNS not only contributes to the outcome of the initial patient for whom he or she consulted but perhaps to that of many patients through the recognition and navigation via a systems issue.

Patient/Client

The CNS functions as a direct caregiver or an indirect caregiver within this sphere. The primary focus of the work for the CNS is on the patient or client within this sphere of influence. In the arena of indirect care, the CNS may ensure implementation of an evidence-based protocol in a particular patient situation or within a population of patients. This can also extend to the formulation of a patient care protocol, an order set, a policy, a procedure, or a program for a group or population of patients. Typically, the CNS will do this through collaboration within an interdisciplinary team. Again, the focus is on a patient problem. The CNS ensures efficiency and quality within this approach to indirect care while carefully integrating the ability for individualization based on caring, diversity, and cultural needs. This work in changing practice or implementing EBP is primarily performed or driven by the CNS. Research focused on patient care is critical within this sphere. The CNS may assist with the integration of conceptual or care delivery models into practice. The work is continually being evaluated for effectiveness, both clinically and from a cost-effective perspective.

Nursing/Multidisciplines

Within this sphere, the CNS works through individuals or groups of individuals to achieve outcomes. It is on a different plane or within a different sphere than that of the direct focus on the patient. Key to CNS practice in this sphere are role modeling, teaching, coaching, collaborating, facilitating, and mentoring.

The CNS functions in staff development within this sphere. While the CNS's foundational concept still lies within patient care, the focus is now on the nursing staff or other disciplines. Examples of activities include monitoring of orientation, evaluation of initial or annual competencies, and staff education. While other roles such as a nurse educator may follow many of these tasks or skills, it is important to ensure that the involvement of CNSs also fully uses their talent, skill, and knowledge. For example, a CNS may not need to teach basic dysrhythmia interpretation; however, an advanced 12-lead electrocardiograph educational offering may fully use the CNS's talent. Similarly, within the arena of initial and annual competencies, the CNS may evaluate a registered nurse's competency regarding a new skill or new patient care device. This line is not always clear; much of what determines the use of CNS talent is dependent on patient population need, facility resources, and skill level of nursing staff.

There are significant gaps within health care that are begging to be addressed. The CNS is skilled at collaboration with physicians and members of other health care disciplines. Much of the CNS's work within providing quality relies not only on nursing but also the work with colleagues in medicine and the myriad of other disciplines. To integrate evidence into practice, it is important to note that in most cases the evidence is not solely within the nursing realm. Integration of EBP has demonstrated reductions in morbidity, mortality, length of hospital stay, rate of readmissions, reductions in hospital-acquired infection, and much more. The CNS carefully integrates evidence into multidisciplinary care with special attention to nursing sensitive outcomes. Facilitation of research also applies.

Organization/System

Facilitation of change plays a significant role for the CNS within the organization and system sphere. The CNS skillfully uses change theory to develop and evaluate programs and ensure implementation and hardwiring of EBPs. These types of changes may include addressing organizationwide or systemwide processes or problems through the implementation of policy, initiatives, or programs (17). Clinical consultation often leads to evaluation of current programs or to the creation of a new program to address particular patient population needs. An example of this occurred at Massachusetts General Hospital, where a multidisciplinary group recommended the creation of a domestic violence program. Within this program, the CNS clearly used an organization or system focus and acted as consultant to the creation of the program and as a consultant to staff who had concerns surrounding particular patients at risk (19).

Also from within the organization/system sphere, the CNS is keenly aware of changes in technology, pharmacology, the health care environment, and practice. Cost-effectiveness within program development is also critically important. In Fort Worth, Texas, a CNS supported the implementation of a fast-track postanesthesia care program (20). This evaluation and implementation of a clinical program added great benefit through increasing operating room throughput capacity (20). As in this program, working within the organization and system sphere can lead to cost-effectiveness gains; however, the CNS may quantify secondary gains in patient, family, nursing, and physician satisfaction. Acting as a change agent is a key attribute of the role; it is imperative that the CNS build, support, and maintain relationships with colleagues of many disciplines. It is this relationship building that allows the CNS to traverse a multitude of process improvements, programmatic changes, and building and integration of evidence-based concepts into practice. The organizational culture itself is often changed and transformed through the work.

It is fairly common that a CNS does not have line authority or administrative authority (13-17). Because the CNS is typically responsible for outcomes, it is imperative that the individual have a set of interpersonal characteristics in place. Zuzelo delineates these skill sets into professional attributes including self-awareness, honesty, self-reflection, and risk taking. She also suggests a strong set of leadership skills, which allows the CNS to maintain a vision and inspire colleagues to move toward and achieve such a vision. Last, the ability to use collaboration skills in concert with consultation skills lends great strength to the CNS role, where often no official authority to coerce others to achieve compliance exists. To function effectively within the spheres of influence, one must have a strong command of several sources of power to include informational, expert, legitimate, referent, charismatic, reward, and self (13). However, the form of coercive power is not usually functional due to the lack of line authority. This places great emphasis on the use of other forms of power. This apparent lack of coercive power also has benefit. It is within this lack of line authority that often leads staff to view the CNS as nonthreatening and can open channels of communication leading to a proactive approach to patient care or system problems.

Implementation and support of initiatives to ensure regulatory requirements are met are fairly common within CNS practice. The talent and skill of CNSs are often tapped because of their focus on quality and quality improvement. Also because of this focus, the CNS is a perfect choice in working with multidisciplinary teams in leading product evaluation. Within the arena of health policy, there are many opportunities for significant use of CNS influence.

CNS Competencies and Spheres of Influence

In 2008, the cumulative work of 22 CNS stakeholder nursing organizations that stemmed from the NACNS, ANA, and the American Board of Nursing Specialties (ABNS) was presented for endorsement (21). This work was a set of CNS core competencies. This group organized the competencies with behavioral statements, and then the behavioral statements were categorized based on the NACNS-defined spheres of influence and on defined nurse characteristics from the American Association of Critical Care Nurses Synergy Model. The model is illustrated in Table 1–2.

Clinical Expert/Direct Care

The provision of direct care is a cornerstone of advanced practice. CNSs provide direct care to patients in many ways. In a 2005 descriptive pilot study that used questionnaires to ascertain the amounts of time spent in the particular roles of a CNS, Darmody found that 30% of CNS time was spent in the patient/client sphere of influence (22). She grouped the trends of these findings into physical or technical care for patients with further description being troubleshooting equipment, monitoring a critically ill patient with highly specialized equipment, and direct patient teaching in preparation for discharge. As Darmody infers within her article, these direct care activities are often intertwined with other competencies. For example, as a CNS consulted to evaluate a particular therapy by a bedside nurse, when assessing and intervening on the situation at hand, the CNS will often guide and teach

(Text continued on page 13)

TABLE 1–2 Organizing Framework and CNS Core Competencies

A. Direct Care Competency: Direct interaction with patients, families, and groups of patients to promote health or well-being and improve quality of life. Characterized by a holistic perspective in the advanced nursing management of health, illness, and disease states.

Behavioral Statement	Sphere of Influence	AACN Synergy Model Nurse Characteristic
A.1 Conducts comprehensive, holistic wellness and illness assessments using known or innovative evidence-based techniques, tools, and direct and indirect methods.	Patient	Clinical Judgment
A.2 Obtains data about context and etiologies (including both non–disease- and disease-related factors) necessary to formulate differential diagnoses and plans of care, and to identify and evaluate of outcomes.	Patient	
A.3 Employs evidence-based clinical practice guidelines to guide screening and diagnosis.	Patient and System	
A.4 Assesses the effects of interactions among the individual, family, community, and social systems on health and illness.	Patient, Nurse and System	
A.5 Identifies potential risks to patient safety, autonomy, and quality of care based on assessments across the patient, nurse, and system spheres of influence.	Patient and System	
A.6 Assesses the impact of environmental/system factors on care.	Patient and System	
A.7 Synthesizes assessment data, advanced knowledge, and experience, using critical thinking and clinical judgment to formulate differential diagnoses for clinical problems amenable to CNS intervention.	Patient	
A.8 Prioritizes differential diagnoses to reflect those conditions most relevant to signs, symptoms, and patterns amenable to CNS interventions.	Patient	
A.9. Selects interventions that may include, but are not limited to: A.9.a. Application of advanced nursing therapies A.9.b. Initiation of interdisciplinary team meetings, consultations, and other communications to benefit patient care A.9.c. Management of patient medications, clinical procedures, and other interventions A.9.d. Psychosocial support including patient counseling and spiritual interventions.	Patient	
A.10 Designs strategies, including advanced nursing therapies, to meet the multifaceted needs of complex patients and groups of patients.	Patient	
A.11 Develops evidence-based clinical interventions and systems to achieve defined patient and system outcomes.	Patient, Nurse and System	Caring Practice

TABLE 1-2 Organizing Framework and CNS Core Competencies—cont'd

Behavioral Statement	Sphere of Influence	AACN Synergy Model Nurse Characteristic
A.12 Uses advanced communication skills within therapeutic relationships to improve patient outcomes.	Patient	Clinical Judgment
A.13 Prescribes nursing therapeutics, pharmacologic and non-pharmacologic interventions, diagnostic measures, equipment, procedures, and treatments to meet the needs of patients, families, and groups, in accordance with professional preparation, institutional privileges, state and federal laws and practice acts.	Patient	
A.14 Provides direct care to selected patients based on the needs of the patient and the CNS's specialty knowledge and skills.	Patient	
A.15 Assists staff in the development of innovative, cost-effective programs or protocols of care.	Patient, Nurse and System	
A.16 Evaluates nursing practice that considers Safety, Timeliness, Effectiveness, Efficiency, Efficacy, and Patient-centered care.	Patient, Nurse and System	
A.17 Determines when evidence-based guidelines, policies, procedures, and plans of care need to be tailored to the individual.	Patient	
A.18 Differentiates between outcomes that require care process modification at the individual patient level and those that require modification at the system level.	System	Systems Thinking
A.19 Leads development of evidence-based plans for meeting individual, family, community, and population needs.	Patient and System	Caring Practices
A.20 Provides leadership for collaborative, evidence-based revision of diagnoses and plans of care, to improve patient outcomes.	Patient, Nurse and System	Clinical Judgment

B. Consultation Competency: Patient-, staff-, or system-focused interaction between professionals in which the consultant is recognized as having specialized expertise and assists consultee with problem solving.

Behavioral Statement	Sphere of Influence	AACN Synergy Model Nurse Characteristic
B.1 Provides consultation to staff nurses, medical staff, and interdisciplinary colleagues.	Patient, Nurse and System	Clinical Judgment
B.2 Initiates consultation to obtain resources as necessary to facilitate progress toward achieving identified outcomes.	Patient	
B.3 Communicates consultation findings to appropriate parties consistent with professional and institutional standards.	Patient	Collaboration
B.4 Analyzes data from consultations to implement practice improvements.	Nurse and System	Facilitation of Learning

Continued

TABLE 1-2 Organizing Framework and CNS Core Competencies—cont'd

C. Systems Leadership Competency: The ability to manage change and empower others to influence clinical practice and political processes both within and across systems.

Behavioral Statement	Sphere of Influence	AACN Synergy Model Nurse Characteristic
C.1 Facilitates the provision of clinically competent care by staff/team through education, role modeling, teambuilding, and quality monitoring.	Nurse and System	
C.2 Performs system level assessments to identify variables that influence nursing practice and outcomes, including but not limited to:	System	Systems Thinking
C.2.a. Population variables (age distribution, health status, income distribution, culture)	Patient and System	Response to Diversity
C.2.b. Environment (schools, community support services, housing availability, employment opportunities)	Patient and System	Systems Thinking
C.2.c. System of health care delivery	Patient and System	
C.2.d. Regulatory requirements	System	
C.2.e. Internal and external political influences/stability	System	
C.2.f. Health care financing	System	
C.2.g. Recurring practices that enhance or compromise patient or system outcomes.	Patient, Nurse and System	
C.3 Determines nursing practice and system interventions that will promote patient, family, and community safety.	Nurse and System	
C.4 Uses effective strategies for changing clinician and team behavior to encourage adoption of evidence-based practices and innovations in care delivery.	Nurse and System	
C.5 Provides leadership in maintaining a supportive and healthy work environment.	System	
C.6 Provides leadership in promoting interdisciplinary collaboration to implement outcome-focused patient care programs meeting the clinical needs of patients, families, populations, and communities.	Patient and System	Collaboration
C.7 Develops age-specific clinical standards, policies, and procedures.	System	Collaboration and Response to Diversity
C.8 Uses leadership, team building, negotiation, and conflict resolution skills to build partnerships within and across systems, including communities.	System	Collaboration
C.9 Coordinates the care of patients with use of system and community resources to ensure successful health/illness/wellness transitions, enhance delivery of care, and achieve optimal patient outcomes.	Patient and System	

TABLE 1–2 Organizing Framework and CNS Core Competencies—cont'd

Behavioral Statement	Sphere of Influence	AACN Synergy Model Nurse Characteristic
C.10 Considers fiscal and budgetary implications in decision making regarding practice and system modifications.	System	Systems Thinking
C.10.a. Evaluates use of products and services for Appropriateness and cost/benefit in meeting care needs		
C.10.b. Conducts cost/benefit analysis of new clinical technologies		
C.10.c. Evaluates impact of introduction or withdrawal of products, system systems thinking services, and technologies		
C.11 Leads system change to improve health outcomes through evidence-based practice:	Patient, Nurse and System	Systems Thinking
C.11.a. Specifies expected clinical and system level outcomes.	Patient, Nurse and System	
C.11.b. Designs programs to improve clinical and system level processes and outcomes.	Patient, Nurse and System	
C.11.c. Facilitates the adoption of practice change	Patient, Nurse and System	
C.12 Evaluates impact of CNS and other nursing practice on systems of care using nurse-sensitive outcomes.	Nurse and System	
C.13 Disseminates outcomes of system-level change internally and externally.	System	

D. Collaboration Competency: Working jointly with others to optimize clinical outcomes. The CNS collaborates at an advanced level by committing to authentic engagement and constructive patient-, family-, system-, and population-focused problem-solving.

Behavioral Statement	Sphere of Influence	AACN Synergy Model Nurse Characteristic
D.1 Assesses the quality and effectiveness of interdisciplinary, intra-agency, and inter-agency communication and collaboration.	Nurse and System	Clinical Inquiry and Collaboration
D.2 Establishes collaborative relationships within and across departments that promote patient safety, culturally competent care, and clinical excellence.	System	Collaboration and Response to Diversity
D.3 Provides leadership for establishing, improving, and sustaining collaborative relationships to meet clinical needs.	Nurse and System	
D.4 Practices collegially with medical staff and other members of the health care team so that all providers' unique contributions to health outcomes will be enhanced.	Nurse and System	
D.5 Facilitates intra-agency and inter-agency communication.	Nurse and System	

Continued

TABLE 1–2 Organizing Framework and CNS Core Competencies—cont'd

E. Coaching Competency: Skillful guidance and teaching to advance the care of patients, families, groups of patients, and the profession of nursing.

Behavioral Statement	Sphere of Influence	AACN Synergy Model Nurse Characteristic
E.1 Coaches patients and families to help them navigate the health care system.	Patient	Advocacy and Moral Agency
E.2 Designs health information and patient education appropriate to the patient's developmental level, health literacy level, learning needs, readiness to learn, and cultural values and beliefs.	Patient	Facilitation of Learning and Response to Diversity
E.3 Provides education to individuals, families, groups and communities to promote knowledge, understanding and optimal functioning across the wellness-illness continuum.	Patient	Diversity
E.4 Participates in pre-professional, graduate, and continuing education of nurses and other health care providers:	Nurse	
E.4.a. Completes a needs assessment as appropriate to guide interventions with staff;	Nurse	
E.4.b. Promotes professional development of staff nurses and continuing education activities;	Nurse	
E.4.c. Implements staff development and continuing education activities.	Nurse	
E.4.d. Mentors nurses to translate research into practice.	Nurse	Facilitator of Learning and Clinical Inquiry
E.5 Contributes to the advancement of the profession as a whole by disseminating outcomes of CNS practice through presentations and publications.	Nurse	
E.6 Mentors staff nurses, graduate students, and others to acquire new knowledge and skills and develop their careers.	Nurse	Facilitator of Learning
E.7 Mentors health professionals in applying the principles of evidence-based care.	Nurse and System	
E.8 Uses coaching and advanced communication skills to facilitate the development of effective clinical teams.	Nurse and System	Advocacy and Moral Agency
E.9 Provides leadership in conflict management and negotiation to address problems in the health care system.	Patient, Nurse and System	Collaboration

TABLE 1-2 Organizing Framework and CNS Core Competencies—cont'd

F. Research Competency: The work of thorough and systematic inquiry. Includes the search for, interpretation, and use of evidence in clinical practice and quality improvement, as well as active participation in the conduct of research.

I. INTERPRETATION, TRANSLATION AND USE OF EVIDENCE

Behavioral Statement	Sphere of Influence	AACN Synergy Model Nurse Characteristic
F.I.1 Analyzes research findings and other evidence for their potential application to clinical practice.	Patient, Nurse and System	Clinical Inquiry
F.I.2 Integrates evidence into the health, illness, and wellness management of patients, families, communities, and groups.	Patient	
F.I.3 Applies principles of evidence-based practice and quality improvement to all patient care.	Patient and System	
F.I.4 Assesses system barriers and facilitators to adoption of evidence-based practices.	System	
F.I.5 Designs programs for effective implementation of research findings and other evidence in clinical practice.	Patient, Nurse and System	
F.I.6 Cultivates a climate of clinical inquiry across spheres of influence:	Patient, Nurse and System	Clinical Inquiry and Systems Thinking
F.1.6.a. Evaluates the need for improvement or redesign of care delivery processes to improve safety, efficiency, reliability, and quality.	Patient, Nurse and System	
F.1.6.b. Disseminates expert knowledge;	Patient, Nurse and System	Facilitation of Learning

II. EVALUATION OF CLINICAL PRACTICE

Behavioral Statement	Sphere of Influence	AACN Synergy Model Nurse Characteristic
F.II.1 Fosters an interdisciplinary approach to quality improvement, evidence-based practice, research, and translation of research into practice.	Nurse/Team	Collaboration
F.II.2 Participates in establishing quality improvement agenda for unit, department, program, system, or population.	System	Clinical Inquiry
F.II.3 Provides leadership in planning data collection and quality monitoring.	System	
F.II.4 Uses quality monitoring data to assess the quality and effectiveness of clinical programs in meeting outcomes.	Patient, Nurse and System	
F.II.5 Develops quality improvement initiatives based on assessments.	System	
F.II.6 Provides leadership in the design, implementation, and evaluation of process improvement initiatives.	System	
F.II.7 Provides leadership in the system-wide implementation of quality improvements and innovations.	System	

Continued

TABLE 1–2 Organizing Framework and CNS Core Competencies—cont'd

III. CONDUCT OF RESEARCH

Behavioral Statement	Sphere of Influence	AACN Synergy Model Nurse Characteristic
F.III.1 Participates in conduct of or implementation of research which may include one or more of the following: F.III.1.a. Identification of questions for clinical inquiry F.III.1.b. Conduct of literature reviews F.III.1.c. Study design and implementation F.III.1.d. Data collection F.III.1.e. Data analysis F.III.1.f. Dissemination of findings	Patient, Nurse and System	Clinical Inquiry

G. Ethical decision-making, moral agency, and advocacy: Identifying, articulating, and taking action on ethical concerns at the patient, family, health care provider, system, community, and public policy levels.

Behavioral Statement	Sphere of Influence	AACN Synergy Model Nurse Characteristic
G.1 Engages in a formal self-evaluation process, seeking feedback regarding own practice, from patients, peers, professional colleagues, and others	Nurse	Clinical Inquiry
G.2 Fosters professional accountability in self or others.	Nurse and System	Advocacy and Moral Agency
G.3 Facilitates resolution of ethical conflicts: G.3.a. Identifies ethical implications of complex care situations G.3.b. Considers the impact of scientific advances, cost, clinical effectiveness, patient and family values and preferences, and other external influences. G.3.c. Applies ethical principles to resolving concerns across the three spheres of influence	Patient, Nurse and System	Response to Diversity
G.4 Promotes a practice climate conducive to providing ethical care.	Nurse and System	Moral Agency
G.5 Facilitates interdisciplinary teams to address ethical concerns, risks or considerations, benefits and outcomes of patient care.	Nurse and System	Advocacy and Collaboration
G.6 Facilitates patient and family understanding of the risks, benefits, and outcomes of proposed health care regimen to promote informed decision making.	Patient	Facilitator of Learning
G.7 Advocates for equitable patient care by: G.7.a. Participating in organizational, local, state, national, or international level of policy-making activities for issues related to their expertise G.7.b. Evaluating the impact of legislative and regulatory policies as they apply to nursing practice and patient or population outcomes	Patient and System	Advocacy and Moral Agency

TABLE 1-2 Organizing Framework and CNS Core Competencies—cont'd

Behavioral Statement	Sphere of Influence	AACN Synergy Model Nurse Characteristic
G.8 Promotes the role and scope of practice of the CNS to legislators, regulators, other health care providers, and the public:	Nurse and System	Advocacy and Facilitator of Learning
G.8.a. Communicates information that promotes nursing, the role of learning the CNS and outcomes of nursing and CNS practice through the use of the media, advanced technologies, and community networks.	Nurse and System	
G.8.b. Advocates for the CNS/APRN role and for positive legislative response to issues affecting nursing practice.	Nurse and System	

the nurse through the process of troubleshooting and correcting the problem. This, in turn, promotes staff development and enhanced competency and develops confidence within the nursing staff involved.

There are a multitude of examples of CNS-led EBP initiatives within the literature. Identification of a gap and implementation of the EBP is a key component of the direct care role of the CNS. Just a few of those examples include implementation of an EBP alcohol withdrawal syndrome protocol at Froedtert Hospital in Milwaukee, Wisconsin, and the CNS-led process of implementing a rapid response team at both Pinnacle Health System in Harrisburg, Pennsylvania, and Shawnee Mission Medical Center in Shawnee Mission, Kansas (23-25).

Direct patient care affords the CNS many opportunities to directly influence quality issues. As previously mentioned, the opportunities for care delivery improvement are unfortunately many. CNSs are perfectly positioned to immerse themselves in care processes and see the potential disconnects that need to be addressed. The direct care component allows for correction or creation of processes to ensure that "never events" do not occur and that nursing sensitive indicators are established to ensure only the best in quality.

This direct care competency also allows for the use of caring practices. Enuring that the psychosocial needs of patients and families are met in an EBP manner is essential. The CNS guides and facilitates staff into ensuring that along with the science of nursing, the art is also retained. This can also be accomplished within the realm of the community and differing population needs.

Consultation

Consultation in its strictest sense can be a difficult and problematic competency in which to engage. The CNS often consults with physicians, nurse practitioners, and

other colleagues within the realm of her or his individual expertise. At the patient level, the attending physician may consult a CNS regarding the best approach to care for a wound or the best approach to ensure true compliance with medications and regimens needed for care of a complex cardiac problem. Physicians and other licensed independent providers often recognize the knowledge and experience of a strong CNS.

Nurses may consult the CNS for difficult patient situations, either clinical or psychosocial in nature. When a bedside nurse has exhausted her or his efforts and is not achieving the desired outcome, a CNS provides strength and support to both the nurse and the particular patient situation.

At the system level is where consultation can become quite complicated. Participation on multiple committees is not an uncommon expectation of the CNS. Participation within the committees often entails leadership of the CNS in imparting expert knowledge into the very problem or issue that has given the committee its purpose. The difficulty lies within a lack of organizational understanding of the strength of the CNS consultation role. The CNS is often charged with providing expert knowledge surrounding an issue or problem yet is often charged with creating and implementing its solution. The larger question remains: Is this the best use of the talent and expertise of the CNS, or would the organization be better served to continue with the CNS consultation ability to lead and guide multiple initiatives rather than focus on one or a small number of issues? The additional accountability lies also within the CNS in the ability to clearly articulate expectations.

Systems Leadership

Systems leadership is a key component of CNS practice as well. Because of the depth and breadth of knowledge and experience, and the ability to navigate through multiple disciplines and thick layers of bureaucracy, the CNS is positioned to create and maintain large scale change. Knowledge of the current landscape of the health care environment often comes with participation in professional organizations and a significant competence in maintaining knowledge current with relevant literature. These facets of knowledge combined with clinical expertise help to guide the CNS through creating and/or maintaining systems of care delivery to a vast array of populations through a health care system.

The quality initiatives mentioned earlier in this chapter driven by a multitude of regulatory agencies and organizations provide the CNS with opportunities to drive processes at the system or organizational level. Through the knowledge and experience within the direct care competency, the CNS is uniquely positioned for comprehensive program development at a higher level, and with careful planning and a broad overview of system intricacies, there may be less opportunity for disconnects downstream that become problematic.

Knowledge of regulatory requirements is a must, and the CNS is often consulted to ensure that nursing and other processes are compliant with current and evolving requirements. Patient safety is a high priority in this realm. The CNS is vigilant in ensuring that at the highest level within the system, the context of the patient and family is always in the forefront of decision making. Cost-effectiveness is also a significant theme within systems leadership. It boils down to effectiveness. Effectiveness is a true measure of the CNS's ability to assess and synthesize data and to frame it within the complex and matrixed delivery system where the actual care is delivered. The CNS must be skilled at creating, articulating, and communicating a cost-effective analysis when suggesting system-level change. Changes often occur in the form of the creation of a policy, procedure, or order set to ensure the use of current and pertinent evidence, while ensuring continuity and consistency of care within particular patient populations.

Collaboration

Collaboration takes many forms and is most often a competency used in combination with other competencies. *Team competency* is a term becoming much more common, and it makes sense that in today's complex environments it takes many people and often many disciplines to accomplish a particular goal. The CNS is a wonderful advocate for change, an active change agent, and a skilled facilitator.

A CNS has mature clinical and professional judgment and has built on significant working relationships to accomplish collaboration (26). In 2005, the American Association of Critical Care Nurses published the AACN Standards for Establishing and Sustaining Healthy Work Environments (27). This landmark document was intended to address situations in which unhealthy work environments were leading to medical errors and ineffective care delivery in addition to conflict and stress among health care workers. There are six essential standards. These standards have been well recognized, used, and adopted by many other professional organizations and institutions since its publication. Disch, Walton, and Barnsteiner described how the CNS could, through the use of collaboration in conjunction with other competencies, implement the standards in their own professional environments (26). These authors report that key partnerships are necessary for the CNS. These are partnerships with staff where the CNS models expert practice and coaching abilities and appropriately frames issues so that staff can gain a full sense of the context of a pressing situation and fully value nursing's contributions. Partnership with the nurse manager is also essential. This partnership assists in gaining momentum within a unit where the CNS focuses on clinical care and other appropriate issues, allowing the nurse manager to focus on operations and acquiring needed resources. Disch et al.'s suggestion of CNS collaboration does not stop with nursing staff and the nurse manager, however; the partnerships with physicians and across the system or community are also highlighted, allowing the CNS a full and complete process of collaboration to accomplish goals within a unit or an environment (Table 1–3).

Coaching/Teaching/Mentoring

Coaching, guiding, and teaching are frequently used competencies. The CNS intuitively teaches in almost every interaction. Education may be provided through formal presentation; however, it probably is most often performed at the bedside with staff in a just-in-time fashion. These competencies are usually used in concert with other competencies. They allow the CNS to expand her or his reach through the development of staff.

Another key element within the realm of coaching, guiding, and teaching is the dissemination of EBP. The CNS uses EBP dissemination models to guide staff through the process of practice change. There are a myriad of conceptual models used for the dissemination of EBP; a small sample of these are found in Table 1–4. It is well known that moving evidence into practice often takes some time. The need for movement into the practice setting is critical to ensure clinical outcomes and quality of care. Ervin communicates in her 2005 article that the CNS role is critical in achieving the integration of and maintenance of EBP elements into the care setting (28).

From bedside just-in-time training to teaching within formal seminars or within internship or residency programs, the CNS has a key role in the education of others. The integration of these competencies into practice allows for the continual improvement of patient care. Though the CNS is critical in the education and professionalization

TABLE 1–3 American Association of Critical-Care Nurses Standards for Establishing and Maintaining Healthy Work Environments

Standard	Description
Skilled Communication	Nurses must be as proficient in communication skills as they are in clinical skills.
True Collaboration	Nurses must be relentless in pursuing and fostering true collaboration.
Effective Decision Making	Nurses must be valued and committed partners in making policy, directing and evaluating clinical care, and leading organizational operations.
Appropriate Staffing	Staffing must ensure the effective match between patient needs and nurse competencies.
Meaningful Recognition	Nurses must be recognized and must recognize others for the value each brings to the work of the organization.
Authentic Leadership	Nurse leaders must fully embrace the imperative of a healthy work environment, authentically live it, and engage others in its achievement.

From: Crit Care Nurse December 2009, Vol 9, No. 6, pp. 20–27.

TABLE 1–4 Models of Evidence-Based Practice Dissemination

Model	Brief Description
Stetler Model	APRN typically described as the leader in making changes. Uses a 5-step approach that includes preparation, validation, decision making, translation or application, and evaluation
Johns Hopkins Model	Global model and somewhat complex. Uses internal/external factors to determine what approach should be taken from an education, practice, and research perspective.
Iowa Model	Uses an algorithmic approach including feedback loops to drive practice change. Can easily be used for driving practice, quality improvement projects, and nursing research.
CURN (Conduct and Utilization of Research in Nursing) Model	A process of defining a patient care problem, exploration of the problem followed by a decision to adopt, alter, or reject and innovation. The model also includes movement from a trial to maintenance of the new innovation over time.

of nursing staff, expert knowledge and practice supported by evidence reach well into other health care disciplines, leading to positive patient outcomes.

Research/Evidence-Based Practice

Along with the integration of EBP into the clinical setting, the CNS has a key role in the practice of nursing research. The research possibilities within today's health care settings are endless. There are a multitude of possibilities for clinically based research and for those that affect the care environment. Moffitt and Butler used research to address the problems of a unit in chaos after a merger. After this merger occurred, marked differences in unit culture became evident, with a negative impact on patient,

staff, and physician satisfaction along with a growing trend in failing to meet national benchmarks for certain patient care outcomes. The researchers used a descriptive study with a convenience sample to determine the effect of their four-pronged approach to changing the environment. The researchers instituted walking rounds. During the rounds the CNS monitored the rounds and provided feedback as required. Hourly rounds by staff in visiting patients and families to ensure that needs were met followed. The last two interventions addressed staffing issues. The unit practiced a closed staffing model to allow for staff who were willing to work additional shifts to cover patient needs. The outcomes were markedly positive. The CNS was able to facilitate great change in this environment through research that resulted in positive increases in each of the identified areas of need (29).

There are multiple models of nursing research. The CNS may be the principal investigator within a project at a particular facility, while other models of research mentoring are also in existence. Some models include the CNS as a research mentor to staff driven research projects. Facilities such as Providence St. Vincent Medical Center in Portland, Oregon, have used this model and successfully completed multiple projects simultaneously within the institution. The projects in this case are unit driven, in which nurses from particular units define a clinical problem or question and follow it through the full research process, including dissemination of the findings to the health care community.

Ethical Decision-Making/Moral Agency/Advocacy

Within today's health care settings, there are many opportunities for the CNS to share expertise, experience, and knowledge in addressing situations in which there are ethical decisions and moral agency and advocacy implications. These situations are often difficult, stressful, and quite timely for staff caring for patients and families. The CNS's expertise allows for staff to move forward with their care activities while allowing opportunities for coaching and mentoring through these tenuous situations to better prepare the care provider for situations to come.

In times past, many of these situations often presented exclusively within critical care units. This is not necessarily the case any longer as patients are of much higher acuity and maintained with the support of various kinds of technology within the acute care setting. Advances in medicine and nursing have provided us with many more ethical questions to be addressed. Puntillo and McAdam completed a literature review to specifically examine the communication between physicians and nurses in an effort to identify the challenges and opportunities for caring for patients at the end-of-life (30). The researchers identified the contribution of critical care nurses to the process and found that joint grand rounds, patient care educational opportunities, and interprofessional dialogue can greatly enhance care and improve communication. These are wonderful opportunities for CNS-led initiatives, given the preparatory advanced education. Frontline nurses are often concerned about ethical aspects of patient care; however, the concerns are often passed over due to the complex hospital milieu, competing demands for time and other resources, and attention to clinical care (31).

It is not uncommon for the CNS to be consulted in working with families in difficult situations. Those situations include where proposed or continued treatment is of a concern, where there are questions about risk, and where there is a need to ensure informed consent occurs at the most fundamental level. The CNS is well equipped to provide such family consultation and ensure that the full interdisciplinary team is involved to address these concerns, risks, and considerations.

Advocacy is a significant area of interest for the CNS, as it is for all APRNs. It is well known that APRNs contribute significant positive outcomes to the care of patients and their families. To continue to contribute to this process in a meaningful way, it is critically important for CNSs to be an advocate for the role. This can be accomplished in a number of ways; involvement within professional organizations and ensuring that the voice of CNSs is heard during legislative processes are two key ways. As CNSs, we need to continue to communicate our significant contributions to patient outcomes and process improvement. This should be done at multiple levels, including within our institutions but also through a wider dissemination of process improvement, research, and other key initiatives in which we are involved.

While this work seems to be focused on articulation of the importance of APRN and CNS roles, this work is critical when thought of in the context of access to our unique skill set. Continued movement within the legislative arena will only improve access to care and assist us in articulating the great value of CNS practice to facilities in need of our talent.

Another key set of elements that falls within this set of competencies is that of formal self-evaluation. The CNS genuinely and frequently seeks feedback surrounding her or his own practice. This practice is markedly significant in the journey of a CNS's development. In order to role model learning as a process, self-evaluation, and professional accountability, it is profoundly necessary that a CNS engage in continual evaluation. As a CNS, it is sometimes felt that one should know everything within the field. A CNS is after all, a clinical expert. Unfortunately, as medical knowledge increases at an exciting, yet alarming rate, the expectation of a CNS knowing everything is simply unrealistic. It is the practice of inquiry and questioning that should be role modeled, and this practice will hopefully be seen as an example for nurses and members of other health care disciplines.

CNS Practice
AACN Synergy Model

There are multiple care delivery and practice models that have been historically used in providing care to patients and families. Each of these models is unique and provides opportunity for CNSs to examine the appropriateness of use within individual institutions. Shirey asserts that the evaluation of these delivery models provides us with a foundation to evaluate future methods of care delivery for both acute and critical care (32). The evolution of nursing care delivery has called for change or modification within these models. We are in a time of great change.

The AACN Synergy Model for Patient Care is a conceptual model of care delivery developed to describe and guide care delivered to patients and families based on a set of patient needs or characteristics. These characteristics drive the care delivered and "synergy results when the needs and characteristics of a patient, clinical unit or system are matched with a nurse's competencies" (24).

The eight patient characteristics each have three levels that describe the patient's particular need on a continuum. The characteristics are resiliency, vulnerability, stability, complexity, resource availability, participation in care, participation in decision-making, and predictability. The patient can be described or conceptualized by need, set of needs, and individual levels within each continuum. Just as there are levels within the needs of patients, the nurse characteristics can be described by levels of competence within each of the nurse characteristics. The eight nurse characteristics include clinical judgment, advocacy and moral agency, caring practices, collaboration, systems thinking, response to diversity, facilitator of learning, and clinical inquiry.

In its simplest terms, matching patient needs with appropriate nurse characteristics is when care delivery is at its best. The AACN Synergy Model for Patient Care provides a relatively simple, yet remarkably descriptive and appropriate model for guiding delivery of patient care. The use of this model has many applications. The model has been described in the literature as a method of illuminating the APRN or, more specifically, the CNS role in contemporary practice (33).

Variance in CNS Practice

There is often significant ambiguity within actualization of the CNS role in both its understanding and operationalizing within organizations. Organizational need may also influence CNS practice. Early authors identified this variance as both a bane and a benefit in that flexibility within the role allows a fluid movement between competencies or roles (7). Traditionally, the CNS had been described in terms of five subroles: clinical expert, educator, consultant, leader, and researcher. There has also been great variance in actualization of all or some of the subroles within the CNS practice in institutions. In 1999, Scott completed a study of activity within these roles to quantify practice within them in addition to facilitating CNSs' inability to explicate value in economic terms (34). There were 23 psychosocial and 44 medical skills listed within the findings, a summary of which is included in Table 1–5. Some professional organizations have made efforts to assist in adding clarity to the role. An example

TABLE 1–5 CNS Roles and Activities

Role	Percentage of Time Spent in Role
Educator Role	24-89%
Consultant Role	18-96%
Researcher	15-93%
Clinical Leadership	34-85%
Clinical Expert	Top 10 psychosocial activities: Family therapy Grief therapy Psychotherapy Crisis intervention Marriage counseling Sex/sex abuse therapy Relaxation therapy Substance abuse therapy Depression therapy Smoking cessation therapy Most Frequent Advanced Medical Skills: Pacemaker programming, management, and discontinuation Suturing and stapling Wound debridement Pelvic/rectal/prostate examination Central line and chest tube insertion and discontinuation Invasive arterial and venous sheath removal Pulmonary artery catheter management and discontinuation Cardiac arrest management

of this is the publication of *Scope of Practice and Standards of Professional Performance for the Acute and Critical Care Clinical Nurse Specialist* by the American Association of Critical Care Nurses in 2002 (7, 18). These standards allow for variances within practice and may contribute to the confusion and lack of understanding of the CNS role. On the other hand, it may be just that flexibility, fluidity, and interplay of roles that make the CNS successful in achieving positive patient and family outcomes within divergent practice settings.

Specialty Practice

Another hallmark of CNS practice is the specialist component and repertoire of skills. Specialization builds on the baccalaureate foundation of knowledge with a generalist focus. After attending a CNS program and with additional practice, the CNS is then moved toward a specific, specialty practice. This specialty practice has great possibilities. The specialization may exist within the form of a setting, focusing on a single or group of diseases or pathology, an even more defined focus such as cardiac medicine, a type of care such as wound care, or a more broad population. This practice is most often population based; however, the specificity or breadth of the population varies greatly. Examples of population include cardiology, heart failure, medical, critical care, surgical, obstetrics, orthopedics, psychiatric/mental health, and many more.

In practice, CNSs may also be unit based or service based, which often takes the CNS through the facility, in and out of units and service areas. In either case, because many units tend to focus on a specific population, the CNS's focus remains on a specific patient population. However, it is easy for the organization to place demands on the CNS with a significant percentage of her or his role acting exclusively as an educator. This can be a gross misuse of the CNS's talent, skill, and training. At the University of Iowa Hospitals and Clinics, role restructuring occurred, leading the CNS role to become unit based (35). The aims of the restructuring were to affect specific patient populations, allowing the CNS to directly affect clinical care, enhance and expand understanding of the CNS role, and enhance measurement of clinical efficacy and outcomes. One of the most interesting aims was to increase unit efficiency by allowing shared responsibilities by the nurse manager and CNS roles. This process allowed the nurse manager to focus on operations, while the CNS maintained focus on clinical activities.

APRN REGULATION

There is inconsistency in the regulation of APRNs between states and jurisdictions. This has been a source of significant debate in the APRN arena for many years, as forms of regulation, licensure, and certification requirements differ greatly. Although this is the current reality, there has been a groundswell for change. Organizations and agencies representing APRNs have made significant contributions in creating a model for regulatory consistency.

The LACE Model

In 2005, the National Council of State Boards of Nursing (NCSBN) released the *Vision Paper on the Future of APRN Regulation*. This report was the result of the NCSBN's APRN Advisory Committees work from the prior few years. The report created significant dialogue within the advanced practice community because there was a recommendation to exclude CNSs as APRNs. Along the same timeline, the Advanced Practice Nursing Consensus Group was working on a similar product and goal. After much dialogue, the two groups worked collaboratively to create one common document. This collaboration resulted in *Consensus Model for APRN Regulation: Licensure, Accreditation, Certification and Education* (36). The process was aided by a third group formed from members of each of the two major groups. The focus of this group was to facilitate communication, and it became known as the APRN Joint Dialogue Group (36).

This consensus model has far-reaching implications for advanced practice nursing. The report was the result of a significant amount of work, collaboration, and compromise. It has been approved by essentially all nursing organizations representing APRNs. The model sets a clear direction for the future of APRN practice. *Key elements of the mode include licensure, accreditation, certification, and education, referred to by the acronym the LACE model.* This group represents members of nursing organizations and regulatory bodies and is pushing to ensure that the model is implemented by 2015.

Because of the vast differences in licensure and regulation across the United States, it can be quite difficult for APRNs to move from one state to another. Another problem for APRNs results from differences in education programs, which contributes to differences in licensure, recognition, and requirements for national certification within the states. These inconsistencies have an end result of decreasing access for patients and families to expertise and services that APRNs provide.

The LACE model clearly delineates the four roles. Within the model, the roles are grouped within the title of APRN. The APRNs are then licensed by specific role and within specific population foci. These population foci include family and individuals across the life span: adult/gerontology, neonatal, pediatrics, women's health/gender related, and psychiatric and mental health. The adult population focus is a continuum from the young adult through the older adult. This change from the previous separate designation of gerontology is intended to meet the needs of the aged as a population. The model is illustrated in Figure 1–1.

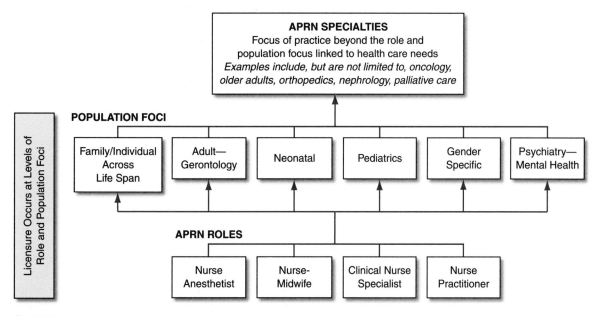

FIGURE 1–1: APRN Regulatory Model. From: APRN Consensus Work Group, National Council of State Boards of Nursing, APRN Advisory Committee, Consensus model for APRN Regulation: Licensure, Accreditation, Certification, and Education, 2008, p. 9.

Broad-based APRN education is required. The requirements are intended to support the elements and context of the model. Among other requirements, it ensures graduate-level preparation and inclusion of a core of comprehensive courses. This core includes advanced pathophysiology, advanced physical assessment, and advanced pharmacology.

The model mandates that national certification is required for all APRNs. The certification must meet the requirements within the licensure scheme of the model. That is, the role and a population focus must be addressed within the certification exam. Another important change is the movement to accountability for the continuum from health promotion and maintenance to the assessment, diagnosis, and management of problems. A key point in this process includes the use of both pharmacologic and nonpharmacologic interventions. This holds importance meaning for many CNSs who, in the past, did not have an opportunity for prescriptive authority for pharmacologic agents and a significant portion of the CNS workforce lacks prescriptive authority to this day.

Licensure

Licensure as awarded by states or jurisdictions indicates completion of an educational program. In addition to completion of the educational program, it generally indicates successful completion of an exam that is intended to ensure safe, entry-level practice. The state boards of nursing also vary. Each state has a board of nursing. Some states have two boards of nursing that may represent registered nursing and practical nursing, while other states have separate advanced practice nursing boards.

Application to practice as an APRN may entail two licenses: one registered nurse license and an additional APRN license. Certified registered nurse anesthetists (CRNAs) are not regulated similarly to nurse practitioners in many states. Only 38 states currently recognize the CNS as an APRN.

Prescriptive authority differs between states as well in a number of ways. The ability to prescribe scheduled drugs differs. In some instances, formulary systems exist. An additional example includes limits on days an APRN may prescribe. Even though some states do not recognize the CNS as an APRN, in some of these states, CNSs do have prescriptive authority. Historically, it has been thought that CNS practice did not require the ability to prescribe, although with the changing landscape of health care, it is evident that this can be a significant limitation of patient access to appropriate care.

Accreditation

Accreditation is a process in which a body with authority to do so issues credentials that particular educational or certifying bodies have met or exceeded known standards of performance. These organizations ensure that the processes and standards are followed in a method to ensure quality assurance of an educational program or certifying program. This is the formal review process that "accredits" the educational program and ensures that it has met appropriate standards. The Commission on Collegiate Nursing Education (CCNE), for example, provides accreditation to master's and doctor of nursing practice degrees, two options for CNS educational preparation.

Certification

Certification examinations are intended to be job related in that the examination evaluates knowledge required for current practice versus creating the standard for practice. To accomplish this, certifying organizations follow a process in creating and updating certification examinations. The tests must also be valid and reliable. A job analysis must be completed to ensure that the examination evaluates knowledge for current practice and, that within the test, there is a blueprint that assigns appropriate percentages to each content area. The intent for this rigorous process is that the certification examination is valid, reliable, legally defensible, and psychometrically sound.

In the case of advanced practice nursing, national certification often fulfills the examination requirement. Proof of maintenance of recertification is also often required and can be tied to the license renewal process within states that do require certification for APRN recognition and licensure. It is one proxy measure of competence and is used as such in the process. However, many but not all states require national certification for APRN recognition and licensure or license renewal.

CNS Certification

Because of the myriad of possibilities of specialization within CNS practice, certification has been an area of great debate. Because of differing practices among the states and jurisdictions regarding the requirement of certification for APRN recognition, it has been difficult for some CNSs to find a certification examination that appropriately fits their specialty. Certification examinations are quite expensive to create and maintain due to accrediting requirements. A certification examination must be based on a current study of practice and an associated test plan ensuring minimal competency of the nurse or APRN. Because of the proliferation of specialties and subspecialties, there are not always enough potential certificants to ensure a cost-effective program. This has been quite problematic in the past. The new APRN Regulatory Model will hopefully assist in this process since APRNs will be licensed and certified based on one of the four APRN roles and a population focus. Specialization can occur after this has been achieved.

Education

Over the years, the educational programs for APRNs have not been routinely uniform in curriculum. Not all APRNs have been required to achieve a master's degree and have functioned with certificate program education. Within programs, inclusion of courses considered to be foundational to advanced practice has not been consistently included in the curriculum. There has been lack of uniformity and inconsistency in application of clinical hour requirements. Many of these issues have the potential to prevent graduates and applicants to become

licensed in some states. These issues have been the topic of ongoing work of regulatory and professional organizations. The groups have been placing significant focus on ensuring patient and family access to the APRN.

DOCTOR OF NURSING PRACTICE

The most recent debate over CNS educational preparation relates to the doctor of nursing practice (DNP) as a terminal practice-oriented degree. It should be emphasized that the DNP is a practice doctorate, different from the traditional, research-focused doctor of philosophy (PhD). This new practice doctorate focuses on advanced practice, research utilization, and evaluation of outcomes. The introduction of the DNP brings nursing into the arena of and aligns recipients with other disciplines that have already embraced the practice doctorate concept. Such is the case with medicine, dentistry, psychology, pharmacy, physical therapy, and others. According to the *AACN Position Statement on the Practice Doctorate in Nursing* published in 2004, up until then, there were only two nursing practice–oriented doctoral degrees offered: at the University of Colorado and Case Western Reserve University in Ohio (37).

The AACN task force who assembled prior to the publication of the position statement examined the prospect of the DNP and interviewed administrators, students, and graduates of practice-focused programs and found significant differences that have led to the suggested curriculum elements of the DNP. The findings included less emphasis on theory and less content regarding research methodology, with the focus being on use and evaluation of research (37). Other recommendations included emphasis on practice, clinical practice, or residency requirement; an emphasis on scholarly practice; and, in place of the traditional dissertation with the doctorate, the DNP should require a capstone project (37). A key element of the capstone project is that it should be focused on clinical practice, intended to solve a practice issue or to directly inform practice. The task force also recommended seven essential areas of content. In 2005, the AACN convened two additional task forces—one task force to examine the DNP essentials to focus on and refine content and competencies and the other focused on a roadmap for implementation. Stakeholders meetings occurred involving leaders from a large number of nursing organizations. In 2006, the final report was provided to and approved by the AACN board. Programs began to be planned and implemented quickly. The DNP is an ideal mechanism for APRNs who wish to acquire a terminal degree and remain practice rather than research oriented (DPN essentials are included in Table 1–6). It is the expectation that all advanced practice education programs will move to the achievement of a DNP by 2015 (37).

TABLE 1–6 Essentials of Doctoral Education

1. Scientific underpinnings for practice;
2. Organization and system leadership for quality improvement and system thinking;
3. Clinical scholarship and analytic methods for evidence-based practice;
4. Technology and information for the improvement and transformation of patient-centered health care;
5. Health care policy for advocacy in health care;
6. Interprofessional collaboration for improving patient and population outcomes;
7. Clinical prevention and population health for improving the nation's health; and
8. Advanced nursing practice for improving the delivery of patient care

As the landscape of care continues to evolve and we realize our preferred future within our profession, perhaps the boundaries and distinctions will continue to gain clarity. These are times of great change, and we have been preparing for quite some time. It truly is about looking forward through a new vision for nursing, particularly advanced practice nursing. New and exciting roles, increasing expectations in practice, and implementation of a standard approach to APRN preparation will cumulatively guide us toward a solid future. Our contributions to the health of our patients and families can be maximized.

NEW ROLE: THE CLINICAL NURSE LEADER

In 2007, the AACN released "White Paper on the Education and Role of the Clinical Nurse Leader," which is a new role requiring graduate education and is intended to be an advanced generalist (38). In 2000, the review of published studies citing fragmented care, medical errors, and broken health care systems led to the initial work in defining this role. The report also cites the problems with health care quality and outcomes, the nursing shortage, and the further reality of a global society, technology, and diversity in our population as the impetus for the role. This clinical nurse leader (CNL) is the first nursing role in more than three decades and is based on the acquisition of a master's degree (39).

The educational or core competencies and fundamental aspects of the CNL role are delineated in Table 1–7. The white paper clearly articulates the meaning and components of each of these competencies. The overlap of competencies and roles has created some confusion and concern within the CNS community (40, 41). Despite some overlap within the competencies, it is important to be aware of the critical and distinct differences that delineate CNL from CNS practice. These two roles can clearly complement each other and lead to positive patient and family outcomes. Each of the roles

TABLE 1–7 Clinical Nurse Leader

Core Competencies	Fundamental Aspects of the Role
Critical thinking	Clinician
Communication	Outcomes manager
Assessment	Client advocate
Nursing technology and resource management	Educator
Health promotion/Risk reduction/Disease prevention	Information manager
Illness and disease management	Systems analyst/risk anticipator
Information and health care technologies	Team manager
Ethics	Collaborator
Human diversity	Member of the profession
Global health care	Lifelong learner
Health care systems	
Health care policy	
Provider and manager of care	
Designer/Manager/Coordinator of care	
Member of a profession	

has a focus on management of care based on particular patient and family needs. The roles are also complementary in that they are prepared to provide care for the full continuum of the patient experience including health promotion and disease prevention through disease management.

The first characteristic difference lies within preparation and function. The CNL is intended to be an advanced generalist. This role is typically intended to function at the unit level and not as an expert in a particular population. The CNS is as the title suggests a specialist. The CNL is prepared at the master's level, based on the guiding competencies found in the Essentials of Master's Education for Professional Nursing Practice (42, 43). The APRN Consensus Model clearly defines the APRN as being prepared in one of the four previously mentioned roles (34). The competencies and educational preparation for CNS practice are defined within the new model.

Another significant difference lies within the area of practice. The CNL focuses on the microsystem. Although the CNS practice includes issues within a microsystem, the macrosystem is a key focus. It is noted that even for the CNS who is unit based, there is often participation and involvement at the system or organizational level, far outside the microsystem. Literature is beginning to evolve from those early adopters of the CNL role. A case study of a for-profit facility delineates how the business case for the role can be articulated and a model of care delivery can be designed and implemented using the role effectively (7). These authors note that at the time of their publication, the case study focuses on implementation of the model and outcomes had yet to be measured. However, other literature suggests the role is quite valuable in improving outcomes. The Department of Veterans Affairs in the Tennessee Valley Healthcare System implemented the role in five diverse microsystems: an ambulatory surgery unit, a surgical inpatient unit, a gastrointestinal laboratory, a surgical intensive care unit, and a transitional care unit. In each of these environments, clinical, satisfaction, and financial outcomes were measured. Each of the five outcome measures examined demonstrated statistically significant improvements post implementation of the role (44). This exemplifies the potentially positive impact of the CNL at the microsystem level.

One of the key elements of the CNL role is that of a "lateral integrator." This particular concept and aspect of care that the CNL provides have great benefit in ensuring that gaps in communication are identified and corrected. Matrixed systems and nursing complexity continue to bring rise to the myriad of task-related activities with each patient encounter. Anecdotal evidence continues to emerge supporting this problem. Researchers in 2006 studied six hospitals in the United States through examination of work system failures (45). The findings from this study are startling in that the average number of work system failures in an 8-hour shift was 8.4 (45).

The CNS is prepared for the design and evaluation of comprehensive patient and family programs, which is another distinction between the CNS and CNL roles. While the program design and evaluation may fall on the expertise of the CNS, the CNL may be in the perfect position to implement this macrosystem approach within the microsystem. Another hallmark of CNS practice has long been involvement in research and the generation of nursing knowledge. To compliment the CNS as generator of research, the CNL is prepared as a consumer of research and charged with implementation of EBP. Ultimately, the CNL functions at the point of care. The CNS will likely be a consultant to the CNL through the CNS's unique expertise and experience.

SUMMARY

Since the advent of advanced practice nursing, there has been much change. As the landscape of health care continues to change, the challenge of advanced practice nursing will surely continue to bring significant contributions and positive outcomes to patients and their families. The current environment is riddled with system issues and barriers to accessing appropriately and timely care. There is no greater time of need for promoting CNS practice. There is promise on the horizon with a movement toward consistency in APRN regulation ensuring standardized education, licensure, and practice. Many professional organizations are aligning to bring this consistency to reality and ensure that methods of competency assessment are reliable and valid.

Over the next few years we will surely see more change. The further implementation of new roles in nursing will bring more depth and richness to our practice while augmenting care provided by the bedside nurse. The CNS is at the forefront, uniquely educated and skilled at being a change agent and highly skilled clinician. As the CNS works within the spheres of influence and interweaving a menagerie of perfectly tuned competencies within each situation, we will continue to demonstrate and illustrate our strength.

References

1. Kohn LT, Corrigan J, Donaldson MS. To Err Is Human: Building A Safer Health System. Washington, DC: National Academy Press; 2000:xxi, 287.

2. Institute of Medicine, Committee on Quality of Health Care in America. Crossing the Quality Chasm: A New Health System for the 21st Century. Washington, DC: National Academies Press; 2001:xx, 337.

3. National Quality Forum. About Us. Retrieved July 1, 2009, from http://www.qualityforum.org/about/

4. American Nurses Association. The National Database. Retrieved July 1, 2009, from http://www.nursingworld.org/MainMenuCategories/ThePracticeofProfessionalNursing/PatientSafetyQuality/Research-Measurement/The-National-Database.aspx

5. National Association of Clinical Nurse Specialists. FAQ's: What Is a Clinical Nurse Specialist? 2009 (cited March 29, 2009). Available from http://www.nacns.org/AboutNACNS/FAQs/tabid/109/Default.aspx

6. Hamric A. History and overview of the CNS role. In Hamric A, Spross J, editors. The Clinical Nurse Specialist in Theory and Practice. Philadelphia: WB Saunders; 1989:3-18.

7. McKinley M. Evolution of the clinical nurse specialist in acute and critical care. In McKinley M, editor. Acute and Critical Care Clinical Nurse Specialists: Synergy for Best Practices. St Louis: Saunders; 2007:7-9.

8. DeWitt K. Specialties in nursing. Am J Nursing 1900;1:14-17.

9. Komnenich P. The evolution of advanced practice nursing. In Stanley J, editor. Advanced Practice Nursing: Emphasizing Common Roles. Philadelphia: FA Davis; 2005:2-45.

10. Keeling A. A brief history of advanced practice nursing in the United States. In Hamric A, Spross J, Hanson C, editors. Advanced Practice Nursing: An Integrative Approach. St Louis: Saunders; 2009:3-32.

11. American Nurses Association. Nursing: A Social Policy Statement. Silver Spring, MD: American Nurses Association; 1980.

12. Lyon B. Clinical nurse specialists: Current challenges. In Stanley J, editor. Advanced Nursing Practice: Emphasizing Common Roles. Philadelphia: FA Davis; 2005:xxv-xxviii.

13. DeBourgh GA. Champions for evidence-based practice: a critical role for advanced practice nurses. AACN Clin Iss 2001;12:491-508.

14. Lyon BL. Clinical nurse specialist profile. Interview by Jo Ellen Rust. Clin Nurse Spec 2005;19:124-126.

15. Murray T. Clinical nurse specialist profile. Interview by Jo Ellen Rust. Clin Nurse Spec 2006;20:158-159.

16. NACNS Research and Practice Committee. Statement on Clinical Nurse Specialist Practice and Education. Glenville, IL: National Association of Clinical Nurse Specialists; 1998.

17. Zuzelo PR. Clinical nurse specialist practice: spheres of influence. AORN J 2003;77:361-366, 369-3672.

18. Advanced Practice Work Group; Bell L, editor. Scope of Practice and Standards of Professional Performance for the Acute and Critical Care Clinical Nurse Specialist. Aliso Viejo, CA: American Association of Critical Care Nurses; 2002.

19. Mian P. The role of the clinical nurse specialist in the development of a domestic violence program. Clin Nurse Spec 2000;14:229-234.

20. Harrington L. Program development: role of the clinical nurse specialist in implementing a fast-track postanesthesia care unit. AACN Clin Iss 2005;16:78-88.

21. National CNS Competency Task Force; Filipovich C, editor. Organizing Framework and CNS Core Competencies. Harrisburg, PA: National Association of Clinical Nurse Specialists; 2008.

22. Darmody JV. Observing the work of the clinical nurse specialist: a pilot study. Clin Nurse Spec 2005;19:260-268.

23. Bahr S, Smith J. Improving patient outcomes utilizing an evidence-based alcohol withdrawal protocol. In France M, Urden L, Waldo M, editors. NACNS National Conference Abstracts. Philadelphia: Lippincott Williams and Wilkins; 2007:101-123.

24. Bennett T, Duffy M. The role of the clinical nurse specialist in the implementation of a multidisciplinary rapid response team. In France M, Urden L, Waldo M, editors. NACNS National Conference Abstracts. Philadelphia: Lippincott Williams and Wilkins; 2007:101-123.

25. Curl P, Oberg M. CNS leadership: saving lives with a rapid response team. In France M, Urden L, Waldo M, editors. NACNS National Conference Abstracts. Philadelphia: Lippincott Williams and Wilkins; 2007:101-123.

26. Disch J, Walton M, Barnsteiner J. The role of the clinical nurse specialist in creating a healthy work environment. AACN Clin Iss 2001;12:345-355.

27. American Association of Critical Care Nurses; Barden C, editor. AACN Standards for Establishing and Sustaining Healthy Work Environments: A Journey to Excellence. Aliso Viejo, CA: American Association of Critical Care Nurses; 2005:1-44.

28. Ervin NE. Clinical coaching: a strategy for enhancing evidence-based nursing practice. Clin Nurse Spec 2005;19:296-301.

29. Moffitt B, Butler M. Changing a medical unit culture. Clin Nurse Spec 2009;23:187-191.

30. Puntillo KA, McAdam JL. Communication between physicians and nurses as a target for improving end-of-life care in the intensive care unit: challenges and opportunities for moving forward. Crit Care Med 2006;34(11 suppl):S332-S340.

31. Crawford GW. A commentary: a practical application for a framework for ethical decision making. Dimens Crit Care Nurs 2005;24:80-81.

32. Shirey MR. Nursing practice models for acute and critical care: overview of care delivery models. Crit Care Nurs Clin North Am 2008;20:365-373.

33. Moloney-Harmon PA. The Synergy Model: contemporary practice of the clinical nurse specialist. Crit Care Nurse 1999;19:101-104.

34. Scott RA. A description of the roles, activities, and skills of clinical nurse specialists in the United States. Clin Nurse Spec 1999;13:183-190.

35. Cram E, et al. Restructuring the clinical nurse specialist position to a unit-based role. J Nursing Admin 1996;26:33-38.

36. APRN Consensus Work Group, National Council of State Boards of Nursing APRN Advisory Committee. Consensus Model for APRN Regulation: Licensure, Accreditation, Certification & Education. Silver Spring, MD; 2008:1-40.

37. American Association of Colleges of Nursing. AACN Position Statement on the Practice Doctorate in Nursing. Silver Spring, MD: American Association of Colleges of Nursing; 2004:1-20.

38. American Association of Colleges of Nursing. White Paper on the Education and Role of the Clinical Nurse Leader. Silver Spring, MD: American Association of Colleges of Nursing; 2007:1-40.

39. Gabuat J, et al. Implementing the clinical nurse leader role in a for-profit environment: a case study. J Nursing Admin 2008;38:302-307.

40. Goudreau KA. Confusion, concern, or complimentary function: the overlapping roles of the clinical nurse specialist and the clinical nurse leader. Nursing Admin Q 2008;32:301-307.

41. Thompson P, Lulham K. Clinical nurse leader and clinical nurse specialist role delineation in the acute care setting. J Nurs Admin 2007;37:429-431.

42. American Association of Colleges of Nursing. The Essentials of Master's Education for Professional Nursing Practice. Silver

Spring, MD: American Association of Colleges of Nursing; 2011.

43. Stanley J, et al. Working Statement Comparing the Clinical Nurse Leader and clinical nurse specialist Roles: Similarities, Differences and Complementarities. Silver Spring, MD: American Association of Colleges of Nursing; 2004:1-7.

44. Hix C, McKeon L, Walters S. Clinical nurse leader impact on clinical microsystems outcomes. J Nursing Admin 2009;39:71-76.

45. Tucker AL, Spear SJ. Operational failures and interruptions in hospital nursing. Health Serv Res 2006;41: 643-662.

CHAPTER 2

Phenomena of Concern to the Clinical Nurse Specialist

Cheryl A. Lehman, PhD, RN, CNS-BC, RN-BC, CRRN

INTRODUCTION

Phenomena of concern to the clinical nurse specialist (CNS) are many and include prevention, remediation or alleviation of illness, and promotion of health within a specialty population. The CNS addresses these phenomena in the three spheres of influence: patients, nurses and nursing practice, and organizations and systems. This chapter reviews common problems that occur in acute care, including nondisease causes of illness and complications defined as nursing sensitive indicators of quality of care. The CNS has a special role in addressing these phenomena, be it as the caregiver, clinical expert, educator, collaborator, or researcher.

The National Association of Clinical Nurse Specialists (NACNS) defines *illness* as:

> *the subjective experience of somatic discomfort, including physical discomfort, emotional discomfort, and/or reduction in functional ability below the perceived capability level (1, page 64).*

They then state that the hallmark of CNS practice is the "diagnosis and treatment of illness" (1, page 64).

Nondisease causes of illness are seen in every population including medical, surgical, the acutely or critically ill, pediatric, adult, and geriatric. These problems complicate the healing process and can cause significant morbidity and mortality. They can prolong length of stay and influence discharge planning and are often very difficult to address. The CNS has the ability to have a significant impact on these problems in all three spheres of influence. Addressed in this chapter are delirium, obesity, mobility, sleep, and malnutrition.

Nurses have been recognized as having a significant effect on health care outcomes and patient safety. Recently, organizations such as the American Nurses Association (ANA) and the National Quality Forum have collaborated on the identification of nurse sensitive indicators. These measurements track clinical complications that can be seen as an outcome of the quality of nursing care delivered. This chapter will review three of these indicators: falls, pressure ulcers, and restraints. CNS involvement is integral to preventing these occurrences in the acute and long-term care settings.

DELIRIUM

Delirium has been known by many names, including acute confusional state, acute mental status change, altered mental status, organic brain syndrome, reversible dementia, Intensive Care Unit (ICU) psychosis, sundowning, acute brain failure, and toxic or metabolic encephalopathy (and don't forget subacute befuddlement!) (2, 3). According to the fourth edition of the *Diagnostic and Statistical Manual of Mental Disorders* (*DSM-IV*), key features of delirium include a disturbance of consciousness with reduced ability to focus, sustain, or shift attention, as well as a change in cognition or the development of a perceptual disturbance that is not better accounted for by a preexisting, established, or evolving dementia that develops over a short period of time (hours to days) and that tends to fluctuate during the course of the day. There is also evidence from the history and physical or from diagnostic findings that the disturbance is caused by a medical condition, substance intoxication, or medication side effect (4).

Delirium is the most common psychiatric syndrome found in the general hospital setting (5). It is often mistaken for dementia, depression, mania, or "old age" (6). Delirium affects 11% to 42% of hospitalized patients and is unrecognized in 66% to 84% of patients (5). As many as 60% to 80% of patients in the medical ICU setting may be delirious (5). Mortality rates of hospitalized patients with delirium range from 22% to 76% (7). For patients admitted with delirium, mortality has been documented to range from 10% to 26%; for patients who develop delirium during a hospital stay, mortality jumps to 22% to 76%. The latter group of patients also has a high rate of death in the months after discharge (6). Delirium increases hospital length of stay and costs, particularly in the older adult population (7). Delirium can last 12 months or longer, especially in persons with dementia. Delirium may be the only symptom suggesting acute illness in an older adult. Acute-onset delirium is considered to be a medical emergency.

Etiology

A syndrome rather than a disease, delirium has been found to have both predisposing and precipitating factors. Predisposing factors include age older than 65, male gender, dehydration, dementia, immobility, chronic renal or hepatic impairment, and vision or hearing impairment (5, 7). Precipitants of delirium include admission to the ICU setting, restraints, infection, malnutrition, polypharmacy, electrolyte imbalance, environmental stimuli, hypoxia, hypoglycemia, stroke, hip fracture, hypothermia or hyperthermia, seizures, pain, sleep deprivation, surgery, indwelling urinary catheter, and drug or alcohol withdrawal (5, 7). Drugs believed to induce delirium are many and include antibiotics such as ampicillin, cephalosporins, and gentamicin; antidepressants such as amitriptyline, desipramine, and monoamine oxidase (MAO) inhibitors; cardiac medications such as beta blockers, isosorbide dinitrates (ISDNs), and captopril; and pain medications such as aspirin, codeine, and opiates, as well as hypnotics and sedatives (5).

Pathophysiology

The exact pathophysiology of delirium is not known. It has been hypothesized that there are two basic classifications: direct brain insults and aberrant stress responses. Direct brain insults would include general and regional energy deprivation (hypoxemia, hypoglycemia, stroke); metabolic disorders such as hyponatremia and hypercalcemia; and/or the effects of medications. Aberrant stress responses include inflammation and the activity of the limbic-hypothalamic-pituitary-adrenal axis. These responses are associated with aging and CNS disease, two major predisposing factors for delirium (8).

Clinical Presentation

Patients with delirium present with an acute onset of confusion. One early sign is an inability to sustain attention, usually noticed first by the family or caregiver. The confusion has a fluctuating course, the presence of inattention, and either disorganized thinking or an altered level of consciousness. Patients with delirium may exhibit hyperactive, hypoactive, or mixed behavior. Hyperactive delirium is often associated with alcohol withdrawal or use of PCP, LSD, or amphetamines. The most common subtype of delirium is hypoactive delirium, which can be associated with diseases such as hepatic encephalopathy and hypercapnea. Hypoactive delirium is often unrecognized since the patient is usually subdued, lethargic, or even comatose. Mixed delirium can be associated with daytime sedation and nocturnal agitation (6, 7).

Diagnosis

The first step in diagnosis of delirium is recognition of risk. Delirium is a clinical diagnosis. The American Psychiatric Association recommends use of a valid and reliable scale, such as the Confusion Assessment Method (CAM), for diagnosis. Diagnosis of delirium using the CAM requires the presence of 1 and 2, plus either 3 and 4.

1. Acute change in mental status and fluctuating course
   - Is there evidence of an acute change in cognition from the patient's baseline?
   - Does the abnormal behavior fluctuate during the day (i.e., tend to come and go, or increase or decrease in severity?)
2. Inattention
   - Does the patient have difficulty focusing attention (e.g., being easily distractible or having difficulty keeping track of what is being said?)
3. Disorganized thinking
   - Is the patient's thinking disorganized or incoherent (e.g., rambling or irrelevant conversation, unclear or illogical flow of ideas, or unpredictable switching from subject to subject?)
4. Altered level of consciousness
   - Is the patient's mental status anything besides alert (i.e., hypervigilant [hyperalert], lethargic [drowsy but easily aroused], stuporous [difficult to arouse], or comatose [unarousable]

There is also a CAM-ICU scale available for clinicians in the ICU setting. The CAM or CAM-ICU scales should also be used to routinely screen for development of delirium in high risk groups (9-11).

The CNS should suspect delirium in any patient who:

- Receives orders for restraints or requires restraints for safety
- Receives an order for an as-needed tranquilizer

- Falls or pulls on tubes/catheters
- Wanders/leaves against advice
- Is arguing with staff
- Demonstrates restlessness/insomnia
- Is hallucinating, picking at things in air
- Described as "pleasantly confused" or "cloudy"
- Not moving out of bed/sleeping too much
- Not eating meals
- Unreasonably refusing medications (12)

The differential diagnosis of delirium concerns the presence of dementia and/or depression—are the presenting symptoms due to dementia, due to delirium, or due to delirium superimposed on dementia or is depression present? A detailed history from the family, caregivers, and nurses becomes important in distinguishing these details.

Physical examination is indicated to address the precipitating factors, including new or worsened illness, alcohol withdrawal, sleep deprivation, hypoxia, and pain. Medication review is certainly indicated, paying particular attention to drug-drug interactions and drug-disease interactions. Vital signs and pulse oximetry are included in the physical examination. The physical examination should attempt to rule in or rule out pain, infection, urinary retention, fecal impaction, pressure ulcers, and acute musculoskeletal injury. A focused neurological examination should be included.

Diagnostic studies for work-up of delirium include the following laboratory tests: complete blood count (CBC) with differential, basic metabolic panel (BMP), liver function tests (LFTs), renal function tests, electrolytes, glucose, urinalysis, cardiac enzymes, and cultures as appropriate. Arterial blood gases (ABGs), thyroid function tests, thiamine and B_{12} levels, and sedimentation rate should be considered. Depending on the results of the review of medications, drug levels and toxicology screen might be ordered. Electrocardiogram (ECG) and chest radiograph should be ordered, and head imaging considered if there has been recent trauma or a new focal neurologic finding. A lumbar puncture might be performed if CNS infection is suspected, and electroencephalogram (EEG) may also be indicated (6, 13).

Management

The focus of treatment of delirium is reversal of the cause. This might include treating infection, correcting electrolyte imbalances, calming and quieting the environment, removing tubes and lines, or applying hearing aids and glasses. Medications that could be causing or contributing to the delirium should be discontinued, including such drugs as alcohol, illegal drugs, analgesics, anticholinergics, CNS depressants, cimetidine, and lidocaine. Disorders that may be causing or contributing to the delirium should be addressed, including fecal impaction, myocardial infarction, heart failure, hypoxia, hypercapnea, thyroid disorders, anemia, nutritional disorders, renal failure, hepatic failure, and psychiatric conditions, including depression.

Behavior may need to be managed in the short term. Medications commonly used to manage behaviors associated with delirium include:

Haloperidol (Haldol)

- 1-2 mg every 2-4 hours prn PO, IM, IV (4, 11)
- Elderly: 0.25-0.5 mg every 4 hours prn PO, IM, IV (4, 11)
- Titrate up as needed for continued agitation (4, 11)
  - *Note.* IV form is 2× as potent as PO form
- IV administration is not a U.S. Food and Drug Administration (FDA)-approved route
- Never administer decanoate form IV; IV use of lactate form is an unlabeled use
- Parenteral administration may cause hypotension
- Avoid in parkinsonism due to risk of worsening Parkinson symptoms and motor function, substitute lorazepam
- Monitor for QTc prolongation with ECGs. Use with caution with QTc interval of ≥400 ms; administration of other drugs that may increase QTc interval; or electrolyte imbalance
- Major substrate of cytochrome (CYP) P450 2D6, 3A4
- Inhibits CYP 2D6 and 3A4
- Half-life 18 hours (14)

Risperodone (Risperdal)

- 0.5-2 mg PO daily or bid
- 0.5 mg PO bid for elderly debilitated patients with severe renal failure or hepatic failure or predisposed to hypotension
- *Black box warning*: patients with dementia-related psychosis at high risk of death
- Caution with Parkinson disease due to risk of worsening motor function, cardiovascular (CV) disease (may be associated with orthostatic hypotension and tachyardia)
- Can cause orthostatic hypotension, seizures, hyperprolactinemia, and body temperature abnormalities
- Monitor renal function
- May prolong QT interval
- >2 mg/day may increase extrapyramidal effects in elderly (6)

Benzodiazepines

- Use with great caution, low dose, lorazepam preferred (short acting, high potency)
- For alcohol or sedative-hypnotic withdrawal delirium (12)

- Lorazepam: 0.5-2 mg PO/IV/IM, may need to repeat every 2-4 hours
- For delirium tremens
- Caution with limited pulmonary reserve, elderly, myasthenia gravis, organic brain syndrome, or Parkinson disease (6)

Nurses have an important role in the prevention, early recognition, and treatment of delirium, as many interventions are nursing focused. These include:

1. Addressing sensory problems by ensuring the patient has glasses and hearing aids in place
2. Addressing environmental issues by maintaining a quiet unit, allowing time for uninterrupted sleep, keeping the patient awake during day, hanging wall calendars and clocks, and adjusting lighting to accurately reflect day/night
3. Avoiding restraints and Foley catheters and minimizing the use of "tubes" such as IV lines
4. Optimizing nutrition and hydration
5. Assessing and treating pain
6. Encouraging the family to bring in familiar objects
7. Encouraging the family to stay with patient
8. Providing frequent orientation and a predictable environment
9. Keeping tasks simple and avoiding multiple stimuli
10. Allowing uninterrupted time for sleep at night
11. Encouraging mobility and self-care
12. Considering relaxation tapes, pleasant music, or massage
13. Monitoring and preventing constipation and urinary retention (15)

The most effective treatment for delirium is prevention, including

- Nonpharmacologic sleep protocols
- Emphasis on mobility activities
- Maintaining sensory aids—glasses, hearing aids
- Maintaining hydration
- Maintaining oxygenation
- Monitoring medications

CLINICAL NURSE SPECIALIST COMPETENCIES AND SPHERES OF INFLUENCE

CNSs play an important role in the prevention, recognition, assessment, and treatment of delirium in the clinical setting in the patient, nurse, and systems spheres.

Clinical Expert/Direct Care

Care related to this competency will vary according to the specific role of the CNS in the institution or facility. The CNS who enacts the "mid-level" provider role will combine medical and nursing management. This CNS will recognize the patient's cognitive changes, perform a focused physical and cognitive assessment, order lab work and other tests, interpret findings, and order interventions. Follow-up to ensure clearing of delirium and preventive measures will be performed and the environment examined for needed changes such as staff education, unit practices, or edits in documentation practices. The CNS in a direct caregiving, bedside role will have recognized risk factors for a population of patients and this patient in particular, implemented preventive strategies, recognized early symptoms, performed a focused assessment, and collaborated with the assigned provider to relate findings and recommend tests and interventions. Since delirium is often misdiagnosed or not recognized at all, the CNS plays an important role as a clinical expert who is knowledgeable in care of the patient at risk for delirium.

Consultation

Fulfillment of this competency in relation to delirium again depends on the exact role of the CNS in the setting. The mid-level provider may initiate consultation with other professional providers when performing the workup for delirium, if the cause of delirium is not clearly found in the tests ordered. The CNS may also, however, act as the consultant if recognized by others as an expert in care of the confused patients. Any member of the professional team may consult the clinically expert CNS, including physicians, nurses, therapists, and others.

Systems Leadership

The leadership competency of the CNS is important in the care of the patient population who is at risk for delirium. The CNS leadership skills may be beneficial in systems analysis in which the overall care of the delirious patient is examined in relation to evidence-based practice protocols. The CNS may lead a team of interdisciplinary professionals in assessing systemwide care of delirious patients and recommending changes to administration to improve care such as medication reviews, changes in mealtime routines, and infection control practices. The CNS may also initiate examination of the complications related to delirium and develop interventions and system "fixes" to decrease these complications (e.g., falls). The CNS is key in assessing and revising the structure affecting these patients—for example, nurse education, documentation, policies, and procedures.

Collaboration

The CNS will collaborate with many others in care of the patient with delirium, including those consulted, nurses and other team members, and departments such as risk management. The delirious patient should not exist in isolation, but through collaboration with others the CNS will ensure that the best care is given, systems are evaluated, and practices are updated, and the entire

team is knowledgeable about prevention, early identification, and prompt treatment of delirium while maintaining patient safety. Collaboration with the therapists in developing distractional activities for the delirious, restless patient is another way in which the CNS can collaborate with others.

Coaching/Teaching/Mentoring

This CNS competency may be one of the most important in care of the patient with delirium. The CNS has a strong role in educating the entire team, including physicians, on care of the patient population at risk for delirium. The CNS will likely be most involved in nursing staff education in which the entire nursing staff is taught about delirium and mentored in updating unit practices to prevent delirium. CNS interventions might include locating and sharing pertinent articles, assisting nurses to develop and present information to their peers, working with staff to develop education materials for all levels of staff as well as patients and families, and modeling interventions for the agitated patient.

Research/Evidence-Based Practice

This competency becomes evermore key as the importance of evidence-based practice (EBP) grows. The CNS whose population is at risk for the development of delirium will assume responsibility for remaining current on EBP in relation to delirium. This will involve literature searches, participation in online or email chat groups, interpretation of research studies, discussion with experts, attendance at relevant educational offerings, and participating/networking within professional organizations. The CNS will then share this knowledge with the team and ensure that practices are up to date and evidence based.

Ethical Decision Making/Moral Agency/Advocacy

The CNS must be a strong advocate for the confused patient. Although confused, if diagnosed with delirium, the patient still has a right to informed decision making and participation in care as cognition allows. Since delirium can be expected to clear as the cause is addressed, decisions that can be delayed should be delayed. Paperwork requiring the patient's informed consent and legal signatures cannot be processed when delirium is present. Legal requirements for consent and identification of decision-maker must be followed and documented and HIPAA rules adhered to. Ethical standards still apply, such as beneficence, nonmaleficence, justice, veracity, fiduciary responsibilities, and fidelity, and it is the CNS who should take the lead in ensuring that ethical standards are met and maintained.

Patients and Families

In the patient sphere, the CNS uses the competencies of direct care in assessment, diagnosis, planning, intervention, and evaluation. The CNS provides advanced assessment skills for early recognition of delirium, develops differential diagnoses, investigates the patient's problems through initiation of diagnostic studies, and addresses the direct cause of the delirious state. Patient outcomes are evaluated by the CNS and interventions modified as needed.

Teaching/coaching about the importance of hydration, nutrition, and mobility is central to prevention of delirium. The CNS encourages the patient/family to supply and maintain sensory aides such as glasses and hearing aids. Families are encouraged to stay with elder family members to provide a recognizable face in an unfamiliar environment.

Nurses and Nursing Practice

The CNS assesses nurses and nursing staff knowledge about prevention, recognition, and interventions for delirium. The CNS engages in teaching/coaching activities to educate nurses and support staff in evidence-based prevention and early recognition of delirium. The importance of monitoring bowel and bladder function, treating pain effectively and efficiently, and providing a quiet environment for sleep is stressed. Mobility protocols are taught to staff, and interventions for the agitated/delirious patient are developed in conjunction with unit employees. Restraint use is addressed and minimized, and staff is taught about alternatives to restraints. The CNS teaches staff proper documentation of patient assessment, interventions, and outcomes and then reviews the documentation to determine issues and trends in the management of delirium.

Organizations and Systems

At the organization or system level, the CNS assesses need, then plans and intervenes to develop educational programs for units other than his or her own. Activity packs are constructed to aid nurses in channeling the delirious patient's excess energy. The CNS participates in designing safe patient-care units for populations likely to experience delirium and in assisting administrators in developing staffing guidelines for care of the high-risk populations, thus minimizing liability for both facility and staff. The CNS also collaborates with other professionals on the health care team to establish interprofessional guidelines for care of the patient with delirium.

OBESITY

Obesity is at epidemic proportions in the United States. Thirty-three percent of men, 35.3% of women; and 16.3% of children aged 2 to 19 are currently obese according to recent studies (16). Obesity is implicated in many health conditions, including coronary heart disease, type 2 diabetes, cancers (endometrial, breast, and colon), hypertension, dyslipidemia, stroke, liver and gallbladder disease, sleep apnea and respiratory problems, osteoarthritis, and gynecological problems such as abnormal menses and infertility. In 2007, only one state (Colorado) had a prevalence of obesity less than 20%. Thirty states had a prevalence equal to or greater than 25%; three of these states (Alabama, Mississippi, and Tennessee) had a prevalence of obesity equal to or greater than 30% (17).

Healthy People 2020 has two objectives related to obesity:

- To increase the proportion of adults who are at a healthy weight
- To reduce the proportion of children and adolescents who are considered obese

Obesity affects not only the health of the individual but the health care system as a whole. As hospitals strive to meet the needs of morbidly obese patients, the bottom line for hospitals is profoundly affected. The prevalence of obesity is now factored into designs of patient rooms and the purchase of new equipment. Greater Cincinnati Hospital recently spent $6,900 extra per new patient room in constructing bariatric accessible patient rooms. Additional costs of $15,000 per room were needed to install steel reinforcement in each ceiling to support sling devices to lift heavy patients, and $4,000 per room for bariatric beds. There is also added cost for bariatric stretchers and wheelchairs. Doorways have to be wider to accommodate the wider stretchers and wheelchairs, and bathrooms must be specially fitted, at an added expense (18). Imaging equipment requires expensive upgrades to accommodate patients over 300 pounds and still may provide suboptimal diagnostic results, adding to liability issues.

Nurses who must assist the bariatric patient to move put themselves at risk for workplace injuries. The unique activity of moving flexible humans from surface to surface has been difficult to study in real-life situations in which the rooms might be small, the equipment might be unreliable, and the patient might be unpredictable or unable to cooperate. Moving the bariatric patient presents its own unique challenge, and risk of injury to the nurse as well as the patient increases as weight increases. If the nurse is obese, risk factors multiply (19).

Etiology

While the basics of obesity seem to be too much food intake combined with too little exercise, the etiology of obesity is really a complex interaction among body weight, genetics, metabolism, behavior, environment, education, culture, and socioeconomic status. Poverty and lack of education have been found to contribute to obesity. A reliance on modern transportation rather than walking or bicycling contributes to a lack of calorie expenditure. The ever-growing fast-food industry has been blamed for providing busy families with high-fat, high-calorie foods at an affordable price. Certain ethnic groups and races seem to be predisposed to obesity. The Pima Indians of Arizona and other Native American groups have a high prevalence of obesity. Polynesians, Micronesians, Anurans, Maoris, African Americans, and Hispanic populations also have tendencies toward obesity. Some illnesses may lead to obesity or weight gain. These include Cushing disease, hypothyroidism, and polycystic ovary syndrome. Drugs such as steroids and some antidepressants may also cause weight gain (20, 21).

Pathophysiology

The pathogenesis of obesity is complex. Studies of twins, adoptees, and families suggest that genetics plays a role in obesity. Genetics is presumed to explain 40% to 70% of the variance in obesity. For instance, the agouti gene defect has been found to cause obesity in rats. In humans, serum concentrations of the agouti gene are higher in obese males than in nonobese males. The importance of the gene in humans is not yet known.

Proopiomelanocortin (POMC) and alpha–melanocyte-stimulating hormone (alpha-MSH) act centrally on the melanocortin receptor 4 (MC 4) to reduce dietary intake. Genetic defects in POMC production and MC4 genetic mutations have been described as monogenic causes of obesity. As many as 5% of children who are obese have MC4 or POMC mutations. Prohormone convertase is an enzyme that may be involved in the conversion of POMC to alpha-MSH. Rare patients who have been found to have an alteration in this enzyme have also been found to have significant obesity, hypogonadotropic hypogonadism, and central adrenal insufficiency. PPAR-gamma is a transcription factor that affects adipocyte differentiation. Every person with mutations of this receptor has severe obesity (21).

Leptin is also under investigation for its role in obesity. The major role of leptin, a 1-kDa protein that is produced mainly in the white adipose tissue, is to signal satiety to the hypothalamus and thus reduce food intake while modulating energy expenditure and carbohydrate metabolism, preventing weight gain. Most humans who are obese are leptin resistant. While other factors also contribute strongly to obesity, the discovery of leptin in 1994 has added to the knowledge about the factors that contribute to obesity (21).

One recent hypothesis is that an inflammatory and possibly infective etiology may be found for obesity. For example, adenovirus 36 infection is associated with obesity in chickens and mice. Data suggest that humans who are not obese have a 5% prevalence of adenovirus 36 infection, while obese persons have a prevalence of 20% to 30% (21).

Predictors of obesity include a low metabolic rate, increased CHO oxidation, insulin resistance, and low sympathetic activity. Social predictors include lower socioeconomic class, lower education level, and cessation of smoking (22).

Clinical Presentation

The clinical presentation of obesity is obvious, with the patient presenting with complaints of weight management or failure in achieving weight loss. Other patients may present with secondary complications, such as CV disease and diabetes.

The most commonly used method of measuring obesity is the body mass index (BMI). BMI is weight (in kilograms) divided by height (in meters) squared. Class I obesity is defined as BMI of 30 to 34.9 mg/kg^2. Class II obesity is BMI of 35 to 39.9 mg/kg^2, and Class III or morbid obesity is defined as BMI of 40 kg/m^2 or greater (21, 22).

Recent research indicates that regional fat distribution affects the prevalence of comorbidities for an individual. For instance, high abdominal fat is correlated with worse metabolic and clinical consequences of obesity such as CV risk and metabolic syndrome (21).

Diagnosis

The history taken from the bariatric patient should include dietary habits and patterns of exercise. Family history of weight issues should also be explored. Social issues such as socioeconomic status, race, and ethnic and cultural issues must be assessed. Bariatric patients should be screened for depression, eating disorders, and the comorbidities that commonly accompany obesity. See Table 2–1 for a further description of comorbidities associated with obesity.

The CNS should measure the waist and hips as an estimate of visceral fat. Persons with a BMI of 25 to 34.9 mg/kg^2 and/or a waist circumference of more than 40 inches have a greater risk of hypertension, type 2 diabetes, and dyslipidemia. Waist circumferences of 102 cm in males and 88 cm in females require urgent therapeutic intervention (21). Neck circumference is thought to be predictive for sleep apnea and should also be serially measured. A detailed CV and respiratory evaluation is always indicated, as well as an in-depth assessment of endocrine and musculoskeletal systems, nutritional status, and condition of patient's skin.

Differential diagnosis of obesity includes Cushing syndrome, hypothyroidism, insulinoma, hypothalamic obesity, genetic syndrome, growth hormone deficiency, hypogonadism, eating disorders (binge-purge and night-eating disorder), and polycystic ovarian syndrome. Other considerations are sleep apnea, cardiomyopathy, cirrhosis, diabetes, hypertension, and nephrotic syndrome. Medications should be reviewed as possible contributors to weight gain (21). These might include drugs such as steroids, antidepressants, and antipsychotics, among others.

Work-up for obesity includes a lipid panel, LFTs, thyroid function tests, fasting glucose, and renal function, and diagnostics for congestive heart failure (CHF) should be included as well. Standard anthropometric measurements to estimate the degree of visceral and subcutaneous fat are also indicated. A 24-hour urinary free cortisol should be ordered when Cushing

TABLE 2–1 Comorbidities That Commonly Accompany Obesity

System	Manifestation
Cancers	Endometrial, prostate, gallbladder, breast, colon, lung
Cardiovascular	Essential hypertension, coronary artery disease, left ventricular hypertrophy, cor pulmonale, cardiomyopathy, pulmonary hypertension
Central nervous system	Stroke, idiopathic intracranial hypertension
Extremities	Venous varicosities, venous or lymphatic edema
Gastrointestinal	Gallbladder disease, fatty liver infiltration, reflux esophagitis
Genitourinary	Stress incontinence
Metabolic	Insulin resistance, hyperinsulinemia, type 2 diabetes, dyslipidemia
Obstetric	Pregnancy-related hypertension, fetal macrosomia
Orthopedic	Osteoarthritis, joint disease
Psychologic	Depression, social isolation
Respiratory	Obstructive sleep apnea, obesity hypoventilation syndrome, respiratory infections, bronchial asthma
Reproductive	Early puberty, infertility, polycystic ovaries, anovulation, hypogonadotrophic hypogonadism
Skin	Intertrigo, hirsutism, increased risk of cellulitis and carbuncles
Surgical	Increased surgical risk, increased postoperative complications
Other	Impaired mobility, difficulty with personal hygiene

syndrome is suspected. A dietary consult is also indicated (21).

Management

The goals of weight management programs are weight loss and improvement in risk factors for secondary complications. The American College of Physicians has issued guidelines for management of obesity in primary care. There are five recommendations in the guidelines:

- Counsel all patients with BMI ≥30 kg/m² on diet, lifestyle, and goals for weight loss.
- Drug therapy may be offered to patients who have not achieved weight loss through diet and exercise alone.
- Drug options include sibutramine, orlistat, phentermine, diethylpropion, and off-label drugs fluoxetine and bupripion.
- Consider bariatric surgery for patients with BMI ≥40 kg/m² who have failed diet and exercise (with or without medications) and who have obesity-related comorbidities such as hypertension and diabetes.
- Bariatric surgery should be performed at high-volume centers with experienced surgeons (23). Extensive counseling must be part of the program before and after the surgery.

Weight loss should be medically monitored for the bariatric patient. The CNS should monitor for cardiac arrhythmias, electrolyte imbalances, and hyperuricemia. There should be psychological support at all times. Weight loss programs are long term, with prescreening,

weight-loss, and weight-maintenance aspects. Goals are individualized and families should be included in the program. The most important aspect is achieving a calorie deficit. Activity must be maintained throughout the program to ensure good results. The exercise goal is 30 to 60 minutes of aerobic isotonic exercise 5 to 7 times per week (21).

Medications are increasingly available to assist in weight loss programs. They are of three types: (1) those that impair appetite through central action; (2) those that impair dietary absorption; and (3) those that increase energy expenditure. See Table 2–2 for further discussion of medications for obesity. While drug therapy can play a supporting role in weight management, there are legitimate concerns about efficacy, safety, and observations that most patients regain weight when the medications are stopped (22). Antiobesity medications are useful, along with diet and exercise, for patients with a BMI >30 kg/m². There are no published data about drug treatment with sibutramine and orlistat for longer than 2 years and 4 years, respectively. It should be remembered that drug therapy does not cure obesity. Patients prescribed drug therapy for weight loss should be taught that when the maximal therapeutic effect of the drug is achieved, weight loss will cease; and when drug therapy is discontinued, weight is regained (22).

The only proved modality associated with sustained weight loss in the bariatric patient is surgical therapy. On the one hand, it works ... on the other hand, it is expensive, surgical risks are many, and results vary depending on surgeon and the procedure selected. Surgical therapy

TABLE 2–2 Medications for Treating Obesity

Medication	Classification	Comments
Sibutramine (Meridia)	Sympathomimetic	Schedule IV drug Recommended for BMI ≥30, or ≥27 with risk factors like diabetes, hypertension, or dyslipidemia Blocks norepinephrine and serotonin reuptake Inhibits food intake (anorexian) Rapidly absorbed Active metabolite Weight loss associated with decreased low-density lipoprotein (LDL) and triglycerides Increases systolic and diastolic blood pressure (SBP and DBP) Caution with congestive heart disease (CHD), congestive heart failure (CHF), cerebrovascular accident (CVA), arrhythmia Caution with renal impairment, glaucoma, seizures, or liver failure Not within 2 weeks of MAO inhibitors Metabolized by P-450 system (CYP 3A4) Start with 10 mg daily/titrate to effect 15 mg/day max

TABLE 2-2 **Medications for Treating Obesity—cont'd**

Medication	Classification	Comments
Phentermine (Adipex-P)	Sympathomimetic	Schedule IV drug Recommended for BMI ≥30, or ≥27 with risk factors such as diabetes, hypertension, or dyslipidemia Anorexiant For short-term use only (~12 weeks) Low-dose, nonresin complex formulation: 8 mg PO tid, 30 min before meals or 1-2 h after meals High dose, resin complex formulation: 15-37.5 mg PO q AM 30 min ac or 2 hours pc Tolerance to anorexiant effect develops with a few weeks: do not increase dose, but do discontinue drug when this occurs Increases BP Antagonizes antihypertensive agents May enhance hypoglycemic medication action Decreased anorexiant action with tricyclic antidepressants (TCAs) Enhanced cardiovascular (CV) effects with MAO inhibitors Do not give with fluoxetine Potential for abuse Caution with hyperthyroidism, diabetes, arteriosclerosis, renal impairment, glaucoma, drug abuse
Diethylpropion (Tenuate)	Sympathomimetic	Schedule IV drug Recommended for BMI ≥30, or ≥27 with risk factors such as diabetes, hypertension, or dyslipidemia Anorexiant 25 mg PO tid ac or 75 mg sustained release PO qd midmorning Not within 2 weeks of MAOI administration Decreased effect with TCAs Antagonizes antihypertensive effect of guanethidine Caution with history of drug abuse, glaucoma, or CV disease
Orlistat (Xenical) (Alli OTC)	Pancreatic lipase inhibitor	Recommended for BMI ≥30, or ≥27 with risk factors such as diabetes, hypertension, or dyslipidemia Inhibits absorption of dietary fats Increases fecal fat Xenical 120 mg tid with each main meal containing fat (Alli OTC 60 mg dose available). Omit dose if meal skipped or if meal is fat free Decreases LDL and total cholesterol May decrease absorption of fat-soluble vitamins: give multivitamin with vitamins ADEK 2 h before or after orlistat Side effects include cramps, flatus, fecal incontinence, oily spotting Side effects increase if meal is high in fat
Fluoxetine (Prozac)	SSRI	Off-label use For short-term use only Benefit in obese patients with depression Not FDA approved for weight loss Dose = 60 mg daily Weight loss may not be sustained
Bupropion (Wellbutrin)	Dopamine-reuptake inhibitor	Off-label use Trials show promise

has been shown to improve type 2 diabetes, hypertension, heart failure, edema, respiratory complications, asthma, dyslipidemia, and other complications associated with obesity. Surgical therapy is recommended for those with BMI ≥ 40 mg/kg^2 or those with BMI 35 to 40 mg/kg^2 with serious comorbidities (21).

CLINICAL NURSE SPECIALIST COMPETENCIES AND SPHERES OF INFLUENCE

Clinical Expert/Direct Care
The CNS in a mid-level provider role would be expected to monitor the weight of the patients seen, recognize the risks of weight gain and obesity, assess the patient who is gaining weight or who cannot lose weight thoroughly, order laboratory tests and work-up as needed, and collaborate with the patient to develop a weight-management plan. The CNS would be alert for complications and comorbidities related to obesity, such as hypertension and dyslipidemia, and intervene appropriately. The CNS would also, then, address system issues related to the presence of obese patients in the practice or setting—equipment size and safety, staff safety, liability issues, and policies/procedures related to care of the obese patient.

Consultation
The CNS may consult others, for example, the bariatric surgeon or nutritionist, in care of the patient with obesity. The CNS also acts as consultant to those caring for the obese patient, such as nurses, aides, therapists, and physicians. The CNS in the consultant role for the obese patient population would be sharing skills and knowledge in issues such as patient equipment, patient transfers (and staff safety), and prevention of complications.

Systems Leadership
CNS leadership within the system is important in provision of quality care to the obese patient population. The CNS might lead a team in needs assessment for appropriate safe equipment (beds, chairs, bedside commodes), exploration of safety issues related to patient transfers between surfaces, minimizing facility and staff liability, or community prevention practices related to obesity. The CNS might be the system leader in evidence-based practices in care of the obese patient, and emerge as "the one to ask" when there are related concerns for this population of patients.

Collaboration
Collaboration can be important in care of the obese population within a hospital. CNSs in different areas of a facility have different knowledge and expertise that should be shared with others. For example, the CNS in the operating room who assists in bariatric surgery might collaborate with the postanesthesia care nurses and the CNS on the surgical unit to work on ways to minimize postoperative complications. CNSs might collaborate with physical therapists to determine safe methods of transfers for obese patients and also might collaborate with case managers and facility engineers if issues of structural safety emerge for patients being admitted.

Coaching/Teaching/Mentoring
This CNS competency is very important for the obese patient and the staff who care for him or her. New procedures, new equipment, and new knowledge must be shared with the team. The team should be mentored in their skills in working with the obese patient, including development of THEIR roles in teaching/coaching and mentoring the patient and family. Patients must be taught and coached in lifestyle changes. Families must be mentored in their role in the life of the person with obesity.

Research/Evidence-Based Practice
Since obesity is now a major issue in all populations, all CNSs should make the effort to remain up to date on care and management of the patient with obesity. As stated earlier, the CNS will perform literature searches for new research and practice guidelines, evaluate the evidence, and decide on the application of that evidence in the CNS's practice and facility. The CNS then would use leadership skills to work within the system and ensure that EBP is implemented and outcomes evaluated.

Ethical Decision-Making/Moral Agency/Advocacy
The obese patient requires an advocate to help navigating both systems and societal attitudes, and the CNS is the perfect advocate for this population. The CNS can ensure that biases within the institution do not interfere with provision of holistic, quality care. The CNS can advocate for appropriate equipment and other support services within the institution and ensure that ethical standards are met and maintained.

Patients and Families
The CNS uses the competencies of assessment, diagnosis, planning, intervention, and evaluation to manage the care of the bariatric patient. The CNS may directly manage the bariatric patient in a weight-reduction program in the outpatient setting, using clinical CNS competencies. The CNS may also directly affect the care of the bariatric patient in a hospital or long-term care setting through monitoring the care delivered, assessing for complications, and implementing interventions should complications occur. The CNS is involved in teaching and coaching the bariatric patient and family about weight management nutrition, mobility, and prevention of

complications. Often times there are deep-seated issues in the family that contribute to the patient's eating disorders, and comprehensive care in this sphere would be greatly advanced by an all-encompassing family care plan for this patient.

Nurses and Nursing Practice

The CNS assesses nurses and nursing staff knowledge about management of the bariatric patient. The CNS engages in teaching/coaching activities to educate nurses and support staff in evidence-based prevention activities. The physiology and psychological effects of obesity are taught, as are importance of maintaining mobility, ensuring proper nutrition, nurse safety in mobility activities, and safe equipment use, to all nursing staff.

Two types of obese patients may come into a facility or practice—those being seen for another medical or surgical issue and those seeking weight-loss surgery. The CNS ensures that due diligence and appropriate care are provided to each population. The obese patient in general can be expected to have difficulty healing, be prone to the complications of immobility such as pressure ulcers and pneumonia and may have signs of malnutrition. The patient experiencing weight-loss surgery will also be at risk for metabolic disturbances, pain, and fluid imbalance. Staff must be taught population specific signs and symptoms of complications, and protocols should be developed to standardize care.

The CNS also addresses staff biases and attitudes in regard to the obese patient. The CNS helps, through teaching and coaching, to explore staff feelings, model appropriate behaviors, and promote unbiased care.

The CNS participates in development of nursing policies and procedures to ensure the safe care of the bariatric patient. The CNS teaches staff proper documentation of patient assessment, interventions, and outcomes, then reviews the documentation to determine issues and trends in the management of bariatric patients. Finally, the CNS also teaches staff about the importance of personal weight management, including education on nutrition as well as stress management.

Organizations and Systems

The CNS advocates for the safety of nursing staff and bariatric patients through participation in the development of no-lift policies and in equipment purchase and environmental design. Specialized equipment needed for the bariatric patient includes blood pressure measurement equipment, gowns, wheelchairs, commodes, beds, support surfaces, lifts, bedside chairs, and shower chairs. Review and recommendation for special equipment should be based on critical analysis of cost, safety, utility, and quality. The CNS reviews environmental needs of the facility, including door width, toilet height, and weight restrictions of equipment, and makes formal recommendations to administrators on actions needed to ensure patient and staff safety.

The CNS also participates with the interprofessional team to address the needs of the bariatric patient across the facility. This might include physical therapy to collaborate on mobility, staff training, staff safety, and equipment prescription for patients on any unit. Psychological services should be included, aiming at patient and staff support and training. Case managers and discharge planners should be included, so that information can be shared and admissions and discharges flow as smoothly as possible. The CNS also includes the nutritionist, physicians, occupational, and recreational therapists as part of the team and might consider development of an obesity team for facility-wide support and training.

BEDREST AND IMMOBILITY

There is no doubt that bedrest and immobility are nondisease causes of illness and disease. Extended periods of immobility have been shown to cause a variety of problems ranging from deep venous thrombosis to pneumonia, pressure ulcers, urinary tract infection, urinary stones, constipation, confusion, aspiration, depression, postural hypotension, muscle weakness, and exercise intolerance. The CNS has the ability to affect immobility in numerous ways in the three spheres of influence.

Etiology

The etiology of immobility is not the same for all people. Psychiatric illnesses such as depression or cognitive changes can cause withdrawal and refusal to move. Severe cases of illness can be direct causes of immobility. Pain may make it difficult to move, as might morbid obesity. There are also iatrogenic causes of immobility, such as orders for bedrest, sedative medications, traction, casts, limb restraints, ventilators, and tubes/lines.

Through qualitative research, Zegelin (24) describes five phases of becoming bedridden. Phase I encompasses instability, a baseline during which patient has problems with ambulation and balance. Phase II occurs when there is a fall and/or a hospital stay. "They just left me lying there," said one subject. In Phase III, patients are moved between the bed and the chair, and are more inclined to remain in bed. By Phase IV, transferring on one's own is no longer possible. "I can't leave here on my own." And in Phase V, patients are in bed 24 hours per day. They do not leave the bed for elimination, diapers are used, and there is a loss of power and control.

Pathophysiology

The effects of prolonged bedrest have been known since the time of Hippocrates. More recently, bedrest studies were initiated by NASA in the 1960s to learn more about the effects of weightlessness in space flight. The closest that they could get to studying weightlessness was to study enforced bedrest with non–weight-bearing for extended periods of time. Findings from their early studies initiated thought and more study of the effect of bedrest and non–weight-bearing on patients.

Bedrest causes loss of most hydrostatic pressure in the vasculature below the heart, nearly total elimination of longitudinal compression on the shins and the long bones, reduced muscular forces on nearly all bones, and reduced energy utilization (25). During periods of bedrest, there is a decrease in skeletal muscle mass and strength. Muscle mass can decrease by as much as 5% per week during absolute bedrest, while strength decreases by 1% to 1.5% per day and by 40% during the first week (26). Lower extremity muscles lose strength about twice as fast as the muscles of the upper extremities. The quadriceps and the extensor muscles of the back atrophy the most rapidly, affecting the ability to walk and climb stairs (27). There may be as much as 50% loss of muscle strength in 3 weeks of bedrest; while strength recovery is only 10% per week (27).

Joints decrease in range of motion, and contractures may form, affecting the ability to stand, ambulate, and perform activities of daily living (ADLs). The mineral content of bone decreases, which can lead to osteoporosis and pathologic fractures, as well as urinary calculi and heterotopic ossification. There is deconditioning of the heart, resulting in decreased cardiac reserve, decreased stroke volume, decreased cardiac output, decreased oxygen uptake, and resting and postexercise tachycardia. Circulation becomes sluggish, leading to venous stasis and thrombosis. Lungs do not fully expand, leading to atelectasis and pneumonia. There is an increased risk of pulmonary embolism and aspiration pneumonia as well. Effects on the autonomic nervous system lead to orthostasis. Effects on the gastrointestinal tract include anorexia, decreased fluid intake, peptic ulcer disease, constipation, and impaction. The bladder does not fully empty, leading to urinary tract infection. The skin is prone to breakdown. Other changes occur in the hematologic, metabolic, thermoregulatory, immune, and neuroendocrine systems. The patient may experience psychiatric symptoms of anxiety, depression, and confusion (25, 28).

Brown, Friedkin, and Inouye (29) studied mobility and outcomes in hospitalized older patients. They found that low mobility and bedrest are common in hospitalized older adults and are important predictors of bad outcomes. They view the outcomes of low mobility and bedrest as iatrogenic events that lead to complications such as functional decline.

Studies of older adults have found that effects of bedrest extend into the community. Bedrest in the community setting has been found to be associated with decline in ability to perform instrumental ADLs (IADLs), as well as declines in mobility, physical activity, and social activity (30).

ECONOMIC CONSIDERATIONS

Studies have found that decreasing time in bed and increasing mobility in hospitalized patients can decrease the length of stay, and thus costs, in the ICU setting. Morris et al. (31) found that early consults to physical therapy with initiation of a mobility protocol resulted in patients out of bed 6 days earlier than nonprotocol patients, 1.4 fewer ICU days, and lower complication rates. They also found no costs increase with the initiation of the mobility protocol.

Rogers et al. (32) studied predictors of hospitalization for patients in skilled nursing facilities, particularly for urinary tract infection (UTI). They found that the ability to walk was associated with a 69% lower risk of hospitalization for UTI and that improving mobility from baseline for residents with severe mobility problems also resulted in reduction in risk of hospitalization.

Acute Care for Elders (ACE) and Geriatric Evaluation and Management (GEM) units have a core philosophy of implementing early mobilization and rehabilitation interventions with acutely ill older adults as one component of an interprofessional team intervention. Studies about these units have found decreased mortality, decreased costs, decreased length of stay, and improved function (33, 34).

While there are no cost estimates for the complications of immobility, one can examine the reported costs of pressure ulcer treatment and imagine the costs for the above mentioned complications as a whole. The Centers for Medicare and Medicaid Services (CMS) will no longer reimburse hospitals for several conditions that can be related to immobility and bedrest, including pressure ulcers, falls, UTI, deep venous thrombosis, and pulmonary embolism (the latter two in relation to total knee replacement and hip replacement).

Management

The prevention of the complications of immobility is an interprofessional team effort. Early mobilization is a key intervention that will likely involve orders for physical therapy intervention. Weight-bearing and ambulation are key activities. Occupational therapy can assist with assessment and treatment of impairments in ADLs such as dressing, grooming, and bathing. Nursing's important role includes supporting therapy by enforcing out-of-bed activities such as up in the chair for meals and ambulation to the bathroom for personal care. Nurses aid in ambulation in the hall, range-of-motion exercises, and patient education. The dietitian can help the patient through a dietary assessment, monitoring of nutritional health, and provision of attractive food and snacks. The pharmacist, through medication review, can screen for medications and medication interactions that may cause fatigue and sedation, while ensuring that pain is controlled and depression is addressed.

CLINICAL NURSE SPECIALIST COMPETENCIES AND SPHERES OF INFLUENCE

Clinical Expert/Direct Care
The CNS as a clinical expert understands the dangers of immobility and directly intervenes through recognition of risk factors, assessment, planning, and intervention. The CNS monitors the patient for complications of immobility with the goal of prevention of pressure ulcers, postural hypotension and falls, constipation, incontinence, and malnutrition, among others.

Consultation
The CNS consults others as necessary to address immobility, including the physical and occupational therapist. The CNS as consultant offers knowledge and skills to families, patients, nurses, aides, and other unit staff members to prevent the complications of immobility.

Systems Leadership
The CNS works within the system to minimize immobility in patient populations. This is accomplished through increasing awareness of the effect of immobility on the system's bottom line—increased costs of managing complications, increased length of stay as patients are unable to go home secondary to deconditioning, and increased need for case managers to coordinate complicated discharge plans. The CNS stresses to managers the importance of staffing in preventing patient immobility and works to acquire adequate mobility equipment for the nursing units. The CNS also stresses the importance of the therapists—physical and occupational—in assisting the facility with maintaining/improving patient mobility. The CNS might develop an interprofessional team to address immobility in the institution, which could include staff education, equipment assessment and purchase, and outcomes monitoring in conjunction with the Quality Department.

Collaboration
The CNS collaborates with many departments and personnel in prevention of immobility in patients in the facility, including therapists, physicians, other nursing units/departments, and even transportation. Collaborative relationships with others will facilitate gaining assistance for nurses in mobilizing patients, acquiring formal orders for therapist consultation for individual patients, and sharing knowledge and skills in difficult-to-mobilize cases.

Coaching/Teaching/Mentoring
The CNS has ongoing opportunities to educate, coach, and mentor for the prevention of patient immobility with patients, families, nurses, and the rest of the team. Patients and families require extensive education of potential complications, methods of increasing mobility, and mobility equipment. Nursing staff requires ongoing emphasis on the importance of mobilizing patients, and training in accessing resources, equipment use, and encouragement to monitor for complications. The CNS can model appropriate interventions for mobility, as well as assist staff in maintaining patient activity out of bed.

Research/Evidence-Based Practice
This competency is an important one for the CNSs managing patients with impaired mobility. The CNS stays abreast of developments in mobility products, including support surfaces and positioning aids. The CNS also monitors advances in prevention of the complications of mobility and networks with other CNSs and professionals through online and email communication to share best practices.

Ethical Decision-Making/Moral Agency/Advocacy
The CNS advocates for the patient at risk for complications of immobility through modeling caring behaviors, developing interventions for immobility, and training staff. The CNS also ensures that ethical practices are in place, in particular related to the fine line between honoring the patient's wishes for continued immobility and the importance of encouraging out-of-bed activities. This will involve patient and family education, coaching and educating staff on the philosophy of restorative nursing, and monitoring unit activities and patient outcomes.

Patients and Families
The CNS implements the direct care role through evaluation of the reasons for bedrest and immobility. Thorough and careful assessment facilitates the development of a plan for mobility and patient and family teaching regarding the importance of activity. There are often many barriers to facilitating mobility for patients. The interference from ancillary departments, pain management, safety issues, and staff availability can prove to be detrimental to the process. The CNS works to maintain patient mobility as a priority for the unit where possible and improve it where necessary. The CNS initiates consults to physical, occupational, and

recreational therapy and collaborates on the coordination of patient interventions.

Nurses and Nursing Practice

The CNS teaches nurses about the effects of immobility and the importance of nursing intervention. Working with the nursing staff, the CNS develops unit protocols for ensuring effective patient mobility practices and consults with nursing administration about appropriate staffing, along with valid data on patient outcomes to support the practices. The CNS monitors adherence to unit protocols and documentation of interventions. The CNS also tracks patient complication rates and collaborates with staff to evaluate patient outcomes.

Organizations and Systems

The CNS uses leadership skills to engage the interprofessional team in development of protocols and practices that ensure patient mobility is appropriately addressed across the facility. The CNS engages research skills to find and assess data on length of stay, costs, and complications attributable to immobility and bedrest and presents this data to health care team members and administrators with a cost-effective, evidence-based plan to improve these outcomes.

The CNS also maintains current knowledge on national safety standards, so that interventions that are implemented meet the standards and thus minimize facility liability for the complications of immobility. These include CMS guidelines on hospital-acquired conditions, The Joint Commission (TJC) standards, state health department standards, and national patient safety goals.

SLEEP

Sleep is another significant, nondisease cause of illness. Sleep deprivation has been shown to have adverse effects on health, including impaired glucose utilization, diabetes, obesity, hypertension, CV disease, depression, and exacerbation of pain. Sleepiness can also lead to cognitive impairment, increasing the risk for accidents (35).

Approximately 70 million people in the United States have a sleeping disorder. The number of people reporting sleep problems rose by 13% between 2001 and 2009. Fifty-four percent of adults in a recent sleep poll have driven when drowsy at least once in the past year, while 28% have nodded off or fallen asleep while driving. Twenty percent of people in this poll sleep less than 6 hours per night. The National Highway Traffic Safety Administration estimates that 100,000 police-reported car crashes are caused by drowsy drivers, resulting in more than 1,500 fatalities and 71,000 injuries for an estimated $12.5 billion in diminished productivity and property damage (36).

Daley et al. (37) found that insomnia was associated with significant morbidity, health care utilization, work absenteeism, reduced productivity, and risk of nonvehicle accidents. Patients with symptoms of insomnia were more likely to have a diagnosis for a mood disorder or anxiety and higher rates of chronic illness compared to good sleepers. Their chronic health problems included arthritis, ulcers, chronic pain, sinusitis, headaches, and hypertension. More people with insomnia used medications for mood, anxiety, and sleep problems. They were also more likely to use alcohol to sleep than the good sleepers.

Patients in hospital suffer from sleep deprivation for a number of reasons, not the least of which is the environment. Cmiel et al. (38) found that one significant problem was the noise level in hospitals due to patient care procedures, monitoring and diagnostic equipment, conversation among providers, and background noise from air conditioning and heating systems. The Environmental Protection Agency recommends that hospital noise not exceed 45 dB(A) during the day and 35 dB(A) during the night. Cmiel et al. found that night-time noise at their facility exceeded 45 dB(A) in empty rooms and 53 dB(A) in semiprivate occupied rooms. Sound peaks up to 113 dB(A) occurred at change of shift.

Apart from noise, the routine activities of the hospital interrupt sleep. Medication administration, vital signs, turning and positioning, hourly checks, treatments, blood draws, and even early morning bathing affect sleep and sleep quality in patients. Roommates, televisions, and bright lights can be added to this list (39).

Pathophysiology

It is not yet known why we sleep, but it is thought that sleep is a restorative function. Sleep is divided into two stages: rapid eye movement (REM) and non–rapid eye movement (NREM) sleep.

REM sleep has three main features:

- Low-voltage, fast-frequency EEG pattern that resembles an awake EEG pattern
- An atonic electromyogram (EMG) consistent with relaxation of all voluntary muscles except the extraocular muscles
- The presence of REMs

The three characteristics are not always present simultaneously. It is thought that REM sleep might be a trigger for CV and cerebrovascular ischemic events.

Abnormalities in REM sleep may be the cause of narcolepsy. The atonia of REM sleep is thought to exacerbate sleep apnea. REM sleep can be suppressed by alcohol, MAO inhibitors, tricyclic antidepressants, stimulants, and some hypnotic/sedative medications. Drugs with anticholinergic properties may also suppress REM sleep.

NREM sleep has three stages:

Stage 1 = transition from wakefulness to deeper sleep.
Stage 2 = true physiologic sleep, accounting for 40-50% of sleep time.
Stage 3 = 20% of sleep time in young adults, is deep sleep.

The purpose of NREM sleep is uncertain.

SLEEP ARCHITECTURE

Sleep stages typically last 90 to 120 minutes. In the first half of the night, the person passes briefly through Stage 1 sleep, to Stages 2 and 3. Stages 2 and 3 cycle again, into REM sleep. REM and Stage 2 sleep alternate through the second half of the night. Deep sleep declines with age, while light sleep increases (40).

Any medication that passes the blood-brain barrier can alter the quality of sleep, including the speed of sleep onset, the continuity of sleep, and the duration of sleep. See Table 2–3 for further information.

SLEEP DEPRIVATION

Sleep deprivation can result in cognitive impairment. Symptoms include difficulty with short-term memory, motor skills, impaired attention, depression, anxiety, irritability, low energy, and poor judgment. Symptoms like these disappear when sleep is restored. Excessive

TABLE 2–3 Medications That Affect Sleep Quality

Category	Medication	Comments
CNS DRUGS		
	Benzodiazepines	Improve sleep quality
		May reduce wakefulness in sleep period
		Reduce Stage 1 sleep (therapeutic effect)
		Suppress Stage 3 sleep (significance not known)
		Little effect of REM sleep
	Melanin receptor agonists	Reduce latency to sleep onset
		Increase sleep duration
		No effect on sleep architecture
	Antiepileptics	Increase total sleep time
		Increase Stage 3 sleep
		Suppress REM sleep
	Antidepressants	SSRIs—stimulating
		SARIS—sedating
		TCAs—sedating
		MAOIs—sedating
		All except SARIs suppress REM sleep
	Analgesics	Opioids increase wake time, reduce slow wave and REM sleep
		NSAIDS associated with increase time awake
	CNS stimulants	Increase Stage 1 sleep
		Reduce Stage 3 sleep
		Suppress REM sleep
CARDIOPULMONARY		
	Beta blockers	Increase number of awakenings
		Suppress REM sleep
		Effects limited to lipophilics (metoprolol, pindolol, propranolol)
		Increase daytime sleepiness
	Central alpha agonists	Induce more shifts to Stage 1 sleep
		Suppress REM sleep
		Increase daytime sleepiness
	Theophylline	Delays sleep onset
		Increases wake time after sleep onset
		Increases Stage 1 sleep
	Corticosteroids	Supress REM sleep
	Tobacco	Longer sleep latency
		Less total sleep time
		Less slow wave sleep

sleepiness is the second major cause of automobile accidents in the United States. Poor judgment due to sleep deprivation has been implicated in the tragedies at Three Mile Island and Chernobyl, in the Exxon Valdez oil spill, and in the Space Shuttle Challenger disaster. Quality of life declines as sleepiness increases; that is, people who are sleep deprived report a lower quality of life.

Sleep deprivation is thought to depress respiratory responses to hypercapnea and hypoxia and possibly contribute to hypoventilation in hospitalized patients. Sleep deprivation can also affect immune function, resulting in increases in plasma levels of soluble tumor necrosis factor-alpha and interleukin-6. Sleep restriction has also been shown to result in a decrease in serum leptin (an anorexigenic hormone) and increase in serum ghrelin (an orexigenic hormone), resulting in increased hunger and appetite (41).

Sleep problems increase with age. Older adults tend to have increased sleep latency (time to fall asleep), changes in sleep maintenance (ability to stay asleep), and early awakening. They also spend more time in Stage 1 and Stage 2 of sleep, with a decrease in Stage 3 sleep, REM, and total sleep time. Insomnia in older adults often leads to daytime sleepiness and napping. Chronic insomnia in older adults has been shown to be an independent predictor of falls, cognitive decline, and 2-year mortality. The presence of dementia further complicates the problems with sleep in older adults, accentuating the normal changes in sleep and increasing the burden on caregivers (42).

Diagnosis

A careful history of usual sleep patterns should be documented, including prevalence of daytime napping, usual sleep and wake times, amount of light exposure, intake of caffeine and alcohol, prescription and over-the-counter medications, and sleep hygiene habits. Asking the patient to complete a sleep log for a 2-week period will aid in diagnosis. Screen for medical, psychiatric, and environmental conditions that could be affecting sleep, including heart failure, restless leg syndrome, chronic obstructive pulmonary disease (COPD), gastroesophageal reflux, chronic or recurrent pain, depression, posttraumatic stress disorder (PTSD), anxiety, bereavement, shift work, and sleep environment temperature and noise levels. The physical examination should include measurements of neck circumference. A neck circumference greater than 43 cm in males and greater than 41 cm in females has been associated with obstructive sleep apnea.

Differential diagnoses include alcoholism, anxiety disorders, asthma, bipolar disorder, chronic disease, COPD, depression, hyperthyroidism, hyperparathyroidism, menopause, nocturia, obstructive sleep apnea, opioid abuse, pain, PTSD, restless leg syndrome, and stimulant abuse (43, 44).

Work-up includes CBC, arterial blood gases, thyroid function tests, and drug and alcohol toxicity screening. Monitored polysomnography in a sleep lab is the standard for evaluating sleep.

Management

Teach good sleep hygiene: use the bed for sleep only; avoid caffeine and stimulating activities late in the day; practice relaxation techniques at bedtime; exercise daily; avoid naps; and maintain a regular sleep and wake schedule. Weight loss may help sleep apnea, as will continuous positive airway pressure (CPAP). Surgery may also be useful in obstructive sleep apnea from enlarged palate or uvula. Light-phase therapy can be used when there are circadian rhythm disturbances. Cognitive-behavioral therapy and hypnotic medication may help in the short term.

In the hospital, monitor for and control environmental noises and routines that interrupt patient sleep. Educate staff on sleep hygiene techniques to aid patients in sleep. Reschedule medications, vital signs, and treatments to daytime hours when possible. Dim unit lights and enforce quiet zones. Question patients about their ability to sleep, and identify the problems that are preventing them from resting. Consider designating an uninterrupted period for sleep that is consistent every night.

Medications used short term for sleeplessness are outlined in Table 2–4 (44).

Use all of these medications with caution in the elderly; document patient teaching on avoiding operating heavy machinery or driving while taking these medications (44). Educate the nursing staff regarding the adverse reactions and side effects of the medications so they can offer first-line interventions when needed.

CLINICAL NURSE SPECIALIST COMPETENCIES AND SPHERES OF INFLUENCE

Clinical Expert/Direct Care

CNS practice within this competency will vary depending on the role of the CNS in question. The CNS as mid-level provider will assess sleep in assigned patients, including eliciting assessments from staff, family, and patient on quality of sleep. The CNS will plan and implement pharmacologic and nonpharmacologic therapies to assist with normalization of the sleep pattern, will assess patient outcomes, and plan accordingly. The CNS in a direct care role will also assess sleep quality and implement interventions as outlined earlier. CNSs in both roles will assess staff knowledge, unit routines, and other system issues that could affect sleep and work to address these issues as well.

TABLE 2-4 Medications for Short-term Use for Sleeplessness

Medication	Classification	Comments
Temazepam (Restoril)	Benzodiazepine	For initial and middle insomnia 15-30 mg PO at bedtime Minimal grogginess next day Not with glaucoma, untreated obstructive sleep apnea, history of substance abuse, uncontrolled pain Multiple drug interactions Caution with COPD, hepatic disease, elderly; Long-term use may result in cognitive dysfunction and rebound insomnia
Zolpidem (Ambien)	Imidazopyridine	Fast onset, good for sleep induction, decreases sleep latency and increase sleep time 5-20 mg PO at bedtime Increases toxicity of alcohol and CNS depressants Give only 5 mg in elderly Caution with pulmonary dysfunction
Zaleplon (Sonata)	Pyrazolopyrimidine	Take immediately before bedtime; Decreases time to sleep onset 10 mg PO HS (½ or 2× dose depending on patient weight and response) Multiple drug interactions Taking drug while awake and active may cause hallucinations, memory impairment, impaired coordination, and dizziness For short-term use—do not prescribe in quantities exceeding 1 month supply Reduce dose to 5 mg in hepatic dysfunction
Ezsopiclone (Lunesta)	Pyrrolopyrazine	Decreases sleep latency and improves sleep maintenance Lower dose for difficulty falling asleep; higher doses for sleep maintenance Adults 2 mg HS, increase to 3 mg if needed Elderly—1 mg HS—do not increase to more than 2 mg PO HS Hepatic impairment—do not increase to more than 2 mg PO HS Multiple drug interactions Alertness may be affected the next day
Ramelteon (Rozerem)	Melatonin receptor agonist	For difficulty with sleep onset 8 mg PO 30 min before bed on empty stomach Multiple drug interactions Not with severe hepatic impairment
Trazodone (Desyrel)	Antidepressant	50 mg PO HS to start, increase as needed to 400 mg max May enhance response to alcohol, barbiturates and CNS depressants Multiple drug interactions Monitor for hypotension, syncope, dizziness, priapism

Consultation

As with other conditions, the CNS may consult other professionals to assist with sleep issues or be consulted by other staff for CNS input and assistance in dealing with sleepless patients and related system issues. Consultants whom the CNS may ask to see the patient include sleep specialists, bariatric specialists, pulmonary specialists, gerontologists or internal medical specialists, and other advanced practice nurses.

Systems Leadership

The CNS will recognize the importance of sleep in the patient population and will lead within the system to address associated issues. This might include working with a different team of professionals than with other conditions. For instance, if nighttime noise is an issue, then the CNS might assemble a team of nurses as well as staff from departments contributing to nighttime noise: central supply/materials management, respiratory therapy, transportation or perhaps pharmacy. The CNS will adjust communication skills and personal interactions to encourage full and equal participation of these departments in problem solving on behalf of the patients. The CNS will also work within the system to evaluate patient outcomes related to sleep, such as patient satisfaction or falls, and to develop and evaluate a plan for intervention.

Collaboration

As mentioned earlier, the CNS may have to collaborate with nonmedical professionals to address sleep issues in the patients, particularly those with an environmental cause. The CNS might team with pharmacists to evaluate the appropriateness of medication-ordering practices related to sleep and then collaborate with prescribers if issues are found. The CNS might also team with such diverse departments as nutrition, recreation therapy, engineering, and accounting to explore novel ways of promoting sleep, such as nutritional sleep aids, quiet music, and dim lighting.

Coaching/Teaching/Mentoring

Medical professionals often relate tales of their experiences as a patient in their own system, including remarking upon the noise at night. While working with diverse departments to address sleep issues, the CNS might initiate a program in which workers from these departments room-in on a unit at night to experience "sleep" firsthand. This would be a novel method of teaching non-medical professionals about the environmental issues associated with sleep. The CNS also must educate her team members on the physical and psychological aspects of poor sleep, including the potential for longer lengths of stay from poorer or delayed healing related to sleeplessness. The CNS plays a special role in intervening with nighttime staff, which will include spending time at night on the unit with staff to observe, coach, and mentor them in addressing patient sleep.

Research/Evidence-Based Practice

As with other conditions, the CNS must remain up to date in the literature, research, and clinical practice guidelines associated with sleep. The CNS must also apply this information to her or his specific patient population; for instance, if the CNS is working with a geriatric population, then the CNS will be aware of the link between sleeplessness, delirium, and/or falls in that population. The CNS might consider subscription to a service that alerts the user to new articles on the topic.

Ethical Decision Making/Moral Agency/Advocacy

The CNS has a strong role to play in advocating for patient sleep, enacted through use of the above competencies in all spheres of influence. This advocacy can be considered a core role, in fact, as sleep issues affect all ages and populations of patients in all settings.

Patients and Families

The CNS uses direct care competencies to assess, diagnose, plan, and intervene for patients with sleep problems. Depending on area of practice, the CNS may prescribe medications to aid in the sleep process. Patients are taught and coached about sleep hygiene practices and encouraged to maintain a sleep log. Families are counseled and educated on the signs and symptoms of sleep deprivation and its implications for the patient. Caregivers also should be made aware of concerns relative to sleep deprivation and potentials for the patient's well-being.

Nurses and Nursing Practice

The CNS monitors the literature for updates in EBPs related to patient sleep. The CNS teaches nursing staff about the importance of facilitating sleep for all patients. The CNS collaborates with staff to plan nursing activities and medications to allow each patient the most sleep possible. The CNS monitors documentation to search for trends in patient sleep habits so that she may most effectively intervene.

Organizations and Systems

The CNS works with administrators for various departments to ensure that the importance of noise abatement at night is emphasized and encourages the ancillary and support personnel to plan delivery of supplies at times least likely to interfere with patient sleep. When the opportunity arises, the CNS consults on unit architectural designs to emphasize the importance of keeping patient rooms and noisy areas like supply rooms and medication rooms at a distance from one another. As always, it is important to collaborate with the interprofessional team to advocate for patient sleep when diagnostic tests and other interventions can be delayed until waking times.

MALNUTRITION

Malnutrition is both a cause and a consequence of illness. Unfortunately, it can also be a cause and a consequence of hospitalization. As many as 69% of inpatients demonstrate declining nutritional status during admission (46). Malnutrition affects every body system, impairs healing, increases morbidity and mortality, lengthens hospital stays, increases costs, and increases the risk of hospital readmission. There are several faces of malnutrition in the hospital. These include the patient who is admitted with malnutrition, the patient whose nutritional status worsens during hospitalization, and the patient who develops malnutrition in the hospital.

An estimated 13% to 69% of hospitalized patients worldwide are malnourished (47). A study in St. Louis found that 91% of patients admitted to subacute care were either malnourished or at risk for malnutrition (48). TJC has developed nutrition screening and assessment requirements. All patients, with few exceptions, should be screened for nutritional issues on admission to the hospital. Those deemed to be at risk should have a more formal nutrition assessment, ideally by a dietitian. It has been noted that TJC guidelines do not address those patients admitted to hospital who go to surgery within 24 hours of admission—there is not enough time before surgery for those patients to be fully assessed for nutritional needs and thus no time for preoperative intervention in which need would be assessed (49).

Etiology

There are many causes of malnutrition as seen in the hospital setting. Social causes outside of the hospital include socioeconomic, environmental, and transportation issues. Pirlich et al. (50) identified risk factors that included age greater than 60, polypharmacy, isolation, less education, and malignancy as risk factors for malnutrition. Chronic medical or psychiatric illnesses can dampen the appetite. Functional problems such as dysphagia can also interfere with adequate intake. Iatrogenic malnutrition can be caused by NPO orders for tests and procedures, dislike for the taste and variety of hospital-supplied foods, and side effects from medications. Malnutrition in the hospital can also be caused by missed meals when testing and procedures interrupt the meal schedule, the inability to access the tray, cold or unappetizing foods, and the inability to open cartons or feed oneself due to fatigue or generalized weakness. Test preparation may involve liquid diets or medications that interfere with appetite. Illness itself increases metabolic requirements. Enteral feedings and parenteral feedings may not supply adequate calories. Oral feedings may not be nutritionally adequate for promotion of healing and management of disease effect on intake.

Older adults are particularly at risk for changes in nutritional status because of normal changes of aging. These include changes in taste and smell, early satiety, and delayed gastric emptying. Older adults are more likely to eat alone and more likely to have chronic or undiagnosed illnesses that affect intake (51).

Pathophysiology

Malnutrition initially causes loss of fat, muscle, and skin. Eventually there is loss of bone and visceral tissue with overall weight loss. This dramatic loss of cellular structures causes fluid shifts and a resulting increase in extracellular fluid volume (52). There is an associated susceptibility to infection, altered wound healing, increased risk of pressure ulcers, as well as bacterial overgrowth in the gastrointestinal tract. Critical illness exaggerates these problems with catecholamine-mediated hypercatabolism, resulting in a negative nitrogen balance and a shift to the metabolism of fat as an energy source (52).

Diagnosis

Identification of malnutrition is key to prevention of complications. The first step in the hospital is nutrition screening to identify those patients who might benefit from a more thorough nutritional assessment. At-risk populations, such as older adults, should be aggressively screened. Nutrition screening parameters identified by The American Society of Parenteral and Enteral Nutrition (ASPEN) include height, weight, changes in weight, primary diagnosis, and comorbidities. Periodic rescreening should be standard care.

Nutritional assessment parameters include medical, nutrition, and medication history; physical examination; anthropometric measurements; and laboratory data (53). Body mass index (BMI) is calculated. The history should include recent weight changes, usual dietary intake and patterns of intake, gastrointestinal symptoms, and functional abilities. The physical includes assessment for edema, ascites, cachexia, obesity, skin problems, wounds, and assessment of the oral cavity. The clinician should look for the presence of subcutaneous fat and muscle wasting and calculate BMI.

Laboratory tests are not always good indicators of nutritional status, due to the effect of illness and inflammation on the tests. Serum albumin levels do have prognostic value. Low albumin levels are associated with poor clinical outcomes and are an independent risk factor for mortality in older persons, but they have been found to be poor indicators of the adequacy of nutritional support, due to the long half-life and the effect of illness on albumin. Serum albumin levels may be altered in dehydration, sepsis, trauma, and liver disease, no matter what the nutritional status is. Serial measurements of prealbumin can be used to track nutrition changes in response to nutrition therapy, although, like albumin, the serum concentration is affected by renal or hepatic disease.

Laboratory tests that may be useful for a full work-up include fasting lipid profile, blood glucose, hemoglobin A1C, CBC, CRP, hematocrit, renal function tests, and electrolytes. Other possible labs, depending on differential diagnosis, include PTT, iron, magnesium, calcium, and phosphate. Cellular immunity can be tested with a total lymphocyte count or delayed type hypersensitivity testing (52). Screening for celiac disease may be indicated, as well as colitis, Crohn disease, and other disorders that require dietary intervention.

ASPEN notes that "the only clinical method [of nutritional assessment] that has been validated as reproducible and that evaluates nutrition status (and severity of illness) by encompassing patient history and physical parameters is the subjective global assessment (SGA)" (53). The SGA is available online at http://www.hospitalmedicine.org/geriresource/toolbox/howto.htm.

Differential diagnoses related to malnutrition and/or weight loss include hyperthyroidism, new-onset diabetes, dental conditions, heart failure, COPD, renal insufficiency or failure, celiac disease, liver or pancreatic disease, infections, rheumatoid arthritis, Parkinson disease, inflammatory bowel disease, drug or alcohol abuse, and side effects of medications (51).

Management

Should ongoing screening indicate nutritional problems, and nutritional assessment supports these findings, interprofessional intervention is indicated. Nursing staff can assist in monitoring and documenting the patient's nutritional intake and in ensuring that food is served and assistance with feeding offered. Dietary consult is certainly necessary as nutrition may need to be supplied enterally or parenterally. The dietitian may also have the ability to specially craft a diet that suits the patient's tastes and preferences if oral feedings can be continued. Occupational therapy can assist with assessment and intervention for functional problems, such as arm weakness or hand contractures. They can also aid in evaluation of food preparation abilities for the home setting. Speech-language pathologists (SLPs) can aid in diagnosis and intervention for swallowing and cognition problems. Social workers can assess for problems with attaining food in the home and help set up home nutrition support services such as Meals on Wheels.

Easing of dietary restrictions to improve dietary intake should be strongly considered. Supplements should be ordered, and special effort made to improve the taste and variety of food. Cultural preferences should be honored and the family encouraged to bring in food from home. Medications useful in appetite stimulation include megestrol (Megace) and dronabinol (Marinol). Megestrol is a progestin appetite stimulant used in palliative treatment of breast and endometrial cancer, as well as treatment of anorexia and cachexia. It is thought to stimulate appetite through antagonizing the metabolic effects of catabolic cytokines. Megace has been linked to the new onset of diabetes with chronic use and is used with caution is patients with liver disease or thromboembolic disease. Vaginal bleeding may occur in elderly women who take this drug. Dronabinol has been found to work in AIDS-associated anorexia. It is a Schedule III drug and should be used with caution in hepatic disease or seizure disorders. There is a potential for abuse as the active drug is a cannabinoid. Dronabinol is also used as an antiemetic with chemotherapy-related nausea and vomiting (14).

It is beyond the scope of this chapter to discuss enteral and parenteral feeding, but more information can be found at the website homes of the American Society of Parenteral and Enteral Nutrition and the American Dietetic Association. Overnutrition is another face of malnutrition—see earlier in this chapter for discussion of obesity.

CLINICAL NURSE SPECIALIST COMPETENCIES AND SPHERES OF INFLUENCE

Clinical Expert/Direct Care

The CNS in a mid-level provider role will remain alert for the risk of malnutrition in the patient population. Patients deemed at risk, or who the CNS suspects of malnourishment, will be holistically assessed, including not only medical assessment, but social, economic, functional, cognitive, and psychiatric assessments as well. The CNS in a direct care role will screen all patients for malnutrition, and recommend a more formal work-up to the ordering practitioner as indicated. CNSs in both roles will monitor intake of food and fluids and include the nursing staff and the system in the assessment of conditions that could affect patient intake and nutrition.

Consultation

Consultants employed by the CNS for this patient population might include the nutritionist, the gastrointestinal specialists, psychiatrist or psychologist, internal medicine physician, occupational therapist (OT), SLP, and social worker. The CNS might be consulted by all of these professionals as well as nursing staff and families to address issues of malnutrition.

Systems Leadership

With any patient complication, such as malnutrition, the CNS should always look outside of his or her assigned space and role to explore the possibility that the complication is present systemwide. This expands the influence of the CNS and may result in added responsibilities and duties, but it is the CNS who is most able to assess the system and lead interventions to address conditions that cross real or imagined boundaries. The CNS is thus a valuable leader in addressing not only the patient problem, but the system's liability, costs, and outcomes. So, if nutritional issues on the CNSs unit are related to environmental issues, for example, the CNS should suspect that these same issues are present on other units and act for the good of the system.

Collaboration

Continuing the preceding thought, CNS as systems leader, the CNS would then collaborate with a wide range of professionals to address nutrition in the institution. Collaborators might include the dietary department and the nutritionist, physicians, CNSs and other advanced practice nurses, occupational therapists, nursing staff, and nurse managers from the affected units.

Coaching/Teaching/Mentoring

As with other conditions mentioned previously, the CNS employs the competencies of coaching, teaching, and mentoring in addressing patient nutrition. A wide audience of professionals might benefit from coaching and teaching—not only the nurses the CNS personally works with but also nurses in other areas of the facility. Novice CNSs can also benefit from coaching and teaching; the problem of nutrition could easily be missed by the novice who is overwhelmed with the multiple roles and responsibilities of the CNS.

Research/Evidence-Based Practice

This competency related to nutrition does not differ from the conditions mentioned earlier. What might be added is concentration on assessment tools used for nutritional status and the reliability and validity of those instruments. Instruments must measure what they are expected to measure and must have equivalent scores from practitioner to practitioner. The CNS will always anticipate the need for adequate documentation in the literature of reliability and validity of any instrument and may engage a statistician or researcher to assist with validation of the instrument with the CNS's patient population and nursing staff.

Ethical Decision Making/Moral Agency/Advocacy

Nutrition can be a difficult issue to deal with in some situations, such as end of life. The CNS ensures that decisions related to continuing or ending nutrition in complex patient cases adheres to ethical principles and consults the ethics service as needed for guidance. The CNS advocates for both individual patients and entire populations of patients regarding provision of adequate nutrition by the appropriate route, be it enterally or parenterally.

Patients and Families

The CNS in the direct care role assesses for malnutrition of the hospitalized patient and for contributing factors to the malnutrition. It is critical that specialists such as OT and SLP are consulted and recommendations of the specialists are implemented. Meetings with the patient and family to discuss issues related to food intake allows for planning more effective interventions. The CNS will sometimes need to initiate conversations with the family about nutritional support in cases where invasive nutritional support will not change the outcomes—for instance, with the patient with end-stage dementia.

Nurses and Nursing Practice

The CNS ensures that staff has the necessary knowledge and tools to provide nutritional support in the hospital setting. Assisting the staff in the identification of at-risk patients and in the formulation of nursing goals and interventions will be important to the patient's outcomes. The CNS collaborates with nursing administration in documenting the need for nutritional support, as well as support staff to feed patients. Monitoring of nursing documentation for evidence of ongoing nutritional screening, trends indicating the need for intervention, and response to therapy will provide important data to support the efforts. The CNS will need to support the nursing staff in communication with the nutritional support team regarding availability of meals and snacks supplied to patients on the unit. It will be important to develop mechanisms for obtaining meals at alternative times for patients returning from procedures, transferring between units, and completing admission and discharge procedures. The CNS should use optimal communication skills to break down barriers to anticipating and meeting nonroutine patient needs regarding nutrition, especially for high-risk patients. Collaboration with the nutritional support staff will ensure that diets supplied to patients are well presented, at the right temperature, and to the patients' liking.

Organizations and Systems

The CNS collaborates with the interdisciplinary team in setting facility standards for nutritional support of patients. Most important is the facilitation of an attitude encompassed by the entire health care team that focuses on high-risk patients and their nutritional needs. The utilization of valid data regarding patient outcomes associated with nutritional needs can be instrumental in obtaining cooperation from all members of the team and with evaluation of adherence to TJC requirements on nutritional screening and assessment. The same valid data will also be invaluable in planning goals and interventions for high-risk patients. Conversely, the CNS will participate in ethics discussions for patients who refuse nutrition and for whom invasive nutritional support would not change the outcomes.

NURSING-SENSITIVE INDICATORS

The ANA defines *nursing sensitive indicators* as those indicators that are closely linked with changes in quantity or quality of nursing care. "Nursing-sensitive indicators identify structures of care and care processes, both of which in turn influence care outcomes. Nursing-sensitive indicators are distinct and specific to nursing, and differ from medical indicators of care quality" (54). The ANA has developed the National Database of Nursing Quality Indicators (NDNQI) to assist with the collection of data to further knowledge of factors that affect the quality of nursing care. More than 1,100 facilities contribute data to the NDNQI, from which conclusions are beginning to be drawn about these factors.

The National Quality Forum (55) has identified the "NQF 15", or 15 voluntary consensus standards for nursing sensitive care. These include patient-centered outcome measures such as pressure ulcer prevalence, falls prevalence and failure to rescue; nursing-centered intervention measures such as smoking cessation counseling; and system-centered measures, including skill mix, nursing hours per patient day, and voluntary turnover rates (55). This section will address a select group of patient-centered outcome measures identified as important by the ANA and the NQF that the CNS can directly affect through assessment, intervention, and monitoring.

FALLS

Falls are a significant source of morbidity and mortality. In 2009, TJC recognized this as outlined in the 2009 National Patient Safety Goal No. 9: Reduce the risk of patient harm resulting from falls through implementation of a fall reduction program (56).

More than one third of adults aged 65 and older fall each year in the United States. Falls are the leading cause of injury deaths among older adults and are a common cause of nonfatal injuries and hospital admissions. In 2005, 15,800 older adults died from injuries sustained during an unintentional fall; 1.8 million older adults were treated in emergency departments for nonfatal injuries from falls, and of those, more than 433,000 were hospitalized (57). Between 3% and 20% of inpatients fall at least once during their hospital stay (58). The rate of fall-related deaths among older adults has risen significantly over the past 10 years (57).

Between 20% and 30% of the people who fall suffer moderate to severe injuries such as hip fracture, bruises, and brain trauma. The most common fractures from falls are of the spine, hip, forearm, leg, ankle, pelvis, upper arm, and hand. Many people who fall develop an incapacitating fear of falling, which may affect their mobility, living arrangements, and community involvement. The risk of being seriously injured in a fall increases with age. Nearly 85% of fall deaths in 2004 were among people aged 75 and older (59).

More than 90% of hip fractures in people aged 65 and older are caused by falls. In 2004, there were more than 320,000 hospital admissions for hip fractures. One in five persons with hip fracture dies within 1 year of their injury (59). Falls in the hospital setting account for as much as 40% of incident reports, and it has been found that up to 10% of falls in the hospital lead to serious injury. Eighteen percent of deaths from falls occur in the institutional setting, including nursing homes and hospitals (60), making prevention of falls of central interest to hospitals and nursing homes.

Falls are of interest to a number of government agencies. The Centers for Disease Control and Prevention (CDC) developed an interagency agreement with the Administration on Aging (AoA). The AoA currently is funding four grants that concern the implementation of evidence-based fall prevention models. Under this interagency agreement, the CDC is conducting three activities related to falls in older adults. The CDC has also funded a randomized controlled trial in Wisconsin to assess the effectiveness of fall intervention in community dwelling older adults, as well as funding fall studies in California and Washington State and studies concerning medications and falls (61).

Medicare and many state Medicaid agencies have included falls as 1 of 10 conditions on its "no-pay" list. Injuries or added costs that are due to a fall during hospitalization will not be reimbursed by Medicare as falls are seen to be preventable. While this point can be argued, the "no-pay" rules offers added incentives for institutions to prevent falls, especially falls with injury. It has been estimated that this will cost hospitals in excess of $2.4 billion annually, as they will not be allowed to pass the costs onto the patients (62).

What Medicare does not consider is that falls occur even when the best of care is given in an institution: not all falls are preventable (58). Consider the statistics on community falls—as many as one third of persons aged 65 and older and 50% of those 80 and older fall in the community setting annually. These people enter the hospital at high risk for falls—the hospital does not cause the higher risk. Inouye notes that only about 20% of falls in the hospital can be prevented.

CAUSES OF FALLS

Falls are a multifactorial problem. It is easy to identify the cause after a fall; it is not always so easy to identify and quantify risk so that a fall can be prevented. Intrinsic factors that increase risk for falls include older age, neurologic diagnosis, cognitive impairment, history of falls, sensory deficits, mobility impairment, musculoskeletal effects of immobility, CV instability, medical interventions such as medications, elimination disturbances, and acute and chronic illness. Extrinsic factors include the environment: poor lighting, obstacles in walkways, lack of appropriate footwear, lack of sensory aids, bedrails, unsafe floor surfaces (wet, slick, and/or uneven), medical tubes and restraints, and presence of adaptive equipment (canes, walkers, handrails). Nurse staffing has also been found to affect fall rates, with fewer falls occurring as registered nurse care hours increase (60). Falls in health care institutions are also suspected to be associated with nursing unit activity, with fewer falls during visiting hours and more at midnight (60). Aizen et al. (63) found that risk factors for falls differed among different groups of patients, such as those with stroke and those with hip fracture.

One difficulty with assessing risk is that single risk factors may interact to exponentially increase risk overall. It is difficult to quantify whether the patient with uncorrected visual deficits in a poorly lit room is at more risk than the same patient in a well-lit room who has urinary urgency. Fall etiology tends to differ from institution to institution and setting to setting. Multiple fall risk scales have been developed, but as with any scale, interrater reliability may suffer if training is inadequate and ongoing monitoring of reliability is not performed.

The Morse Fall Scale scores six variables: history of falling, secondary diagnosis, intravenous therapy, use of ambulatory aids, gait, and mental status. Although widely used, there is conflicting evidence of the validity and reliability of this scale (60, 64, 65). The Hendrich Fall Risk model is also widely used. This scale scores 8 factors: confusion/disorientation, depression, altered elimination, dizziness or vertigo, gender, prescribed antiepileptics/benzodiazepines, and ability to rise from a chair. Kim et al. (65) found the Hendrich II Fall Risk Model to be comparable to the Morse scale regarding sensitivity (the ability to correctly identify patients at high risk for falls) with scores of 88% and 70%, respectively. The Hendrich II model, however, had higher specificity (the ability to correctly identify low risk) than the Morse scale, with scores of 48.3% and 61.5%, respectively.

One common problem that hospital nurses complain about is the overidentification of fall risk (poor specificity) that results in extensive interventions for persons who may not actually be at risk for falls. Poor sensitivity results in a decreased likelihood of high-risk fallers being identified as high risk; they may therefore not receive appropriate interventions. The ideal risk scale would have high sensitivity and specificity. Another unaddressed problem with fall risk scales are the legal and safety implications of cut-off scores. Rutledge et al. (60) recommend that institutional administration be included in all decisions about cutoff scores.

Although risk assessment scales may not perfectly quantify fall risk, they do increase the staff's awareness of the presence of specific risk factors in each patient. The staff can then implement appropriate interventions such as ensuring that adaptive equipment is within reach, regular toileting schedules, and so on.

INTERVENTIONS

Many studies have focused on the evaluation of focused interventions on fall rates. Focused interventions studied have included timed toileting, chart stickers and colored dots on name bands indicating risk, individualized patient education, low beds, bed alarms, environmental assessments, and staff education. While many of these interventions have shown some improvements in fall rates, the multifactorial causes of falls necessitate institution-specific and patient-specific identification of risk factors and appropriate interventions.

Interventions should be aimed at addressing identified risk factors. Thus, the patient with poor vision should be supplied with good lighting and assurance that glasses are in reach or in place. The confused patient should be offered added supervision; the weak patient should have the call light in reach and assistance with activity. Anticipating needs is critical to providing a safe environment.

CLINICAL NURSE SPECIALIST COMPETENCIES AND SPHERES OF INFLUENCE

Clinical Expert/Direct Care

CNSs working with a specific population are knowledgeable in the health risks of their patients. Thus, the CNS with a pediatric specialty has a different view of falls than the CNS working with older adults. Falls are very worrisome in the older population, and the CNSs working with these adults are aware of the risks, assess for specific risk factors, and intervene as necessary. The CNS in the mid-level provider role pays special attention to the ongoing status of the older adult patient, including cognition, balance, functional status, nutritional and fluid status, and social and home environment as related to falls. Special care will be taken to avoid polypharmacy and unnecessary medications, and home visits may be initiated to ensure home safety. The CNS in a direct care role will initiate, monitor and maintain physical out-of-bed activity for muscle strengthening, ensure adequate dietary and fluid intake, and ensure safety of the environment. Attention will be paid to sensory input with use of proper lighting and application of visual aids such as glasses. Adaptive equipment such as walkers or canes will be recommended to promote good balance and safety.

Consultation

The CNS may use several specialists in fall prevention for the older adult, physical and occupational therapy in particular. These include physical therapy for lower extremity strengthening, gait evaluation, transfer training, and equipment prescription. The OT will assess self-care abilities, prescribe equipment to aid in self-care and work with the upper extremities for strengthening. Both therapists may perform a home safety evaluation, assessing the safety of the home environment for gait and self-care and making recommendations to the family on needed structural adaptations such as grab bars in the bathroom and removal of throw rugs.

Systems Leadership

The CNS plays a key role in fall prevention in the hospital setting. As mentioned, the CNS has the ability to assess the entire system and lead a team of professionals in addressing issues important to the institution, such as falls. Falls with injury add to a hospital's liability, and the new CMS view of nonpayment for injuries related to falls ensures that hospitals are very interested in fall prevention as well as injury prevention.

Collaboration

The CNS as a system leader will collaborate with risk managers, quality improvement managers, therapists. and others to address system issues related to falls. One of the most important is identification of risk factors specific to the institution that can be addressed on the system level.

Coaching/Teaching/Mentoring

As for other conditions, the CNS uses this competency throughout the system to address fall prevention.

Research/Evidence-Based Practice

This competency is extremely important for fall prevention. The CNS must ensure that the fall risk instrument selected for the institution is both valid and reliable. The CNS must also maintain a current level of knowledge of the requirements of regulating agencies such as CMS for fall prevention, current research findings about risk factors, measurement of risk, and fall prevention strategies and the best practices of other institutions that may be applicable to the CNS's own institution.

Ethical Decision Making/Moral Agency/Advocacy

The CNS advocates throughout the spheres of influence for best practices related to fall prevention.

Patients and Families

In the patient sphere, the CNS uses the competencies of direct care in assessment, diagnosis, planning, intervention, and evaluation. The CNS provides advanced assessment skills for early recognition of fall risk and addresses the direct causes of fall risk. Patient outcomes are evaluated by the CNS and interventions modified as needed.

Teaching/coaching about the importance of fall prevention is of utmost importance. The CNS encourages the patient/family to supply and maintain sensory aides such as glasses and hearing aids. Families are encouraged to stay with elder family members to help with fall prevention activities. The importance of calling for help with mobility out of bed, scheduled toileting, and safety are emphasized.

Nurses and Nursing Practice

The CNS assesses the knowledge of nursing staff relative to prevention and interventions for falls. The CNS engages in teaching/coaching activities to educate nurses and support staff in evidence-based prevention of falls. The importance of risk assessment with appropriate interventions is stressed. Planning individualized care for patients includes fall prevention interventions for high-risk patients, including scheduled toileting, environmental modifications, and interprofessional team involvement. The staff is also included in critically evaluating fall risk factors on the unit and in designing unit-based and patient-focused interventions for fall prevention. The CNS ensures that staff is included in critical analysis of monthly data and fall trends over time. Analysis of fall events should be made available to nursing staff and others on the patient care team. The CNS also teaches staff proper documentation of patient assessment, interventions, and outcomes and then reviews the documentation to determine issues and trends in the management of falls.

Organizations and Systems

At the organization or system level, the CNS assesses need, then plans and intervenes to develop educational programs for fall prevention on units other than his or her own. The CNS identifies and critically evaluates evidence-based guidelines for fall prevention and assesses the need for implementation of EBP guidelines in the institution. Fall risk scales are critically evaluated, and the CNS assists in selecting a scale with acceptable sensitivity and specificity. Leadership skills are employed in assisting the department and institution in designing facility-specific, evidence-based fall prevention strategies and assists in the critical evaluation of fall prevention equipment (such as low beds). The CNS also participates in designing safe patient-care units for populations likely to experience falls and in assisting administrators in developing staffing guidelines for care of the high-risk populations. The CNS collaborates with other professionals on the health care team to establish interprofessional guidelines for care of the patient with high risk for falls. As a member of the interprofessional team, the CNS also assists the institution in evaluating the outcomes of the fall prevention program and designing changes in the program as indicated by the outcomes. The CNS ensures that, as a nursing-sensitive indicator, falls are appropriately defined, reported, tracked, and analyzed and that results and trends are acted upon.

PRESSURE ULCERS

Stage III and IV pressure ulcers are another "no-pay" complication in the Medicare system (66). Seen as preventable, pressure ulcers are one of the nursing sensitive indicators tracked by many health care systems. Healthy People 2010 objectives included reduction of pressure ulcers in nursing homes, while TJC's goal is to prevent health care–associated pressure ulcers (67, 68).

Pressure ulcers can cause significant morbidity and even death. Pressure ulcers are skin lesions caused primarily by unrelieved pressure, usually over a bony prominence. They are among the most common complications of an acute hospital stay or a stay in the long-term care setting (69). While exact numbers are unknown, an estimated 2.5 million pressure ulcers are treated annually in acute care facilities in the United States (69). Most patients with pressure ulcers are over the age of 65, and their pressure ulcers are commonly a hospital-acquired condition. Prevalence rates for pressure ulcers are estimated to range from 3% to 15% in acute care facilities, and units such as ICUs will have a higher incidence than units such as postpartum. As many as 50% of patients in one recent study in an ICU developed a Stage 1 or worse pressure ulcer (69). Pressure ulcers also occur in long-term care facilities. Studies have reported that 4% to 8% of nursing home residents develop a Stage II or greater pressure ulcer within 6 months of admission. Other studies have reported incidence rates of pressure ulcers as high as 24%, with over 70% of high-risk patients developing a wound (69). A review of data from the Healthcare Cost and Utilization Database (HCUP) found that hospital stays related to pressure ulcers were more likely to be discharged to a long-term care facility (~54% compared to ~16% of the general hospital population) and more likely to result in death (11.6% of stays with pressure ulcers as a secondary diagnosis compared to 4.2% of stays with a primary diagnosis of pressure ulcers and 2.6% for all other conditions) (70).

Patients with orthopedic conditions, such as hip fracture, have been found to be at higher risk for pressure ulcers than the general medical/surgical population. Pressure ulcers also occur more frequently in the frail elderly, immobile, and obese patients. Underweight and malnourished people are at risk, as are those who use equipment such as wheelchairs and braces and those with uncontrolled moisture or incontinence. Pressure ulcers increase length of stay to between 10.2 and 14.1 days, compared with the average of 4.6 days (68). Costs to treat a single pressure ulcer can range up to $40,000 or more, depending on severity and associated costs such as hospital room and dressings.

Pressure ulcer severity is defined through staging. These stages as defined by the National Pressure Ulcer Advisory Panel (NPUAP) include the following.

SUSPECTED DEEP TISSUE INJURY

A suspected deep tissue injury is a purple or maroon localized area of discolored intact skin or blood-filled blister. This type of injury may be difficult to see in patients with dark skin tones. A suspected deep tissue

injury can progress rapidly and quickly involve exposure of several skin layers (71).

Stage I: Intact skin with nonblanchable redness of a localized area, usually located over a bony prominence. Darkly pigmented skin may not have visible blanching; its color may differ from the surrounding area (71).

Stage II: Partial-thickness loss of dermis presenting as a shallow open ulcer with a red or pink wound bed, without slough. This stage may also present as an intact or open/ruptured serum-filled blister (71).

Stage III: Full-thickness tissue loss. Subcutaneous fat may be visible but bone, tendon, or muscle is not exposed. Slough may be present but does not obscure the depth of tissue loss. It may include undermining and tunneling (71).

Stage IV: Full-thickness tissue loss with exposed bone, tendon, or muscle. Slough or eschar may be present on some parts of the wound bed. This wound often exhibits undermining and tunneling (71).

Unstageable: Full-thickness tissue loss in which the base of the ulcer is covered by slough (yellow, tan, gray, green or brown) and/or eschar (tan, brown, or black) in the wound bed (71).

CAUSES OF PRESSURE ULCERS

While caused primarily by unrelieved pressure, many factors contribute to the development of a pressure ulcer.

Pressure damage tends to be greatest over bony prominences, where soft tissue can become trapped between the underlying bone and the source of pressure. Pressure applied to the skin in excess of the arteriolar pressure (32 mm Hg) blocks blood supply to the tissue, cutting off delivery of oxygen and nutrients to the tissues (69). Metabolic wastes then accumulate, and free radicals are generated. Berlowitz reports that in animal models, just 2 hours of compression will cause irreversible muscle damage while damage from a tourniquet is more reversible. Both situations induce hypoxia, so there may be other factors associated with pressure that play an important role in pressure ulcer development. Lying on a standard hospital mattress can induce pressure of 150 mm Hg; sitting in a chair, up to 300 mm Hg (69). Pressure is transmitted to underlying tissues in an iceberg configuration, with more damage incurred but invisible at the deeper levels.

Other external factors contributing to pressure ulcer development are shearing forces, friction, and moisture. Shearing forces, such as those caused by sliding down in bed, stretch and traumatize underlying blood vessels. Friction forces abrade the outermost layers of skin and are most often related to Stage II pressure ulcers.

Moisture macerates the outer layers of skin, helping to predispose to superficial ulceration (69).

Internal factors also contribute to pressure ulcer development in varying degrees. These are many and include immobility, incontinence, nutritional deficits, skin perfusion, neurologic disease, diabetes, peripheral arterial disease, sepsis, and hypotension. A study in Belgium in the ICU setting identified history of vascular disease, treatment with dopamine or dobutamine, intermittent hemodialysis, and mechanical ventilation as strongly associated with the development of Stage II to IV ulcers (72).

Assessment of risk of pressure ulcer development is recommended, and several scales have been developed to assist nurses in assessment, including the Braden and the Norton scales. The Norton scale uses a 1 to 4 rating scale that rates the patient on physical condition, mental condition, activity, mobility, and incontinence. A score less than 14 indicates high risk for pressure ulcer development (73). The Braden scale rates patients in six subscales, including sensory perception, moisture, activity, mobility, friction and shear, and nutrition. A score of 16 or less indicates pressure ulcer risk. Both scales are widely used in practice and have been found to be valid; however, issues of interrater reliability have been identified, as have issues of positive predictive value. Also, there have been no studies that evaluate the effects of the use of risk identification on pressure ulcer incidence (73).

Interventions

The first intervention for pressure ulcer prevention is to follow evidence-based national guidelines in employing a risk assessment tool for pressure ulcers. Interventions should not be aimed at just the total score from an instrument; rather, the subscales should be analyzed so that interventions could be more efficiently and effectively targeted. Thus, if a nutritional deficit exists, nutritional interventions should be found in the documentation, including referral to a dietitian.

External Factors

Pressure on bony prominences cannot be eradicated, but it can be reduced through use of specialty devices. These include specialized mattresses, chair and wheelchair cushions, heel boots, pillows, and foam wedges. Basic nursing care also plays an important role—regularly turning and positioning off of the bony prominences, encouraging time out of bed, and assisting in weight shifts in chairs. Turning schedules should be posted and turning and repositioning well documented in the care plans and nurse's notes. Orthotics and prosthetics should be specially fitted and padded to avoid pressure.

Friction and shear are reduced through keeping the head of bed below 30 degrees and lifting instead of dragging when repositioning. The simple application of cotton socks and draw sheets can help protect heels and tailbones from friction and shear. Nurses must ensure adequate staff is available for turning, repositioning, and transferring in and out of bed. Use of gait belts and positioning aids can also assist in reducing friction and shear.

Moisture is controlled through bowel and bladder programs, consistent skin checks and cleaning, timed toileting, and use of moisture barriers. Diapers should be disposable and up to date, with fluid-absorbing properties that limit the amount of moisture near the skin.

Internal Factors

Pressure ulcer risk assessment should trigger a dietary consult if nutritional deficits are identified. These can include underweight or overweight, poor chewing or swallowing abilities, self-care and self-feeding concerns, dehydration, or the presence of a Stage III or IV ulcer.

Immobility is to be minimized. If identified as a risk factor, it should be addressed through a consult to physical therapy for assessment and recommendations. Medications should be reviewed to look for medications that may contribute to the immobile state. Equipment should be provided to assist with out-of-bed mobility, including gait belt, transfer board, comfortable bedside chair or wheelchair, and chair cushion. Hydraulic patient mobility equipment may be necessary for the obese or agitated patient.

The patient with hemodynamic instability in the ICU can be difficult to turn, position, or mobilize. Vasosupportive medications such as dopamine may further compromise skin perfusion. In these cases, rotating beds may be a viable option. A last resort for the patient who severely desaturates with the slightest movement would be to manually place small soft pads and pillows under bony prominences and then gently removing them, gently massaging the bony prominence with lotion, and replacing the pads and pillows at set intervals.

The patient with metastatic disease can also be difficult to turn and reposition due to pain. If it fits with the patient's goals, the patient can be premedicated before any activity. Physical therapy may also be a useful consult in these situations to advise on padding and cushioning.

Facility Activities

Most facilities have implemented routine, regular pressure ulcer surveys. During these surveys, pressure ulcer prevalence, incidence, and severity are ascertained. Some facilities submit this data to the NDNQI so that they may be compared to like facilities.

Pressure ulcer prevalence is defined as the number of patients with pressure ulcers present in a facility at a given time. For instance, if a survey is done on May 5 and 80 patients with pressure ulcers are found when the entire population of 800 patients is assessed, then the prevalence would be 10% (80/800).

Pressure ulcer incidence is the number of patients with new ulcers that have developed since admission at a particular facility. So if 10 of the above patients developed pressure ulcers after admission, then the incidence is 1.25% (80-70/800). This means that 70 of the patients had pressure ulcers on admission. This does not measure how many of these patients developed pressure ulcers at your facility, were discharged, and then readmitted.

Many facilities have also developed skin care teams. These teams of nurses meet regularly to learn about skin and wound care, perform prevalence and incidence surveys, analyze findings of surveys, and plan institutional and unit-level interventions. Nurses on these teams make wonderful resources for the staff on the units.

CLINICAL NURSE SPECIALIST COMPETENCIES AND SPHERES OF INFLUENCE

Clinical Expert/Direct Care

This competency can be one of the most important in pressure ulcer prevention. The CNS as clinical expert holistically assesses the patient for risk, including not only items on a prediction scale, but assessing quality of nutritional intake, functional status, social status, caregiver issues, and medications. The CNS also expertly assesses wounds, recommends or orders wound care, and monitors outcome. Factors complicating would healing are addressed, such as obesity, comorbidities, concomitant injuries, and vasopressive support.

Consultation

Depending upon CNS expertise, the CNS may consult the wound care specialist, the plastic surgeon, or the physical therapist for assistance with pressure ulcer prevention or wound care. The CNS may also be consulted by others for his or her expertise.

Systems Leadership

CNSs have a strong track record of involvement and success in systems leadership for pressure ulcer prevention and wound care. Skin care teams exist at most institutions, led by CNSs. Wound care products, support surfaces, and positioning devices are ideally selected by the CNS in conjunction with the interprofessional team. Risk managers often consult CNSs for advice on managing pressure ulcer incidence at facilities, and it is usually the CNS who leads quarterly pressure ulcer incidence and prevalence surveys. CNSs also alert risk managers of particularly concerning cases of incident pressure ulcers so that the institution can examine the problem on both an individual patient and a system level.

Collaboration

Successful pressure ulcer prevention and skin team function depends on interprofessional collaboration. The CNS leads the efforts, involving nursing unit champions, physicians, therapists, nutritionists, and even pharmacists in the systemwide effort.

Coaching/Teaching/Mentoring

Unit champions for pressure ulcer prevention must be mentored by the CNS, taught about the current guidelines for skin and wound care, and coached into becoming leaders in their own right. The aim of the CNS should be that bedside nurses gradually accept the lead in pressure ulcer prevention, with the CNS playing a background role to ensure that best practices are implemented and standards of care are up to date.

Research/Evidence-Based Practice

This competency is consistent for all conditions and complications that the CNS may encounter, no matter the role of the CNS or the characteristics of the population. That is, actions and interventions must be research-based, evidence-based, and defensible through science.

Ethical Decision Making/Moral Agency/Advocacy

Many of the newer dressings and interventions for pressure ulcer prevention and wound care are cost-intensive. One can never know how many pressure ulcers were prevented with a particular piece of equipment, so justifying an expensive intervention can be difficult. Risk and benefit must be weighed carefully, and CNSs must ensure that ethical principles are followed in the delivery of preventive services and wound care to all patients, particularly the principles involving equitable distribution of care. The CNS also must advocate for the at-risk patient, ensuring that all possible mechanisms of prevention have been employed.

Patients and Families

The CNS employs the competencies of direct care in assessment, diagnosis, planning, intervention, and evaluation. The CNS assesses risk factors, skin and wound condition and identifies contributing medical conditions. The CNS plans and implements interventions for pressure ulcer prevention as well as treatment. The CNS participates in development of patient and family education materials about pressure ulcers and pressure ulcer prevention. The CNS assists in evaluating financial resources for preventive equipment, including bed surfaces, chair cushions, and positioning devices.

Nurses and Nursing Practice

The CNS assesses nurse knowledge about pressure ulcer prevention and provides education where indicated. The CNS engages in teaching and coaching activities with nurses to improve knowledge and skills related to pressure ulcer prevention and wound care. The CNS aids staff in planning individualized pressure ulcer prevention activities for patients, and in analysis of unit-specific practices and outcomes. The CNS also acts as consultant to staff in complicated skin and wound care cases. The CNS reviews documentation to identify trends and needs related to pressure ulcer prevention and wound care, including individualized patient interventions based on risk-assessment scale subscores.

Organizations and Systems

The CNS acts as the institutional liaison to the skin and wound care product vendors, critically evaluating and recommending products based on quality, availability, cost, and outcomes. The CNS leads the institution in data collection, analysis, and interpretation for pressure ulcer prevalence and incidence. The CNS identifies, evaluates and interprets evidence-based practices for pressure ulcer prevention and wound care for the institution. The CNS employs leadership skills in initiating an interprofessional skin care team and helps to develop individual skin care champions for each unit. The CNS helps maintain institutional expenditures through critical analysis of costly interventions such as specialty beds and wound vacuum systems. The CNS also advocates for the patient population in terms of equipment and staffing required for optimal pressure ulcer prevention in the institution.

RESTRAINTS

Use of physical restraints occurs in all treatment settings and in all patient age groups. As far back as 1992 the FDA issued a safety alert on potential hazards with restraint devices. The FDA included safety vests, lap and wheelchair belts, and body holders in this warning. They issued the warning because reports of deaths and injuries related to the use of restraint devices was increasing and noted that many restraint-related injuries and deaths are probably not reported at all. At that time, the FDA estimated that there were at least 100 deaths or injuries annually associated with restraints as the patient tried to get out of the restraint. They also noted that many injuries seemed to be related to improper use of the devices, including inappropriate patient selection, incorrect restraint selection, errors in correctly applying the devices, and inadequate monitoring of the patients while restrained (74).

The Patients' Rights Conditions of Participation (CoP) (2006) that hospitals must meet to participate in Medicare and Medicaid programs contains two standards for the use of restraint and seclusion in hospitals: restraint for acute medical and surgical care and restraint and seclusion for behavior management. CMS defines restraint as either physical or chemical. A physical restraint is any manual method or device used to restrict freedom of movement or access to one's body, while a chemical restraint is a medication not standard for the patient's medical or psychiatric condition that is used to control behavior or restrict freedom of movement (75).

The final regulation from CMS includes, among other criteria, a strong staff training standard.

Mion (76) estimates that approximately 27,000 people are physically restrained every day in hospitals in the United States. Hospitals in Mion's study varied in rates, from a low of 4.7 to a high of 94 restraint-days/1,000 patient-days. Intensive care units accounted for 56% of all restraint days despite having only 16% of the patient-days. Differences in rates were found among types of ICU, with pediatric units using fewer restraints. The author believes that the major concern of critical care personnel is the risk of the patient's premature termination of live-saving therapies such as ventilators and medications. She notes, however, that studies of individual devices such as endotracheal tubes have found that up to 74% of patients who disrupt the device are restrained at the time.

Causes

Restraints have historically been used to meet a variety of perceived needs in acute and critical care. The above-mentioned reason of preventing the patient from removing tubes and lines is one. Restraints have been thought to prevent falls, to prevent injury to patient or staff, to remind the patient to stay in bed or to remain seated, and to maintain a body part in a required position. Staff uses restraints to prevent wandering, to manage violent behavior, and to maintain sitting balance (77). Unfortunately, restraints have also been used as a staff-replacement, a staff timesaver, as punishment, and for behavior modification. When restraints are used, the staff becomes the powerful and the restrained become the powerless.

Restraints have been shown to be a significant cause of morbidity and mortality in the hospital setting. Restriction of movement enforces immobility, potentially elevating the risk of pneumonia, aspiration, flexion contractures, deep venous thrombosis, and pulmonary emboli, as well as incontinence, muscle weakness, and skin breakdown. Patients who try to loosen or escape from restraints can incur friction burns, skin wounds, and impedance of circulation. Strangulation is not unheard of, as again the patient tries to "escape." Restraints can contribute to cardiac death due to the cascade of physiologic responses that occur with states of hyperarousal (78). Behavioral arousal with the stress reaction has been shown to induce malignant cardiac rhythms, and an outpouring of catecholamines can sensitize the heart and contribute to disturbances in rhythm (78). And do not forget the psychological effects of restraints, including social isolation, PTSD, nightmares, and mistrust of health care personnel.

As NINR (77) points out, the nurse is the primary health professional who decides whether restraints will be used. Studies have found that restrained patients tended to be older, had higher morbidity and mortality rates, and had longer lengths of stay compared to nonrestrained patients. Studies have also found that abnormal mental status, organic brain syndrome, surgery and the presence of at least one restrictive device (such as oxygen or IV tubing) predicted restraint use. Potential risk factors for restraint use include a room change, surgery, and the number of restrictive tubes, lines, and pieces of equipment that are used with an individual patient (77).

Nurses who care for patients in restraints also suffer distress. There is a basic cognitive dissonance between valuing patient autonomy and dignity and restraining an individual against his will. Federal regulations have generally held that a patient has the right to be free from physical and chemical restraints. Legally, restraint use in acute care is not clear. While CMS and TJC have clear rules concerning restraint use, the courts have not been as clear in their rulings concerning liability for falls in non-restrained patients. The ethical concern related to restraint use is the conflict between the principles of beneficence and autonomy. Nurses are meant to "do good," but yet the individual has the right to choose his or her own course of action.

Alternatives to restraints do exist. No, they may not be "easy," but when balancing the risk-to-benefit ratio, the alternatives win. Many nursing units are restraint-free. With a change in unit philosophy emphasizing the value of NOT using restraints, these units have developed protocols for managing wandering behaviors, falls, equipment, and agitation. The geriatric field has been the leader in restraint-free environments.

What does it take? The CNS as leader must consider the:

- Ethics, values, attitudes, and beliefs of staff
- Physical environment
- Care needs and medical profiles of the patient population
- Options available to maintain a restraint-free environment

Interventions

Staff education is the core of a restraint-free environment. Staff should participate in examining their own ethics, values, attitudes, and beliefs concerning the patient population and the perceived need for restraints. Staff involvement in evaluation of evidence-based restraint alternatives, formulation of unit policy and standard practices for elimination of restraints, and education of other health care team members, patients, and families is vital. The administration may wish to consider the placement of staff who do not share the new restraint-free philosophy of the unit.

The physical environment needs to support a restraint-free philosophy. Patient rooms with a window view onto the hall, where staff can easily view patients, is a time-saving method of patient observation. Activity baskets or packets with recreational activities for patients should be available when distraction is needed. These baskets might include crossword puzzles, coloring books, jigsaw puzzles, and yarn crafts. Staff should be available for assisting with distractive activities; for instance, a unit secretary can watch a patient who is seated in a geriatric chair, interact verbally with the patient, and monitor the patient while he completes activities such as folding towels. Floors should be made of newer, flexible materials to prevent injury if a patient falls; low beds can be purchased for the same reasons; clutter and equipment should be kept in formal service areas.

The patient population should be profiled, so that the administrator can plan on appropriate staffing. Is the patient population older, with frequent delirium and dementia among the diagnoses? Or is it pediatric, with risk takers or toddlers? What equipment is currently used? Are other equipment options available that would negate the need to restrain individuals for whom the equipment is used? Do your patients have family members who usually accompany them and who could help with restraint-free tactics?

Sitters have been used by some facilities in an attempt to prevent falls in lieu of restraints. Although a logical solution, studies have questioned the effectiveness of sitters in reducing institutional fall rates. Hospitals have found the cost of sitters to outweigh the benefits. Since the majority of sitters are typically not professionally trained, and since the quality, capabilities, and responsibilities of sitters may vary widely even within a single institution, sitter use is losing favor as an "easy fix" for fall prevention (79).

CLINICAL NURSE SPECIALIST COMPETENCIES AND SPHERES OF INFLUENCE

Clinical Expert/Direct Care

The CNS in the expert clinician role maintains a practice that encourages alternatives to restraints. This would include expert assessment of and intervention for factors leading to the need for restraints such as dementia, delirium, or medications.

Consultation

In advocating for a restraint-free environment, the CNS may need to consult experts to manage behaviors. These could include the psychiatrist, internal medicine physician, occupational or recreational therapist, and nurse's aides. The CNS might act as consultant not only on the unit, but to other units as well.

Systems Leadership

An increased focus on restraint use by regulating agencies has necessitating an increased awareness of restraint use at the institutional level. The CNS can emerge as a leader in reducing restraints through sharing knowledge and skills related to alternatives to restraints throughout the institution.

Collaboration

The CNS collaborates with many others in restraint reduction, including risk managers, nursing staff, therapists, patients, and families.

Coaching/Teaching/Mentoring

Long-held beliefs can be a barrier to reducing restraint use, and the CNS is an expert in teaching others about the topic. The CNS uses multiple strategies to teach alternatives to restraints, including sharing best practices and modeling appropriate behaviors.

Research/Evidence-Based Practice

Remaining up to date in the literature about reducing restraint use is the best way to ensure that best practices are used.

Ethical Decision-Making/Moral Agency/Advocacy

One must consider both ethical and legal implications of restraint use. The CNS advocates for the patient by introducing alternatives to restraints and ensuring that ethical principles are employed when restraints are used.

Patients and Families

The CNS uses the competencies of direct care in holistically assessing the factors involved in the consideration of restraint use. Often, families request restraints to keep the relative safe. After assessing the patient and the situation, the CNS uses teaching competencies in educating the family on restraint alternatives, which may include roles for the family members. The CNS teaches the family methods of managing behaviors that may lead the family into requesting restraints for their loved ones. The CNS participates in the development of patient-family teaching materials about alternatives to restraints.

Nurses and Nursing Practice

The CNS evaluates the ethics, values, and beliefs of the staff, as well as their knowledge of restraint effects and restraint alternatives. The CNS shares evidence-based information with the staff to reinforce the necessity of a restraint-free environment and in teaching staff alternatives to restraints. The CNS encourages staff to collaborate with other health care practitioners in individualizing patient care—including collaboration with occupational, physical, recreational, and music therapists. The CNS acts as a consultant to staff in difficult situations requiring advanced knowledge, judgment, and skills. The CNS reviews documentation to identify trends and needs related to restraint use and compares data to like units and to evidence-based practice guidelines.

Organizations and Systems

The CNS collaborates with other nursing professionals in ensuring institutional compliance with national guidelines and with accrediting agency recommendations. The CNS identifies, evaluates, and shares evidence-based information concerning restraint reduction with administrators and risk managers. The CNS assists nurse managers in evaluating individual plans of care for challenging patients, including the recommendation of staffing levels to ensure patient safety.

References

1. National Association of Clinical Nurse Specialists. Statement on Clinical Nurse Specialist Practice and education. Harrisburg, PA: National Association of Clinical Nurse Specialists; 2004.

2. Dart RC, editor. Medical Toxicology (3rd ed.). New York: Lippincott, Williams and Wilkins; 2004.

3. Ely EW, Siegel ND, Inouye SK. Delirium in the intensive care unit: an under-recognized syndrome of organ dysfunction. Semin Resp Crit Care 2001;22(2). Retrieved May 22, 2009, from www.medscape.com/viewarticle/410883

4. American Psychological Association. Diagnostic and Statistical Manual of Mental Disorders, Fourth Edition. Arlington, VA: American Psychological Publishing; 2001.

5. Maldonado JR. Delirium in the acute care setting: characteristics, diagnosis and treatment. Crit Care Clin 2008;24:657-722.

6. Alagiakrishnan K, Blanchette P. Delirium. In Emedicine Clinical Knowledge Base, Institutional Edition, 2007. Retrieved May 21, 2009, from http://www.imedicine.com.libproxy.uthscsa.edu/DisplayTopic.asp?bookid=6&topic=3006

7. Miller MO. Evaluation and management of delirium in hospitalized older patients. Am Fam Physician 2008;78:1265-1270. Retrieved May 22, 2009, from www.afp.org/afp

8. MacLullich AMJ, Ferguson KJ, Miller T, deRooik SEJA, Cunningham C. Unraveling the pathophysiology of delirium: a focus on the role of aberrant stress responses. J Psychosomatic Res 2008;65:229-238.

9. Ely EW, Margolin R, Francis J, et al. Evaluation of delirium in critically ill patients: validation of the Confusion Assessment Method for the Intensive Care Unit (CAM-ICU). Crit Care Med 2001;29:1370-1379.

10. Inouye S, van Dyck C, Alessi C, et al. Clarifying confusion: The confusion assessment method. Ann Intern Med 1990;113:941-948.

11. Malone M, Danto-Nocton E. ACE cards: Identifying delirium in hospitalized older patients, 2003. (Available from Aurora Sinai Medical Center/UW Medical School, 945 N 12th Street, Milwaukee, WI 53233.)

12. Francis J, Young GB. Diagnosis of delirium and confusional states, 2009. UpToDate Online 17.1. Retrieved May 22, 2009, from http://www.utdol.com/online/content/topic.do?topicKey=medneuro/2425&selectedTitle=1~150&source=search_result

13. American Psychiatric Association. Practice guideline for the treatment of patients with delirium. Am J Psych 1999;156(5 suppl):1-20.

14. Turkoski BB, Lance BR, Bonfiglio MF. Drug Information Handbook for Advanced Practice Nursing (9th ed.). Hudson, Ohio: Lexi-Comp; 2009.

15. Tullman DF, Mion LC, Fletcher K, Foreman MD. Delirium: Prevention, early recognition, treatment. In Evidence-Based Geriatric Nursing Protocols for Best Practice (3rd ed.). New York: Springer Publishing Company; 2008;111-125.

16. Overweight and Obesity. Retrieved May 25, 2009, from http://www.cdc.gov/nccdphp/dnpa/Obesity/

17. Overweight and Obesity. Retrieved May 25, 2009, from http://www.cdc.gov/nccdphp/dnpa/obesity/trend/maps/index.htm

18. Ritchie J. Nation's soaring obesity impacts hospital construction. Birmingham Business Journal, August 24, 2007. Retrieved May 25, 2009, from http://www.bizjournals.com/birmingham/stories/2007/0August 27/focus6.html

19. Humphreys SL. Obesity in patients and nurses increases the nurse's risk of injury lifting patients. Bariatr Nurs Surg Pt Care 2007;2:3-6.

20. Understanding Adult Obesity. Retrieved May 25, 2009, from http://win.niddk.nih.gov/publications/understanding.htm#cultural

21. Uwaifo GI, Arioglu E. Obesity. In Emedicine Clinical Knowledge Base, Institutional Edition. Retrieved May 21, 2009, from http://www.imedicine.com.libproxy.uthscsa.edu/DisplayTopic.asp?bookid=6&topic=1653

22. Bray GA. Drug therapy of Obesity. In UpToDate online 17.1. Retrieved May 25, 2009, from http://www.utdol.com/online/content/topic.do?topicKey=obesity/5774&selectedTitle=22~150&source=search_result

23. Snow V, Barry P, Fitterman N, et al. Pharmacologic and surgical management of obesity in primary care: a clinical practice guideline from the American College of Physicians. Ann Intern Med 2005;142:525-531.

24. Zegelin A. 'Tied down': the process of becoming bedridden through gradual local confinement. J Clin Nurs 2008;17:2294-2301.

25. Convertino VA, Bloomfield SA, Greenleaf JE. An overview of the issues: physiological effects of bed rest and restricted physical activity. Med Sci Sports Exerc 1997;29:187-190.

26. Choi JY, Tasota FJ, Hoffman LA. Mobility interventions to improve outcomes in patients undergoing mechanical ventilation: a review of the literature. Biol Res Nurs 2008;10:21-33.

27. Spellman NT. Prevention of immobility complications through early rehabilitation. In Belandres PV, Dillingham TR, editors. Rehabilitation of the Injured Combatant (Vol. 2). Washington, DC: Borden Institute: 1999:741-777.

28. Corcoran PJ. Use it or lose it: the hazards of bedrest and inactivity. Rehabil Med 1991;154:536-538.

29. Brown CJ, Friedkin RJ, Inouye SK. Prevalence and outcomes of low mobility in hospitalized older patients. J Am Geriatr Soc 2004;52:1263-1270.

30. Gill TM, Allore H, Guo Z. The deleterious effects of bed rest among community-living older adults. J Gero 2004;59A:755-761.

31. Morris PE, Good A, Thompson C, et al. Early intensive care unit mobility therapy in the treatment of acute respiratory failure. Crit Care Med 2008;36:2238-2243.

32. Rogers MAM, Fries BE, Kaufman SR, et al. Mobility and other predictors of hospitalization for urinary tract infection: a retrospective cohort study. BMC Geriatr 2008;8. Retrieved May 28, 2009, from BioMed Central: www.biomecentral.com

33. Saltvedt I, Opdahl E-S, Fayers P, et al. Reduced mortality in treating acutely sick, frail older patients in a geriatric evaluation and management unit: a prospective randomized trial. J Am Geriatr Soc 2002;50:792-798.

34. Landefeld CS, Palmer RM, Kresevic DM, et al. A randomized trial of care in a hospital medical unit especially designed to improve the functional outcomes of acutely ill older adults. N Eengl J Med 1995;332:1338-1344.

35. Neubauer DN. Difficulties with sleep or wakefulness. Prim Psych 2009;16:23-25.

36. National Sleep Foundation. (2009). Sleep Stats and Facts. Retrieved May 28, 2008, from http://www.sleepfoundation.org/site/c.huIXKjM0IxF/b.2419253/k.7989/Sleep_Facts_and_Stats.htm

37. Daley M, Morin CM, LeBlanc M, et al. Insomnia and its relationship to health-care utilization, work absenteeism, productivity and accidents. Sleep Med 2009;10:427-438.

38. Cmiel CA, Karr DM, Gasser DM, et al. Noise control: a nursing team's approach to sleep promotion. J Neurol 2004;104:40-48.

39. Southwell MT, Wistow G. Sleep in hospitals at night: are patient needs being met? J Adv Nurs Pract 1995;21:1101-1109.

40. Pressman MR. (2009) Stages and Architecture of Normal Sleep. UpToDate online 17.1. Retrieved May 25, 2009, from http://www.utdol.com/online/content/topic.do?topicKey=sleepdis/8234&selectedTitle=1~150&source=search_result

41. Pressman MR. (2009). Definition and Consequences of Sleep Deprivation. UpToDate online 17.1. Retrieved May 25, 2009, from http://www.utdol.com/online/content/topic.do?topicKey=sleepdis/9502&selectedTitle=6~150&source=search_result

42. Shub D, Darvishi R, Kunik ME. Non-pharmacologic treatment of insomnia in persons with dementia. Geriatrics 2009;64:22-26.

43. Panossian LA, Avidan AY. Review of sleep disorders. Med Clin North Am 2009;93:407-425.

44. Lubit RH, Bonds CL. (2009). Sleep disorders. In Emedicine Clinical Knowledge Base, Institutional Edition. Retrieved May 21, 2009, from http://www.imedicine.com.libproxy.uthscsa.edu/DisplayTopic.asp?bookid=6&topic=609

45. Roehrs T, Roth T. (2009). The Effect of Drugs on Sleep Quality and Architecture. UpToDate online 17.1. Retrieved May 25, 2009, from http://www.utdol.com/online/content/topic.do?topicKey=sleepdis/6893&selectedTitle=15~150&source=search_result

46. Medical Laboratory Observer. (2000). Nutrition Assessment Outcomes: A Protocol for Native American Hospitals. Retrieved June 1, 2009, from http://entrepreneur.com/tradejournals/article/68743431_1.html

47. Fessler TA. Malnutrition: a serious concern for hospitalized patients. Today's Dietitian 2008;10:44.

48. Thomas DR, Zdrowski CD, Wilson M-M, et al. Malnutrition in subacute care. Am J Clin Nutr 2002;75:308-313.

49. Kudsk KA, Reddy SK, Sacks GS, Lai H-C. Joint Commission for Accreditation of Health Care Organizations guidelines: too late to intervene for nutritionally at-risk surgical patients. J Parental Enteral Nutr 2003;27:288-230.

50. Perlich M, Schutz T, Kemps M, et al. Social risk factors for hospital malnutrition. Nutrition 2005;21:295-300.

51. Ritchie C. (2008). Geriatric Nutrition: Nutritional Issues in Older Adults. UpToDate online. Retrieved May 25, 2009, from http://www.utdol.com/online/content/topic.do?topicKey=geri_med/8473&selectedTitle=6~150&source=search_result

52. Bellini LM. (2004). Assessment of Nutrition in the Critically Ill. Up toDate online 17.1. Retrieved May 25, 2009, from http://www.utdol.com/online/content/topic.do?topicKey=cc_medi/17912&selectedTitle=10~150&source=search_result

53. American Society for Parenteral and Enteral Nutrition. (n.d.). Nutrition Screening. Retrieved June 1, 2009, from www.nutritioncare.org/lcontent.aspx?id=550

54. American Nurses Association (2009). The National Database of Nursing Quality Indicators™ (NDNQI®). Retrieved August 11, 2009, from http://www.nursingworld.org/MainMenuCategories/ANAMarketplace/ANAPeriodicals/OJIN/TableofContents/Volume122007/No3Sept07/NursingQualityIndicators.aspx

55. National Quality Forum. (2009). Tracking NQF-Endorsed™ Consensus Standards for Nursing-Sensitive Care: A 15-Month Study. Retrieved August 11, 2009, from http://www.qualityforum.org/Projects/s-z/Tracking_Nursing-Sensitive_Care_Consensus_Standards_%282O07%29/Tracking_Nursing-Sensitive_Care_Consensus_Standards.aspx

56. The Joint Commission. (2009). National Patient Safety Goals. Retrieved August 11, 2009, from http://www.jointcommission.org/NR/rdonlyres/F71BC4E9-FEB6-495C-99D8-DB9F0850E75B/0/09_NPSG_General_Presentation.ppt#286,31,Reduce Falls

57. Centers for Disease Control and Prevention (2009). Falls Among Older Adults: An Overview. Retrieved August 11, 2009, from http://www.cdc.gov/HomeandRecreationalSafety/Falls/adultfalls.html

58. Inouye SK, Brown CJ, Tinetti ME. Medicare nonpayment, hospital falls, and unintended consequences. N Engl J Med 2009;360:2390-2393.

59. Centers for Disease Control and Prevention (2009). Hip Fractures Among Older Adults. Retrieved August 11, 2009, from http://www.cdc.gov/HomeandRecreationalSafety/Falls/adulthipfx.html

60. Rutledge DN, Donaldson NE, Pravikoff DS. Update 2003: fall risk assessment and prevention in hospitalized patients. Online J Clin Innov 2003;31:1-55.

61. Centers for Disease Control and Prevention (2009). Fall Prevention Activities. Retrieved August 11, 2009, from http://www.cdc.gov/HomeandRecreationalSafety/Falls/FallsPreventionActivity.html

62. Free Press Release. (2008). Patient Falls, Medicare Changes Could Cost Hospitals Billions. Retrieved August 11, 2009, from http://www.free-press-release.com/news/200806/1213324809.html

63. Aizen E, Shugaev I, Lenger R. Risk factors and characteristics of falls during inpatient rehabilitation of elderly patients. Arch Gerontol Geriatr 2006;44:1-12.

64. O'Connell B, Myers H. The sensitivity and specificity of the Morse Fall Scale in an acute care setting. J Clin Nursing 2002;11:134-136.

65. Kim EAN, Mordiffi SZ, Bee HW, et al. Evaluation of three fall risk assessment tools in an acute care setting. J Adv Nursing 2007;60:427-435.

66. Mattie AS, Webster BL. Centers for Medicare and Medicaid Services' "Never Events": an analysis and recommendations to hospitals. Health Care Manager 2008;27:338-349.

67. Healthy People 2010 Objective 1-16. Retrieved August 11, 2009, from http://www.npuap.org/archive/HP2010.htm

68. Van Gilder C, MacFarlane G, Lachencruch C. Body mass index, weight and pressure ulcer prevalence. J Nurs Care Qual 2008;24:127-135.

69. Berlowitz D. (2009). Pressure Ulcers: Epidemiology, Pathogenesis, Clinical Manifestations and Staging. UpToDate online 17.1. Retrieved August 15, 2009, from http://www.utdol.com/online/content/topic.do?topicKey=gensurg/6909&selectedTitle=3~75&source=search_result

70. Russo CA, Steiner C, Spector W. (2008). Hospitalizations Related to Pressure Ulcers Among Adults 18 Years and Older, 2006. Retrieved August 15, 2009, from http://www.hcup-us.ahrq.gov/reports/statbriefs/sb64.pdf

71. National Pressure Ulcer Advisory Panel. Pressure Ulcer Stages Revised by NPUAP. Retrieved August 15, 2009, from http://www.npuap.org/pr2.htm

72. Nijs N, Toppets A, Defloor T, et al. Incidence and risk factors for pressure ulcers in the intensive care unit. J Clin Nursing 2008;18:1258-1266.

73. Berlowitz D. Prevention of Pressure Ulcers. UpToDate online 17.1. Retrieved August 14, 2009, from http://www.utdol.com/online/content/topic.do?topicKey=gensurg/7182&selectedTitle=2~75&source=search_result

74. Food and Drug Administration. FDA Safety Alert: Potential Hazards with Restraint Devices. Retrieved August 24, 2009, from http://www.fda.gov/downloads/MedicalDevices/Safety/AlertsandNotices/PublicHealthNotifications/ucm063107.pdf

75. CMS Issues New Restraint and Seclusion Regulations: More Training Mandated. Retrieved August 24, 2009, from http://www.medlaw.com/healthlaw/HOSPITAL/6_2/cms-issues-new-restraint-.shtml

76. Mion LC. Physical restraint in critical care settings: will they go away? Geriatr Nursing 2008;20:421-423.

77. National Institute of Nursing Research. Chapter 5: Problems Associated With the Use of Physical Restraints. Retrieved August 24, 2009, from http://ninr.nih.gov/ninr/research/vol3/Restraints.html

78. Mohr WK, Petti TA, Mohr BD. Adverse effects associated with physical restraints. Can J Psychiatry 2003;48:330-337.

79. Tzeng HM, Yin CY, et al. Effective assessment of use of sitters by nurses in inpatient care settings. J Adv Nursing 2008;64:176-184.

CHAPTER 3

Pain

Paul Arnstein, PhD, APRN-BC, FAAN,
Hannah Felton Lyons, MSN, RN, AOCN,
and Yassaman Khalili, MSc, RN

INTRODUCTION

Pain is encountered daily in acute care settings and is one of the most pervasive and expensive health care problems of the twenty-first century (1). This year, close to 50 million Americans will have surgical pain, and 80% of those will experience severe pain during their recovery. The importance of effective pain management cannot be understated given that pain intensity in acute care is the best predictor of patients who still have pain a year after major surgery or trauma (2). Recent estimates hold that 25% of the general population is living with chronic pain, with the proportion of those living with pain for more than a year increasing over time (1). Therefore, in addition to the pain associated with acute conditions and diagnostic and therapeutic procedures, chronic pain is increasingly a comorbid condition that must be controlled to facilitate healing and recovery.

Despite remarkable progress in the prevention, diagnosis, and treatment of acute pain, the challenges of easing it are increasingly complex. Although the know-how is available, the consistent application of evidence-based interventions to prevent and treat acute pain is lacking (3). Even when these techniques are used, the need to reevaluate the plan of care while tailoring assessments and therapies to the individual's needs is often lacking. The clinical nurse specialist (CNS) is in an ideal position to improve the way pain is managed because of her or his ability to work directly with patients, clinical staff, and organizational systems where the barriers to optimal care reside. To do this, CNSs need to update and maintain their own knowledge, skills, and attitudes in this clinical area to be able to role model best practices.

The first priority is to ensure that the minimum standards of care that have been adopted by regulators (Medicare/Medicaid) and accreditors (The Joint Commission) are met. These are often misunderstood. For example, meeting the standards for pain assessment and reassessment can be difficult because nurses do not use pain assessment methods consistently and/or they fail to reassess pain in a timely manner. Standardizing algorithms to guide critical thinking for nurses is even more challenging. In addition, the way nurses choose drugs when multiple "as needed" (prn) orders exist or the selection of a dose within a range order is a controversial area of practice. Indeed, nurses in some areas may be functioning beyond their scope of practice if prescribed orders and related policies are not clear and aligned with laws in their particular state. Those in many acute care settings, however, erroneously believe permitted practices are illegal and restrict the role of nurses more than is necessary.

A useful starting point is to clearly define terms and concepts related to pain (Table 3-1), including different pain types, because the goals of care and treatment strategies may differ based on these classifications. Treatment options often vary depending on whether the patient has an acute, a chronic, or a life-threatening condition. Treatment responses also vary based on whether the patient has nociceptive, neuropathic, or mixed types of pain.

Historically, beliefs about the nature of pain have evolved from being a purely mystical or spiritual phenomenon, to being viewed as either an entirely emotional or a purely physical state but not both (4). This is referred to as the "Cartesian split," which assumes pain without a measurable physical explanation represents a psychological illness. Often this failure to objectify pain is more an indication of the limits of current technology rather than a valid way to determine whether a patient has a mental illness. Advanced imaging methods confirm that common emotional responses such as fear, anxiety, or anger can amplify pain and

TABLE 3–1 Terms and Concepts Related to Pain

PAIN: An unpleasant experience affecting the mind, body, spirit, and social interactions; associated with actual or potential harm to the person. By nature it is subjective, therefore best defined by the patient; however, behaviors can indicate its presence in those unwilling or unable to inform others that it is being experienced.

- ACUTE PAIN: Pain that lasts for seconds, minutes, hours, days, or weeks until healing occurs and the pain resolves
- CHRONIC PAIN: Pain that lasts well beyond the expected healing time and/or is present for longer than 6 months
- NOCICEPTIVE PAIN: Pain related to injury or illness transmitted by intact, properly functioning nerves
    - SOMATIC PAIN: Pain related to an injury or illness of skin, muscle, bone, connective and soft tissues. It is generally well localized and the intensity often correlated with the amount of tissue damage.
    - VISCERAL PAIN: Pain related to injury or illness of visceral tissues. The location and intensity may not correlate with the tissue damage.
    - INFLAMMATORY PAIN: Pain associated with an inflammatory process
    - NEUROPATHIC PAIN: Abnormal pain related to damaged or malfunctioning nerves

ALLODYNIA: Perception of innocuous stimuli (light touch, warmth) as pain
HYPERALGESIA: A phenomenon of a heightened perception of and response to pain

- PRIMARY HYPERALGESIA: An exaggerated pain response (primary hyperalgesia) resulting from lower firing thresholds of peripheral nociceptors and central interneurons
- SECONDARY HYPERALGESIA: The extension of an area of hyperalgesia to adjacent body parts so that an uncomfortable stimulus applied near injured tissue evokes an exaggerated pain response

that amplified pain intensifies these emotions (5). Thus, it is better to treat both the underlying cause of the pain and co-occuring emotions that amplify it, rather than failing to treat either by labeling the patient as mentally ill or having "psychogenic" pain. As a clinical leader, the CNS can help clinicians better understand and attend to patient-centered needs in a more comprehensive fashion.

CONCEPTUAL MODEL

One way of conceptualizing pain that a CNS may find useful for guiding therapy and teaching others about pain has been described as the "gain control" model. This model (Figure 3-1) delineates factors in the body, mind, spirit, and social interactions that control the strength of pain impulses, which can act as amplifiers and dampeners of the pain experience. Using this model nursing interventions can target the enhancement of dampeners and blocking amplifiers (Figure 3-2) of pain (6) using multimodal approaches.

In the body, factors capable of amplifying pain include inflammation, hypoxia, muscle tension, or spasms. Therefore, pain can be cut by minimizing inflammation or further tissue damage while promoting nutrition, oxygenation, and relaxation in order to facilitate tissue repair. Pain itself when severe or allowed

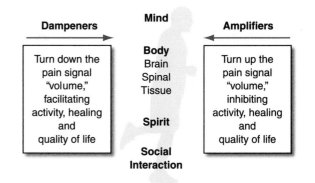

FIGURE 3–1: Gain Control Model of Pain. *(Adapted from Arnstein PM. Clinical Coach for Effective Pain Management. Philadelphia: FA Davis; 2010.)*

to persist without relief can produce changes in the peripheral and central nerves through processes known as sensitization, wind-up, and neuroplasticity. These in turn produce structural changes in the nerves that increase their permeability to sodium and calcium ions, which, along with other nerve alterations, can amplify, spread, and prolong the transmission of pain signals. Thus, preventing and controlling pain effectively can limit its amplification and spread.

Dampeners →		← Amplifiers
Strong faith Unchanged essence Sense of purpose Sense of connecting Balanced energy flow	**Spirit**	Spiritual disturbance Loss of connections Dire meaning Suffering Energy imbalance
Emotionally stable Love Self-sufficient, optimistic Feelings of acceptance Realistic beliefs/expectations Mental distraction Effective coping	**Mind**	Emotional distress • Anxiety, fear, depression, etc. High or prolonged stress Unhelpful thoughts • Catastrophising • Self doubts • Helplessness, hopelessness
Tissues Tissue repair, healing Tissue stimulation Optimal nutrition, O_2 Position support (brace) Muscle relaxation **Nervous system** Gentle dermatome stimulation • A-Beta-fiber activity (warm, cool, touch) Endorphin release Avert hyper excitability	**Body**	**Tissues** Ongoing tissue damage Inflammation/infection Hypoxia Muscle tension/spasm **Nervous system** Irritation/overstimulation of area surrounding pain Sensitization (peripheral/central nerves) Maladaptive neuroplasticity Neuronal inflammation
Socially engaged Pursuit of meaningful, pleasurable activities Effective communication Work, volunteering	**Social Interaction**	Socially isolated Relationship/role conflict Over dependency Dysfunctional relationships

FIGURE 3–2: Gain Control Model of Pain. *(Adapted from Arnstein PM. Clinical Coach for Effective Pain Management. Philadelphia; FA Davis; 2010.)*

The importance of pain assessment is often overlooked, as it provides insight into what is happening within the the patient's mind and body at a given moment. The patient's verbal report of pain remains the gold standard for assessing and reassessing pain. Overreliance on a scale as a single measure of pain may be counterproductive when the patient cannot understand or use these scales effectively. Therefore, time is well spent having a conversation with the patient about their pain and about how it can be measured in a meaningful way.

For those with impaired cognition or difficulty with communicating their pain verbally, other assessment methods are available. In those cases, functional or behavioral indicators of pain are used. Several examples of validated tools are indentified in Table 3-2 for both verbal and nonverbal populations. Although the tools themselves may be simple, sometimes clinical conditions make the selection process complex (Figure 3-3).

Clinical measurement tools aside, the CNS should also consider how psychosocial, existential, and environmental factors affect pain, which in turn can interfere with overall health, functioning, and individualized therapeutic goals.

As important as the initial assessment of pain, the reassessment can be equally challenging. Many clinicians reassess pain solely on the basis of pain intensity fluctuations. Whenever analgesics are used, reassessment parameters also need to include medication side effects and technology-related complications. However, an improvement in mood, sleep pattern, activity level, and ability to feel connected (socially or spiritually) can be indicators of treatment success, even if the pain intensity remains unchanged (7). Sometimes, despite a significant change in pain intensity, the patient stays focused only on the unresolved fraction of pain that remains. In these cases, the patient's expectations (e.g., for complete pain relief) may be unrealistic or the physical pain is being amplified

TABLE 3-2 **Examples of Commonly Used Pain Assessment Tools**

Patient Population	Type of Measure	Assessment Tool*
Pediatric* behavioral	Behavioral observation	FLACC (Face, Legs, Activity, Cry, Consolability)
		COMFORT Behavior Scale
		CHEOPS (Children Hospital of Eastern Ontario Pain Scale)
Pediatric	Self-report	FACES
Adult	Self-report	Numeric "0-10" Scale
		Verbal Descriptor Scale
		Brief Pain Inventory-SF
		McGill Pain Questionnaire-SF
Adult	Self-report & observation	Functional Pain Scale
Nonverbal Adult	Behavioral observation	CNPI (Checklist of Non-verbal Pain Indicators)
		FLACC-a (Face, Legs, Activity, Cry, Consolability – adult)
Adult with Dementia	Behavioral observation	PAINAD (Pain Assessment in Advanced Demetia)
		ADD (Assessment of Discomfort in Dementia)
		PACSLAC (Pain Assessment Checklist for Seniors with Limited Abililty to Communicate)
		NOPAIN
Intubated Adult	Behavioral observation	BPS (Behavioral Pain Scaled)
		CPOT (Critical Care Pain Observation Tool)

*Tools used in the neonatal population are not listed.

by other factors. Thus, getting to know what the patient expects and values is an important but often overlooked step in the process of establishing meaningful and realistic therapeutic goals.

Analgesic therapy targets the physiologic pain mechanisms of the body. It is optimal when it balances concerns for safety and efficacy. This starts by selecting analgesia based on the individual's risk factors as well as the type and severity of pain. When using monotherapy, generally nonopioids (e.g., ibuprofen or acetaminophen) are appropriate for mild to moderate pain and opioids (e.g., morphine or oxycodone) are considered better for moderate to severe pain. For certain types of neuropathic pain, adjuvant drugs such as anticonvulsants (gabapentin) or antidepressants (nortriptyline) may be most effective.

Among the nonopioids, nonsteroidal antiinflammatory drugs (NSAIDs) like ibuprofen are considered better for many types of pain than acetaminophen, which lacks antiinflammatory activity. However, this lack of activity affords acetaminophen the distinction of being the safest and best tolerated analgesic drug if the maximum daily dose is adhered to.

In 1986, the World Health Organization recommended a stepped approach: starting with nonopioids before moving to opioids, then continuing to titrate doses up, with or without nonopioids and/or adjuvants until relief was achieved. We now know that high doses of opioids over long periods of time can produce a paradoxical increase in pain known as opioid-induced hyperalgesia. Therefore, whenever opioids are used now, the addition of a nonopioid, an adjuvant drug, and/or nondrug methods are recommended to keep the dose and duration of opioid therapy as low as possible (8).

Using anti-inflammatory pain relievers to reduce tissue inflammation as well as centrally acting drugs (e.g., opioids, anticonvulsants) to dampen pain levels is one

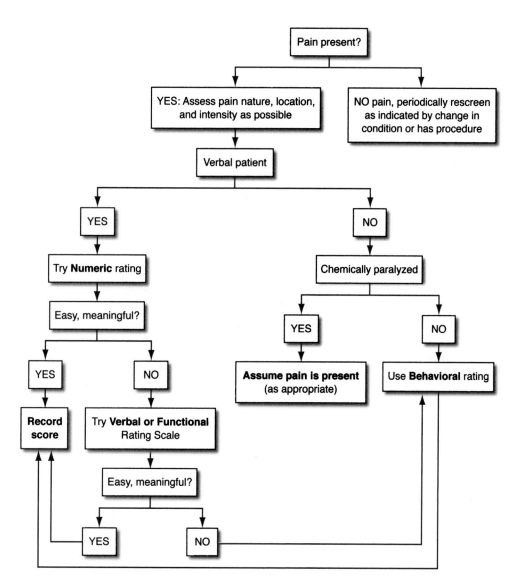

FIGURE 3–3: Selecting pain assessment tools based on patient ability and preferences.

example of multimodal therapy. This is consistent with the "Gain Control" concept of targeting multiple receptors (6). Pain signals are dampened when:

- NSAIDs reduce the inflammation that irritate and sensitize (lowers firing thresholds) peripheral nerves
- Local anesthetics raise the pain threshold by blocking sodium ion channels
- Opioids inhibit the transmission of pain primarily by blocking the release of presynaptic calcium and escape of post synaptic potassium
- Anticonvulsants quiet overactive ion channels that transduce or modulate pain
- Antidepressants increase spinal serotonin and norepinephrine modulators of pain

Combined, the transduction, transmission, modulation, and ultimately perception of pain can be reduced by using the additive and/or synergistic effects of these medications. Although the stability of neuronal activity is affected by these medications, there are many other factors that contribute to the perception of pain.

Although focusing on the body is an essential part of developing a treatment plan, inportant psychosocial or spiritual factors (e.g., attention, mood, motivation, personality, culture, and meaning) that may be amplifying pain are frequently not assessed. These factors (Figures 3-2 and 3-3) involving the mind, spirit, and social interactions should be included in the assessment and treatment plan. With these insights, nursing interventions such as fostering optimism, reducing anxiety, restoring faith, and promoting effective coping can be tailored to the individual to lower pain and distress.

Nondrug adjuvants can also be incorporated into the treatment plan to dampen the pain and help the patient think, feel, and do better. Thus, facilitating access to ice packs, mental distraction, therapeutic touch, and pet therapy can help minimize pain by turning down the "gain" at physical, mental, spiritual, and social levels, respectively. Not all patients will need all of these targets addressed; however, through a comprehensive assessment and conversations that help the clinician know the patient, a variety of these methods can be incorporated into the treatment plan. Using this perspective, the CNS

can help the treatment team, patient, and family use multimodal approaches to best control the pain, improving functioning and enhancing quality of life.

The CNS can discuss with the treatment team a variety of options, some of which are listed in Table 3-3, that tailor interventions to treat multiple simultaneous targets. Nurses may know and wish to use many of the simple nondrug pain relief methods listed there but are prevented from doing so due to the culture or policies of the organization. The CNS is ideally situated to work at the institutional level to help nurses learn and be able to use these simple nondrug pain-relieving techniques. The CNS is also in a position to identify resources and

TABLE 3–3 Spectrum of Pain Control Options Adopted

Self-initiated or "Low-tech" Approaches	Common Medications	Professional-initiated or "High-tech" Approaches
IMMEDIATE AREA OF PAIN		
Massage, rubbing		Physical therapy (modalities)
Moist heat	NSAIDs	Electric stimulation (TENS)
Application ice	Cause-directed	Specialize massage techniques
Positioning	Capsaicin or menthol cream	Trigger point Injections
Braces, orthotics, compression		Laser therapy
Treat cause/source of pain		Surgery
REGION OF PAIN OR SPINE		
Reduce dermatonal stimuli		Nerve blocks (sensory, autonomic)
Contralateral stimulation	Opioids,	Cryotherapy, radiofrequency
Proximal/distal stimulation	anticonvulsants	Prolotherapy (sugar injected in tendons)
	Antidepressants	Peripheral nerve stimulation
	Other co-analgesics	Spinal cord stimulation
	(e.g. Muscle relaxants, alpha	Epidural/spinal analgesia
	blockers, etc.)	Physical manipulation, traction
WHOLE BODY		
Diet, nutritional supplements		Acupuncture, acupressure
Exercise, pacing activities		Work hardening
Herbal or aroma therapy		Functional restoration
Breathing techniques		Multidisciplinary rehabilitation
BRAIN OR MIND-BODY FOCUSED		
Relaxation, imagery, hypnosis		Biofeedback training
Knowledge about condition	Opioids	Counseling
Music, distraction	Anticonvulsants	Electroconvulsive therapy
Journal writing	Antidepressants	Deep-brain stimulation
Change thinking, attitudes	Other co-analgesics	Cognitive-behavioral therapy
Reduce fear, anxiety, stress		
Reduce sadness, helplessness		

TABLE 3–3 Spectrum of Pain Control Options Adopted—cont'd

Self-initiated or "Low-tech" Approaches	Common Medications	Professional-initiated or "High-tech" Approaches
SPIRITUAL OR ENERGY-FOCUSED		
Prayer, meditation		Spiritual healing
Self-reflection, re: life/pain		Magnetic therapy
Meaningful rituals		Homeopathic remedies
Energy work (e.g., Therapeutic Touch, Reiki, Chi, quigong)		
SOCIAL INTERACTION–FOCUSED		
Improved communication		Family therapy
Volunteering		Functional restoration
Problem solving		Vocational training
Support groups		Psychosocial counseling
Pet therapy		

Adapted from Arnstein P. Clinical Coach for Effective Pain Management. Philadelphia: FA Davis; 2010.

facilitate access to the specialized therapies listed based on patient need and preferences.

Furthermore, the CNS is in a position to identify groups of patients who are at high risk for having their pain undertreated or untreated. These populations may be identified by age, gender, diagnosis, or lifestyle choices. Rather than providing detailed population-specific activities of the CNS, the following three case studies (using pseudonyms) are given to illustrate the role of the CNS in improving pain management through direct and indirect patient care; acting as role models for nurses and nursing practice; and having an impact on positive changes at different levels of the organization.

Case Report 1 ("Mrs. Massey")

As Dana began her 12-hour shift, she heard a scream from Mrs. Massey's room. Upon entering the patient's room, Dana found the nurse from the previous shift adjusting the pillows and wrist restraints. Mrs. Massey, a 72-year-old hemiplegic, aphasic woman with multiple comorbidities was recovering from a gastrectomy for stomach cancer. When Dana asked about her pain regimen, she learned that her colleagues were attributing her screaming and combativeness to her dementia based on reports from the nursing home where she resided. This behavior was deemed typical for Mrs. Massey according to the nursing home, but her family members were convinced it was from pain. The nurse reported that Mrs. Massey settled down when she is left alone for 30 minutes but needed the wrist restraints to prevent her from pulling out her PEJ tube and from punching the nurses trying to care for her.

Dana discussed these concerns with the CNS on rounds, wondering if the screaming and aggressive behavior represented pain or were really just a result of her dementia. Although the family wanted her medicated, Dana worried that the pain medications would worsen Mrs. Massey's dementia and/or gastrointestinal problems. The CNS stepped into the room to evaluate Mrs. Massey. When she was not screaming, she had periods of rapid, shallow breathing and was grabbing her siderails tightly. When she was moved she started screaming, wincing with tightened lips, and constantly shifted her position. The CNS reviewed with Dana the two pain scales that could be used to assess Mrs. Massey's level of discomfort. Using the Checklist of Nonverbal Pain Indicators (9), the bracing (grasping siderails) counted as the only indicator of pain at rest, with considerably more pain behaviors triggered by movement.

The PAINAD scale (10) was developed for patients with dementia and was considered a more sensitive way to assess pain for Mrs. Massey because it includes assessment of hyperventilation, consolability, and aggressive behavior (Table 3-4) not measured by the other tool. The CNS educated the nurses about her rationale for choosing the PAINAD scale and on how to use it appropriately. Ms. Massey's pain rating on both scales was greater than the midpoint, supporting the appropriateness of an analgesic trial.

The CNS discussed with Mrs. Massey's nurse, Dana, the analgesic options in light of available orders. They discussed risk factors such as age, frailty, cancer, postoperative status, and gastrointestinal problems. The latter ruled out the use of ibuprofen as first-line therapy. The CNS also raised the possibility that allowing Mrs. Massey to endure high levels of pain

TABLE 3–4 Elements of Commonly Used Adult Pain Assessment Tools

Pain Assessment Tool	Self Report	Ability to Function	Facial Expression (e.g., frown, tight lips, brows lowered, grimace)	Body Position or Movements (e.g., rubbing, bracing, writhing, fetal position, rocking)	Sounds (e.g., cry, sigh, moan, scream, say ouch, swearing, calling out)	Muscle Tension	Ability to Console	Breathing Patterns (short, shallow breathing, breath-holding, ventilator asynchrony)	Surrogate Reporting (by those who know patient best)	Atypical Behaviors (e.g., pacing, pulling or pushing away, fidgeting, striking out)
Numeric (0-10) Pain Scale	●									
Verbal Descriptor Scale	●									
Faces Pain Scale-revised	●									
Functional Pain Scale	●	●								
Checklist of nonverbal pain indicators (CNPI)			●	●	●	●				
Faces Legs Activity Cry and Consolability revised r-FLACC			●	●	●	●	●			
Pain Assessment in Advanced Dementia (PAINAD)			●	●	●	●	●		●	●
Critical Care Pain Observation Tool (CPOT)			●	●	●	●		●		

could worsen her hypertension and diabetes and put her at risk for postoperative complications such as atelectasis and pneumonia (11). Using existing orders, the decision was made to start with a low dose of hydromorphone (Dilaudid) rather than the acetaminophen, which might mask a fever. Given a range order of hydromorphone 0.5 to 1.5 mg IV every 3 hours prn, the CNS and Dana decided to try 0.5 mg Dilaudid slow IV push, then reevaluate her in 30 minutes.

During the reevaluation, 30 minutes after the administraion of hydromorphone, Mrs. Massey was visibly less agitated and her PAINAD score was reduced from her preadministration (8/10) score to 4/10. Her respirations remained at baseline, and she was no longer screaming with simple movements. She moaned when her arm was moved to evaluate her level of muscle tension. She tensed up and frowned with routine care but could easily be distracted by soft touch and a calming voice. With success of the intervention, the CNS and Dana discussed the merits of giving the hydromorphone routinely every 3 hours for five doses to achieve a pharmacologic steady state and more consistent pain control (12,13). Dana felt more comfortable trying the acetaminophen (Tylenol) 650 mg rectal suppository every 6 hours routinely and using the hydromorphone 30 minutes before procedures anticipated to be painful. They agreed to testing using scheduled acetaminophen first and if that failed, then scheduled doses of hydromorphone would be tried.

The plan was discussed with the family, who agreed with its appropriateness. They were also asked about nondrug options that may help reduce her pain. They noticed that back rubs and using the music channel had a calming effect. The family agreed to bring in music from her native culture that was soothing to her. Family members who were frequently present also agreed to bring in rosary beads and pray with her, which in the past had a calming effect. Dana agreed to detail the plan, including the use of the PAINAD, in order to promote continuity of care from shift to shift and so the CNS could evaluate the established plan the following day.

The next day, the CNS spoke with both the night and day nurses caring for Mrs. Massey. Although she was combative during the insertion of a rectal suppository, the acetaminophen helped bring the pain at rest down to a 2/10 on the PAINAD scale. The preprocedure hydromorphone reduced some of the screaming and fighting during procedures (PAINAD 6/10), allowing her to return to baseline in 15 minutes. The CNS advised a couple of minor adjustments in the plan of care: first, she recommended administering the hydromorphone 15 minutes rather than 30 minutes before the painful procedures; and second, she advised securing an order to change the route of acetaminophen administration from rectal to her jejunostomy tube.

In anticipation of discharge, the CNS took the opportunity to contact the skilled nursing facility (SNF) where Mrs. Massey resided in order to better understand her baseline behaviors and describe the current plan that effectively managed her pain behaviors. The staff at the nursing home were not familiar with the use of the PAINAD scale. A discussion with the director of education revealed that their facility used the FLACC scale (14,15) to assess pain in nonverbal patients. The director of education at the SNF was resistant to changing the assessment scale used and suggested that patients with dementia did not really feel pain. Besides, she claimed, "Dilaudid just makes these patients delirious." The CNS challenged that belief, pointing out the research that suggests older adults without opioids for postoperative pain have 10 times more delirium that those treated with opioids (16).

The CNS knew that this population was particularly vulnerable, as up to 80% of nursing home residents have pain that is often improperly assessed and either untreated or undertreated (17). However, the CNS pointed out that unrelieved pain has a significant impact on the residents' quality of life and described how Mrs. Massey was calmer and more cooperative with therapeutic and rehabilitative activities when her pain was better managed. Furthermore, she described how Mrs. Massey exhibited all six of the behaviors identified by the American Geriatrics Society as indicators of pain (18). The director evaded the assessment issue and refocused on the difficulty in stocking controlled substances and stated that the facility did not have the resources for around the clock administration of hydromorphone. Anticipating discharge at the end of the week, the CNS arranged for a conference call in 2 days between the director of education and the intake case manager from the nursing home, as well as herself, the primary nurse caring for Mrs. Massey, and the case manager from the acute care setting.

During that time, the CNS considered the limited resources of the SNF and facilitated a switch from hydromorphone and acetaminophen to a transdermal buprenorphine (Butrans) system that has a good safety and efficacy profile in older adults with multisystem disease. This would require only once a week dosing of the scheduled drug (19), with additional acetaminophen available, which was infrequently needed in the hospital. On this regimen, Mrs. Massey demonstrated continued improvement in her sleep, functioning, and cooperation with therapy.

Reflecting on this case, the CNS acted as an expert clinician, patient advocate, as well as a mentor, educator, and consultant to the professionals she worked with. In addition to providing direct care, she influenced the treatment plan and promoted continuity of care both within her setting and in preparation for transfer to the next level of care. One of the greatest challenges she encountered was helping nurses both at her setting and in the nursing home to select the best pain assessment tool for this complex patient. Moreover, the reliable reassessment of pain using the same tool consistently provided the basis for safe, effective adjustment of treatment that could be adapted to the environment of care and available resources. In addition, the CNS addressed staff misconceptions and beliefs about the experience of pain in patients with dementia, a significant barrier to effective pain management in this population.

Case Report 2 ("Karla Gulur")

Ms. Gulur was a 63-year-old patient with a history of metastatic breast cancer to the pelvic bone. She was admitted to the hospital for uncontrolled pain from mucositis to the point where she was not eating, drinking, or able to take oral medications. On admission she reported 9/10 pain in her throat and mouth. Before admission her sacral pain had been well controlled with a combination of short-acting and long-acting oxycodone totaling on average 110 mg oxycodone/day. However, her last dose of sustained release oxycodone was 18 hours ago. Ms. Gulur was given 2 mg of IV push morphine in the emergency department with minimal effect. Her labwork indicated that she was neutropenic, thrombocytopenic, and dehydrated.

Admission orders included IV and oral antifungal agents for oral candidiasis, "magic mouthwash" swish and swallow q2h prn, and standard patient-controlled analgesia (PCA) orders. During the evening the patient continued to report uncontrolled pain. She was teary, had not slept in five nights, and dozed off frequently. The resident questioned her report of pain because she was not using the PCA doses frequently and was able to doze off despite the pain.

Nursing advocated strongly for the patient and contacted the oncologist for guidance related to pain management, pointing out that her sleepiness was likely due to her lack of sleep. When she was awake, she remained awake and did not drift off mid-sentence as is the pattern with opioid-induced sedation. Her respiratory rate was the same as before the PCA was started, supporting the safety of increasing her doses of opioids. The CNS also pointed out that her home regimen of oxycodone was equipotent to 1.8 mg morphine/hr. A basal rate of 2 mg/hr was started and the PCA dose was increased to 1 mg q6min with a 1 hr lockout of 5 mg of IV morphine. A clinician-activated bolus of 4 mg (5%-15% of daily dose) every 2 hours was also available if needed (20).

In the morning, the treatment team met to discuss the uncontrolled pain. The CNS noted that Ms. Gulur had used 124 mg IV morphine the prior day without relief or respiratory depression. Her pain remained severe, she was visibly uncomfortable, and it interfered with eating, drinking, sleeping, and talking. Her sacral pain was a moderately intense (4/10) gnawing, aching feeling that limited her ability to transfer to a chair and sit for longer than 30 minutes. She wanted to be able to sit while visitors came, but the pain cut those visits short. According to guidelines issued by the National Cancer Coalition Network and the American Pain Society (21-23), it would be safe to increase the basal rate to 5 mg/hr (120 mg/day) and increase the bolus by 50% to 100% given the current pain crisis.

Other adjuvant medications such as NSAIDs were not recommended because of the risk of exacerbating thrombocytopenia and renal dysfunction and the potential to increase GI irritation if the mucositis extended the length of the GI tract. The team established that a pain goal of 3-4/10 would allow the patient to tolerate liquids, pureed foods, and sitting for at least 1 hour. Psychosocial interventions addressed Ms. Gulur's

expressed fears that mucositis meant her disease was progressing. The CNS offered to provide Therapeutic Touch and arranged for a social work consult, a visit from clergy, and a dietary consult to address weight loss. Ms. Gulur was discharged 7 days after admission on a soft diet and an oral analgesic regimen with her pain well controlled.

Several key factors were present in this case. As the expert consultant, the CNS intervened to address the clinicians' lack of knowledge related to equianalgesia and how to safely titrate opioids for effect. Pharmacotherapy included opioids, cause-directed antifungal agents; and adjuvants like topical local anesthetics combined with soothing Maalox-diphenhydramine that comprised the "magic mouthwash." She guided the interdisciplinary treatment team to consider psychosocial, spiritual, and social aspects of Ms. Gulur's comfort needs. Given the difficulties in managing an acute pain crisis in an opioid-tolerant patient; the CNS turned to evidence-based guidelines for options most likely to help Gulur meet her comfort and function goals.

Case Report 3 ("Bill Cutler")

A nurse-nurse consult was received to evaluate Bill Cutler, a 25-year-old man who is admitted for cellulitis, believed secondary to drug abuse. The nurse was concerned about the abnormal presentation of pain and his increasingly angry demands for medication. The cellulitis involved the left foot; but his primary reports of pain involved his right neck, shoulder, and arm. His angry demands for more medication were based on his experience that hydrocodone (Vicodin) as ordered was not enough to manage his pain. The question posed to the CNS was, is his pain real or is he drug-seeking?

The assessment revealed a moderate (4/10) intensity "tense, throbbing" pain at the site of his left foot cellulitis. The more bothersome pain in his neck and right upper extremity was attributed to a motor vehicle accident 9 years earlier and was an intense (8/10), deep ache and annoying tingling. Occasionally if he stood too long or moved his right arm in a certain way, sudden stabbing pain would shoot down that arm. He was increasingly concerned about aching all over, abdominal pain, and nausea that developed since his admission.

The CNS conducted a complete assessment. The focused neurologic examination revealed hyperalgesia involving his right arm with allodynia in a 10 × 6 cm area extending from the right side of his neck to his right scapula. Motor weakness with muscle atrophy was noted in his right (dominant) upper extremity. His pupils were dilated and he had severe cramping and involuntary leg movements and elevated vital sign readings and developed vomiting. These signs fit the clinical picture of active opioid withdrawal complicated by verified acute and chronic conditions known to be painful. For the past month he had been using a "stamp bag" of heroin to control his pain and prevent withdrawal. In the past, trials of ibuprofen, hydrocodone, Tramadol, anticonvulsants, antidepressants, epidural steroid injections, and lidocaine patches failed. He developed a craving for the hydrocodone, used it compulsively when available, and continued to use them despite knowing they were bad for him.

The CNS explained to the treatment team the different types of pain that Bill was experiencing, A pain treatment regimen of intermittent Vicodin was insufficient to address the different types of pain Bill was experiencing and his opioid withdrawal. The inflammatory pain related to cellulitis is more appropriately treated with an analgesic that has antiinflammatory properties, like ibuprofen. The neuropathic pain manifests as a constant aching with evoked "shooting" characteristics that typically responds to one or more adjuvant (e.g., anticonvulsant, antidepressant, local anesthetic, etc.) drug.

For the suspected withdrawal-mediated pain, stronger opioids were likely going to be needed. Although his drug misuse likely had some elements of pseudo-addiction (drug-seeking behaviors motivated by desperation for pain control), some features of a true addiction disorder were also present. Therefore, it was clear the treatment team needed to be expanded to include a professional with expertise in substance abuse. The prescriber was not familiar with a substance abuse specialist on staff at the hospital but agreed to contact the community-based professional that the CNS recommended.

Working with the expanded treatment team, the CNS recommendations to use a stronger opioid and add ibuprofen and adjuvant medications were agreed upon. The substance abuse specialist determined that 50 mg IV morphine per day was needed daily to prevent withdrawal symptoms. She warned that if opioid replacement therapy was not begun within 12 hours, his withdrawal symptoms would escalate to the point where they would threaten his recovery from the cellulitis. She also advised that transdermal clonidine could help the opioid withdrawal symptoms and perhaps also his neuropathic pain.

Working with the treatment team, the CNS convinced the prescriber to start a 2 mg/hr morphine drip, with ibuprofen, gabapentin, and a lidocaine 5% dermal patch for the sensitive right shoulder area. Meanwhile, the CNS and explored with Bill from a variety of other pain relief and coping skills what additional nondrug methods could be used. Physical therapists taught him exercise and pacing techniques; the CNS taught him imagery techniques; the nurses caring for him used gentle massage and therapeutic communication. Bill's mother was very concerned and remained close to him through his 9-year ordeal, but other family members were estranged. His mother was coached to provide distraction and caring presence, while avoiding either punishing or overprotective responses.

Within a couple of days Bill stabilized. His pain was manageable and he could participate with therapy. He verbalized willingness to follow-up with substance abuse and psychological counseling after discharge. The prescriber agreed to an oral methadone regimen but would only provide a 2-week supply with refills contingent on several factors. First, Bill's mother would need to be in control of securing the supply, locking and administering the medications every 8 hours. Second, Bill must adhere to a treatment agreement that includes periodic urine drug testing and making and keeping appointments with the community-based prescriber and

substance abuse counselor. Third, Bill was required to keep a daily record of his pain, medications taken, and the self-initiated nondrug techniques he used to control his pain and improve his functioning while he mastered coping skills. The health care team, Bill, and his mother agreed to this treatment plan.

The next challenge was to convert Bill off the morphine drip to oral methadone without sacrificing the treatment gains made. The CNS helped the prescriber determine a proper starting dose using an equianalgesic conversion equation (Box 3-1). The transition to methadone is known to be problem-prone, because of accumulating drug that influences its safety and efficacy during the first week or two of therapy. To facilitate the transition, the morphine drip was lowered to 1 mg/hr for 12 hours after the oral methadone (2.5 mg q8h) was started. Bill responded well to this regimen and expressed to the nurse discharging him that he would like help coping with the anger he still feels towards the drunk driver who caused his neck injury. He also expressed an interest in reconnecting with the people and places that were important to him before his life took a downward spiral.

The case of Bill Cutler raised awareness of gaps in the treatment team's training and the systems barriers that made it hard to effectively care for him. Subsequent activities included the development of educational programs for health professionals to help them differentiate clinical phenomenon of physical dependence, tolerance, addiction, and pseudo-addiction, without labeling the patient as drug-seeking. Inservice and continuing education programs integrated elements of this case to inform professionals about neuropathic pain, opioid withdrawal, methadone prescribing, and safeguards that should be in place when prescriptions for opioids are provided to patients on discharge.

The fact that this acute care setting had no substance abuse specialist on staff (or with clinical privileges) seemed like an important void in light of the growing prevalence of substance abuse problems in the community. The case also raised awareness of the complexities associated with starting patients on oral methadone as an analgesic agent. The CNS subsequently led a team of physicians, nurses, and pharmacists to develop and gain approval of both a policy and a clinical guideline for the initiation of methadone therapy.

The case also reinforced a growing awareness that nurses and other professionals needed training and clarity regarding which nondrug interventions like Therapeutic Touch, relaxation techniques, and positioning could be done without a medical order; what could be done if a protocol were developed; and what therapies like craniosacral massage or acupuncture were available in the community when opioid-sparing treatments are needed.

Pain is a pervasive clinical phenomenon that benefits from the clinical knowledge and systems savvy of the CNS. Their impacts on patients and families, nursing and nursing practice, and the system of care comprise their major spheres of influence (24). In all three of the case reports presented, the CNS touched on all three of these areas to varying degrees and demonstrated many of the CNS core competencies.

BOX 3–1 Equianalgesic Conversion—Example: Switching Mr. Cutler to Methadone

---

Step 1 Determine daily oral morphine requirement:

24 mg IV morphine

A) Can use the ratio technique

1:3 ratio 24 mg IV = <u>72 mg oral morphine</u>

-OR-

B) Can use equation method

<u>Equianalgesic table dose of current drug</u>   <u>Daily dose needed of current drug</u>
Equianalgesic table dose of desired drug   Equipotent daily dose of new drug

$$\frac{10 \text{ mg}}{30 \text{ mg}} = \frac{24 \text{ mg}}{N \text{ mg}}$$

$$10 \, N = 30 \times 24 \ldots N = 30/10 \times 24 \ldots N = 3 \times 24 \ldots \underline{N = 72 \text{ mg oral morphine}}$$

72 mg oral morphine need to approximate the effect of 24 mg IV morphine

Step 2 Consider the methadone requirement based on the amount of daily oral morphine needed:

Calculated 24 hour oral morphine requirement (mg/day)	Equianalgesic ratio oral morphine to oral methadone
<90	4:1
90-300	8:1
>300	12:1

Given <90 mg oral morphine a 4:1 ratio is used

72 mg oral morphine = 18 mg methadone

Step 3 Consider a 25% to 50% dose reduction (to 9 mg to 13.5 mg/day) for limited cross tolerance.

Step 4 Consider how medication is supplied to determine a daily regimen.

Step 5 Consider making short-acting analgesics available for breakthrough pain.

In this case acetaminophen was used. Often medication for breakthrough pain is 10% of daily amount made available at intervals tailored to the needs of the individual and the drug used.

Step 6 Plan for monitoring patient and refining the plan. Based on long and variable half-life of methadone, dose adjustments would be considered on a weekly basis.

---

1. Adopted from American Pain Society. Principles of Analgesic Use in the Treatment of Acute Pain and Cancer Pain. 6th edition. Glenview, IL: APS Press; 2008.

CLINICAL NURSE SPECIALIST COMPETENCIES AND SPHERES OF INFLUENCE

Clinical Expert/Direct Care

In all of the cases described, the CNS was consulted to help in the assessment and development of a plan of care for complex pain patients who were at high risk for under treatment of their pain. The CNS was instrumental in identifying a valid and reliable pain assessment tool that met the individual's needs. The assessments also included the assessment of preexisting and co-existing pain, the preadmission medications, efficacy of pharmacologic and nonpharmacologic interventions for both the chronic and acute pain, a psychosocial/spiritual assessment, and the setting of a goal for pain management that was acceptable to the patient. The value of a comprehensive pain assessment was stressed as a key factor in the successful management and prevention of complications related to unrelieved pain.

Coaching/Teaching/Mentoring

The CNS also acted as a role model and mentor for nursing in the care provided for these complex pain patients. By acting as facilitator for interdisciplinary collaboration, each plan of care was optimized. The CNS was able to address barriers and misconceptions that could have resulted in suboptimal care for the patients by incorporating national guidelines for pharmacologic interventions, including appropriate titration, route, and dose of analgesics. Evidence-based nursing interventions such as oral rinses for mucositis and complementary interventions such as music therapy were also recommended by the CNS and implemented as part of the care plan. In addition, consults to other disciplines were obtained to round out the plan of care. The CNS was also responsible for ensuring that the plan of care was reevaluated and side effects of treatment were managed and for guiding any adjustments in the plan of care that were needed. In each case, the CNS also had the opportunity to mentor staff in identifying the most salient aspects of the pain assessment and demonstrating how to present data in a clear, concise, while effective manner when advocating for patients. This included the need to access resources to help the nurse evaluate the appropriateness of the changes in the plan of care.

Systems Leadership

Last, within the organizational and systems sphere of influence, the CNSs in all three cases educated other health care professionals by bringing evidence-based information on pain management to the interdisciplinary team. In addition, all the cases were then incorporated into organizational continuing education programs. Therefore, the CNSs were able to not only work at the micro level but also address the need of the greater system to better manage pain in complex patients.

CNSs MAKE THE DIFFERENCE

Pain in acute care settings continues to be increasingly pervasive and costly. The importance of effective pain management is greater than ever since pain intensity in acute care is the best predictor of patients developing chronic pain a year after their trauma or surgery. There is much progress in prevention, diagnosis, and treatment of acute pain, however, and the CNS is in an ideal position to help tailor assessment and therapies to meet individual's needs. The CNS has the ability to work directly with patients and clinical staff and the organization to help remove the barriers that prevent effective pain management in complex patients.

References

1. IOM (Institute of Medicine) 2011. *Relieving Pain in America: A Blueprint for Transforming Prevention, Care, Education and Research,* Washington, DC; The National Academies Press.

2. Rathmell JP, Wu CL, Sinatra RS, et al. Acute post-surgical pain management: a critical appraisal of current practice. Reg Anesth Pain Med 2006;31:1-42.

3. Rivara FP, Mackenzie EJ, Jurkovich GJ, et al. Prevalence of pain in patients 1 year after major trauma. Arch Surg 2008;143:282-287.

4. Arnstein PM. Theories of pain. In St. Marie B, editor. Core Curriculum for Pain Management Nurses. Philadelphia: WB Saunders; 1992:107-119.

5. Tracey I. Imaging pain. Br J Anesth 2008;101:32-35.

6. Arnstein P. Clinical Coach for Effective Pain Management. Philadelphia: FA Davis; 2010.

7. Arnstein PM. Lessons from Mrs. Tandy: learning to "live with" chronic pain. Top Adv Pract Nursing 2007;7(1). Retrieved August 29, 2010, from http://www.medscape.com/viewarticle/557719_4

8. Chou R, Fanciullo GJ, Fine PG, et al. Clinical guidelines for the use of chronic opioid therapy in chronic noncancer pain: American Pain Society & American Academy of Pain Medicine Opioids Guidelines Panel. J Pain 2009;10:113-146.

9. Feldt, K. The checklist of nonverbal pain indicators (CNPI). Pain Manage Nursing 2000;1:13-21.

10. Warden V, Hurley AC, Volicer L. Development and psychometric evaluation of the Pain Assessment in Advanced Dementia (PAINAD) Scale. J Am Med Dir Assoc 2003;4:9-15.

11. Desai PM. Pain management and pulmonary dysfunction. Crit Care Clin 1999;15:151-166.

12. Arnstein P. Balancing analgesic efficacy with safety concerns in the older patient. Pain Manage Nursing 2010;11(2 suppl):S11-S22.

13. Pasero C, McCaffery M. Pain Assessment and Pharmacologic Management. St Louis: Mosby; 2011.

14. Malviya S, Voepel-Lewis T, Burke C, et al. The revised FLACC observational pain tool: improved reliability and validity for pain assessment in children with cognitive impairment. Pediatr Anesth 2006;16:258-265.

15. Manworren RCB, Hynan LS. Practice applications of research: clinical validation of FLACC—preverbal patient pain scale. Pediatr Nursing 2003;29:140-146.

16. Morrison RS, Magaziner J, Gilbert M, et al. Relationship between pain and opioid analgesics on the development of delirium following hip fracture. J Gerontol Ser A Biol Sci Med Sci 2003;58:76-81.

17. Arnstein P, Herr K. Pain in the older person. In Fishman SM, Ballantyne JC, Rathmell JP, editors. Bonica's Management of Pain. 4th edition. Philadelphia: Lippincott Wiliiams & Wilkins; 2010:782-790.

18. American Geriatrics Society. AGS panel on persistent pain in older persons. Clinical practice guidelines: the management of persistent pain in older persons. J Am Geriatr Soc 2002;50 (6 suppl):S205-S224.

19. Pergolizzi J, Boger RH, Budd K, et al. Opioids and the management of chronic severe pain in the elderly: consensus statement of an international expert panel with focus on the six clinically most often used World Health Organization Step III opioids (buprenorphine, fentanyl, hydromorphone, methadone, morphine, oxycodone). Pain Pract 2008;8:287-313.

20. Fine PG, Portenoy RK. A Clinical Guide to Opioid Analgesia. New York: Vendome Group; 2007.

21. American Pain Society. Principles of Analgesic Use in the Treatment of Acute Pain and Cancer Pain. 6th edition. Glenview, IL: APS Press; 2008.

22. Miaskowski C, Cleary J, Burney R, et al. Guideline for the Management of Cancer Pain in Adults and Children, APS Clinical Practice Guideline Series, No. 3. Glenview, IL: American Pain Society; 2005.

23. National Comprehensive Cancer Network. Clinical Practice Guidelines: Adult Cancer Pain. 2010. Retrieved August 29, 2010, from http://www.nccn.org/professionals/physician_gls/PDF/pain.pdf

24. Duffy M, Dresser S, Fulton JS, editors.. Clinical Nurse Specialist Toolkit: A Guide for the New Clinical Nurse Specialist. New York: Springer; 2009.

4

Health Problems Associated with Aging

Paul Netzel, MSN, RN, ACNP

INTRODUCTION

Clinical nurse specialists (CNSs) use a broad skill base to deliver expert nursing care across the adult continuum. CNSs must be cognizant of current evidence-based practices, health care policies, and costs containment approaches, as well as the needs and demands that each patient group presents in the acute care setting. This is especially true with patients greater than 65 years of age. This chapter will provide a discussion of some unique age-related physiologic and psychological changes expected in this patient population, as well as the impact of hospital-associated functional decline and pharmacologic interventions.

NATIONAL STANDARDS AND COMPETENCIES FOR ADULT-GERONTOLOGY CLINICAL NURSE SPECIALISTS

In 2008, the APRN Consensus Workgroup and the National Council of State Boards of Nursing APRN Advisory Committee, published a *Consensus Model for APRN Regulation*, which addresses licensure, accreditation, certification, and education, frequently referred to as the *LACE Model* (1). One of the most important new standards included in this model is the expectation that all programs that educate, certify, and license adult registered advanced practice nurses (APRNs), including CNSs, must also include specific content related to the care of geriatric clients.

After the LACE model was published and endorsed by 45 national nursing organizations, a second expert panel convened to develop *Adult-Gerontology Clinical Nurse Specialist Competencies*, published in 2010 (2). Both of these processes and the documents that were published as results confirm the importance of the role of the CNS in responding to the unique needs of geriatric clients. In most American acute care facilities, the elder cohort is the largest inpatient population. Yet these environments present considerable risks for this patient population. CNSs can make major contributions to safeguard and improve the quality of care for these patients.

DEMOGRAPHICS OF THE AGING POPULATION

The cost of health care in the United States is among the highest of all developed countries. Estimates of national health expenditures from the Centers for Medicare and Medicaid Services (CMS) for 2009 reached $2.5 trillion, or 17.6% of the nation's gross domestic product (3). Hospital care accounted for $759 billion, or 30% of total health care expenditures, and $502 billion were paid by Medicare during 2009. Total health care cost is expected to reach $4.6 trillion in 2019 according to CMS (September 2010 Projections), and Medicare payments are projected to increase nearly 76% above 2009 estimates to $891 billion (4).

The significance in these statistics is that a majority of Medicare costs reflect health care utilization from patients over the age of 65, while the remaining cost is used by other Medicare eligible patients, such as those with qualifying disabilities and end-stage renal failure. In 2009, there were approximately 37.8 million elderly U.S. citizens, or 12.5% of the total U.S. population; yet that group generated approximately 20% of health care costs in the same year (5). This population was estimated to be 40.2 million for 2010; it will 46.8 million by 2015 and will reach 54.8 million in 2020 (6). The growth rate will be significantly higher for this population beginning in 2011, as the Baby Boomer generation begins to pass age 65. This higher growth rate will continue through 2030, when the elderly will nearly double to 70 million, in comparison to the 2000 census (7).

Trends in hospitalization rates for the elderly population have continued to remain significantly higher than in all other groups. According to the National Hospital Discharge Survey for 2007, there were 34.3 million hospital discharges and elderly patients accounted for 37% of those, as well as 43% of all hospital days (8). The average length of stay for elderly patients was 5.6 days compared to an average of 4.5 days for the three remaining groups (8). These trends suggest that as the population of elderly patients begins to increase proportionate to the overall population over the next decade, acute care facilities will see a corresponding increase in hospital bed occupancy by elderly patients.

CNSs in the acute care setting must understand these trends and recognize the changing demographics of the acute care patient population to meet the needs of hospitalized patients, especially those who are elderly. In anticipation, this increase of hospital utilization will shift current patient case mixes to higher levels of acuity and potentially extend lengths of stay. At the very least, these changes will make transitions in levels of care and the discharge process more complex. This will increase the demand for more highly skilled and specialized staff to care for the elderly patients. These challenges can best be handled through utilization and integration of organized frameworks and CNS core competencies. A systematic approach to meeting the individualized health care needs of patients and families will facilitate optimal care.

AGE-RELATED PHYSIOLOGIC CHANGES

It is important to understand the physiologic differences between patient populations in the acute care setting. As the body ages, normal physiologic processes, functions, and structures gradually change. These changes are the result of many internal and external influences on the cells, tissues, organs, and systems. These influences may include physical or chemical stressors; genetic or cellular alterations and abnormalities; nutritional and environmental factors; and the severity of acute or chronic illnesses or injuries over time. Age-related physiologic changes affect individuals differently throughout their lives, and the severity of chronicity of illness, functional decline, or disability varies widely as people reach age 65 and beyond.

Using the framework for CNS core competencies and the spheres of influence, most CNSs in the acute care setting directly engage in the central competency: Direct Care (9). Most often, they are in the best position as experts to influence and direct appropriate care. Understanding these changes allows CNSs to facilitate, coordinate, and direct care for the elderly population in the acute care setting. This section will provide an overview of the major systems that are affected by age-related changes and a brief discussion of the integration of CNSs' core competencies to facilitate care in relation to these changes. A more detailed discussion of major systems is covered in later chapters.

Neurologic

The central nervous system is a complex system that is responsible for maintaining normal homeostasis throughout the body. This is accomplished through its primary functions of neuronal transmissions in the central and peripheral nervous systems that regulate neurologic functions of the brain, as well as vital organ systems essential for life. This complex system is not immune to age-related changes and plays a more significant role in the functional decline experienced by the elderly than most other biologic systems.

The structural changes within the brain that occur are global. The number and production of neuron cells decrease with the aging process, which results in a generalized loss of brain mass. This resulting atrophy of the brain and its reduced mass contributes to a shift in the normal occupied volume within the skull and potentiates change in other brain structures. Surface structures such as the gyri narrow and the sulci widen increasing the subarachnoid space. Atrophy of the brain also increases adherence between the dura mater and the skull, increasing the potential of stress on the bridging vessels (10). Changes are also noted in the cerebral vasculature in the basal ganglia and an increase in ventricle size to accommodate loss of neuronal mass (11). Decreases in neuron size and number does not necessary indicate loss of cognitive function. However, with the cellular changes that occur within the neurons, there is a loss of neurotransmission to the effector organs through the autonomic nervous system (10, 11). These changes disrupt the normal homeostasis within the body and contribute to the increased risks associated with the ability to recover from physiologic stressors (10).

Cerebrovascular disease leading to stroke is the third leading cause of death in the United States. There were 829,000 hospital discharges in 2007 with stroke as the first-listed diagnosis. Approximately 67% of theses discharges were elderly patients over the age of 65 with an average acute care length of stay of 5.4 days (8, 12). Although lifestyle behaviors and associated risk factors are major contributors to the development of cerebrovascular disease, age-related changes do occur within cerebrovascular systems. Studies have shown that cerebral blood flow diminishes with physiologic aging that can be associated with global or regional affects on the brain (13, 14). Another study suggests that while there is an overall decrease in cerebral blood flow that contributes to localized or regional atrophy, gray or white matter changes still occur independently from reduced cerebral blood flow (15). The significance of these findings is the relationship that exists between cerebrovascular impairment and the development of pathologic conditions such as strokes and vascular dementia.

The degree of functional impairment as result of age-related changes may differ among patients, but nonetheless, these patients experience common neurologic deterioration in several motor and sensory abilities that are exhibited in the acute care setting. These patients may experience deficits that affect reaction times in performing daily tasks. This can be cause for their concern as a matter of safety and a source of stress or frustration in completing simple normal activities. This change is often associated with an increasing loss of independence.

Another sensory impairment that is expected with physiologic aging is diminished proprioception and balance. Patients begin to lose sensory transmissions from the peripheral receptors to the cerebral cortex and cerebellum. These functional areas are responsible for balance and coordination and may increase the patient's risks for injuries as a result of disequilibrium and falling. Notably, patients with balance difficulties may have marked gait disturbances that are being affected by peripheral and central sensory and motor deficits that may be indicative of advanced physiologic aging or other pathologic conditions (10).

Elderly patients also often complain of dizziness. This complaint is sometimes difficult to assess due to variability among patients' abilities to describe what exactly they are experiencing. Dizziness may be associated with several physiologic conditions but it can be a normal age-related symptom that results from a decrease in sensory input peripherally (eyes, ears, hands, feet) or centrally. Dizziness can be categorized into four types: vertigo—rotational sensation generally related to vestibular conditions; presyncope—lightheadedness typically associated with orthostatic hypotension, hypoglycemia, arrhythmia, or hypoxia; disequilibrium—an unsteadiness with standing or walking originating from sensory loss, vestibular impairment, or motor or cerebellar lesions; and nonspecific dizziness—vague descriptions of dizziness unrelated to physiologic changes (10).

This brief description of the neurologic age-related changes lends itself to the role that the CNS may play in the care of elderly patients in the acute care setting. This role often focuses on the prevention of further neurologic impairment through the implementation of evidence-based practices. Stroke patients can benefit from the clinical expertise and efforts of CNSs in ensuring up-to-date

protocols for acute stroke management are initiated and followed facility wide. These are fundamental quality improvement core measures that have demonstrated significant improvements in patient outcomes.

Barrere, Delaney, Peterson, and Hickey (16) describe the steps needed to implement an effective Stroke Management Program to meet criteria established by The Joint Commission (TJC). This stroke program has received national recognition for the overall effectiveness. The theoretical framework of Structure, Process and Outcomes served as the basis for development of The Stroke Nurse Education Program of The Hospital of Central Connecticut (THOCC) (16). This was an interdisciplinary approach that included a stroke coordinator, oversight clinician team, nursing leadership, CNSs and staff nurses who evaluated the existing protocols, educational needs of staff, and available and required resources. The stroke coordinator and the oversight team with support of nursing leaders took advantage of the clinical expertise, creative education tools, and clinical mentorship to address the needs of each specialty area in preparing for them for the delivery competent, high-quality, and efficient stroke care. The effectiveness of this program was measured using three perspectives: (a) before, during, and after The Joint Commission Core Education Measures; (b) annual Defect-Free Care data; and (c) nurses' experience—caring for stroke patients (16). The outcomes measures demonstrated significant improvements in all three perspectives with the results of each measure supporting the others (Table 4–1).

This program underscores the importance of the collaborative approach necessary to improve the delivery of care and subsequent patient outcomes. The CNSs involved in the implementation of this program provided a foundation representative of Hamric's Model of Advanced Practice Nursing. A primary criterion of the model is that the CNS establishes the foundation for clinical practice changes. Table 4–2 identifies the CNS competencies that were used to implement this program, which engaged CNSs, staff, and clinicians to improve patient outcomes for this population (9).

Cardiovascular

Heart disease continues to be the number one leading cause of death in the United States. While there are many factors related to the development of heart disease, advanced age is widely recognized as one of the most important factors. In 2007, there were 616,067 deaths reported from cardiovascular diseases, accounting for 25.4% of all deaths that year. Elderly persons over the age of 65 years represented 89.3% of all deaths reported and 30% of them died from cardiovascular diseases (17).

It is often difficult to differentiate pathologic versus age-related changes within the cardiovascular system. However, what is known is the importance of reducing

TABLE 4-1 Quality Measures on the Effectiveness of the Stroke Nurse Education Program of the Hospital of Central Connecticut (THOCC)

Outcome Perspective	Quality Measure	Before	After
Before, During, and After		First Quarter 2008 (Jan-Mar)	Fourth Quarter 2009 (Oct-Dec)
	Stroke education	42%	86%
	NPO until dysphagia	47%	90%
	Smoking cessation	100%	100%
Defect-Free Care		2008	2009
	Percent of stroke patients who receive care without missing core measures	46%	79%
Nurses' Experiences		2008	2009
	Number of patients who received tPA in emergency department	2	12

Adapted from Barrere C, Delaney C, Peterson D, Hickey K, 0101215 Primary Stroke Center education for nurses: improving core measures Journal of Nursing Administration. 40:515-521, Dec 2010.

TABLE 4-2 CNS Competencies and Spheres of Influence Related to the Stroke Nurse Education Program of the Hospital of Central Connecticut (THOCC)

Competency	Behavioral Statement	Sphere of Influence	Practice Domain
A. Direct Care	A3—Employs evidence-based clinical practice guidelines to guide screening and diagnosis.	Patient, System	Clinical Judgment
A. Direct Care	A5—Identifies potential risk to patient safety, autonomy, and quality of care based on assessment across the patient, nurse, and system spheres of influence	Patient, Nurse, System	Clinical Judgment
A. Direct Care	A18—Provides leadership for collaborative, evidence-based revision of diagnosis and plans care, to improve patient outcomes	Patient, Nurse, System	Clinical Judgment
B. Consultation	B1—Provides consultation to staff nurses and interdisciplinary colleagues	Patient, Nurse, System	Clinical Judgment
B. Consultation	B5—Assists staff in the development of innovative, cost-effective programs or protocols of care	Patient, Nurse, System	Facilitation of Learning

Continued

TABLE 4-2 CNS Competencies and Spheres of Influence Related to the Stroke Nurse Education Program of the Hospital of Central Connecticut (THOCC)—cont'd

Competency	Behavioral Statement	Sphere of Influence	Practice Domain
C. Systems Leadership	C1—Facilitates the provision of clinically competent care by staff/team through education, role modeling, teambuilding, and quality monitoring	Nurse, System	Caring Practices
C. Systems Leadership	C4—Develops clinical standards, policies, and procedures	System	Collaboration
D. Collaboration	D1—Assesses the quality and effectiveness of interdisciplinary, interagency, and interagency communication and collaboration	Nurse, System	Clinical Inquiry & Collaboration
D. Collaboration	D2—Establishes collaborative relationships within and across departments that promote patient safety, culturally competent care, and clinical excellence	System	Collaboration
D. Collaboration	D3—Provides leadership for establishing, improving, and sustaining collaborative relationships to meet clinical needs	Nurse, System	Collaboration
E. Coaching	E4—Addresses the professional educational needs of nurses and other health care professionals	Nurse	Facilitation of Learning
E. Coaching	E4a—Completes a needs assessment as appropriate to guide interventions with staff	Nurse	Facilitation of Learning
E. Coaching	E4e—Mentors nurses to translate research into practice	Nurse	Facilitation of Learning
F. Research I—Interpretation, Translation and Use of Evidence	FI1—Critically analyzes research findings for the potential application to clinical practice	Patient, Nurse, System	Clinical Inquiry
F. Research II—Evaluation of Clinical Practice	FII4—Uses quality monitoring data to assess the quality and effectiveness of clinical programs in meeting outcomes	Patient, Nurse, System	Clinical Inquiry

some of the pathologic risk factors such as diet, smoking, lack of exercise, and stress in the development of atherosclerosis, hypertension, and diabetes. Modifying these risk factors can enhance cardiovascular responses to adapt to the age-related changes expected to occur even in the presence of chronic conditions. The development of vascular disease affects not only the heart but also other vital organs such as the brain, kidneys, and lungs, thereby increasing the risk for mortality the elder population.

Structural changes within the heart contribute to development of left ventricular hypertrophy. Fatty accumulation in the myocardial fibers increases muscular stiffness, which results in deceased cardiovascular compliance. Fibrotic changes and thickening increase the stiffness and decrease the compliance of the aortic and mitral valves. This allows blood to flow back into the ventricles, which may be noted as systolic ejection murmurs. Aortic calcification is a common finding and further reduces elasticity of the aorta. These changes in the valves and aorta increase the afterload of the left ventricle, further contributing to enlargement of the left ventricle. The peripheral arterial walls also develop decreased elasticity and increased wall stiffness. This produces increased peripheral arterial pressure that must be overcome by increased left ventricular pressure and systolic pressures. The resultant increase in left ventricular pressure contributes to the thickening of the musculature seen with left ventricular hypertrophy (18).

Structures that autoregulate cardiac functions such as heart rate and blood pressure undergo age-related changes as well. There is a gradual loss of myocardial cells that make up the sinoatrial node, which reduces the electrical pacing function of these specialized cells. This affects heart rate regulation and elderly persons often may develop increased rates and dysrhythmias. Baroreceptor activity is diminished, which reduces timely compensation and regulation of blood pressure. Alterations in neurohormonal influences on the heart are demonstrated by increased catecholamine levels with corresponding decreases in cardiac beta-adrenergic sensitivity (19).

Pulmonary

Age-related physiologic changes that affect the respiratory system typically involve chest wall muscular skeletal alterations, structural parenchyma, and alveolar surface changes. Chest wall compliance is diminished due to ossification of the costal cartilage and ribs producing stiffness and loss of elastic recoil. Osteoporosis plays a role in the disintegration of bony support of the ribs and vertebral spaces. This results in an increased anteroposterior diameter of the chest wall, which also contributes to the loss of elastic recoil. Changes in the muscular fibers of the diaphragm and intercostal muscles decrease muscular strength and endurance (20, 21).

A decline in the glandular epithelial cells reduces mucous production necessary to fight pulmonary infections. Elastin and collagen support of the airways diminish, allowing for an accelerated collapse during expiration. Although there is no reduction in the number of alveoli, there is a loss in elastic fibers around the alveoli and alveolar ducts, resulting in enlargement of these structures. Overall, the surface area for oxygen exchange is decreased. These parenchymal changes contribute to increased air trapping and diminished gas exchange (21, 22). The relationship between physiologic and functional age-related pulmonary changes is illustrated in Table 4–3.

Renal and Genitourinary

The kidney decreases in size and weight in both the cortical and renal areas, with an overall reduction in the number of nephrons and glomeruli. With this reduction in numbers, existing glomeruli increase in size in an attempt to compensate and maintain filtration homeostasis.

TABLE 4–3 Physiologic and Functional Changes of the Lungs

	Physiologic Change	Functional Change
MUSCULOSKELETAL		
	• Increased anteroposterior diameter • Decreased chest wall compliance • Decreased muscular strength • Ossification of ribs	• Decreased ventilatory capacity • Decreased vital capacity • Increased residual volume • Decreased ventilatory-perfusion ratio
LUNG TISSUE		
	• Decreased elasticity • Increased compliance	• Decreased ventilatory capacity • Decreased vital capacity • Increased residual volume

Continued

TABLE 4-3 Physiologic and Functional Changes of the Lungs—cont'd

	Physiologic Change	Functional Change
AIRWAYS		
	• Decreased glandular cells • Alteration in elasticity and collagen • Early collapse during expiration	• Decreased mucus production • Reduced immune response • Increased closing volume
ALVEOLI		
	• Breakdown of alveolar septa • Enlargement of alveoli and ducts • Decreased surface area	• Air trapping • Decreased gas exchange • Increased ventilatory-perfusion mismatch

Adapted from Brashers VL. Structure and function of the pulmonary system. In McCance KL, Huether SE, editors. Pathophysiology: The Biologic Basis for Disease in Adults and Children. 5th edition. St Louis, MO: Mosby; 2006: p1181-1204.

Renal blood flow is thought to contribute to these changes. As with other systemic vascular changes, renal arteries loss elasticity and become stiff, thus reducing blood flow to the renal structures and filtration processes within the nephrons. As glomerular structures diminish, alterations in vascular pathways between afferent and efferent vessels shunt blood away from damaged glomeruli to healthy glomeruli to maintain filtration. As a result of glomerular and vascular changes, there is a generalized decline in the ability to concentrate urine and decreased glomerular filtration rate and creatinine clearance in the elderly population (23-25). Some studies suggest that cellular changes as a result of genetic defects can contribute to the aging process and the decrease in glomeruli, thus negatively affecting the renin-angiotensin system (26).

Changes occur in the tubules in the form of mass loss and shortening. This has an impacts on the tubular functions of acid base balance and electrolyte control. Water and sodium regulation, as well as aldosterone production and renin secretion, are impaired. As a result, elderly patients are subject to hypervolemic or hypovolemic states; potassium regulation dysfunction; and a decrease in vitamin D activation and the absorption of calcium (23, 24).

Ureter and bladder dysfunction are common age-related changes in the elderly. Urinary reflux occurs as a result of changes in the vesioureteral junctions that allow urine to flow back into the renal pelvis. Smooth muscles surrounding the bladder weaken and are replaced by fibrous connective tissues. Neurologic deficits occur in response to bladder stretching. These changes effect the micturition cycle, the capacity of the bladder is diminished, and older patients frequently experience frequency, urgency, and nocturia. Difficulty starting a urine stream, a slow or weak stream, or intermittent dribbling or incontinence may also be due to loss of muscular strength around the bladder and urethra. Bladder obstruction may occur with urethral and prostate changes in both females and males (23, 24).

Gastrointestinal

Age-related changes within the gastrointestinal system begin in the mouth. Teeth and teeth surfaces lose dentine and enamel, which encourages tooth decay and cavity formation. Gradual regression of gingival tissue further exposes dentine surface and tooth root systems that weaken the soft tissue support structure of the tooth. This increases risk for cracking, loosening, and mobility, which contribute to the decay of root systems and abscess formation (27). These changes have an impact on the patient's ability to chew and eat, thus affecting their oral intake and general nutritional status. The oral mucosa thins and there is a reduction in the number of taste buds, contributing to less tasteful meals and a decrease in appetite. The salivary glands decrease saliva production, making the oral mucosa drier and leading to swallowing difficulties (27-29).

The esophagus undergoes mild decreases in motility and upper esophageal sphincter muscular contractions, which give rise to swallowing difficulties and esophageal reflux. The stomach experiences a decrease in gastric motility and acidity. This reduction in the number of parietal cells and other secretory cells is thought to be caused in part to infection with *Helicobacter pylori*. A consequence of the destruction of these glands and cells is a decrease in the production of intrinsic factor (28, 29).

Age-related changes within the intestinal tract have been limited in the small intestines. Absorption of nutrients in the small intestines may be diminished by the decreasing surface area due to broadening and shortening of the villa. However, the effects of aging on the large intestine are related to cellular changes that reduce the muscular contractility, slowing gastrointestinal transit time, and decreasing sphincter muscle tone in the anus and rectum (29). Woo et al. (30) reported that colorectal cancer development is associated with a greater number of genetic alterations of normal stem cells and is more common in older patients. These findings suggest that age-related cellular mutations contribute to chronologic aging associated with colorectal cancers.

Liver and pancreatic structural changes occur with aging. The liver decreases in size and weight due to a reduction in hepatocytes. Reduced hepatic blood flow diminishes the first-pass metabolism of many drugs, contributing to higher serum accumulation of many drugs. The pancreas structure changes due to fibrosis and fatty deposits, and the pancreatic duct becomes wider. Exocrine secretions, such as bicarbonate and digestive enzymes, tend to decrease with age (28, 29).

Integumentary

The effects of aging are clearly evident in the appearance and functionality of the skin. Some of the external signs of aging are a result of decreased elasticity and loss of subcutaneous connective tissue that may appear as skin wrinkling or sagging (31). In addition to these internal structural changes, skin appearance may also be affected by external factors such as sun exposure that contribute or accelerate normal physiologic changes of aging. Photoaging, primarily as a result of ultraviolet light exposure, is the most common cause of premature aging of the skin. This exposure degrades the dermal connective tissues, collagen, and other matrix proteins that impair the appearance and function of the skin (32-34).

The undermining of the epidermal and dermal structures seriously degrades the protective, sensory, and thermoregulatory functions of the skin. As the epidermis becomes thinner and the dermis thickens, there is a loss of melanocyte production, reducing the protection against ultraviolet radiation. Decreased blood flow, lymphatic drainage, atrophy of glands in the skin, and decreased dermal immune response contribute to skin tearing, dryness, cracking, and impaired wound healing (31). Age-related changes of the skin also may affect vitamin D production, thus increasing the patient's risk for osteomalacia (35). Whether through chronologic aging or external factors, the decreased functionality of the skin increases the patient's susceptibility to skin disorders, infection, and skin breakdown.

Competency Application

It is important for CNSs to recognize the potential risks that the aging process has on the integumentary system to minimize complications in the acute care setting. The prevention and early identification of skin breakdown and the development of pressure ulcers need to be top priorities for nursing staff. The CNS can play a vital role in this nursing priority and may demonstrate several core competencies that influence the patient, nurse, and system spheres, by identifying the potential risks associated with age-related skin changes.

By identifying this potential risk, the CNS can be involved in the assessment, either primarily or as a consultant, of elderly patients at risk for potential skin breakdown. This assessment should include a thorough physical examination, health history, and nutritional status assessment of the patient. These assessment findings can be individualized to develop a plan of care to prevent skin breakdown. Evaluation and assessment of nursing staff competencies are important to identify discrepancies in training that might contribute to the risk of skin breakdown for these patients. Staff unfamiliar with risk factors or conditions contributing to age-related changes may inadvertently overlook key signs or symptoms indicating early stages of skin breakdown. CNSs often take the lead in the application of evidence-based practices and protocols to decrease the potential for skin breakdown. As the proportion of elderly patients increases, this role takes on even greater importance. A systemwide approach can improve the outcomes of these patients through standardized prevention and treatment protocols that can be tailored to individual patient needs. This clinical problem provides ample opportunities for the CNS to demonstrate proficiency in direct care, consultation, systems leadership, coaching, and research competencies, as illustrated in Table 4–4.

Musculoskeletal

Bone structure and density decline with age. A generalized decease in bone density evolves from an increase of bone absorption and a loss of spongy bone, which affects women more than men beginning with menopause. The bones become brittle, losing stiffness and strength, increasing the potential for fractures with minimal stress. The gradual loss of height and postural changes in elders are by-products of this bone loss. Spongy bone loss in the vertebral bodies causes compression of the vertebra and shortening of the vertebral height. These compromised vertebral bodies are particularly at risk for compression fractures due to increased stress (36). Dietary and nutritional changes that occur in this process have an impact on the degree and rate of bone demineralization that occurs. Reduced intake or absorption of vitamin D, calcium, phosphorus, and other essential dietary or environmental elements, as well as hormonal changes of the parathyroid, decrease new bone formation and accelerate the rate of bone decline, both contributing to the development of osteoporosis (37).

Similar to the heart and other muscular organs, the skeletal muscles decrease in mass due to a decrease in the

TABLE 4-4 Application of CNS Core Competencies Related to Age-Related Integumentary Changes

Competency	Behavioral Statement	Sphere of Influence	Practice Domain
A. Direct Care	A3—Employs evidence-based clinical practice guidelines to guide screening and diagnosis	Patient, System	Clinical Judgment
A. Direct Care	A5—Identifies potential risk to patient safety, autonomy, and quality of care based on assessment across the patient, nurse, and system spheres of influence	Patient, Nurse, System	Clinical Judgment
B. Consultation	B1—Provides consultation to staff nurses, and interdisciplinary colleagues	Patient, Nurse, System	Clinical Judgment
C. Systems Leadership	C4—Develops clinical standards, policies, and procedures	System	Collaboration
E. Coaching	E4—Addresses the professional educational needs of nurses and other healthcare professionals	Nurse	Facilitation of Learning
F. Research I—Interpretation, Translation, and Use of Evidence	FI1—Critically analyzes research findings for the potential application to clinical practice	Patient, Nurse, System	Clinical Inquiry
F. Research II—Evaluation of Clinical Practice	FII4—Uses quality monitoring data to assess the quality and effectiveness of clinical programs in meeting outcomes	Patient, Nurse, System	Clinical Inquiry

number of muscle fibers, with the fast twitching (Type II) fibers undergoing more rapid decline than slow twitching (Type I) fibers. This results in bulk muscle mass loss known as muscle wasting. Unlike bone, muscles still maintain much of their regenerative capabilities throughout the latter part of the aging process, although there is a notable decline in remodeling. Declining muscle strength and endurance are directly related to the loss of bulk muscle mass and inactivity. Muscle motor functions and reflexes are diminished due to the loss of motor neurons and shortened muscle fibers. Cartilage and tendons become brittle and inflexible. Synovial fluid production and synovial membrane mass both decrease, resulting in joint pain, stiffness, deformity, and immobility (36, 37).

Endocrine

The role of aging on the endocrine glands is not very clear. There are conflicting data regarding the contributions of cellular changes from aging, stress and adaption,

diseases, genetic programming, and decreased uptake by target organs, as the causes of endocrine glandular dysfunction over time. Nevertheless, it is certain that neurohormonal regulation and function are altered through the aging process (38). These alterations can occur in the thyroid, parathyroid, adrenal glands, pituitary glands, and pancreas, as well as the reproductive organs, with hormonal dysfunctions.

The thyroid gland develops atrophy, fibrosis, and inflammatory changes that may be related to aging or from autoimmune causes. There is an overall decrease in thyroid-stimulating hormone (TSH), thyrotropin-releasing hormone (TRH), and T_4 secretion with a reduction in serum T_3 levels. The development of hypothyroidism is common in elderly patients. The regulation and maintenance of calcium is primarily controlled by the parathyroid gland. Aging increases serum parathyroid hormone concentrations, which is thought to be consistent with age-associated decreasing vitamin D levels, increased resorption of calcium from bone, and the development of osteoporosis (39). Pancreatic secretion of insulin is reduced due to cellular changes. Reduced insulin levels, increased insulin resistance, and altered uptake of glucose are contributors to the development of type 2 diabetes mellitus.

Other hormonal variations occur as a result of aging. A reduction in the size and mass of the adrenal cortex contributes to a decrease in the metabolic clearance of cortisol resulting in higher serum cortisol and decreased androgen production. There is some change in the secretion and feedback mechanisms of aldosterone and antidiuretic hormone (ADH) attributed to aging of the adrenal cortex; however, alterations in these hormones are thought to be primarily caused by pathologic renal disease as opposed to endocrine gland dysfunction (38, 39).

The onset of menopause is associated with a reduction in gonadotropin sensitivity and estrogen production. Follicle-stimulating hormone (FSH) and luteinizing hormone (LH) levels gradually increase early in the menopause cycle and then decline. As estrogen levels decrease, the reproductive organs, the uterus and ovaries, begin to shrink in size and the feedback mechanism of hormone release is diminished. Testosterone levels decline from structure changes of the testes and prostate gland, resulting in decreased sperm production with an increase of estrogen-to-testosterone ratio (39).

Immunologic

Age-related changes that occur within the body affect the body's innate and adaptive immunologic response. Innate immunity is considered the first line of defense and comprises physical barriers such as the skin and mucus membranes, phagocytosis, and the complement system. Degradation of some of these physical barriers was discussed earlier in the chapter; however, there is a decrease in the number of circulating immunosurveillance cells that are essential for early recognition of pathogens. The number of phagocytes, neutrophils, macrophages, monocytes, and natural killer cells responsible for digestion of pathogens diminishes with age (40). There is a decline in the number of T cells and their function in cell-mediated response. B cells remain relatively stable, but there are increases in antibodies IgG and IgA. Cytokines, especially interleukin (IL)-6, increase with aging and are thought to play a role in the metabolic changes contributing to frailty (40).

These immunologic changes enhance the susceptibility to infection, development of cancers, and other autoimmune disorders. Elderly patients need vaccinations for pneumonia and influenza due to this blunted immune response. Fever may not be present during the early onset of an infection and can increase the risk of mortality if not recognized. With these decreased immunologic responses and increased potential for infections, it is important to identify any subtle changes in the patient's history and assessment to prevent mismanagement of potentially life-threatening conditions.

Psychosocial

Understanding the impact of aging on the psychosocial aspect of elderly life is complex, since so many factors contribute to well-being and quality of life, particularly as people progress through the aging process. The biologic, psychological, and social aspects of life are influenced by constantly changing conditions and unique experiences, creating the opportunity to maintain balance, well-being, and quality of life, despite a variety of insults that can lead to negative psychosocial consequences.

The psychological changes related to aging must be evaluated in the context of a person's personality, their cognitive abilities, their attitudes, as well as their physical and psychological stressors. The development of personality is generally thought to evolve over time influenced by individual experiences and interactions. Several models of this development offer differing perspectives on how these experiences are viewed, internalized, and translated in how the individual personality evolves. For example, in the stage model, it is proposed that the individual goes through different stages in their life and that personality is a reflection of how they view themselves and manage the experiences within those stages. In these models, the common developmental theme elderly individuals go through is a reflection on their past and drawing meaning from those experiences. This helps shape their present perspective on how meaningful their contributions were to those around them and the impact that was left during those experiences. Regardless, these reflections on the meaning of life can influence behaviors as people progress through the aging process (41).

Cognitive ability tends to decline in the aging process. Whether physiologic in origin or evolving from life experiences, cognitive ability plays a major role in the psychosocial well-being of an elderly individual. Memory loss, perceived loss of intelligence, impaired learning, and the ability to maintain attention have a tremendous impact on the individual's ability to interact with others in a meaningful way. This can result in the development of inappropriate behaviors and a threat to the individual's feeling of security and well-being and may lead to isolation from family and friends (41). Another influence of age-related change is in the development of extreme attitudes of elderly individuals toward certain aspects of life. These attitudes influence behaviors and interactions around social aspects of life such as retirement, religion, relationships, and death, to name a few, that can reinforce positive or negative stereotypes of the elderly. More important, as people age, there may be a loss in achieving or maintaining social interactions that have provided a source of community and support. This loss may contribute to behaviors and interactions that further isolate an elderly individual from loved ones or activities (42).

Social isolation is a common contributor to impaired psychological health; and the problem is frequently exacerbated by hospitalization.

Waite and Das discuss findings of the National Social Life, Health, and Aging Project (NSHAP [43]). In Wave I of this project, focus on partnerships, relationship quality, sexuality, nonsexual intimacy, social isolation and health, social networks, and mistreatment were evaluated to understand some of the components that make up biopsychosocial health of the elderly persons. The findings suggest that family involvement throughout the life span is important to the health and well-being as people reach the later years. Despite the changes in family dynamics during this time, whether positive or negative, the ongoing social and emotional support that family brings to the situation tends to provide a positive influence on health and well-being. Relationships and partnerships that maintain a level of intimacy, either sexual or nonsexual, contribute to high levels of emotional and physical satisfaction resulting in increased happiness.

Functional Decline

Nurses apply a holistic approach in understanding the patient's overall well-being. This is accomplished through the health assessment that evaluates a patient's physical and psychological health and medical history, as well as their normal daily activities, and ability to provide self-care, generally referred to as the patient's functional status. Lach and Smith suggest that a patient's functional status is an integration of three domains of function: biologic, psychological, and social (44). This integration is dependent on the older person's ability to adapt to daily stressors in maintaining his or her daily activities; however, functional status typically declines with advanced age.

Functional decline is the limitation or inability to perform activities of daily living (ADLs), such as mobility, toileting, bathing, dressing, and feeding, and instrumental ADLs (IADLs), such as shopping, meal preparation, housework, laundry, transportation, medication management, and managing finances (45, 46). Most often, the normal physiologic changes contribute to these limitations and can be accentuated by a chronic or an acute medical event. These age-related changes such as decreased muscular strength, bone density, or sensory capacity can affect the elderly person's physical capabilities in performing routine tasks. These physical states can be further impacted by acute or chronic medical conditions such as stroke, heart disease, pulmonary diseases, or arthritis, which then increases the severity of functional decline. A person's cognitive abilities, whether from an acute event such as a stroke or a chronic progression of dementia, often play a major role in their functional status. Social isolation and depression are often associated with physical and psychological impairment for these patients, further contributing to functional decline (44-46).

Understanding the functional abilities of elderly patients can be difficult to determine for nurses in the acute care setting. Often, nurses do not have the benefit of the patient's complete medical history or social circumstances prior to admission and must rely on admission assessment input data. These data may or may not be comprehensive or complete depending upon the patient's condition or the availability of family providers, which often leads to a lack of understanding of the patient's needs. Many institutions have implemented age-specific competencies to help nurses understand the needs of elderly patients, to reduce potential negative outcomes. However, this is not always the case. Many acute care staff members have minimal educational preparation on the unique characteristics and needs of the geriatric population. This can result in increased hospital stays from preventable complications and increased hospital morbidity and mortality (47-49).

Mudge, O'Rourke, and Denaro (49) evaluated timing and risk factors for functional changes associated with hospitalization. They reported that 64% of patients 65 years or older admitted to a general medical unit experienced prehospital functional decline. Of this group, 42% were able to return to preadmission levels of activity upon discharge, while only 7% experienced an in-hospital decline. These findings suggest that interventions should focus on recovery of function rather, as well as prevention of decline prior to discharge (49). The degree to which functional decline occurs during the hospitalization is relative to the patient's current medical state, level of cognitive function, and iatrogenic measures to prevent injuries. Bed rest and subsequent reduced mobility, medications to promote sleep and pain relief, and use of safety devices to prevent falls for those with dementia or other cognitive impairment all reduce the chances of successful rehabilitation and recovery efforts (45, 50).

Discharge planning for elderly patients must be considered early in the hospitalization; because successful transition from hospital to home is an indicator of the quality of acute care delivered to elderly patients. Tanaka, Yamamoto, Kita, and Yokode (51) found that elderly patients, particularly those 75 years and older with documented functional decline, are in need of early screening for discharge. The use of a screening sheet at admission (SSA) that focused on functional and social issues was determined to be a valuable tool in identifying patients who will require a more intensive discharge planning. Arora and colleagues (52) demonstrated a relationship between the quality of care of hospitalized vulnerable elderly and postdischarge mortality. This study evaluated the delivery of quality care, as indicated by the Assessing Care of Vulnerable Elders (ACOVE), in predicting 1-year mortality rates. The Vulnerable Elder Survey (VES-13) was used as a means to identify those patients with a score of 3 or greater in functional decline. When comparing the ACOVE scores for those vulnerable elders, 1-year posthospitalization death rates were higher in those vulnerable elders who had lower ACOVE scores (52). This finding suggests that identification of vulnerable elders using an assessment tool such as the VES-13 may be useful in improving the inpatient hospital quality of care for these patients in order to improve long-term outcomes.

Dementia

Dementia is a condition resulting in nerve cell degeneration and atrophy, affecting the cerebral cortex, diencephalon, and basal ganglia and ultimately causing a progressive loss of cognitive abilities and function. Dementia has many causes, classified as organic, genetic, traumatic, and environmental (Table 4–5) (53). By far, Alzheimer's disease is the most common cause of dementia in elderly adults, representing 60% to 80% of all dementia cases (54).

Deterioration of cognitive function is progressive and can often be treated to slow or reverse the effects of dementia. However, with some diseases, such as Huntington's disease or Parkinson's disease, there are no widely accepted treatments that are effective in halt-ing the cognitive decline or improving dementia. The clinical manifestations of dementia vary and are often confused with other acute cognitive impairments such as delirium or depression. Patients with dementia may exhibit progressive memory impairment, aphasia, apraxia, decreases in higher cognitive function skills (such as mathematics, planning, or organizing), loss of motor function (scuffling gait, tendencies for falls), apathy, and depression (53, 54).

Dementia is frequently underdiagnosed, underestimated, or poorly documented in patients upon admission to acute care facilities. This increases a patient's risk for further cognitive decline and injury during hospitalization (55, 56). Assessment for dementia in the acute care setting is essential to establish the underlying level of cognitive function and abilities and to monitor changes during the course of care. The most commonly used screening tool in acute care facilities is the Mini-Mental State Examination (MMSE). This examination assesses memory, orientation, concentration, language, and praxis and is a reliable method to determine dementia and

TABLE 4–5 General Groupings and clinical manifestations of Dementia.

Group	Illness	Clinical Manifestations
ORGANIC		
	• Alzheimer's • Parkinson's • Vascular • Lewy body • Normal pressure hydrocephalus • Frontal lobe	• Loss of memory • Apraxia • Agnosias • Decreased math skill • Deceased language comprehension • Apathy
GENETIC		
	• Huntington's chorea	• Depression
TRAUMATIC		
	• Punch-drunk (repeated head injuries) • Traumatic brain injury • Slow growing tumors	• Slow thought process • Personality changes • Loss of motor functions
ENVIRONMENTAL		
	• Alcohol abuse • Wilsons • Syphilis • AIDS • Creutzfeldt-Jakob • Vitamin deficiencies	

Adapted from Boss BJ, Wilkerson RR. Concepts of neurologic dysfunction. In McCance KL, Huether SE, editors. Pathophysiology: The Biologic Basis for Disease in Adults and Children. 5th edition. St Louis, MO: Mosby; 2006, p. 491-546.

levels of cognitive impairment (54-46). Additionally, the Short Nocturnal Activity Scale (SNAS) is a simple and reliable tool used to assess the nocturnal activity of geriatric patients with dementia (57). Since the cognitive status of hospitalized elders frequently changes at night, this tool can be helpful to assess nighttime behaviors and implement strategies to minimize the risk for falls.

Appropriate management of dementia in the acute care setting includes understanding the patient's cognitive status, preserving function, and preventing injury. However, communication is often difficult with those patients with advanced dementia and poses challenges to their care. An inability to understand the patients' needs or care requirements increases the risk for potential injury (58). Patients with decreased cognition and physical function are particularly at risk for falls at home and when hospitalized. Welmerink, Longstretch, Lyles, and Fitzpatrick (59) reported that many patients hospitalized for a fall demonstrated decreased cognitive function and vision problems and exhibited difficulties with one or more ADL at the time of admission. When planning acute care of elderly patients with dementia, their current medical state, medications, and the impact of unfamiliar environments are all risk factors to consider. Strategies must be applied to identify risks and intervene for these patients to prevent falls, functional and cognitive decline, and other negative outcomes of hospitalization.

Delirium

Delirium is defined as an acute onset of confusion and cognitive impairment. It is characterized by an altered level of consciousness and an inability to focus attention, disorientation, perceptual disturbances, such as illusion, delusion or hallucinations, and disruptions in emotional stability (60, 61). This is a common presentation in elderly patients with existing chronic medical conditions, as well as cognitive and functional impairments. Delirium can be difficult to diagnose, particularly in patients with underlying dementia. The onset of delirium may be an early manifestation of a more serious condition that requires prompt diagnosis and treatment. Medication side effects and interactions, infection, dehydration, drug and alcohol withdrawal, metabolic or electrolyte disorders, and worsening of a chronic medical condition can all be underlying causes of the delirium (60, 61).

Careful attention should be given to elderly patients who present or are admitted with these symptoms, as well as those demonstrating signs and symptoms after admission. Delirium occurs in up to 24% of elders at time of admission, 56% during hospitalization, 53% postoperatively, and 70% to 87% of intensive care elderly patients (62). Early assessment is essential to identify these patients through standard screening tools such as the MMSE, Confusion Assessment Method (CAM), and depression screens to establish baseline cognitive functions in the acute care setting (63). The use of modern technology such as personal digital assistants (PDAs) has demonstrated fast, efficient, and effective bedside assessment tools to track and monitor cognitive functions of hospitalized elderly patients (63).

Interventions are directed to identify, prevent, and reverse cognitive decline from delirium. Models of care designed to reduce the morbidity and mortality of the affects from delirium have been successfully implemented in several acute care environments. The Hospital Elder Life Program (HELP) was developed to target the several risk factors in hospitalized elderly patients, which contribute to the onset or worsening of delirium (62). Disorientation, therapeutic activities, immobilization, sensory impairment, dehydration, malnutrition, and sleep disturbances have been documented as causes of delirium that can be managed by nursing interventions (63-66).

Delirious patients have difficulty communicating their pain, particularly in the postoperative and intensive care settings. This may complicate interventions for pain management and contribute to increased cognitive decline and delirium from undermedication or overmedication (67). Nonpharmacologic measures, as well as appropriate pharmacologic selections, are advocated in nursing care to optimize pain control while minimizing their impact on delirium. Increased family involvement as an extension to formal delirium prevention programs has been helpful in reducing delirium in the acute care setting (68).

GEROPHARMACOLOGY

The complexities of acute and chronic illness on elderly patients pose challenges to health care providers. The use of medications plays an important role in this management but not without concern. Many factors need to be considered in relation to prescribing and administering medications to this population. These decisions are based on the individual elderly patient's needs and physical state of health, rather than the generalization of use for all patients.

Germane to the principles of individualized care is the understanding and appreciation for physiologic changes within the target organs and the metabolic variations that occur with aging. Routine prescribing and administration of medication are not at all routine in geriatric care. The pharmacokinetic properties of drugs, including absorption, distribution, metabolism, and elimination rates are all affected either by age-related changes or through existing pathologic processes of illness or disease in elders (69) (Table 4–6).

Pharmacodynamics (what the drug does to the body) is affected by the receptor sites of target organs. With age-related changes, enhanced and/or diminished sensitivity to some drugs may occur. This may result in increased therapeutic values at lower doses or decreased effects even at higher dosage. Management may be

TABLE 4–6 Pharmacokinetics Issues to Consider with Elderly Patients

Pharmacokinetic Properties	Age-Related Physiologic Effects
ABSORPTION	
	• Increased gastric pH • Decreased gastric empting • Decreased splanchnic blood flow
DISTRIBUTION	
	• Body water volume fluctuations • Body fat distribution • Plasma protein binding
METABOLISM	
	• Hepatic volume
ELIMINATION	
	• Reduced renal mass, size and number of nephrons • Renal blood flow • Glomerular filtration rate • Tubular secretion

Adapted from Linton AD. Pharmacological considerations. In Linton AD, Lach HW, editors. Matteson & McConnell's Gerontological Nursing; Concepts and Practice. 3rd edition. St Louis, MO: Saunders; 2007, p. 138-168.

troublesome in achieving the desired effects and benefits of these medications without the potential risk of adverse side effects (69).

Elderly patients often have multiple providers involved in the management of their conditions or diseases. However, with limited communication between these individual specialists, patients are often prescribed medications that may interact, potentiate, reduce, or negate the effects of another medication. Polypharmacy, which is common among elders, is associated with increased risk of adverse drug reactions, medication errors, impaired patient medication adherence, increased cognitive and functional impairment, toxicity, and potentially life-threatening outcomes (70).

Another prescribing practice that is a major safety concern is prescribing potentially inappropriate medications (PIMs). PIMs are medications with potential risks that outweigh the potential benefits and where a good alternative is available (70). Safeguards have been developed and instituted to prevent use of these medications. The Beers list was developed as a specific list of PIMs that should not be prescribed for elderly patients (71). This list was first established by consensus of a panel of experts in 1991. The list has been modified over time and is currently widely used in acute care settings. (See Table 4–7.) Additionally, the Screening Tool of Older Persons' potentially inappropriate Prescriptions (STOPP) is used to identify patients who were hospitalized as a result of PIM-related adverse drug reactions (72).

Medication review is imperative for each elderly patient admitted to the acute care setting. Management of multiple medications, PIMs, and potential adverse drug reactions is a high-priority nursing intervention for these patients. Literature is abundant documenting relationships between elder medications and unanticipated side

TABLE 4–7 Beers List of Drugs to Avoid in Patients Aged 65 Years and Older

Analgesic/anti-inflammatory	*Psychotropics*
Indomethacin	Amitriptyline, and amitriptyine combinations
Ketorolac	Amphetamines, anorexic agents
Long-term use of full-dose, non–COX-selective NSAIDs: naproxen, oxaprozin, and piroxicam	Barbiturates (except phenobarbital), except for seizures control
Meperidine	Benzodiazepines (short-acting):
Pentazocine	doses >3 mg lorazepam; >60 mg, oxazepam;
Propoxyphene and propoxyphene	>2 mg alprazolam;>15 mg, temazepam;
Combination products	>0.25 mg triazolam
	Benzodiazepines (long-acting): Chlordiazepoxide, chlordiazepoxide-amitriptyline
Cardiovascular	Clidinium-chlordiazepoxide
Amiodarone	Diazepam
Clonidine	

Continued

TABLE 4–7 Beers List of Drugs to Avoid in Patients Aged 65 Years and Older—cont'd

Digoxin	Quazepam
Disopyramide	Halazepam
Doxazosin	Chlorazepate
Guanadrel	Doxepin ergot mesyloids
Methyldopa	Cyclandelate
Hydrochlorothiazide	Fluoxetine, daily dose
Reserpine, >0.25 mg	Flurazepam
Short-acting dipyridamole	Guanethidine
Short-acting nifedipine	Meprobamate
Ticlopidine	Mesoridazine
	Thioridazine

Diabetic agents Chlorpropamide

Gastrointestinal

Cimetidine

Gastrointestinal antispasmodic drugs: dicyclomine, hyoscyamine, propantheline, belladonna alkaloids, and clindinium-chlordiazepoxide

Long-term use of stimulant laxatives: bisacodyl, *Cascara sagrada*

Neoloid, except when used with opiate analgesic

Mineral oil

Trimethobenzamide

Respiratory

Anticholinergics

Antihistamines:

Chlorpheniramine

Diphenhydramine

Hydroxyzine

Cyproheptadine

Promethazine

Tripelennamine

Dexchlorpheniramine

Diphenhydramine

Muscle relaxants

Ditropan XL

Muscle relaxants, antispasmodics: Methocarbamol

Carisoprodol

Chlorzoxazone

Metaxalone

Cyclobenzaprine

Oxybutynin

Orphenadrine

Adapted from Fick DM, Cooper JW, Wade WE, et al. Updating the Beers Criteria for potentially inappropriate medication use in older adults: results of a US consensus panel of experts. Arch Intern Med 2003;163:2716-2724.

effects, drug interactions, functional decline, alterations in mental status, delirium, falls, and other iatrogenic complications (73-75). These hazards offer another opportunity for CNSs to model comprehensive assessments and evidence-based interventions to yield optimal outcomes for hospitalized elders.

References

1. APRN Consensus Work Group and the National Council of State Boards of Nursing APRN Advisory Committee. Consensus Model for APRN Regulation: Licensure, Accreditation, Certification, and Education. 2008. Retrieved May 24, 2011, from http://www.aacn.nche.edu/Education/pdf/APRNReport.pdf

2. American Association of Colleges of Nursing. Adult-Gerontology Clinical Nurse Specialist Competencies. 2010. Retrieved May 24, 2011, http://www.aacn.nche.edu/Education/curriculum/adultgeroCNScomp.pdf

3. Centers for Medicare & Medicaid Services, Office of the Actuary, National Health Statistics Group (CMS1). Retrieved March 19, 2011, from http://www.cms.gov/NationalHealthExpendData/02_NationalHealthAccountsHistorical.asp#TopOfPage

4. Centers for Medicare & Medicaid Services, Office of the Actuary, National Health Statistics Group (CMS2). Retrieved March 19, 2011, http://www.cms.gov/NationalHealthExpendData/downloads/NHEProjections2009to2019.pdf

5. U.S. Census Bureau, Current Population Survey, Annual Social and Economic Supplement. 2009. Retrieved March 19, 2011,

http://www.census.gov/population/www/socdemo/age/older_2009.html

6. U.S. Census Bureau, Population Division. Projections of the Population by Selected Age Groups and Sex for the United States: 2010 to 2050 (NP2008-T2). Retrieved March 19, 2011, http://www.census.gov/population/www/projections/summarytables.html

7. He W, Sengupta M, Velkoff VA, et al. U.S. Census Bureau, Current Population Reports, P23-209, 65+ in the United States. Washington, DC: U.S. Government Printing Office; 2005. Retrieved March 19, 2011, from http://www.census.gov/prod/2006pubs/p23-209.pdf

8. Hall MJ, DeFrances CJ, Williams SN, et al. National Hospital Discharge Survey: 2007 summary. National Health Statistics Report No 29. Hyattsville, MD: National Center for Health Statistics; 2010.

9. Hamric AB. A definition of advanced practice nursing. In Hamric AB, Spross JA, Hanson CM, editors. Advanced Practice Nursing: An Integrated Approach. 4th edition. St Louis, MO: Saunders; 2009:75-94.

10. Millsap P. Neurological system. In Linton AD, Lach HW, editors. Matteson & McConnell's Gerontological Nursing: Concepts and Practice. 3rd edition. St Louis, MO: Saunders; 2007:406-441.

11. Sugerman, RA. Structure and function of the neurologic system. In McCance KL, Huether SE, editors. Pathophysiology: The Biologic Basis for Disease in Adults and Children. 5th edition. St Louis, MO: Mosby; 2006:411-446.

12. Internet Stroke Center at UT Southwestern Medical Center. Stroke Statistics. Retrieved August 31, 2011 from http://www.strokecenter.org/patients/stats.htm.

13. Chung CP, Wang PN, Wu YH, et al. More severe white matter changes in the elderly with jugular venous reflux. Ann Neurol 2011;69:553-559.

14. Iseki K, Hanakawa T, Hashikawa K, et al. Gait disturbances associated with white matter changes: a gait analysis and blood flow study. NeuroImage 2010;49:1659-1666.

15. Chen JJ, Rosas HD, Salat DH. Age-associated reductions in cerebral blood flow are independent from regional atrophy. NeuroImage 2011;55:468-478.

16. Barrere C, Delaney C, Peterson D, et al. Primary stroke center education for nurses: improving core measures. J Nursing Admin 2010;40:515-521.

17. Xu JQ, Kochanek KD, Murphy SL, et al. Deaths: final data for 2007. National Vital Statistics Reports Vol. 58, No. 19. Hyattsville, MD: National Center for Health Statistics; 2010.

18. McCance KL. Structure and function of the cardiovascular and lymphatic systems. In McCance KL, Huether SE, editors. Pathophysiology: The Biologic Basis for Disease in Adults and Children. 5th edition. St Louis, MO: Mosby; 2006:1029-1079.

19. House-Fancher MA, Lynch RJ. Cardiovascular system. In Linton AD, Lach HW, editors. Matteson & McConnell's Gerontological Nursing: Concepts and Practice. 3rd edition. St Louis, MO: Saunders; 2007:313-352.

20. Brashers VL. Structure and function of the pulmonary system. In McCance KL, Huether SE, editors. Pathophysiology: The Biologic Basis for Disease in Adults and Children. 5th edition. St Louis, MO: Mosby; 2006:1181-1204.

21. Linton AD. Respiratory system. In Linton AD, Lach HW, editors. Matteson & McConnell's Gerontological Nursing: Concepts and Practice. 3rd edition. St Louis, MO: Saunders; 2007:353-405.

22. Sharma G, Goodwin J. Effect of aging on respiratory system physiology and immunology. Clin Interv Aging 2006;1:253-260.

23. Linton AD. Genitourinary system. In Linton AD, Lach HW, editors. Matteson & McConnell's Gerontological Nursing: Concepts and Practice. 3rd edition. St Louis, MO: Saunders; 2007:484-524.

24. Huether SE. Structure and function of the renal and urologic systems. In McCance KL, Huether SE, editors. Pathophysiology: The Biologic Basis for Disease in Adults and Children. 5th edition. St Louis, MO: 2006:1279-1300.

25. Martin JE, Sheaff MT. Renal ageing. J Pathol 2007;211:198-205.

26. Perico N, Remuzzi G, Benigni A. Aging and the kidney. Curr Opin Nephrol Hypertens 2011;20:312-317.

27. De Rossi SS, Slaughter YA. Oral changes in older patients: a clinician's guide. Quint Int 2007;39:773-780.

28. Linton AD. Gastrointestinal system. In Linton AD, Lach HW, editors. Matteson & McConnell's Gerontological Nursing: Concepts and Practice. 3rd edition. St Louis, MO: Saunders; 2007:442-483.

29. Huether SE. Structure and function of the digestive system. In McCance KL, Huether SE, editors. Pathophysiology: The Biologic Basis for Disease in Adults and Children. 5th edition. St Louis, MO: Elsevier Mosby; 2006:1353-1383.

30. Woo YJ, Siegmund KD, Tavare S, et al. Older individuals appear to acquire mitotically older colorectal cancers. J Pathol 2009;217:483-488.

31. Nicol N, Huether SE, Weber R. Structure, function, and disorders of the integument. In McCance KL, Huether SE, editors. Pathophysiology: The Biologic Basis for Disease in Adults and Children. 5th edition. St Louis, MO: Mosby; 2006:1573-1623.

32. Amano S. Possible involvement of basement membrane damage in skin photoaging. J Invest Dermatol Symp Proc 2009;14:2-7.

33. Quan T, Qin Z, Xia W, et al. Matrix-degrading metalloproteinases in photoaging. J Invest Dermatol Symp Proc 2009;14:20-24.

34. Fisher GJ. The pathophysiology of photoaging of the skin. Cutis 2005;75(2 suppl):5-8; discussion 8-9.

35. Linton AD. Integument system. In Linton AD, Lach HW, editors. Matteson & McConnell's Gerontological Nursing: Concepts and Practice. 3rd edition. St Louis, MO: Saunders; 2007:225-254.

36. Crowther CL. Structure and function of the musculoskeletal system. In McCance KL, Huether SE, editors. Pathophysiology: The Biologic Basis for Disease in Adults and Children. 5th edition. St Louis, MO: Mosby; 2006:1471-1495.

37. Linton AD. Musculoskeletal system. In Linton AD, Lach HW, editors. Matteson & McConnell's Gerontological Nursing: Concepts and Practice. 3rd edition. St Louis, MO: Saunders; 2007:259-312.

38. Huether SE. Mechanisms of hormonal regulation. In McCance KL, Huether SE, editors. Pathophysiology: The Biologic Basis for Disease in Adults and Children. 5th edition. St Louis, MO: Mosby; 2006:655-681.

39. Linton AD, Hooter LJ, Elmers CR. Endocrine system. In Linton AD, Lach HW, editors. Matteson & McConnell's Gerontological Nursing: Concepts and Practice. 3rd edition. St Louis, MO: Saunders; 2007:525-571.

40. Linton AD. Immune system. In Linton AD, Lach HW, editors. Matteson & McConnell's Gerontological Nursing: Concepts and Practice. 3rd edition. St Louis, MO: Saunders; 2007:572-599.

41. Carroll DW, Linton AD. Age-related psychological changes. In Linton AD, Lach HW, editors. Matteson & McConnell's Gerontological Nursing: Concepts and Practice. 3rd edition. St Louis, MO: Saunders; 2007:631-684.

42. Zukerberg CL, Linton AD. Age-related sociological changes. In Linton AD, Lach HW, editors. Matteson & McConnell's Gerontological Nursing: Concepts and Practice. 3rd edition. St Louis, MO: Saunders; 2007:685-711

43. Waite L, Das A. Families, social life, and well-being at older ages. Demography; 2010; 47-Supplement; S87-S109.

44. Lach HW, Smith CW. Assessment: focus on function. In Linton AD, Lach HW, editors. Matteson & McConnell's Gerontological Nursing: Concepts and Practice. 3rd edition. St Louis, MO: Saunders; 2007:25-51.

45. Kleinpell RM, Fletcher K, Jennings BM. Reducing functional decline in hospitalized elderly. In Hughes RG, editor. Patient Safety and Quality: An Evidence-Based Handbook for Nurses. (Prepared with support from the Robert Wood Johnson Foundation.) AHRQ Publication No. 08-0043. Rockville, MD: Agency for Healthcare Research and Quality; March 2008.

46. Ang YH, Au SY, Yap LK, et al. Functional decline of the elderly in a nursing home. Singapore Med J 2006;47:219-224.

47. Stolley J. Caring for hospitalized older adults. J Gerontol Nursing 2010;36:3-5.

48. Hickman LD, Rolley JX, Davidson PM. Can principles of the Chronic Care Model be used to improve care of the older person in the acute care sector? Collegian 2010;17:63-69.

49. Mudge AM, O'Rourke P, Denaro CP. Timing and risk factors for functional changes associated with medical hospitalization in older patients. J Gerontol A Biol Sci Med Sci 2010;65:866-872.

50. Boltz M, Capezuti E, Shabbat N, et al. Going home better, not worse: older adults' views on physical function during hospitalization. Int J Nursing Pract 2010;16:381-388.

51. Tanaka M, Yamamoto H, Kita T, et al. Early predictions of the need for non-routine discharge planning for the elderly. Arch Gerontol Geriatr 2008;47:1-7.

52. Arora VM, Fish M, Basu AN, et al. Relationship between quality of care of hospitalized vulnerable elderly and postdischarge mortality. J Am Geriatr Soc 2010;58:164-168.

53. Boss BJ, Wilkerson RR. Concepts of neurologic dysfunction. In McCance KL, Huether SE, editors. Pathophysiology: The Biologic Basis for Disease in Adults and Children. 5th edition. St Louis, MO: Mosby; 2006:491-546.

54. Millsap P. Neurological system. In Linton AD, Lach HW, editors. Matteson & McConnell's Gerontological Nursing: Concepts and Practice. 3rd edition. St Louis, MO: Saunders; 2007:406-441.

55. Mazlow K, Mezey M. Recognition of dementia in hospitalized older adults. Am J Nursing 2008;108:40-50.

56. Douzenis A, Michopoulos I, Gournellis R, et al. Cognitive decline and dementia in elderly medical inpatients remain underestimated and underdiagnosed in a recently established university general hospital in Greece. Arch Gerontol Geriatr 2010;50:147-150.

57. Banerjee S, Corte G, Moulin P, et al. A short nocturnal activity scale used by nurses to evaluate hospitalized patients with dementia. J Am Geriatr Soc 2009;57:1953-1955

58. Jootun D, McGhee G. Effective communication with people who have dementia. Nurs Stand [serial online]. 2011;25:40-47.

59. Welmerink DB, Longstretch WT, Lyles MF, et al. Cognition and the risk of hospitalization for serious falls in the elderly: results from the Cardiovascular Health Study. J Gerontol Ser A Biol Sci Med Sci 2010;65A:1242-1249.

60. Boss BJ, Wilkerson RR. Concepts of neurologic dysfunction. In McCance KL, Huether SE, editors. Pathophysiology: The Biologic Basis for Disease in Adults and Children. 5th edition. St Louis, MO: Mosby; 2006:491-546.

61. Millsap P. Neurological system. In Linton AD, Lach HW, editors. Matteson & McConnell's Gerontological Nursing: Concepts and Practice. 3rd edition. St Louis, MO: Saunders; 2007:406-441.

62. Inouye SK. Delirium in older persons. N Engl J Med 2006;354:1157-1165.

63. Zalon ML, Sandhaus S, Valenti D, et al. Using PDAs to detect cognitive change in the hospitalized elderly patient. Appl Nursing Res 2010;23:e21-e27.

64. Inouye SK, Baker DI, Fugal P, et al. Dissemination of the hospital elder life program: implementation, adaption, and successes. J Am Geriatr Soc 2006;54:1492-1499.

65. Vidan MT, Sanchez E, Alonso M, et al. An intervention integrated into daily clinical practice reduces the incidence of delirium during hospitalization in elderly patients. J Am Geriatr Soc 2009;57:2029-2036.

66. LaReau R, Benson L, Watcharotone K, et al. Examining the feasibility of implementing specific nursing interventions to promote sleep in hospitalized elderly patients. Geriatr Nursing 2008;29:197-206.

67. Schreier AM. Nursing care, delirium, and pain management for the hospitalized older adult. Pain Manage Nursing 2010;11:177-185.

68. Rosenbloom-Brunton DA, Henneman EA, Inouye SK. Feasibility of family participation in a delirium prevention program for hospitalized older adults. J Gerontol Nursing 2010;36:22-33

69. Linton AD. Pharmacological considerations. In Linton AD, Lach HW, editors. Matteson & McConnell's Gerontological Nursing: Concepts and Practice. 3rd edition. St Louis, MO: Saunders; 2007:138-168.

70. Ferrario CG. Geropharmacology: a primer for advanced practice acute care and critical care nurses, part I. Adv Crit Care 2008;19:23-35.

71. Fick DM, Cooper JW, Wade WE; et al. Updating the Beers Criteria for potentially inappropriate medication use in older adults: results of a US consensus panel of experts. Arch Intern Med 2003;163:2716-2724.

72. Gallagher P, O'Mahony D. STOPP (Screening Tool of Older Persons' potentially inappropriate Prescriptions): application to acutely ill elderly patients and comparison with Beers' criteria. Age Ageing 2008;37:673-679.

73. Mamun K, Lim JK. Association between falls and high-risk medication use in hospitalized Asian elderly patients. Geriatr Gerontol Int 2009;9:276-281.

74. Thornlow DK, Anderson R, Oddone E. Cascade iatrogenesis: factors leading to the development of adverse events in hospitalized older adults. Int J Nursing Stud 2009;46: 1528-1535.

75. Dahlke S, Phinney A. Caring for hospitalized older adults at risk for delirium: the silent, unspoken piece of nursing practice. J Gerontol Nursing 2008;34:41-47.

CHAPTER 5

Palliative and End-of-Life Care

Amy Brin, MSN, MA, APRN, CNL, and Suzanne Prevost, RN, PhD

INTRODUCTION

Of the 307 million Americans, approximately 133 million live with at least one chronic disease, and 7 of 10 deaths are the result of chronic diseases, such as heart disease and cancer (1). Approximately, one quarter of Americans living with a chronic disease have, at least, one impairment in their activities of daily living (2). This is the somber reality of the U.S. health status. It is diseased. It is broken. It is suffering.

Providers, working within this reality, struggle to adjust practice norms to address the truth that exists—one cannot fix, cure, or mend all that is broken. However, a parallel health care perspective, aimed at comforting and supporting the natural processes involved with living with a life-threatening or limiting chronic condition is growing rapidly across the United States. This emerging subspecialty is palliative care.

Palliative care—which stems from the Latin term *palliare*, "to cloak"—is a model of health care delivery focused on relieving distressing symptoms that are part of a patient's disease trajectory (3). It is appropriately intended to accompany other more traditional health care approaches targeted at curing or reversing illness, whereas a patient should have both: cure and comfort (4). Distressing symptoms addressed by palliative care include physical (i.e., pain, nausea, dyspnea, anorexia, fatigue), as well as social (i.e., relationships, work, financial strain) and spiritual symptoms (i.e., feelings of grief, uncertainty, powerlessness). According to the World Health Organization, *palliative care* is "an approach that improves the quality of life of patients and their families facing the problems associated with life-threatening illness, through the prevention and relief of suffering by means of early identification and impeccable assessment, and treatment of pain and other problems, physical, psychosocial and spiritual" (4).

Founded from clinical curiosity, palliative care began in late 1950s as two physicians—Cicely Saunders and John Bonica—began observational studies to illicit insights into patients living with and dying from life-threatening or life-limiting diseases and the medical management these patients were receiving (5, 6). Both Saunders from the United Kingdom and Bonica from United States acknowledged pain and suffering as natural parts of advancing disease and the responsibility of medical professionals to address (7). From these studies, Saunders published a proposed care model based on the following criteria:

- A physician should have an active role throughout a patient's dying process.
- A patient's entire medical team should engage in supporting the patient's own sources of comfort.
- Physicians and nurses should use the best available evidence-based practices to manage and relieve physiologic symptoms affecting a patient's comfort (8).

Through the impetus of this publication, Saunders integrated such a care model into St. Christopher's Hospice in London in 1958. During her work at St. Christopher's, Saunders embraced clinical research regarding pain protocols, especially the use of opioids to effectively treat a patient's pain, while maintaining alertness. This work led to future collaboration with researchers in the United States at Memorial Sloan-Kettering Cancer Institute in New York City (9). Outcomes from this collaboration served as the bedrock for the initial World Health Organization (WHO) clinical guide on cancer-related pain management. The WHO framework still today serves as the cornerstone to adult and pediatric pain management protocols for cancer and noncancer diagnoses (10) (Figure 5-1).

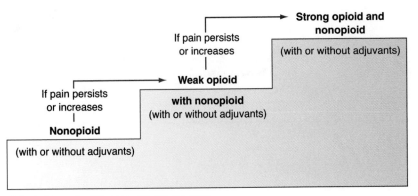

Adapted from the World Health Organization.

FIGURE 5–1: WHO's Pain Relief Ladder.

Saunders' research findings also highlighted to practitioners around the globe the importance of effectively using opioids to treat pain in various settings. This discovery fueled many to train with Saunders and then return to their own communities to integrate these new therapies. The translocation of this evidence-based practice contributed to the establishment of the first U.S. hospice in Connecticut in 1974.

PALLIATIVE CARE VERSUS HOSPICE CARE

Palliative care and hospice are commonly used interchangeably in today's practice, yet their clinical implications are different. Palliative care's parallel approach to cure allows it to be introduced early in a patient's life-threatening/limiting trajectory, as well as being incorporated into end-of-life (EOL) care. It is an interdisciplinary approach that accompanies the patient throughout his or her illness. This requires palliative care to be optimally accessible wherever the patient is physically with his or her disease, including in the community or in a tertiary care setting. It is a fluid, dynamic model of care, as illustrated in Figure 5-2 (11).

Conversely, hospice is a model of care focused on the EOL phase of care. Originating from Saunders' work in symptom management, the intent is to provide patient-focused EOL care to those living with a terminal illness to include psychosocial and spiritual care, as well as the management of physical symptoms. To employ this holistic approach, the hospice model of care bridges the strengths of multiple disciplines, including medicine, nursing, social work, and clergy. This interdisciplinary team fuels the patient-focused, EOL plan of care.

In 1982, the U.S. Congress saw benefit in the hospice model of care and developed a specific Medicare hospice benefit (12). This benefit allows Medicare recipients to elect its coverage for hospice services once a physician certifies that a patient's disease process—if it follows the typical disease trajectory—will most likely result in death within 6 months. State Medicaid and private insurance plans also offer hospice benefits that are designed similar to the Medicare hospice benefit but do have individual nuances regarding services covered. The hospice benefit's time parameter—established on loose prognostic data from an oncology model in the early 1980s—is what logistically separates the provision of palliative care from hospice. Palliative care can be part of a patient's care plan regardless of prognosis, and hospice services must be certified as appropriate at the end of a patient's illness trajectory.

PALLIATIVE CARE AND THE U.S. HEALTH CARE SYSTEM

The present U.S. health care system is designed to focus primarily on acute care management. This design leads to fragmentation of services and duplication of care and often acts in discord to individual patient and family goals of care, particularly for patients with complex chronic illnesses and those at the EOL. In recent years, persons living with life-threatening/limiting conditions have become the most frequent consumers of health care services, with 68% of Medicare spending used to provide care for patients living with five or more chronic conditions (i.e., heart disease, diabetes, pulmonary disease, etc.) (13). Site of death also affects health care spending. Medicare estimated that 44% of its recipients died in a hospital setting, which costs twice as much as a death in an alternative setting, such as a home, where most patients prefer to die (14). In 2006, 5.3 million Americans were

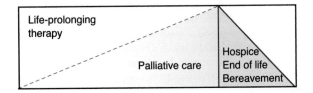

FIGURE 5–2: Palliative and hospice care trajectory.

over the age of 85; this group is projected to grow to 21 million by 2050 (15), which will further stress our health care system's capacity to deliver high-quality EOL care.

Chronically ill and dying patients and their families often report overwhelming dissatisfaction with both the provider communication and the physical care they receive. However, caregivers of chronically ill patients who received palliative care consultation reported more positive perceptions of the information and communication received, emotional and spiritual support, care around the time of death, patient well-being and dignity, and care consistent with the patient's preferences (16). Such data are a reminder of the need for health care delivery to be patient-focused, not solely directed toward treatment of disease.

SETTINGS FOR PALLIATIVE CARE

Since a goal of palliative care is to provide accessible support to a patient wherever he or she is in the disease trajectory, palliative care programs exist in a variety of settings, including ambulatory care clinics, long-term care facilities, and community-based and home-based programs, in addition to hospital-based services. The Center to Advance Palliative Care (CAPC) hosts a current national registry of all programs (17). These varying models are created to match the needs of local communities with available palliative care resources. For example, a hospital-based program may also provide palliative care services to affiliated ambulatory clinics.

Currently, the most prevalent types of palliative care programs in the United States are those based in hospitals. In 2008, 58.5% of U.S. hospitals had a palliative care consult service (18).

These consult service teams are interdisciplinary in nature, loosely based on a hospice model, and tend to include physicians, advanced practice nurses (who may be clinical nurse specialists [CNSs]), registered nurses, social workers, chaplains, and case managers. This interdisciplinary approach enables the palliative care team to address the patient's needs from a holistic perspective. Hospital-based teams are generally available for consultation throughout the entire facility, partnering with trauma, burn, and surgical intensive care teams to address highly acute patient episodes, as well as the chronic illness scenarios encountered with pulmonary, neurology cardiology, and oncology patients.

Acute care settings are naturally designed to deliver the most advanced and intensive interventions. Therefore, the most medically fragile patients typically receive care in these settings. Critical care units provide an even higher intensity of care, allowing the sickest patients to receive precisely the right treatment at the right time, usually with the goal of sustaining life.

Critical care units are also the setting for approximately 540,000 deaths per year in the United States. It is estimated that one in five Americans are admitted to an intensive care unit (ICU) prior to his or her death (19). Therefore, while critical care units are a vital entity for treatment and maintenance of life, they are also a clinical setting actively involved in EOL care. This dichotomy in clinical practice perspectives and goals is often difficult for providers to navigate, thus providing an optimal context for palliative care consultation and integration and for care coordination by CNSs.

In recent years, the presence of palliative care in ICUs has emerged in an attempt to facilitate a seamless transition from intensive treatment to supportive treatment. Research has indicated palliative care consultation on an ICU patient can result in establishment of goals of care, reduction of duplicative or nonbeneficial tests and treatments, completion of advance directives, education and support to family and staff, and overall improved care coordination (20-22). Moreover, palliative care intervention in ICUs has produced remarkable cost-savings for such units. Among patients admitted to an ICU, who received palliative consultation and who were discharged alive from the unit, associated costs were approximately $5,178 lower than those for similar patients who did not receive palliative consultation. For patients admitted to the ICU, who also received palliative care consultation but who died during their hospitalization, the decrease in spending approximated $6,613 (23). Whether for improved patient outcomes, family satisfaction, or cost-savings, palliative care consultations and interventions have demonstrated significant impact within acute and critical care settings.

By definition, CNSs are trained to be "clinical experts in the application of theoretical principals and research-based knowledge in regard to a chosen area of specialization in setting and practice" (24), and most CNSs practice in acute care settings. This role description positions CNSs in a unique relationship with palliative care providers. The CNSs charge to serve as a clinical expert in delivery of direct patient care, as well as a leader in systems management, provides a dynamic opportunity to facilitate the integration of palliative care. Therefore, a CNS's understanding of palliative care is critical to optimize the delivery of quality care, enhance delivery systems, and reduce costs. The following case report illustrates a typical example of a patient and family member in need of palliative intervention and includes a description of one way that a CNS might engage in this process.

Case Report (Part I): "Meeting Jed"

Jed Whitaker is a 70-year-old, Caucasian man who presents to a rural emergency department with respiratory distress. He presents on a gurney, ashen, diaphoretic, and not oriented to person or place. His 65-year-old wife, Nora, is at his side. She reports that he "was fine" and then all of a sudden "he started breathing hard and fell to the ground." Nora does not recall any precipitating signs, except "he just seems so much weaker these days."

Jed has a past medical history of congestive heart failure (CHF), chronic obstructive pulmonary disease (COPD), peripheral vascular disease (PVD), and diabetes mellitus type 2 and a history of laparoscopic cholecystectomy 5 years earlier. His daily medication regimen includes an angiotensin-converting enzyme (ACE)-inhibitor, beta-blocker, bronchodilator, oral antihyperglycemic, statin, aspirin, diuretics, and oxygen via nasal cannula as needed. According to Nora, Jed enjoys "reading the newspaper every morning over breakfast" and light-gardening "he can only handle about an hour." He and Nora live alone, with her managing all of his medication refills and physician appointments. They have three grown children: two live out of state and one lives one hour's travel time away. Jed does not have any orders limiting resuscitation efforts.

Immediately following intake, Jed experiences a cardiac arrest, and the emergency department staff initiates cardiopulmonary resuscitation (CPR). After resuscitation, Jed continues to have difficulty maintaining effective respirations, so he is intubated and placed on a ventilator. He is transferred to the ICU, where labs and radiographs reveal that Jed has developed bilateral bacterial pneumonia. Intravenous fluids and antibiotics are initiated. Nora remains at Jed's bedside continuously. After the initial rounds of antibiotics, Jed's pneumonia does appear to be responding to therapy; however, his overall respiratory status continues to be compromised, and he has difficulty with weaning from mechanical ventilation. His interdisciplinary team members are concerned about his ability to tolerate extubation, even with a successful wean from the ventilator. The team continues planning and monitoring his care. At day 7 of his ICU stay, the intensivist consults the hospital's palliative care team.

The palliative care physician and CNS respond to the initial consult and receive telephonic report from the attending physician regarding the patient's status and plan of care. He has requested palliative care consultation to help understand the preferences of the patient (who is sedated and cannot articulate his wishes) and the family's goals of care. At this time, symptom management is not a high priority for the ICU team.

The palliative care physician and CNS meet with Nora and review Jed's current medical status, the process of extubation, and the possibility of his inability to tolerate extubation or "breathe on his own." They describe how Jed's chronic conditions, combined with the recent pneumonia, influence his potential to maintain a healthy pulmonary status. The CNS asks Nora if Jed and she had ever discussed what his choices would be for his care. What interventions would he want? If he could speak now, which ones would he not want?

Nora expresses that they have briefly talked about care decisions and that Jed never "wants to be a bother." She discusses how he "loves life, especially his grandchildren and garden," and that she cannot imagine him not being able to enjoy those things again. Nora expresses, "I want everything done for Jed to allow him a chance to garden at least one more time and hug those grandbabies. I owe him that."

The palliative care physician and CNS review what they have heard from Nora about their desired goals of care, including full treatment with a goal of returning home. They explain the possibility that he may not survive extubation. Nora affirms. The palliative care team reviews with Nora that they will convey her goals to the ICU team and that they will continue to visit her and Jed throughout his stay to assist with symptom management and offer her support. Over the next 10 days, Jed is successfully weaned and extubated. When it becomes clinically evident that Jed will be going home, the CNS and palliative care team facilitate discharge planning to ensure the necessary support and equipment is in the home, since Nora will continue to serve as Jed's primary caregiver.

Clinical Presentation and Diagnoses

Guidelines often recommend the introduction of palliative care services for any patient with a life-threatening condition (4, 7). However, the confirmation of the presence of a life-threatening condition can prove difficult to translate to practice. Examples of diagnoses that are appropriate for the application of palliative care interventions, yet may be overlooked, include:

- Dementia
- Congestive heart failure
- Chronic obstructive pulmonary disease (COPD)
- Chronic renal failure
- Cancer
- Liver failure and/or cirrhosis
- Neurodegenerative disease
- Sepsis
- Multiorgan system failure
- Human immunodeficiency virus (HIV) infection/ acquired immune deficiency syndrome (AIDS)
- Major trauma (7, 8)

The need for palliative intervention increases exponentially when patients present with a combination of the diagnoses on this list. Dementia is one diagnosis that is frequently overlooked, in terms of the potential for improving outcomes through palliative intervention.

Other contributing and complicating factors include the presence of comorbidities, frequent readmissions to hospitals for exacerbations, a decline in overall function related to a life-threatening condition, the need for organ transplantation, a lack of support systems, and forthcoming significant health care decisions, such as the need for a tracheostomy or feeding tube (8). It is important to note that palliative care interventions can be appropriate at all stages of the life span. The applicability of palliative care in the pediatric population parallels that of adults, with unique nuances outlined throughout pediatric palliative care literature. In some settings, age-related biases may inhibit the full application of palliative interventions for elders. For each of these populations, the CNS can serve as a patient and family advocate by proactively identifying patients that can benefit from palliative intervention.

Management and Palliative Care Interventions

An initial palliative care consult should be multidimensional, comprehensive, and interdisciplinary in nature. This process should include assessing the physical, social, psychological, and spiritual components of the case.

Physical: The physical assessment includes the primary diagnosis, presence of comorbidities, current level of function, current status on the projected disease trajectory related to employed therapies, present symptoms, anticipated symptoms (related to therapies or further disease progression), and resuscitation status. Physical symptoms assessed for and commonly managed by palliative care providers include pain, dyspnea, nausea and vomiting, anorexia, insomnia, pruritus, anxiety, agitation, delirium, depression, fatigue, candidiasis, fever, diarrhea, constipation, cough, and hiccups (25). If symptom management recommendations are generated by the palliative care provider, he or she will suggest treatment options to the primary team managing the patient's care. Palliative care consultants work collaboratively with other health care providers, never becoming the primary service of management.

Social/Psychological: The second component of assessment would include current support systems, coping strategies related to the disease or injury, presence of anticipatory grief, bereavement needs, at-risk behaviors, and the community resources being used and those that are needed. While CNSs may participate in these assessments, they are supported by social or psychologically focused team members, including social workers or psychologists, as well as the appropriate family and caregivers actively involved in patient's care (25). Counseling and other supportive therapies are frequently offered, as well as assistance in coordinating community resources as needed throughout the patient's stay and in preparation for discharge. Often these patients' high acuity levels contribute to greater resource and counseling needs, which require effective collaboration with social and psychological resource personnel among hospital staff, beyond those on the palliative care team.

Spiritual: The spiritual history and assessment includes religious or spiritual beliefs, questions and doubts about stated religious or spiritual beliefs, accessed or needed religious or spiritual resources or groups, performance of religious or spiritual rituals, and bereavement needs. The chaplain on a palliative care team lends another level of overall, holistic support to the patient and his or her family. Patients receiving palliative care intervention are likely to have significant spiritual needs, yet those needs are often perceived to be secondary by acute care staff, and they may ignore them, if a patient is physically unstable. The CNS and other palliative care providers can encourage and remind direct care staff to consider the patient's needs from a holistic perspective, so that religious and/or spiritual interventions are not deferred until a time that may be too late. The chaplain provides an outlet for patients and families/caregivers to discuss how their religious or spiritual beliefs intersect with pending medical decisions, health, and death. They may serve as a liaison for collaborating with the patient's established religious/spiritual figure. The palliative care chaplain also aims to work in collaboration with other hospital-based chaplains.

BARRIERS TO PALLIATIVE CARE

Several barriers exist that inhibit access to and effectiveness of palliative care. They can be grouped into two categories: infrastructural and attitudinal barriers. Barriers related to infrastructure have garnered much attention and have prompted the development of protocols, research projects, and legislative activity. Attitudinal barriers are equally present but tend to be more covert and difficult to address.

INFRASTRUCTURAL BARRIERS

Organizing systems of care to integrate palliative care, so that its provision is easily accessible, collaborative, credible, and financially feasible, demands creativity, ingenuity, and strong leadership. Potential infrastructural barriers that tend to impede the effectiveness of palliative care teams are:

- Recruitment challenges and limited availability of appropriately trained staff
- Sufficient financial support from the institution, considering that palliative care is cost-effective, but not revenue-generating
- Nuances with procedural terminology, coding, and reimbursement and the interface with palliative care practice (i.e., time-intensity, location, consultation)

- Existing information-technology templates may not encompass the details of palliative care triggers, assessments, interventions, and referrals
- Standard quality improvement data collection methods may not appropriately acknowledge palliative care outcomes (i.e., death as an expected outcome)
- Limited physical space for palliative care team members, since they do not tend to be aligned with a specific department or group of patients (7, 26, 27)

ATTITUDINAL BARRIERS

Despite administrative support, appropriate financial resources, and the presence of skillful, credible providers, many palliative care teams experience resistance to their clinical practice daily. Palliative care team involvement in a patient's case signifies the presence of a disease or such significant demise that providers may not be able to fix, cure, or heal the problem; therefore, these patients, their families, and their health care providers are particularly vulnerable. When faced with an uncomfortable, uncontrollable situation, due to tragedy or the unknown, coping mechanisms begin to manifest. In palliative care cases, these coping strategies frequently arise in the form of avoidance, anger, denial, or confrontation. These behaviors often produce barriers to the palliative care team's inclusion or effectiveness, often until death is imminent.

Moreover, the frequent use of palliative care as a synonym for hospice is also problematic. This misconception can inhibit palliative care referrals early in a patient's disease trajectory, when a therapeutic rapport can more easily be initiated, thus allowing for support throughout the illness trajectory as health care decisions arise. Many palliative care teams employ a host of educational interventions in their attempts to decrease these barriers, through daily conversations with unaware providers or through other more formal marketing campaigns (28). The CNS can function as an advocate and a powerful facilitator to promote effective working relationships between the front line acute care staff and the members of the palliative care consultation team.

Case Report (Part II): "Seeing Jed Again"

Jed was readmitted to the rural hospital 4 months later, directly from an office visit with his primary care provider. Nora explains their visit with Dr. Berger was "just to check on Jed's breathing and all his medications." Apparently, upon presentation, Jed was wheezing with an oxygen saturation of 88% on a 4 LPM nasal cannula. He experienced a cardiac arrest in the emergency department, where resuscitation was initiated; since he was still on full resuscitation status. Jed presented to the ICU requiring full ventilatory support. His initial cultures and lab reports were clear; however, within his first week of admission, he developed bowel incontinence and a urinary tract infection. All attempts to wean ventilatory support were futile, requiring 100% oxygen on day 10 of his stay. His lab results began to indicate renal and liver failure.

Since Jed had a previous palliative consult, on readmission, the palliative care team was automatically reconsulted via a trigger mechanism in the hospital's electronic health record. On reexamination, the palliative care CNS noted that Jed had lost 20 pounds in 4 months, had significant muscular atrophy, and required a significant increase in oxygen support. Nora explained that Jed stopped being able to "work in the garden about a month ago," decreased his food intake to "maybe half of a plate on a good day," and required assistance with dressing, bathing, and toileting. She reported that "he needed that walker to move around, but couldn't really do that so good anymore either."

From the previous admission, the palliative care social worker was able to collaborate with community-based resource personnel to provide Nora with additional home support two times per week, as well durable medical equipment that would appropriately support Jed's daily functional level. Nora expressed how helpful the support had been and then became tearful: "It's still really hard."

The palliative care physician and CNS reviewed with Nora their assessments of Jed's medical status—including his lack of acute symptoms needing management—and how his functional decline was related to his existing life-threatening condition and comorbidities. They reviewed their past goals-of-care discussion, where Nora indicated, "I want everything done for Jed to allow him a chance to garden at least one more time and hug those grand-babies. I owe him that." Nora became tearful and said, "I remember that conversation. I mentioned it to Jed when we got home. He just shook his head and said, 'Don't leave me on those machines.' I don't know what to do. He'd never want to live like this." The palliative care team expressed that these decisions are difficult, and need time. They offered to call Jed and Nora's adult children to update them on his status, and Nora said the children would be arriving later that evening. She requested a visit from the team again the next day.

The following day the palliative care CNS entered the room after reviewing the record and confirming that there was no improvement. She engaged the family in a discussion, noting goals of care that had been mentioned previously, and educating the family on Jed's current medical status involving prolonged ventilation, multiorgan failure, and his potential for survival after extubation. Then she explained to the family what extubation looks like and discussed possible symptoms and the interventions that could be used to ensure comfort. The palliative care chaplain explored the family's religious beliefs and discussed how those beliefs might affect their decision-making process. The family thanked the palliative care team and said they wanted to go to lunch "to think about all this." The palliative care team let them know they would be available and checking on Jed daily.

CLINICAL NURSE SPECIALIST COMPETENCIES AND SPHERES OF INFLUENCE

CNSs have a unique opportunity to translate and facilitate the infusion of palliative care philosophies and interventions with many acute and critical patient populations (24). Due to the CNS's dynamic practice scope, there are several ways an individual practitioner can provide and support palliative care. As stewards of a holistic perspective from direct patient care to education to system leadership—CNSs are positioned to support the goals of aggressive symptom management, patient and family satisfaction, and cost-effectiveness. The growing evidence-base supporting palliative care interventions provides an innovative and encompassing care concept for the CNS to embrace.

Several options exist for specialty preparation in palliative care. As of 2010, there were 15 graduate level nursing programs in the United States offering palliative care specialization (personal communication with J. Pace, Coordinator—Palliative Care Focus, Vanderbilt University, School of Nursing, September 6, 2010). Meanwhile, 74 U.S. universities offer palliative care medical fellowship programs. (29). Additionally, the American Association of Colleges of Nursing sponsors the End-of-Life Nursing Education Consortium (ELNEC), which offers continuing education workshops and certification programs throughout the United States each year (30). The Hospice and Palliative Nursing Association (HPNA) also offers specialty credentialing programs for advanced practice nurses, as well as registered nurses, licensed practical nurses, and nursing assistants (31).

Clinical Expert/Direct Care

As part of the interdisciplinary palliative care team, a CNS administers care via an advanced practice nursing scope. Such practice includes assessing and monitoring symptoms, managing symptoms through pharmaceutical and nonpharmaceutical therapies, leading or participating in family care conferences, initiating discussions on advance directives (i.e., Do Not Resuscitate orders, placement of feeding tubes, etc.), and offering support (24). While every palliative care team operates in a unique manner, CNSs who work with palliative care teams often provide follow-up consults after the initial interdisciplinary assessment and consultation. In another model used by some teams, the nature of follow-up consultation and the choice of follow-up provider are driven by the patient's or family's most pressing needs.

Consultation

Palliative care offers the CNS a host of ways to use consultation competencies: as a patient advocate who identifies the need for palliative care consultation and intervention, as a member of a palliative care team, or as an expert clinician being consulted by a palliative care team. If a CNS has received specialty training in palliative care, he or she may be in a position to consult with other providers about the appropriateness for palliative care interventions on a given patient. This type of consultation is especially prudent in communities with minimal access to palliative care providers and services. This type of consultation demands a high degree of professional awareness of the appropriate timing to make such consultations, as well as ensuring accurate information and recommendations are given (32).

As a member of a palliative care team, each interdisciplinary specialist approaches the patient as a consultant. Recommendations for the patient's care are crafted through the palliative care lens (i.e., symptom management or discussion of medical futility) and then offered to the primary team of health care providers managing the patient's care. This collaboration requires professional, competent communication, an understanding of roles, and respectful acknowledgment of the norms of the practice setting (33).

Since palliative care teams tend to function independent of specific departments and services, it is often helpful for those providers to have accessible experts in the various settings where they provide services. A palliative care provider approaches a case with a general understanding of the complexities of the patient and family and then applies palliative care expertise to the situation. A CNS who practices in the setting can provide expert consultation to enhance the team's understanding of the specific patient population and protocols of that setting (24). Again, this type of consultation requires a high degree of respect for roles, differing perspectives and practice norms, as well as strategic communication.

Systems Leadership

The pioneering nature of palliative care requires strong leadership to promote acceptance in clinical settings. A CNS is uniquely qualified to serve as such a leader due to his/her acknowledgement of how systems management affects patient care. CNSs can support the adoption and effectiveness of palliative care programs by implementing protocols or "triggers" for palliative care consultations for appropriate patient populations, identifying and facilitating electronic health record functionalities to support palliative care, developing budgets and pursuing funding for a palliative care team that are mindful of the cost-saving benefits, and articulating the relationship between palliative care and quality improvement. From establishing a palliative care program to managing its daily integration in a clinical unit or department, there are many opportunities for CNS leadership in palliative care practice.

Collaboration

Palliative care is a consultative service. A consult or referral must be made for a palliative care provider to deliver care. This relationship is dependent upon effective collaboration. To sustain healthy provider-to-provider relationships, larger, more systematic collaboration must also take place. A CNS's ability to identify palliative care needs in a system, work within that system to gain resources and decrease barriers, and establish processes for application, all require collaboration. A CNS competent in the art and skill of collaboration will be most effective in promoting the adoption and infusion of palliative care into a practice setting to meet patient needs and improve outcomes.

Coaching/Teaching/Mentoring

The coaching, teaching, and mentoring roles of the CNS also support palliative care. The CNS can employ these roles to assist individual patients and their families, to help staff understand palliative interventions, or to promote the translation of palliative care into practice. A CNS coaching a family through EOL decision-making or advance care planning discussions employs palliative care concepts. Teaching colleagues about specific palliative care interventions or appropriate timing for consults and referrals promotes further integration into practice. Mentoring younger colleagues about specialized interventions used during EOL or bereavement care can help engage more providers into the practice of palliative care. Often, times of choosing to escalate or withdraw therapies produce tremendous conflict. A CNS's ability to effectively coach families and/or colleagues through that process can be critical in resolving the scenario. The CNS as coach, teacher, and mentor can be a tremendous asset in promoting and enhancing the effectiveness of palliative care.

Research/Evidence-Based Practice

The evidence-base supporting palliative care is expanding, but additional research is needed regarding interventions, settings, and unique patient populations. The CNS research role is multidimensional in supporting palliative care. First, the CNS is a consumer of palliative care research by staying abreast of the latest developments in hospice and palliative care literature, as well as palliative or EOL research within other specialties, such as oncology, critical care, or pain management. The CNS serves as a teacher, mentor, and role model to other staff in promoting the application of evidence-based practice guidelines for palliative care. The CNS can also provide leadership in the collection and synthesis of data to document effectiveness of palliative interventions for individuals and patient populations, as well as the impact on overall quality of care and cost-effectiveness. Through critical analysis and synthesis of research findings the CNS can help make the case for implementing or promoting palliative care interventions and services. Finally, CNSs can be integral members of a palliative care research team, and may serve as principal investigators.

Ethical Decision-Making/Moral Agency/Advocacy

Clinical palliative care scenarios often involve ethical discussions, such as withdrawal of therapies or medical futility. These cases typically evoke tremendous emotion, as well as require high utilization of physical and financial resources. Palliative care consultation helps patients, families, and providers weigh the benefit versus burden of related interventions. Such insight is helpful in guiding decision-making, as well as eliciting goals of care (7). A CNS's familiarity and comfort with introducing and discussing these concepts, or facilitating collaboration with palliative care providers around these concepts, can support the patient, family, and team through the decision-making process.

Not only do such clinical issues fuel ethical considerations, but when they do arise, they often illuminate chasms in micro and macro systems. Advocates are needed to give voice to these chasms and champion these issues to improve practice environments. Advocacy on the legislative front is necessary to inform policy-makers on controversial issues such as narcotic management and advance care planning for these special patient populations. Additionally, internal advocacy efforts to initiate or sustain palliative care programs within an institution require consistency and diligence. CNSs are situated to be effective advocates on all levels due to their expert knowledge of patient needs.

Case Report (Part III): "Helping Jed Live until He Dies"

Jed's family returned to the unit and notified his nurse that they wanted to prevent any further resuscitation efforts and begin withdrawal of therapies. The nurse who attended a staff development program on EOL communication the month prior actively listened and offered reassurance to the family. The primary medical team notified the palliative care team of the family's decision. The palliative care social worker and chaplain revisited the family the same day to offer further support and explore the family's wishes for the time of extubation. The family, already aware of the mechanics of extubation due to the earlier explanation by the CNS, decided that Nora and all three children would stay in the room. They made plans to bring the grandchildren in tonight to say goodbye to Jed, and the palliative care social worker provided guidance on age-appropriate communication strategies to use. Additionally, the palliative care social worker provided bereavement counseling information for the family to use later. Nora requested a specific religious ritual prior to extubation. The palliative care team assured the family that they would return to provide additional support.

Working together, the primary health care team and palliative care team planned an extubation time to accommodate Nora's wishes. The CNS provided recommendations for control of pain, dyspnea and secretions, including the use of an opioid, a benzodiazepine, and anticholingerics. These medications were ordered, with appropriate titration parameters outlined for the nursing staff. An hour prior to the time for extubation, the family's religious leader arrived and performed the ritual. The family said their goodbyes, alone and with as much privacy as possible. At the scheduled time, the CNS, physician, respiratory therapist, and primary nurse entered the room. All monitors were turned off, electrodes were removed, and intravenous fluids were stopped with only access remaining for medication administration. Appropriate doses of symptom management medications were administered, and Jed was extubated.

Jed lived for another 2 hours, requiring additional medication to manage his dyspnea and secretions. The staff nurse managed those needs using the established medication orders. Jed's family remained in the room until his last breath. The palliative care chaplain escorted them to a private conference room to wait until postmortem care was completed. Then he accompanied Nora back into the room for a final private goodbye. "I'm going to miss him so," she said as she rejoined the rest of the family at the unit's exit.

While the palliative care chaplain is with the family, the CNS offered support to the nursing staff and affirmed the manner in which they served Jed and his family. The registered nurse responded, "Doesn't matter how often you observe a death, they are just hard. You want to make sure you do everything right. The anxiety can stay with you." The CNS offered additional reassurance and then made notes to include in her quarterly quality improvement meeting.

CLINICAL NURSE SPECIALIST COMPETENCIES APPLIED TO THE CASE

Clinical Expert/Direct Care

This case report illustrates the process and the importance of providing palliative care consultation and intervention early in a chronic disease trajectory, in an acute care setting, rather than merely providing palliation at the EOL. Jed's life-threatening diagnoses were his chronic conditions and comorbidities. While he presented both times to tertiary care in acute crisis, an assessment of his functionality and maintenance medications suggested that his disease was progressing. His poor capacity for tolerating his ventilatory wean revealed his overall poor pulmonary status and lack of reserve. Assessment of Jed's complete medical picture indicated a need for palliative care consultation.

The initial palliative care consultation provided the palliative care team with a baseline summation of Jed's disease state, function, as well as past and current medical interventions. Even though symptom management was not needed initially, the early meeting provided both the team and Nora with an opportunity to initiate rapport, and a framework to initiate the goals of care conversation. The repeated visits and conversations gave the family time to process their wishes, so that decisions did not have to be made in a hurry or out of reaction. This gradual approach is often more malleable for family members and caregivers than the typical rapid decision-making conversation often presented to families in acute and critical care settings.

The latter palliative care consultation was geared more toward EOL. Death was imminent due to the multiorgan system failure. While extubation and correlating clinical interventions were clearly indicated, the palliative care team's presence assisted in adding appropriate symptom management interventions, as well as coordinating valued religious rituals. These strategies supported the family's goals of care for comfort and honoring Jed's religious beliefs. This holistic coordination demonstrates the art of palliative care; it is both patient and family-centered.

Systems Leadership

This case study demonstrated an evolved system for palliative care integration. Examples of leadership interventions to support palliative care included electronic record functionality to generate a palliative care consult, an electronic trigger for palliative consult on readmission, telephonic means for collaboration between the primary medical team and palliative care team, quality improvement measurements capturing the impact of palliative care, and an overall collaborative environment. In order for such processes to be in place, and in such an inclusive culture, strong leadership is essential.

Coaching/Teaching/Mentoring

While the primary focus of palliative intervention was Jed, there were several opportunities for coaching, teaching, and mentoring throughout the case study. The entire palliative care team coached Jed's family through the decision-making process. It was implied that the palliative care team and system leaders had partnered to offer unit teaching sessions on EOL communication techniques, which Jed's nurse used. Finally, the palliative care CNS mentored the staff registered nurse by facilitating a brief and informal debriefing session about Jed's death and the role the nurses played. It is important for a CNS to consider any professional communication as an opportunity for coaching, teaching, or mentoring.

Collaboration

Collaboration between multiple participants was depicted throughout the case study. Examples included:

- The primary health care team and the palliative care team
- The palliative care chaplain with the community-based religious leader
- The palliative care CNS with the staff nurses
- Among the palliative care team members
- And with all members of Jed's family

Effective collaboration demands good communication, understanding of roles, and shared consensus. Collaboration is a vital tool for ensuring all efforts are focused on meeting a patient's goals of care.

AN EVOLVING FIELD

The field of palliative care is evolving. Recent research indicates palliative care not only alleviates symptoms and aids in decision-making but can actually extend the life of some patients, such as those living with non–small cell lung cancer (34). Such findings generate tremendous implications for the entire health care system, including CNSs working in acute and critical care settings. CNSs are well positioned to use palliative interventions to help individual patients and families, and to enhance overall quality of care by supporting palliative care programs and providers throughout their institutions. Regardless of role, CNS support for palliative care indicates a commitment to patient-centered care and acknowledgement that patients should fully live until they die.

References

1. Centers for Disease Control and Prevention. Chronic Diseases and Health Promotion. 2009. Retrieved January 28, 2011, from http://www.cdc.gov/chronicdisease/overview/

2. Anderson G. Chronic Conditions: Making the Case for Ongoing Care. Baltimore, MD: John Hopkins University Press; 2004.

3. Stephenson R. Palliative care: more than just care from a friendly relative. N C Med J 2004;65:4.

4. World Health Organization (WHO), National Cancer Control Programmes. Policies and Managerial Guidelines: Policies and Managerial Guidelines. 2nd edition. Geneva: World Health Organization; 2002.

5. Meldrum M. The ladder and the clock: Cancer pain and public policy at the end of the twentieth century. J Pain Sympt Manage 2005;29:41-54.

6. Wall PD. The generation of yet another myth on the use of narcotics. Pain 1997;73:121-122.

7. Davis MP, Kuebler KK. Palliative and end-of-life care perspectives. In Kuebler K, Heidrich D, Esper P, editors. Palliative & End-of-Life Care: Clinical Practice Guidelines. 2nd edition. St Louis, MO: Elsevier Health Sciences; 2007.

8. Seymour J, Clark D, Winslow M. Pain and palliative care: the emergence of new specialties. J Pain Sympt Manage 2005;29:2-13.

9. Clark D. Cicely Saunders: Founder of the Hospice Movement Selected Letters 1959-1999. Oxford, UK: Oxford University Press; 2002.

10. World Health Organization. WHO's Pain Relief Ladder. Retrieved January 28, 2011, from http://www.who.int/cancer/palliative/painladder/en/

11. National Consensus Project for Quality Palliative Care. Clinical Practice Guidelines for Palliative Care. 2nd edition. Retrieved January 28, 2011, from http://www.nationalconsensusproject.org/guideline.pdf

12. Lynn J. Serving patients who may die soon and their families: the role of hospice and other services. JAMA 2001;285:325-332.

13. Anderson GF. Medicare and chronic conditions. N Engl J Med 2005;353: 305-309.

14. Raphael C, Ahrens J, Fowler N. Financing end-of-life care in the USA. J R Soc Med 2001;94: 458-461.

15. Federal Interagency Forum on Aging Statistics. Population. Retrieved January 28, 2011, from http://www.aoa.gov/agingstatsdotnet/Main_Site/Data/2008_Documents/Population.aspx

16. Cassaret D, Pickard A, Bailey A, et al. Do palliative consultations affect patient outcomes? J Am Geriatr Soc 2008;56:593-599.

17. Center to Advance Palliative Care. National Palliative Care Registry. Retrieved January 29, 2011, from http://www.getpalliativecare.org/providers

18. Center to Advance Palliative Care. Palliative Care Programs Continue Rapid Growth in U.S. Hospitals: Becoming Standard Practice Throughout the Country. Retrieved January 29, 2011, from http://www.capc.org/news-and-events/releases/04-05-10

19. Angus D, Barnato A, Linde-Zwirble W, et al. Use of intensive care at the end of life in the United States: an epidemiologic study. Crit Care Med 2008;32:638–643.

20. Gade G, Venohr I, Conner D, et al. Impact of an inpatient palliative care team: a randomized controlled trial. J Palliat Med 2008; 11:180-190.

21. Ahrens T, Yancy V, Kolleef M. Improving family communication at the end-of-life: implications for length of stay in the intensive care unit and resource use. Am J Crit Care 2003;12:317-323.

22. Campbell ML. Palliative care consultation in the intensive care unit. Crit Care Med 2006;34:S355-S358.

23. Morrison RS, Penrod JD, Cassel JB, et al. Cost savings associated with US hospital palliative care consultation programs. Arch Intern Med 2008;168:1783-1790.

24. Kuebler KK, Pace JC, Esper P. The advanced practice nurse in palliative care. In Kuebler K, Heidrich D, Esper P, editors. Palliative & End-of-Life Care: Clinical Practice Guidelines. 2nd edition. St Louis, MO: Elsevier Health Sciences 2007.

25. Ferrell BR, Coyle N. Textbook of Palliative Nursing. 2nd edition. Oxford, UK: Oxford University Press; 2006.

26. Bendaly EA, Groves J, Juliar B, et al. Financial impact of palliative care consultation in a public hospital. J Palliat Med 2008;11: 1304-1308.

27. Rodriguez KL, Barnato AE, Arnold RM. Perceptions and utilization of palliative care services in acute care hospitals. J Palliat Med 2007:10:99-110.

28. Center to Advance Palliative Care. Making the Case for Hospital-Based Palliative Care. Retrieved January 28, 2011, from http://www.capc.org/building-a-hospital-based-palliative-care-program/case

29. American Academy of Hospice and Palliative Medicine. (2010, January). Fellowship directory. Retrieved January 28, 2011, http://www.aahpm.org/fellowship/default/fellowshipdirectory.html

30. American Association of Colleges of Nursing. End of Life Nursing Consortium. Retrieved January 28, 2011, from http://www.aacn.nche.edu/ELNEC/factsheet.htm

31. Hospice and Palliative Care Nurses Association. Certification information. Retrieved January 28, 2011, from http://www.hpna.org/DisplayPage.aspx?Title=Certification%20Preparation

32. Dahlin CM, Giansiracusa T. Communication in palliative care. In Textbook of Palliative Nursing, 2nd edition. Oxford, UK: Oxford University Press; 2006.

33. Meier DE, Beresford L. Consultation etiquette challenges palliative care to be on its best behavior. J Palliat Med 2007;10:7-11.

34. Temel JS, Greer JA, Muzikansky A, et al. Early palliative care for patients with metastatic non–small-cell lung cancer. N Engl J Med 2010;363:733-742.

Psychosocial Health Problems

Laura G. Leahy, MSN, APN, CRNP, PMH-CNS/FNP, BC,
and Julie Rosof-Williams, MSN, APRN, FNP-BC, SANE-P, SANE-A

INTRODUCTION

Nurses' holistic bio-psycho-social-spiritual approach to patient care makes them well suited to address the health and forensic needs of patients who experience family violence. These patients must be identified and offered health care with forensic services and safety planning so the longer-term sequelae associated with violence may be reduced or even ameliorated. Advanced practice nurses (APRNs)'s knowledge and skills associated with clinical assessment, diagnosis, communication techniques, patient education, case management, and compassionate care make them ideal front line providers who enhance an individual patient's health and well-being.

Family violence involves one family member harming or putting another family member in imminent threat of harm through overt acts of violence or abuse (e.g., hitting, name calling) or acts of omission (e.g., withholding nutrition). Family violence includes child maltreatment, intimate partner violence (i.e., domestic violence), and elder mistreatment.

Family violence is a hidden, stigmatized, criminal act. Victim dynamics and offender tactics are powerful. Often the abuse is kept a secret for extended, if not indefinite, periods of time (1, 2). While patients may experience obvious signs of victimization (e.g., physical injury), these signs are often transient and no individual outside the family may witness the violence or signs associated with victimization. Unless a victim is willing to tell a non-family member, the abuse may never be detected. This makes family violence very difficult to identify and manage from the perspective of the health care system, health and human services, and criminal justice system. These challenges cannot prevent health care providers from responding to violence as a health care issue.

FAMILY VIOLENCE IS A HEALTH CARE ISSUE

In 1985, Surgeon General Koop recognized violence as a health care issue (3). In 2006, Surgeon General Carmona reaffirmed violence as a public health issue and recognized that federal, state, and local resources are necessary to identify abuse, implement safety measures, and offer a continuum of services to limit the negative sequalae associated with victimization (4). In 1991, the American Nurses Association (ANA) affirmed a nursing role in the management of intimate partner violence. In 2000, ANA published a Position Paper on Violence Against Women that supported the following (5):

1. Performing universal, routine assessment and further targeted screening of patients at increased risk for victimization (e.g., pregnant women, trauma victims, etc.).
2. Supporting patient autonomy by fostering a partnership between nurse and patient that allows for patient choice and safety planning.
3. Fostering the development of coordinated community systems to address abuse.
4. Educating all patients about the cycle of violence, the potential for homicide, and community resources for primary, secondary and tertiary prevention, and subsequent care.
5. Supporting research on violence against women.
6. Supporting the development of nurses who specialize in the care of patients who experience sexual assault.

COSTS ASSOCIATED WITH FAMILY VIOLENCE

The societal costs for violence are significant with respect to lost productivity and resource utilization; for intimate partner violence, including rape, physical assault, and stalking, they exceed $5.8 billion a year (6). Approximately $4.1 billion is for direct medical and mental health services, which accounts for more than two-thirds of the total societal costs (6). These figures are likely an underestimate of costs because of the under-reporting of intimate partner violence. Patients who are victims of intimate partner violence require services and should receive high-quality health care services. However, if our society could prevent violence and/or limit the negative outcomes associated with violence, the health care dollar savings could be impressive.

DEFINING FORMS OF FAMILY VIOLENCE

Family violence is complex and difficult to define, which, in turn, makes it difficult to identify. The labels people apply to individuals who experience violence (Box 6-1) can have profound meaning to patients, families, investigators, and agents of the criminal and civil justice systems. State legal definitions tell clinicians what kinds of cases must be reported and investigated by authorities. Nurses must know and correctly interpret their local state definitions of various forms of family violence. This chapter's content does not replace state statutes and does not offer legal advice in the interpretation of legal definitions of various forms of violence.

Generally, nurses provide care to "patients" or "clients." These terms connote a legal duty to provide services within a standard of care and scope of clinician practice. The provider-patient relationship is recognized by the criminal justice system as unique and special. In the criminal and civil justice systems the nurse's work product (e.g., medical record and its components) may become a form of evidence. This evidence can aid law enforcement (LE) and adult/child protective services (APS/CPS) in their investigations. In criminal proceedings the evidence may be presented by prosecution and/or defense during legal proceedings (e.g., preliminary hearings, trial, etc.) (7, 8).

Another term commonly used for individuals who experience violence is "survivor." In the author's clinical experience, this is a powerful term used in consideration of the patient's perception of her or his own situation. Some patients are ready and willing to believe

they survived their violent experience(s) while other patients are not as prepared to identify themselves as survivors.

"Victim" is a term that connotes a wronged individual or an individual without power or control. Agents associated with the criminal and civil justice systems may use the term to identify crime victims. In the author's clinical experience, the journey from victim to survivor is a complex one that takes time and/or professional counseling services.

Generally, society's legal interventions for family violence include but are not limited to reporting, investigation, mandated safety planning for victims, mandated treatment for victims and/or offenders, and criminal prosecution. Unfortunately, these interventions are not accessed by all reported cases, any nonreported cases, and are insufficient to treat the effects of family violence. Therefore, clinical definitions of family violence based on legal definitions and violence dynamics allow clinicians to more broadly identify cases and develop treatment plans not limited by legal interventions (7).

Family violence addresses violence across the life span and includes child, adult, and elder victims. The offenders are family members in the sense they have an intimate current or past relationship with the victims. The term "violence" includes overt acts of violence, abuse, and neglect.

Child Maltreatment

Child maltreatment affects children of all ages, backgrounds, and types of families. The common theme is that children and adolescents are not protected by parents or other caregivers. As a result these children are harmed or put in imminent risk of harm. Clinicians who serve adolescents will care for patients who have been and/or are currently victims of child maltreatment.

All states have laws defining child maltreatment, reporting mandates, and how the state will respond to

---

BOX 6–1 Labels and Meaning for Health Care Professionals in the Legal System

- Nurses provide care to "patients" or "clients": Connotes a legal duty to provide services within a standard of care and scope of clinician practice.
- Nurse's work product: The criminal and civil justice systems (e.g., medical record and its components) may become a form of evidence and can aid law enforcement and adult/child protective services in their investigations.
- In criminal proceedings the evidence may be presented by prosecution and/or defense during legal proceedings (e.g., preliminary hearings, trial, etc.).
- "Survivor": A powerful term used in consideration of the patient's perception of her or his own situation. Some patients are ready and willing to believe they survived their violent experience(s) while other patients are not as prepared to identify themselves as survivors.
- "Victim": A term that connotes a wronged individual or an individual without power or control. Agents associated with the criminal and civil justice systems may use the term to identify crime victims. In the author's clinical experience, the journey from victim to survivor is a complex one that takes time and/or professional counseling services.

allegations of abuse and neglect. Laws pertaining to definitions and reporting of family violence are listed in Box 6-2 (8). The individual state laws are derived from the federal Child Abuse Prevention and Treatment Act (CAPTA) and its subsequent amendments. The federal legislation defines child abuse and neglect as (1) any recent act or failure to act on the part of a parent or caretaker that results in death, serious physical or emotional harm, or sexual abuse or exploitation; or (2) an act or failure to act that presents an imminent risk of serious harm (9).

This definition recognizes child maltreatment does not have to be violent or result in harm before the state can investigate, provide services, and/or prosecute. Also, this definition allows for variation among individual states' legal definitions of child maltreatment. Clinicians must know and correctly interpret their local state's definitions of child maltreatment, which in turn will influence when they are mandatory reporters of crimes involving pediatric victims. While an individual case may not meet local state definitions of maltreatment, clinical interventions may strengthen families, thereby improving child safety and health outcomes.

Child maltreatment includes but is not limited to neglect, physical abuse, sexual abuse, emotional/ psychological abuse, and abandonment. Table 6-1 outlines conceptual definitions and examples of various forms of child maltreatment in adolescents (10, 11). Hopefully, this will help clinicians identify cases

---

BOX 6–2 Reporting Family Violence

- The Child Welfare Information Gateway is a service of the Children's Bureau, Administration for Children and Families, US Department of Health and Human Services that provides information about individual state statutes and child maltreatment (http://www.childwelfare.gov).
- The American Prosecutors Research Institute provides information about state statutes and reporting relevant to:
  1. Intimate partner violence, http://www.ndaa.org/apri/programs/vawa/dv reporting requirements.html
  2. Rape, http://www.ndaa.org/apri/programs/vawa/state rape reportings requirements.html
- The American Bar Association provides annual summaries of state legislation amending Adult Protective Services laws, which clarify definitions of elder mistreatment, http://www.abanet.org/aging/elderabuse.shtml

---

TABLE 6–1 Clinical Definitions of Child Maltreatment and Examples

Forms of Child Maltreatment	Conceptual Definitions	Examples in Adolescent Patient Population
PHYSICAL ABUSE		
	Nonaccidental physical injury or otherwise harm to a child that is inflicted by a parent, caregiver, or other person who has responsibility for the child. The injury is considered abuse regardless of whether the caregiver intended to hurt the child (9).	• Parent slaps teenage daughter in face after breaking curfew. • A grandfather pushes teenage grandson to ground during an argument.
CHILD SEXUAL ABUSE		
	Sexual activities intended for sexual stimulation and the presence of at least one abusive condition. Activities: • Contact sexual activities (e.g., genital fondling, oral-genital contact, child being made to touch offender's genitals) • Noncontact sexual activities (e.g., exposure to pornography) • Excludes activities related to caregiving and health care services	• A grandfather inserts his penis in his teenage granddaughter's vagina. • Teenage male performs cunnilingus on his adult aunt. • Teenage female's breasts are fondled by her mother's boyfriend.

TABLE 6–1 Clinical Definitions of Child Maltreatment and Examples—cont'd

Forms of Child Maltreatment	Conceptual Definitions	Examples in Adolescent Patient Population
CHILD SEXUAL ABUSE		
	Abusive condition: • Offender has a maturational advantage • Offender is in a position of authority (e.g., teacher, clergy) • Offender has a caregiving role (e.g., parent, grandparent, custodian) • Activities are carried out using force, bribery, or trickery (e.g., alcohol ingestion)	
RAPE		
	One person does not consent to sexual activity with another person. Consent is not obtained under any of the following conditions: • Overt use of force (e.g., hitting, restraining) • Threat of force (e.g., I will kill your mother if you don't do this) • Patient indicates she or he does not want to engage in sexual activity (e.g., patient says "no" or "stop" or tries to physically leave). • Patient is intoxicated during sexual contact. • Offender abuses power to gain patient's compliance for sexual activity. • Sexual activity is misrepresented as a therapeutic intervention by a helping professional (e.g., therapist).	• Teenage female reports her boyfriend made her "have sex" with him. • Teenage male has penile-anal intercourse with the "house father" of his residential treatment center. • Teenage female is forced to perform fellatio when she is told "do it or I will kill you" by her adult male "date." • Teenage female has penile-vaginal intercourse with peer while intoxicated by alcohol.
STATUTORY RAPE		
	The teenager is not competent to give consent and engages in sexual activity with an older person. The teen may volunteer and cooperate with sexual activity. Individual state statute outlines the age of consent for teenagers and when the age difference between a teenager and another person makes the sexual activity illegal.	• Teenage male has intercourse with adult male.
NEGLECT		
	Act's commission or omission committed by parent/caregiver so that a child does not receive adequate nutrition, shelter, medical care, clothing, education, supervision, and/or other. Note—poverty, cultural values, and community standards will influence interpretation of neglect cases.	• Teenage diabetic does not have opportunity to receive adequate nutrition. • Teenage male comes out to his parents as a homosexual and he is told to leave the family home.

Continued

TABLE 6–1 Clinical Definitions of Child Maltreatment and Examples—cont'd

Forms of Child Maltreatment	Conceptual Definitions	Examples in Adolescent Patient Population
EMOTIONAL/PSYCHOLOGICAL ABUSE		
	Impairs child emotional development and sense of self-worth. May include overtly critical caregivers, threats, rejection, and/or withholding love, support, or guidance. Note—emotional/psychological abuse is co-morbid with other forms of child maltreatment	• Teenage female has been told "all her life" she is fat and lazy. • Teenage male is told to "man up" when his fear of crowded spaces triggers a panic attack.
ABANDONMENT		
	When parents' identity and/or location is unknown OR child is not adequately supervised and suffers serious harm OR parent does not maintain contact or provide reasonable support	• While teenage female was on "runaway," she was raped by strangers while on the street. Parents refuse to come to emergency department to assist with evaluation and take teen home after evaluation.

so treatment plans can reflect referrals, reporting activities, monitoring, and family support.

Intimate Partner Violence

Intimate partner violence involves physically assaultive and coercive behaviors used by one individual to control another individual. Behaviors can involve obvious physical acts of violence (e.g., hitting, slapping, pulling hair, etc.) to the more subtle coercion and manipulation that demeans, demoralizes, and isolates an individual. The intimate relationships involve adolescents, adults, and elders in a variety of relationships (e.g., dating, married, divorced, separating, and broken-up) (12). The partners are generally peers, but violence between adults and adolescents may be a form of child maltreatment. The partners can be of the same sex. Both individuals may engage in some form of violence and manipulation. Women abuse men.

The seminal work by Lenore Walker proposed that violence between intimate partners is cyclical and each stage or phase can be characterized by offender and victim behaviors (13). Note this is a theory and does not fit all cases of intimate partner violence. However, this theory can be helpful for defining intimate partner violence because a spectrum of behaviors and tactics can be identified and discussed. This theory proposes that couples involved in violent relationships will go through phases that promote the offender's control and the victim's entrapment. Table 6-2 outlines the phases, offender tactics, and partner responses.

Elder Mistreatment

Elders have a lifetime of knowledge and experience, which allows them to care for themselves in a manner they enjoy and/or desire. However, over time, many elders (but not all) will experience functional decline and increased dependency. These elders' vulnerabilities will place their daily care, longer term well-being, and financial resources in other's hands (14). The elders' vulnerabilities put them at risk for many of the forms of abuse and neglect seen in childhood. Elders experience neglect, physical abuse, sexual abuse, and emotional/psychological abuse at the hands of their caregivers, family members, or strangers (15, 16). In almost 90% of the elder abuse and neglect cases, the perpetrator is a family member (17). The elders may be neglected or abused in their home or institutional setting. As opposed to child maltreatment, many elders have resources, including Social Security, retirement funds, an owned home, medications, etc., that can be exploited or stolen (15, 16). This is a form of financial exploitation that is seen less commonly in childhood or adolescence. In addition, elder adults experience intimate partner violence and the violent relationship may have been

TABLE 6-2 Characteristics of Intimate Partner Violent Relationships

Phases	Offender Tactics	Partner Responses
1. Tension Building. The pressure builds between the offender and partner. The partner may try to placate the offender to avoid abuse/violence or the partner may provoke the offender to release the stress and move forward to the calmer phase.	• Display negative emotions (e.g., moody, angry, jealous) • Display possessive behaviors (e.g., jealous of time spent with others, accuse partner of flirting/infidelity) • Scornful of partner's perspective, knowledge, skills, etc. • Use/abuse substances (e.g., alcohol, prescribed drugs) • Isolate partner (e.g., take phone, hide car keys, chase away family/friends) • Control access to resources (e.g., money, insurance card, passport) and social network (e.g., family, friends, work colleagues, and health care providers)	• Manage offender's emotions (e.g., placate) • Keep the home calm and quiet (e.g., children quiet, visitors out of home) • Exhibit fear of offender • Express fear/concerns for personal safety, safety of children, safety of pets, etc.
2. Crisis/Violence. The tension breaks and the offender hurts the partner through emotional/ psychological abuse, sexual abuse, and/or physical violence.	• Physical abuse—pushing, slapping, restraining • Verbally abuse partner (e.g., "you are too stupid to work," "nobody will believe you," "you are too ugly ... nobody wants you") • Sexual abuse—forced/coercive sex acts, unprotected sex • Psychological/emotional abuse—threatening family pets, family members, destroying favored items	• Survival mode • Become quiet/passive • Become physically aggressive • Call for help • Seek health care services
3. Calm. Offender may become contrite, romantic, apologetic, and/or demonstrate guilt. The offender and victim may believe the crisis/violence won't happen again.	• Explain away/rationalize the violence. • Be vague about violence • Apologize/ask for forgiveness • Purchase gifts • Engage in romantic/courting behaviors • Have offensive wounds on body from partner defending her/himself.	• Minimize/deny the violence/abuse • Forgive/remain with batterer • Forgive/return to batterer • Feel valued/loved • Blame self for the violence/abuse • Experience somatic and psychological health problems

ongoing for decades. Table 6-3 summarizes forms of elder mistreatment and provides examples.

INCIDENCE OF FAMILY VIOLENCE

The real prevalence and incidence of family violence are not known. The criminal nature of the acts, the pressures to not report, and the methodologic difficulties in studying family violence make it impossible to obtain an accurate count of incidents. However, current rates of family

violence (Box 6-3) indicate that if providers choose to identify victims, these patients will be seen in all health care settings.

The U.S. Bureau of Justice Statistics report from the National Crime Victimization Survey indicates that U.S. residents over the age of 12 years experience approximately 23 million crimes per year (18, 19). Seventy-six percent of the crimes were against property, and 23% were violent crimes against a person (19). Teens and young adults experienced the highest rates of violent crimes, which included homicide, rape,

TABLE 6–3 Clinical Definitions of Elder Mistreatment and Examples

Forms of Elder Mistreatment	Conceptual Definitions	Examples
PHYSICAL ABUSE		
	The use of physical force that results in or may or may not result in bodily injury, physical pain, or impairment	• Caregiver restrains elder who is getting up too much. • Son threatens to hit his father if he "doesn't shut-up."
SEXUAL ABUSE		
	Elder experiences sexual activities with another who is responsible for health, safety, or well-being Sexual Activities: • Contact sexual activities (e.g., genital fondling, oral-genital contact, elder being made to touch offender's genitals) • Noncontact sexual activities (e.g., elder not draped appropriately, sexual language used in front of elder)	• Elder woman's son fondles his mother's breasts during visits to the nursing home.
RAPE		
	One person does not consent to sexual activity with another person	• Male elder has penile-vaginal intercourse with his wife against her will.
NEGLECT		
	The refusal or failure to fulfill any part of obligations or duties to an elder	• Granddaughter has financial responsibility for her grandfather and does not pay his bills in a timely manner.
SELF-NEGLECT		
	The behaviors of an elderly person that threaten his or her own health or safety Note: The definition of self-neglect excludes situations in which a mentally competent person who understands the consequences of his or her decisions makes a conscious and voluntary decision to engage in acts that threaten his or her health or safety	• Elder does not bathe for 7 days when she or he has the ability and means to practice sound hygiene. • Elder does not eat when she or he has the resources and ability to prepare food.
EMOTIONAL/PSYCHOLOGICAL ABUSE		
	The infliction of anguish, pain, or distress	• A vulnerable adult in a residential facility is told she or he will be punished "real bad" if she or he does not stop yelling and crying.

TABLE 6–3 Clinical Definitions of Elder Mistreatment and Examples—cont'd

Forms of Elder Mistreatment	Conceptual Definitions	Examples
ABANDONMENT		
	• An individual who had physical custody or otherwise had assumed responsibility for providing care for an elder deserts elder • A person with physical custody of an elder deserts elder	• Elder is left in day care center hours after closing time.
FINANCIAL OR MATERIAL EXPLOITATION OR ABUSE		
	• The illegal or improper use of an elder's funds, property, or assets	• Adult grandson moves in with grandparents and starts selling unused household goods without permission. • Adult daughter gains access to her mother's bank accounts and starts paying her household expenses from her mother's account without permission.

BOX 6–3 Important Statistics and Family Violence

• Family violence accounted for 11% of all reported and unreported violence between 1998 and 2002.
• About 22% of murders in 2002 were family murders.
• National child maltreatment estimates report 794,000 children were victims of maltreatment in 2007. The rate of victimization was 10.6 per 1,000 children in the US in 2007.
• In a national survey to estimate the incidence of intimate partner violence, 25% of women and 7.6% of surveyed men reported they were raped and/or physically assaulted by a current or former intimate partner at some time during their lifetime.
• Approximately 1.5 million women and 834,732 men are raped and/or physically assaulted by an intimate partner annually in the United States.
• The National Elder Abuse Incidence Study reported approximately 450,000 elderly in domestic settings were abused and/or neglected during 1996. When self-neglect is added, approximately 551,000 elderly were mistreated in 1996. Elders over 80 years of age are mistreated two to three times their proportion of the elderly population.
• In a more recent national sample, 9% of adults between 57 and 85 years of age reported verbal mistreatment, 3.5% financial mistreatment, and 0.2% physical mistreatment in the past year.

---

robbery, and assault (19, 20). While any age patient may be sexually abused or raped, statistics indicate that sex crimes predominantly involve adolescents and young adult victims (21, 22).

SOCIETAL RESPONSE TO FAMILY VIOLENCE

Multiple agencies are involved in the investigation, safety and treatment planning, plan implementation, and prosecution of offenders. Clinicians will interact with these agencies during all phases of a case if the allegations or concerns of family violence are reported to authorities. This interaction will be influenced by institutional policies related to patient confidentiality, release of medical records, and procedures to facilitate testimony in criminal and civil court systems. The key stakeholders in the management of family violence include, but are not limited to, APS, CPS, LE, and agents of the criminal and civil justice system. Since nurses are not routinely educated about these agencies, the following is a brief discussion of these agencies' duties. How clinicians interface with these agencies will be outlined in more detail when the health care provider's response to family violence is discussed later in the chapter.

Adult Protective Services

Individual state APS were established under Title XX of the Social Security Act in 1975. The federal legislation was essentially an unfunded mandate (23). The legislation required states to develop programs to protect and serve older adults and adults with disabilities who were being mistreated or in danger of being mistreated (24). As a result each state has developed APS programs given individual states' definitions of elder and vulnerable adult mistreatment, the state elder and vulnerable adult populations' needs, and state resources (24). States have passed laws that mandate development of a centralized system to receive reports of adult/elder abuse and neglect; investigate reports; intervene with victims by offering them services; and deliver services to adults/elders with diminished capacity through involuntary interventions (23). APS programs are the first responders to reports of abuse, neglect, and exploitation of vulnerable adults.

Child Protective Services

In 1974 the Child Abuse Prevention and Treatment Act (CAPTA) was enacted. It was recently amended and reauthorized by the Keeping Children and Families Safe Act of 2003. This federal legislation provides funding to states to support of prevention, assessment, investigation, prosecution, and treatment for children and families. Thus CAPTA provided the mandate and support to develop CPS in all 50 states (25).

Children are exceptionally vulnerable due to their dependency on caregivers for all of the necessities of life, health, and happiness. Generally, parental/legal guardian's caregiving responsibilities do not legally cease until a child turns 18 years of age. As children progress to adolescence, their vulnerabilities change given their personal development and needs. If parents/legal guardian's actions or inactions leave their child injured or at serious risk of harm, then CPS is one of the mandated agency that responds.

CPS's societal intervention is based on the concept of *parens patriae*, which is the legal term that asserts the government's role in protecting minors (17 years or younger). If parents or other legal guardians fail to protect or harm a minor, then the government will intervene. CPS is but one agency that intervenes, but it is the one with key responsibilities for investigating allegations of child maltreatment, developing safety plans, implementing safety and treatment plans, and monitoring children's and families' response to interventions. More specifically, CPS is responsible for (1) receiving reports of suspicion or concern regarding child maltreatment; (2) conducting initial assessments and investigations from reports; (3) assessing families' strengths, resources, and needs; (4) developing case plans to enhance children's safety and well-being; and (5) implementing plans by providing direct services, coordinating services by other professionals, and completing case management functions (25).

LAW ENFORCEMENT

Police officers are one of the most commonly identified LE officials. However, LE officials may work for city, county, state, or federal agencies and are not limited to police departments. The LE agency that investigates a crime will be determined, for the most part, by jurisdiction. An LE agency's jurisdiction is the geographic location where the agency can apply its powers. Also, LE's involvement in initial assessment and investigation of family violence will vary across states and communities due to the nature of family violence (e.g., child abuse, intimate partner violence, sex crime, etc.), state and federal statutes and regulations, and local resources. Box 6-4 describes the primary responsibilities of LE officials when investigating crimes associated with family violence.

When child maltreatment cases are reported, frequently CPS and LE both respond and participate in the investigation. While each agency may seek out similar information, they use the information for very different

---

BOX 6–4 Primary Responsibilities of Law Enforcement and Investigating Sex Crimes

- Identifying and reporting suspected cases of child maltreatment to other agencies (e.g., CPS)
- Receiving reports of child maltreatment
- Conducting investigations when a crime may have been committed
- Managing physical evidence (e.g., identification, collection, preservation, and storage)
- Identifying and investigating evidence that can support prosecution
- Protecting victims and family members
- Providing protection to CPS staff when necessary
- Supporting the victim through processes of the criminal justice system

reasons. During the initial investigation phase, CPS is focused on minors' current and future safety, measures to keep minors safe, injuries/harm suffered by the minor, risk of future maltreatment, and what community services are needed to address maltreatment or risk of future maltreatment. LE focuses on determining if a crime occurred, identifying potential offenders, managing physical evidence, identifying and interviewing witnesses, and determining if there is enough evidence to arrest a suspect. Finally both agencies evaluate the evidence to determine if the allegations can be corroborated by other sources (e.g., witnesses, physical evidence), identify other victims, and determine if the minor should be separated from parents/legal guardians (25).

Forensic Nurses

Forensic nurses' practice interfaces or potentially interfaces with the legal system (26). Nurses from a wide variety of backgrounds work in a variety of clinical and nonclinical settings (e.g., attorney's offices). Forensic nurses' scope of practice includes health care services for patients with emphasis on the identification, retrieval, storage, and release of a variety of forms of evidence (26). The evidence includes the documentation of the medical history, which can be a form of evidence in legal proceedings, documentation of physical injury (e.g., bruising, abrasions, penetrating wounds, etc.), physical evidence (e.g., seminal products, bullets, urine and blood samples for drug screens), and establishing and maintaining the chain of evidence (27-29). In addition, forensic nurses address patient short- and longer-term health care needs by either directly providing care (e.g., cleaning wounds after documentation, prescribing pregnancy prophylaxis) and/or referring for additional services (e.g., emergency physician for more advanced assessment and treatment, mental health professionals for counseling and support, etc.).

In cases of family violence, forensic nurses often work closely with CPS, APS, LE, and attorneys associated with the civil and criminal justice systems. Forensic nurses contribute key information so each agency can more effectively perform its duties. As a result of the nursing and forensic services they provide, forensic nurses testify in a wide variety of legal proceedings including but not limited to depositions, preliminary hearings, civil and criminal trials, postconviction relief hearings, and probation hearings (30). Forensic nurses educate others about the nursing profession, topics related to forensic services and findings (e.g., evidence management, injury patterns consistent with inflicted injury, etc.), and characteristics of individual cases. Forensic nurses are an invaluable resource to health care providers and patients alike because of their specialized knowledge and skills.

CLINICAL PRESENTATION

Family violence is not a quickly resolved or easily managed clinical situation. However, when clinicians know family violence is a component of the chief complaint or the primary reason for the patient's visit, the agenda for the clinical visit is obvious. For example, a father is shot by his son, a patient reports she was raped by her boyfriend last night, or an elderly woman reports her nephew is selling her pain medication. Both patient and clinician know family violence must be addressed during the clinical visit.

In the second situation, a patient presents and wants the provider to figure out she or he is a victim of family violence. The patient wants help. However, the patient will not voluntarily disclose unless asked and/or supported through the disclosure process. Thus, if the provider does not consider family violence part of the clinical picture, the victimization will be missed. For instance, a clinician asks an elderly male patient if he feels safe at home and after a long pause and no eye contact he denies being fearful. The clinician reviews with the patient his repeated patterns of injury and gently suggests there is more to his story. The clinician lets the patient know she or he is willing to listen if the patient would like to talk about his home life.

In another situation, the patient does not want to address the family violence during her or his clinical visit. For example, the patient's physical exam suggests she is a victim of strangulation but she will not report the details. The clinician may discover the abuse and the patient is unprepared and/or unwilling to address the abuse.

Finally, the discovery of abuse can be a surprise to everyone, including care providers and clinicians. For instance, an elderly woman in a secure dementia unit is diagnosed with a sexually transmitted infection when the laboratory reports indicate she has gonorrhea.

All of these situations require different clinical approaches and finesse. The following will help improve clinicians' knowledge about signs/symptoms of family violence and clinical approaches for all presentation types.

Signs and Symptoms Associated with Family Violence

Signs and symptoms of family violence must be considered in the context of the patient's culture, current situation, and physical and cognitive development. Identifying signs and symptoms requires clinicians to ask questions in a skillful and sensitive manner. The most important "sign" of family violence is the patient's disclosure or statement about the abuse. Often there is no other sign or symptom other than the history describing the violence, abuse, and/or neglect.

Patients who experience family violence often have chaotic and unpredictable lives. They are trying to maintain "normal lives" while keeping a painful secret. The nature and severity of symptoms will vary across patients and during a single patient's lifetime as the nature of the violence and abuse alter and the patient's coping mechanisms adapt or fail to adapt. It is important to note that the majority of signs and symptoms of family violence are nonspecific and are seen in the nonabused patient population. In addition, some patients who experience family violence may report no significant signs and symptoms, while other patients will experience multiple signs and symptoms. The severity of symptoms may not be related to the severity of the violence. Abuse severity is subjective, which means what is considered "bad" will vary by individuals. Finally, clinicians cannot judge the veracity of patients' history based on clinical signs and symptoms.

Emotionally, adolescents and adults who experience family violence may appear evasive and noncompliant as they miss appointments; evade discussions about their living situation, partners, and/or caregivers; do not follow-up with clinicians' recommendations; and hesitate to explain patterned injuries and patterns of injury (31). Patients may report insomnia, sadness, or fearfulness. Patients may present with clinical diagnoses of depression and/or anxiety as well as the symptoms of depression and/or anxiety. Patients' unpredictable home life, isolation, and emotional pain may cause them to seek pain and/or psychotropic medications. If the abusive family member accompanies the patient during the evaluation, she or he may attempt to or will successfully accompany the patient during the entire visit. Thus, the patient may never have a chance to disclose and discuss her or his options.

Medically, patients who experience family violence report an increase in symptoms compared to nonabused population (32, 33). Patients can repeatedly report vague complaints with multiple body systems involved, yet no definitive cause for complaints can be identified despite all the clinician's and patient's efforts. Table 6-4 outlines potential signs and symptoms associated with intimate partner violence by systems (34-36).

Signs and Symptoms Associated with Physical Abuse

The physical signs associated with physical violence focus on on patterns and patterned injuries that indicate the injuries are inflicted rather than accidental. Evaluators must consider other causes (e.g., congenital, infectious process) associated with findings to adequately address differential diagnoses and correctly attribute findings to specific cause. In addition, many inflicted injuries heal without lasting physical changes. If the acute findings are not documented while acute or healing, then valuable physical evidence will be lost to investigators (e.g., CPS, APS, and LE) and the district attorney's office. All findings must be considered in the context of the patient's history, when available, and given the individual patient's development and capabilities. Box 6-5 lists characteristics that typify nonaccidental injury. Box 6-6 provides descriptions of injury patterns commonly found in nonaccidental injury.

Bruising is a common physical finding, especially in individuals who are mobile. The appearance of bruises is influenced by a wide variety of factors described in Box 6-7.

Bruising *cannot* be dated by its color based on simple physical examination. Furthermore, bruises that occurred at the same time can have different coloration at the same point in time and over time (37).

Signs and Symptoms of Sexual Abuse and Rape

If the sexual abuse or rape involved physical violence, then many of the injury patterns seen in physical

TABLE 6-4 Signs and Symptoms Associated With Intimate Partner Violence

System	Signs/Symptoms
General/constitutional	Poor general sense of health and well-being, chronic pain
Skin	Unexplained bruising/injury
HEENT	Headaches, dental pain, oral injuries, neck stiffness/pain, injury
Cardiovascular	Palpitation, dyspnea, pain
Respiratory	Shortness of breath, dyspnea
Gastrointestinal	Changes in appetite, abdominal pain
Genitourinary	Dysuria, vaginal discharge, changes in libido, genital injury, discharge, dysmenorrheal, postmenopausal bleeding, pregnancy, spontaneous and therapeutic abortions, repeated urinary track complaints and infections
Musculoskeletal	Pain, limitation in range of motion, injury
Neurologic/psychiatric	Mood disorders, anxiety, depression, memory problems

BOX 6–5 Characteristics of Nonaccidental Injury

- Injury without explanation or the "magical injury"
- Injury history substantively changes over time
- Injury is implausible given patient's development and capabilities
- Injury is implausible given the provided history
- Injuries seen over generally well-protected body surfaces
- Delay in seeking medical care for injuries that warrant care
- Patterned injury or the injury appearance suggests the implement that caused the injury
- Patterns of injury that indicate an event (e.g., defensive wounds to hands and forearms)
- Patterns of injury that are repeatedly inconsistent with history over time
- Patient and/or caregiver unconcerned about significant injury

BOX 6–6 Injury Patterns Suggestive of Nonaccidental Injury

Injury to head, neck, chest, posterior torso breasts, abdomen, buttocks, and/or genitals

Variety of injuries in different stages of healing

Ligature marks indicating restraint (e.g., cord or rope marks around wrists, neck, ankles)

Grasp marks suggesting restraint (e.g., 4 circular-oval "finger tip" bruising on forearm)

Slap marks (e.g., tramline bruising where the fingers leave imprint with bruising between the digits and sparing where digits impacted body)

Bite marks

Linear, curve-linear, and loop mark injuries (e.g., bruising, abrasions) over trunk or extremities

Physical injury during pregnancy, especially on the breasts and abdomen

BOX 6–7 Considerations in Assessment of Bruises

- Surface of impacting object (or surface)
- Force of the impact
- Depth of injury
- Available space for the blood to collect
- Vascularity of the impacted area
- Fragility of the blood vessels
- Location of the bruise—resilient areas (not over boney area) less likely to injure
- Individual patient characteristics—e.g., weight, skin color, chronic illnesses, medications, etc.

abuse can be seen in sexual abuse and assault. It is important to note many patients may have no physical findings after sexual abuse or rape (38). The presence of injury and other forms of transient trace physical evidence diminishes over time. Therefore, the most important "sign and symptom" of sexual abuse or rape is the patient's disclosure of the event. Other signs and symptoms of sexual abuse or rape are outlined in Box 6-8.

Signs and Symptoms of Neglect

Generally, neglect involves a caregiver not providing for the patient's needs, including but not limited to nutrition, hydration, hygiene, shelter, clothing, medical care, education, and emotional and psychological well-being. As a result, the signs and symptoms of neglect involve signs of malnutrition, dehydration, malodorous body odor, poor dentition, lack of clothing, clothing inappropriate for weather, truancy for adolescents, patient's mobility inappropriately limited, skin break down (e.g., pressure ulcers), depression, and anxiety. It is important to note that the cause of these signs and symptoms is not limited to neglect and may be seen in a wide variety of conditions and situations.

Signs and Symptoms of Self-neglect

"Self-neglect" is a term generally applied to adults and elders who do not provide adequate care for themselves, thereby jeopardizing their well-being, health, and safety. Self-neglect is difficult to address because it is neither a health care problem nor a social problem but rather both (39). Generally, adults who neglect themselves have deficits in multiple domains, including physical, cognitive, and/or functional abilities, and live in squalid situations (17, 41). In a study of the medical records of 460 patients over the age of 65 years

---

BOX 6–8 Signs and Symptoms Associated With Sexual Abuse and Assault

- Patient reports she or he was raped
- Injury to breast, buttocks, anal and/or genital areas without adequate history
- Presence of ano-genital injury, sexually transmitted infections, pregnancy and/or seminal products with an individual who cannot consent to sexual activity
- Ano-genital and/or urinary tract complaints (e.g., dysuria, pain) without etiology
- Repeated diagnosis of sexually transmitted infections and patient reports compliance with treatment

---

identified as neglecting self, 50% demonstrated impaired mental status, 15% had abnormal depression scores, 76.3% had impaired physical performance test scores, and 95% had poor to moderate social support (40). The authors developed a model postulating that impaired executive functioning leads to functional impairment in the setting of inadequate medical care and social support (40).

The signs and symptoms of self-neglect are similar to those of neglect. In addition, self-neglectful adults and elders often refuse to leave their homes (39). These elders have limited opportunities to interact with systems that detect their self-harm. Thus, elders who do not keep their appointments, are lost to follow-up, report a diminished or diminishing social support, or have an exacerbation of medical conditions may require home visits to assess their living situation and ability to care for themselves.

Signs and Symptoms of Financial Abuse and Exploitation

Financial exploitation is generally used to describe the abuse of elders and vulnerable adults. To gain insight into the signs of financial exploitation, 164 professionals with extensive experience investigating and addressing elder financial abuse reached consensus on the common elements seen in financial exploitation. The common elements seen in cases of financial exploitation are summarized in Box 6-9.

DIAGNOSIS

Diagnostics focus on interviewing techniques to screen for family violence. Additional diagnostic tests and lab studies are often used given presentation (e.g., unconscious patient, aggressive/noncompliant patient) and injury patterns. This chapter will not address these additional studies.

Screening for family violence is required by institutions accredited by The Joint Commission (TJC). TJC standards require institutions to identify and respond to victims of physical assault, rape and sexual molestation, domestic abuse, elder neglect/abuse, and child neglect/abuse (42). As a result, health care staff must be educated about interpersonal violence, including family violence, screening techniques, and procedures for responding to negative and positive screens (42).

BOX 6–9 Common Elements Seen in Financial Exploitation

An elder or vulnerable adult is impaired due to medical, pharmacologic, psychological, and/or social problems

Another individual establishes a trusting relationship with elder through variety of means, including deceit, intimidation, becoming overly involved in elder's life, or creating dependency so that the elder becomes vulnerable and/or compliant

The perpetrator gains access to and uses the elder's assets and resources (e.g., cash, trust funds, valuables, and material goods)

The elder is kept isolated and controlled and/or the transactions are kept secret

An unbiased, qualified expert did not assess elder's mental capacity and self-determination or the situation to determine if undue influence was exercised to gain access to elder's resources

If assets are transferred, the benefit to elder is not proportional to the value of assets to the perpetrator or the transfer is inconsistent with elder's previous behaviors or beliefs

Common business or personal ethics are not followed; including no written agreements, no full disclosures, no means for elder to change his or her mind, and no assessment for conflicts of interest

The perpetrator does not consider the effects of the transaction on others, including elder, family members, beneficiaries, or the public welfare system

The institution must develop and implement a standard for screening that is met when patients enter the system and when repeated periodic screenings are performed thereafter.

SCREENING FOR FAMILY VIOLENCE

Screening for child maltreatment, intimate partner violence, and elder mistreatment requires sound clinical interviewing techniques and a compassionate, unflappable demeanor. Screening is not limited to the triage nurse asking, "Do you feel safe in your home?" Rather a clinician must be sensitive to the signs and symptoms of family violence and follow up on cues presenting during chief complaint, past medical history, review of systems, physical exam, and/or by reviewing the entire medical record to gain insight into patterns over time.

There is some controversy in screening for family violence. In 2004, the U.S. Preventive Services Task Force (USPSTF) published recommendations pertaining to the efficacy of family violence screening. "The USPSTF found no direct evidence that screening for family and intimate partner violence leads to decreased disability or premature death. The USPSTF found no existing studies that determine the accuracy of screening tools for identifying family and intimate partner violence among children, women, or older adults in the general population" (44). However, TJC requires accredited institutions to screen for violence, including family violence. Other key professional organizations including the American Medical Association, American Academy of Pediatrics, American College of Obstetricians and Gynecologists, American Academy of Family Physicians (43), and American Nurses Association (5) support screening. The absence of evidence does not equate a recommendation for no screening but rather further study weighing the benefits and costs of screening need to be performed. Given current professional recommendations and TJC requirements, health care professionals must be prepared to screen for family violence.

Along with screening, providers must identify cases they are required to report to authorities by local state statute. TJC requires providers to refer victims of violence to local public and private community agencies for services related to treatment and promotion of safety and well-being. Institutions will identify advocacy and support services within health care settings and refer to community advocacy and support services for all types of patients (e.g., elder, hearing impaired, vision impaired, etc.). Finally, data suggest patients perceive screening for violence as part of the health care provider's role (43-46). Thus, clinicians are expected to ask patients about their "private lives," including experiences with violence.

Screening for intimate partner violence should be avoided only in rare exceptions: when private space cannot be used to screen, when screening will make the patient and/or provider unsafe (e.g., potential offender will not allow for privacy), or when an appropriate interpreter cannot be found (12).

Screening Techniques

Screening for family violence begins with asking patients questions. The setting, how the questions are asked, and the clinician's approach will influence the victim's disclosure process. Ideally, patients are screened repeatedly over time as their intimate relationships and their readiness to disclose family violence will vary over their lifetime. Suggestions for when to screen for intimate partner violence are provided in Box 6-10.

When screening for any form of family violence, the patient must be interviewed or complete a questionnaire alone. Patients will have a wide variety of reasons for not disclosing maltreatment in front of family members and caregivers. Some reasons include embarrassment, retribution by the perpetrator if she or he finds out about the disclosure, hopelessness, fear of not being believed, and/or fear the disclosure of abuse will result in other negative outcomes (e.g., negative reactions to homosexuality, drug abuse, mental illness, or remaining with offender). The forces preventing disclosures are impressive.

How patients are screened for family violence is often dictated by available resources and feasibility of implementing screening protocols. Screening for family violence can be conducted via paper and pencil tools, computer-facilitated screening, and interviews. Screening techniques will be shaped by patient literacy and patient-provider shared understanding of language. Data support that while women perceive that

---

BOX 6–10 When to Screen for Intimate Partner Violence

- During every new patient encounter
- As part of the routine health history
- As part of the standard health assessment (or at every encounter in urgent care)
- During periodic comprehensive health visits (assess for current victimization only)
- During a visit for a new chief complaint (assess for current victimization only)
- At every new intimate relationship (assess for current victimization only)
- When signs and symptoms raise concerns
- Other times at the provider's discretion

clinicians should screen for family violence, it may be easier for patients to make the initial disclosure via a paper and pencil questionnaire or form (44, 47). There are numerous questionnaires available for screening for family violence (49-55) and examples are outlined in Table 6-5.

Screening children and adolescents for child maltreatment is complicated because the offender is often a parent and informant. The parent/caregiver will be hesitant to answer direct questions about abusive and neglectful behaviors (48). Therefore, it is vital to interview adolescents alone. The adolescent may provide a history relevant to child maltreatment, intimate partner violence, or some other form of interpersonal violence.

While paper and pencil tools will be used in some settings, it is acceptable to screen for family violence by

TABLE 6–5 Examples of Screening Tools for Family Violence

Name	Target Audience/Information	Notes
ELDER ABUSE SCREENING TEST (EAST)		
	Elder mistreatment	15 items Completed by a health care provider based on the patient's responses Limited because of the small unrepresentative samples used to test it, the low internal consistency, and a relatively high false-negative rate [50]
ELDER ASSESSMENT INSTRUMENT (EAI)		
	Reviews signs, symptoms, and subjective complaints of elder abuse, neglect, exploitation, and abandonment	• 41-item scale • Used by variety of health care providers in variety of settings • Free online video demonstrating – http://links.lww.com/A321
ELDERS' PSYCHOLOGICAL ABUSE SCALE (EPAS)		
	Screening for psychological abuse in elders	• 32 items
FAMILY VIOLENCE QUALITY ASSESSMENT TOOL		
	Screens for child abuse, intimate partner violence, and elder mistreatment in primary care setting	• 111 items with 9 categories
INDICATORS OF ABUSE (IOA)		
	Discriminating abuse and nonabuse cases elder mistreatment	• 22 items • Completed by a health care professional after home assessment
SELF-NEGLECT SEVERITY SCALE (SSS)		
	Based on observation and interview with elder and is administered in the home to include an environmental assessment	• Research measure • Developed with APS workers and national experts. • First self-neglect measure

TABLE 6-5 Examples of Screening Tools for Family Violence—cont'd

Name	Target Audience/Information	Notes
WOMAN ABUSE SCREENING TOOL (WAST)		
	Victims of intimate partner violence	• Long version— • Short version—1st two questions from WAST • Clinicians and patient report comfortable using the short version.
WOMEN'S EXPERIENCE WITH BATTERING (WEB) SCALE		
	Victims of intimate partner violence	• 10-item scale

asking questions of patients and/or other informants. Clinical interviewing allows clinicians to use familiar skills to gather information in a sensitive manner while reducing the potential for compromising an investigation (56). Table 6-6 outlines interviewing techniques and implications in cases of family violence.

In addition to the aforementioned interviewing techniques, framing questions and direct questions can help clinicians build rapport and elicit accurate information from informants (12, 57). Informants may include the patient, their caregivers, other family members, investigators, etc. These interviews can help clinicians determine if they should be concerned about family violence and clarify the nature of the violence and abuse. Framing questions does not presume the informant's response will support a scenario of abuse. Framing questions should not lead or suggest a specific answer or scenario to informant. Finally, framing questions can help set the stage to improve patient (and clinician) comfort discussing sensitive topics, including family violence. Examples of framing questions relevant to informant are summarized in Table 6-7.

While the more general and less leading questions may help patients feel more comfortable with disclosing family violence, direct verbal questions can be very helpful to clarify questionable situations or attempt to verify a negative screen. When using direct questioning, clinicians need to avoid an accusatory tone and a

TABLE 6-6 Interviewing Techniques and Family Violence

Interviewing Technique	Interviewing Technique Explanation	Implications in Cases of Family Violence
ACTIVE LISTENING		
	A process of closely attending to patient's verbal and nonverbal communication. Listener is aware of, noting, and responding to patients emotions. Listener is present with patient rather than thinking of the next question or formulating diagnosis and treatment plan.	Listening to patient's account of violence, abuse, and neglect can be very difficult because the history can highlight clinician's vulnerabilities or clinician's personal experiences with violence and can be painful as a form of vicarious distress/trauma. Forensically, it is important to objectively document patient's emotional affect. Sometimes the patient's emotive statements can be evidence in legal proceedings under hearsay exceptions.

Continued

TABLE 6-6 Interviewing Techniques and Family Violence—cont'd

Interviewing Technique	Interviewing Technique Explanation	Implications in Cases of Family Violence
GUIDED QUESTIONING		
	• Moving from open-ended to focused questions (e.g., "Please tell me about last night." To more focused . . . "Did he touch your breast?"	Ideally, patients would provide a narrative about their abusive experiences without guidance from clinicians.
	• Offering multiple choices (e.g., Did he touch your over your clothes, under your clothes, both or neither?)	This would avoid the possibility of suggesting answers or leading patients.
	• Clarifying what patient means (e.g., "When you say she touched your privates, what body part are you talking about?")	Good guided questioning supports patients through the disclosure process while avoiding leading and suggestive questions.
	• Encourage with continuers (e.g., "I am listening, can you tell me more?")	
	• Echoing (e.g., Pt—"He hit me with his fist"; Clinician—"His fist?")	
NONVERBAL COMMUNICATION		
	Communication that does not involve spoken, written, or signed words.	Patients can be very sensitive to clinician's nonverbal communication. It is vital clinicians are willing to receive a disclosure and do not indicate any discomfort with all forms of family violence. A calm, soothing demeanor is helpful.
	Provides cues to both patient and clinician about each others emotional state.	
EMPATHIC RESPONSE		
	Empathy can strengthen patient-clinician rapport and patient trust.	Counter intuitively, patients are often calm and cooperative when reporting family violence.
	Clinician identifies and clarifies patient's emotional state and indicates acceptance of patient's feelings.	However, it may take little probing to elicit an emotional response. Acknowledging the patient's emotions demonstrates a clinician is attending to patient's situation and can indicate clinician comfort with variety of emotions. Hopefully the patient will believe the clinical setting is a "safe place."
	Example: Patient becomes tearful during interview. Clinician responds "I can see you are crying. This is difficult and what you are telling me is something people cry about."	

TABLE 6-6 Interviewing Techniques and Family Violence—cont'd

Interviewing Technique	Interviewing Technique Explanation	Implications in Cases of Family Violence
VALIDATION		
	To affirm a patient's emotional reaction as real and acceptable.	There is NO EXPECTED emotional reaction to experiencing family violence. Affirming patient's current emotional reaction as "normal" or "not unexpected" is a therapeutic intervention. Also, educating patient that they may experience very different emotions in a short period of time serves as anticipatory guidance.
SUMMARIZATION		
	Providing a brief summary of patient's account • Helps patient understand clinician was listening. • Highlights what the clinician does not know or has gotten wrong • Verifies clinician understands events and patient's history.	• Patient's account of violence, abuse, and neglect are not only relevant to medical management but also to investigators and the civil and criminal justice systems. • The patient history is a form of evidence; thus, verifying patient accounts of events is helpful. • Clinician verification of patient's history will avoid clinician errors or highlight inconsistencies, which will aid the investigation.

TABLE 6-7 Framing Questions by Informant Relevant to Family Violence

Informant	Framing Questions
PARENT/CAREGIVER	
	• I ask all parents about violence in their children's lives. Are you worried about violence or some form of abuse? • Violence is such a common event in our society and my practice. I want the families to know it is OK to talk about violence. Have you ever been worried about your child/teenager/elder family member?
ADOLESCENT/ADULT PATIENT	
	• Because violence is so common, I ask all my patients about violence in their lives. Have you experienced any form of violence or abuse? • Can you tell me how you got this injury? • Some of my patients have been hurt by someone in their lives. Has this ever happened to you?

Continued

TABLE 6–7 Framing Questions by Informant Relevant to Family Violence—cont'd

Informant	Framing Questions
ADOLESCENT/ADULT PATIENT	
	• Violence is a health problem I am worried about, and I want to help my patients who have been hurt. If you want to talk to me about any abuse or violence in your life, I am here to listen and help.
	• I don't understand what I am seeing here. You have injuries that do not fit with what you have told me about how you got them. Can you help me understand?
ELDER PATIENT	
	• Same as Adolescent/adult patient.
	• I ask all my patients about different health problems. Since it is so difficult to know who needs help, I ask everyone about abuse and neglect. Do you have any concerns about abuse or neglect?
	• When elders need help sometimes they don't get the help that they need. Is this happening to you?
	• Sometimes people get taken advantage of financially. Are you worried about being taken advantage financially?

confrontational demeanor. Clinicians need to simply ask the question so the informant is not confused or unsure of the topic. Box 6-11 provides examples of direct questions.

Positive Screens for Family Violence

Once a clinician becomes suspicious or concerned a patient is a victim of family violence, the clinician must

---

BOX 6–11 Examples of Direct Questions for Discussing Violence With Patients

Have any of your (family members, partners, ex-partners) hurt or threatened you?

Has your (family member, partner, or ex-partner) physically hit you?

Has your (family member, partner, or ex-partner) scared you will her or his temper, words, or actions?

Do you feel controlled by your (family members, partner, ex-partner)?

Have you ever been forced to have any kind of sex and you did not want to?

Have you not been able to or allowed to practice safer sex or use birth control and you wanted to?

Are you afraid or do you feel like you are in danger?

Do you feel safe to go home today?

---

respond. Clinician responses will be dictated by the patient's vulnerabilities (e.g., minor, incompetent elder, unconscious adult), local state statute, workplace policies, clinician's knowledge and skills, and breadth and depth of community services. The time needed for assessment may be considerable given patient condition. All interventions including reporting, triaging, and referrals serve to protect the patient and promote health and well-being.

If the patient is a competent adult, not at risk of imminent harm, and able to address her or his own needs, then the clinical assessment may occur over a period of time, in multiple visits, and/or with a specialist who is trained in the medical and forensic care of patients who report family violence (12). This allows the patients to address the violence at their own pace. While clinicians may not agree with patients' choices, this process demonstrates the clinician's respect for the patient's autonomy. If patients do not feel comfortable returning to the clinician's practice, then the patient has lost key resources and support for improving her or his life over time. In addition, other specialists (e.g., forensic nurse, social worker, advocate, etc.) can be included in the evaluation process, which can improve patient rapport with providers, provide clinical support during the disclosure process, and allow specialists to develop safety and treatment plans given local resources.

If a patient discloses any experiences with family violence over her or his lifetime, then an expanded assessment is warranted (12). A full medical, social, and family history should be collected, and a physical examination should be performed. The providers who participate in this evaluation can be identified by the patient (e.g., primary health care provider) or by the referring clinician when she or he consults with or sends the patient to a specialist trained in forensic and medical management of family violence. If the evaluation occurs over time and with multiple clinicians, collaboration and information sharing are required. The following provides an overview and highlights key issues in the clinical management of family violence.

MANAGEMENT

Patient Confidentiality

Before starting an evaluation, patients should be informed about the limits of patient confidentiality. Patient confidentiality cannot be maintained when patients are a harm to themselves, may harm others (e.g., duty to warn) (58), are victims of certain types of crime, and/or have reportable conditions (e.g., botulism, gonorrhea, syphilis) (59).

Thus, health care providers should never offer unconditional confidentiality to their patients. If patients are informed about confidentiality limits prior to their evaluation, then rapport and the therapeutic bond are less likely suffer damage when clinicians report without patient consent in cases of mandatory reporting.

Maintaining patient confidentiality promotes patient safety. Perpetrators who learn about clinician's concerns of family violence may attempt to alter or destroy evidence, intimidate witnesses, and/or retaliate against the patient, who may or may not disclose the abuse and violence. Finally, if the allegations prove to be false or the original suspected perpetrator is innocent, confidentiality with the report and allegation may protect the innocent or promote the identification of other perpetrators. Investigators may find it easier to believe suspects if they have no time to prepare their "stories."

Finally, the storage and release of information relevant to family violence need to be carefully considered by clinicians and administrative staff. Like HIV and genetic test results and mental health records, careful consideration should be given to who has access to family violence data in the medical record and under what conditions.

Medical Stability

The patient's stability will depend on recent injuries, emotional/psychological functioning, and current medical diagnoses (60). For example, a neglected elder with uncontrolled diabetes could present with acute complaints of rape by a caregiver. Obviously, the patient's hydration, nutrition, and blood glucose levels will need to be assessed before the acute rape can be managed. Life

and limb will always come before the management of evidence.

The primary survey of patients with significant trauma will identify all potential injuries and prioritize those that are threats to life and limb. As clinicians manage the patient's urgent and nonurgent needs, evidence or potential evidence will be lost or altered as time lapses and the medical evaluation progresses. If the patient's clothing is removed and patient's body cleaned for inspection and treatment without thought given to stains, tears, or bullet holes in clothing, valuable evidence that corroborates the patient's history and/or facilitates crime scene re-creation will be lost (29, 61). The first collected urine and blood samples could later be tested for drugs, which in turn could indicate the patient was vulnerable or incompetent to participate in sexual activities. Many forms of transient trace physical evidence (e.g., seminal products, saliva, blood, fibers, etc.) could be lost if invasive procedures (e.g., urine catheterization) are conducted before a forensic examiner evaluates a patient.

If a patient is medically stable and the patient may be a victim of a crime, then every effort should be made to preserve evidence and consult with a forensic health care provider, such as a forensic nurse.

Consent

A patient's ability to participate in care will be determined by age, competency, and severity of injury.

Consenting for health care services is one of the first patient directed activities in the provider-patient encounter. Patients who have had little to no control over their bodies and interpersonal interactions can benefit from clinicians who demonstrate respect for the patient's autonomy and choice. A patient may regain a sense of some control over her or his body and an increased sense of self-determination when a clinician goes through the *process* of gaining informed consent. Obtaining consent is not only a key legal/ethical issue but also a potential therapeutic intervention.

In many clinical settings, the general consent obtained for treatment may be insufficient for managing the forensic care of a patient who may be a victim of child maltreatment, intimate partner violence, or elder mistreatment. Facility administrators will be helpful in outlining additional consents that may needed before reporting to authorities when there is no mandate to report; identifying and collecting physical evidence (e.g., drug testing, sexual assault evidence kit, or pictures of injuries); releasing medical and forensic reports and images to authorities; and permission to follow up with patient after she or he leaves the health care setting (61).

Minors or incompetent adults' legal guardians' consent is not required to evaluate the patient when there are concerns of violence, abuse, or neglect. In addition, adolescents' ability to consent for their family planning services, including medical/forensic evaluations for sex crimes, varies across states. The Guttmaker Institute periodically summarizes state laws relevant to adolescents' consent and health care services (62).

Unresponsive or Unconscious Patient

If a patient is unable to participate in care, then interventions to preserve life and limb can be instituted without written or verbal consent from patient, legal guardian, or other proxy. Ideally, an individual with power to make health care decisions will be available to consent for procedures and interventions that are not required to save life and limb. In instances when a patient is unresponsive or unconscious and may be a victim of a crime, health care providers have limited choices with respect to evidence collection. Evidence management does not save life or limb so this author does not recommend collecting evidence without consent or court order. Ideally, evidence external to the body (e.g., bed linens, gauze to clean wounds, etc.) will be saved by staff and turned over to LE if an investigation is initiated.

Imminent Risk of Physical and/or Psychological Harm

Physical and/or psychological harm can progress as injuries, chronic illnesses, and mental health and emotional issues are left untreated or become resistant to treatment. Detection of family violence is the first step to prevent worsening of patients' health and well-being.

Physical and/or psychological harm can progress if the offender discovers the victim has disclosed abuse. In many situations, the victim can and will return home and the offender will have access to her or him. It is *vital* that patients are screened alone for family violence. If the patient takes referral information with her or him that the offender can identify as a sign of disclosure, then the patient's safety may be in jeopardy. Therefore, all discharge planning and patient educational materials need to take into account patient privacy.

Physical and/or psychological harm can progress to life-threatening conditions or death when the violence itself progresses. While the lethality and danger vary greatly, tools may help clinicians and patients recognize when the threat to life is increasing.

The Danger Assessment

Developed by nurse Jacquelyn Campbell, the Danger Assessment offers clinicians and patients a method to review a patient's risk of severe injury or death from intimate partner violence (63). Patients and clinicians assess the severity and frequency of battering by asking women to review a calendar and report the incidence of violence (e.g., slap, pushing, use of a weapon) and evaluate risk factors associated with intimate partner homicide (63). The forms, psychometric properties, and training to administer and score the tool are available at www.dangerassessment.com.

The site includes English, Spanish, Portuguese, and French Canadian danger assessment translations. No single assessment can guarantee a patient's safety. Clinicians cannot discount safety issues even if the patient does not report warning signs of escalating violence in her or his relationship. Patients need to know there are no guarantees of safety. Box 6-12 provides some questions that may facilitate a discussion that helps identify areas of significant concern (12). If the patient states that there has been an escalation in the frequency and/or severity of violence, that weapons have been used, or that there has been hostage taking, stalking, or homicide or suicide threats, providers should conduct a homicide/suicide assessment.

THE NATURE OF VIOLENCE/ ABUSE

Clinicians must identify what kind of family violence they are addressing in the clinical setting. The nature of the abuse/violence will influence reporting to authorities, triaging the urgency of medical and forensic services, and formulating the treatment plan. When patients choose to disclose they are often concerned about the reaction they will receive from clinicians, family members, and others. Patients must not be shamed (e.g., "Why didn't you tell me sooner?"); their veracity questioned (e.g., "Are you sure that is what happened?"); or shut down before they disclose (e.g., "Wait a minute, let me get the social worker before you say anything else."). Clinician responses to disclosures should be nonjudgmental, calm, and matter of fact. Ideally, the clinician and patient are alone and

---

BOX 6–12 Questions for Assessment of Patient's Immediate Safety Intimate Partner Violence

- "Are you in immediate danger?"
- "Is your partner at the health facility now?"
- "Do you want to (or have to) go home with your partner?"
- "Do you have somewhere safe to go?"
- "Have there been threats or direct abuse of the children (if she or he has children)?"
- "Are you afraid your life may be in danger?"
- "Has the violence gotten worse or is it getting scarier? Is it happening more often?"
- "Has your partner used weapons, alcohol, or drugs?"
- "Has your partner ever held you or your children against your will?"
- "Does your partner ever watch you closely, follow you, or stalk you?"
- "Has your partner ever threatened to kill you, him/herself or your children?"

in a quiet place where they will not be interrupted. The clinician should listen quietly (active listening) and then follow up with questions as necessary.

Clinicians should inform patients when a report to authorities and/or other health care staff is necessary. Some helpful phrases to tell patients when family violence must be reported to authorities include:

I am so glad you told me about this. It can be very hard to talk about, and I am grateful you trusted me. I want to help you (and your other family members) stay safe. To do this, I must tell a few people what you have told me. These people can help find services and treatment that might help you feel better, help you be safer, and help your family. I am going to tell (list who you need to report to and other health care staff who can evaluate and contribute to the treatment plan). I will not tell the person who brought you here unless you tell me it is OK. I won't tell people who do not need to know, like my co-workers who are not taking care of you, your teachers, or your boss. Do you have any questions?

If the clinician is not a mandatory reporter of a specific form of family violence, certain issues are helpful to the individual when discussed. Box 6-13 summarizes key points to address when patients disclose intimate partner violence.

To accurately triage the urgency of the forensic medical evaluation, clinicians need to know (a) the nature of the family violence; (b) the age and gender of patient; (c) the age and gender of alleged offender(s); (d) the date and time of last episode of violence; (e) patient activities after the most recent of episode of abuse; and (f) other activities that remove evidence from patient's body and clothing.

Ideally, a forensic clinician manages evidence collection and chain of evidence in the health care setting. Transient, trace evidence will be lost over time, and the crime scene (i.e., patient's body) changes with medical interventions.

Currently, guidelines for sex crimes suggest an emergency forensic evaluation should be performed if the last

episode of sexual contact occurred within the past 72 to 120 hours (64). This timeframe is dictated by the chance of recovering transient evidence from the patient's body and clothing. Examples of evidence include seminal products, saliva, intoxicating substances, fibers, and injuries. Obviously the nature of the sexual contact will dictate what kinds of evidence may be present on the patient's body and clothing.

In cases of sexual assault/abuse, the time-sensitive medical interventions include pregnancy (65) and HIV (66) prophylaxis, both of which need to be initiated within 72 hours of the last episode of sexual abuse/assault.

Other forms of family violence will dictate if evidence is time sensitive. For example, documenting dehydration secondary to neglect includes identifying factors contributing to neglect (e.g., patient is dependent on others for nutrition) and documenting the absence or presence of organic causes for dehydration. The timeliness of the forensic medical evaluation will affect not only patient health and well-being but also the clinician's ability to attribute dehydration to neglect rather than other causes.

The first step in the assessment for injuries is a complete survey of the patient's body to document the presence and absence of injuries, including sparing of specific body surfaces or areas. The patient's general physical characteristics (e.g., gender, age, light/dark skin, balding, etc.), physical condition (e.g., nourishment, hydration, etc.), and physical and cognitive developmental capabilities (e.g., able to communicate, primary spoken and written languages, mobility, aids for mobility, etc.) should be documented as well. All of these factors contribute to an increased understanding of the context for injuries, including patients' day-to-day activities, risk factors for family violence, and clinician interpretation of physical exam findings.

The interpretation of physical exam findings, including patterned and patterns of injury and attributing conditions to inflicted mechanisms, requires a high level of clinical skill. Generally, clinicians trained in forensics will be well versed in the differential diagnoses of findings associated with injury and in the process of attributing findings to an inflicted or nonaccidental mechanism. An in-depth discussion of this process is beyond the scope of this text. However, all clinicians should be able to identify and describe physical exam findings because the findings themselves change over time. Different bodies of professional literature describe injuries. It is important a clinician remain consistent in her or his labeling of injury across patients and over time. Table 6-8 identifies and describes findings associated with injuries from the forensic literature (67).

Injury documentation includes describing the wound in reference to the standard anatomical position (standing, facing examiner with palms forward and flaccid penis

---

BOX 6–13 Issues to Discuss When Responding to a Disclosure

- Concerns about patient and other family members' (children) safety, health, and well-being.
- Help is available and won't be forced on patient and family.
- If patient discloses victimization, patient is not at fault for the violence/abuse.
- The violence can affect your health negatively and in many ways.
- Patient questions and concerns about reporting violence/abuse.

TABLE 6-8 Findings Associated With Injuries

Findings	Descriptions
ABRASIONS	
	• Superficial injuries caused by friction or rubbing of the skin against a surface or object. • Debris or trace evidence can be trapped in abrasions. • Called "scrapes" by lay public.
AVULSIONS	
	• Skin or other tissue that has been torn away by blunt and/or shearing forces. • Frequently occurs over bony prominences, forearms, and hands. • Debris or trace evidence can be trapped in avulsions.
BRUISES OR CONTUSIONS	
	• Discoloration of skin or other organs when blunt or compression forces push vascular contents out of ruptured blood vessels. • Discoloration will evolve over time, sometimes becoming more impressive as deep tissue bruising and discoloration develop. • CANNOT date bruising by appearance
ECCHYMOSIS	
	• Subcutaneous, hemorrhagic blotching under the skin often caused by medical/hematologic conditions or indirectly caused by trauma. • Forensically, accurate to describe the spread of discoloration from injury from one site to another (e.g., Battle sign, raccoon eyes) • Ecchymosis is not synonymous with bruises/contusions.
ERYTHEMA	
	• Redness of the skin • Blanches with pressure • Usually diffuse and does not have a pattern • No leakage of intravascular contents into surrounding tissue
FACTURES INCISIONS/CUTS	
	• Lacerations of bone (68) • Caused by sharp instrument or object • Edges are smooth • Depth of wound is consistent. • If uncertain if injury is an incision or laceration, refer to the finding as a wound.
LACERATIONS	
	• Tearing or splitting of tissue from blunt and/or shearing forces. • Margin abrasion, bridging vessels, and connective tissue seen • Jagged edges • Undermining, especially over bone, and debris (evidence) can be trapped. • Depth of wound can vary. • Occur most often over bony prominences. • Skin and other organs can be lacerated.

TABLE 6–8 Findings Associated With Injuries—cont'd

Findings	Descriptions
PATTERNED INJURY	
	• Any injury that gives an indication of object that caused injury
PETECHIAE	
	• Tiny, nonelevated purplish hemorrhagic spots • Often found secondary to a variety of medical conditions, vigorous activities (e.g., vomiting, vaginal child birth), and strangulation
SHARP FORCE INJURIES INCISED WOUNDS	
	• Caused by tangential impact with sharp-edged object • Typically longer on skin surface than deep (exceptions occur) • "Cuts" or "slashes"
STAB WOUNDS	
	• Caused by roughly perpendicular or puncture-type impact with a pointed object • Usually deeper than they are long on skin (exceptions occur)
CHOP WOUNDS	
	• Intermediate between sharp force and blunt force wounds • Typically inflicted by heavy object with relatively sharp edge striking body
TRAUMATIC ALOPECIA	
	Traumatic loss of hair associated with being pulled by hair

Adapted from Sheridan D, et al. Forensic implications of intimate partner violence. In Hammer R, Moynihan B, Pagligario E. Forensic Nursing a Handbook for Practice. Burlington, MA: Jones & Bartlett Learning; 2006. pp. 265-271.

in males). The findings (e.g., wounds, tattoos, stains on skin) would be described in reference to bony landmarks. Finally, Box 6-14 outlines how to describe and document wound or injury characteristics.

Documentation aids include bodygrams or body maps, which allow clinicians to draw the findings on a human figure representing a specific body area (e.g., genitalia, feet, head) and whole body. The bodygrams allow clinicians and investigators to understand relationships among injuries and affected and spared body areas.

Images and Injury Documentation

Documentation of injuries often includes photographic documentation. These photographs may be taken with colpscopes (used to examine ano-genital areas in cases of sex assault/abuse), cameras that use film, and digital cameras. Clinicians and/or investigators can take images. It is important to note who takes the images, not only for

---

BOX 6–14 Documentation of Wounds and Injury Characteristics

- Areas of body involved and spared—forensic interpretation of injuries often benefit from understanding which areas of the body were spared as much if not more from which areas of the body were wounded
- Size—length, width, depth of wounds
- Shape—liner, ovoid, etc.
- Surrounds
- Color
- Contour/Edges
- Contents—many wounds (e.g., abrasions, lacerations, etc.) will have trace evidence that will be reviewed as contaminants by clinicians. It is important to collect and give this evidence to the law enforcement that has jurisdiction
- Pattern(s)

evidence management and chain of evidence but also regarding who owns the images. If clinicians take the images, it is most likely they will become part of the medical record and subject to all policies and procedures for medical records.

Briefly, taking images of injuries requires adequate lighting, appropriate focus, and steady equipment. Take images before and after injuries are evaluated and cleaned, record with images the patient's unique identifying information (e.g., medical record number), date and time images taken, a scale (e.g., ruler, coin), and color standard (e.g., Macbeth ColorChecker or Kodak Gray Card) and include images with and without scale and color standard to document that those instruments do not hide anything (68). Injury images should include overviews, mid-range views, and close-up views (68).

Finally, documenting injuries with images alone is insufficient. A clinician's professional evaluation is required to verify what the images capture and to document any findings images cannot or did not capture.

Diagnosis

Clinician diagnoses are not the results of a legal process. If a clinician's evaluation leads to a diagnosis associated with family violence, then it is the clinician's opinion based on education, training, currency in literature, and professional skills. If the clinician is asked to testify during legal proceedings, including criminal proceedings, clinicians need to clearly identify themselves as a health care provider and explain how they reached their conclusions.

To reiterate, the analysis and interpretation of physical exam findings, medical conditions (e.g., malnutrition, dehydration, pressure sores), historical data, labs, and studies are high-level clinical skills. Concluding a patient's injuries or condition is caused by abuse and/or neglect requires evaluating the likelihood of differential diagnoses and discarding them as clinical data dictate. Clinicians trained in forensics are well versed in this process. The analysis and interpretation of findings in cases of family violence are beyond the scope of this text.

Management

The clinical plan to address family violence includes the clinical management of wounds and conditions, reporting to authorities when mandated, safety planning and referral for medical forensic evaluation when possible, and referral for longer-term mental health and social services.

Family violence is associated with negative health outcomes. Health issues associated with intimate partner violence include multiple injuries over time, chronic pain, sexually transmitted infections, vaginal and urinary tract infections, sexual dysfunction, peptic ulcers, irritable bowel syndrome, insomnia, depression, posttraumatic stress disorder (PTSD), anxiety, stress, suicide, and substance use/abuse (12). Moreover, pregnant women are at an increased risk for miscarriages, low weight gain, anemia, infections, first and second trimester bleeding, and low-birth-weight babies (12).

The urgency of patient care will be dictated by each patient's individual case. One, more than one, or none of these conditions may be seen in survivors of intimate partner violence. Only through evaluation can patients' health care needs be identified. A variety of clinicians can assist in this process and may become involved in patient care over time.

Reporting and Adolescent Victims of Family Maltreatment

All 50 states and territories have laws mandating certain individuals as mandatory reporters of suspected child maltreatment (9). Generally, health care providers (e.g., physicians, nurses, counselors, etc.) are mandatory reporters. Clinicians need to know and correctly interpret their local state statues with respect to reporting child maltreatment. If an adolescent presents with allegations of parental abuse or neglect, it is clear the clinician must report to the local authorities, usually CPS and/or LE. The Child Welfare Information Gateway (11) provides information about individual state statutes relevant to reporting child maltreatment.

The mandate to report adolescent victims of rape and statutory rape is less clear. If the sex crime does not meet the definition of child maltreatment and/or child sexual abuse, then the adolescent may refuse to report to authorities in some states and territories. Moreover, adolescent victims of sex crimes may seek and receive medical and forensic services without reporting to authorities (69).

Reporting and Adult Victims of Family Violence

Generally, competent adults have the right to privacy and control who has access to their health information. Several states (e.g., California, Colorado, Kentucky, New Hampshire, Rhode Island, and New Mexico) at one point in time have mandated reporting of intimate partner violence suspicions to authorities. This reporting mandate is controversial and has resulted in unintended consequences (70). Data suggest women value their autonomy and privacy even when they are living in harmful and dangerous situations (71, 72).

Many states require reporting of injuries caused by weapons and/or injuries, caused by violations of criminal laws, as the result of violence, or through nonaccidental mechanisms (12). Patients may be victims of family violence and have an injury that is reportable by state statue. If there is a conflict between patient wishes about nonmandatory reporting of family violence and mandatory reporting injuries, it is most likely the clinician will be required to report. However, clinicians should consult their institutions' legal counsel, privacy offers, and/or risk management if they have any questions or concerns.

If an adult victim of sex crime is not a victim of intimate partner violence as well, then it is likely the patient not only has the right to privacy but also may seek forensic and medical services without reporting to authorities. The Violence Against Women and Department of Justice Reauthorization Act of 2005 ("VAWA 2005"), 42 U.S.C. § 3796gg-4(d), states jurisdictions may not require victims of sex crimes to participate in the investigation and prosecution of sex crimes in order to receive a forensic medical examination (69).

Reporting Elder Victims of Family Violence

If an elder is abused or neglected in an institutional setting, all 50 states require reporting to authorities (73). Many states require reporting elder mistreatment in all settings as well. The mandatory reporters include but are not limited to health care providers. Depending on local state laws, reports may be made to APS and/or LE officials. The American Bar Association provides annual summaries of state laws pertaining to elder mistreatment.

Patient Does Not Want to Report

When patients do not want to report their victimization, clinicians must explore patients' concerns and explain the benefits and costs associated with reporting and not reporting (12, 64). Furthermore, if the clinician is a mandatory reporter of the patient's case of abuse/neglect, further patient education and support will be necessary. Hopefully, before the clinician became concerned about family violence, the patient was educated about the limits of provider-patient confidentiality. The provider can explain, "This is a situation that needs more help than I can provide. I am required by law to report so that you receive the help you need." Box 6-15 outlines, in no particular order, concerns patients may have about reporting their victimization (73).

BOX 6–15 Patients' Concerns About Reporting Victimization

- Being believed by family members, investigators, friends, and others
- Involuntary removal from their home
- Retribution from offenders and/or family members who support offender
- Discovery of homosexuality, drug use, mental illness, etc.
- Fear of investigative process
- Feelings of hopelessness and helplessness

Clinicians can address some of the patient's concerns by explaining the investigative process, including how the investigators generally interact with victims. Fears about safety and retribution will have to be addressed through community resources, including restraining orders, orders of protection, shelter placement, kinship placements, etc. Finally, understating how the dynamics of family violence will be helpful for patient anticipatory guidance and crisis counseling.

Ultimately patients will need to be told if they choose not to report, then valuable evidence may be lost, offenders may have more opportunities to abuse them, and their life may be in danger. Then the clinician must support the patient's decision and be prepared to provide the same counseling in the future if the patient returns. The hope is that the more times the patient prepares to leave, listens to the clinician's counseling, and learns about her or his inner resources, then she or he will ultimately make the choice to live in a healthier setting with people who do not hurt her or him.

Reporting and Health Insurance Portability and Accountability Act (HIPAA)

HIPAA was enacted in 1996 to "assure that individuals' health information is properly protected while allowing the flow of health information needed to provide and promote high quality health care and to protect the public's health and well-being" (74). The Act causes confusion and concern over what information can be released to investigators when allegations about family violence arise and a patient does not consent to release of protected information or the clinician is a mandated reporter of some form of violence (e.g., child maltreatment). The U.S. Department of Health and Human Services allows for exception so covered entities (e.g., hospitals, clinics, etc.) can share protected health information with LE and social service agencies (e.g., APS and CPS) (75). HIPAA legislation allows covered entities to share protected information without patient's or legal guardian's consent in cases when a covered entity reasonably believes the patient to be a victim of abuse, neglect, or domestic violence (76).

Reporting family violence requires clinicians to understand their local state laws and workplace policies related to reporting. Generally, health care institutions' privacy officers, risk management, legal counsel, administrators, and clinicians (e.g., social workers, nurses, and physicians) will have vital roles in developing, reviewing, and refining these policies so staff can be in compliance with local reporting and privacy laws.

Report Content

Individual state laws will outline what information must be shared with investigators. Often, CPS, APS, and LE officials will continue their investigation after a patient has been seen by a clinician and will interview victims, witnesses, suspects, and others after the patient has left the health care setting. Reporting may precede full evaluation, and the additional key history and physical exam findings can be shared with investigators later. Table 6-9 outlines the contents frequently included in reports to authorities.

SAFETY PLANNING

Safety planning begins with assessment and it is addressed episodically. Safety planning requires monitoring by clinicians and APS, CPS, and LE officials when they are involved in a patient's case. When a mandatory report is required, that report is the first step in safety planning because state agencies can remove a patient from a dangerous situation without patient consent and/or bring resources to the patient and family.

Clinicians assist with safety planning by helping patients identify personal resources (e.g., employment, savings); family resources (e.g., places to stay, emotional support); supportive social networks (e.g., friends, co-workers, church members, etc.), and community resources (e.g., shelters, Food Stamps, childcare, fostering for pets, etc.) that can help patients seek safer situations. Sometimes a patient leaves an abuser, goes back to an abuser, or continues to live with an abuser while she or he develops and implements a safety plan. In cases of intimate partner violence, clinicians must tolerate patients' choices after options have been discussed and evaluated. In case of child maltreatment and adult/elder mistreatment, depending on state statues, state agencies may intervene and provide services. In those cases, if clinicians become concerned state-developed safety plans are not being followed, then a report must be made to authorities.

Often, printed materials about safety planning, family violence, and community resources are given to patients. This can be a dangerous intervention if the offender discovers the materials. Allow patients to determine if it is safe to take materials with them. Some shelters put their telephone numbers on innocuous objects like nail files and pens, which patients may feel more comfortable taking. When possible, give

TABLE 6–9 Information Shared With Authorities When Reporting a Form of Family Violence

Type of Information	Examples
Patient's identifying information	Name, date of birth, Social Security number, current location, and anticipated future locations (e.g., going to shelter, staying with family/friends, going home, etc.)
Caregiver and/or legal guardian's identifying information	Name, phone numbers, home address, work address
Description of the nature of the concerns/allegations	Type of violence, abuse, and/or neglect
	Details about why reporter is concerned (e.g., patient statement, concerning injury, etc.)
	Last known contact between patient and alleged offender
	Last known episode of violence or abuse
Physical exam findings or potential findings	Injuries
	Possible transient, trace physical evidence (e.g., torn clothing, drug screen, seminal products, etc.)
Alleged offender' identifying information	Name, phone numbers, home address, work address
Factors that enhance risk of harm	Other victims identifying information
	Witness's identifying information
	Alleged offender's access to patient
	Alleged offender's access to other vulnerable individuals
Reporter's identifying information	Name, phone number
	Note—anonymous reporting is an option in many states.

patients information about advocacy and support groups. Refer patients to organizations that work with specific populations (i.e., specific ethnic or cultural groups, hard of hearing, teens, or lesbian, gay, transgendered, or bisexual clients) when appropriate. Offer patients information about the national Domestic Violence Hotline (800) 799-SAFE, TTY (800) 787-3224.

Finally, schedule follow-up appointments with health care providers and follow up if patient does not keep appointment. Remember to discuss and document patient's safe numbers to call and/or leave messages, times of day to call, and safety of making appointment reminder calls. The monitoring and opportunities for further evaluation and counseling can be invaluable. Box 6-16 outlines materials patients may want to collect if they decide to leave a dangerous relationship or situation (77).

The medical record provides a permanent record for documentation of the data collected during assessment, diagnosis, and treatment. It is vital that all health care providers gather information about the patient's evaluation and care and record information accurately and in an unbiased manner.

Clinicians should avoid subjective statements (e.g., "patient disheveled") and pejorative or judgmental statements (e.g., patient not cooperative) when documenting information from any informant or from physical examination. Objective descriptions like "leaves and twigs in patient short, dark head hair; without over coat; front right shirt pocket torn off, and half of black sliver studded belt partially threaded around light blue jeans" or "patient states 'don't need a checkup' and 'no need to call police because he will just get madder'" are better.

Given that health care providers are offering health care services, relevant clinical data should be recorded in the usual manner. Data relevant to the violence or abuse should be carefully described and quotes used when possible. Table 6-10 outlines information relevant to forensic issues.

NEGATIVE SCREENS FOR FAMILY VIOLENCE

When patients do not report family violence, clinicians should document they screened the patient and the patient's response was negative, and let the patient know the clinician is a safe person to tell if she or he should ever be in a violent situation (12). If the clinician is seriously concerned about family violence but the patient will not disclose, then specific risk factors in the patient's life may

---

BOX 6–16 Safety Planning List

IDENTIFICATION FOR YOURSELF AND YOUR CHILDREN
- Birth certificates
- Social Security cards (or numbers written on paper if you can't find the cards)
- Driver's license
- Photo identification or passports
- Welfare identification
- Green card

IMPORTANT PERSONAL PAPERS
- Marriage certificate
- Divorce papers
- Custody orders
- Legal protection or restraining orders
- Health insurance papers and medical cards
- Medical records for all family members
- Children's school records
- Investment papers/records and account numbers
- Work permits
- Immigration papers
- Rental agreement/lease or house deed
- Car title, registration, and insurance information

FUNDS
- Cash
- Credit cards
- ATM Card
- Checkbook and bankbook (with deposit slips)

KEYS
- House
- Car
- Safety deposit box or post office box

A WAY TO COMMUNICATE
- Phone calling card
- Cell phone
- Address book

MEDICATIONS
At least 1 month's supply for all medicines you and your children are taking, as well as a copy of the prescriptions

A WAY TO GET BY
Jewelry or small objects you can sell if you run out of money or stop having access to your accounts

THINGS TO HELP YOU COPE
- Pictures
- Keepsakes
- Children's small toys or books

TABLE 6–10 Information Included in Medical Record

Characteristics of alleged offender	Name, relationship to patient, contact information, current location
Characteristics of violence/ abuse	Onset, most recent episode, frequency, trigger(s), use of weapon, access to weapon
History of current and/or past violence	How injuries occurred (e.g., "He pushed me into the door. He held me on the floor and put it in me.")
	Clarification about violence (e.g., "When I was on the floor he pushed my night shirt up and stuck his thing in my vagina.")
	Location, date, and time of violent acts (e.g., "In my house in the living room." "Last night about 9:30 at night.")
	Threats, use of weapons/force (e.g., "He told me he would beat the kids if I didn't do what he wanted.")
	Witnesses to the abuse (e.g., "The kids where in their bedrooms. I don't think they saw it happen, but I think they heard something and they saw me after.")
Physical exam findings	Ability to participate in care
	Wounds
	Intoxication
	General physical health
Report to authorities (if made)	Who received report, title, and phone number, and date and time report made
Report not made to authorities	Discussions about safety
	Evidence management
	Patient's decision
Supportive services	Referrals to community resources (e.g., shelters, counseling, etc.)
	Safety planning—follow-up visits, "checking in," etc.
	Patient's decisions to accept, consider, or reject services.

be identified and discussed, incongruences between history and physical exam should be discussed, and an open invitation should be left with the patient to discuss the topic in the future. If the clinician remains concerned about family violence, the concerns should be addressed (e.g., reporting if mandated) and documented despite the patient's negative screen.

CLINICAL NURSE SPECIALIST COMPETENCIES AND SPHERES OF INFLUENCE

Clinical Nurse Specialists (CNSs) can play a key role in raising patient and provider satisfaction, improving quality of care, and potentially improving patient outcomes through managing their institution's response to family violence.

Administrative support, including adequate staffing, staff education and training, and pragmatic tools, can improve the provider's compliance with protocols addressing intimate partner violence (12). If CNSs lead and/or

project manage the development of institutional specific policies and procedures relevant to screening, negotiating reporting, safety planning, and referrals, then the patient care will meet TJC standards and best practices. The implementation of policies will require training and support for front line clinical staff and periodic identification and updating of community resources, including social services, mental health services, and medical forensic services. Given institutions' pressure to perform, CNSs can identify the unique issues for implementing interventions to detect and treat family violence. In addition, CNSs can facilitate communication with investigators (e.g., LE, APS, and CPS) and other key agents (e.g., shelter supervisors, mental health clinicians) who address family violence in the community. The efficacy of institutions' response is based on coordination and management of clinician interventions, for which the CNS is ideally suited.

Monitoring and assisting with quality improvement in the management of family violence can be key roles for the CNS. The CNS can bench mark screening success rates based on local community or national rates of family violence. Clinician response to screening efforts and interpersonal skills may influence disclosure rates. However, disclosure rates cannot be the sole mark of a successful program because patient disclosure is not controlled by the health care provider. Evaluating patient satisfaction with screening programs and interventions and evaluating patient health outcomes and safety planning for cases that report family violence can help programs develop and improve services (12). Suggestions for monitoring compliance for family violence protocols and procedures include (1) reviewing random samples of medical records for screening documentation; (2) reviewing all positive screens, including cases where patients disclosed and/or clinicians were concerned about family violence, to assess quality of documentation relevant to assessment, intervention, and follow-up; and (3) reviewing cases during morbidity and mortality review (12).

Monitoring reporting efforts should include the percent of (1) patients who were assessed for family violence during a specific time period, (2) patients who disclosed information relevant to family violence, and (3) clinicians who implemented family violence protocols (12). Box 6-17 outlines topics the CNS could consider when evaluating the medical records of patients who were assessed positive for family violence.

Finally, CNSs can obtain additional training and education in forensic nursing so they become the forensic clinician in their institution. The International Association of Forensic Nurses (www.iafn.org) maintains a list of resources to assist clinicians in identifying educational opportunities and program development.

HELP RESOURCES

For a list of resources for assistance with family violence, see the end of this chapter under Help Resources: Family Violence.

Family violence affects all members of our society directly or indirectly. Health care providers must address family violence to promote patient safety, health, and well-being.

SUBSTANCE USE AND ABUSE DISORDERS

Substance use and abuse disorders present very challenging issues for CNSs practicing in the acute care setting. Some may present with obvious symptoms of intoxication, whether drug or alcohol induced. Others may not present in such an overt manner, but rather the symptoms of the substance abuse disorder may manifest themselves as unusual complications in treating medical conditions when withdrawal symptoms arise or when a family member or friend or the patient decides to "come clean" and admit that there is an underlying contributor to the symptoms. The CNS plays an important role in working with the patient to realistically face his or her substance abuse/dependence. The CNS can also assist in identifying strategies to manage the potential withdrawal symptoms, educate nursing staff on the symptoms and therapies available, collaborate with other members of the health care team to coordinate treatments while the patient is experiencing withdrawal, and work with the patient, family, and friends to coordinate therapies on the patient's discharge from the acute care setting.

Stigma continues to surround disorders such as alcohol or drug dependence. Our society tends to stereotype substance abusers as those who make a conscious choice to "do this to themselves." As health care providers, we know that this is untrue. Over the past decade, "the decade of the brain," clinicians involved in treating patients with substance abuse disorders understand that, like psychiatric disorders, substance abuse disorders are also "diseases of the brain." The brain neurochemistry is altered; in particular, the neurotransmitter dopamine is depleted. Additionally, the neurotransmitters serotonin and norepinepherine may play a critical role in the comorbid symptoms of disorders such as anxiety and depression. In relation to those with a substance abuse disorder and comorbid psychiatric illness, we often infer that those who abuse substances are "self-medicating." This term may, in fact, be true, as many who abuse or become dependent on drugs or alcohol are using these substances to alter the neurochemistry of the brain, which contributes to their symptoms of depression,

---

BOX 6–17 Topics for Medical Records Review

Safety assessment, including suicide and homicide assessment when warranted

Reporting when mandated or patient allows as directed by local state statutes

Abuse history relevant to the medical management of patient's health, well-being, and safety

Safety planning efforts and patient response to safety planning

Consultations with other services including forensic health care providers

Crisis counseling and interventions, including conversations with advocates, hot line staff, etc.

Review health risks associated with family violence for patient and other dependent family members

Review of discharge instructions

anxiety, and even psychosis. In this chapter, we will explore the substance use and abuse disorders, the contributing factors and symptoms, their presentation in the acute care setting, as well as potential treatment options and the role of the CNS in treating the patient who presents with symptoms of a substance use or abuse disorder.

Incidence of Substance Abuse Disorders in Acute Care Settings

Substance use disorders constitute a major public health care problem in the United States, costing our society greater than $300 billion in direct and indirect costs on an annual basis (78). Disorders related to substance use can result in multiple levels of impairment in the individual, including conflicts within relationships, impairment in the work setting, comorbid medical illnesses, injuries, disability, and possible death. Approximately 14 million Americans abuse alcohol, and more than half of American adults have a close family member who has suffered from alcohol dependence (79). Similarly, approximately 2.4 million adults in the United States abuse opioid analgesics, making it increasingly likely that health care providers in the acute care setting will be faced with the decision on how to treat pain in a patient with current opioid abuse. Unfortunately, undertreatment of pain is a more typical scenario in the acute care setting when faced with a patient who actively abuses the opioids, which may result not only in discomfort for the patient but also the complication of withdrawal symptoms (80).

To best understand the substance abuse and dependence disorders, we must first define the terms "abuse" and "dependence." Table 6-11 offers an overview of abuse and dependence terminology.

Clinical specialists within the acute care setting must also familiarize themselves with the definitions of substance intoxication and substance withdrawal. Table 6-12 provides an overview of substance intoxication and substance withdrawal.

Withdrawal from substance such as alcohol, opioids, or benzodiazepines can present serious, potentially life-threatening effects. It requires immediate medical intervention to insure that the patient does not develop complications such as seizures, delirium tremens, and respiratory failure, to name a few. The CNS is prepared to work with the patient and health care team to manage the patient's withdrawal symptoms in an effective and safe manner.

Health Care Costs and Etiology of Substance Abuse Disorders

In 2007, patients with alcohol and substance–related disorders accounted for 12.6% of all hospital discharges against medical advice (AMA), but only 1.1% of all hospital stays. Those patients who were either uninsured or insured through Medicaid accounted for nearly one-half of all AMA discharges, but less than 20% of all other discharges. Patients with alcohol and substance-related disorders were 11.6 and 10.8 times more likely, respectively, to leave the acute care setting AMA than were other patients. Although AMA discharges involved a shorter hospital stay (2.7 versus 5.1 days) and were about half as expensive ($5,300 versus $10,400) than all other hospital stays, the frequency with which those who abuse drugs and alcohol return to the acute care setting is also greater (83).

The National Institute on Drug Abuse (NIDA) estimates that the total overall costs of substance abuse in the

TABLE 6–11 Abuse and Dependence Terminology

Term	Definition
Abuse	to use wrongly or improperly, misuse
Tolerance	Normal neurobiological process characterized by the need to increase the dose over time to obtain the original effect
Cross-tolerance	Tolerance to effects of medications within the same drug class
Dependence/addiction	Chronic neurobiological disorder as a pattern of maladaptive behaviors, including loss of control over use, craving, and preoccupation with non-therapeutic use and continued use despite cognitive, behavioral, legal, social, and/or physiologic problems
Physical dependence	Normal physiologic adaptation defined as the development of withdrawal with abrupt dose reduction or discontinuation
Pseudo-addiction	Behavior similar to those in patients with opioid addiction but is secondary to inadequate pain control
Drug-seeking behaviors	Directed or concerted efforts on the part of the patient to obtain opioid medication or to ensure an adequate supply of medication; may be an appropriate response to inadequately treated pain

TABLE 6–12 Intoxication and Withdrawal Terminology

Intoxication	Recent overuse of a substance that results in a reversible substance-specific syndrome; it can occur with just one use of a substance; there are significant behavioral, psychological, and physical changes (for example: alcohol; slurred speech, impaired memory/"black out," ataxia, stupor, and/or coma)
Withdrawal	Specific physical and emotional manifestations (anxiety, restlessness, irritability, fatigue, depression, and insomnia, etc)unique to the individual substance when that substance is discontinued after frequent use
Physical withdrawal	Physiologic response to the abrupt cessation or drastic reduction of a substance used over a prolonged period of time; again the symptoms are specific to the substance used

United States—including health and crime–related costs as well as losses in productivity—exceed half a trillion dollars annually. Almost 20 million (8.3%) of Americans 12 years of age and older are current users of illicit drugs and close to 7 million Americans are abusing prescription drugs (84). In 2003, over 200,000 direct hospitalizations and about 1.1 million concomitant stays were for alcohol abuse disorders, totaling about $2 billion in aggregate charges annually (79). Similarly, in 2005, close to $10 billion in hospital costs were charged for the 1.3 million hospital stays related to drug abuse (85). Over the past few years, the United States has experienced a growing trend of individuals who are abusing psychotherapeutic medications for nonmedical purposes. These medications include pain relievers (such as OxyContin and Vicodin), tranquilizers (such as Xanax and Valium), stimulants (such as Ritalin and Adderall), and sedatives (such as Ambien). The abuse of prescription drugs is increasing among our nation's adolescents. The ease of availability (e.g., via the medicine cabinet, the Internet, and physicians) and the misperception that prescriptions medications are safer than illegal drugs have contributed to the rise in abuse of prescription medications (86).

Screening Tools for Substance Use and Abuse Disorders in the Acute Care Settings

When screening for substance use and/or abuse disorders in the acute care setting, we must first define the term "substance." Substances of abuse include prescription medications, over-the-counter medications (such as cough and cold preparations), alcohol, nicotine, caffeine, illegal drugs (such as cocaine, heroin, marijuana, PCP, LSD, etc.), "designer/club" drugs (e.g., ecstasy, ketamine, rohypnol, etc.), opioid pain relievers (e.g., oxycodone and Vicodin), sedatives/hypnotics (e.g., the benzodiazepines and sleep medications), stimulants, and other agents that may alter the individual's mood, thoughts, and/or behaviors. The

CNS in the acute care setting who encounters a patient who has been using and/or abusing substances faces many challenges. First, a determination must be made as to what substance or substances the individual may be using. Second, the CNS must determine whether the patient is under the influence of or intoxicated by the substance. Third, an evaluation for dependency must be performed, as dependency on various substances may present with significant health risks, including possible death if not immediately and adequately managed from a medical perspective. Fourth, the patient must be assessed for withdrawal symptoms. Once the patient is detoxified or withdrawn from the substance of abuse, coordination of further substance abuse treatment must occur. This final phase in the acute care setting may involve not only the patient but also the patient's family and friends who may support the patient in obtaining the resources needed to decrease and ultimately eliminate the abuse and/or substance dependence.

Furthering the challenges faced by the CNS in treating a patient with a substance use/abuse disorder in the acute care setting is society's view that certain substances—alcohol, nicotine, caffeine, and even the opiates, when used for pain management—are viewed as acceptable in moderation. The definition of "moderation," however, remains in question and varies from person to person. For example, one patient may be able to drink three 20-ounce cups of coffee per day without any effects such as anxiety, shaking, sweating, tachycardia, or sleep disturbance, whereas another patient may experience tremors, insomnia, palpitations, and headaches if he misses his one 16-ounce cup per day.

The substance use screening tool known as ASSIST (Alcohol, Smoking and Substance Involvement Screening Test), modified by the National Institute on Drug Abuse (http://drugabuse.gov/nidamed/screening/nmassist.pdf), was developed by the World Health Organization to identify not only the substances an individual is using/abusing but also the extent to which the individual is ingesting the substance (87, 88). The overall score allows the CNS to better define the patient's risk for tolerance, dependence, addiction, and withdrawal. This comprehensive screening tool is in the public domain and readily available through various government web sites. Although it appears rather lengthy, it does not require more than about 30 minutes to complete and provides a very comprehensive overview of the patient's risk for substance use and/or abuse.

Medical and Laboratory Studies

It is well known that those who abuse nicotine, drugs, and alcohol are at greater risk for physical health problems. The CNS practicing in the acute care setting is in a position to observe and assess and to treat the medical conditions related to the patient's substance abuse. A thorough physical examination, focusing on the neurologic, circulatory, respiratory, gastrointestinal, and integumentary systems, should be conducted on the substance abusing patient. The symptoms associated with each bodily system are outlined in Table 6-13 (89).

Laboratory studies should also be completed to assess for any cardiac, hepatic, pancreatic, renal, or thyroid dysfunction as well as pregnancy and infection. Table 6-14 will also offer insights into the patient's physical health and risk factors (89).

Other medical studies might include a computed tomography (CT) scan or magnetic resonance (MR) image of the brain and/or an electroencephalogram

TABLE 6–13 Physical Symptoms and Health Risks Related to Substance Abuse

Physical Symptoms	Potential Health Risks
Yellow skin, yellow eyes, right-sided abdominal pain, increased abdominal girth	Jaundice, hepatitis, liver damage
Swelling of lower extremities	Edema, cardiac disease/failure, cellulitis
Coughing, wheezing, shortness of breath	COPD, pneumonia, asthma, cardiac disease, emphysema, respiratory failure
Chest pain, dizziness, tachycardia, lightheadedness	Cardiac disease/failure
Ataxia, numbness, weakness, severe headache, visual changes, difficulty speaking	Transient ischemic attack, stroke
Pain, redness, swelling, discharge, and possibly fever	Cellulitis, MRSA, infection
Severe abdominal pain	Pancreatitis, appendicitis, GERD, opiate withdrawal, peptic ulcers
Tremors, involuntary movement of extremities	Seizure
Confusion, hallucinations, disorientation	Delirium, alcohol withdrawal

TABLE 6–14 Laboratory Studies to Assess Health Risks in Substance Abusers

Laboratory Study	Potential Health Risks if Abnormal
Complete blood count with differential	Infection, anemia
Comprehensive metabolic panel	Electrolyte imbalance, cardiac/respiratory issues, dehydration, diabetes, renal function
Liver function tests	Hepatic dysfunction, liver failure, hepatitis
Thyroid function tests	Hypothyroid or hyperthyroid conditions
Amylase and lipase	Pancreatitis
β-hCG	Pregnancy
HIV titer	HIV/AIDS
Urinalysis and urine drug screen	Dehydration, UTI, and substances ingested

(EEG) if the gross neurologic examination is positive or the patient exhibits seizure activity. A chest radiograph might be prudent if the patient is a heavy cigarette or marijuana smoker and exhibits symptoms such as coughing, shortness of breath, or other respiratory ailments. Finally, a nutrition consult would be helpful, as patients presenting with substance-related disorders often exhibit poor dietary and nutrition habits.

Substance Abuse

According to the *Diagnostic and Statistical Manual of Mental Disorders, Fourth Edition, Text Revision (DSM-IV-TR)*, substance abuse is characterized by a maladaptive pattern, occurring within a 12-month period, of the use of the substance contributing to significant clinical impairment or distress without meeting the criteria for substance dependence (90). This impairment is manifested by one or more of the following:

1. Recurrent use of the substance resulting in the failure to fulfill major role obligations at work, school, or home
2. Recurrent substance use in situations where it is physically hazardous (e.g., driving while impaired, in workplaces involving machinery, in environments where others lives are under the individual's care)
3. Recurrent substance-related legal problems
4. Continued use of the substance(s) despite having persistent or recurrent social or interpersonal problems caused or exacerbated by the effects of the substance(s)

These criteria are consistent regardless of whether the substance in question is alcohol, a prescribed medication, an over-the-counter drug, an inhalant, an illegal drug (e.g., marijuana/cannibus, heroin, cocaine), a "club drug" (e.g., ecstasy, ketamine [aka Special K], rohypnol (aka "the date rape drug")), a hallucinogenic (e.g., LSD or PCP), caffeine, nicotine, amphetamines, opioids (e.g., morphine, Percocet, OxyContin, Vicodin, or heroin), or sedatives-hypnotics-anxiolytics (SHAs). The key factor in substance abuse is the significant decrease in the individual's level of functioning.

Substance Dependence

Substance dependence is defined by the *DSM-IV-TR* as a maladaptive pattern of substance use, leading to clinically significant impairment or distress, as manifested by three or more of the following, occurring at any time in the same 12-month period (90):

1. Tolerance, as manifested by either of the following: a need for more of the substance to achieve intoxication or desired effect; or a markedly diminished effect with continued use of the same amount of the substance.
2. Withdrawal, as manifested by either of the following: characteristic withdrawal syndrome for the substance, or greater amounts of the substance (in the same or different form) are ingested to relieve or avoid withdrawal symptoms.
3. The substance is consumed in larger amounts or over a longer period than intended.
4. There is a persistent desire or unsuccessful efforts to cut down or control the use of the substance.
5. Large amounts of time are spent in activities necessary to obtain the substance (e.g., visiting multiple practitioners or driving long distances to obtain the substance).
6. Use the substance (e.g., for "weekend binges," chain smoking, etc.) or recover from its effects.
7. Social, occupational, or recreational activities are reduced or given up because of the substance.
8. The consumption of the substance continues despite knowledge of having a persistent or recurrent physical or psychological problem that is likely to have been caused or exacerbated by the use of the substance.

Again, like substance abuse, substance dependence contributes to a significant decrease and impairment in the person's level of functioning in various areas of life and may also affect the individual's physical health due to the effects of intoxication and withdrawal. In the following sections, we will explore the symptoms of intoxication and withdrawal from, the clinical presentation of, and the management of patients who present with abuse and/or dependence on the substances—alcohol, opioids, SAHs, and nicotine—most commonly presenting for treatment in the acute care setting.

Alcohol Use and Induced Related Disorders

About 30% of U.S. adults drink at levels that elevate their risk for physical, mental health, and social problems. Of this population of "heavy drinkers," about one in every four has alcohol abuse or dependence issues (91). Physically, these individuals may suffer from hypertension, sleep disturbances, depressive disorders, seizures, "black outs," cirrhosis of the liver, pancreatitis, several forms of cancer, gastrointestinal bleeding, and malnutrition, among many other health risks. Unfortunately, heavy drinking often goes undetected and therefore untreated. In fact, only about 10% of these patients receive the recommended assessment and referral for treatment (92).

Alcohol Intoxication

Alcohol intoxication is one of the more frequently encountered conditions in patients admitted to acute care facilities through the emergency department. The patient typically presents after recent ingestion of substantial amounts of alcohol, which contribute to changes in mood and behavior. The patient may exhibit slurred speech, ataxia, nystagmus, lack of coordination, and difficulty in paying attention or remembering. Physical changes for the alcohol-intoxicated patient may include stupor, seizures, or coma as well as nausea, vomiting, and potential loss of bladder function. If the alcohol-intoxicated patient also presents with chronic alcohol abuse, he will be a much greater risk for alcohol withdrawal syndrome and the serious medical complications, including death that may arise.

Alcohol Withdrawal

Alcohol withdrawal results from a drastic reduction in or abrupt discontinuation of the consumption of alcohol in the patient who has been a chronic, heavy drinker. Alcohol withdrawal symptoms may develop within several hours to a few days after the reduction or discontinuation of ingestion of alcohol. According to the *DSM-IV-TR* (90), two or more of the following symptoms are present during withdrawal: autonomic hyperactivity (sweating, tachycardia); increased hand tremors; insomnia; nausea/vomiting; psychomotor agitation; anxiety; transient visual, tactile, or auditory hallucinations or illusions (delirium tremons); or grand mal seizures. The patient will likely be very uncomfortable during this period of time if left untreated or undertreated. Should the patient experience grand mal seizures as a manifestation of alcohol withdrawal, additional medical and safety risks may evolve, with the potential of coma and/or death. Alcohol withdrawal and detoxification are medical issues, and the CNS is in a prime position to assist the patient in safely and effectively withdrawing from the alcohol and beginning the interventions that will aid the patient in moving toward a life of sobriety.

Case Report

Joe is a 54-year-old man who presents to the emergency department via ambulance after his girlfriend found him "passed out" on the floor of the bedroom when she returned home from work at 11:30 p.m. Joe had urinated on himself and was disheveled; he was difficult to arouse and was mumbling and slurring his speech. The emergency medical responders found Joe's blood pressure to be elevated; he was diaphoretic and stuporous. Upon arriving at the emergency department, Joe suddenly "woke up," attempting to get himself off the gurney and straining his body against the restraint straps used for transport. He was screaming and yelling, still slurring his speech. Abruptly, Joe fell back on the gurney and his upper and lower extremities began to convulse. He was having a seizure. Once Joe was stabilized for the seizure and intubated for airway management, blood samples were drawn, including a blood alcohol level, which was 348, almost 5 times the legal limit of 0.08 or 80 (93). See Box 6-18 for blood alcohol levels and psychomotor effects.

Joe was admitted to the intensive care unit, and the CNS was called to consult for alcohol withdrawal, detoxification,

BOX 6–18 Blood Alcohol Levels and Psychomotor Effects	
BLOOD ALCOHOL CONTENT (BAC) G/100 ML BLOOD	**SYMPTOMS AND EFFECTS AT VARIOUS BLOOD ALCOHOL LEVELS**
0.02 to 0.03 BAC RELAXED	• Slight euphoria, loss of shyness • Depressant effects are not apparent • Mildly relaxed and may be a bit lightheaded
0.04 to 0.06 BAC BUZZED	• Euphoria, feeling of well-being, relaxation, lowered inhibitions and caution • Sensation of warmth • Exaggerated behaviors • Intensified emotions • Minor impairment in reasoning and memory
0.07 to 0.09 BAC LEGALLY DRUNK	• Slight impairment of balance, speech, vision, reaction time, and hearing • Reduced judgment and self-control • Impaired caution, reason, and memory • Belief that they are functioning better than they really are • Euphoria • **0.08 is legally impaired . . . it is illegal to drive at this level**
0.10 to 0.125 BAC EUPHORIC	• Speech may be slurred • Loss of good judgment • Significantly impaired motor coordination • Euphoria • Impaired balance, vision, reaction time, and hearing

BOX 6–18 Blood Alcohol Levels and Psychomotor Effects—cont'd

BLOOD ALCOHOL CONTENT (BAC) G/100 ML BLOOD	SYMPTOMS AND EFFECTS AT VARIOUS BLOOD ALCOHOL LEVELS
0.13 to 0.15 BAC IMPAIRED	• Gross motor impairment and lack of physical control • Blurred vision • Ataxia/loss of balance • Severely impaired judgment and perception • Reduced euphoria and dysphoria • Anxiety/restlessness begin to appear
0.16 to 0.19 BAC VERY DRUNK	• Dysphoria predominates • Nausea may occur • Drinker has the appearance of a "sloppy drunk"
0.20 BAC CONFUSION	• Feeling dazed, confused, and disoriented • May need help to stand or walk • If injured, may not feel pain • Nausea and vomiting • Impaired gag reflex • "blackouts"
0.25 BAC DAZED	• Severely impaired mental, physical, and sensory functions • Increased risk of asphyxiation from choking on vomit • Increased risk of serious injury by falls/accidents
0.30 BAC STUPOR	• Stupor • Little comprehension of where they are • May pass out suddenly and be difficult to awaken
0.35 BAC COMA	• Level of surgical anesthesia • Coma is possible
0.40+ BAC DEATH	• Onset of coma possible

and treatment options. As alcohol withdrawal presents serious risks for potential life-threatening conditions and Joe has already had at least one seizure, the CNS must determine the extent of Joe's drinking, to adapt the hospital's standardized orders to his specific needs. The CNS meets with Joe's girlfriend and determines that he has recently lost his job and over the past few months he has been consuming at least a six-pack of beer and a pint of vodka on a daily basis, mainly in the evening. His girlfriend is concerned because she found an empty liter-sized bottle of vodka in the kitchen trash before leaving to follow the ambulance. Given this level of alcohol abuse and dependence, coupled with Joe's acute intoxication and risk for withdrawal, the CNS must act quickly to minimize further seizures, the risk of coma, and/or death. Joe's diagnoses would be Alcohol Intoxication, Alcohol Dependence, and Alcohol Withdrawal. The following section will offer guidelines for the management of alcohol-related disorders in the acute care setting.

Management

As alcohol intoxication is not an uncommon diagnosis in patients presenting to the emergency department, whether as a primary presentation or secondary ailment, each acute care facility should be prepared with standardized protocols as guidelines for management of alcohol-related disorders. Alcohol detoxification is a medical procedure typically conducted in the acute care setting or detoxification unit of a substance abuse rehabilitation facility. In order to determine the most appropriate course of treatment, the clinical specialist must first assess/predict the severity of the patient's alcohol withdrawal. Predictors that increase the severity and risk for adverse events include previous withdrawal, particularly with a history of withdrawal seizures or delirium; number of previous detoxifications; quantity and duration of alcohol abuse or dependence; high blood alcohol level without signs of intoxication; current withdrawal signs with high blood alcohol level; concurrent use of sedative-hypnotics or opioids; and/or coexisting medical conditions (94). Symptoms of alcohol withdrawal generally begin within 4 to 12 hours after the cessation or reduction of alcohol use, peak in intensity during the second day of abstinence, and typically resolve within 4 to 5 days (95). The goal of alcohol detoxification is to safely minimize the potential adverse outcomes (discomfort, seizures, Wernicke's encephalopathy, delirium, and mortality) and to avoid the adverse effects of the withdrawal medications (excessive sedation) (94). Using the Clinical Institute Withdrawal Assessment for Alcohol–Revised (CIWA-Ar) (96) shown in Box 6-19, the CNS is able to determine and monitor the severity of the patient's withdrawal symptoms. Based on the patient's score on the CIWA, appropriate adjustments to the medical detoxification protocol can be made. Box 6-20 provides an example of a Standardized Alcohol Withdrawal Protocol (97).

Management of alcohol intoxication and withdrawal in an acute care setting involves a multidisciplinary approach including the patient, the patient's family or supports (if available), nursing, social work, and a general medical practitioner (APRN/clinical specialist or physician), among others. During the medical withdrawal phase, the nursing staff is responsible for observing the signs and symptoms of withdrawal, conducting the withdrawal assessment or CIWA-Ar, monitoring vital signs, and alerting the medical practitioner/clinical specialist of any changes in the patient's status. The medical practitioner/CNS is responsible for providing adequate pharmacologic meas-

---

BOX 6–19 Clinical Institute Withdrawal Assessment of Alcohol Scale–Revised (CIWA-Ar)

Clinical Institute Withdrawal Assessment of Alcohol Scale, Revised (CIWA-Ar)

Patient: _____ Date: _____ Time: _____ (24 hour clock, midnight = 00:00)
Pulse or heart rate, taken for one minute: _____ Blood pressure: _____

NAUSEA AND VOMITING — Ask "Do you feel sick to your stomach? Have you vomited?" Observation.

0 no nausea and no vomiting
1 mild nausea with no vomiting
2
3
4 intermittent nausea with dry heaves
5
6
7 constant nausea, frequent dry heaves and vomiting

TACTILE DISTURBANCES — Ask "Have you any itching, pins and needles sensations, any burning, any numbness, or do you feel bugs crawling on or under your skin?" Observation.

0 none
1 very mild itching, pins and needles, burning or numbness
2 mild itching, pins and needles, burning or numbness
3 moderate itching, pins and needles, burning or numbness
4 moderately severe hallucinations
5 severe hallucinations
6 extremely severe hallucinations
7 continuous hallucinations

TREMOR — Arms extended and fingers spread apart. Observation.

0 no tremor
1 not visible, but can be felt fingertip to fingertip
2
3
4 moderate, with patient's arms extended

5
6
7 severe, even with arms not extended

AUDITORY DISTURBANCES — Ask "Are you more aware of sounds around you? Are they harsh? Do they frighten you? Are you hearing anything that is disturbing to you? Are you hearing things you know are not there?" Observation.

0 not present
1 very mild harshness or ability to frighten
2 mild harshness or ability to frighten
3 moderate harshness or ability to frighten
4 moderately severe hallucinations
5 severe hallucinations
6 extremely severe hallucinations
7 continuous hallucinations

PAROXYSMAL SWEATS — Observation.

0 no sweat visible
1 barely perceptible sweating, palms moist
2
3
4 beads of sweat obvious on forehead
5
6
7 drenching sweats

VISUAL DISTURBANCES — Ask "Does the light appear to be too bright? Is its color different? Does it hurt your eyes? Are you seeing anything that is disturbing to you? Are you seeing things you know are not there?" Observation.

BOX 6–19 Clinical Institute Withdrawal Assessment of Alcohol Scale–Revised
(CIWA-Ar)—cont'd

---

0 not present
1 very mild sensitivity
2 mild sensitivity
3 moderate sensitivity
4 moderately severe hallucinations
5 severe hallucinations
6 extremely severe hallucinations
7 continuous hallucinations

ANXIETY — Ask "Do you feel nervous?" Observation.

0 no anxiety, at ease
1 mild anxious
2
3
4 moderately anxious, or guarded, so anxiety is inferred
5
6
7 equivalent to acute panic states as seen in severe delirium or acute schizophrenic reactions

HEADACHE, FULLNESS IN HEAD — Ask "Does your head feel different? Does it feel like there is a band around your head?" Do not rate for dizziness or lightheadedness. Otherwise, rate severity.

0 not present
1 very mild
2 mild
3 moderate

4 moderately severe
5 severe
6 very severe
7 extremely severe

AGITATION — Observation.

0 normal activity
1 somewhat more than normal activity
2
3
4 moderately fidgety and restless
5
6
7 paces back and forth during most of the interview, or constantly thrashes about

ORIENTATION AND CLOUDING OF SENSORIUM — Ask "What day is this? Where are you? Who am I?"

0 oriented and can do serial additions
1 cannot do serial additions or is uncertain about date
2 disoriented for date by no more than 2 calendar days
3 disoriented for date by more than 2 calendar days
4 disoriented for place/or person

Total **CIWA-Ar** Score _____
Rater's Initials _____
Maximum Possible Score 67

---

*The **CIWA-Ar** is not copyrighted and may be reproduced freely. This assessment for monitoring withdrawal symptoms requires approximately 5 minutes to administer. The maximum score is 67 (see instrument). Patients scoring less than 10 do not usually need additional medication for withdrawal. Sullivan JT, Sykora K, Schneiderman J, et al. Assessment of alcohol withdrawal: the revised Clinical Institute Withdrawal Assessment for Alcohol scale (**CIWA-Ar**). Br J Addict 1989;84:1353-1357.*

BOX 6–20 Alcohol-Benzodiazepine (Sedative-Hypnotic) Withdrawal Protocol—Sample
Order Set

Place X in box next to Diagnosis and Patient Orders . . . . Orders left Blank WILL NOT be Transcribed

DIAGNOSIS: ☐ Alcohol ☐ Benzodiazepine ☐ Sedative ☐ Hypnotic Withdrawal ☐

Date/Time and Amount of Last Ingestion of Substance of Abuse: _____
VITAL SIGNS:

☐ **Monitor patient every 4 hours using CIWA-Ar until score if less than 10 for 24 hours while awake (include: BP, pulse, respiratory rate, temperature)**
☐ **Reassess patient 1 hour after each dose of Ativan; STAT page practitioner if symptoms not controlled** (CIWA-Ar still 20 or more or score is worsening)
☐ **STAT page practitioner if patient experiences any of the following: respiratory distress, change in mental status, oral temperature: >101.5°F, urine output <250cc/shift, heart rate <50 or >120, systolic blood pressure ≥180 or ≤110 or diastolic blood pressure ≥100**

Continued

BOX 6–20 Alcohol-Benzodiazepine (Sedative-Hypnotic) Withdrawal Protocol—Sample Order Set—cont'd

---

MEDICATIONS:

☐ **Use CIWA-Ar (Clinical Institute Withdrawal Assessment for Alcohol-Revised) to determine doses below:**

CIWA-Ar Score	DO NOT EXCEED 4mg in any 4-hour period without practitioner order
9 or less	None
10 to 19	Ativan 2mg PO or IM or IV
20 to 29	Ativan 3mg PO or IM or IV
30 or more	Ativan 4mg PO or IM or IV

OTHER MEDICATIONS:

☐ Thiamine 100mg IM STAT × 1 dose on admission then
☐ Thiamine 100mg PO Daily × 3 days
☐ Folic Acid 1mg PO STAT on admission then
☐ Folic Acid 1mg PO Daily × 3 days
☐ Multivitamin with Iron PO Daily
☐ Maalox or Mylanta 30cc PO Every 6 hours PRN for abdominal discomfort
☐ Ibuprofen 400mg PO every 4 hours PRN for muscles aches/pains or headache
☐ _____

DIET:

☐ Clear Liquids
☐ Regular
☐ Other (specify) _____
☐ Dietary/Nutrition Consult

ACTIVITY:
Bedrest with Bathroom Privileges

☐ Up and
☐ Up and Out of Bed ad lib
☐ Other (specify) _____

DIAGNOSTIC STUDIES (if not previously completed):

☐ CBC with Differential _____ Liver Functions Studies _____ βhCG
☐ Comprehensive Metabolic Panel _____ Amylase and Lipase

---

ures to ensure that the patient does not experience any adverse events such as seizures or delirium during the withdrawal phase as well as monitoring the patient's condition and reducing the withdrawal medications as indicated to avoid adverse effects such as sedation. Along with the clinical specialist, the social worker, patient, and patient's family/supports coordinate the aftercare plan on when the patient completes the withdrawal phase and is determined to be medically stable.

Many options exist for the treatment of the alcohol-related disorders after the completion of medical detoxification. Typically, some form of treatment program is recommended to aid in the prevention of relapse. Such programs might include an inpatient rehabilitation facility stay of 14 to 28 days (or longer), a partial hospitalization program, an intensive outpatient program, or attendance at community-based self-help groups such as Alcoholics Anonymous. Other treatment options for the alcohol-related disorders include pharmacotherapy. Box 6-21 illustrates the most common medication therapies for prevention of relapse (98-104). More often than not, however, after successful medical detoxification in an acute care setting, the patient with an alcohol-related disorder uses a combination treatment approach to move toward a life of sobriety. Relapse and a return to the abuse of or dependence on alcohol as a way to manage life's stressors are often part of the individual's struggle and should certainly be discussed prior to discharge from the acute care setting. Given the clinical specialist's

BOX 6–21 Medications for Treating Alcohol Dependence

	Naltrexone (102, 103) (Depade, ReVia)	Extended-Release Injectable Naltrexone (Vivitrol) (100, 101, 102)	Acamprosate (102, 103) (Campral)	Disulfiram (Antabuse)	Topiramate (Topamax) OFF LABEL
Action	Blocks opioid receptors, resulting in reduced craving and reduced reward in response to drinking.	Same as oral naltrexone; 30-day duration.	Affects glutamate and GABA neurotransmitter systems, but its alcohol-related action is unclear.	Inhibits intermediate metabolism of alcohol, causing a buildup of acetaldehyde and a reaction of flushing, sweating, nausea, and tachycardia if a patient drinks alcohol.	Thought to work by increasing inhibitory (GABA) neurotransmission and reducing stimulatory (glutamate) neurotransmission
Contraindications	Currently using opioids or in acute opioid withdrawal; anticipated need for opioid analgesics; acute hepatitis or liver failure.	Same as oral naltrexone, plus inadequate muscle mass for deep intramuscular injection; rash or infection at the injection site.	Severe renal impairment (CrCl ≤30 mL/min).	Concomitant use of alcohol or alcohol-containing preparations or metronidazole; coronary artery disease; severe myocardial disease; hypersensitivity to rubber (thiuram) derivatives.	Hypersensitivity to topiramate.
Precautions	Other hepatic disease; renal impairment; history of suicide attempts or depression. If opioid analgesia is needed, larger doses may be required and respiratory depression may be deeper and more prolonged. Pregnancy Category C. Advise patients to carry a wallet card to alert medical personnel in the event of an emergency. For wallet card information, see *www.niaaa.nih.gov/guide.*	Same as oral naltrexone, plus hemophilia or other bleeding problems.	Moderate renal impairment (dose adjustment for CrCl between 30 and 50 mL/min); depression or suicidal ideation and behavior. Pregnancy Category C.	Hepatic cirrhosis or insufficiency; cerebrovascular disease or cerebral damage; psychoses (current or history); diabetes mellitus; epilepsy; hypothyroidism; renal impairment. Pregnancy Category C. Advise patients to carry a wallet card to alert medical personnel in the event of an emergency. For wallet card information, see *www.niaaa.nih.gov/guide.*	Narrow-angle glaucoma, kidney stones, renal or hepatic impairment, severely underweight, use of CNS depressants. Pregnancy Category C.
Serious adverse reactions	Will precipitate severe withdrawal if the patient is dependent on opioids; hepatotoxicity (although does not appear to be a hepatotoxin at the recommended doses).	Same as naltrexone, plus injection site reactions that may be severe (click here for FDA alert). Instruct patients to closely monitor site and seek care immediately if reaction is worsening. Also depression and rare events including allergic pneumonia and suicidal ideation and behavior.	Rare events include suicidal ideation and behavior.	Disulfiram-alcohol reaction, hepatotoxicity, optic neuritis, peripheral neuropathy, psychotic reactions.	Metabolic acidosis, acute myopia and secondary narrow-angle glaucoma, oligohydrosis, and hyperthermia

Continued

BOX 6–21 Medications for Treating Alcohol Dependence—cont'd

	Naltrexone (102, 103) (Depade, ReVia)	Extended-Release Injectable Naltrexone (Vivitrol) (100, 101, 102)	Acamprosate (102, 103) (Campral)	Disulfiram (Antabuse)	Topiramate (Topamax) OFF LABEL
Common side effects	Nausea, vomiting, decreased appetite, headache, dizziness, fatigue, anxiety.	Same as oral naltrexone, plus a reaction at the injection site; joint pain; muscle aches or cramps.	Diarrhea, somnolence.	Metallic after-taste, dermatitis, transient mild drowsiness.	Paresthesias, taste perversion, anorexia and weight loss, somnolence, cognitive dysfunction.
Examples of drug interactions	Opioid medications (blocks action).	Same as oral naltrexone.	No clinically relevant interactions known.	Anticoagulants such as warfarin; isoniazid; metronidazole; phenytoin; any nonprescription drug containing alcohol.	Other anticonvulsants, other carbonic anhydrase inhibitors, hydrochlorthiazide, metformin, pioglitazone, lithium, amitriptylene
Usual adult dosage	Oral dose: 50 mg daily. Before prescribing: Patients must be opioid-free for a minimum of 7 to 10 days before starting. If you feel that there's a risk of precipitating an opioid withdrawal reaction, administer a naloxone challenge test. Evaluate liver function. Laboratory follow-up: Monitor liver function.	IM dose: 380 mg given as a deep intramuscular gluteal injection, once monthly. Before prescribing: Same as oral naltrexone, plus examine the injection site for adequate muscle mass and skin condition. Laboratory follow-up: Monitor liver function.	Oral dose: 666 mg (two 333-mg tablets) three times daily; or for patients with moderate renal impairment (CrCl 30 to 50 mL/min), reduce to 333 mg (one tablet) three times daily. Before prescribing: Evaluate renal function. Establish abstinence.	Oral dose: 250 mg daily (range 125 mg to 500 mg). Before prescribing: Evaluate liver function. Warn the patient (1) not to take disulfiram for at least 12 hours after drinking and that a disulfiram-alcohol reaction can occur up to 2 weeks after the last dose and (2) to avoid alcohol in the diet (e.g., sauces and vinegars), over-the-counter medications (e.g., cough syrups), and toiletries (e.g., cologne, mouthwash). Laboratory follow-up: Monitor liver function.	Oral dose: Initial dose 25 mg at bedtime, increasing the dose by 25-50 mg daily each week, divided into morning and evening doses. Faster titration is more likely to cause adverse reactions. Target dose is 200 mg per day total dose, but patients unable to tolerate that dose may respond to lower doses Before prescribing: Evaluate renal function, obtain serum electrolytes and bicarbonate Laboratory follow-up: Monitor renal function, serum electrolytes and bicarbonate.

Adapted from US Department of Health and Human Services National Institutes of Health National Institute on Alcohol Abuse and Alcoholism Helping Patients Who Drink Too Much: A Clinician's Guide NIH Publication 07–3769 Update October 2008. www.niaaa.nih.gov/guide

Note—This chart highlights some of the properties of each medication. It does not provide complete information and is not meant to be a substitute for the package inserts or other drug reference sources used by clinicians. For patient information about these and other drugs, the National Library of Medicine provides MedlinePlus (http://medlineplus.gov). Whether or not a medication should be prescribed and in what amount is a matter between individuals and their health care providers. The prescribing information provided here is not a substitute for a provider's judgment in an individual circumstance, and the NIH accepts no liability or responsibility for use of the information with regard to particular patients. Also note that while topiramate may be prescribed **"off-label"** by a practitioner, it has not yet been approved for the treatment of alcohol dependence by the FDA holistic training in not only the medical and physical sequelae resulting from chronic alcohol-related disorders but also the social, psychological, and interpersonal aspects that affect the patient's life, she or he is in a prime position to discuss the potential for relapse, the stressors that may trigger the patient to drink, as well as the need to adhere to all aspects of treatment—pharmacotherapy, social supports, individual, group, and family therapies—in order to lead a better quality of life as a sober individual.

Sedative, Hypnotic, or Anxiolytic Use and Induced Disorders

Throughout history, humans have sought agents to relieve the effects of stress and ameliorate the feelings of discomfort, tension, and anxiety; as a result, the SHAs were created. The benzodiazepines were synthesized in the late 1950s with the creation of Librium (chlordiazepoxide). Today there are over 3,000 known benzodiazepines, of which 50 are currently marketed (105). The SHA class of drugs is composed of the barbiturates, benzodiazepines, and alcohol, as previously discussed in this chapter (Table 6-15). The benzodiazepines are the most commonly prescribed and abused sedatives-hypnotics. The long-acting metabolites often cause intoxication that lasts for days. They are most lethal in overdose in combination with other sedatives-hypnotics and alcohol (106).

Even though up to 90% of hospitalized patients are given one of the SHAs and more than 15% of all American adults use these medications during any given year, less than 1% of individuals are identified as having abuse or dependence problems associated with their use. In the United States, it is reported that greater than 50% of these medications are prescribed in the primary care setting (106). Given these statistics, it is prudent for the CNS in the acute care setting to evaluate for

SHA abuse, intoxication, dependence, and withdrawal and to work with the multidisciplinary health care team to provide safe and effective treatment and management to those patients entrusted to our care.

Sedative, Hypnotic, or Anxiolytic Intoxication

The recent use of an SHA is necessary to diagnose intoxication, coupled with maladaptive behavioral and psychological changes (e.g., inappropriate sexual or aggressive behavior, mood lability, impaired judgment, impaired social or occupational functioning) that developed during, or shortly after, the use of the substance, according to the *DSM-IV-TR* (90). One or more of the following signs must also be present during or shortly after the use of the SHA: slurred speech, incoordination, unsteady gait, nystagmus, impaired attention or memory, stupor, and/or coma. The individual intoxicated on an SHA may be at risk for serious and life-threatening withdrawal symptoms that may require immediate medical intervention.

Sedative, Hypnotic, or Anxiolytic Withdrawal

Withdrawal from heavy and prolonged use of an SHA may be caused by the cessation or reduction in the amount of substance being abused. The withdrawal symptoms contribute to clinically significant distress or impairment in social, occupational, and other areas of functioning. According to the *DSM-IV-TR* (90), two or more of the following symptoms develop within several hours to a few days after the cessation or reduction in the substance: autonomic hyperactivity (e.g., sweating or pulse rate >100 beats per minute); increased hand tremor; insomnia; nausea/vomiting; transient visual, tactile, or auditory hallucinations or illusions; psychomotor agitation; anxiety; and/or grand mal seizures. Given these symptoms, the CNS must be acutely aware of the signs of intoxication and withdrawal from the SHAs.

TABLE 6–15 Sedative, Hypnotic, and Anxiolytic Medications and Their Equivalencies

Generic Name	Brand Name	Dosage
alprazolam	Xanax, Xanax XR	1 mg
chlordiazepoxide	Librium	25 mg
clonazepam	Klonopin	0.5-1 mg
diazepam	Valium	10 mg
lorazepam	Ativan	2 mg
oxazepam	Serax	30 mg
temazepam	Restoril	20 mg
zolpidem	Ambien	10 mg
zolpidem CR	Ambien CR	12.5 mg

Case Report

Sandy is a 39-year-old woman whose divorce was finalized 6 months earlier after 4 years of severe physical abuse. Approximately 13 months ago, Sandy discussed her situation with her primary care practitioner, who prescribed Xanax (alprazolam) 1 mg qid (4 times daily) for "anxiety, stress, and tension." Due to the side effect of sedation, Sandy began by taking only one-half tablet twice a day, but she began to relax and experience a bit of euphoria, which "took her mind off her day-to-day problems." Unfortunately, this feeling began to wear off and Sandy began increasing her dose up to the dose prescribed by her practitioner. Over the next few months, the stress of divorce proceedings exacerbated Sandy's anxiety and she began using more of the benzodiazepine to obtain relief. She would frequently run out of her prescription prior to the renewal date and began seeking prescriptions from other practitioners and using various pharmacies, paying cash, to obtain the drug. On the day that Sandy presented at the emergency department of the local hospital, the CNS discovered three empty prescription bottles for alprazolam, all filled within the last 45 days, totaling 120 of 1-mg tablets and 150 of 0.5-mg tablets. Sandy had been out of alprazolam for about 2 days and was trembling, sweating, complaining of nausea, and experiencing episodes of "memory loss." Sandy was admitted to the acute medical care unit and placed on a benzodiazepine withdrawal protocol. Her CIWA score was 51. Sandy's diagnoses are Benzodiazepine Dependence and Benzodiazepine Withdrawal. The following section will offer management strategies for treating the SHA-related disorders.

Management

Clinical management of SHA-related disorders in the acute care setting is very similar to that of the management of alcohol-related disorders. Overdose, whether intentional (i.e., a suicide attempt) or unintentional, constitutes the need for medical detoxification. The acute care CNS must first determine the amount of substance ingested over what period of time and the time since last ingestion. As most SHA medications fall under the drug category of the benzodiazepines, for simplicity, from here on they will be referred to as such. Low-dose benzodiazepine withdrawal is characterized by anxiety, irritability, insomnia, panic, mood lability, and neurologic-like symptoms (intolerance to bright light, bright colors, or noise). On the other hand, high-dose benzodiazepine withdrawal syndrome occurs after abrupt discontinuation of the drug and can result in very serious adverse events such as seizures, delirium, coma, and death (96). Benzodiazepine withdrawal may occur within hours of the ingestion of the last dose of drug. The abrupt cessation of drug intake progresses rapidly and depending on the half-life of the benzodiazepine ingested; withdrawal symptoms may occur over a period of 3 to 5 days up to 2 weeks or more from the last ingestion. Withdrawal from the benzodiazepines is considered a medical procedure and is typically conducted in the acute care setting of a hospital or the detoxification unit of a rehabilitation facility. The CIWA-Ar can be adapted to assess and monitor the severity of the patient's benzodiazepine withdrawal symptoms. The clinical specialist can use the score from the CIWA to adjust and personalize the standard benzodiazepine withdrawal protocol, which is typically available in acute care settings (a sample standardized Alcohol-Benzodiazepine Withdrawal Protocol was shown in Box 6-19 [94-96]).

Although detoxification can be conducted on an outpatient basis, the process of gradually reducing the amount of benzodiazepine while simultaneously monitoring the potential for serious adverse events requires a commitment from both the patient and clinician to effectively promote abstinence over a period of months or even years. The general "rule of thumb" for outpatient detoxification from the benzodiazepines tends to be a reduction by 0.5 mg per month; thus, for example, if the patient is prescribed Klonopin (clonazepam) 1 mg tid (3 times per day), it will take a minimum of 6 months to safely and comfortably detoxify the patient from the drug.

Similar to the management of the alcohol-related disorders in the acute care setting, management of the SHA (benzodiazepine)-related disorders require a multidisciplinary approach. The CNS can coordinate the team and facilitate the withdrawal procedures as well as offer treatment options to the patient and family/supports as the patient is ready to be discharged. Upon release from an acute care setting, the patient might enter a short- or long-term rehabilitation program, a partial hospital program, an intensive outpatient program, or one of the many self-help groups or individual or family therapy programs available in the community. Many times patients who have abused or developed dependence on the benzodiazepines have been prescribed the medication for treatment of an anxiety-related disorder. A psychiatric consultation or outpatient evaluation might prove helpful to address the patient's underlying anxiety and offer alternative pharmacologic agents that would not promote abuse or dependence.

Opioid Use and Induced Disorders

Opioid drugs, also called opiates or narcotics, have been used since the beginning of recorded history. Opium, derived from a white liquid produced by the poppy plant, was used therapeutically in ancient cultures to induce calm and to relieve pain and recreationally to induce euphoric dream states. Today, opioid drugs are prescribed for pain relief. The opiates bind to certain pain-reducing sites in the brain and, over time, build up and block the production of the brain's natural pain-killing chemicals, the endorphins (107). The most commonly prescribed opioid medications include codeine, oxycodone (e.g., OxyContin, Vicodin, Percocet), or morphine. The opioid analog medications are often more potent and therefore more likely to contribute to dependence than the opioids themselves. For example, fentanyl, used as a surgical anesthetic and pain-relieving transdermal patch, is 50 times more potent than heroin, and meperidine, marketed under the brand name of Demerol, can rapidly stop respiration (108). Recently, these Controlled Dangerous Substances (CDS) Schedule II prescription medications have surged in their nonmedical use or abuse. This is a serious and growing public health problem in the United States, with an estimated 48 million people, ages 12 and older, using prescription drugs for nonmedical reasons over the course of their lifetimes. This represents approximately 20% of the U.S. population. Even more alarming is the fact that in 2004, the National Institute on Drug Abuse found that almost 15% of 12-graders reported taking either Vicodin or OxyContin, making the opioids among the most commonly abused prescription drugs by adolescents (109).

Individuals who take the opioid pain relievers for pain management have a potential to also experience reward. The opioids produce reward by binding to the GABAergic receptors, which normally inhibit dopamine production in the limbic reward system and prevent them from doing so (110). The resulting increase in dopamine and the cascade of secondary effects produce feelings of reward. Unfortunately, when the reward or euphoria becomes the focus of the patient's opioid use, it may undermine the individual's pain treatment and become a problem in and of itself (111).

Opioid Intoxication

Similar to the criteria for alcohol intoxication, the *DSM-IV-TR* defines Opioid Intoxication as the recent use of an opioid that contributes to clinically significant maladaptive behavioral or psychological changes (e.g., euphoria followed by apathy, dysphoria, psychomotor agitation or retardation, impaired judgment, or impaired social or occupational functioning) that developed during or shortly after opioid use. Physical symptoms are also present in opioid intoxication and include constriction (or dilation due to anoxia from severe overdose) and one (or more) of the following signs, developing during or shortly after opioid use: drowsiness or coma, slurred speech, and/or impairment in attention or memory.

Opioid Withdrawal

Withdrawal from opioids can be severe and life-threatening and requires medical intervention. The *DSM-IV-TR* (90) characterizes opioid withdrawal as either (1) the cessation of (or reduction in) opioid use that has been heavy and prolonged (several weeks or longer) or (2) the administration of an opioid antagonist after a period of opioid use. To diagnose opioid withdrawal, the patient must also demonstrate three (or more) of the following signs developing within minutes or days after the ingestion of the opioid: dysphoric mood, nausea/vomiting, muscle aches, lacrimation or rhinorrhea, papillary dilation, piloerection or sweating, diarrhea, yawning, fever, and/or insomnia. Like withdrawal from other substances, opioid withdrawal causes significant distress in the individual's level of functioning.

Case Report

Alan is a 22-year-old college graduate and retail sales manager. He began taking Vicodin (acetaminophen-hydrocodone) following a skiing injury in which he herniated his L4-L5 lumbar disc. The Vicodin was initially prescribed on an as-needed basis for pain. Alan found that not only did the Vicodin relieve the pain in his lower back, but it also gave him a bit of a "high." He began seeking similar medications when he was unable to obtain the Vicodin and would often be late for work or meetings, especially on Mondays, after a weekend of binging on various opioid derivatives when "hanging out" with his college buddies. One Monday morning Alan was quite late for work and his supervisor summoned him to his office, where he expressed concern regarding Alan's behaviors over the past few months. Alan recognized this as his one and only warning and presented to the emergency department seeking detoxification and treatment for opioid abuse. Alan's urine drug screen was positive for opiates and marijuana, although he did not appear intoxicated and did not appear to have symptoms of withdrawal. He was evaluated by the CNS and referred to an after-work intensive outpatient program, which provides individual, group, and family therapy as well as psychiatric evaluation and medication management. Alan's diagnosis is Opioid Abuse and Cannibus Abuse. The following section will offer management strategies for treating the opioid-related disorders in the acute care setting.

Management

Addiction to the opioids is very difficult to overcome without support. Medications are often prescribed as part of the treatment plan for opioid dependence as they help to reestablish normal brain function, prevent relapses, and decrease cravings. The first step in managing opioid-related disorders is to assist the patient in detoxing from the drug(s) as safely and comfortably as possible. Medically assisted detoxification is typically conducted in either an acute care setting or the detox unit of a substance abuse rehabilitation facility. Studies have shown that patients who go through medically assisted withdrawal but do not receive further treatment show drug abuse patterns similar to those who were never treated (113). Withdrawal from the opioids is less dangerous than alcohol or SHA withdrawal; it is rarely fatal. Medications such as Catapres (clonidine) and Suboxone (buprenorphine) have helped to minimize the symptoms of withdrawal, which usually peak within 48 to 72 hours after the last dose of the opioid and subside within 1 week. Some individuals may show withdrawal symptoms for a month or longer, and cravings, especially for heroin, can last for years after drug cessation (108). Many acute care and detoxification units have standardized opioid withdrawal protocols and medication orders. A sample of opioid withdrawal orders can be found in Box 6-22 (113).

In addition to treating the withdrawal symptoms related to opioid dependence, medications become an important part of maintaining abstinence. The cravings related to the opioids can last for months to years depending on the drug, severity of use, and length of dependence. If the patient is unable to disengage from the drug-seeking behaviors, he or she will not be receptive to the behavioral interventions used to maintain abstinence and, thus, often relapses. Methadone is the mostly widely known and used medication to treat opiate addiction. It has been used for more than 30 years. Methadone is a synthetic opiate medication that, when taken orally, has a gradual onset of action and sustained effect. It is not intoxicating or sedating and its effects do not interfere with ordinary daily activities. Methadone maintenance usually occurs in specialized opiate treatment programs that also provide therapies, medical, psychological, and social services

---

BOX 6–22 Opioid Withdrawal Protocol—Sample Order Set

Place X in box next to Diagnosis and Patient Orders . . . . Orders left Blank WILL NOT be Transcribed

DIAGNOSIS: ☐ **Heroin Withdrawal**   ☐   **Prescription Opioid Withdrawal**

Date/Time and Amount of Last Ingestion of Substance of Abuse: _____

VITAL SIGNS:

Monitor patient every 4 hours (include: BP, pulse, respiratory rate, temperature)

☐ **STAT page practitioner if patient experiences any of the following: respiratory distress, change in mental status, oral temperature >101.5°F, urine output <250cc/shift, heart rate <50 or >120, systolic blood pressure ≥180 or ≤110 or diastolic blood pressure ≥100**

MEDICATIONS:

☐ Monitor blood pressure before and 20 minutes after each Clonidine dose
  Day 1: Clonidine 0.1-0.2mg every 4 hours not to exceed 1mg in 24 hours
  Day 2 to Day 4: Clonidine 0.1-0.2mg every four hours not to exceed 1.2mg in 24 hours
  Day 5 to d/c: Reduce dose by one-half every 24 hours not to exceed reduction of >0.4mg/day
☐ Vistaril (hydroxyzine) 25-50mg every 4 hours as needed for anxiety, nausea, or insomnia
☐ Ibuprofen 400mg PO every 4 hours PRN for muscles aches/pains or headache
☐ Bentyl 20 mg PO every 6 hours as needed for abdominal cramping
☐ Lomotil 2 tablets every 6 hours as needed for diarrhea
☐ Multivitamin PO Daily
☐ _____

DIET:

☐ Clear Liquids, encourage adequate fluid intake
☐ Regular
☐ Other (specify) _____
☐ Dietary/Nutrition Consult

ACTIVITY:

☐ Bedrest with Bathroom Privileges
☐ Up and Out of Bed ad lib

DIAGNOSTIC STUDIES (if not previously completed):

☐ CBC with Differential _____ Comprehensive Metabolic Panel _____ Liver Functions Studies _____ βHCG

(112). More recently, Suboxone (buprenorphine) has been used for both opiate withdrawal and maintaining abstinence. Buprenorphine is less likely to contribute to overdose and withdrawal and produces a lower level of physical dependence than methadone; thus, patients experience fewer withdrawal symptoms when they discontinue this medication compared to discontinuing methadone. Buprenorphine is available in authorized practitioner's offices, making it less stigmatizing to opioid-addicted patients seeking treatment (114). Both methadone and buprenorphine act on the same receptors in the brain as heroin and morphine and not only suppress withdrawal symptoms but also relieve cravings. The last medication approved for treatment of opioid dependence is naltrexone. As an opiate antagonist, naltrexone blocks the effects of the opiates on the receptor sites. It is shorter acting and has been used to treat cases of opiate overdose. Naltrexone has been used for maintaining abstinence once patients have been detoxified and has also been used as a "rapid detox" medication in some addiction specialists' offices.

Behavioral therapies are equally as important in assisting the patient with an opioid-related disorder to maintain a drug-free life. The CNS can assist in determining the most appropriate treatment setting to which the patient can be referred on being detoxified in the acute care setting. Such treatment settings may include rehabilitation facilities, after-work intensive outpatient programs, or community-based self-help organizations such as Narcotics Anonymous. Rehabilitation facilities offer programs that last from 2 weeks to 12 months. The objectives of enrolling the patient in behavioral therapies are to reinforce healthy life skills, modify attitudes related to drug abuse, and engage in the treatment process. The therapies work in tandem with the medications and aid the patient in learning ways to cope with their cravings and life stressors that may have exacerbated their opioid addiction. After-work intensive outpatient programs offer group and individual therapies similar to those in the rehabilitation facility but are not nearly as comprehensive as an inpatient rehab. Support groups, such as Narcotics Anonymous, have been long-standing programs of individuals who have conquered their addiction and are maintaining abstinence. They typically consist of a stepwise program offering a treatment philosophy and guidance that the patient adopts to a clean and sober lifestyle.

A Note on Pain Management

A chapter on addiction in the acute care setting would not be complete without addressing pain management in our society. It is estimated that over 50 million Americans suffer from chronic pain. Given this statistic, health care providers have long struggled with the dilemma: how to adequately relieve the patient's pain, while avoiding the potential for the patient to become addicted to the pain medication. Unfortunately, many practitioners allow the fear (known as "opiophobia") of their patient becoming addicted to the pain medication to override their better judgment in adequately managing their patient's pain syndrome. Many practitioners underprescribe the opioid pain relievers, and their patients continue to suffer and may seek ways to relieve their pain through other potentially illegal avenues (115). The risk of addiction in a patient who experiences chronic pain is very low and the risk-to-benefit ratio must be carefully weighed and monitored to allow our patients to receive the most appropriate treatments available without judgment or stigmatization.

Untreated acute pain causes unnecessary suffering, prolonged hospital stays, and increases medical costs and may actually progress to chronic pain (116). Chronic pain, then, decreases the patient's quality of life and work productivity. The societal costs of untreated (or undertreated) chronic pain are extremely high, with the economic burden in the United States estimated to be more than $100 billion per year (117). As CNSs, we must educate our patients as to the risks and benefits of the opioid pain relievers as well as the very real potential for physiologic dependence on the medication. Practitioners must discuss with their patients and families/supports the need to take the medication as prescribed and to not skip or miss doses due to the potential for withdrawal. CNSs, as educators and holistic health care providers, treat the whole patient, their pain, and their dependence on the medication, whether physiologic or psychological in nature. They will educate their patients in a manner that will minimize adverse effects and events and maximize pain relief and consistently monitor the patient related to dependency and potential for withdrawal.

Nicotine Use and Induced Disorders

According to a 2001 study published by the Centers for Disease Control and Prevention, every year, tobacco-related illnesses kill 440,000 U.S. citizens, more Americans than were killed in World War II and the Vietnam Conflict combined (118). Tobacco is the only product in the United States that causes death and disability when used as intended—the single, most preventable cause of death in America (119). It is well known that smoking and use of tobacco products increase the risk of many diseases such as cardiovascular disease; emphysema; bronchial disorders; stroke; lung cancer; cancer of the kidney, larynx, head, or neck; and oral cancers, as well as breast cancer in both men and women. It is also well known that the risk of secondhand smoke is equally as harmful as if the individual were the smoker.

Each year, nearly 35 million people make a concerted effort to quit smoking. Sadly, less than 7% succeed in abstaining for longer than 1 year, and most start smoking again within days of quitting (120). About half of all people who do not quit smoking will die of smoking-related health problems. Despite these grim statistics, soon after an individual quits smoking, their circulation begins to improve, blood pressure stabilizes and returns to normal, the person's sense of taste and smell return, and breathing becomes easier. Additionally, the risk of getting cancer decreases with each year the patient remains smoke free (121).

For the CNS to assist patients in the process of smoking cessation over the long term, it is important to understand the nature of nicotine addiction. Smoking is not just a "bad habit"; it is an addiction with a very real impact on the brain's neurochemistry. As the nicotine in a cigarette is inhaled, it moves through the lungs, into the bloodstream, and circulates through the smoker's brain in less than 10 seconds, causing the release of adrenaline. This release of adrenaline signals the body to dump excess glucose into the bloodstream; however, nicotine inhibits the release of insulin from the pancreas, leaving the smoker in a slightly hyperglycemic state, which reduces hunger. Upon reaching the brain, nicotine activates the reward pathways through an increase in dopamine in the brain, creating a temporary feeling of pleasure for the smoker. Unfortunately, these pleasurable sensations are short-lived and subside within minutes leaving the smoker feeling edgy and agitated—this is how rapidly nicotine withdrawal begins. In order to avoid and relieve these uncomfortable feelings, the smoker lights up another cigarette, and another, and another. This is the vicious cycle of nicotine addiction (122).

Nicotine Withdrawal

According to the *DSM-IV-TR* (91), Nicotine Withdrawal is characterized by the following:

1. Daily use of nicotine for at least several weeks;
2. Abrupt cessation of nicotine use or reduction in the amount of nicotine used, followed within 24 hours by four (or more) of the following signs: dysphoric or depressed mood, insomnia, irritability, frustration or anger, anxiety, difficulty concentrating, restlessness, decreased heart rate, and/or increased appetite or weight gain;
3. The symptoms cause clinically significant distress or impairment in social, occupational, or other important areas of functioning.

Case Report

As a majority of health care facilities have adopted a "smoke-free facility" policy in recent years, nurses are on the front lines attempting to assist those patients who present to the acute care setting as active smokers. Take the case of Jane, for example, a 58-year-old woman who has smoked a minimum of one pack of cigarettes per day for over 35 years. At times she smoked as much as two packs per day and has attempted to quit smoking on at least four occasions. Her longest period of abstinence was during her pregnancy with her eldest child 26 years ago. Her most recent period of abstinence was 2 years ago after being hospitalized for "chest pain." This period of smoking cessation lasted 3 months. Jane presents today with shortness of breath, chest pressure, a deep wracking cough, elevated blood pressure, loss of appetite, and fatigue. She has been smoking about one pack per day over the past 21 months. The CNS is called to consult on smoking cessation protocols to assist Jane with obtaining and maintaining nicotine abstinence. Jane's diagnosis would be Nicotine Dependence. The following section will outline management strategies to treat nicotine-related disorders in the acute care setting.

Management

As many hospitals, public facilities, and even bars and restaurants are now maintaining "smoke-free" environments around the country, the management of a patient with nicotine addiction presents quite a challenge in the acute care setting. First, the patient is likely experiencing an increase in anxiety related to his or her hospitalization. Second, under stress, the patient is more likely to crave cigarettes and the pleasurable feeling resulting from the effects of the nicotine. Finally, the patient is unlikely to be prepared to quit "cold turkey." Fortunately, there are a variety of formulations of nicotine replacement therapies that exist to reduce the discomfort, anxiety, and irritability common to nicotine withdrawal. The various delivery systems for nicotine replacement include the patch, a spray, gum, and lozenges; thus, if the patient is NPO, they may still be treated for nicotine withdrawal by using the transdermal patch formulation of nicotine replacement while waiting for their testing or surgery in an acute care setting.

The CNS in an acute care setting can provide the patient and family with information on smoking cessation, the costs, risks, and benefits to the patient's health due to continued smoking as well as offer various treatment options that may be started while the patient is in the hospital. The most successful smoking cessation programs include not only nicotine replacement therapies and or medications but also behavioral interventions, group and/or individual therapy, and telephone quit-lines.

Support to aid the patient in abstaining from smoking is extremely important, just as it is with all of the other substance use and abuse disorders discussed in this chapter. The cravings and desire are powerful urges that weaken even the most committed smoker in the early phases of quitting. The U.S. Food and Drug Administration (FDA) has approved two prescription medications for the treatment of nicotine/tobacco dependence/addiction: bupropion (Wellbutrin) and varenicline (Chantix). Although these two medications have very different mechanisms of action in the brain, they both help to prevent relapse in individuals attempting to quit smoking.

The dopamine-norepinepherine reuptake inhibitor antidepressant bupropion, marketed under the brand names Wellbutrin and Zyban, is used to treat both depression and nicotine dependence. Its effectiveness as an aid to quit smoking was discovered when smokers taking the medication to treat depression lost interest in smoking and found themselves quitting with relative ease. Bupropion blocks the reuptake of dopamine, thus allowing the individual to experience similar effects to the pleasure they experience when smoking. When used with other nicotine replacement therapies, the patient increases their chances for long-term success related to smoking cessation (123). Varenicline, marketed under the brand name Chantix, on the other hand, is a nonnicotine medication that targets the nicotine receptors in the brain by binding to them and blocking the nicotine in cigarette smoke from reaching them. By attaching to the nicotine receptors in the brain, a signal is sent out to a different part of the brain to release dopamine, the pleasure-enhancing neurochemical. It is believed that varenicline, unlike nicotine from cigarettes, causes less dopamine to be released; thus, the pleasurable sensations are not as great and the cravings for more nicotine are reduced, allowing the patient to stop smoking (124). Both of these medications can be managed on an outpatient basis and need to be monitored regularly due to the potential risk for increased suicidal thinking, agitation, and other changes in thought, mood, or behavior. Medications used for treatment of nicotine dependence are described in Table 6-16 (124-126).

CLINICAL NURSE SPECIALIST COMPETENCIES AND SPHERES OF INFLUENCE

The CNS in the acute care setting offers many competencies in treating patients with substance-related disorders. These patients often require immediate treatment interventions related to intoxication and withdrawal symptoms that may be life threatening. The effective management, through the CNS's direct expert clinical care, of substance-related disorders requires a timely, comprehensive, collaborative approach to achieve optimal patient outcomes within the acute care setting. Once the patient is detoxified, the CNS can assist in collaborating with social work in coordinating community-based resources to aid the patient in their quest to lead a clean and sober life.

As many patients with substance-related disorders relapse, the CNS may provide education to the patient, and family/support system, that focuses on recovery and abstinence. The CNS may provide educational materials related to various pharmacologic and therapeutic interventions that are indicated to provide the best patient outcomes and abstinence. Patients may also receive education related to their medication management, insight into the life stressors that lead to substance abuse, the nature of psychological versus physiologic dependence, and ways to cope with their addiction by using supports. Connecting the patient with supportive therapies on discharge from the acute care setting is one of the most important functions that the CNS can provide. Without behavioral and pharmacologic treatments, the patient with a substance-related disorder is highly likely to continuing abusing the substance(s) and will continue to be admitted to the acute care setting for detoxification as well as treatment for the various health conditions that result from a life of substance abuse.

Admission to an acute care setting is often the gateway for substance abusers to obtain the rehabilitation services they require to detoxify prior to engaging in the significant process of recovery and abstinence. The patient's interaction with the health care team in the acute care setting may influence the patient's decision to continue into the next phase(s) of recovery. The CNS can provide education to the medical, nursing, and allied health care staff on ways to appropriately interact with the patient to avoid stigma and personal biases. As substance abusers may be "well known" to the health care staff due to multiple admissions for intoxication and medical conditions related to their abuse, it is critical that the staff approach the patient in a positive, professional manner so that this admission may prove to be the one in which the patient engages in treatment and the road to abstinence. With a holistic approach to the patient and his or her treatment, the CNS may serve as the point person for the treatment team in responding to questions related to the patient's management in the acute care setting and beyond.

Successful management of substance-related disorders commonly treated in the acute care setting, such as intoxication, withdrawal, and dependence on the various substances, requires a comprehensive, collaborative, pharmacologic, and therapeutic approach to obtain the most successful patient outcomes. The acute care setting is the first step in the patient's journey toward a clean and sober life of abstinence and may "make or break" the patient's engagement and investment in the treatment process. The CNS caring for patients with substance-related disorders collaborates with the health care team, provides education to the patient and the family/support system, and offers a comprehensive treatment plan including medication and therapeutic interventions, all while ensuring that the patient is treated in an appropriate professional manner free of stigma and biases. The role of the CNS in treating patients with substance-related disorders in the acute care setting is extremely important in offering these patients a new approach to managing their addiction and move toward a life of sobriety and abstinence.

TABLE 6–16 Medications for Treating Nicotine Dependence

	Nicotine Gum/Lozenge	Nicotine Inhaler	Nicotine Nasal Spray	Nicotine Transdermal Patch	Bupropion (Zyban, Wellbutrin)	Varenicline (Chantix)
ACTION	Rapid absorption through oral mucosa approximates time course of plasma nicotine levels observed with cigarette smoking	Same as nicotine gum and lozenge	Rapid absorption through nasal mucosa approximates time course of plasma nicotine levels observed with cigarette smoking	Absorbed through the skin Most appropriate for those who smoke more than 10 cigarettes per day	Inhibits neuronal dopamine reuptake and blocks norepinephrine reuptake in the brain	Binds to and blocks nicotine receptors signaling release of dopamine in the brain
CONTRAINDICATIONS	Hypersensitivity, nonsmokers, children, pregnancy, life-threatening arrhythmias, angina pectoris	Same as nicotine gum and lozenge	Same as nicotine gum and lozenge	Same as nicotine gum and lozenge	Hypersensitivity, seizures, anorexia nervosa, concurrent use with MAOIs or other bupropion products	Hypersensitivity, severe renal impairment, angioedema, use caution if psychiatric illness
PRECAUTIONS	Pregnancy Category D No smoking cigarettes Peptic ulcers, CAD, angina, HTN, PAD, DM, renal dysfunction, Hepatic dysfunction	Same as nicotine gum and lozenge	Same as nicotine gum and lozenge	Same as nicotine gum and lozenge	Pregnancy Category B Renal/hepatic insufficiency, doses >450 mg/day ↓ seizure threshold, possible HTN	Pregnancy Category C Mania, psychosis, aggression, depression, anxiety, homicidal and suicidal ideation

INTERACTIONS

| ↓ effects of diuretics, ↓ cardiac output, ↓ absorption of glutethimide, ↑ cortisol and catecholamines, other nicotine products ↑ toxicity | Same as nicotine gum and lozenge | Same as nicotine gum and lozenge | Same as nicotine gum and lozenge | Carbamazepine, cimetidine, phenytoin, and phenobarbital may ↓ effects, toxicity ↑ with levodopa and MAOIs | ↓ in renal clearance with cimetidine, ↑ AEs with nicotine replacement therapy |

COMMON SIDE EFFECTS

| Tingling sensation, peppery taste, numbness of cheek/gum | Rhinitis, throat and mouth irritation | Coughing, worsening of asthma, burning or irritation of nasal passages | Skin irritation, insomnia (if persistent remove patch at bedtime) | Headache, nausea, anxiety, insomnia, potential ↑ suicidal thinking, worsening of depression, agitation | Nausea, GI upset, constipation, insomnia, headache, abnormal dreams |

USUAL ADULT DOSING

| GUM: chew 1 piece every 1-2 hours while awake × 6 weeks then, ↓ to 1 piece every 2-4 hours for 2 weeks, then ↓ to 1 piece every 4-8 hours × 2 weeks LOZENGE: dissolve 1 every 1-2 hours while awake × 6 weeks, then ↓ to 1 every 2-4 hours × 2 weeks, then ↓ to 1 every 4-8 hours × 2 weeks | Most effective with continuous puffing over 20 minutes using 6-16 cartridges daily, gradually ↓ dose over 6-12 weeks | 1-2 sprays per hour intranasally not to exceed 10 sprays per hour or 40 sprays in 24 hours Each spray = 0.5 mg nicotine | Apply highest dose patch daily × 6 weeks then ↓ to middle dose patch × 2 weeks then ↓ to lowest dose patch × 2 weeks | 150 mg daily × 3 days then increase to 300 mg daily in the morning | Days 1-3 0.5 mg once daily Days 4-7 0.5 mg twice daily Day 8: End of treatment 1 mg twice daily Treatment is 12 weeks If abstinent at 12 weeks an additional 12 week course is recommended to maintain abstinence |

HELP RESOURCES
For a list of resources for substance-related disorders for patients, families, and caregivers, see the end of this chapter under Help Resources: Substance-Related Disorders.

Anxiety and Depression

Two-thirds of patients who are high users of acute medical care suffer from a psychiatric disturbance: 23% suffer from depression, 22% suffer from anxiety, and 20% experience various somatic complaints (127-129). This is an extraordinary number of individuals who come into contact with nurses and APRNs in an acute care hospital setting. APRNs are educated and trained as licensed independent practitioners who collaborate with patients, their families, physicians, nurses, and other members of the health care team to provide holistic care to the hospitalized individual. Psychiatric APRNs have specialized training in mental health care and are in the prime position to work with patients in an acute care setting who suffer from symptoms of anxiety and depression.

Anxiety disorders are among the most common of the psychiatric/mental health disorders. They are characterized as the pathologic counterpart of normal fear and are manifest by disturbances of mood, thought, behavior, and physiologic activity (130). Patients in acute care settings may suffer not only from a primary anxiety disorder such as generalized anxiety disorder, obsessive compulsive disorder, panic disorder, acute stress disorder, PTSD, and phobias but also anxiety disorder related to their medical condition. Anxiety disorders are both common and chronic. They contribute to both distress and disability. When left untreated, they are costly to both the individual and society. The treatment of anxiety disorders in the acute care setting is not only prudent but warranted, as this may be the only opportunity for the patients to obtain the needed mental health care. Working with the anxious patient in an acute care setting may prove less threatening than if the patient were to seek treatment from a psychiatric or mental health provider. Additionally, as stress and anxiety are known to contribute to diminished levels of health, treatment within the acute care settings allows the practitioner the opportunity to educate the patient regarding the effects of anxiety on physical health and ways to improve overall quality of life.

Similarly, depressive disorders contribute to the growing cost of health care. In the first study to examine the connection between depression and acute care hospitalizations, researchers reviewed the records of more than 60,000 depressed, chronically ill patients and found that they were twice as likely to use the emergency department or to have a preventable hospitalization compared to their nondepressed, chronically ill counterparts (131). Depression is also a common and chronic illness. It contributes to both distress and disability and if left untreated can prove costly to both the individual and society. Whenever and wherever patients present with depressive symptoms, it is in everyone's best interest to begin treatment. The sooner the symptoms are treated, the better are the potential outcomes for the individual's physical and mental health as well as quality of life.

It is generally accepted that patients in an acute care setting experience stress/anxiety on entering the hospital. The impact of chronic stress may prove to exacerbate the individual's physical symptomatology; should the patient's acute hospitalization, unfortunately, take an extended course, depression may result. When iatrogenic depressive symptoms emerge in hospitalized patients, nurses, the primary care providers, are typically the first to observe such changes in the patient. It is critical that nurses have an understanding not only of physical disease processes and symptoms but also of psychiatric disturbances that may have an impact on the patient and contribute to potentially poor outcomes or prolonged hospitalization. The APRN is able to provide this education and knowledge when consulting to nurses staffing acute care medical units. Given the continued stigma toward mental illness in the United States, the identification and treatment of anxiety and depression during an acute care hospitalization may be the only opportunity for the patient to receive the psychiatric care and treatment that he or she requires. APRNs, again, play a leading role in offering holistic care to patients with physical as well as emotional symptoms that have an impact on and potentially decrease their overall quality of life.

Incidence of Anxiety and Depression in Acute Care Setting

In any given 1-year period, 44 million adults, or about 23% of the general population, suffer from a diagnosable psychiatric disorder. Of those individuals, almost 18% suffer from an anxiety-based disorder and roughly 7% suffer from a mood disorder. To complicate the diagnostic picture, approximately 15% of the population suffers from not only one but two or more co-occurring mental health conditions (130).

Individuals suffering from anxiety and/or depression may visit their primary care practitioners and, possibly acute care facilities, many times before they are diagnosed with a psychiatric condition. They will often present with physical complaints of pain, headaches, insomnia, as well as racing heart, shortness of breath, and gastrointestinal upset. Suicidal thinking may or may not be part of the presenting symptom profile when the patient presents to the acute care setting. Additional complaints of feeling overwhelmed, helpless, and hopeless and having difficulty coping are also frequently heard. There may be lateness or absence from work; the individual may begin to isolate from family and friends; the individual may seek to relieve discomfort through alcohol or drugs, including over-the-counter medications such as headache and pain relievers. It behooves practitioners of all disciplines and specialties to further explore such complaints with their patients so that treatment may be initiated as soon as possible.

Of the 40 million plus American adults diagnosed with anxiety disorders, 2.2 million are diagnosed with obsessive-compulsive disorder, 7.7 million suffer from PTSD, 15 million are affected by social anxiety disorder, 6.8 million suffer from generalized anxiety disorder, and approximately 6 million are diagnosed with panic disorder. Women are almost twice as likely as are men to be diagnosed with an anxiety disorder (132). Anxiety disorders frequently occur along with other physical and mental illnesses as well as substance abuse, which may mask the symptoms of anxiety and worsen the symptoms of the anxiety and/or the patient's physical illness. Fortunately, with treatment most individuals suffering from an anxiety disorder can lead healthy and productive lives.

It is not uncommon for individuals who suffer from anxiety to also suffer from comorbid depression. Depression also coexists with substance abuse and other serious medical illnesses such as heart disease, cancer, HIV infection/AIDS, stroke, diabetes, and Parkinson disease. Not only do these disease states coexist with depression, but the individual's symptoms tend to be more severe, the individual may struggle to adapt and cope with their medical condition, and greater medical costs are expended by depressed individuals than by those who do not have a coexisting depression (133). According to the Web site of the National Institute of Mental Health, depression is the leading cause of disability among Americans between the ages of 15 and 44. During any given calendar year, statistics show that 14.8 million adults, or 6.7% of the U.S. population, are affected by major depression, 3.3 million adults are diagnosed with dysthymic disorder, and 5.7 million are diagnosed with bipolar disorder (including bipolar depression) (134).

About 90% of completed suicides are committed by those individuals diagnosed with a mental illness, most commonly depression and/or substance abuse. Despite the fact that women attempt suicide two to three times more frequently than men, four times as many men die by suicide. The highest rates of suicide in the United States are found among elderly men over the age of 85

(134). We can again hypothesize that, in the elderly, the impact of physical illness on depression and depression on physical illness may contribute to these unfortunate statistics. Although suicide is a potential grim reality associated with mental illness and depression in particular, depression is a highly treatable disorder with very favorable outcomes allowing the individual to lead a fulfilling and productive life.

Societal Stigmatization of Anxiety and Depression

An estimated 50 million Americans experience a mental disorder in any given year, yet less than 25% of them actually receive mental health treatment and other services. Why, you ask? STIGMA (135). Stigmatization of people with mental disorders has persisted throughout history. It is manifested by bias, distrust, stereotyping, fear, shame, embarrassment, anger, and/or avoidance. Stigma is about disrespect, the use of a negative label to identify a person living with mental illness (130). In the United States, the news media and entertainment industry play a critical role in forming society's opinion related to mental illness. In a 2005 study of 70 major U.S. newspapers, 39% of all stories published about the mentally ill focused on dangerousness—the single largest area of the media's coverage of mental health. Similarly, Hollywood has greatly benefitted from its long-standing and lurid fascination with psychiatric illness reflected by such characters as Norman Bates in Alfred Hitchcock's *Psycho;* Dr. Hannibal Lecter in *Silence of the Lambs;* Glenn Close's portrayal of Alex, the spurned and psychotic lover in *Fatal Attraction;* and others (136). The reality is, however, that these characters are exaggerated and fantastical, which sells at the box office but unfortunately portrays those with mental illness as threatening, deviant, dangerous individuals.

On a more positive note, history has provided us with many notable public figures and celebrities who have revealed their own experiences with psychiatric illness yet continue to thrive and achieve at the highest levels of their fields: Abraham Lincoln's depression was thought to be a source of his greatness; Vincent van Gogh's hypothesized struggle with psychotic depression/bipolar may have accounted for his creative genius; the Nobel Prize–winning economist John Forbes Nash struggled with schizophrenia; actress and talk-show host Roseanne Barr has had experiences with anxiety, obsessive-compulsive disorder, PTSD, and multiple personality disorder, among others (136, 137).

To assist our acute care patients who present with symptoms of anxiety, depression, or another mental illness, we as health care providers must be very conscious of the language we use to describe our patient's symptoms and to be sure we are not attributing the symptom to the person. Per the Substance Abuse and Mental Health Administration's efforts to dispel the stigma of mental illness, "words can be poison or words can heal" (138). Therapeutic words for people with anxiety are found in Table 6-17.

Health Care Costs of Anxiety and Depression

Due to the stigmas described in the last section, individuals may feel discouraged and ashamed to seek mental health treatment for fear of being the victim of further discrimination. This is extremely troubling as mental health disorders rank as one of the top five most costly conditions in the United States. From 1996 to 2006, direct medical expenditures related to mental illness rose from $35.2 billion (in 2006 dollars) to $57.5 billion, and the number of individuals with expenditures associated with mental health disorders rose from 19.3 million in 1996 to 36.2 million in 2006 (139). According to a 1999 study commissioned by the Anxiety Disorders Association of America (140), anxiety disorders cost the United States more than $42 billion a year, almost one-third of the country's $148 billion total mental health bill. Almost $23 billion of those costs are associated with the repeated use of health care services for anxiety symptoms that mimic physical illness.

Over the past 25 plus years there has been a growing body of evidence showing that individuals suffering from depression have a greater utilization of general medical care services than those without depressive symptoms. Likewise, general medical pharmaceutical costs for patients diagnosed with depression were greater than general medical pharmaceutical costs for nondepressed patients. Inpatient costs for treatment of coronary artery disease, epilepsy, and congestive heart failure among depressed patients were $1,890, $2,560, and $13,900 greater, respectively, than treatment for the same medical conditions in nondepressed patients (141).

Although these trends have been explored for almost a quarter century, the reasons for the discrepancies and increased health care expenditures among individuals diagnosed with anxiety and depression remain uncertain. We can hypothesize that patients' behavior plays a role in their overall level of wellness. Given that depressed individuals generally are less compliant with their treatment regimen, may have poor self-care skills, and experience poor overall coping skills, the likelihood of an individual suffering from depression adhering to their medication and therapies, whether for mental or physical illness, is poor. As compliance and adherence decrease, the likelihood of their physical disease states worsening increases proportionately, thus contributing to greater utilization of acute care services by the depressed individual. Similarly, in a study exploring the relationship between anxiety and poor perceived health in patients with an implantable defibrillator, patients suffering from anxiety may avoid behaviors that they believe may trigger shocks, thus limiting the frequency and intensity of their former activities of daily life (142). This avoidance behavior may, again, contribute to a decline in the patient's physical health as the individual may not exercise, follow healthy nutritional guidelines, or engage in social activities they may experience as stressful in order to avoid triggering the implantable defibrillator. Unfortunately, avoidant behaviors may also contribute to worsening of anxiety and/or depressive symptoms, especially when the patient is confronted with a situation they have avoided. To say the physical and emotional impact of anxiety and depression on a patient's overall health and well-being are tremendous would be an understatement.

Anxiety Disorders in the Acute Care Setting

Anxiety disorders are a category of psychiatric disorders with the common characteristics of excessive, irrational fear and dread. They tend to overwhelm the individual and may permeate the individual's relationships socially as well as at home and work. These disorders are chronic conditions, unlike the episodic feelings of anxiety experienced when an individual is faced with a stressful event. The following disorders all fall under the heading of the anxiety disorders, yet each is unique and distinct in its manifestation and level of debilitation to the individual.

TABLE 6–17 Therapeutic Words for Those With Anxiety

Words That Poison	Words That Heal

1. Don't portray successful persons with disabilities as superhuman
2. Don't use generic labels such as retarded or mentally ill
3. Don't use terms like crazy, schizo, lunatic, slow, retarded, or normal
	1. Do use respectful language such as:
	  a. -a person with depression
	  b. -she has a psychiatric disability
	  c. -he suffers from anxiety
	2. Do emphasize abilities, not limitations
	3. Do tell someone if they express a stigmatizing attitude

Generalized Anxiety Disorder

Generalized anxiety disorder (GAD) is characterized by at least 6 months of a constant state of exaggerated tension or worry unrelated to any particular situation, problem, or event. Many times the worries focus on family, health, employment, and/or money. The individual who suffers from GAD typically views life as if the glass is half empty; he is always anticipating disaster or catastrophe. Many physical symptoms accompany the worry, including headache, muscle aches, fatigue, insomnia, tension, twitching, trembling, poor concentration, shortness of breath, excessive sweating, nausea, diarrhea, and irritability. They simply cannot seem to relax.

Although quite distressing to the individual, the worries may or may not be evident to those with whom they have contact. Women tend to be twice as likely to suffer from GAD, which can occur at any age across the life span. GAD rarely occurs alone but rather with a comorbid second anxiety disorder, depression, or substance abuse disorder.

GAD is commonly treated with cognitive-behavioral therapy (CBT) and/or medication therapy. With treatment those suffering from GAD can finally relax and experience a better quality of life.

Panic Disorder With or Without Agoraphobia

Panic disorder is one of the most common yet highly unrecognized psychiatric disorders in medical settings. Approximately one-third to one-half of the patients presenting in acute care settings with panic disorder do not manifest the key trademark of "fear of dying," "fear of going crazy," or "fear of losing control" that typically distinguishes the patient's symptoms as those of an anxiety-based mental health condition (143, 144). The common symptoms of panic disorder include racing heart, irregular heartbeat, shortness of breath, pressure in the chest, sweating, dizziness, lightheadedness, weakness, numbness and tingling in the extremities, nausea, and/or chest pain. Some have described their symptoms as similar to those of an individual experiencing a heart attack and frequently seek acute medical care multiple times before being diagnosed with panic disorder. The physical symptoms are often accompanied by an impending sense of dread or doom and the fear of impending death. The "panic attack" can last from 2 to 20 minutes with an average of 10 minutes before the physical symptoms subside. The attacks can occur anytime, day or night, even during sleep, and are not typically related to any particular activity, situation, or stressful event. It is the worry and fear of having another attack and the fear of embarrassing one's self in a public forum that drive the individual suffering from panic attacks to begin to isolate and avoid social situations and previously enjoyed activities. When the individual with panic disorder restricts activities and avoid contact outside of the home, the diagnosis is Panic Disorder with Agoraphobia, fear of the outside.

Adolescence and young adulthood are the most common periods of onset for panic disorder and seem to exacerbate during transitional life phases such as high school to college or the work force, marriage, birth of a child, etc. Again, females are twice as likely as males to be diagnosed with Panic Disorder. Fortunately, panic disorder, whether or not agoraphobia is present, is highly treatable. Relaxation techniques, behavioral modification, exposure, and medication are the most widely used treatment modalities in assisting those diagnosed with panic disorder to lead healthy and productive lives.

Obsessive-Compulsive Disorder

Obsessive-compulsive disorder (OCD) is arguably one of the most debilitating of the anxiety disorders. Often first occurring in childhood and afflicting over 4 million Americans, OCD does not distinguish between males and females as they are equally as likely to be diagnosed with this disorder. The individual who experiences obsessive thoughts and/or compulsive behaviors understands and realizes that the thoughts and actions are irrational, yet feels incapable of controlling the anxiety resulting from the obsession without completing the compulsive behavior. The person with OCD is literally held captive by his symptoms. When untreated, patients with OCD often are late for work or appointments, may miss important events, may experience physical health concerns, and may find it difficult to lead a healthy social life.

Obsessions are recurrent, persistent thoughts, impulses, or images that exacerbate feelings of anxiety in the individual. These intrusive thoughts cannot be resolved by logic or reasoning; thus, most people try to rid themselves of the thoughts by trying to ignore them or suppress them with some other thought or action. The most common obsessions concern worries about contamination with germs; excessive concerns about being injured or a loved one being injured or harmed; the need for order, symmetry, and exactness; and obsessions about "forbidden" sexual, religious, or racial thoughts.

Compulsions, on the other hand, are repetitive behaviors or mental exercises that the individual feels compelled to perform in response to an obsession. The purpose of the compulsive behavior is to reduce or extinguish the distress, worry, and concerns produced by the obsessive thoughts. The individual, again, realizes that the compulsive behaviors are irrational and unfounded, yet must complete the ritual or behavior to "undo" the obsessive thought. The most common compulsions are outlined in Table 6-18 (145).

OCD is very disruptive to one's familial and social relationships. Studies have shown that some women experience an acute onset of OCD during pregnancy or within the first few weeks after giving birth (146, 147). The most common symptoms of "postpartum OCD" are intrusive, ego-dystonic, anxiety-evoking obsessional thoughts about

TABLE 6–18 Obsessive Compulsive Disorder

Compulsion	Behavior	Rationale
CHECKING		
	Retracing steps/routes Checking locks, stoves, lights	Reduce fear of harming oneself or others if behaviors not completed
ORDERING/ARRANGING		
	Aligning items symmetrically Things "have to be perfect"	Reduce discomfort of perceived chaos
CLEANING		
	Repetitive washing, use of sanitizers or chemicals May take hours May cause irritation to skin	Reduce the fear of germs contaminating one's being or surroundings
REPEATING/COUNTING		
	Must repeat phrases, names, numbers, etc. Ritualized number patterns, e.g., chewing, brushing teeth	Dispel anxiety if behavior not completed Reduce fear of harm
HOARDING		
	Collecting items (newspaper, scraps, old worn clothing, etc.) such that piles are formed "just in case"	Reduce anxiety related to disposing of an item one might potentially need in the future

harming the newborn and avoidance of situations that evoke those cognitions (i.e., carrying the baby down the steps, allowing the dog to be in the house, etc.). In a case report by Abramowitz and Moore (147), they found that four male patients also experienced an acute onset of significant anxiety and ego-dystonic thoughts about responsibility for harm coming to their newborn child or their wife. None of these individuals had any prior mental health history, yet they experienced excessive worry that they may act on their obsessions or not complete a compulsion and harm would come to their wife or child. Fortunately, OCD, whether acute onset such as the postpartum scenario described here, or chronic, is treatable with a combination medication and CBT approach.

Posttraumatic Stress Disorder

PTSD manifests itself after an individual has experienced or witnessed a life-threatening or traumatic event such as natural disasters, terrorist incidents, war, violent personal assault, traumatic injury, or abuse. Individuals relive the trauma through flashbacks or nightmares, suffer from significant sleep disturbance, and may feel detached or estranged both from themselves as well as those around them. PTSD can occur at any point across the life span, with a higher number of females being diagnosed than males. The symptoms of PTSD typically occur within 3 months of the traumatic event but can be delayed and appear later when least expected. This anxiety-based disorder often occurs with other related disorders such as depression, substance abuse, memory deficits, as well as other physical and mental health disorders.

The symptoms of PTSD fall into three categories as illustrated in Table 6-19 (148).

Fortunately, with medication and psychotherapy, the symptoms of PTSD, which interrupt and interfere with the individual's quality of life, can be reduced if not alleviated. Treatment of the individual with PTSD may also involve the family and loved ones who are affected by the devastation that trauma creates in an individual's life.

Anxiety Disorder Due to General Medical Conditions

When an individual is diagnosed with an acute or a chronic medical condition, it is generally accepted that the patient may initially experience anxiety. Should those anxiety symptoms persist and prevail solely within the context of the medical condition, a diagnosis of Anxiety Disorder Due to General Medical Condition is warranted. The predominant characteristics of this disorder include excessive anxiety, panic attacks, obsessions related to the medical condition, and compulsions to dispel the perceived harm arising from the obsessive thoughts (149). One example might be a 56-year-old woman status post kidney transplantation who continues to require dialysis and experiences severe panic attacks on the way to dialysis and continues to worry and obsess about her renal status. She is otherwise able to function without anxiety, worry, or panic. She would be diagnosed with Anxiety Disorder Due to Chronic Renal Failure.

Again, many of the patients seen in the acute care medical setting experience anxiety; this disorder manifests itself in persistent debilitating anxiety symptoms solely due to the medical condition and no other stressor or life event. As with the previously discussed anxiety disorders, this disorder also contributes to significant distress and/or impairment in the individual's ability to function in social, occupational, educational, and/or other important areas. A multidisciplinary treatment approach is necessary to optimize the outcomes for patients with an anxiety disorder due to their medical condition. First, the physical disorder must be stabilized; then, the emotional disturbances and anxiety can be treated with psychoeducation regarding their mental illness, health education regarding their medical condition, and psychotherapeutic interventions and possibly medications to minimize the discomfort of the anxiety.

Case Report

A 24-year-old man is hospitalized after presenting to the emergency department with complaints of chest pressure causing tingling and numbness in his right arm, racing heart with occasional irregular heartbeat, shortness of breath, and sweating. "I feel like I'm having a heart attack, I was just sitting there surfing the net and next thing I know I can't breathe, I'm dizzy, the room's spinning . . . my girlfriend was scared so she brought me here." All blood work and laboratory studies (complete blood count [CBC] with differential, comprehensive metabolic screen, urine drug screen, and thyroid function tests) returned within the normal range. His electrocardiogram was normal. A chest radiograph was normal, and his vital signs indicated mild tachycardia with a pulse rate of 88 and mildly elevated blood pressure of 138/86 mm Hg. He was admitted for observation.

Further evaluation by the CNS reveals a family history of anxiety on the maternal side. The patient also reports that he has experienced similar symptoms in the past but not to the current extent. He reports that he has awakened at times from a sound sleep with his heart pounding and rapid breathing lasting about 5 to 10 minutes. "This episode was the worst. I'm too young to have a heart attack, and there's no history in my family. I work out, I watch my diet, what's going on with me?" As the CNS on the unit, you are able to provide your patient with the reassurance that there are no medical findings indicating any physical cause for his symptoms. He is still unconvinced. As a clinical specialist, you are also able to share with your patient that his symptoms are consistent with a diagnosis of Panic Disorder without Agoraphobia. Further, you offer that this is a highly treatable anxiety-based disorder that typically manifests itself around transitional life phases (the patient shared that he plans to ask his girlfriend to marry him this month). You review the symptoms of the disorder with your patient and his girlfriend and family, as they too are concerned that he has some undiagnosed cardiac condition. You offer him referrals to a local psychiatric APRN for a medication evaluation and a local therapist for CBT to assist him in better coping with this new diagnosis.

Diagnosis

Although the exact mechanisms of action are generally unknown, anxiety disorders are thought to be caused by dysregulation of the neurotransmitters norepinepherine

TABLE 6–19 Symptoms Related to PTSD

Intrusion	Avoidance	Hyperarousal
Flashbacks	Avoids close emotional ties	Act as if constantly threatened
Sudden vivid memories	Feelings of numbness	Sudden irritability
"Feel" painful emotions	Diminished emotions	Sudden explosiveness
Diminished attention	Labile emotions	Poor concentration
	Flood to Devoid	
Reliving trauma in real time	Depression	Insomnia and hypervigilence
Dissociation	Survivor guilt	Exaggerated startle reflex

(NE), serotonin (5-HT), and gamma-aminobutyric acid (GABA). Other contributors to anxiety include activation of the autonomic nervous system and norepinepherine release in the limbic system (150). There is also a strong genetic/hereditary component to all of the anxiety disorders except PTSD. Various medications such as the steroids, medications used to treat asthma, hormonal treatments, oral contraceptives, over-the-counter cold and flu preparations, diet and weight loss pills, energy drinks, and even some herbal supplements, among others, can contribute to and mimic symptoms of anxiety. There are also some medical conditions that mimic symptoms of anxiety. The most common include hyperthyroidism, pheochromocytoma, electrolyte imbalances, hormonal imbalances, infections, substance abuse disorders (including caffeine and nicotine abuse), as well as other anxiety disorders. A routine physical examination, laboratory studies (including CBC with differential, comprehensive metabolic panel, T_3, free T_4, total T_4, and thyroid-stimulating hormone, a urinalysis, and urine drug screen) and an electrocardiogram are typically sufficient to rule out gross medical etiology (150). Additionally, a psychiatric evaluation including mental status examination and suicide risk assessment are necessary diagnostic tools to evaluate and determine the appropriate course of treatment for the patient.

Anxiety Rating Scales

Although there are a myriad of anxiety rating scales that can be used to determine not only if a patient suffers from anxiety but also to what extent, the most commonly used and most reliable, consistent, and valid scales seem to be the Zung Self-rating Anxiety Scale, developed in 1971 (150), and the Hamilton Anxiety Rating Scale (HAM-A), which was developed earlier, in 1959 (151).

Hamilton Anxiety Rating Scale

Available in the public domain, the HAM-A, shown in Box 6-23, was one of the first rating scales developed to measure the severity of anxiety symptoms. It remains

---

BOX 6–23 Hamilton Anxiety Rating Scale (HAM-A)

Below is a list of phrases that describe certain feelings that people have. Rate the patient's by finding the answer which best describes the extent to which he/she has these conditions.

Individual Item Score: 0 = Not Present   1 = Mild   2 = Moderate   3 = Severe   4 = Incapacitating

HAM-A score level of anxiety: <17 mild; 18 - 24 mild to moderate; 25 - 30 moderate to severe

1 Anxious Mood   0   1   2   3   4
Worries, anticipation of the worst, fearful, anticipation, irritability

2 Tension   0   1   2   3   4
Feelings of tension, fatigability, startle response, moved to tears easily, trembling, restlessness Inability to relax

3 Fears   0   1   2   3   4
Of dark, of strangers, of being left alone, of animals, of traffic, of crowds

4 Insomnia   0   1   2   3   4
Difficulty falling asleep, broken sleep, dreams, unsatisfying sleep, fatigue on waking, nightmares, night terrors

5 Intellectual   0   1   2   3   4
Difficulty in concentration, poor memory, premature ejaculation

6 Depressed Mood   0   1   2   3   4
Loss of interest, lack of pleasure in hobbies, depression, early waking, diurnal swing

7 Somatic (muscular)   0   1   2   3   4
Aches and pains, twitching, stiffness, myoclonic jerks, grinding of teeth, unsteady voice, increased muscular tone

8 Somatic (sensory)   0   1   2   3   4
Tinnitus, blurring of vision, hot and cold flushes, feelings of weakness, pricking sensation

9 Cardiovascular symptoms   0   1   2   3   4
Tachycardia, palpitations, pain in chest, missing beats, throbbing of vessels, fainting feelings

10 Respiratory symptoms   0   1   2   3   4
Pressure or constriction in chest, choking feeling, sighing, dyspnea

11 Gastrointestinal symptoms   0   1   2   3   4
Difficulty swallowing, abdominal pain, nausea, burning sensations, bloating, loose bowels, weight loss, constipation, borborygmi

12 Genitourinary symptoms   0   1   2   3   4
Urgency and/or frequency of micturition, frigidity, loss of libido, impotence, amenorrhea, menorrhagia

13 Autonomic symptoms   0   1   2   3   4
Dry mouth, flushing, pallor, giddiness, sweating, tension headache, raising of hair

14 Behavior at Interview   0   1   2   3   4
Fidgeting, restlessness, pacing, tremor of hands, furrowed brow, strained face, sighing, rapid respiration swallowing, etc.

Overall Score: _____   **Rater Signature/Date:** _____

Hamilton M. The assessment of anxiety states by rating. Br J Med Psychol 1959; 32:50-55.

widely used in both clinical and research settings. It measures both psychic anxiety (mental agitation in psychological distress) and somatic anxiety (physical complaints related to anxiety). This clinician-rated scale can be generalized for use with patients across the life span and requires approximately 10 to 15 minutes to complete (151).

Zung Self-rating Anxiety Scale

The Zung Self-rating Anxiety Scale (150, 152) is a compilation of 20 questions rated and scored by the individual. The individual rates his or he or her thoughts, behaviors, and mood over the past week and can then provide the results to a health care provider for assistance in developing an appropriate treatment plan if marked symptoms of anxiety are present. This scale can be accessed online at http://www.psychresidentonline.com/zung%20anxiety.pdf.

Treatment Options for Patients With Anxiety Disorders in the Acute Care Setting

There are various treatment options for the anxiety-ridden patient presenting in an acute care setting. Often an acute care setting is the first and only place that the patient's anxiety disorder may come into focus. An acute care setting may also be the first place in which treatment is initiated. There remains the stigma of mental illness in our society; thus, many patients "suffer in silence" and avoid seeking treatment. Additionally, the multiple barriers (extensive wait lists, paucity of providers, lack of insurance coverage, prohibitive costs of treatments, both therapies as well as medication, are just a few) in obtaining mental health care also contribute to patients' frustration and furthers their anxiety, perpetuating the negativistic outlook, helplessness, and hopelessness, and other symptoms in many of the anxiety disorders. Despite the barriers and stigmas, anxiety disorders as a whole are readily treatable disorders. Many are treated with specific types of psychotherapies or psychotropic medications, or both. In seeking treatment for anxiety, the clinician must gather as detailed a history of prior therapeutic as well as medication interventions as possible to best guide the course of current treatment. Patients who believe they have "failed" at treatment have often either not been in treatment for an adequate length of time or may not have had an adequate trial—either dosage or duration—of medication, or both. Additionally, as psychotherapy is an interpersonal experience, both the practitioner and the patient must agree that "the fit is right" to provide the best treatment outcomes.

Psychotherapies

CBT is the most widely known and evidence-based form of psychotherapeutic intervention for the treatment of anxiety disorders. The success rate of treatment with CBT is 60% to 90% and is theoretically equally as effective in reducing anxiety symptoms as treatment with medication. Typically the practitioner and patient explore the options and choose a treatment course based on the patient's preferences. CBT consists of five fundamentals (153):

1. *Learning:* In this first stage, the therapist, who might be a psychiatric clinical specialist or advanced practice nurse, explains the illness, teaches the patient to identify the symptoms, and outlines the treatment plan.
2. *Monitoring:* Patients keep a diary to monitor panic attacks and record anxiety-inducing situations.
3. *Breathing:* The clinician teaches breathing and relaxation techniques to combat the physical reactions associated with anxiety symptoms and panic attacks.
4. *Rethinking:* The practitioner helps the patient to change his or her interpretation of the physical symptoms of anxiety from catastrophic to realistic.
5. *Exposing:* In this final stage, the clinician helps the patient encounter situations that evoke frightening physical sensations at levels of gradually increasing anxiety.

CBT sessions typically run about 12 weeks. There is frequently "homework" assigned so that the patient can continue to progress between therapy sessions. As the premise of CBT is to change the thought and behavioral patterns that interfere with the individual's level of functioning, there is some evidence that CBT interventions may last longer than pharmacologic interventions for the patient with an anxiety disorder.

Other Forms of Psychotherapy

Although CBT is the most widely used form of psychotherapy in treating anxiety disorders, "talk therapy" or traditional psychotherapy in which the patient meets individually with a trained mental health professional, such as a psychiatric clinical specialist or an APRN, to explore the underlying contributors to the individual's anxiety symptoms and develop strategies to cope with them in daily life is increasingly used. The clinician may offer relaxation techniques, guided imagery, association, or exposure as therapeutic interventions (154). Each of these techniques has shown some efficacy in reducing the symptoms associated with the anxiety disorders.

Medication Therapies

Excessive anxiety and other associated symptoms of the anxiety disorders are hypothetically caused by dysregulation of the neurotransmitters in the limbic system in the brain. With this in mind, it makes sense that psychopharmacologic medications that act on those neurotransmitters would improve the symptoms and level of functioning in the individual with an anxiety disorder. Medications are prescribed by physicians and many APRNs who can either offer psychotherapy themselves or work with other mental health professionals who provide psychotherapy. The primary classes of medications used in the treatment of anxiety disorders include the antidepressants medications, the antianxiety medications, and the beta-blockers.

The antidepressant (154-156) class of medications is not only effective in the treatment of depression but also the anxiety disorders—GAD, panic disorder, OCD, and PTSD, among others. The selective serotonin reuptake inhibitor (SSRI) antidepressants are the first line pharmacologic treatment for the anxiety disorders. They are generally well tolerated with few to no side effects. The most common side effects of the SSRIs include nausea, headache, insomnia/hypersomnia, anorgasmia, or delayed ejaculation (commonly known as sexual dysfunction). Some individuals may also experience increased anxiety or agitation; these symptoms require a discussion with the patient's practitioner if they continue longer than 2 weeks as they may be indicative of a cyclic mood disorder requiring alternative medication therapies. The SSRIs also have a Black Box Warning from the FDA for increased risk of suicidal thoughts among children, adolescents, and young adults up to the age of 25. Unfortunately, when the Black Box Warning was placed on the SSRI antidepressants, a proportionate decrease in the number of prescriptions written correlated with an increase in the number of completed suicides in the United States. One must also note that through all of the retrospective studies reviewed prior to the Black Box Warning, there were no completed suicides among the thousands of study participants.

The newer selective norepinepherine serotonin reuptake inhibitors (SNRIs) are also useful in treating anxiety disorders and have been shown to demonstrate efficacy similar to the SSRIs. The side effect profile of the SNRIs is also very similar to that of its predecessor, as listed earlier. The benzodiazepines are typically used as a short-term adjunct treatment while waiting for the effects of the SSRIs or SNRIs to take effect, about 2 to 6 weeks. They are prescribed for relief of acute anxiety and panic attacks. The benzodiazepines are considered controlled substances due to risk for dependency, abuse, and addiction. The most common side effects include sedation, dizziness, headache, ataxia, and euphoria. They should not be stopped abruptly for risk of withdrawal, which may include seizures or death, depending on the length of time and dosage the patient was prescribed the medication.

Buspar (buspirone) is a nonbenzodiazepine used to treat GAD. Unlike the benzodiazepines, buspirone takes a minimum of 2 weeks, and at times up to 8 weeks, to achieve its antianxiety effect. It is generally well tolerated

with possible side effects of nausea, dizziness, and headaches. The older tricyclic antidepressants are rarely used since the SSRIs and SNRIs entered the market. The side effect profile of the tricyclic antidepressants is less favorable and may include dry mouth, constipation, weight gain, sedation, and potential cardiac arrhythmias. At higher doses, it is prudent to obtain at least an annual electrocardiogram if the patient continues on a tricyclic antidepressant. Finally, the beta-blockers used to treat heart conditions have shown efficacy in relieving the physical (tremors, rapid heartbeat, shortness of breath, etc.) associated with the anxiety disorders. They can also be used on an as-needed basis for short-term relief of anticipatory anxiety when a feared situation can be predicted (such as a speech). The typical side effects of the beta-blockers include fatigue, weakness, orthostatic hypotension, and constipation.

Table 6-20 outlines each of the medications used in treating the anxiety disorders. It identifies the FDA-approved indication for each medication as well as those medications that are used in an off-label capacity. The table also highlights the pregnancy category for each medication.

Depressive Disorders in the Acute Care Setting

The depressive disorders are quite common, affecting over 10% of the adult population in any given year. Although depressive symptoms can occur at any time across the life span, they typically first appear during late adolescence or young adulthood. They are characterized by a wide variety of symptoms such as deep feelings of sadness or a marked loss of interest or pleasure in activities that were once enjoyable to the individual. Other symptoms include insomnia or hypersomnia, increased appetite or reduced appetite, loss of energy, feelings of thoughts of death or suicide, self-injurious behaviors (such as cutting or burning oneself), and suicide attempts. There are multiple theories on the causes of depression. The most common factors are summarized next (156):

1. *Biochemistry*—Dysregulation of the neurotransmitters serotonin and norepinephrine may contribute to the symptoms of depression, anxiety, irritability, and fatigue, while the dysregulation of the neurochemical dopamine may contribute to loss of energy and the lack of pleasure.
2. *Genetics/heredity*—Depression tends to run in families. For example, if an identical twin has depression, the other has a 70% chance of developing the disorder at some time over the life span.
3. *Personality*—Individuals who are generally pessimistic, easily overwhelmed by stress, and suffer from low self-esteem appear to be vulnerable to depression.

TABLE 6-20 An Overview of Medications Used to treat Anxiety Disorders

SSRI Medications	Generalized Anxiety D/O	Panic Disorder	Obsessive-Compulsive D/O	Social Anxiety Disorder	Post Traumatic Stress D/O	Pregnancy Category
Prozac (fluoxetine)		x	x Ages 7 and older			C
Paxil/Paxil CR (paroxetine)	x	x	x	x	x	D
Zoloft (sertraline)	x	x	x Ages 7 and older	x	x	C
Celexa (citalopram)	OFF LABEL					C
Lexapro (escitalopram)	x					C
Luvox/Luvox CR (fluvoxetine)	x		x	x		C
SNRI Medications						
Effexor XR (venlafaxine)	x	x		x		C
Pristiq (desvenlafaxine)	x					C
Cymbalta (duloxetine)	OFF LABEL					C
Common Benzodiazepine Medications						
Xanax/Xanax XR (alprazolam)	x	x				D
Ativan (lorazepam)	x					D
Klonopin (clonazepam)	x OFF LABEL	x				D
Other Agents Used to Treat Anxiety						
BuSpar (buspirone) Nonbenzodiazepine	x					B
Tofranil (imipramine) Tricyclic antidepressant	x	x				C
Anafranil (clomipramine) Tricyclic antidepressant			x			C
Inderal (propranolol) Beta-Blocker	x OFF LABEL For physical symptoms			x OFF LABEL For physical symptoms		C

4. *Environmental factors*—Continuous exposure to violence, neglect, abuse, or poverty may exacerbate the vulnerability of those already susceptible to depression.
5. *Medical conditions and medications*—Chronic, debilitating medical conditions such as heart disease, pulmonary disease, cancer, and diabetes, to name a few, have a high likelihood of comorbidity. Similarly, the medications used to treat some of these chronic medical conditions may exacerbate depressive symptoms.

Depressive disorders place a large strain on acute care hospitals, accounting for nearly 1 in 10 hospital admissions. There is a very high comorbidity among acute care patients with cardiovascular, cerebrovascular, and pulmonary diseases as well as various forms of cancer and patients with depressive disorders. For example, in 2005, hospitalizations involving depression as a comorbid condition accounted for more than 2.9 million hospital admissions and totaled $21.8 billion in hospital costs (157). Symptoms of depression can be viewed as a marker for medical comorbidities. Depressed patients who are hospitalized for heart failure are at two to three times the risk of death and readmission as their nondepressed peers (158). Another study indicates that almost 20% of those diagnosed with heart failure are diagnosed with comorbid depressive and/or anxiety disorders and use twice as many health services as those without a comorbid mental illness (159). Similarly, nearly one-half of all patients diagnosed with chronic obstructive pulmonary disease (COPD) have a comorbid mental health condition that significantly affects the individual's quality of life. Depressive disorders ultimately contribute to persistent feelings of frustration, hopelessness, helplessness, and the additional burden of coping with a chronic medical condition such as COPD (160-162). Fortunately, the depressive disorders are highly treatable conditions, and nursing interventions, among others, have been found to reduce the incidence of major depression among high-risk individuals.

Major Depressive Disorder

Major depressive disorder is an episode disorder characterized by constant, debilitating feelings of sadness, feeling as if you are a burden to others, and loss of interest in activities that affect the level of functioning at work, at home, at school, and in relationships with family and friends. These symptoms persist nearly all day, on most days, and last a minimum of 2 weeks. During this period, the individual also experiences at least four of the following signs of depression: changes in appetite leading to weight loss or gain, insomnia or (less often) oversleeping, restlessness and an inability to sit still, or, conversely, a slowdown in talking and performing tasks, problems concentrating or making decisions, feelings of worthlessness or excessive, inappropriate guilt, thoughts of death or suicide, or suicide plans or attempts. Still other symptoms may include a loss of sexual desire, pessimistic or hopeless feelings, and physical symptoms such as headaches, muscle and joint aches and pains, or gastrointestinal problems (156).

Those suffering from major depressive disorder may find that the symptoms can continue with fluctuations of severity over a period of months or even years and may be exacerbated by life stressors such as the death of a loved one, loss of a job, or financial hardship, among others. This would be diagnosed as Major Depressive Disorder, Recurrent (specify the severity—mild, moderate or severe, with or without psychotic features).

Dysthymic Disorder

Dysthmic disorder is characterized as an emotional depression that persists for at least 2 years in adults, usually with no more than moderate intensity. Although not as debilitating as major depression, dysthymia can keep individuals from experiencing a sense of well-being and may permeate aspects of the individual's social, work, and home life. Its symptoms have been likened to a "black cloud" or a "gray veil." Individuals diagnosed with this depressive disorder describe an overall melancholy or low-level depression lasting most hours of the day, most days of the week. Symptoms may also include overeating or loss of appetite, insomnia or sleeping too much, fatigue or lack of energy, low self-esteem, difficulty concentrating or indecisiveness, and hopelessness. At times an episode of major depression can occur on top of dysthmia; this is known as double depression. In any given year, about 10% of people spontaneously emerge from dysthymic disorder, although more commonly, the symptoms persist for years (156).

Seasonal Affective Disorder

Seasonal affective disorder (SAD) affects 1% to 2% of the population in a given year. It may stand alone or exist as an exacerbation of another mental health disorder. Although SAD is not fully understood, it is hypothesized that the hormone melatonin, which helps to regulate an individual's sleep-wake cycle, plays a role. Given this hypothesis, it makes sense that the symptoms of SAD increase during the fall and winter months when the hours of daylight are more limited and the symptoms subside in the spring and summer months when the hours of daylight are more prevalent (163). The most difficult months for patients diagnosed with SAD tend to be January and February, when the daylight hours are limited, the weather is cold, and the "winter doldrums" set in. Of course, patients living in the western or southern parts of the United States, where the weather is warmer and sunny days are more the norm, may not be susceptible to SAD.

Symptoms of SAD are similar to those of general depression, as described. The CNS treating a patient for symptoms of depression should pay particular attention to the patient's symptoms, especially around the times of year that daylight savings time begins and ends in the eastern part of the United States. Other disruptions (such as crossing time zones) to the patient's circadian rhythm can contribute to an exacerbation of similar symptoms. In treating seasonal affective disorder, the APRN may suggest such holistic treatments as walking or being outdoors during daylight hours, establishing good sleep hygiene patterns, and light box therapy (also known as phototherapy), which involves sitting in front of a very intense specially designed light source for 30 minutes every morning. If these remedies prove ineffective in alleviating the symptoms of SAD, antidepressant therapy and/or psychotherapy may be beneficial (163).

Postpartum Depression

Almost half of women who have recently given birth experience the "baby blues" characterized by weepy, anxious, emotionally labile feelings and lasting no more than a few weeks after birth. Unlike the "baby blues," postpartum depression may occur within 3 to 6 months, and even up to 1 year, after giving birth. It is a devastating disorder that presents at a time when our culture dictates that the mother be filled with joy and excitement after having given birth. Stress, sleep deprivation, hormonal fluctuations, physical discomfort, financial hardship, and limited supports as well as a colicky or sick infant can contribute to a diagnosis of postpartum depression (156).

During the postpartum period, not only might a new mother experience debilitating symptoms of depression but also obsessive thoughts and anxiety about potentially harming the baby or having something catastrophic happen to their infant. These anxiety-based thoughts are often followed by compulsive behaviors to relieve the anxiety and "ward off" any potential threat to the baby. In the worst case scenario, the symptoms become so severe that the new mother is completely unable to function. She is unable to attend to her own activities of daily living, much less the many demands of a newborn infant. She may present as indifferent to her baby and refuse to hold, feed, bathe, or clothe the child. She may also have thoughts of harming herself and/or the baby. These symptoms are commonly referred to as "postpartum psychosis" and require immediate psychiatric intervention due to the potential threat to the safety of the infant and the mother and possibly other family members. Fortunately, very few women experience symptoms of this severity.

A majority of acute care hospital maternity wards screen for postpartum depression. Although this is a very chaotic time in the life of the new mother, she tends to respond openly and honestly to the questions presented. The most widely recognized and reliable screening tool is the Edinburgh Postnatal Depression Scale (164). The APRN nurse in the acute care setting is an ideal provider to offer education, resources, and treatment to the new mother with symptoms of postpartum depression. The clinical specialist can work with the patient to differentiate the symptoms of the "baby blues" from the more serious condition of postpartum depression. With this early intervention, the outcomes for mother, baby, and extended family are quite positive, allowing the new mother to enjoy this truly wonderful time in her life.

Case Report

As discussed throughout this chapter, depressive disorders are quite common in the acute care hospital setting. As an integral member of the health care team, the CNS is called to evaluate a 57-year-old divorced woman who has been hospitalized with diabetic ketoacidosis and pain related to peripheral neuropathy in her lower extremities. Her blood glucose levels remain in the 300s even with fasting blood work. She is overweight and complains of low energy, lack of motivation, difficulty getting out of bed in the morning, and generally feeling depressed. After a period of time, the patient confides in you that she has not been able to adjust to her newly diagnosed diabetes and "all the things that need to be followed, I can't stick myself that many times a day; my fingers feel like pin cushions." She admits that she has been nonadherent to the 1800-calorie diet, especially as it relates to carbohydrates. "I'm a carbohydrate junkie, I guess that's what got me into this mess to begin with." She does report that she has adhered to her medication regimen as prescribed by an endocrinologist and that she wants to get out and walk like she used to but "I just don't have the energy or motivation; besides, my legs really hurt, they feel like they're on fire." Her laboratory studies find no other medical conditions. "I'm just so depressed, I don't know if I can go on living like this. My social life is gone, because I'm divorced now and all my friends are still married; we used to get together as couples to play cards. I'm only working part-time as my employer is laying people off due to the economy. Now this diabetes thing. I don't think I can take much more."

Given the patient's statements implying hopelessness and passive suicidality, the APRN furthers explores the patient's risk for suicide. The patient adamantly insists that although she is depressed and hopeless, she would never commit suicide. "Suicide's the ultimate sin, it's against my Catholic upbringing; besides, I'd never give my ex-husband the pleasure of thinking that I couldn't live without him." The patient agrees to the safety plan of informing the nursing staff if her feelings change and she begins to feel like she is at risk to harm herself. The patient is diagnosed with Major Depressive Disorder, Single Episode, Moderate. In formulating a treatment plan, the CNS discusses the various treatment recommendations with the patient. Those recommendations include an antidepressant medication such as Cymbalta (duloxetine) as it has the FDA indication for both Major Depressive Disorder and Diabetic Neuropathy; thus, it should relieve not only the symptoms of depression but also relieve the peripheral pain the patient is experiencing. The APRN reviews the side effects, risks, and benefits of this medication with the patient, including the Black Box Warning for increased suicidality in children and young adults despite the patient's age, as she was concerned that taking medication might make her want to commit suicide. Additionally, the clinical specialist discusses the need for the patient to engage in psychotherapy as an outpatient given the patient's difficulty coping with her diabetes as well as her overall diminished level of functioning. This scenario illustrates a typical manifestation of an adult patient presenting to the acute care setting with comorbid medical and depressive symptomatology. As you can see, the APRN plays a key role in initiating treatment for this patient while in the acute care setting, and studies have shown that the quicker the onset of treatment for depression, the more favorable are the outcomes.

Diagnosis

The depressive disorders are thought to be caused by dysregulation of the neurotransmitters NE, 5-HT, and dopamine (DA). Other contributors to depressive symptomatology include dysfunction in the hypothalamic region of the brain. There is also a strong genetic/hereditary component to the depressive disorders, with a female-to-male ratio of 3:1 (156, 162).

There are a multitude of medications that contribute to symptoms of depression including the steroids, heart and blood pressure agents, hormonal treatments, oral contraceptives, antimicrobials, antibiotics, antivirals and antifungals, tranquilizers, barbiturates, sleep aids, and sedatives, as well as alcohol, pain relievers, and withdrawal from cocaine or amphetamines and other forms of substance abuse. A thorough review of the patient's medications, including over-the-counter drugs, vitamins, and supplements, can assist the practitioner in ensuring that the symptoms are truly related to depression and not the side effect of the patient's current medications. There are also various medical conditions that mimic the symptoms of depression. It is estimated that 10% to 15% of all depressions can be attributed to a medical condition. The most common medical condition characterized by exhaustion, weight gain, and depression is hypothyroidism, in which the patient's body produces too little thyroid hormone. Although hypothyroidism and a depressive disorder may coexist, hypothyroidism alone affects more than 9 million Americans. Heart disease, diabetes, pulmonary disorders, neoplasms, adrenal dysfunction, vitamin deficiencies (folic acid, B_{12}), and disorders of the central nervous system such as stroke and multiple sclerosis may also mimic the symptoms found in the depressive disorders and must be ruled out to ensure the most appropriate treatment (161).

A routine physical examination, laboratory studies (including CBC with differential, comprehensive metabolic panel, liver function tests, T_3, free T_4, total T_4, and thyroid-stimulating hormone, a urinalysis, and urine drug screen), an electrocardiogram, and a CT scan are typically sufficient to rule out any gross medical etiology mimicking the symptoms of depression (161). Additionally, a psychiatric evaluation including mental status examination and suicide risk assessment is necessary diagnostic tools to evaluate and determine the appropriate course of treatment for the patient.

Suicide

Suicide is the 11th leading cause of death in the United States. Men account for 80% of suicide victims. Whites are twice as likely to commit suicide as Blacks and Hispanics. Elderly men, above the age of 85, have the highest rate of suicides. Suicide is the third leading cause of death among American adolescents, accounting for 14% of deaths for people between the ages of 15 and 24 (162). These are startling statistics and grounds for concern. Any number of factors may contribute to the desperation an individual must experience when he or she commits to this irrevocable step and ends one's life. Suicide may arise from feelings of intense anger, hopelessness, despair, or panic; it may also be carried out under the sway of highly distorted or psychotic ideas. Screening for suicide in the acute care setting is not only necessary but mandatory when patients present with symptoms of anxiety or depression.

The CNS is again in a prime position to conduct the suicide screening evaluation of those patients presenting with anxiety or depressive symptoms, exploring the patient's current life situation to determine if they are experiencing any significant crises or hardships such as the death of a spouse or child, the loss of employment, significant financial hardship, the loss of social supports, a separation or divorce, or a significant or terminal illness. One should determine if they are taking medications known to induce changes in mood or an increase in suicidal thinking (antidepressants, interferon therapy, accutane therapy); are currently in the midst of an episode of psychosis, depression, or anxiety; or have recently experienced or been witness to a traumatic event (return from active duty in a war, rape, witness to event in which people were killed or maimed).

In addition to the above high-risk factors, the APRN should explore the patient's family psychiatric history, including family history of suicide, whether the patient has access to guns or other weapons, whether the patient has made prior suicide attempts and by what means, whether the patient has begun "setting his or her affairs in order" (giving away personal effects, writing "good-bye" letters, writing or revising a will, etc.), and whether the patient self-medicates with alcohol or other substances and to what extent (154). If the patient is assessed to be at imminent risk of suicide or self-harm while in the acute care setting, he or she should be placed on 1:1 observation and coordination of a transfer to an acute psychiatric facility should be initiated. Once the patient is medically stabilized, a transfer to the psychiatric facility should occur for stabilization of the psychiatric symptomatology and suicidality. If the patient is unwilling to enter a psychiatric facility on a voluntary basis and remains a risk for suicide, involuntary commitment proceedings should be initiated to ensure the safety of the patient who is unable to provide the same for themselves. As health care providers, CNSs/APRNs have an obligation to maintain our patient's safety as well as the safety of others. If the acute care patient presents with thoughts of self-harm or thoughts to harm others, we are mandated to report these findings and initiate any and all safety precautions necessary to protect the patient and others.

Depression Rating Scales

Although there are a myriad of depression rating scales that can be used to determine not only if a patient suffers from anxiety but also to what extent, the most commonly used and most reliable, consistent, and valid scales seem to be the Hamilton Depression Rating Scale (HDRS), which was developed in 1960 and the Zung Self-rating Depression Scale developed in 1965. Additionally, the Edinburgh Postnatal Depression Scale (EPDS), developed in Great Britain in 1987, is the most widely used screening tool to evaluate new mothers who may be at risk for postpartum depression.

The Hamilton Depression Rating Scale

The Hamilton Depression Rating Scale (165) in Box 6-24 is the most widely used clinician administered assessment scale to determine the severity of a patient's depressive symptoms. It requires approximately 20 to 30 minutes to complete. With its emphasis on melancholic and physical symptoms of depression, the HDRS was originally developed for hospital inpatients, making it an ideal screening tool to be used in the acute care setting when patients are identified with depressive symptoms. The HDRS does not assess for the atypical symptoms of depression such as

---

BOX 6–24 Hamilton Depression Rating Scale

This scale is to be administered and rated by a health care professional. Administration time is approximately 20 to 30 minutes. The purpose of this rating scale is to rate the severity of depression in patients who are experiencing symptoms of depression. The higher the score, the more severe the depression.

For each item, write the correct number on the line next to the item (only one response per item)

_____ **1. DEPRESSED MOOD** (sadness, hopelessness, helplessness, worthlessness)

0 = Absent
1 = These feeling states indicated only on questioning
2 = These feeling states spontaneously reported verbally
3 = Communicates feeling states nonverbally—i.e., through facial expressions, posture, voice, and tendency to weep
4 = Patient reports VIRTUALLY ONLY these feeling states in his spontaneous verbal and nonverbal communication

_____ **2. FEELINGS OF GUILT**

0 = Absent
1 = Self Reproach, feels he has let people down
2 = Ideas of guilt or rumination over past errors or sinful deeds
3 = Present illness is a punishment. Delusions of guilt
4 = Hears accusatory or denunciatory voices and/or experiences threatening visual hallucinations

_____ **3. SUICIDE**

0 = Absent
1 = Feels life is not worth living
2 = Wishes he were dead or any thoughts of possible death to self
3 = Suicidal ideas or gesture
4 = Attempts at suicide (any serious attempt rates 4)

_____ **4. INSOMNIA EARLY**

0 = No difficulty falling asleep
1 = Complains of occasional difficulty falling asleep—i.e., more than 30 minutes
2 = Complains of nightly difficulty falling asleep

Continued

BOX 6–24 Hamilton Depression Rating Scale—cont'd

_____ 5. **INSOMNIA MIDDLE**

      0 = No difficulty

      1 = Patient complains of being restless and disturbed during the night

      2 = Waking during the night—any getting out of bed rates 2 (except for purposes of voiding)

_____ 6. **INSOMNIA LATE**

      0 = No difficulty

      1 = Waking in early hours of the morning but goes back to sleep

      2 = Unable to fall asleep again once out of bed

_____ 7. **WORK AND ACTIVITIES**

      0 = No difficulty

      1 = Thoughts and feelings of incapacity, fatigue, or weakness related to activities, work or hobbies

      2 = Loss of interest in activities, hobbies, or work—either directly reported by patient or indirect in listlessness, indecision, and vacillation (feels he has to push self to work or activities)

      3 = Decrease in actual time spent in activities or decrease in productivity

      4 = Stopped working because of present illness

_____ 8. **RETARDATION: PSYCHOMOTOR** (slowness of thought and speech, impaired ability to concentrate, decreased motor activity)

      0 = Normal speech and thought

      1 = Slight retardation at interview

      2 = Obvious retardation at interview

      3 = Interview difficult

      4 = Complete stupor

_____ 9. **AGITATION**

      0 = None

      1 = Fidgetiness

      2 = Playing with hands, hair, etc.

      3 = Moving about, can't sit still

      4 = Hand wringing, nail biting, hair-pulling, biting of lips

_____ 10. **ANXIETY (PSYCHOLOGICAL)**

      0 = No difficulty

      1 = Subjective tension and irritability

      2 = Worrying about minor matters

      3 = Apprehensive attitude apparent in face or speech

      4 = Fears expressed without questioning

_____ 11. **ANXIETY (SOMATIC)** Physiologic concomitants of anxiety (effects of autonomic overactivity, "butterflies," indigestion, stomach cramps, belching, diarrhea, palpitations, hyperventilation, paresthesias, sweating, flushing, tremors, headache, urinary frequency). Avoid asking about possible medication side effects (dry mouth, constipation, fatigue)

      0 = Absent   1 = Mild   2 = Moderate   3 = Severe   4 = Incapacitating

_____ 12. **SOMATIC SYMPTOMS (GASTROINTESTINAL)**

      0 = None

      1 = Loss of appetite but eating with encouragement from others; food intake normal

      2 = Difficulty eating without urging from others; marked reduction in appetite and food intake

_____ 13. **SOMATIC SYMPTOMS (GENERAL)**

      0 = None

      1 = Heaviness in limbs, back, or head. Backaches, headaches, muscle aches. Loss of energy, and fatigability

      2 = Any clear-cut symptom rates 2

_____ 14. **GENITAL SYMPTOMS** (loss of libido, impaired sexual performance, menstrual disturbances)

      0 = Absent   1 = Mild   2 = Severe

BOX 6–24 Hamilton Depression Rating Scale—cont'd

_____ **15. HYPOCHONDRIASIS**

0 = Not present

1 = Self-absorption (bodily)

2 = Preoccupation with health

3 = Frequent complaints, requests for help, etc.

4 = Hypochondriacal delusions

_____ **16. LOSS OF WEIGHT** (when rating by history...)

0 = No weight loss

1 = Probably weight loss associated with present illness

2 = Definite (according to patient) weight loss

3 = Not assessed

_____ **17. INSIGHT**

0 = Acknowledges being depressed and ill

1 = Acknowledges illness but attributes cause to bad food, climate, overwork, virus, need for rest, etc.

2 = Denies being ill at all

_____ **18. DIURNAL VARIATION**

Note whether symptoms are worse in morning or evening if NO diurnal variation, mark none

0 = No variation   1 = Worse in morning   2 = Worse in evening

When present, mark the severity of the variation. Mark "None" if NO variation

0 = None   1 = Mild   2 = Severe

_____ **19. DEPERSONALIZATION and DEREALIZATION** (Feelings of unreality, Nihilistic ideas)

0 = Absent   1 = Mild   2 = Moderate   3 = Severe   4 = Incapacitating

_____ **20. PARANOID SYMPTOMS**

0 = None   1 = Suspicious   2 = Ideas of reference   3 = Delusions of reference and persecution

_____ **21. OBSESSIONAL and COMPULSIVE SYMPTOMS**

0 = Absent   1 = Mild   2 = Severe

TOTAL SCORE_____

Signature of Rater/Date:_____

Hamilton M. A rating scale for depression. J Neurol Neurosurg Psychiatry 1960; 23:56-62

---

hypersomnia and hyperphagia; however, this limitation is minor. For the HDRS, a score of 0 to 7 is generally accepted as clinical remission, a score of 20 to 50 is within the moderate range of depressive symptom severity, and a score over 50 is thought to be severe, incapacitating depression likely requiring immediate inpatient psychiatric hospitalization.

Zung Self-Rating Depression Scale

The Zung Self-Rating Depression Scale (166) is a brief, patient-administered rating scale exploring the patient's physical and emotional symptoms of depression over the past several days. This scale provides a snapshot of the individual's symptomatology and quantifies it into an easily understandable score. With the highest possible score of 80, a score of 50 to 69 is where most patients with depression are scored. This screening toll generally takes about 10 minutes to complete. This scale can be found online at http://healthnet.umassmed.edu/mhealth/ZungSelfRatedDepressionScale.pdf.

Edinburgh Postnatal Depression Scale

The Edinburgh Postnatal Depression Scale (164) (Box 6-25) was developed to help acute care practitioners detect mothers suffering from postpartum depression. Postpartum depression affects at least 10% of women, and many depressed mothers remain untreated. Studies have shown that 92.3% of mothers who scored above 13 on the EPDS were likely to be suffering from depression of varying severity. The scale will not detect

BOX 6–25 Edinburgh Postnatal Depression Scale (EPDS)

Please circle the response which most closely represents how you have felt during the **past week.**

1. ***I have been able to laugh and see the funny side of things.***

   As much as I always could — 0
   Not quite so much now — 1
   Definitely not so much now — 2
   Not at all — 3

2. ***I have looked forward with enjoyment to things.***

   As much as I ever did — 0
   Rather less than I used to — 1
   Definitely less than I used to — 2
   Hardly at all — 3

3. ***I have blamed myself unnecessarily when things went wrong.****

   Yes, most of the time — 3
   Yes, some of the time — 2
   Not very often — 1
   No, never — 0

4. ***I have been anxious or worried for no good reason.***

   No, not at all — 0
   Hardly ever — 1
   Yes, very often — 2
   Yes, sometimes — 3

5. ***I have felt scared or panicky for no very good reason.****

   Yes, quite a lot — 3
   Yes, sometimes — 2
   No, not much — 1
   Not at all — 0

6. ***Things have been getting on top of me.****

   Yes, most of the time I haven't been able to cope at all — 3
   Yes, sometimes I haven't been coping as well as usual — 2
   No, most of the time I have coped quite well — 1
   No, I have been coping as well as ever — 0

7. ***I have been so unhappy that I have had difficulty sleeping.****

   Yes, most of the time — 3
   Yes, sometimes — 2
   Not very often — 1
   No, not at all — 0

8. ***I have felt sad or miserable.****

   Yes, most of the time — 3
   Yes, quite often — 2
   Not very often — 1
   No, not at all — 0

9. ***I have been so unhappy that I have been crying.****

   Yes, most of the time — 3
   Yes, quite often — 2
   Only occasionally — 1
   No, never — 0

10. ***The thought of harming myself has occurred to me.****

    Yes, quite often — 3
    Sometimes — 2
    Hardly ever — 1
    No, Never — 0

Taken from the British Journal of Psychiatry June 1987, Vol. 150 by J.L Cox, J.M. Holden, R. Sagovsky mothers with anxiety, phobias, or personality disorder. A full psychiatric assessment should be made to confirm the diagnosis and plan for treatment. Most acute care facilities request a psychiatric consult if the mother scores above 10 on the overall scale or has any response other than NEVER (0) on question number 10 regarding self-harm. Answers are scored 0, 1, 2, or 3 with increasing symptom severity. Items marked with an asterisk are reverse scored (i.e., 3, 2, 1, and 0). The total score is calculated by adding the scores for each of the 10 items. The higher the score, the more likely the new mother is to develop postpartum depression.

Management

One of the many challenges of facing the patient diagnosed with depression in the acute care setting is what treatment options are available once the patient is discharged to home. Another challenge is finding the "right fit" in a treatment provider. When patients enter into psychotherapy to aid them in their struggle to relieve depressive symptoms, it can be overwhelming. The patient is not obligated to continue with the first therapist they obtain an appointment with if they feel the "fit" isn't right. After all, the dynamics in therapy may contribute to the patient's feeling vulnerable and if the trust and comfort level is not sufficient, the treatment will not progress and the patient's symptoms may worsen. Box 6-26 lists some guidelines for the patient when choosing a therapist; of course, CNSs and APRNs with specialized training in the mental health field are among those practitioners who just might provide "the right fit."

CBT is one of the most common of the various forms of psychotherapy. The purpose of CBT is to challenge and change entrenched patterns of negative thoughts and behaviors. The patient is taught to identify the thought distortions and judge the truthfulness of the statements. The patient is then guided by the therapist to transform the automatic thoughts into reality-based positive, productive thoughts and behaviors and to recognize and "let go of" events that are beyond one's control. Through breaking down tasks into smaller, more manageable pieces, the patient is primed for success (162). CBT is an active therapy with "homework" assignments and rehearsals to practice the new coping and social skills, which will ultimately improve the patient's self-esteem and reduce the symptoms of depression. Similarly, Interpersonal Psychotherapy in the treatment of depression usually involves 12 to 16 weeks of in-depth exploration of the patient's current relationships, both at home and within the workplace, and focuses on the impact of conflicts, change, grief, and/or isolation on those relationships with the objective of improving one's interactions to reduce symptoms of depression (162).

Medication Therapies

The antidepressant medications (153, 154) such as the SSRIs are the first line pharmacologic treatment for the depressive disorders. As their name implies, these medications work in the brain to block the reuptake of the neurotransmitters serotonin in the synapse, thereby allowing more serotonin to be available, which, in turn, improves the patient's mood and other symptoms of depression. The SSRIs are generally well tolerated with few to no side effects. The most common side effects of the SSRIs include nausea, headache, insomnia/hypersomnia, anorgasmia, or delayed ejaculation (commonly known as sexual dysfunction). Some individuals may experience increased anxiety or agitation; these symptoms require a discussion with the patient's practitioner if they continue longer than 2 weeks as they may be indicative of a cyclic mood disorder requiring alternative medication therapies. Some practitioners have hypothesized that if the patient becomes "disinhibited," more agitated, more excitable, or

---

BOX 6–26 Guidelines for Choosing a Therapist

The Ingredients of Good Therapy Seek out a clinician who is licensed or certified by their state (such as an Advanced Practice Nurse)

1) You should feel reasonably at ease with your therapist, and both must respect ethical and professional boundaries
2) Treatment goals should be realistic, developed mutually, and addressed within a reasonable timeframe
3) Good therapy should assist you in adjusting, adapting, and functioning in a more effective manner
4) Your practitioner should address your symptoms and issues in a way that's unique to your needs, taking into account your gender, culture, and age as well as individual differences. Therapy is not a "one size fits all" encounter
5) If your clinician is not the individual who prescribes your medication, collaboration between them should occur regularly
6) Don't allow yourself to feel "stuck" for extended periods of time, discuss these feelings with your clinician to adapt the therapeutic techniques to better meet your needs or explore the option of obtaining a second opinion or transitioning to a new practitioner
7) Remember that the process of therapy is to help you to improve your level of functioning while simultaneously reducing your symptoms of anxiety and/or depression. If that's not happening, move on. The "right fit" is out there

otherwise manic, then the patient's symptoms are more consistent with bipolar disorder and should be treated as such.

The SSRIs do have a Black Box Warning from the FDA for increased risk of suicidal thoughts among children, adolescents, and young adults up to the age of 25. While individuals suffering from depression may be suicidal, in psychiatry it is generally accepted that one of the highest times of risk for a patient committing suicide occurs within the first 2 weeks of starting antidepressant therapy and with any dosage change. The Black Box Warning suggests that patients should be monitored frequently, even on a weekly basis, when antidepressant therapy is initiated to continually assess for suicidality.

The newer SNRIs are also useful in treating the depressive disorders and have been shown to demonstrate efficacy similar to the SSRIs. The side effect profile of the SNRIs is also very similar to that of its predecessor, as listed earlier. The atypical antidepressants such as bupropion (a selective serotonin-dopamine reuptake inhibitor) are again equally as efficacious as the other first line treatments for the depressive disorders. Bupropion (Wellbutrin) has a slightly different side effect profile from the SSRIs and SNRIs in that it may lower the seizure threshold in patients. It has also been used for smoking cessation and curbing the cravings for anything from food to cocaine to alcohol.

Since the introduction of the SSRIs and SNRIs in the 1990s, the older tricyclic antidepressants are rarely used in the treatment of the depressive disorders. The side effect profile of the tricyclics is less favorable and may include dry mouth, constipation, weight gain, sedation, and potential cardiac arrhythmias. Additionally, the tricyclic antidepressants are potentially lethal in overdose due to the risk of cardiac arrhythmias. At higher doses, it is prudent to obtain at least an annual electrocardiogram if the patient continues on a tricyclic antidepressant.

Table 6-21 outlines the most common medications used in treating the depressive disorders. It identifies the FDA-approved indication for each medication as well as those medications that are used in an off-label capacity. The chart also highlights the pregnancy category for each medication. None of the medications listed has an FDA-approved indication for dysthymic disorder, though clinical practitioners accept the use of these medications in an off-label capacity for this condition.

CLINICAL NURSE SPECIALIST COMPETENCIES AND SPHERES OF INFLUENCE

The CNS can play a vital role in educating acute care patients regarding the medications used to treat their anxiety and/or depressive disorder symptoms. First, the patient should understand that medications do not cure these disorders, but rather help to alleviate the symptoms so that the patient can lead a better quality of life. Second, the clinical specialist can review the intended effects, risks, benefits, and side effects of the medication with the patient and alert the patient to any Black Box Warnings. Third, the APRN can provide a realistic perspective to the patient that the majority of the medications used to treat anxiety and depression may take 2 to 8 weeks to reduce the patient's symptoms; the exception to this is the use of the benzodiazepines for short-term, immediate relief of acute anxiety and panic symptoms. Fourth, the practitioner should educate the patient that the medications must be taken as prescribed on a daily basis and that the symptoms may recur if adherence is not followed. Finally, the clinical specialist should inform the patient that many of these medications should not be stopped abruptly, but rather tapered slowly due to potential uncomfortable side effects such as dizziness, odd "zapping-like" sensations, and general "flulike" symptoms of aches, pains, nausea, and malaise. Most important for the APRN treating patients with anxiety and depressive disorders in the acute care setting is that her interactions with the patient regarding his symptoms will "set the stage" for the patient's compliance with treatment and progress toward a more fulfilling and productive life free of debilitating symptoms when discharged and moving into the outpatient or primary care setting (155).

The CNS may also provide care to the patient with an anxiety or depressive disorder on discharge from the acute care setting. As APRNs, CNSs use a holistic approach to treatment by obtaining information about the context and etiologies of both non–disease- and disease-related factors that may have an impact on the patient's health, safety, autonomy, wellness, and overall quality of life. In treating the patient with an anxiety or depressive disorder, the CNS with specialized training and state licensing and/or certification may be able to prescribe medications, provide psychotherapy, or both. Both within the acute care setting as well as the outpatient or primary care setting, CNS's collaborate with their peers as well as other members of the health care team, which include the patient, the patient's family members, physicians, other nurses, social workers, case managers, and others, to explore resources and further treatment options available to the patient. By continually monitoring and assessing not only her patient's needs but also her own need for evidence-based knowledge, the APRN assures her patients the most current treatment options available to treat their symptoms of anxiety and depression and to progress toward a more rewarding quality of life free of the debilitating symptoms of depression and anxiety symptoms.

TABLE 6-21 An Overview of the Medications to Treat Depressive Disorders

SSRI Medications	Major Depressive Disorder	Dysthymic Disorder	Seasonal Affective Disorder	Atypical forms of Depression	Adjunctive Treatment of Depression	Pregnancy Category
Prozac/Serafem (fluoxetine)	X Ages 8 and up			X Premenstrual dysphoric disorder		C
Paxil/Paxil CR (paroxetine)	X			X Premenstrual dysphoric disorder Paxil CR only		D
Zoloft (sertraline)	X			X Premenstrual dysphoric disorder		C
Celexa (citalopram)	X					C
Lexapro (escitalopram)	X Ages 12 and up					C
SNRI Medications						
Effexor XR (venlafaxine)	X			X Premenstrual dysphoric disorder OFF LABEL		C
Pristiq (desvenlafaxine)	X					C
Cymbalta (duloxetine)	X					C
Other Medications						
Wellbutrin SR/XL (bupropion HCl)	X		X			B
Aplenzin (bupropion HBr)	X					C
Remeron (mirtazapine)	X					C
Zyprexa (olanzepine)				X Bipolar depression	X	C
Abilify (aripiprazole)					X	C
Seroquel/XR (quetiapine)				X Bipolar depression		C

Various anxiety and depressive disorders manifest themselves in recognizable ways in the acute care setting. Although the symptoms of these mental health disorders may exacerbate the patient's physical ailments (or vice versa), the anxiety and depressive disorders are readily treated with medications, psychotherapy, or both. Given their holistic approach, the CNS practicing in an acute care setting is the ideal health care practitioner to manage both the patient's physical and emotional deviations from wellness. The clinical specialist in the acute care setting can evaluate the patient's physical symptoms, screen for anxiety and/or depression, rule out any underlying physiologic disorder that may mimic anxiety and depressive symptoms, and develop a comprehensive treatment plan to initiate treatment for anxiety and/or depression, offering the patient a "head start" on the road to wellness and recovery.

HELP RESOURCES
For a list of resources for anxiety and depression for patients and caregivers, see the end of this chapter under Help Resources: Anxiety and Depression.

HELP RESOURCES:
FAMILY VIOLENCE
Child Maltreatment
- Childhelp 1.800.4.A.CHILD (1-800-422-4453). National organization that provides crisis assistance and referral services. The Childhelp National Child Abuse Hotline is staffed 24 hours a day, 7 days a week, with professional crisis counselors who have access to a database of 55,000 emergency, social service, and support resources. All calls are anonymous.
- Child Welfare Information Gateway lists contact information for recipients of child maltreatment reports by state: http://www.childwelfare.gov/pubs/reslist/rl_dsp.cfm?rs_id=5andrate_chno=11-11172

Intimate Partner Violence Hotlines (for Women and Girls)
- National Domestic Violence Hotline: 1-800-799-7233/1-800-78-3224 (TTY) (Call this number to find the domestic violence program in your area): http://www.ndvh.org
- National Sexual Assault Hotline: 1-800-656-4673 (You can call the National Sexual Assault Hotline, 24 hours a day, 7 days a week): http://www.rainn.org/counseling.html

Teen Dating Violence Resources
- When Love Hurts. A guide for girls on love, respect and abuse in relationships: http://home.vicnet.net.au/~girlsown/index.htm
- Love Doesn't Have to Hurt American Psychological Association website on teen dating violence: http://www.apa.org/pi/pii/teen/contents.html

- In the Mix: Twisted Love. PBS show on dating violence: with Neve Campbell: http://www.pbs.org/
- National Runaway Switchboard: http://www.nrscrisisline.org/
- Dating Violence Happens: Information from a Portland, OR shelter: http://www.bradleyangle.org/For_Teens/teen_dating_violence.htm
- National Sexual Violence Resource Center, Teen Dating Violence: http://www.nsvrc.org/teendating.html
- Women's Coalition of St. Croix, Teen Dating Violence: http://www.wcstx.com/teendatv.htm

Adult Domestic Violence Resources
- Family Violence Prevention Fund: http://endabuse.org/
- Pennsylvania Coalition Against Domestic Violence: 1-800-537-2238/1-800-553-2508 (TTY) (This website has a link to Domestic Resources by State): http://www.pcadv.org/
- Violence Against Women Online Resources, University of Minnesota: http://www.vaw.umn.edu/library/
- American Bar Association Commission on Domestic Violence: http://www.abanet.org/domviol/home.html
- Office on Violence Against Women, United States Department of Justice: http://www.ojp.usdoj.gov/vawo/
- Rape, Abuse and Incest National Network: 1-800-656-4673 http://www.rainn.org/
- Feminist Majority Foundation: http://www.feminist.org/911/crisis.html#national (for national resources); http://www.feminist.org/911/crisis.html#state (for state by state resources)
- Alberta Council of Women's Shelters: http://www.womensshelter.ca/

Elder Mistreatment
From http://www.apa.org/pi/aging/eldabuse.html

National Center on Elder Abuse
1225 Eye Street NW, Suite 725
Washington, DC 20005
202-898-2586
Fax: 202-898-2583
www.elderabusecenter.org
NCEA is a resource for public and private agencies, professionals, service providers, and individuals interested in elder abuse prevention information, training, technical assistance, and research.

Eldercare Locator is sponsored by the Administration on Aging (AoA). If you know the address and ZIP code of the older person being abused, Eldercare Locator can refer you to the appropriate agency in the area to report the suspected abuse.
1-800-677-1116

Area Agency on Aging
Most states have an information and referral line that can be helpful in locating services for victims or potential perpetrators of elder abuse and neglect. Check your local telephone directory.

Medicaid Fraud Control Units (MFCU)
Each state attorney general's office is required by federal law to have an MFCU that investigates and prosecutes Medicaid provider fraud and patient abuse and neglect in

health care programs and home health services that participate in Medicaid.

Adult Protective Services
In many states, Adult Protective Services is designated to receive and investigate allegations of elder abuse and neglect. Every state has some agency that holds that responsibility. It may be the Area Agency on Aging, the Division of Aging, the Department of Aging, or the Department of Social Services.

National Domestic Violence Hotline
The hotline provides support counseling for victims of domestic violence and provides links to 2,500 local support services for abused women. The hotline operates 24 hours a day, every day of the year.
1-800-799-SAFE
TDD 1-800-787-3224

SUBSTANCE-RELATED DISORDERS
Adult Children of Alcoholics
P.O. Box 3216, Torrance, CA 90510
www.adultchildren.org 1-310-534-1815

Alcoholics Anonymous (AA)
Look up the AA number in your local phone book under "alcoholism"
A.A. World Services, Inc.
Grand Central Station
P.O. Box 459
New York, NY 10163
www.aa.org 1-212-870-3400

Al-Anon/Al-Ateen
For families of alcoholics, look up Al-Anon in your local telephone book or
www.al-anon.alateen.org 1-888-425-2666/1-888-425-2666 (toll-free) to find a meeting
Al-Anon World Services Office
1600 Corporate Landing Parkway
Virginia Beach, VA 23454
www.al-anon.org 1-757-563-1600

National Clearing House for Alcohol and Drug Information
P.O. Box 2345
Rockville, MD 20847-2345
1-877-726-4727 (toll-free)
www.ncadi.samhsa.gov

National Institute on Alcohol Abuse and Alcoholism
5635 Fishers Lane, MSC 9304
Bethesda, MD 20892-9304
www.niaaa.nih.gov 1-301-443-3860

National Institute on Drug Abuse
www.nida.nih.gov 1-301–443–1124

Substance Abuse and Mental Health Services Administration
1 Choke Cherry Road
Rockville, MD 20857
www.samhsa.gov 1-877-726-4727 (toll-free)

Substance Abuse Treatment Facility Locator
www.findtreatment.samhsa.gov 1-800-662-HELP

World Health Organization—The ASSIST Project:
http://www.who.int/substance_abuse/activities/assist/en/index.html

American Academy of Addiction Psychiatry
www.aaap.org 401-524-3076

American Psychiatric Nurses Association
www.apna.org
American Psychological Association 1-800-964-2000

American Society of Addiction Medicine 301-656-3920

NAADAC Substance Abuse Professionals
www.naadac.org 1-800-548-0497

National Association of Social Workers
www.helpstartshere.org

ANXIETY AND DEPRESSION
American Foundation for Suicide Prevention
120 Wall St., 22nd Floor
New York, NY 10005
888-333-2377 (toll free) www.afsp.org
This nonprofit organization supports research on suicide. It also offers information on suicide and its prevention as well as support for survivors.

American Psychiatric Association
1000 Wilson Blvd., Suite 1825
Arlington, VA 22209
703-907-7300 www.psych.org
This medical society's Web site offers fact sheets, booklets, and news articles on a wide range of mental health issues. It also includes a listing of psychiatric societies throughout the United States that can provide referrals to psychiatrists.

American Psychological Association
750 First St., NE
Washington, DC 20002
800-374-2721 (toll free) www.apa.org
The organization's Web site has information and helpful publications on mental illness and many other topics for psychologists, parents, teens, and others. It also carries news on psychology and offers referrals to psychologists in the United States and Canada.

Anxiety Disorder Association of America
8730 Georgia Ave, Suite 600
Silver Spring, MD 20910
240-485-1001 www.adaa.org
This organization's Web site offers a plethora of information related to all of the anxiety disorders. It offers detailed information on the symptoms, diagnosis, and treatment of the anxiety disorders.

Depression and Bipolar Support Alliance
730 N. Franklin St., Suite 501
Chicago, IL 60610
800-826-3632 (toll free) www.dbsalliance.org

Continued

This nonprofit organization provides information, advocacy, and support for people with depression and bipolar disorder, as well as their family members. The Web site has detailed information on suicide prevention strategies for anyone struggling with thoughts of suicide or for concerned family and friends.

National Alliance on Mental Illness (NAMI)
Colonial Place Three
2107 Wilson Blvd., Suite 300
Arlington, VA 22201
800-950-6264 (toll free) www.nami.org
This advocacy group offers information and support groups for people coping with a variety of mental illnesses and for families of people with such illnesses.

National Center for Complementary and Alternative Medicine
NCCAM
Clearinghouse
P.O. Box 7923
Gaithersburg, MD 20898
888-644-6226 (toll free) nccam.nih.gov
This government agency, part of the National Institutes of Health, offers a wealth of publications and fact sheets on a variety of health problems, including mental illness. It also sponsors valuable research on complementary and alternative medicine.

National Institute of Mental Health
6001 Executive Blvd., Room 8184, MSC 9663
Bethesda, MD 20892
866-615-6464 (toll free) www.nimh.nih.gov
This government agency, part of the National Institutes of Health, sponsors research on mental illness. It offers a wide array of free publications. The Web site has educational segments on anxiety and depression, news on studies, and information about clinical trials.

National Mental Health Association
2001 N. Beauregard St., 12th Floor
Alexandria, VA 22311
800-969-6642 (toll free) www.nmha.org
This nonprofit organization supports mental health research, provides advocacy, and offers information on a variety of mental health topics, including depression. The Web site has discussion boards and a free, confidential screening test for depression.

Obsessive Compulsive Foundation (OCF)
676 State St.
New Haven, CT 06511
203-401-2070 www.ocfoundation.org

Screening for Light Treatment and Biological Rhythm (SLTBR)
4648 Main St.
Chincoteague, VA 23336
www.websciences.org/sltbr
This organization's Web site provides information regarding light therapy for the treatment of Depressive and Seasonal Affective Disorders

References

1. Duterte EE, et al. Correlates of medical and legal help seeking among women reporting intimate partner violence. J Womens Health (Larchmt) 2008;17(1):85-95.

2. Smith DW, et al. Delay in disclosure of childhood rape: results from a national survey. Child Abuse Neglect 2000;24(2):273-287.

3. Koop CE. Surgeon General's Workshop on Violence and Public Health Report. Washington, DC: US Government Printing Office; 1986.

4. Carmona RH. Family Violence as a Public Health Issue, in United States Surgeon General U.S. Department of Health and Human Services Symposium on Family Violence: The Impact of Child, Intimate Partner, and Elder Abuse. Washington, DC: Office of the Surgeon General; 2003.

5. American Nurses Association. Position Statement on Violence Against Women. Washington, DC: American Nurses Association; 2000.

6. National Center for Injury Prevention and Control. Costs of Intimate Partner Violence Against Women in the United States. Atlanta, GA: National Center for Injury Prevention and Control; 2003.

7. Schmitt K, Shimberg B. Changes in Healthcare Professions' Scope of Practice: Legislative Considerations 1996. Retrieved from https://www.ncsbn.org/ScopeofPractice.pdf.

8. Myers JEB. Legal Issues in Child Abuse and Neglect Practice. Interpersonal Violence. 2nd edition. Thousand Oaks, CA: Sage Publications; 1998:412.

9. US Department of Health and Human Services Administration on Children Youth and Families. Child Maltreatment. Washington, DC; US Government Printing Office: 2008.

10. Finkelhor D. Current information on the scope and nature of child abuse. Future Child 1994;4(2):31-53.

11. Child Welfare Information Gateway. Definitions of Child Abuse and Neglect. 2007. Retrieved from www.childwelfare.gov/systemwide/laws_policies/statutes/define.cfm

12. Family Violence Prevention Fund. National Consensus Guidelines Responding to Domestic Violence Victimization in Health Care Settings. San Francisco, CA: Family Violence Prevention Fund; 2006.

13. Walker LE. The Battered Woman. First Harper Colophon Edition. New York: HarperPerennial; 1980:xviii.

14. Dong X. Medical implications of elder abuse and neglect. Clin Geriatr Med 2005;21(2):293-313.

15. Muehlbauer M, Crane PA. Elder abuse and neglect. J Psychosoc Nursing Ment Health Serv 2006;44(11):43-48.

16. Reed K. When elders lose their cents: financial abuse of the elderly. Clin Geriatri Med 2005;21(2):365-382.

17. Tatara T. The National Elder Incidence Abuse Study. Washington, D.C.: The National Center on Elder Abuse at The American Public Human Services Association in Collaboration with Westat, Inc. 1998

18. National Aging Resource Center on Elder Abuse (US), Tatara T. NARCEA's Suggested State Guidelines for Gathering and Reporting Domestic Elder Abuse Statistics for Compiling National Data. Washington, DC: National Aging Resource Center on Elder Abuse; 1990.

19. US Department of Justice Office of Justice Programs Bureau of Justice Statistics. Criminal Victimization. 2009. Retrieved from http://www.ojp.usdoj.gov/bjs/cvictgen.htm

20. US Department of Health and Human Services Children's Bureau. Child Maltreatment. 2007. Retrieved from www.acf.hhs.gov/programs/cb/pubs/cm07/index.htm.

21. Tjaden PG, et al. Extent, Nature, and Consequences of Intimate Partner Violence. Research Report. Washington, DC: US Dept of Justice, Office of Justice Programs, National Institute of Justice; 2000:xii.

22. Laumann EO, Leitsch SA, Waite LJ. Elder mistreatment in the United States: prevalence estimates from a nationally representative study. J Gerontol Psychol Sci 2008;63(4):S248-S254.

23. Koenig RJ, DeGuerre CR. The legal and governmental response to domestic elder abuse. Clin Geriatr Med 2005;21(2):383-398.

24. Teaster PB, et al. The 2004 Survey of State Adult Protective Services: Abuse of Adults 60 Years of Age and Older. Washington, DC: National Center on Elder Abuse; 2006.

25. Goldman J, US Office on Child Abuse and Neglect. A Coordinated Response to Child Abuse and Neglect: The Foundation for Practice. Washington, DC: US Dept of Health and Human Services, Office on Child Abuse and Neglect; 2003.

26. International Association of Forensic Nurses and American Nurses Association. Forensic Nursing: Scope and Standards of Practice. Silver Spring, MD: American Nurses Association; 2009.

27. Evans MM, Stagner PA, Rooms R. Maintaining the chain of custody: evidence handling in forensic cases. AORN J 2003; 78(4):563-569.

28. Goll-McGee B. The role of the clinical forensic nurse in critical care. Crit Care Nursing Q 1999;22(1):8-18.

29. Hoyt CA. Evidence recognition and collection in the clinical setting. Crit Care Nursing Q 1999;22(1):19-26.

30. Perry SE. The CNS as expert witness. CNS 1992;6(2):122-127.

31. Ferrea PC, Colucciello SA, Marx J, Verdile VP, and Gibbs MA (eds.). Trauma Management: An Emergency Medicine Approach. St Louis; Mosby; 2000.

32. Campbell J, Jones AS, Dienemann J, et al. Intimate partner violence and physical health consequences. Arch Intern Med 2002;162(10):1157-1163.

33. Nicolaidis C, McFarland B, Curry M, et al. Differences in physical and mental health symptoms and mental health utilization associated with intimate-partner violence versus childhood abuse. Psychosomatics 2009;50(4):340-346.

34. Covington C. Health Care Problems in Abusive Relationships. Presented at the American Academy of Nurse Practitioners Annual Conference, Dallas, TX, 2006.

35. Leserman J, Li Z, Hu YJ, et al. How multiple types of stressors impact on health. Psychosom Med 1998;60(2):175-181.

36. Wiglesworth A, Wiglesworth A, Austin R, et al. Bruising as a marker of physical elder abuse. J Am Geriatr Soc 2009;57(7):1191-1196.

37. Kaczor K, Pierce MC, Makoroff K, et al. Bruising and physical child abuse. Clin Pediatr Emerg Med 2006;7:153-160.

38. Hilden M, Schei B, Sidenius K. Genitoanal injury in adult female victims of sexual assault. Forens Sci Int 2005;154(2-3):200-205.

39. Dyer CB, Franzini L, Watson M, et al. Future research: a prospective longitudinal study of elder self-neglect. J Am Geriatr Soc 2008;56(suppl 2):S261-S265.

40. Dyer CB, Goodwin JS, Pickens-Pace S, et al. Self-neglect among the elderly: a model based on more than 500 patients seen by a geriatric medicine team. Am J Public Health 2007;97(9):1671-6.

41. Kemp BJ, Mosqueda LA. Elder financial abuse: an evaluation framework and supporting evidence. J Am Geriatr Soc 2005;53(7):1123-1127.

42. Family Violence Prevention Fund. Comply with JCAHO Standard PC.3.10 on Victims of Abuse. 2009. Retrieved from http://endabuse.org/section/programshe or health_care/_jcaho

43. US Preventive Services Task Force. Screening for Family and Intimate Partner Violence Recommendation Statement. 2004. Retrieved from http://www.ahrq.gov/clinic/3rduspstf/famviolence/famviolrs.pdf

44. Houry D, Kaslow NJ, Kemball RS, et al. Does screening in the emergency department hurt or help victims of intimate partner violence? Ann Emerg Med 2008;51(4):433-442.

45. Hurley KF, Brown-Maher T, Campbell SG, et al. Emergency department patients' opinions of screening for intimate partner violence among women. Emerg Med J 2005;22(2):97-98.

46. Wendt EK, Lidell EA, Westerstahl AK, et al. Young women's perceptions of being asked questions about sexuality and sexual abuse: a content analysis. Midwifery 2009.

47. MacMillan HL, Wathen CN, Jamieson E, et al. Approaches to screening for intimate partner violence in health care settings: a randomized trial. JAMA 2006;296(5):530-536.

48. Faller KC. Screening for Child Maltreatment. Retrieved from http://www.ssw.umich.edu/public/currentProjects/icwtp/childParent/e-cmquest.pdf

49. Meeks-Sjostrom D. A comparison of three measures of elder abuse. J Nursing Scholar 2004;36(3):247-250.

50. Wang JJ, Tseng HF, Chen KM. Development and testing of screening indicators for psychological abuse of older people. Arch Psychiatric Nurs 2007;21(1):40-47.

51. Zink T, Fisher BS. Family violence quality assessment tool for primary care offices. Qual Manage Health Care 2007;16(3):265-279.

52. Dyer CB, Kelly PA, Pavlik VN, et al. The making of a self-neglect severity scale. J Elder Abuse Neglect 2006;18(4):13-23.

53. Brown JB, Lent B, Schmidt G, et al. Application of the Woman Abuse Screening Tool (WAST) and WAST-short in the family practice setting. J Fam Pract 2000;49(10):896-903.

54. Brown JB, Lent B, Brett PJ, et al. Development of the Woman Abuse Screening Tool for use in family practice. Fam Med 1996;28(6):422-428.

55. Smith PH, Earp JA, DeVellis R. Measuring battering: development of the Women's Experience with Battering (WEB) Scale. Womens Health 1995;1(4):273-288.

56. Bickley LS, Szilagyi PG. Bates' Guide to Physical Examination and History Taking. 8th Edition. Philadelphia: Lippincott Williams and Wilkins; 2003.

57. Salber PR, Taliaferro EH. The Physician's Guide to Intimate Partner Violence and Abuse: A Reference for All Health Care Professionals: How to Ask the Right Questions and Recognize Abuse—Another Way to Save a Life. Volcano, CA: Volcano Press; 2006.

58. Geiderman JM, Moskop JC, Derse AR. Privacy and confidentiality in emergency medicine: obligations and challenges. Emerg Med Clin North Am 2006;24(3):633-656.

59. Centers for Disease Control and Prevention. Nationally Notifiable Infectious Diseases. 2005. Retrieved from http://www.cdc.gov/ncphi/disss/nndss/phs/infdis2005.htm

60. Polsky SS, Markowitz J (eds). Color Atlas of Domestic Violence. St Louis: Mosby; 2004.

61. Hoyt CA. Integrating forensic science into nursing processes in the ICU. Crit Care Nursing Q 2006;29(3):259-270.

62. Guttmacher Institute. State Policies in Breif: An Overview of Minor's Consent Laws. 2009. Retrieved from http://www.guttmacher.org/statecenter/spibs/spib_OMCL.pdf

63. Intimate Partner Violence Risk Assessment. Retrieved from http://www.dangerassessment.org/WebApplication1/

64. US Dept of Justice, Office on Violence Against Women. A National Protocol for Sexual Assault Medical Forensic Examinations: Adults/Adolescents. Washington, DC: US Dept of Justice, Office on Violence Against Women; 2004.

65. Hatcher RA. Contraceptive technology. 19th Revised Edition New York: Ardent Media; 2007.

66. Centers for Disease Control and Prevention. Sexually Transmitted Disease Treatment Guidelines. 2006. Retrieved from http://www.cdc.gov/std/treatment/2006/toc.htm

67. Froede RC. Handbook of Forensic Pathology. 2nd Edition. Northfield, IL: College of American Pathologists; 2003.

68. Hammer RM, Moynihan B, Pagliaro EM. Forensic Nursing: A Handbook for Practice. Sudbury, MA: Jones and Bartlett; 2006.

69. US Department of Justice Office of Violence Against Women. Frequently Asked Questions: Anonymous Reporting and Forensic Examinations. 2008. Retrieved from http://www.ovw.usdoj.gov/docs/faq-arfe052308.pdf

70. Iavicoli LG. Mandatory reporting of domestic violence: the law, friend or foe? Mt Sinai J Med 2005;72(4):228-231.

71. Gielen AC, Campbell J, Garza MA, et al. Domestic violence in the military: women's policy preferences and beliefs concerning routine screening and mandatory reporting. Milit Med 2006;171(8):729-735.

72. Gielen AC, O'Campo PJ, Campbell JC, et al. Women's opinions about domestic violence screening and mandatory reporting. Am J Prev Med 2000;19(4):279-285.

73. Abbey L. Elder abuse and neglect: when home is not safe. Clin Geriatr Med 2009;25(1):47-60, vi.

74. US Department of Health and Human Services. Summary of the HIPAA Privacy Rule. 2003. Retrieved from http://www.hhs.gov/ocr/privacy/hipaa/understanding/summary/privacysummary.pdf

75. Podrid A. HIPAA: Exceptions Providing Law Enforcement Officials and Social Service Providers Access to Protected Health Information. Update. Arlington, VA: American Prosecutors Research Institute; 2003.

76. US Department of Health and Human Services Office for Civil Rights. HIPAA Administrative Simplification 45 CFR Parts 160, 162, and 164; 2006. Retrieved from http://www.hhs.gov/ocr/privacy/hipaa/administrative/privacyrule/adminsimpregtext.pdf

77. The National Women's Health Information Center. Safety Planning List. 2008. Retrieved from http://www.womenshealth.gov/violence/planning/

78. American Psychiatric Association. Treatment of Substance Use Disorders in Practice Guidelines for the Treatment of Psychiatric Disorders. Washington, DC: American Psychiatric Association; 2000.

79. Russo CA, Elixhauser A. Hospitalizations for Alcohol Abuse Disorders 2003. Rockville, MD: Healthcare Cost and Utilization Project (HCUP), May 2006.

80. Grant MS, Cordts GA, Doberman DJ. Acute pain management in hospitalized patients with current opioid abuse. Topics Adv Pract eJournal 2007(7):1. Retrieved from http://www.medscape.com/viewarticle/557043

81. Abuse. Retrieved from http://www.thefreedictionary.com/abuse

82. Pedersen DD. Psych Notes: Clinical Pocket Guide. Philadelphia: FA Davis; 2005.

83. Stranges E, Wier L, et al. Hospitalizations in Which Patients Leave the Hospital Against Medical Advice (AMA) 2007. Rockville, MD: Healthcare Cost and Utilization Project (HCUP), August 2009.

84. National Institute on Drug Abuse (NIDA). Understanding Drug Abuse and Addiction, NIDA InfoFacts. June 2008. Retrieved February 22 2009, from http://www.nida.nih.gov/PDF/InfoFacts/Understanding08.pdf

85. Kassed CA, Levit KR, et al. Hospitalizations Related to Drug Abuse 2005. Rockville, MD: Healthcare Cost and Utilization Project, October 2007.

86. National Institute on Drug Abuse. Topics in Brief: Prescription Drug Abuse. March 2008. Retrieved from www.drugabuse.gov

87. National Institute on Drug Abuse. Screening for Drug Use in General Medical Settings: A Resource Guide. Retrieved from www.drugabuse.gov.

88. National Institute on Drug Abuse. NIDA-Modified ASSIST. Retrieved from http://www.drugabuse.gov/nidamed/screening/nmassist.pdf

89. Daly KP, et al. eMedicine Health: Substance Abuse. 2005. Retrieved from http://www.emedicinehealth.com/substance_abuse/page3_em.htm

90. American Psychiatric Association. Diagnostic and Statistical Manual of Mental Disorders, Fourth Edition, Test Revision. Washington, DC: American Psychiatric Association; 2000.

91. National Institute on Alcohol Abuse and Alcoholism. Unpublished data from the 2001-2002 National Epidemiologic Survey on Alcohol and Related Conditions (NESARC), a nationwide survey of 43,093 US adults aged 18 or older 2004.

92. McGlynn EA, Asch SM, Adams J, et al. The quality of health care delivered to adults in the United States. N Engl J Med 2003;348(26):2635-2645.

93. Bailey WJ. Drug Use in American Society. 3rd Edition. Minneapolis, MN: Burgess; 1993. Retrieved from http://www.gdcada.org/statistics/alcohol/bac.htm

94. Kasser C, Geller A, Howell E, Wartenberg A. Detoxification: Principles and Protocols. Chevy Chase, MD: American Society of Addiction Medicine; 2004.

95. National Guideline Clearinghouse 2007. Practice Guideline for the Treatment of Patients With Substance Abuse Disorders. Retrieved from http://www.guideline.gov/summary/summary.aspx?doc_id=9316andnbr=004985andstring=treatment+AND+patients+AND+substance+AND+abuse+AND+disorders

96. Sullivan JT, Sykora K, Schneiderman J, et al. Assessment of alcohol withdrawal: the revised Clinical Institute Withdrawal Assessment for Alcohol scale (CIWA-Ar). Br J Addict 1989;84:1353-1357.

97. US Department of Health and Human Services, National Institutes of Health, National Institute on Alcohol Abuse and Alcoholism. Helping Patients Who Drink Too Much: A Clinician's Guide. NIH Publication 07–3769, Update October 2008. Bethesda, MD: US DHHS.

98. Johnson BA, Rosenthal N, Capece JA, et al; Topiramate for Alcoholism Advisory Board and the Topiramate for Alcoholism Study Group. Topiramate for treating alcohol dependence: a randomized controlled trial. JAMA 2007;298(14):1641-1651.

99. Kranzler HR, Armeli S, Tennen H, et al. Targeted naltrexone for early problem drinkers. J Clin Psychopharmacol 2003;23(3):294-304.

100. Garbutt JC, Kranzler HR, O'Malley SS, et al. Efficacy and tolerability of long-acting injectable naltrexone for alcohol

dependence: a randomized controlled trial. JAMA 2005; 293(13):1617-1625.

101. Bouza C, Angeles M, Munoz A, Amate JM. Efficacy and safety of naltrexone and acamprosate in the treatment of alcohol dependence: a systematic review. Addiction 2004;99(7):811-828.

102. Johnson BA, Ait-Daoud N, Bowden C, et al. Oral topiramate for treatment of alcohol dependence: a randomized controlled trial. Lancet 2003;361(9370):1677-1685.

103. Mann K, Lehert P, Morgan MY. The efficacy of acamprosate in the maintenance of abstinence in alcohol-dependent individuals: Results of a metaanalysis. Alcohol Clin Exp Res 2004;28(1): 51-63.

104. Fuller RK, Gordis E. Does disulfiram have a role in alcoholism treatment today? Addiction. 2004;99(1):21-24.

105. Sola CL, Chopra A. Sedative, Hypnotic, Anxiolytic Use Disorders: Treatment and Medication. 2010. Retrieved from http://emedicine.medscape.com/article/290585-treatment

106. Akinsoto OPA. Sedative, Hypnotic, Anxiolytic Use Disorders. eMedicine. October 2004. Retrieved from http://www.mdguidelines.com/sedative-hypnotic-or-anxiolytic-dependence

107. Larson K, Swierzewski SJ. Narcotic Abuse. Retrieved from http://www.mentalhealthchannel.net/narcotic/index.shtml

108. National Institute on Drug Abuse. Research Report: Heroin Abuse and Addiction. 2009. Retrieved from http://www.nida.nih.gov/ResearchReports/Heroin/heroin5.html#treatment

109. National Institute on Drug Abuse. Research Report: Prescription Drugs: Abuse and Addiction. 2009. Retrieved from http://www.nida.nih.gov/ResearchReports/Prescription/Prescription.html

110. Hurd YL. Perspectives on current directions in the neurobiology of addiction disorders relevant to genetic risk factors. CNS Spectrums 2006;11(11):855-862.

111. Savage SR, Kirsh KL, Passik SD. Challenges in using opioids to treat pain in persons with substance abuse disorders. Addict Sci Clin Pract June 2008.

112. National Institute on Drug Abuse. NIDA Info Facts: Treatment Approaches for Drug Addiction. 2009. Retrieved from http://www.drugabuse.gov/Infofacts/treatmeth.html

113. Kleber HS. Opioids: Detoxification. In: Galanter M, Kleber HD, editors. Textbook of Substance Abuse Treatment. 2nd edition. Washington, DC: The American Psychiatric Press; 1999: 251-269. Retrieved from http://www.txpsych.org/guidelineopiates.htm

114. National Institute on Drug Abuse. NIDA Info Facts: Heroin. 2010. Retrieved from http://www.drugabuse.gov/Infofactshe or heroin.html

115. National Institute on Drug Abuse. Preventing and Recognizing Prescription Drug Abuse. 2009. Retrieved from http://www.nida.nih.gov/ResearchReports/Prescription/Prescription.html

116. Young C, Greenberg MA, Nicassio PM, et al. Transition from acute to chronic pain and disability: a model including cognitive, affective, and trauma factors. Pain 2008;134(1-2):69-79.

117. McCarberg BH, Billington R. Consequences of neuropathic pain: quality of life issues and associated costs. Am J Managed Care 2006;12(9 Suppl):S263-S268.

118. Centers for Disease Control and Prevention. Cigarette smoking among adults: United States 2001. MMRW 2003;52(40):953-956.

119. National Center for Chronic Disease Prevention and Health Promotion. Statistics and Facts. 2009. Retrieved from Tobacco, Smoking and Nicotine Addiction at MyAddiction.com

120. The Search for a Safe Cigarette, NOVA (PBS), October 2001. Retrieved from Tobacco, Smoking and Nicotine Addiction: Statistics and Facts 2009 at MyAddiction.com

121. Quitting Smoking on Medline Plus. Retrieved from http://www.nlm.nih.gov/medlineplus/quittingsmoking.html

122. Martin T. Understanding Nicotine Addiction: Nicotine's Effects on the Brain. Retrieved from http://quitsmoking.about.com/od/nicotine/a/nicotineeffects.htm/

123. Martin T. Using Bupropion (Zyban) as a Quit Smoking Aid. Retrieved from http://quitsmoking.about.com/od/nicotine/a/nicotineeffects.htm

124. Pfizer. July 2009. Chantix (Varenicline) Revised Medication Guide/Package Insert.

125. Grigsby DG, Rager KM, Cheever TR. Substance Abuse, Nicotine: Treatment and Medication. 2009. Retrieved from http://emedicine.medscape.com/article/917297-treatment

126. Katon W, Von Korf M, Lin E, et al: A randomized trial of psychiatric consultation with distressed high utilizers. Gen Hosp Psychiatry 1992;14:86-98.

127. Von Korf M, Ormel J, Katon W, et al: Disability and depression among high utilizers of health care. Arch Gen Psychiatry 1992;49:91-99.

128. US Department of Health and Human Services. Mental Health: A Report of the Surgeon General. Rockville, MD: US DHHA; 1999.

129. Himelhoch S, Weller WE, Wu AW, et al. Chronic medical illness, depression, and use of acute medical services among Medicare beneficiaries. Med Care 2004;42(6):512-521.

130. Anxiety Disorders. Retrieved from http://www.athealth.com/index.html.

131. National Institute of Mental Health. Depression. Publication No. 08 3561 Revised 2008. Retrieved from http://education.ucsb.edu/hosford/documents/Depression.pdf.

132. National Institute of Mental Health. The Numbers Count: Mental Disorders in America 2008. Retrieved from http://www.nimh.nih.gov/health/publications/the-numbers-count-mental-disorders-in-america/index.shtml

133. Substance Abuse and Mental Health Services Administration. Discrimination and Stigma. Retrieved from http://mentalhealth.samhsa.gov/STIGMA/

134. Friedman RA. Stigma: What Hollywood and the Media Teach Us About Mental Illness. 2008. Retrieved from http://www.alternet.org/story/92401/

135. Stahl S. Psychiatric Cases of Famous Faces. 2009. Retrieved from http://www.neiglobal.com

136. Substance Abuse and Mental Health Services Administration. Stigma and Mental Illness. 1996. Retrieved from http://www.samhsa.gov

137. Soni A. The Five Most Costly Conditions 1996 and 2006: Estimates for the US Civilian Noninstitutionalized Population. Rockville, MD: Agency for Healthcare Research and Quality; July 2009.

138. Anxiety Disorders Association of America. Statistics and Facts About Anxiety Disorders. 2009. Retrieved from http://www.adaa.org

139. Welch CA, Czerwinski BS, et al. Depression and health care costs. Psychosomatics 2009;50(4):392-401.

140. van den Broek KC, Nyklicek I, Denollet J. Anxiety predicts poor perceived health in patients with an implantable defibrillator. Psychosomatics 2009;50(5):483-492.

141. Fleet RP, Martel JP, et al. Non-fearful panic disorder: a variant of panic in medical patients? Psychosomatics 2000;41(4):311-320.

142. American Psychiatric Association. Healthy minds. Healthy lives. Obsessive-Compulsive Disorder 2006. Arlington, VA: American Psychiatric Association.

143. Sichel D, Cohen L, Rosenbaum JF, et al. Postpartum onset of obsessive-compulsive disorder. Psychosomatics 1993;34:277-279.

144. Sichel D, Cohen L, Dimmock JA, et al. Post partum obsessive-compulsive disorder: a case series. J Clin Psychiatry 1993;54: 156-159.

145. Abramowitz J, Moore K, Carmin C, et al. Acute onset of obsessive-compulsive disorder in males following childbirth: case reports. Psychosomatics 2001;42(5):429-431.

146. American Psychiatric Association. Posttraumatic Stress Disorder. 2009. Retrieved from http://www.healthyminds.org/ Main-Topic/Anxiety-Disorders

147. American Psychiatric Association. Diagnostic and Statistical Manual of Mental Disorders, Fourth Edition, Text Revised. Washington, DC: American Psychiatric Association; 2000.

148. Pedersen DD. Psych Notes: Clinical Pocket Guide. Philadelphia: FA Davis; 2005.

149. Hamilton M. The assessment of anxiety states by rating. Br J Med Psychol 1959;32:50-55.

150. Zung WWK. A rating instrument for anxiety. Psychosomatics 1971: XII:371-379

151. American Psychiatric Association. Healthy Minds, Healthy Lives: Panic Disorder. Arlington, VA: American Psychiatric Association; 2006.

152. National Institute of Mental Health. Anxiety Disorders. NIH Publication No. 09-3879. Washington, DC: National Institute of Mental Health; 2009.

153. National Institute of Mental Health. Mental Health Medications. NIH Publication No. 08-3929.Washington, DC: National Institute of Mental Health; 2008.

154. Pedersen DD, Leahy LG. Pocket Psych Drugs: Point-of-Care Clinical Guide. Philadelphia: FA Davis; 2010.

155. Organizing Framework and CNS Core Competencies. Retrieved from http://www.nacns.org/LinkClick.aspx? fileticket=22R8AaNmrUI%3Dandtabid=94

156. American Psychiatric Association. Healthy Minds, Healthy Lives: Depression. Arlington, VA: American Psychiatric Association; 2006.

157. Russo CA, Hambrick MM, Owens PL. Hospital Stays Related to Depression. 2005. Retrieved from http://www. hcup-us.ahrq.gov/reports.jsp.

158. Powell LH, Catellier D, Freedland KE, et al. Depression and heart failure in patients with a new myocardial infarction. Am Heart J 2005;149(5);851-855.

159. Cully JA, Johnson M, Moffett ML, et al. Depression and anxiety in ambulatory patients with heart failure. Psychosomatics 2009;50(6);592-298.

160. Cully JA, Graham DP, Stanley MA, et al. Quality of life in patients with chronic obstructive pulmonary disease and comorbid anxiety or depression. Psychosomatics 2006;47(4);312-319.

161. de Jonge P, Bel Hadj F, Boffa D, et al. Prevention of major depression in complex medically ill patients: preliminary results from a randomized, controlled trial. Psychosomatics 2009;50(3); 227-233.

162. Understanding Depression. 2009. Retrieved from http://www. healthline.com/sw/hr-sr-understanding-depression.

163. American Psychiatric Association. Healthy Minds, Healthy Lives: Seasonal Affective Disorder. Arlington, VA: American Psychiatric Association; 2006.

164. Cox JL, Holden JM, Sagovsky R. Edinburgh Postnatal Depression Scale (EPDS). Br J Psych 1987;150.

165. Hamilton M. A rating scale for depression. J Neurol Neurosurg Psychiatry 1960;23:56-62.

166. Zung WWK. A self-rating depression scale. Arch Gen Psychiatry 1965;12:63-70.

Skin Problems and Wound Care

Karen C. Lyon, PhD, APRN, ACNS, NEA

INTRODUCTION

Any first-semester nursing student would be able to tell you that skin is the largest organ in the body, comprising approximately 10% of the total body weight of the average adult. It is one of the first anatomical facts we teach to our young protégés. From the moment we are born, this organ is exposed to physical, mechanical, chemical, and environmental assaults that can have either temporary or permanent consequences. Skin serves as a barrier to these attacks, preventing pathogens from entering the body and attacking internal organs. Besides protection, the skin has five other functions: sensation, thermoregulation, immune processing, metabolism, and the establishment of body image. We feel pain, pressure, heat, and cold through nerve endings in the epidermis. Skin is essential in our regulation of heat and cold through vasoconstriction/vasodilatation mechanisms and the sweating process. There are important resident immune cells in both the epidermis and dermis, and synthesis of vitamin D by skin exposed to sunlight is an important component of metabolism. Finally, the skin's appearance and individual attributes are essential aspects of how we view ourselves and what others think about us.

As we age, the functions of this vital organ decline. The effects of repetitive environmental assaults, chronic disease, poor nutrition, infection, acute and chronic inflammation, and inadequate blood and oxygen supply can combine to transform any acute break in the skin into a chronic, nonhealing wound. The accompanying physical, emotional, and economic toll of these "problem wounds" is incalculable.

CHALLENGING WOUNDS

In the healthy patient without comorbid conditions, healing proceeds through the normal processes of wounding, hemostasis, inflammation, angiogenesis, granulation tissue formation, epithelialization, and remodeling. Chronic wounds do not proceed through that orderly process. Why do some wounds become chronic and nonhealing? There are a variety of factors, all of which can be categorized as either local or systemic. The local factors include ischemia, infection, edema, scarring, radiation injury, topical steroids, local toxins, trauma, pressure, foreign bodies, and local malignancy. The systemic factors involve the presence of diseases such as diabetes mellitus, connective tissue disease, renal failure, hereditary and immunologic disorders, and hepatic failure. Other systemic complications include tobacco and alcohol abuse, nutritional deficiencies, distant malignancy, chemotherapeutic agents, extremes of age, and systemic steroids (1-3). Mustoe presents a unifying hypothesis for the pathogenesis of chronic wounds including the coexistence of the cellular and systemic effects of aging, bacterial colonization and inflammatory host response, and chronic ischemia, hypoxia, and reperfusion injury in the presence of local ischemia (4). The most common chronic wound types—venous leg ulcers (VLE), diabetic foot wounds, and pressure ulcers—present a huge health care cost, both in terms of dollars and in terms of human suffering. Hospital costs alone have been estimated at $50,000 to $100,000. For the more than 5 million Americans suffering with chronic wounds, this represents $250 to $500 billion annually (5). The cost in human suffering is incalculable.

VENOUS ULCERS

Etiology

Chronic venous insufficiency (CVI) is reported as a causative factor in 70% to 90% of chronic leg ulcers (3,6). They are some of the most recalcitrant wounds to deal with and present a particular challenge to the Clinical

Nurse Specialist (CNS) whether hospital or community based. The recurrence rate is high and the financial impact has been estimated at 1% to 3% of total health budget in developed countries including over $3 billion annually in treatment costs and the loss of 2 million working days just in the United States (6). There is significant impact on quality of life including pain, impaired mobility, depression, compromised self-image, and social isolation.

Pathophysiology

Venous leg ulcers are a direct result of prolonged venous hypertension. To understand how this hypertension develops, it is important to review the physiology of venous circulation. The venous system consists of superficial and deep systems based on their position relative to the fascia (3). The superficial system consists of the greater and lesser saphenous veins and branches, while the deep system consists of the femoral and popliteal veins. Connecting these two systems are the perforators. Retrograde blood flow is prevented in all these systems by valves. When the veins, valves, and calf muscles are healthy, venous circulation is maintained. In the presence of disease and dysfunction, chronic venous hypertension develops. This can be related to deep vein obstruction from thrombosis, scarring, obesity or malignancy, valvular incompetence secondary to trauma, thrombus formation or congenital anomalies, and calf dysfunction resulting from paralysis, muscle atrophy, or anatomical abnormalities (6-10). Eventually, the chronic increase in hydrostatic pressure overcomes the tissue osmotic gradient, leading to capillary leakage into surrounding tissue and the hallmark clinical sign of CVI, the edematous leg.

Three distinct hypotheses have been presented for venous ulceration. The first, fibrin cuff development, postulates that the chronic venous hypertension distends the capillary bed with leakage of macromolecules such as fibrinogen into the tissue. This prevents normal oxygenation of tissue ultimately leading to ulceration. A second hypothesis involves blood cell deposition in capillaries leading to local ischemia. Proteolytic enzymes are released, causing a local inflammatory reaction. The final hypothesis theorizes that macromolecules like fibrin trap growth factors and other proteins, making them unavailable for tissue repair (3, 6). The end result of all these processes is ulceration.

Clinical Presentation

Venous ulceration is rarely spontaneous. The usual precipitating event is trauma to the ankle or calf, particularly in patients suffering from lipodermatosclerosis, an inflammation of the layer of fat under the epidermis. These wounds usually fail to heal in an orderly and timely manner, leading patients to seek medical care. Generally, they are found above the medial malleolus, but they can also be lateral, tibial, or calf ulcers. Wound margins are irregular and undermining is not a common feature. The wound will generally be flat, approximately even with the skin edges. The patient usually reports copious amounts of drainage, often malodorous. The wound bed may appear purplish in color with yellowish fibrin slough and epithelial islands. The skin around venous ulcers is generally hyperpigmented with hemosiderin deposits and may be eczematous, inflamed, and indurated (Figure 7-1).

Diagnosis

Recommended tests for evaluating the patient with suspected venous ulcers include the following:

- **Ankle-Brachial Index:** The ankle-brachial index (ABI) is a simple, noninvasive test for determining blood pressure differences between upper and lower extremities. It is important for determining arterial insufficiency. The test should be done with a handheld 5- to 10-MHz Doppler and blood pressure cuff. Have the patient lie supine and palpate for the brachial pulse. Apply the conductivity gel over the brachial artery and listen for the whooshing sound. Pump up the cuff to 20 mm Hg above where the sound is no longer heard. Slowly release the air and listen for the sound to return; the point at which you first hear the sound is the systolic blood pressure. Repeat the procedure on the other arm and record the highest reading. Repeat the sequence for the posterior tibial pulse at the medial aspect of the patient's ankle. To determine the ABI, divide each ankle systolic pressure by the brachial pressure. An ABI less than 0.9 signals arterial insufficiency, which helps to differentiate venous and arterial insufficiency and, in many cases, suggests the presence of both conditions. Additionally, an ABI less than 0.9 contraindicates the use of compression therapy for venous ulcers until more sophisticated tests for arterial function can be performed.
- **Duplex Venous Scan:** A noninvasive ultrasound that detects and quantifies venous reflux.

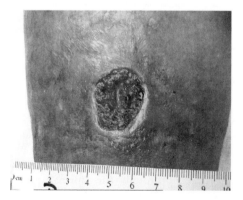

FIGURE 7–1: Venous ulcer with granulation tissue.

- **Biopsy:** Useful for evaluating an atypical ulcer. Basal cell carcinomas can arise from chronic wounds and malignant melanomas have been missed when biopsy of chronic wounds is not performed.

Management

Chronic wounds must be managed according to the mechanisms underlying their development. For venous ulcers, this means controlling venous hypertension, edema, and ulceration. Compression therapy is considered the hallmark of treating venous ulcers. It consists of applying external pressure to promote return of blood flow from peripheral to systemic circulation. In addition to its effect on venous circulation, compression has been reported to improve lymphatic drainage, stimulate fibrinolysis, increase local oxygenation, reduce reflux in the deep veins, and reestablish an environment that is conducive to healing (3, 6, 9). Compression bandages should be used in patients with CVI or CVI with ulcers. Gradient compression stockings can be used for maintenance of patients without ulceration or whose clinically significant edema has been controlled with compression. Both paste bandages like the Unna boot and multilayered long-stretch bandages such as Smith & Nephew's Profore or Johnson and Johnson's DYNA-FLEX can be used for compression therapy (Figure 7-2). Paste bandages are impregnated with medications such as zinc oxide, calamine, glycerin, or sorbitol and applied with a 50% overlap. When they dry, they apply resistance and pressure over the wound. The pressure can be maintained with the outer application of Coban or an Ace wrap. Multilayered wraps are elastic in nature and are available in different pressure gradients. They consist of an initial layer of padding followed by layers of elastic and cohesive bandaging. Both paste and multilayered systems can be left in place for up to 7 days.

Wound debridement is an important aspect of venous ulcer management. This can be accomplished through chemical, mechanical, or sharp techniques. Chemical debridement uses enzyme debriding agents such as collagenase santyl ointment. Collagenase is capable of digesting collagen and facilitates the removal of slough, promoting granulation, and subsequent epithelialization. Mechanical debridement can be accomplished through the use of wet-to-dry dressings, hydrotherapy, or irrigation. The most effective and fastest mechanism for debriding venous ulcers, however, is sharp debridement, which can be accomplished with through curettage or scalpel. Sharp debridement removes slough and senescent cells and is particularly important before applying bioengineered skin like Apligraf (Organogenesis) or Dermagraft (Advanced BioHealing).

Topical dressings for ulcers vary according to the characteristics of the wound, and there are a variety of dressings that can be used depending on exudates, wound size, presence of infection, need for enzymatic debridement, and condition of the periwound. For wounds with light or moderate drainage, hydrocolloid dressings can be used for their moisture retention qualities (e.g., MPM Excel, 3M Tegaderm Hydrocolloid). Absorbent dressings like alginates, foams, and specialty absorptive dressings should only be selected for wounds with copious amounts of drainage (e.g., Mepilex, Optifoam, 3M Foam, Aquacel, CarraSorb H, Kalginate, SilverCel).

DIABETIC FOOT WOUNDS

Etiology

It is estimated that 1 in 10 Americans has diabetes mellitus (DM) (3, 11, 12). It is a disease that has become endemic in the U.S. population. Unhealthy eating habits coupled with an increasingly sedentary lifestyle and obesity are major contributing factors. Additionally, a familial link in Hispanics, African Americans, and Native Americans complicates the epidemiology in these groups. It is well known that these populations have a higher incidence of diabetes than Anglos, Asians, and other Europeans.

Currently, cardiovascular complications are the most common sequelae that result in death and disability for diabetic patients. In the lower extremities, these cardiovascular complications result in decreased blood flow and

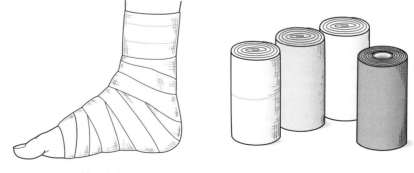

FIGURE 7–2: Unna boot and Smith & Nephew's Profore Multi-Layer dressing.

Unna's boot   Multilayer dressings neuropathy (loss of protective sensation), leading to chronic foot and leg wounds.

Pathophysiology

The pathogenesis of diabetic foot wounds depends on the specific etiology. Most investigators agree that there are three major risk factors that underlie the development of ulceration: neuropathy, foot structure and anatomic deformity, and a pivotal event. Peripheral arterial disease (PAD) also contributes to the problem, as do ischemia and previous history of ulceration.

Peripheral neuropathy is a critical factor in the development of diabetic foot ulcers and is the singular most common complication of type 2 DM. Patients commonly overlook this problem until pain, paresthesias, and the loss of protective sensation (LOPS) develop. At this point, wounding and subsequent amputation become a serious risk.

Diabetic neuropathy involves the sensory, motor, and autonomic nervous systems. The sensory loss causes patients to lose the sensation of pain. In fact, patients may lose all sensation, with total numbness of the foot developing. Patients have been reported to walk across hot cement barefooted, play a round of golf with rocks or other objects in their shoes, or step on needles or pins without any awareness of trauma and subsequent tissue damage. Motor neuropathy leads to changes in the actual biomechanics of walking. Weakness in the anterior tibial compartment and pedal muscular atrophy lead to imbalance in weight bearing with resultant foot deformities. Autonomic deficiencies develop as neuropathy affects smooth muscle, glands, and visceral organs. Foot complications include insufficient sweat gland activity leading to dry, cracked skin; decreased arterial tone with vasodilatation; and impaired response to infection (3, 6, 13, 14).

Foot and other anatomical deformities lead to gait alterations that must be recognized immediately. Diabetic foot ulcers generally develop because the compressive and frictional forces around areas of deformity exceed what the soft tissue can bear. These deformities include bunions, hammer toes, and prominent metatarsals. While patients may see the anatomical changes, because of LOPS, they do not *feel* the changes until a foot ulcer has actually developed. The most serious anatomical deformity in the diabetic patient is Charcot foot, a neuroarthropathy that presents with erythema, swelling, bounding pulses, and increased skin temperature (Figure 7-3). In the long term, there is actual osseous destruction with stress fractures, arch destruction, and the development of the classic rocker-bottom shape (Figure 7-4). Ulcerations are common in patients with Charcot foot but also develop in the absence of this condition. Common sites for diabetic foot ulcer include the plantar surfaces of the metatarsals, especially four and five; the talocalcaneal joint; and the phalanges (3, 6, 13-15).

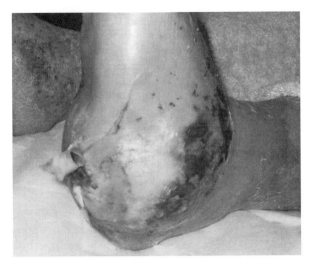

FIGURE 7–3: Infected diabetic ulcer in Charcot foot.

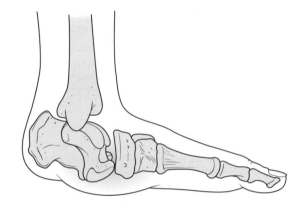

FIGURE 7–4: Charcot deformity.

Pivotal can be defined as vitally important, of critical significance, especially in determining the outcome of an event. In the case of diabetic patients faced with neuropathy, impaired peripheral circulation, and anatomical foot changes, the pivotal event for ulceration is any physical event, trauma, or infection that sets off the cascade. Such events can include cuts, abrasions, burns, mechanical trauma from ill-fitting shoes, soft tissue injury from foreign objects, bumps, callous formation, blister formation, hematomas, and any local infection. Additionally, it will be imperative to ascertain the presence of other risk factors than can complicate ulcer development, including LOPS, history of foot ulceration, previous amputations, limited joint mobility, obesity, and lack of glycemic control. Infections can be limb and life threatening because bacteria spread rapidly through the foot's compartments, through the plantar fascia, and often into the bone. All of these factors play a critical role in failure to heal with subsequent amputation and require the clinician's full armamentarium of wound management tools in order to provide optimal outcomes.

Clinical Presentation

Diabetic ulcers occur on the foot, heel, or toes, or between the toes. They are often preceded by callus formation. The loss of protective sensation and neuropathy also precede foot ulceration. Patients often complain that they have no feeling in their feet or they may have numbness and tingling. Edema is often present and can be dependent or pitting, localized or generalized, and bilateral or unilateral. Perfusion will depend on the presence of associated PAD and can be ascertained through assessing skin temperature, color changes, venous refill, capillary refill time, and paresthesias. If a wound is present, it will be assessed by size, location, visualization of wound base and sidewalls, presence or absence of tunneling or undermining, periwound skin condition, presence of slough, debris, or necrotic material, and assessment for pain. Additionally, complications such as gangrene, cellulitis, and osteomyelitis or Charcot fractures must be determined.

Diagnosis

Causative and contributive factors for the development of diabetic foot ulcers must be evaluated. These include assessing for risk factors for ulceration, identifying infection, screening for neuropathy, and screening for peripheral vascular disease (PVD).

- Risk factors for ulceration
  - Previous history of ulceration or amputation
  - Foot deformities
  - LOPS with autonomic neuropathy
  - Limited joint mobility
  - Obesity
  - Poor/absent glycemic control
  - Impaired vision
- Presence of infection
  - Wound with swelling, redness, pain, malodorous discharge
  - High blood glucose levels
  - Elevated white blood cell count, erythrocyte sedimentation rate, and C-reactive protein
  - Magnetic resonance imaging for definitive diagnosis of osteomyelitis
- Screening for neuropathy
  - Semmes-Weinstein monofilament test
  - Assess for Charcot joint deformity
- PVD screening
  - Palpate all lower extremity pulses
  - Presence/absence of claudication
  - Lower limb angiography

Management

The essence of management for diabetic foot wounds lies in prevention. Clinicians must work with patients and their families to educate diabetics on preventing callus and wound formation. This requires a multidisciplinary approach for identification of any patient at risk for ulcer development, including those with insensate feet, previous ulcerations or amputations, and long-standing diabetes. Surveillance is lifelong and includes at least annual foot screening, patient education, proper selection of footwear, daily patient self-examination of the feet, and management of common skin conditions (16, 17).

In the presence of wounds, treatment is focused on minimizing current damage and preventing complications such as amputation with a focus on preserving as much anatomical function as possible. Nonsurgical treatment of wounds focuses on cleaning and removing slough and necrotic tissue, providing a proper wound-healing environment and eliminating pressure. Surgical interventions include aggressive debridement to convert chronic, nonhealing wounds into acute, inflammatory wounds, managing infections, including osteotomy for removal of infected bone and revascularization to reestablish microcirculation to the foot and toes. Debridement allows for the removal of devitalized tissue and foreign material. Additionally, it removes senescent cells that impede healing and interfere with the deposition of growth factors. While it can be accomplished through the use of autolytic debriding agents and mechanical instrumentation, the quickest and most effective method is sharp debridement with a scalpel whenever significant necrotic or gangrenous tissue is present in the wound (3, 6, 16).

Once wounds are clean, they are ready for dressings that promote a moist environment while controlling exudates. What types of dressings are selected will depend on the cause of the wound and the amount and type of exudates. The most common dressing types include:

- Alginates: Partial- and full-thickness wounds with moderate to heavy exudate
- Antimicrobials: Topical dressings with silver, iodine, and other antibacterial agents for use with draining wounds with evidence of bacterial contamination
- Collagens: Protein laden dressings for use with partial- and full-thickness wounds, infected wounds, tunneling, and with burns or donor sites
- Hydrocolloids: Occlusive or semiocclusive to manage partial- and full-thickness wounds with necrosis and slough and light to moderate drainage
- Hydrogels: Water- and glycerin–based dressings that maintain a moist healing environment and promote granulation (6)

Advanced therapies to supplement traditional wound care include hyperbaric oxygen therapy, bioengineered skin equivalents, regenerative tissue matrix, growth factor therapy, negative pressure, vacuum-assisted closure, and total contact casting. Pain management will be directed at controlling the chronic burning and tingling of diabetic neuropathy. Agents such as gabapentin may be useful. A regular exercise regimen should also be established with care taken to exercise caution in view of LOPS and insensate extremities. Finally, nutrition can never be overlooked. Diet is managed to control serum glucose, hyperlipidemia, and hypertension. Multivitamins and protein supplements may be necessary, especially in the elderly population (16, 18).

PRESSURE ULCERS

Etiology

A pressure ulcer is any lesion caused by unrelieved pressure, which results in damage to the underlying tissue. These are generally located over bony prominences and can also involve shearing and friction forces. Shearing is caused by tissue layers sliding against one another, resulting in disruption or angulation of blood vessels, usually at the fascial level. The purplish discoloration of the skin should be suspect for deep tissue injury, indicating that the wounding starts deep and works its way toward the surface. This type of injury can be difficult to assess in darker-skinned races.

In addition to pressure, many wounds that end up classified as pressure ulcers started with skin breakdown from a different etiology. This can include skin maceration from incontinence, superficial skin tears from friction, and tearing of blood vessels from shear. Terms such as decubitus ulcers and bedsores are still used commonly, although they are inappropriate since they infer an etiology related to being confined to bed when, in fact, these ulcers develop in acute and chronic care settings, in all age groups, and in concert with a variety of diagnoses (3, 5).

Pathophysiology

Pressure ulcers develop when soft tissue is compressed between a surface and a bony prominence. Almost always, immobility is part of the equation. The pressure may be applied with great force for a short period of time or with lesser force over an extended time. The result is the same. When capillary filling pressures exceed the normal 12 to 32 mm Hg for longer than 2 hours, blood supply is disrupted resulting in local ischemia, hypoxia, edema, and inflammation. Ultimately, tissue death occurs (3, 6). The wound often starts with only a small skin defect, but muscle and fat are more susceptible to damage from pressure and a small cutaneous defect can be associated with major tunneling, undermining, and subcutaneous damage. The most common sites for pressure ulcers are the sacrum and the heels, but they can also develop over ischial tuberosities, spinous processes, iliac crests, medial and lateral condyles, greater trochanters, and the malleolus. In addition, they have been noted in areas that do not include bony prominences, like the ears.

As previously noted, shearing and moisture also contribute to the development or worsening of pressure ulcers. Shearing causes mechanical destruction of deep tissues as skin and underlying tissues are pulled in opposite directions, tearing blood vessels and leading to local ischemia. Moisture secondary to incontinence or diaphoresis leads to skin maceration. When skin integrity is disrupted due to maceration, the tissue can tear and erode more easily. This insult to the epidermis is complicated by chemical changes from the acidic nature of urine and feces in incontinent patients and subsequent ulcer development (3, 5, 19).

Clinical Presentation

Pressure ulcers are staged in accordance with recommendations from the National Pressure Ulcer Advisory Panel (5) (Figure 7-5).

> **Stage I:** Intact skin with nonblanchable redness of a localized area, usually over a bony prominence. The area may be painful, firm, soft, warmer, or cooler compared to surrounding tissue.
> **Stage II:** Partial-thickness loss of dermis presenting as a shallow, open ulcer with a red, pink wound bed, without slough
> **Stage III:** Full-thickness tissue loss; subcutaneous fat may be visible, but muscle, tendon, or bone is not exposed. Slough may be present.
> **Stage IV:** Full-thickness skin loss with extensive destruction, tissue necrosis, or damage to muscle, bone, or supporting structures such as tendons or joint capsules

Diagnosis

There are no specific diagnostic tests for pressure ulcers. There are several risk-assessment tools including the Braden Scale and the Norton Scale, which are important tools in evaluating risk factors. The Braden Scale evaluates sensory perception, moisture, activity, mobility, nutrition, and friction/shear. The Norton Scale evaluates physical condition, mental condition, activity, mobility, and continence (3, 5, 6, 19). Unfortunately, neither scale evaluates actual factors that caused the ulcer in the first place. The critical factors that must be assessed include perfusion, tissue oxygenation, cellular effects of aging, cellular reparative processes, and vascular response to stress. At present, there are no practical diagnostic tests to evaluate these factors.

Management

Management of pressure ulcers revolves around prevention and treatment. Obviously, prevention is the priority.

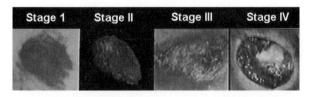

FIGURE 7–5: Pressure ulcers: Stages I to IV. (Photographs courtesy of Dr. Tamara D. Fishman and Dr. Allan D. Freedline.)

The following are prevention recommendations of the Wound, Ostomy and Continence Nurses Society (WOCNS) as published in the National Guideline Clearinghouse in 2003 (19).

1. Clean and dry skin after every incontinence episode.
2. Use turning or lift sheets to turn or transfer patients.
3. Maintain head of bed at or below 30 degrees or the lowest elevation consistent with the patient's medical condition to optimize venous return.
4. Avoid vigorous massage over bony prominences.
5. Schedule regular and frequent turning—at least every 2 hours if on non–pressure-reducing surface and every 2 to 4 hours if on pressure-reducing mattress.
6. Place "at-risk" patients on pressure-reduction surfaces.
7. Avoid foam rings, donuts, and sheepskin to reduce pressure.
8. Use pressure-reducing surfaces in the operating room for high-risk patients.
9. Relieve pressure under heels by using pillows or other devices.
10. Establish a bowel/bladder program for incontinent patients.
11. Use incontinence skin barriers to protect skin.
12. Maintain adequate nutrition to maximize healing.
13. Educate patients and their care providers about causes and risk factors for pressure ulcers.

Treatment protocols have also been published by WOCNS as national guidelines and include the following (19):

1. Reduce friction and shear.
2. Turn patients every 2 hours.
3. Use positioning devices to avoid placing patients on an ulcer.
4. Maintain head of bed at or below 30 degrees for supine and side-lying patients.
5. Use low–air loss and air-fluidized beds for pressure relief in patients with stage III or IV ulcers.
6. Shift weight for chair-bound patients every 15 minutes.
7. Limit time in chair and use pressure-relief cushions in the presence of ulcers on sitting surfaces.
8. Manage urinary/fecal incontinence.
9. Select under pads, diapers, or briefs that wick moisture away from the skin.
10. Ensure adequate nutrient intake: 30 to 40 kcal/kg body weight/day and 1 to 1.5 g protein/kg body weight/day.
11. Cleanse wound at every dressing change with noncytotoxic agent.
12. Debride ulcer of devitalized tissue.
13. Perform wound care using topical dressings determined by wound, patient needs, cost, and caregiver availability.
14. Manage wound infections.
15. Reassess the wound with each dressing change to determine whether modifications are needed as the wound heals or deteriorates.

NECROTIZING FASCIITIS

Necrotizing fasciitis is a severe skin infection caused by bacteria, most commonly group A streptococci, either alone or in combination with other species, often *Staphylococcus aureus* (3). In the lay literature, it is often referred to as "flesh-eating" bacteria. It is a rare but extremely morbid condition with an approximately 40% mortality rate. The progression of the disease is rapid and along the fascial planes. There is usually significant undermining with necrosis of overlying skin. While it can affect any part of the body, it usually affects the extremities, particularly the legs. It is also often seen along the abdominal wall, in the perianal area, and around postoperative wounds.

The portal of entry is usually a site of trauma, burn, laceration, or insect bite. Wounds that come in contact with ocean water or raw fish or oysters can be infected, as can an intestinal surgery site, gunshot wound, and muscle strain or bruise, even if there is no break in the skin. Predisposition exists in immune-compromised hosts such as those with DM, alcoholism, intravenous drug abuse, and obesity.

Clinical presentation is acute with pain from an injury that becomes better over 24 to 36 hours and then gets worse, much worse than the seriousness of the wound would seem to warrant. Chills and fever may or may not be present early on. There will be erythema and cellulitis around the wound. Nausea, vomiting, and diarrhea may also develop. Over the course of 3 to 5 days, the erythematous skin changes will transform to patches of blue-gray, skin breakdown will occur, and cutaneous gangrene is evident. At this point, thrombosis of blood vessels has occurred along with destruction of superficial nerves and necrosis of subcutaneous tissue.

Early diagnosis is the most important step in effective treatment. Outcomes will depend on early surgical debridement, resuscitation, and stabilization. If shock and multiple organ failure develop during the first 24 to 36 hours, streptococcal toxic shock syndrome (TSS) should be suspected. Therapy will include appropriate antibiotics for the identified strains of bacteria, aggressive surgical debridement of the wounds, and adjunctive hyperbaric oxygen therapy (HBO). It has been reported that the use of HBO along with radical surgery and multiple antibiotics such as ampicillin-sulbactam, ticarcillin-clavulanate, piperacillin-tazobactam, or the combination of any of these with a fluoroquinolone or aminoglycocide aztreonam has reduced the mortality rate to as low as 12.5% (3).

CLINICAL NURSE SPECIALIST COMPETENCIES AND SPHERES OF INFLUENCE

Clinical Expert/Direct Care

The CNS for wound care is an essential member of the multidisciplinary team for wound management. In either the hospital or the outpatient clinic, they provide direct care including developing prevention strategies, assessing patient risk, minimizing environmental risk, and providing topical management of wounds. The advanced practice nurse can prescribe autolytic and enzymatic debridement agents such as papain-urea and collagenase santyl, perform mechanical debridement with electrical stimulation, pulse-evac, and whirlpool, and, with advanced training under the direction of a surgeon, perform limited sharp debridements. The CNS will also obtain cultures to diagnose local or systemic infection, prescribe antibiotics, apply protective dressings, prescribe growth factor therapy, and apply skin substitutes such as Apligraf and Dermagraft.

Consultation/Collaboration

The consultative role is one of the most important carried out by the wound care CNS. With the advent of wound development as one of the Centers for Medicare and Medicaid Services Centers for Medicare and Medicaid Services (CMS)-defined "never events," consultation with wound experts has become essential. Staff nurses are often viewed as expert in all things nursing, including wound care. Unfortunately, these nurses are usually laser-focused on issues related to cardiovascular, neurologic, and respiratory function. What they know or remember about wound healing is significantly lacking in current data and their approach to wound care remains surrounded in ritual. This is not meant as a criticism, just an observation about a natural response to the overwhelming demands on today's nurse. This lack of a sound knowledge base related to wound healing and wound care continues to contribute to a hit-or-miss approach to wound management on the traditional medical-surgical floor. The expertise provided by the wound CNS contributes the best evidence and science available to assist staff nurses with assessment, risk factor evaluation, and dressing selections for patients with problem wounds.

In addition to consultation, collaboration is an essential element of the CNS role in wound management. Medical collaboration includes discussion of treatment options with general, plastic, and cardiovascular surgeons; interventional cardiologists; endocrinologists; podiatrists; and infectious disease specialists. Additionally, the CNS consults with nutritionists/dietitians to establish an appropriate dietary plan of care for wound healing. This will include body measurements, evaluation of related laboratory tests, and dietary review. Together, this collaboration will assist in determining patients' nutrient needs for calories, protein, and fluids. Additional collaborations with physical therapy to design an appropriate exercise regimen and orthotists/prosthetists for evaluation of offloading devices, walking boots, and related paraphernalia are also essential.

Coaching/Teaching/Mentoring

Patient education and compliance form the bedrock of wound healing. Staff education and mentoring are essential to ensure that this education takes place. The CNS will have to evaluate the current knowledge level of staff nurses related to wound risk assessment, wound prevention, wound evaluation, and wound treatment. Principles of adult learning should be used to identify barriers to learning, evaluate current knowledge level in regard to wound management, identify staff learning styles and learning goals, and provide ongoing documentation of staff wound care skills. In assisting staff nurses to provide patient education, the CNS provides oversight for patient assessment, identification of patient's wound care needs, documentation of treatment goals and objectives, development of clinical pathways for wound healing and evaluation of patient compliance and rehabilitation.

Research/Evidence-Based Practice

The essence of comprehensive wound management is the development of a wound program based on the best and most current science. Chronic, nonhealing wounds are a challenge for a variety of reasons, not the least of which is their multifactorial etiology. The availability of advanced treatment modalities and clinical expertise of the wound care CNS can positively influence wound healing. These nurses are experts in recognizing initial infection, managing edema through the use of compression wraps, stockings, and pumps and consulting with the attending physician to plan for the proper specialty dressings. They are also the foundation of the educational plan that hospitals must have in order to provide evidence of best practices for wound prevention, management, and healing.

Systems Leadership

The CNS in wound care provides broad leadership on both a local and systems level. On the local level, s/he serves as the expert clinician for developing care maps and clinical pathways for wound care that are based on best evidence. The CNS will provide leadership in designing assessment tools that track a wound's progress and bench mark outcomes based on current knowledge of wound healing.

On the systems level, the CNS serves as the wound expert on hospitalwide or systemwide committees related to clinical practice. For the Pharmacy and Therapeutics Committee, s/he can help design the skin and wound formulary, which provides a process-driven approach for skin and wound care in the hospital. For financial and regulatory control, the CNS manages the development of documentation tools that ensure proper payment for wound care and establishes policies and procedures to implement staff compliance in wound prevention and treatment.

The development of a formalized wound care program directed by a CNS is desirable for most hospitals and health care systems. The challenges of treating problem wounds mandate a multidisciplinary approach, and the CNS is the perfect partner for directing the holistic approach to assessing the patient, not just the wound. Problem wounds are a major cause of human suffering and a financial drain on hospital and national resources. When we fail to manage these wounds with the same sense of importance that we give our patients' cardiovascular, respiratory, and neurologic status, we fail our patients. The overarching goal of effective wound care in any setting should be assessing and treating systemic illness, evaluating nutritional status and correcting deficiencies, identifying and treating infections, and developing an evidence-based protocol for wound healing. Provision of these services directed by a CNS with wound management expertise facilitates improved healing outcomes for our patients and a better quality of life for all who suffer from these debilitating conditions.

References

1. Broughton G, Janis JE, Attinger CE. Wound healing: an overview. Plas Reconstr Surg June supplement, 2006;117(7S):1ES-30ES.

2. Harding KG, Moore K, Phillips TJ. Wound chronicity and fibroblast senescence: implications for treatment. Int Wound J 2005; 2(4):364-368.

3. Sheffield PJ Fife CE, eds. Wound Care Practice. Flagstaff, AZ: Best Publishing; 2004.

4. Mustoe T. Understanding chronic wounds: a unifying hypothesis on their pathogenesis and implications for therapy. Ame J Surg 2004;187(5 suppl):65S-70S.

5. National Pressure Ulcer Advisory Panel. Pressure ulcer prevalence, cost, and risk assessment consensus development conference statement. 1994-1995 edition.

6. Hess CT. Clinical Guide: Skin & Wound Care , 6th ed. Ambler, PA: Lippincott Williams & Wilkins; 2008.

7. Bailey BB, Hurley DD, Wilcox JR. Venous ulcers. A Physician's Guide to Problem Wound Management, Diversified Clinical Services. 2006; 2.

8. Bergan JJ, Schmid-Schonbein GW, et al. Chronic venous disease. N Engl J Med 2006;355:488-498.

9. European Wound Management Association. The use of compression therapy in the treatment of venous leg ulcers: a recommended management pathway. EWMA J 2002;2(1):3-6.

10. Heinen MM, van Achterberg T, Scholte op Reimer W et al. Venous leg ulcer patients: a review of the literature on lifestyle and pain-related interventions. J Clin Nurs, 2004;13:355-366.

11. Bailey BB, Hurley DD, Wilcox JR. Diabetic foot ulcers: A Physician's Guide to Problem Wound Management, Diversified Clinical Services. 2006; 3.

12. Sheehan P. An overview of peripheral neuropathy in diabetes. Wounds 2009;21(4):103-107.

13. Oyibo SO, Jude EB, Tarawneh I, et al. comparison of two diabetic foot ulcer classification systems. Diabetes Care 2001;24(1):84-88.

14. Warriner RA. Diabetic wound of the lower extremity. Grand Rounds, Diversified Clinical Therapies. 2006; 5.

15. Wu SC, Armstrong DG. The role of activity, adherence, and off-loading on the healing of diabetic foot wounds. Plas Reconstr Surg June supplement: 2006;117(7S)248S-252S.

16. Wound, Ostomy and Continence Nurses Society. Guideline for management of wounds in patients with lower-extremity neuropathic disease. WOCN Clinical Practice Guideline. 2004; 3:1-14.

17. Wraight PR, Lawrence SM, Campbell DA, Colman PG. Creation of a multidisciplinary, evidence based, clinical guideline for the assessment, investigation and management of acute diabetes related foot complications. Diabe Med 2004;22:127-136.

18. Arnold M, Barbul A. Nutrition and wound healing. Plas Reconstr Surg June supplement 2006:117(7S)42S-58S.

19. Wound, Ostomy, and Continence Nurses Society. Guideline for prevention and management of pressure ulcers. WOCN Clinical Practice Guideline. 2003;2:1-13.

Neurologic Problems

Sarah Livesay, MS, APRN, CNS

INTRODUCTION

The 1990s were declared the "Decade of the Brain" by then president of the United States, George Bush. Indeed, research findings during the 1990s revealed new treatment strategies for acute neurologic illness that shifted the paradigms of management of neurologic disease. Care provided to patients with neurologic disease shifted from supportive to curative and timeliness of care became essential, particularly for patients with stroke and brain trauma. During the past several decades, the mortality associated with several acute neurologic illnesses has dropped significantly in part due to new treatment modalities. Insights provided during the decade of the brain have led to the explosion of neurologic programs throughout the nation in the past decade (1).

With advancement in medical management of neuroscience patients has come advancement in nursing management of these patients. Neuroscience intensive care management has developed into a highly specialized area for neuroscience physicians and nurses. This has brought about new roles for advanced practice nurses in the care of neuroscience patients as well. This chapter will focus on general concepts that guide the care of the hospitalized neuroscience patient as well as explore current management strategies for many common neurologic diseases.

General Concepts Guiding Neuro-Acute Care and Neuro-Critical Care

Several concepts are central to the understanding of diseases that affect the brain. Regardless of the cause of injury to the brain, whether stroke, trauma, seizure, or another pathology, understanding primary and secondary injury in the brain and the role of elevated intracranial pressure (ICP) and herniation syndromes is essential to providing quality care. In addition, several themes are common regardless of the cause of injury to the brain. The cellular processes that result in tissue damage and death are highly sensitive to temperature and glucose.

Therefore, aggressive glucose and fever management are common themes throughout multiple disease processes and will therefore be reviewed as a foundational building block of providing care. Finally, brain death may be the result of multiple disease processes and will be reviewed as another foundational topic in the hospital management of the neurologically injured patient.

Elevated Intracranial Pressure
Etiology

In a healthy adult, normal ICP is less than 10 to 15 mm Hg. An ICP exceeding 20 to 30 mm Hg is considered mild intracranial hypertension and sustained levels greater than 40 mm Hg is considered severe and life threatening (2). However, the brain's ability to compensate for elevated ICP has to do with how quickly the intracranial hypertension develops as well as the etiology. Therefore, ICP values must be considered in the clinical picture with the patient's neurologic exam. Some patients tolerate a higher ICP level, whereas herniation can occur at ICP levels lower than 20 mm Hg when it develops acutely in certain areas of the brain (2-4).

The concept of ICP is guided by the Monroe-Kelly doctrine (2, 3), which states that because the cranial contents are contained in a fixed, rigid structure (the skull), an increase in the volume of one of the skull contents must be offset by a decrease in another skull content or the pressure inside the skull will rise. The cranial vault contains cerebrospinal fluid (CSF), blood, and brain tissue, which exist in consistent volumes in a healthy individual. The area inside the skull has only a small degree of reserve to accommodate increased volume. In addition to the Monroe-Kelly doctrine, the concepts of cranial compliance, autoregulation, cerebral blood flow (CBF), and cerebral perfusion pressures (CPPs) are critical to the understanding of elevated ICP. Compliance is the change in ICP related to the change in intracranial volume (3). In a healthy individual, the brain is compliant and a change in volume results in only a small change in pressure. However, as pressure builds and cranial compliance is lost, a small change in volume results in a large change in pressure (3).

Autoregulation is a process of vascular constriction and dilation of the vessels in the brain in order to maintain a constant CBF regardless of the CPP. In a healthy brain, as the systemic blood pressure varies, the cerebrovasculature vasodilates or vasoconstricts to maintain a constant CPP to the brain tissue (2). This is necessary because the brain requires a constant blood flow to meet metabolic demands. Brain tissue also has a low energy and glucose reserve and so must rely on constant blood flow (3).

Carbon dioxide, oxygen, and the cerebral metabolic rate of oxygen also influence CBF and ICP. In patients with decreased intracranial compliance, elevated CO_2 results in cerebral vasodilation, increased CBF, and increased ICP. Decreased CO_2 results in vasoconstriction, decreased CBF, and decreased ICP (3).

An increase in any of the three elements inside the skull (CSF, brain tissue, or blood) will result in increased pressure inside the skull. Examples of pathologies that may result in increased ICP include hydrocephalus (increased CSF inside the skull), any type of hemorrhage inside the brain (resulting in increased blood volume inside the head), hyperemia (increased blood flow to damaged tissue in the brain), or cellular edema (cytotoxic, vasogenic edema resulting in increased tissue volume). Abnormal growth inside the brain such as a tumor also increases the volume inside the skull and can lead to an increased pressure (2, 3). Often, cerebral injury results in several factors contributing to increased ICP. For example, in a patient with trauma, they may have a combination of hemorrhage such as traumatic intracerebral hemorrhage (ICH) and subarachnoid hemorrhage (SAH), cerebral edema, hyperemia to the injured tissue as a result of decreased autoregulation, and hydrocephalus as a result of CSF outflow obstruction from the edema and blood in the CSF.

Within brain tissue, there are several etiologies behind the formation of cerebral edema. Cytotoxic edema is a result of increased intracellular water from damage to the cell itself. Cytotoxic edema may result from ischemic stroke, anoxic brain injury, fulminant hepatic failure, lead intoxication, and Reye's syndrome (3). Vasogenic edema is the result of increased extracellular water in the interstitium from a vascular origin. Vasogenic edema may result from hypertensive encephalopathy, eclampsia, posterior reversible encephalopathy syndrome, brain tumors, abscesses, encephalitis, or high altitude cerebral edema (3). Transependymal edema results from CSF shifting from high pressures in the ventricles to lower pressures in the brain interstitium due to hydrocephalus (3). Osmotic edema results from rapid shifts in serum osmolarity and may be associated with hyponatremia, reverse urea syndrome, rebound effect from

osmotherapy, diabetic ketoacidosis, and hyperglycemia nonketotic coma during the correction phase (3).

Venous outflow obstruction may also be the cause of increased ICP. Examples of disease states that result in obstructed cerebral venous outflow include sinus venous thrombosis and jugular vein thrombosis.

Diagnosis

Computed tomography (CT) scanning is generally the imaging test of choice as it can be obtained quickly. Noncontrast CT of the brain may show cerebral edema, sulcal effacement resulting in loss of gyri, midline shift, compressed basal cisterns, hydrocephalus, or mass effect (2, 3). However, lack of these findings does not exclude the development of elevated ICP (2, 3).

Clinical Presentation

The clinical presentation of elevated ICP can range on a continuum from lethargy to stupor and coma as pressures rise. Headache, nausea, vomiting, and diplopia (cranial nerve VI palsy) are associated with elevated ICP. Downward deviation of the eyes may develop with hydrocephalus as a result of damage to the upgaze centers in the midbrain. Papilledema is a sign of increased ICP but may not be present in the setting of trauma (2). A reflex motor exam (flexor or extensor posturing) may also be seen in elevated ICP (2).

If elevated ICP is not treated, it results in the shifting of brain tissue around the static structures in the cranium (bone and dural tissue), resulting in herniation. Several herniation syndromes may be evident depending on the degree and location of elevated ICP (3). Uncal herniation results from the inferior displacement of the temporal lobe past the tentorium cerebella. Symptoms include ipsilateral oculomotor nerve palsy (dilated poorly responsive pupil), posterior cerebral artery infarction, and/or Kernohan's notch phenomenon (trapping of the contralateral cerebral peduncle against the tentorium resulting in hemiplegia that is ipsilateral to the side off the mass effect) (3). Subfalcine herniation results from the cingulated gyrus being compressed under the falx cerebri. Symptoms include altered mentation, contralateral leg weakness, and/or anterior cerebral artery infarction (3). Central (transtentorial) herniation results from the downward displacement of the midbrain and brainstem. This results in coma and brainstem dysfunction, and brain death if uncorrected (3). Tonsillar herniation results from the downward displacement of the cerebellar tonsils through the foramen magnum. Medullary dysfunction and cardiorespiratory arrest and brain death are the result of tonsillar herniation (3).

Cushing's triad is evident at the time of terminal brain herniation. Hypertension, bradycardia and irregular respirations are generally evident in the setting of severe elevations in ICP and signal impending herniation and brain death (3).

ICP monitoring may reveal waveform changes that are indicative of elevated ICP. ICP waveform changes can be seen on individual waveforms as they correlate to arterial blood flow as well as over time. The ICP waveform is a reflection of the arterial blood arriving in the brain and echoing throughout the intracranial cavity. In a healthy brain, with each systolic beat of the heart, the ICP waveform contains three peaks that occur in succession with decreasing amplitude and are named P1, P2, and P3, respectively. As the ICP rises and intracranial compliance is lost, P2 amplitude may increase and be greater than P1. Another sign of lost compliance may be a flattened P1 upslope (3). Pathologic ICP waveform includes the formation of Lundburg A, Bs, and C waves. Lundberg A waves (also known as plateau waves) signal impending herniation and brain death. They are waves that last 5 to 20 minutes with an amplitude of 50 mm Hg or greater. Lundburg B waves (pulse waves) last 2 to 5 minutes with amplitude of greater than 20 mm Hg. Less is known regarding the role of Lundberg B waves, but they may be related to loss of intracranial compliance. The significance of Lundburg C waves is unknown (2, 3).

Management

When treating elevated ICP, the management goal is to decrease the ICP into a normal range while maintaining CPP greater than 60 mm Hg (2). Ideal CPP range is debatable, especially in the setting of damaged brain tissue with loss of autoregulation; however, a minimum of 60 is necessary for adequate cerebral perfusion. Additional goals include minimizing exacerbation of any factors that may contribute to elevated ICP (2).

Hypotension should be avoided as it decreases CPP and CBF (2, 3). In patients who are hypertensive, the elevated blood pressure is generally not treated. Hypertension serves to increase CPP and CBF but may contribute to edema formation and lung injury (2, 3). Hypertension may be the reflexive action of the body to maintain CPP in the setting of elevated ICP. Blood pressure may drop as a result of treatment of ICP with sedatives or other measures (2). Therefore, it is important to put the clinical picture together and exercise caution when managing elevated ICP. Blood pressure and CPP must be a consideration in each treatment decision. To accurately measure CPP, blood pressure transducers should be zeroed at the foramen of Monroe (2).

Initial management measures include head elevation greater than 30 degrees and maintaining head in neutral alignment (2, 3). This promotes jugular venous outflow from the brain. Some studies have suggested that a head-down position is advantageous as it promotes CBF; however, consensus is that there is a benefit to elevating the patient's head. In patients in whom blood pressure is an issue, a minimum elevation of 15 degrees is beneficial (2). The endotracheal tube is carefully secured so as not to compress jugular veins (3). Elevated abdominal pressures from abdominal compartment syndrome can also increase ICP by obstructing cerebral venous outflow. Patients who are at risk should be monitored and promptly treated if abdominal hypertension is present (2).

Patients with elevated ICP generally require rapid sequence endotracheal intubation and mechanical ventilation. Previously, hyperventilation was recommended to induce cerebral vasoconstriction and decrease ICP. While this is effective in decreasing ICP, it causes a decreased CBF, which can lead to ischemia. Its effects are also short lived. This is no longer recommended except in the setting of extreme elevations as a temporizing measure while other interventions are instituted (2). Oxygenation should be maintained in a normal range and positive end-expiratory pressure (PEEP) should be used carefully as it may increase ICP (2, 3).

Fever increases the metabolic rate and induces cerebral vasodilation, which increases CBF and ICP. Fever is associated with poor outcomes in multiple acute neurologic diseases and should be aggressively controlled (2, 3).

Seizures increase ICP and should be avoided in patients with elevated ICP. In the past, many patients with acute neurologic illnesses were placed on seizure prophylaxis. However, studies have emerged showing seizure prophylaxis, particularly with phenytoin, is associated with decreased long-term cognitive function. Further, the actual incidence of seizure in diagnoses other than traumatic brain injury (TBI) is low. Seizure prophylaxis is still considered standard of care in TBI patients but is falling out of favor in other diseases. The risk of seizure should be assessed against the benefit of prophylaxis on a case-by-case basis. At a minimum, seizure activity in a patient with elevated ICP must be promptly recognized and treated emergently (2, 3).

Additional interventions to manage elevated ICP include CSF drainage, sedation, and corticosteroids. CSF drainage through external ventricular drain decreases ICP and also allows for ICP value and waveform monitoring (2, 3). Agitation and pain increase ICP and sedation and pain relief should be provided with care not to drop the blood pressure. Ideally, drugs with short half-life and minimal effect on the blood pressure should be used (2, 3). Corticosteroids should be used only if vasogenic edema is contributing to elevated ICP. Corticosteroids have no benefit in decreasing ICP beyond the setting of vasogenic edema and may contribute to adverse outcomes such as hyperglycemia (2, 3).

If ICP remains elevated despite these interventions, it is considered refractory and several additional interventions may be instituted. Heavy sedation and paralysis may be necessary to control agitation and elevated ICP to decrease metabolic rate (2). Osmotic therapy such as mannitol or hypertonic saline may be used to induce osmotic dieresis, thereby decreasing ICP. Mannitol has a rapid onset and begins to decrease ICP within minutes of administration, with a peak effect at 20 to 60 minutes and duration of 1.5 to 6 hours (2). Mannitol is dosed between 0.25 and 1 mg/kg (2). In critical situations, a dose of 1 mg/kg should be used; smaller doses may be given every 2 to 6 hours if necessary (2). Fluid should be replaced to avoid volume depletion, which may result in hypotension as well as renal failure (2, 3). Side effects of mannitol therapy include hypotension and electrolyte disturbances as well as rebound elevations in ICP if used over longer periods of time (2-4).

Hypertonic saline is another osmotic agent that may be used to decrease elevated ICP (2-4). Hypertonic saline may be given in concentrations between 3% and 23.4% in bolus doses or an infusion. Hypertonic saline works by drawing fluid from the interstitium to the intravascular compartment and is preferred over mannitol in patients who are hypovolemic or hypotensive. Side effects include fluid overload, pulmonary edema, and electrolyte disturbances (2-4).

Barbiturate coma may be induced in patients with elevated ICP refractory to other treatment but is less commonly used as other options have gained favor (2, 3). Pentobarbital is administered in a bolus of 10 mg/kg followed by 5 mg/kg every hour for 3 hours, then maintained at a dosage of 1 to 2 mg/kg/hr, which is titrated to achieve a serum level of 30 to 50 micrograms per milliliter or until electroencephalography (EEG) shows burst suppression (2). Pentobarbital coma is associated with serious complications such as hypotension. Pentobarbital also has a half-life of several days, making neurologic examination and prognostication very difficult.

Induced hypothermia is very effective in decreasing elevated ICP. This therapy is not recommended for routine use to prevent elevated ICP in stroke or trauma patients. However, it is an effective option to control elevated ICP that is refractory to medical therapy. Hypothermia requires cooling blankets or intravascular catheters in order to induce and maintain hypothermia. Patients must be intubated and managed with sedatives and possibly paralytics to minimize shivering and discomfort (2, 3). The rewarming phase in hypothermia is critically important in the injured brain. Rewarming the brain too quickly results in a rebound increase in ICP. Rewarming should be slow and controlled and titrated to the effect on ICP. Side effects of induced hypothermia include increased risk of infection, platelet dysfunction, and electrolyte shifts (2, 3). When done by a practitioner familiar with the effects of induced hypothermia, it is both effective and safe. However, hypothermia affects each body system and should be undertaken with care.

Surgical interventions for elevated ICP include resection of mass lesion (hematoma when appropriate, tumor, abscess, pneumocephalus) and decompressive hemicraniectomy. Decompressive hemicraniectomy involves removing a part of the skull to relieve the pressure on the brain tissue. It is effective in relieving pressure so long as the skull resection is large enough to allow for expansion of the brain tissue. There is debate as to the role of decompressive hemicraniectomy and long-term outcomes. A majority of the data regarding hemicraniectomy originate in the setting of ischemic stroke, showing improved survival as well as improved neurologic outcomes. The timing of hemicraniectomy is important to ensure the damage from edema and elevated ICP has not rendered the tissue unsalvageable. However, when other measures to control ICP have failed, this is an effective means to relieve pressure.

Fever Management

The understanding of the role that temperature has on the brain when injured has evolved through a century of clinical inquiry. Neurons arrive at cell death through multiple pathways depending on the cause of damage in the brain. Many of these pathways are temperature dependent, exacerbated when the body is febrile and minimized when body temperature drops (5). The beneficial role of hypothermia in the damaged brain was validated in two clinical studies on cardiac arrest patients where mild hypothermia was shown to improve mortality and functional recovery in comatose patients following cardiac arrest, and research is ongoing to identify the role of induced hypothermia in other areas of neurologic injury and medicine (5, 6).

Fever is commonly defined as an elevation in body temperature above normal body temperature of 98.6°F. Fever is a common occurrence in patients with neurologic injury, with as many as 70% of patients with brain injury having a fever episode (7, 8). Fever origin may be infectious or drug related but also may be directly related to neurologic injury. The cause of 20% to 35% of fever episodes in the neurologically injured patient remains unclear after extensive diagnostic evaluation (7). This phenomenon has been called "central fever," meaning a fever of unknown origin thought to be directly related to the neurologic injury (7).

Regardless the cause of the fever, there is a large body of research that shows that fever independently increases morbidity and mortality in multiple neurologic diseases and has been shown to increase length of stay and cost associated with caring for these patients (6, 7). In ischemic stroke, normothermia stabilizes the blood-brain barrier and decreases metabolism, ischemic depolarization, and oxidative stress, all processes that result in decreased cell death in the ischemic penumbra. Fever in SAH is related to the size of the bleed and presence of blood in the ventricles and is thought to play a role in the development of vasospasm and secondary injury following hemorrhage (7). There is also some evidence that therapeutic normothermia is associated with improved short-term and long-term functional outcomes (7). In TBI, the presence of fever is associated with increased ICP, neurologic decline, and length of stay (7). Further, fever exacerbates the elevation of ICP in patients with intracranial hypertension from any cause (7). The detrimental effects of fever are evident after an elevation of only 1°C above normal body temperature, thereby challenging the conventional definition of a fever being 101.1°F (6, 7).

There are no randomized controlled trials to date showing that by controlling fever, the poor outcomes and increased length of stay related to the fever are ameliorated. However, the plethora of literature detailing the damage associated with fever in brain injury has led to a general consensus that fever should be aggressively controlled in any patient with acute neurologic damage (5-7). This area of medicine has been termed "therapeutic normothermia" or "controlled normothermia" (6, 7, 9). Further research is needed to guide treatment decisions in the areas of fever prevention and intervention.

Of particular concern has been the lack of translation of the literature on fever management into bedside care. In a study evaluating nursing interventions for fever in patients with TBI, 79% of TBI patients had at least one febrile episode while in the neurologic intensive care unit (ICU). However, only 31% of the fever events had nursing interventions implemented to control for the fever (10). In a national survey of neurocritical care nurses, fewer than 20% of those who responded reported having a fever management protocol in place to help care for their patients (11).

Interventions aimed at decreasing or even preventing fever include pharmacologic interventions, prompt use of cooling blankets and advanced water circulating cooling blankets or intravascular catheters, and the use of newer techniques such as infusion of cold saline (7, 12). In addition to using acetaminophen to treat fever episodes, some centers routinely administer acetaminophen as a scheduled medication to try to lower overall body temperature. With appropriate monitoring of liver enzymes, this practice appears to be safe and mildly effective in decreasing baseline temperature. However, the benefit of routine administration is debated and studies evaluating this intervention are currently under way (6, 9, 10). Cooling blankets should be used to control fevers. There are several models available for use, including those that circulate air or water and adhesive pads with water circulation meant to mimic water immersion (9). Studies have shown the water circulating blankets to be more effective than air blankets (9). Intravascular catheters are also available and may have a role in fever management that is refractory to other interventions (9). In addition, infusing a large volume bolus (30 mL/kg) of cold saline has been shown to be effective in decreasing fever that are refractory to other treatments in one small study (12). Further, the infusion of the cold saline bolus increased the likelihood of the patient remaining afebrile (12). This technique is routinely used in therapeutic hypothermia following cardiac arrest to rapidly decrease body temperature (12).

The major complication associated with induced normothermia is shivering. Shivering is the body's natural defense to increase heat production. Because the body's thermostat is reset to a higher number during fever, efforts to decrease the temperature to normal body temperature may be met with shivering and patient discomfort (5). Fever increases the metabolic rate of the body, theoretically negating the benefits conferred by induced normothermia, and can be a treatment-limiting side effect (5). A bedside shiver assessment scale is available to help the health care team quantify and treat shivering (13). Pharmacologic treatments of shivering include meperidine and buspirone. Surface counterwarming of the face and extremities may also serve some benefit to decrease shivering as most of the cold sensors are located on the extremities (10). Magnesium is also beneficial in controlling against shivering and may be used in bolus doses to maintain normal or slightly elevated levels of serum magnesium (10).

Glucose Control

As the paradigm has shifted in the treatment of hyperglycemia in cardiac surgery patients and general medical-surgical ICU patients over the past decade, the paradigm has also shifted in the management of hyperglycemia for patients with brain injury, stroke, and other neurologic diseases (14). There is an increased understanding of the detrimental role hyperglycemia plays in the ischemic penumbra in stroke and in secondary injury in TBI. Increases in serum glucose greater than 125 mg/dL are associated with increased mortality and larger infarct size in ischemic stroke patients (14). Mild elevations in glucose have also been correlated to worse outcomes in patients with hemorrhagic stroke or TBI. However, few randomized controlled trials have been conducted to identify the ideal glucose range for patients with neurologic injury and ideal treatment modality (14). Retrospective studies have shown improved outcomes in stroke and TBI with control of glucose to normal or near-normal levels (14). Current evidence suggests that aggressive glucose control is reasonable in patients with neurologic disease (14). Brain tissue has a very low tolerance for hypoglycemic episodes. Hypoglycemia is a known complication of aggressive glucose control, particularly with insulin drips (14). Particular attention should be paid to titration of insulin drips and avoidance of hypoglycemic episodes in patients with neurologic illness (14).

Brain Death and Organ Donation

Concept of death has changed as we developed the ability to keep people alive through artificial means such as mechanical ventilation (15). As a result, the basic, vital functions of the body can be artificially maintained even after the brain is no longer functioning (15). The advances in medical care of the critically ill resulted in the need for a new definition of *death* (16, 17). In 1984, the Harvard Ad Hoc Committee on Brain Death released recommendations for the definition of *brain death* (17). Their recommendations were later adapted into the Uniform Determination of Death Act (UDDA) published in 1981 (16, 17). The UDDA and other publications on brain death medical standards have served as the guidelines for states to determine legislation for the declaration of brain death (18). Hospital policy is then determined based on state legislation. Therefore, consult state and institutional guidelines regarding brain death determination as they may vary (18).

The American Academy of Neurology published a summary statement in 1994 to help guide the clinician in determining brain death considering the consensus on brain death determination, with an updated literature review published in 2010 (16, 19). To pursue a diagnosis of brain death, the patient must have no clinical findings of brain activity and a known cause that is thought to be irreversible (16). Neuroimaging should confirm the cause of brain death. In addition, there should be no findings on assessment of any confounding factors such as severe electrolyte imbalance, acid-base imbalance, or endocrine disorders that could interfere with the diagnosis of brain death (16). Finally, the patient should not have any drug intoxication, poisoning, or hypothermia, defined as a core body temperature less than 90°F (16).

The clinician should then perform a clinical exam to determine the appropriateness of further diagnostic testing to determine brain death (16). A clinical exam consistent with brain death would reflect a patient in a coma with the absence of brainstem reflexes (16). Pupils will show no response to bright light and be midposition or dilated (16). There would be no oculocephalic reflex and no response to cold caloric testing (16). Facial sensation and motor response will be absence in brain death as evidenced by an absent corneal reflex, absent jaw reflex, and no motor movement of the face to deep pain (16). Pharyngeal and tracheal reflexes will also be absent. If the clinical exam is consistent with brain death, further diagnostic testing is then ordered to confirm the clinical assessment (16). The cornerstone diagnostic exam for brain death is the apnea test (16). During the apnea test, the patient is removed from the ventilator for 8 to 10 minutes and the $PaCO_2$ is measured before and after the period of apnea (16). The patient is placed back on the ventilator after apnea testing while the clinician waits for the blood gas results (16). Prior to the apnea test, the health care team ensures the patient is not hypothermic (core body temperature greater than 97°F) and the patient has normal $PaCO_2$ and PaO_2 values (16). The patient may be preoxygenated prior to the test with 100% oxygen (16). A $PaCO_2$ greater than 60 mm Hg or an increase in $PaCO_2$ greater than 20 mm Hg is indicative of brain death (16).

In the event the patient is unable to tolerate an apnea test due to hypotension, hypoxia, or any other confounding variable or in the event the apnea test is indeterminant, confirmatory testing may be obtained to diagnose brain death (16). Confirmatory testing includes cerebral angiography, EEG, transcranial Doppler (TCD), somatosensory evoked potentials (SSEP), and cerebral perfusion exam (16). Findings on angiography that are consistent with brain death include lack of cerebral arterial blood flow at the level of the circle of Willis or above (16). Specific guidelines have been published for EEG, SSEP, and TCD interpretation related to brain death (16). A cerebral perfusion exam in a patient with brain death will show no uptake of the isotope into the cerebral tissue—also called the "hollow skull phenomenon" (16).

Organ donation should be considered as an option in all patients who progress to brain death or who undergo withdrawal of care because of a devastating neurologic illness (20). As the current need for organs largely outweighs the supply, there has been a national initiative to improve organ donation awareness and options available to patients and families of those who suffer devastating neurologic illness. In 2003, the national Organ Procurement Breakthrough Collaborative was launched with a goal of achieving organ donation rates of 75% or higher at all hospitals throughout the nation (20). The collaborative encouraged partnership between hospitals and organ procurement organizations (OPOs) to develop policies, procedures, and education for health care personnel to improve organ donation rates. It is often the responsibility of the bedside nurse and advanced practice nurse to work with the OPO to determine patients who could be donors (20). While determining brain death status, failing organ function should be optimized while the family contemplates organ donation decisions (21).

NEUROLOGIC DISEASE PROCESSES

Stroke
Etiology
Nearly 800,000 ischemic and hemorrhagic strokes occur annually in the United States, (22). It is estimated that 600,000 of these strokes are new strokes, whereas 180,000 are recurrent strokes, and more than 150,000 people die from stroke-related causes (23, 24, 25). In the United States, a stroke occurs every 40 seconds and nearly 1 of every 16 Americans will die from a stroke (22). Approximately 80% to 87% of all strokes that occur in the United States are ischemic in nature. The remaining 13% to 20% of strokes in the United States are hemorrhagic strokes, with 10% being ICH and the rest being SAH. Stroke is the third leading cause of death in the nation but the leading cause of illness-related disability. Twenty percent of ischemic stroke survivors require institutional care 3 months after their stroke, and a third of stroke survivors are permanently

disabled (22). Although stroke is the third leading cause of death, the general public reports great fears of having a stroke. More than half those at risk for ischemic stroke report stroke being viewed as worse than death (22). Stroke is associated with a large economic burden with an estimated $65.5 billion directed to the direct and indirect cost of stroke between 1979 and 2005. Overall, stroke is a disease that disproportionally affects women and minority races. Annually, women experience more strokes than men, and American Indian, Alaskan Native, African American, and Hispanic or Latino populations have higher prevalence of stroke than do Caucasians (24).

The meaning of the term "stroke" is often misunderstood by the public. Stroke results in the lack of oxygenated blood being delivered to brain tissue. However, there are multiple mechanisms by which a person can have a stroke. This chapter will provide an overview of the diagnosis and management of ischemic stroke, SAH, and ICH, respectively. While ischemic stroke, ICH, and SAH are all strokes, they are separate but related disease entities with differing pathophysiolgy, diagnosis, and management strategies.

Advancements in the care of stroke patients brought a 60% decline in ischemic stroke–related mortality between 1970 and 2000 (22). However, in the past decade, there has been a plateau in mortality. Further, stroke incidence is on the rise and stroke-related hospitalizations have increased by 40% in recent years (22). Recent advancements and an explosion of research in the area of neurovascular care have led to major developments in the development of neurology and neurosurgery programs. Increasing recognition of the importance of stroke treatment within the minutes to hours after the stroke event has led to the development of regional stroke networks using new technology such as telemedicine to provide much needed care.

Phases of Stroke Care

Regardless of whether a stroke is ischemic or hemorrhagic, stroke is a medical emergency. A two-phase continuum of care has been proposed in the acute management of the patient who has had a stroke patient (24). Phase 1 consists of the hyperacute phase of stroke management including the prehospital (emergency medical services [EMS]) activation and care, the emergency department care of the stroke patient, as well as any acute intervention provided. Phase 2 is defined as stroke acute care and includes the care the patient receives between 24 and 72 hours. During this phase, management is focused on identifying the etiology of the ischemic or hemorrhagic stroke, preventing complications, coordinating hospital discharge, and instituting secondary prevention measures to prevent another stroke event (24).

Stroke Assessment Scales

Several scales have been developed to aid emergency response and emergency department personnel in the identification and triage of stroke patients. The National Institutes of Health Stroke Scale (NIHSS) is a scale that is used widely in stroke trials and particularly useful in the assessment of ischemic stroke. No single scale or score is recommended over another, and they all may be useful in the initial recognition of stroke. Scales include the Cincinnati Pre-hospital Stroke Scale, the Los Angeles Pre-hospital Stroke Screen, the Los Angeles Motor Scale, and the Face Arm Speech Test. A shortened version of the NIHSS is also available for the initial screening of the stroke patient. Each institution should assess each scale for usefulness within the organization in the assessment of stroke patients (23). The NIHSS or the abbreviated version is recommended as useful in stroke prognosis and discharge planning. Patients with an NIHSS score of less than 10 had more favorable outcome 1 year after stroke than did those with an NIHSS score of greater than 20. Patients with an NIHSS score greater than 22 have a higher rate of hemorrhagic conversion, and patients who had an NIHSS of less than 5 at 24 hours of hospital admission were far more likely to be discharged home than were those with an NIHSS greater than 5 (24).

Ischemic Stroke

The incidence of ischemic stroke is estimated to be 5.2 per 1,000 person-years (25). Prevalence of stroke varies according to race and ethnicity in the United States, with a prevalence of 6% among American Indian/Native Americans, 4% among blacks, 2.6% among Hispanics, 2.3% among Caucasians, and 2.6% among Asians (25). The largest risk for having a stroke is having had a previous stroke. Recurrent stroke risk is 2% after 7 days and 4% at 30 days. One year risk of recurrent ischemic stroke is 12%, and 5-year risk is 29%, with the highest risk related to large artery extracranial or intracranial disease (25). Ischemic stroke is the cause of 80% to 90% of strokes nationwide (24).

At its most basic level, ischemic stroke can be divided into thrombotic or embolic sources (26, 27). Ischemic stroke is most commonly caused by atherosclerosis resulting in thrombosis in the large or small vessels of the brain (25). Twenty percent of ischemic strokes are caused by atherosclerosis of the large cerebral vessels while 25% of ischemic strokes are caused by atherosclerosis of small vessels (also called lacunar or subcortical stroke). Thirty percent of strokes are embolic in nature (25). The most common source of embolic stroke is the heart. Of clots that form in the heart, they are most often from the turbulent atrial flow when the heart is in atrial flutter or fibrillation. However, clots may form in the heart from other causes such as valvular disease (endocarditis, mitral valve stenosis or prolapse), heart failure, dilated cardiomyopathy, and recent myocardial infarction (25, 26). In addition, extracranial atherosclerosis arising from the aorta, carotid arteries, or vertebral arteries may rupture and embolize to the cerebral vasculature.

There are many less common causes of ischemic stroke. In patients who do not exhibit typical risk factors of cardioembolic or atherosclerosis, the presence of a hypercoaguable state should be investigated (26, 27). Polycythemia vera, lupus erythematosus, disseminated intravascular coagulation, and antiphospholipid syndrome can all contribute to ischemic stroke. In cases where rapid head or neck motion with severe headache accompanying stroke, symptoms should causes suspicion of arterial dissection. Sickle cell disease can cause both overt and silent ischemic stroke and is often a cause of stroke in younger patients (28). Despite the current knowledge and advanced diagnostics available to determine the cause of stroke, no cause is evident in a third of stroke patients. Strokes with no attributable cause are conventionally termed "cryptogenic" (25).

Several stroke classification scales have been proposed to help classify ischemic stroke subtypes. These include the Stroke Data Bank Subtype Classification, Oxfordshire Community Stroke Project Subtype Classification, Trial of ORG 10172 in Acute Stroke Treatment (TOAST) Classification, and, most recently, the ASCO Phenotypic Stroke Classification system. Of the classification scales, the ASCO system is usable at the bedside and incorporates degree of uncertainty and diagnostic instrument used in stroke diagnosis (26, 27).

Risk factors for the development of ischemic stroke can be divided into modifiable and nonmodifiable causes. Nonmodifiable causes of stroke include age, sex, race, and a family history of stroke (25). The risk of stroke increases with each decade of life, and a majority of strokes occur in patients over the age of 65. Ischemic stroke is more prevalent in men than in women (25). However, women are more likely to have ischemic stroke at a younger age and are more likely to die as a result of their stroke (25). A parental history of ischemic stroke, transient ischemic attack (TIA), or myocardial infarction is associated with an increased risk of stroke (25).

Many modifiable risk factors are attributed to the formation of ischemic stroke. Hypertension is the most significant modifiable risk factor and is considered an independent cause of ischemic stroke. Hypertension contributes to the atherosclerotic process, and there is evidence that modest elevations in blood pressure (high normal blood pressure of 130 to 139/85 to 89 mm Hg) is associated with an increased risk of heart disease and stroke compared to those with a blood pressure less than 120/80 mm Hg (25).

Diabetes and hyperglycemia are considered an independent risk factor in the development of ischemic stroke (25). Hyperglycemia impact on stroke is two-fold. Hyperglycemia accelerates the atherosclerosis process and also increases the probability of other risk factors such as obesity and hyperlipidemia (25). However, the presence of elevated glucose at the time of the stroke event also exacerbates neurologic illness regardless of diabetes history (25). There appears to be a synergistic risk when diabetes and hypertension are present together, and it is estimated that 40% of strokes can be attributed to diabetes or diabetes and hypertension together (25).

Smoking has long been linked to the development of atherosclerosis (29). Smoking is an independent risk factor for the development of ischemic stroke. Smoking accelerates atherosclerosis formation as well as increases vasoconstriction, platelet dysfunction, and clot formation (29). Smoking is associated with a 2- to 4-fold increased risk of stroke. Environmental exposure to smoke (second-hand smoke or passive smoking) is also a risk factor in the development of ischemic stroke. Risk of stroke decreases significantly within 2 years of tobacco cessation (29).

Atrial fibrillation is an independent risk factor for the development of ischemic stroke and is the most common cause of cardioembolic stroke (25). Atrial fibrillation results in the left atrium pumping inefficiently, which causes turbulent blood flow. This flow can lead to clot formation and embolism. Stroke as a result of atrial fibrillation is more common in the elderly and is associated with higher mortality and functional deficits compared to other causes of stroke (29). Those who sustain a cardioembolic stroke as a result of atrial fibrillation are also at higher risk of stroke recurrence (29).

Multiple cardiac conditions and carotid artery disease are associated with the development of ischemic stroke. Carotid stenosis greater than 80% is associated with an increased risk of stroke. There is an increased risk of stroke following myocardial infarction as well as in the setting of ventricular dysfunction such as heart failure, cardiomyopathy, and any other disease process that results in a decreased ejection fraction (29). The presence of a patent foramen ovale (PFO) or an atrial septal aneurysm is associated with shunted blood flow that can lead to clot formation and embolic stroke (29).

Elevated total cholesterol is a risk factor in the development of ischemic stroke (29). Elevated high-density lipoprotein (LDL) cholesterol appears to confer a protective benefit against stroke (29).

Several disease states place patients at increased risk for ischemic stroke. Sickle cell disease results in a decreased oxygen carrying capability and a prothrombotic state that results in ischemic stroke, particularly in younger patients. Hypercoaguability associated with factor V Leiden mutation, thrombophilias, lupus, and antiphospholipid syndrome all increase the risk of stroke. Both viral and bacterial infections are suspected to play a role in inflammation and are casually associated with the development of ischemic stroke (29). Hyperhomocysteinemia and elevated C-reactive protein

(CRP) both appear to be markers of inflammation and elevated levels are associated with ischemic stroke (29).

Several lifestyle factors are associated with the development of stroke. Obesity is a risk factor for ischemic stroke (29). Both elevated body mass index (BMI) and abdominal adiposity appear to play a role in the development of atherosclerosis and stroke. Increased physical activity is linked to a decreased risk of stroke, and physical inactivity leads to obesity. A diet high in sodium and saturated fat is associated with stroke, whereas a diet high in fruit and vegetable consumption decreases the risk of stroke (29). Moderate alcohol intake may be protective against ischemic stroke, whereas high alcohol consumption is a risk factor for ischemic stroke.

The role of hormone replacement therapy (HRT) in the development of ischemic stroke has been debated in the literature. Studies have been mixed, with several studies indicating an increased risk with HRT while others are unable to replicate the association.

There are geographic and socioeconomic variations in the prevalence of ischemic stroke. The southeastern United States with increased stroke prevalence and mortality was conventionally termed the "stroke belt." The exact reason for the geographical variation is unknown. However, modifiable risk factors such as hypertension, obesity, smoking, and diet likely play a large role in the variation (29). Lower educational levels and socioeconomic status are associated with the development of ischemic stroke and are thought to reflect poor access to health care and modifiable risk reduction (29).

Mortality at 30 days after a stroke averages 26% worldwide, with estimates in the United States between 12% and 16% (25). The most common causes of death after an ischemic stroke are death from cardiovascular event, respiratory infection, and immediate stroke-related complications (25). Of those who survive their stroke, 40% will require subacute care and 10% will require care in a nursing home (25). From 68% to 74% of ischemic stroke survivors will eventually require at a minimum the care of a family member (25).

Stroke is associated with a considerable economic burden. While it is the third leading cause of death, stroke is the leading cause of disability in the United States. When measured in 1991, the lifetime cost of ischemic stroke was greater than $90,000 per individual (30). The direct and indirect costs associated with stroke are estimated to be $65 billion, and cost is expected to continue to rise (25). When estimating the cost of stroke in the next 50 years, stroke costs are expected to exceed $1.5 trillion (30). The staggering cost of stroke is in part exacerbated by the fact that stroke is the leading cause of disability compared to any other disease (25). Stroke cost must consider the economic burden of long-term disability, the cost of caregiving, lost wages, drugs, and rehospitalization (30).

Pathophysiology

An ischemic stroke results in the loss of oxygenated blood flowing to brain tissue (31, 32). It is essential to understand that ischemia exists on a continuum ranging from mild ischemia that is reversible to severe ischemia that leads to infarction. Ischemic stroke will generally result in some cells experiencing severe ischemia and infarct and other cells experiencing a degree of ischemia and suffering a degree of injury. Within moments of brain tissue ischemia, a series of processes develop that ultimately lead to cell death. They include neurotransmitter excitotoxicity, acidotoxicity, ionic imbalance, and peri-infarct depolarizations. Cell death results as a result of oxidative and nitrative stress, inflammation, and apoptosis. In the direct territory of ischemia, cell death occurs rapidly, primarily as a result of excitotoxic and necrotic cell death. However, areas of the infarct that are supplied by collateral circulation or partially compromised blood flow (ischemic but not yet infarcted) are commonly referred to as the ischemic penumbra. The penumbral tissue is at risk for cell death, but the degree and timing of actual cell failure are widely variable and depend on the degree of revascularization and ischemia as well as other factors such as hyperglycemia and fever. If the cells in the penumbral area die, they generally do so through a process of inflammation and apoptosis (31, 32).

Within moments of loss of oxygenated blood flow, neurons begin to experience energy failure that leads to depletion of ATP stores. This depletion leads to membrane depolarization and ion shifts that result in either direct necrosis of the cell due in part to intracellular calcium overload or severe damage and excitatory neurotransmitter release. Of the excitatory neurotransmitters, glutamine appears to play a central role in the ischemic pathway. Concurrently, a process of acidosis develops that further threatens cell stability. This acidosis is exacerbated by the presence of hyperglycemia and other correctable metabolic states (31, 32).

Cortical spreading depression is a process of cellular depolarization, neuroelectrical depression, glutamine release, and loss of membrane gradients (31, 32). This process occurs and is tolerated in healthy brains but occurs at an increased frequency and magnitude in the injured brain and contributes to neuronal ischemia. As cells are damaged, they release reactive oxygen species that can contribute to cellular apoptosis. The brain is more sensitive to oxidative stress than other organs as it does not have nearly the degree of protective endogenous antioxidant activity that is present in other areas of the body. The process of oxidative and nitrative stress continues even once the brain is reperfused (31, 32). The oxidative and nitrite stress, along with cell damage already detailed, mobilizes an inflammatory response to the damaged area of the brain. While some aspects of the inflammatory process certainly play a beneficial role, the inflammatory response also plays a role in the continued stroke-related brain injury. The activation of cytokines and Toll-like receptors contributes to cellular apoptosis.

Clinical Presentation

Clinical presentation of ischemic stroke includes the sudden onset of neurologic deficit that correlates to the area of ischemia in the brain (24). A hallmark of stroke is the sudden onset of symptoms. This is not a disease where symptoms develop gradually over time. There are several classic stroke syndromes; however, it must be noted that the neurologic deficit seen correlates to the amount of brain tissue with ischemia (24). Patients with ischemia on the left side of the brain generally will have some degree of left gaze preference, right visual field deficit, right hemiparesis, and right hemisensory loss (24). They also may have some degree of aphasia if the language centers of the brain are involved in the area of ischemia. Conversely, those with right-sided ischemia will have a right visual gaze preference, left visual field deficit, left hemiparesis, and left hemisensory loss with or without neglect or inattention (24). Brainstem stroke may present with nausea or vomiting, diplopia, disconjugate gaze or gaze palsy, dysarthria, dysphagia, vertigo, hemiparesis, hemisensory loss, and decreased level of consciousness. Infarcts in the cerebellum are associated with a truncal or gait ataxia or limb ataxia (24).

Diagnosis

Several common "stroke mimickers" must be considered when making the diagnosis of stroke—specifically, ischemic stroke (23). Hypertensive encephalopathy can mimic a stroke as cerebral edema develops with the significant hypertension. Hypoglycemia must be ruled out as it can also mimic the symptoms of an acute stroke. Hypoglycemia can cause decreased level of consciousness and unilateral weakness or other neurologic findings that resolve once hypoglycemia is treated. A complicated migraine can cause unilateral findings similar to a stroke and should be ruled out as a differential. A seizure, or a patient in a postictal state, can be mistaken for an ischemic stroke. However, some strokes may present with seizure activity. Therefore, seizure should be carefully ruled out in a patient with expected ischemic stroke. Finally, conversion disorder should be considered in any patient with an examination inconsistent with onset story or vascular distribution or with a lack of cranial nerve involvement on physical exam (23).

Neuroimaging is paramount in the patient with stroke symptoms to differentiate between ischemic and hemorrhagic stroke and to guide treatment decisions. Noncontrast CT imaging of the brain is the most commonly used neuroimaging technique because of the ease and speed of obtaining the images as well as the accuracy of identifying ICH (23). CT imaging also may be helpful in ruling out other nonvascular causes of neurologic symptoms. Acute ischemia is often not visible on CT imaging unless a large territory is involved in the stroke. In some cases, large arterial occlusion will be visible and is called the "hyperdense vessel sign." In cases of large vessel stroke, loss of the gray-white differentiation in the cortical ribbon or lentiform nucleus or sulcal effacement is visible within the first several hours of ischemia. Presence of these signs is associated with increased risk of hemorrhagic transformation of the stroke, particularly after treatment with thrombolytic therapy. However, presence of these findings does not preclude thrombolytic treatment (23). Some centers are now able to perform CT angiography (CTA) and CT perfusion imaging. These tests require contrast administration as well as additional radiation exposure. Research is currently under way as to the role of these imaging modalities in acute ischemic stroke. They may be used on a case-by-case basis according to the needs of the patient.

Magnetic resonance imaging (MRI) that includes diffusion-weighted and perfusion-weighted imaging is useful in the diagnosis of ischemia (23). Diffusion-weighted imaging is able to detect ischemic changes within minutes of ischemia occurring. In a few select centers, MRI can be rapidly obtained and is used instead of CT for initial diagnostic imaging. However, most centers are unable to conduct MRI quickly to keep from delaying thrombolytic therapy. Therefore, MRI is more commonly used after the hyperacute diagnostic period as a means to better identify the stroke region (23). Research is currently under way to identify MRI signs that may aid in thrombolytic decision making. MR angiography (MRA) is a noninvasive test often used to image large intracranial and extracranial vessels to identify narrowing or occlusion as well.

Additional diagnostic workup in addition to neuroimaging includes several serum tests and additional testing to aid in the diagnosis of acute stroke and elimination of stroke mimickers from the differential (23). All patients should undergo blood glucose testing. Low glucose can mimic a stroke and elevated glucose levels should be addressed with some urgency as hyperglycemia is associated with worse outcomes in patients treated with thrombolytics (23). All patients should have electrolyte and renal function testing to identify any electrolyte disturbances that may be contributing to the patient's neurologic deficit (23). ECG and cardiac enzyme testing should be completed as a myocardial infarction may precipitate a stroke and a stroke may precipitate a myocardial infarction (23). All patients should have a complete blood cell count evaluation with platelet count as well as coagulation studies. These tests are necessary as the results may influence thrombolytic treatment decisions. In certain patient situations, hepatic function tests, toxicology screening, blood alcohol level, and pregnancy testing may be helpful in arriving at a diagnosis or treatment decision (23). Arterial blood gas testing may be helpful if hypoxia is present, and a chest radiograph may be necessary in patients with a history of lung disease. Chest radiography is no longer considered necessary for all acute stroke patients. Finally, a lumbar puncture (LP) or EEG may be useful in certain patients (23).

After the initial diagnosis of acute ischemic stroke is made, several additional diagnostic tests are useful in determining the etiology of the ischemic event (24). Carotid duplex ultrasonography is used to screen patients for the presence of carotid stenosis. (24) The test is accurate in diagnosing stenosis greater than 60% but it is not completely reliable in differentiating between severe and complete occlusion. Angiography is the 'gold standard' test to diagnose carotid stenosis and may be used if ultrasound or MRA is inconclusive (24). Ischemic stroke patients may undergo transeophageal or transthoracic echocardiography (TEE or TTE) to identify cardiac sources of embolic ischemic events. TEE or TTE may detect ventricular thrombus, motion abnormalities leading to clot formation, aortic atherosclerosis, or PFO, which all are potential sources of emboli (24). TTE is less invasive than a TEE and may be ordered first with TEE as a secondary test if necessary (24).

Management

The management of acute ischemic stroke is best described in three phases: hyperacute management constituting interventions within the first 6 hours of stroke, acute management that includes interventions within the first 24 hours of the stroke, and subacute management that constitutes secondary prevention measures undertaken after the first 24 hours through hospital discharge.

Hyperacute Management

In the hyperacute treatment window, the goal is reperfusion of the ischemic brain tissue through either intravenous thrombolytic agents or intra-arterial intervention (24). Obviously, this must be done concurrently with any acute stabilization of the patient. Any interventions aimed to stabilize airway, breathing, or circulation, particularly in larger strokes, should be followed immediately by a neurologic assessment and consideration for reperfusion (23). Recombinant tissue plasminogen activator (tPA) is a thrombolytic that was approved for treatment of acute ischemic stroke in 1996. Studies showed a statistically significant improved outcome at 3 months after stroke for those treated with the thrombolytic within 3 hours of the onset of the stroke (24). Benefits were sustained at 1 year after the stroke event. Intravenous tPA is the standard of care for patients with ischemic stroke who are eligible to receive the medication. The greatest

risk of tPA administration is symptomatic ICH (defined as a decline in NIHSS score by more than 4 points), which occurred in approximately 6% of patients treated with thrombolytics compared to less than 1% of patients who received placebo (24). Other risks associated with tPA administration include systemic hemorrhage, myocardial rupture if the thrombolytic is administered within several days of an acute myocardial infarction, and anaphylaxis or angioedema reaction to the drug (23). Angioedema occurs in 1% to 2% of patients treated with tPA and is more common in patients with infarcts involving the frontal lobe cortex or the insula (24). Angioedema is also more common in patients who are also taking angiotensin-converting enzyme (ACE) inhibitors (24). If angioedema occurs, the infusion should be immediately stopped and angioedema treated with antihistamines, corticosteroids, or epinephrine (24). While tPA is beneficial in patients when administered within 3 hours of symptom onset, multiple studies show that the sooner the patient receives the medication after the stroke event, the better is the patient outcome.

Between 1996 and 2009, several studies were performed to evaluate the safe upper time limit for the administration of tPA. Most studies showed that outside of 3 hours, the risk of tPA administration outweighed the benefit of recovery. However, in 2008 a large trial showed that tPA could safely be administered up to 4.5 hours after the acute ischemic stroke (23). Based on this trial, both the European Stroke Association and the American Stroke Association have endorsed extending the treatment window for intravenous tPA to 4.5 hours after the onset of the ischemic stroke. The only other thrombolytic to be studied in a rigorous manner for the treatment of acute stroke is streptokinase. Trials were stopped early because streptokinase was associated with a high rate of ICH and is not recommended for the treatment of acute ischemic stroke. Trials are currently under way to evaluate other thrombolytics in the treatment of ischemic stroke. To date, the only medication with approval for ischemic stroke is tPA (23).

Central to the decision to treat with thrombolytic therapy is establishing the stroke onset time. In order to distinguish the amount of time that has lapsed and eligibility for tPA, the patient, family, and any witnesses must be questioned as to when the patient was last seen with normal neurologic function (24). The last time the patient is verified as at his or her neurologic baseline is the beginning of the clock for the thrombolytic window. For patients who awoke with stroke symptoms, the time they went to bed is generally accepted as the time they were last at their neurologic baseline (24).

tPA dosing is weight based at 0.9 mg/kg up to a maximum dose of 90 mg. Ten percent of the total dosage is administered in a bolus dose over 2 minutes and the remaining amount is administered over 60 minutes

(23). Blood pressure should be closely monitored (every 15 minutes for 2 hours, every 30 minutes for 6 hours, and then hourly until 24 hours after treatment) to monitor for acute hypertension (23). Blood pressure greater than 180/105 mm Hg should be treated aggressively as a blood pressure above this threshold within the first 24 hours after thrombolytic administration is associated with an increased risk of intracranial hemorrhage (23). Patients should be monitored in either an ICU or a stroke unit. Because of the risk of hemorrhage with thrombolytic administration, unnecessary procedures should be delayed. Current guidelines suggest CT imaging of the brain 24 hours after thrombolytic administration prior to the administration of antiplatelet or anticoagulants to evaluate for hemorrhage (23).

Current guidelines for the treatment of ischemic stroke list the original inclusion/exclusion criteria used in the initial tPA trial to guide the decision on thrombolytic therapy (23). Those criteria specifically stated that to be eligible for tPA treatment:

- There had to be a diagnosis of acute ischemic stroke with a measurable neurologic deficit, and the deficit should not be minor or clearing spontaneously.
- ICH and SAH are ruled out on neuroimaging.
- Symptoms must have started within 3 hours of treatment (now extended to 4.5 hours based on more recent data).
- There was no head trauma or prior stroke, myocardial infarction, or gastrointestinal or urinary tract infection in the past 3 months.
- There was no major surgery in the past 14 days.
- There was no arterial puncture at a noncompressible site in the past 7 days.
- There was no history of ICH.
- Blood pressure is less than 185/110 mm Hg.
- There is no evidence of active bleeding or trauma on exam.
- The INR is less than 1.5 if on anticoagulation or the aPTT in a normal range if the patient recently received heparin.
- The platelet count is greater than 100,000 mm^3.
- Blood glucose is above 50 mg/dL.
- There is no seizure with residual postictal neurologic impairment.
- CT does not show multilobar infarction (as evidenced by a hypodensity greater than one-third the cerebral hemisphere).
- And the patient and/or family understand the risks and benefits of treatment (23).

Over the last decade of thrombolytic treatment, several of the above criteria have developed into more relative contraindications that are taken into consideration with the clinical picture of the patient (23). It is no longer

considered necessary to require written consent for treatment with tPA. But family should be counseled regarding the risks and benefits as stated, and the conversation should be noted in the practitioner's documentation. Patients treated with thrombolytic agents should have access to neurologic expertise 24 hours a day. A great deal of fear has been associated with thrombolytic treatment in past years, and it has been the topic of many formal and informal publications. Subsequent tPA studies have supported the treatment of ischemic stroke with thrombolytic agents and it is considered the standard of care according to stroke guidelines worldwide. Litigation surrounding thrombolytic treatment in the past decade has been far more focused on patients who did not receive thrombolytic therapy when it was appropriate rather than patients experiencing complications associated with thrombolytic treatment (33). In a majority of litigation cases involving thrombolytic agents in ischemic stroke, injury was claimed to have resulted from failure to provide thrombolytic treatment when necessary (33). Despite tPA being the standard treatment for acute ischemic stroke, less than 5% of patients nationwide receive this standard treatment. Many patients do not mobilize to the hospital immediately and therefore are ineligible for thrombolytic therapy. However, when patients do arrive at the hospital within time to receive tPA, many still do not receive treatment. The gap in treatment has been a major impetus for the development of stroke centers and certification as well as the use of telemedicine to aid in treatment of stroke patients (23). These concepts are discussed elsewhere in the chapter.

There are several neurointerventional radiology procedures that may be considered in the setting of acute ischemic stroke (34). Thrombolytic agents such as tPA can be administered intra-arterially in a highly concentrated manner directly into the clot in large vessel occlusions (34). Several mechanical clot removal devices are currently being tested to remove clots or break up clots in large vessels in conjunction with thrombolytic agents or alone (34). Stenting and/or angioplasty may also be used in select cases of acute ischemic stroke, again in conjunction with thrombolytic agents or alone. Intra-arterial therapies should not be substituted for intravenous tPA in patients who arrive within the treatment window and are eligible for thrombolytic therapy. However, these measures may be used in patients who arrive to the hospital between the 4.5- and 6-hour time-frame or for patients who are ineligible to receive thrombolytic agents at any time in the 6-hour time window (34). There is some evidence that patients who are ineligible for thrombolytic therapy because of recent minor surgery may benefit from intra-arterial thrombolytic agents. Some centers use intra-arterial measures as an adjunct to intravenous tPA, particularly in patients who have a large vessel occlusion and who show no improvement following intravenous thrombolytic agents. This is a rapidly expanding field of acute stroke care that requires treatment at a specialty stroke center with neurointerventional radiology capabilities. An area of continued debate regarding endovascular therapies is the appropriate time window for therapy (34). Studies in this field must be critically evaluated as repeat cannulization rates do not always correspond with neurologic improvement. Therefore, the time the brain has been hypoxic must be considered when pursuing endovascular therapies. Further, success in opening the occluded vessel through endovascular intervention may not improve the patient's clinical exam or functional outcome if the cells are no longer viable (34). Further research is necessary to better guide the use of these interventions in the acute ischemic stroke setting.

Subacute Management

In addition to the efforts to reperfuse the brain in the hyperacute phase of stroke care, several additional interventions should be a priority in the first 24 hours of stroke care to aggressively support the ischemic stroke patient (24). Hypoxia should be avoided as it may worsen cerebral ischemia. Interventions to avoid hypoxia include noninvasive supplemental oxygen and, if necessary, artificial airway with mechanical ventilation(23). Oxygen saturation should be maintained at greater than 92% (23). Aspiration pneumonia is a common complication of stroke and contributes to hypoxia. Therefore, strict aspiration precautions are necessary for stroke patients. As already mentioned, fever in the setting of ischemic stroke worsens outcomes and should be avoided. Temperature should be monitored often and managed aggressively in patients with ischemic stroke. In addition, hyperglycemia is associated with worse outcomes after ischemic stroke and should be managed aggressively regardless of prestroke diabetes status. Stress hyperglycemia is present in as many as 50% of stroke patients and the excess extracellular glucose, regardless of cause, contributes to cell death in the ischemic penumbra. Trials are underway to establish ideal glucose ranges for those with cerebral injury (23). Current standard of care is to use rapid-acting insulin to decrease glucose if blood glucose levels exceed 140 mg/dL (24).

Hypertension (systolic blood pressure greater than 160 mm Hg) is present in more than 60% of patients with acute ischemic stroke (23). There are theoretical reasons to allow blood pressure to remain high in ischemic stroke as well as concerns regarding hypertension in the injured brain. In ischemic stroke, an elevated blood pressure may support collateral circulation to the damaged areas as well as support vessels in the ischemic penumbra that have impaired autoregulation (23). Further, many patients are hypertensive prior to their stroke and there is some concern that by dropping the blood pressure in the setting of ischemic stroke, ischemic injury may worsen. However, elevated blood pressure

may contribute to the formation of cerebral edema in the injured brain and several studies have correlated elevated blood pressure in the initial hours after stroke to poor patient outcomes. Conversely, low blood pressure following an ischemic stroke is also associated with poor patient outcomes. Unfortunately, there is a lack of quality data to drive the decision of how to manage hypertension in acute ischemic stroke. Current guidelines suggest that if the patient is a candidate for thrombolytic therapy, blood pressure should be treated if it exceeds 180/110 mm Hg. If the patient is not a candidate for thrombolytic therapy, blood pressure should be treated if it exceeds 220/120 mm Hg only. Preferred agents for the treatment of hypertension include labetalol and nicardipine. As with any other recommendation, this must be tailored to the needs of the patient, particularly if there are cardiac comorbidities. However, current consensus is to allow the blood pressure to remain elevated according to these parameters (23).

There is a lack of data to guide the duration of permissive hypertension (23). However, once medication is instituted to begin lowering blood pressure, it should be done gradually over several days. In the days to weeks following a stroke, the goal should be to obtain a normotensive blood pressure as hypertension is a major risk factor for ischemic stroke and recurrent stroke (23).

Because of the need to monitor for hypertension as well as the risk for developing cardiac dysrythmia following ischemic stroke, current recommendations are that all ischemic stroke patients are monitored on telemetry for the first 24 hours after the ischemic event (23).

Hypotension (systolic blood pressure less than 100 mm Hg) is associated with poor outcomes after ischemic stroke and should be identified and investigated promptly (23). The source of hypotension should be addressed and corrected through either fluid administration or adjunctive vasopressors. The question remains regarding the role of inducing hemodilution or the use of vasopressors to induce hypertension following ischemic stroke. Studies of excess fluid administration to induce hemodilution were associated with lower overall oxygen delivery. Hemodilution should be avoided in ischemic stroke; fluid resuscitation should be undertaken with a goal of euvolemia, not hypervolemia. Small studies have supported the use of vasopressors to induce hypertension and support cerebral blood flow in ischemic stroke patients. However, inducing hypertension after a stroke is also associated with risk of myocardial ischemia and cerebral edema formation. Studies evaluating the benefit of induced hypertension titrated the therapy to either clinical improvement at higher pressures, perfusion MRI, or both. Because limited data exist to support its use, induced hypertension is not standard for stroke patients. If it is used, it must be on a case-by-case basis with close neurologic and cardiac monitoring (23).

Acute anticoagulation in ischemic stroke has been a subject of controversy over the past 50 years (23). Acute anticoagulation as a necessary treatment was initially based on data that suggested that patients with ischemic stroke, particularly embolic ischemic stroke, were at risk for recurrent stroke in the immediate hours and days following the initial stroke. Some studies suggested as many as 12% of patients were at risk for a subsequent stroke within the first week after the event. However, subsequent studies have shown the rate of recurrence is likely much lower than was initially suspected (less than 0.5%). Early treatment with both low-molecular-weight heparin and heparin infusion has been studied in ischemic stroke (23). Both are associated with higher rates of ICH and do not appear to significantly decrease the risk of recurrent stroke. Based on these data, the current recommendation is not to use heparin or heparinoids in acute ischemic stroke patients. No anticoagulation should be administered within 24 hours of thrombolytic therapy and anticoagulation should not be substituted for thrombolytic therapy (23).

Antiplatelet medication, specifically aspirin, has been studied in ischemic stroke and is proved to decrease the risk of initial stroke as well as recurrent stroke (23). Following an ischemic stroke, all patients who do not have hemorrhagic conversion should have an antiplatelet regimen started within 48 hours of hospital admission. The preferred starting dose is 325 mg in the setting of acute ischemic stroke (23).

Subacute Hospital Management and Secondary Prevention

Telemetry monitoring and frequent vital signs and neurologic assessment should be performed during the first 24 hours and then tapered as the patient progresses (23). There is some evidence that receiving this care in a stroke unit improves patient outcomes. While many patients admitted to the hospital with acute ischemic stroke are initially placed on bed rest, they should be mobilized as soon as their condition is considered stable (23). Nursing interventions such as range of motion and positioning will help prevent joint contracture and muscle atrophy of paretic limbs (24). Because stroke patients often have sensory loss, motor loss, vision loss, and/or decreased coordination, they are at high risk for falls and should be mobilized with caution (23). Patients with right hemisphere strokes and resulting neglect or inattention are at particular risk for fall (24). Hip fracture related to fall is the most common injury after stroke (24). Fractures occur most commonly on the paretic side.

All stroke patients should receive nutritional support as well as hydration. Malnutrition is associated with delayed recovery, and dehydration may decrease cerebral perfusion as well as place the patient at increase risk for venous thromboembolism formation (24). One study found that as many as 50% of stroke patients are malnourished when evaluated 2 to 3 weeks after their stroke (24). Patients should remain euvolemic and supported with intravenous fluid when necessary. Consultation with a nutritionist should be considered if the patient is not meeting his or her caloric needs. All stroke patients should have their swallow ability assessed by either the bedside nurse or speech therapy prior to initiating oral feeding and hydration. Impaired swallow reflex, lack of involuntary cough, lack of gag reflex, and cranial nerve palsies place the patient at increased risk for aspiration. If necessary, nutrition may be provided through an enteral route until the patient is safe to swallow or a percutaneous endoscopic gastrostomy is placed for long-term enteral feeding (24).

Generally, patients are positioned with the head of bed elevated to 30 degrees to decrease the risk of edema formation as well as to minimize aspiration (24). There is some suggestion based on studies using TCD that having the head of bed flat increases cerebral blood flow in ischemic stroke. Patients who are at risk for dysphagia or development of cerebral edema should remain with their head elevated. Head-down positioning may be appropriate for some patients on an individual basis. However, patients should be mobilized out of bed as soon as they are hemodynamically stable (24).

Constipation and incontinence may occur after ischemic stroke and should be managed with a bowel regimen and bladder catheterization (24). Because of the risk of urinary tract infection with indwelling bladder catheters, intermittent catheterization should be instituted as early as feasible (24).

Ischemic stroke patients are at increased risk for the development of deep vein thrombosis (DVT), in part because of the immobility from the stroke event and paresis of lower extremities. Sequential compression devices and low-molecular-weight heparin have been studied in ischemic stroke patients. Sequential compression devices are effective in decreasing the formation of DVT, but best protection comes from a combination treatment with sequential compression devices as well as subcutaneous low-molecular-weight heparin (24).

Interventions aimed at the secondary prevention of recurrent stroke should be started promptly during the hospitalization for ischemic stroke. These changes should be incorporated into the patient's discharge plan and follow-up.

If imaging reveals severe carotid stenosis (greater than 70% stenosis) on the ipsilateral side of the ischemic stroke, either surgical intervention or neurointerventional radiology should be considered to address the atherosclerosis (34). Intervention should be done in the weeks following the stroke rather than delaying due to the risk of recurrent stroke. Carotid endarterectomy has been studied more extensively than carotid artery stenting in treating carotid stenosis. However, no clear data suggest either to be superior (34). Therefore, a decision is made on a case-by-case basis according to the patient situation. Endovascular treatment is preferred if the patient has vertebral artery stenosis causing the stroke despite maximum medical therapy. There are no clear data to guide the use of intracranial stenting versus medical management in cerebral vascular atherosclerosis (34). Several trials are currently under way to try to address this issue.

If the cause of the stroke is thought to be cardioembolic, the patient may require long-term anticoagulation. If the source is thought to be atrial fibrillation or paroxysmal atrial fibrillation, patients receive anticoagulation therapy with warfarin to decrease the risk of recurrent stroke. The goal INR in these patients is between 2 and 3, ideally 2.5. If the decision is made that the patient is not a candidate for anticoagulation, aspirin should be administered daily at a dose of 325 mg. If the stroke is related to dilated cardiomyopathy, either warfarin with a target INR of 2 to 3 or antiplatelet therapy could be considered to prevent another stroke event (35). If the stroke is thought to be related to rheumatic heart disease or mitral valve prolapse, antiplatelet therapy should be adequate in preventing a recurrent stroke. If mitral annular calcification is found but no regurgitation is evident, antiplatelet therapy is appropriate secondary prevention. However, if regurgitation is noted, either warfarin or antiplatelet therapy would be considered appropriate. Patients with aortic valve disease without atrial fibrillation may be treated with antiplatelet medication, whereas the presence of a mechanical heart valve may necessitate anticoagulation with warfarin (35). Aspirin in combination with Coumadin has been studied in clinical trials, and the combination of the two drugs found to greatly increase the risk of ICH. Warfarin and aspirin should not be used together as secondary prevention of ischemic of stroke (35).

In noncardioembolic strokes, patients should be started on a long-term antiplatelet regimen. As mentioned, aspirin should be started within 48 hours of acute ischemic stroke admission. Aspirin alone is effective in preventing another stroke in patients who have had an ischemic stroke. Several studies have evaluated the ideal dose of aspirin for stroke prevention and generally found that 81 mg is as effective as 325 mg in preventing stroke. However, a daily dose between 50 and 325 mg is considered acceptable. Several other antiplatelet medications are currently available, including aspirin with extended release dipyridamole and clopidogrel. There are no data that show any one drug to be more effective than another and decision for treatment must be individualized to patient needs. In general, aspirin or aspirin plus dipyridamole is appropriate for initial antiplatelet therapy. Clopidogrel may be used but should not be administered concurrently with aspirin as it increases the risk of ICH (35). If the patient has an ischemic stroke while on aspirin, there is no evidence that increasing the aspirin dose will prevent subsequent strokes. In clinical practice, a patient who has a stroke while taking a daily aspirin is often switched to clopidogrel. However, data are not available to validate or refute this treatment (35).

Less common causes of ischemic stroke such as arterial dissection, PFO and cerebral venous sinus thrombosis all require specific treatment. Arterial dissection should be managed initially with warfarin anticoagulation for 3 to 6 months and then long-term with antiplatelet medication. In certain situations, endovascular or surgical management of the dissection may be necessary (35). If a PFO is thought to be the cause of the ischemic stroke, it can be managed with antiplatelet therapy or warfarin in high-risk patients. Surgical closure may be considered in patients who continue to have strokes despite medical management. In patients with no apparent risk factors or for stroke in the young, a hypercoaguable workup should be completed and treatment initiated accordingly. Recurrent strokes are often a complication of sickle cell disease, and strokes may occur despite medical management (35). In general, sickle cell patients should be treated according to the guidelines above. Surgical intervention or bypass surgery may be considered in severe sickle cell with recurrent strokes refractory to medical management (35). Patients with cerebral sinus venous thrombosis should be managed with acute anticoagulation followed by long-term warfarin for 3 to 6 months. In women with a history of stroke, postmenopausal hormone therapy should not be instituted or restarted (35).

After the initial period of permissive hypertension after ischemic stroke, blood pressure should be slowly controlled with an overall goal of following the Joint National Committee (JNC) guidelines for blood pressure less than 120/80 mm Hg (35). Blood pressure goals should be individualized to the patient according to their cerebrovascular status and comorbid conditions. There is some evidence that a blood pressure regimen that includes a diuretic or a diuretic in combination with an ACE inhibitor may be of benefit in stroke patients. If the patient also has diabetes, more aggressive control of blood pressure is recommended (35).

Diabetes is a risk factor for the development of recurrent stroke, and patients should be encouraged to continue aggressive glucose control on hospital discharge. There is no suggestion that certain medications or diabetes treatment plans are more or less helpful in stroke patients. Oral antihyperglycemic agents and insulin in combination with diet and exercise are recommended to control hyperglycemia (35).

Hypercholesterolemia and hyperlipidemia are associated with the development of ischemic stroke. Elevated LDL in particular is associated with ischemic stroke. Medication should be instituted to control hyperlipidemia with a goal of reduction of LDL to less than 100 mg/dL in patients with low risk and less than 70 mg/dL in patients with high risk (35). Statin drugs are the medication of choice in stroke patients as they decrease LDL as well as decrease overall inflammation and appear to decrease the risk of recurrent stroke independent of their effect on LDL. There is evidence that patients who have a stroke of suspected atherosclerotic etiology and have no prior indication for statin therapy (normal LDL, no additional cardiovascular risk factors) may still benefit from statin therapy (35).

A stroke scoring system, such as the scale developed by the National Institute of Neurologic Disorders and Stroke (http://www.ninds.nih.gov/doctors/NIH_Stroke_Scale.pdf), may be helpful to the clinician during the initial onset and throughout the trajectory for weeks to months for assessment of functional recovery from stroke. Patients should be counseled by the health care team regarding several lifestyle modifications to reduce the risk of recurrent stroke. All patients who smoke or use excessive alcohol should be counseled regarding tobacco and alcohol cessation (35). Appropriate referrals to community programs to support tobacco cessation and/or alcohol cessation or reduction should be made upon hospital discharge. Weight reduction should be encouraged in those with a BMI greater than 25 kg/m^2 or a waist circumference greater than 35 inches in women and 40 inches in men. Physical activity, regardless of weight or obesity, decreases the risk of recurrent stroke. All stroke patients should be encouraged to exercise at least 30 minutes most days of the week as they are able (35).

Throughout the hospital management of ischemic stroke, prevention and management of complications are priorities of medical and nursing care. The formation of cerebral edema, hemorrhagic transformation of ischemic infarct, seizures, and infection are complications of ischemic stroke (24). Cerebral edema may develop after stroke in as many as 25% of patients with anterior circulation stroke and possibly more often in posterior circulation stroke (24). Large territory infarcts and particularly those involving the middle cerebral artery are most likely to develop edema. Edema generally forms 2 to 5 days after the initial infarct and is rarely a complication in the first day after stroke. Younger patients who have less cerebral atrophy have less tolerance for cerebral edema and may decline quickly (24). In the anterior circulation, early signs of ischemia on CT as well as an infarct that involves more than 50% of the middle cerebral artery territory are associated with early edema formation (24). The term "malignant edema" is associated with cerebral edema in a large territory infarct that develops quickly and results in herniation symptoms. In the posterior circulation, cerebellar infarcts are associated with edema formation (24). Due to the location and proximity to the brainstem, edema in the cerebellum may lead to rapid neurologic decline and compromise of respiratory status.

Management of cerebral edema should follow the algorithm for elevated ICP. Specifically in cerebellar infarcts, decompressive craniectomy and management of obstructive hydrocephalus with external ventricular drainage are the standard of care (24). Decompressive hemicraniectomy may be necessary in patients with anterior circulation infarct and edema (specifically middle cerebral artery–associated edema), and there may be a benefit from early surgical intervention prior to acute neurologic decline in these patients (24).

Hemorrhage into the area of ischemic infarct is a common complication of ischemic stroke. There is some evidence that most ischemic strokes will have small areas of petechial hemorrhage (23). However, less than 5% of patients spontaneously develop clinically significant hemorrhage defined as a decline in NIHSS score of 4 points or greater. However, the use of thrombolytic agents, antithrombotic agents, and significantly elevated blood pressure all increase the risk of hemorrhagic transformation. Large territory infarcts are more likely to develop hemorrhage than are smaller volume strokes (23). Management of a clinically significant hemorrhage is covered in the ICH section of this chapter.

Seizures may develop in a small percentage of patients with ischemic stroke (23). If seizure develops, it generally occurs within the first 24 hours of stroke most commonly as partial seizures. Patients with preexisting dementia are at increased risk for the development of late-onset seizure after ischemic stroke. Little data exists regarding the management of stroke-related seizures. Currently, these seizures are managed according to standard of care for seizure in general (23).

Pneumonia and urinary tract infection (UTI) are some of the most common infectious complications in patients with acute ischemic stroke. Interventions aimed at preventing aspiration pneumonia as well as UTI are an integral part of quality nursing and medical care. Ischemic stroke patients should be monitored for the presence of infection and antibiotics started promptly if they are identified. However, prophylactic antibiotic use is not recommended (23).

Development of Stroke Centers

The approval of thrombolytic treatment for acute ischemic stroke changed the face of stroke care throughout the nation and the world. No longer was stroke a disease for which only supportive care was available. With the research showing the benefit of rapid tPA treatment along with the development of time-sensitive neurointerventional radiology procedures, stroke quickly became a disease process that could be reversed under the right circumstances (33, 36). Despite these advances, a vast majority of patients with ischemic stroke go without these treatments. Reasons for low treatment rates have been attributed to patients not recognizing stroke and activating the EMS system or mobilizing to the hospital, a lack of neurologic expertise available to treat stroke patients, as well as a lack of system organization allowing for efficient treatment once the patient presents (33, 36). Research has repeatedly shown that a majority of the public cannot name the symptoms of stroke, nor do they recognize stroke as a medical emergency (24). Many areas of the nation have no neurologist availability, and those areas of the nation that have neurologists still struggle with maintaining 24-hour availability of those neurologists. Many centers are struggling with neurologists opting-out of acute stroke call in the hospital where they provide care (33). Finally, when patients do arrive at the hospital within the hyperacute treatment window, many hospitals are ill-equipped to rapidly triage, provide diagnostic workup, and administer thrombolytic therapy (36).

To address these concerns, the Brain Attack Coalition has published several guidelines to help guide the formation of Primary Stroke Centers (PSCs) and Comprehensive Stroke Centers (CSCs) (33, 37). These documents outline the infrastructure necessary to provide rapid and thorough stroke care. In 2002, The Joint Commission launched a disease-specific certification program whereby a hospital could apply for certification as a "Primary Stroke Center." To be certified, the hospital must meet certain standards and show evidence of compliance with quality indicators. The Primary Stroke Center certification addresses acute stroke management with intravenous thrombolysis as well as subacute management and secondary prevention but does not address intra-arterial management of the hyperacute stroke patient. Quality measures for PSC certification include DVT prophylaxis, patients receiving antithrombotic therapy during the hospital stay as well as at discharge, patients with atrial fibrillation or flutter receiving anticoagulation therapy, thrombolytic therapy administered if the patient is eligible, statin therapy prescribed at hospital discharge, dysphagia assessment performed prior to any oral nutrition or hydration, stroke education provided to the patient and family, smoking cessation, education/advice/counseling provided to patients who have smoked within the past year, and patients considered for rehabilitation therapy. In addition to quality measures, The Joint Commission PSC designation requires stroke team personnel to maintain stroke continuing education annually, educate staff on stroke care and process, participate in community programs to improve awareness of stroke symptoms and treatments, and provide timely care of acute stroke patients as they arrive to the hospital.

In 2005, guidelines for the program administration of a CSC were published (37). This guideline recognized the role of the PSC in treating most acute stroke patients and introduced the concept of a CSC. The CSC is defined as a facility with the program personnel, infrastructure, expertise, and programs to manage high-acuity hemorrhagic and ischemic stroke patients. The comprehensive stroke center has the ability to perform intra-arterial treatment of acute ischemic stroke as well as SAH, advanced research programs, and fellowship programs, among other program attributes. To date, no certifying body exists to formally recognize CSCs (37).

Development of Telemedicine and Stroke Networks

In the past decade, several groups were also addressing the needs of stroke centers on a regional and even national scale. Because of the barriers to receiving stroke care listed above, it was recognized that systems of hospitals capable of providing stroke care at varying levels would be necessary to allow all people access to stroke treatment (33). The American Stroke Association developed the Task Force on the Development of Stroke Systems, which recommended the Stroke System of Care Model (SSCM). The SSCM endorses the use of telemedicine and aeromedical transport to increase the reach of stroke teams to underserved areas (33, 37). This concept has been supported by several guidelines and has led to the most recent development of stroke telemedicine (also called "telestroke") implementation guidelines (33). Many stroke systems have moved toward a "hub and spoke" model where the hub is the established stroke program and the spokes are hospitals that lack around-the-clock stroke expertise and access services of the hub. Initial telestroke networks have focused on effectively providing acute stroke management. Studies have shown that telestroke models can effectively treat acute stroke patients with morbidity and functional outcomes similar to that of well-established programs. Further, these networks are effective in providing thrombolytic therapy at rates similar to those of established programs (33).

Research has shown that patients have improved outcomes when stroke care is provided by a neurologist both in the acute and the subacute phases. Research has shown that stroke misdiagnosis rates are higher among general practitioners and emergency physicians compared to a neurologist. Research has also shown that inpatient stroke care provided by a neurologist is associated with improved patient outcomes (lower mortality and morbidity) as well as improved financial outcomes (33, 38).

Safety

Several publications have addressed the specific safety needs of stroke patients while in the hospital. One retrospective study evaluated reported miss and near miss errors in stroke patients (39). Evaluation of 176 errors occurring in the care of more than 1,400 stroke patients over 3.5 years revealed 86 preventable errors, 30 unpreventable errors, and 60 indeterminant errors. Errors identified included documentation and transcription errors, errors in communication and handoff, failure to perform a clinical task, and error in calculation and checks (39). A recent publication by the American Heart Association (AHA) identified common errors in patients with stroke. Underuse of tPA is a major safety concern for ischemic stroke patients. In addition, other medications such as heparin and hypotonic saline, warfarin, and corticosteroids are often misused in stroke patients and place them at risk for hemorrhage and edema formation (40).

Clinical Nurse Specialist Competencies and Spheres of Influence

The role of the Clinical Nurse Specialist (CNS) within stroke care has developed as stroke care has developed over the past 15 years. Several publications evaluate the role of the CNS as it relates to emergency department care of the acute stroke patient, secondary prevention of complications, and risk factors for a recurrent stroke and patient education on their disease process, although no experimental studies have been conducted in this area.

Systems Leadership

As care of the acute stroke patient turned from supportive to acute treatment and intervention, the CNS established a place of influence on the acute stroke team (41, 42). The CNS acting as expert clinician can help to assess patients with acute stroke for thrombolytic care and help coordinate the team to work in an efficient and effective manner when under time constraints of stroke care (41, 42). A postgraduate fellowship has been designed to train advanced practice nurses to respond as a part of the acute stroke team. This is the first program of its kind mirroring the postgraduate fellowship that is standard in medical training (43).

Clinical Expert/Direct Care, Consultation, Coaching/Teaching/Mentoring

In the educator role, CNSs are also instrumental in patient education and maintaining patient movement through the hospital system and minimizing length of stay (42). Several publications have outlined the role of the CNS in educating patients and families in their disease process, risk factor modification, and disease management (44, 45). As a consultant and expert clinician, the CNS is instrumental in the development of care pathways and order sets to standardize care and ensure minimum care standards are met (42).

Major complications associated with stroke are dysphagia and aspiration pneumonia (46). In one stroke program, the CNS uses all subroles as a dysphagia CNS (46). The dysphagia CNS assesses, diagnoses, and treats patients with dysphagia as an expert clinician. In addition, the CNS role models behavior for bedside nurses and educates the patient, nursing staff, and multidisciplinary team. The dysphagia CNS is a consultant for the team. The CNS assessment and management occur in addition to the bedside nurse dysphagia team and as an adjunct to speech therapy. The dysphagia CNS is in a unique position to conduct research on dysphagia and oral care (46).

Transient Ischemic Attack
Etiology

As the understanding of ischemia in the brain and ischemic stroke has evolved, so has the understanding of transient ischemia and TIA. Cerebral ischemia exists along a continuum-based on degree and time of loss of blood flow, with TIA being a precursor or a major warning for an ischemic stroke (47). Unfortunately, because the symptoms resolve, much of the general public fails to recognize that TIA, much like ischemic stroke, is a medical emergency that warrants a diagnostic evaluation and treatment to prevent an impending stroke. An estimated 200,000 to 500,000 TIAs occur yearly in the United States. However, this is likely underestimated as many people experiencing TIA do not seek care. Incidence, prevalence, and risk factors mirror those of ischemic stroke (47). Pathophysiology is discussed in the ischemic stroke section.

Clinical Presentation

The clinical presentation of TIA is an acute neurologic deficit just as in ischemic troke. However, in TIA the deficits resolve quickly (47). TIA has traditionally been defined as an ischemic event with symptoms lasting less than 24 hours. However, the definition of TIA has recently been reevaluated. Most transient attacks with no radiographic evidence of infarct resolve within minutes. Transient ischemia that occurs longer than 1 hour are generally associated with tissue infarct and could theoretically be classified as an ischemic stroke (47). Therefore, a recent consensus panel agreed on a new definition of TIA based on tissue death and not time to symptom resolution. Based on their recommendation, TIA is now considered a transient episode of neurologic dysfunction caused by focal brain, spinal cord, or retinal ischemia without acute infarction (47).

Diagnosis

The diagnostic evaluation of TIA mirrors that of ischemic stroke (47).

Management

The major concern with TIA is the alarming number of patients who have a stroke in the days or weeks following the TIA. In patients who present with ischemic stroke, as many as 40% of patients have had a TIA prior to their stroke (47). Greater than 10% of TIA patients will have an ischemic stroke within 90 days of the TIA event, and a majority of the strokes occur within the 2 days following the TIA (47). Risks of cardiac events such as myocardial infarction are also elevated in the days and weeks following TIA. Therefore, the goal of management in the TIA patient is to rapidly institute primary prevention for stroke to mitigate the risk of a major ischemic event (47).

The diagnostic management of TIA mirrors that of ischemic stroke (47). Hospital admission rates tend to vary according to areas of the nation, but general consensus is that TIA is a medical emergency that warrants immediate diagnosis and treatment. Recently, several studies have evaluated the role of risk stratification to evaluate patients for hospital admission versus rapid assessment and discharge with a plan for timely outpatient follow-up (47). The California score and the ABCD score both accurately predict short-term risk of stroke. The ABCD score and the more recent ABCD2 score evaluate patients based on age, blood pressure, focal weakness and speech impairment, duration of TIA, and presence of diabetes. If the patient has a high score, he or she is at high risk for a stroke in the following days and should be admitted to the hospital for full workup and treatment. If the patient has a lower score, there is some evidence that they can be fast-tracked through a program of diagnostic tests and initial management with a plan for discharge and subsequent outpatient management in the following days. Additional evidence is needed regarding programs that successfully implement risk stratification in their TIA management. Regardless, the risk of ischemic stroke following TIA is real and cost-utility analysis has shown that overall there is a benefit of hospital admission and treatment (47).

Subarachnoid Hemorrhage
Etiology
SAH is a devastating disease process that disproportionally affects younger patients compared to other forms of stroke (48). While SAH is a less common form of stroke in the United States and results in only 5% of stroke deaths, SAH results in over 27% of stroke-related potential years lost before the age of 65 because of the high mortality rate and relatively young age of the SAH patient (49). SAH incidence has been stable over the past 30 years at 10 per 100,000 person-years. Prior to CT imaging, SAH was likely overestimated and any trend toward change in incidence is thought to be related to improvements in imaging capabilities allowing differentiation between SAH and ICH (50, 51). SAH affects approximately 30,000 people in the United States annually. However, actual prevalence may be higher as an estimated 12% of patients experience such a severe hemorrhage that they do not survive to seek care or in whom the SAH is misdiagnosed (48).

The average age of SAH peaks in the sixth decade of life, which is lower than any other type of stroke (50, 51). Women have a higher rate of SAH than do men, and African Americans are at higher risk than Caucasians (50). Worldwide, the highest rates of SAH occur in Finland and Japan (50).

Pathophysiology
SAH is simply defined as blood that has left the vasculature and entered the subarachnoid space where CSF circulates around the brain and spinal cord and into the ventricular system. The mechanism by which blood enters the subarachnoid space varies and comprises the cause of SAH. SAH is initially divided into traumatic and atraumatic causes.

Traumatic
Traumatic SAH will be discussed in more detail within the context of TBI. Because traumatic SAH often occurs in the context of other brain trauma, it is hard to isolate the effect that the subarachnoid blood has on the trauma patient (50). However, it is important to note that the presence of subarachnoid blood following trauma has repeatedly proved to be a negative prognostic indicator (50).

In determining the pathophysiology behind traumatic SAH, meticulous history should be obtained surrounding the trauma. The practitioner must discern if it was the trauma that caused the SAH or the SAH that caused the trauma (50). For the purpose of a discussion of SAH, this section will focus on nontraumatic aneurysmal SAH and highlight differences in patient management as it relates to the trauma patient.

Atraumatic
Atraumatic SAH is divided into aneurysmal SAH and perimesencephalic SAH. Aneurysmal SAH comprises 85% of nontraumatic SAH; perimesencephalic, 10%; and other causes, 5% (50).

Aneurysms are an outpouching of a vessel that generally develops at the areas of arterial branching at the base of the brain in the Circle of Willis or arteries arising from the Circle of Willis (51). Initial belief held that many aneurysms were congenital and present at birth. Research has shown that aneurysms are almost never present in neonates and very rarely in children. Newer literature suggests that most cerebral aneurysms develop slowly over the course of years (48, 50,).

Risk factors that play a factor in the development of cerebral aneurysms can be grouped into nonmodifiable and modifiable. Nonmodifiable risk factors largely include hereditary patterns and genetic contributions to aneurysm formation (50, 51). There is some evidence that first-degree relatives of someone who had an aneurysm may have a 3- to 7-fold increased risk of also developing an aneurysm. However, in second-degree relatives, this risk appears to subside and risk of aneurysm development matches that of the general population.

There is a strong link between certain genetically linked connective tissue disorders and the development of cerebral aneurysms (50, 51). However, the presence of an aneurysm does not necessarily translate into the rupture of the aneurysm and development of an SAH. The actual incidence of SAH in relation to aneurysm formation in patients with these disease processes is quite low. Regardless, diseases such as autosomal dominant polycystic kidney disease, Ehlers-Danlos type IV, and neurofibromatosis type II are associated with the development of cerebral aneurysms (50, 51). There is a theoretical risk that patients with Marfan syndrome are also at risk of developing cerebral aneurysms, although the actual link to SAH remains unclear in current studies (50, 51).

Hypertension is considered the strongest modifiable risk factor associated with aneurysm formation and SAH (50, 51). Smoking is also associated with the development of aneurysms, both by contributing to hypertension and causing vessel wall changes that predispose the artery to weakening and developing an aneurysm. Excessive alcohol intake, generally defined as more than five drinks daily, is also associated with aneurysm formation. The use of oral contraceptives and hormone replacement was associated with SAH in some analyses but not replicated in follow-up studies. Therefore, the actual risk associated with these factors is unclear.

Related to the actual SAH event, several situational risk factors emerge in the literature. Drug use, particularly stimulant drugs like cocaine, is associated with SAH and is an important risk factor to consider in a patient who presents with no other apparent risk of developing SAH (50, 51). Participation in a strenuous activity immediately preceding the headache is present in as many as 20% of patients. However, as many as 40% of patients are at complete rest at the time of aneurysm rupture (50, 51). There is a somewhat higher incidence of SAH in the winter and spring months and with changes in atmospheric pressure (49).

Perimesencephalic, or nonaneurysmal, nontraumatic SAH comprises 10% of all nontraumatic SAH and two thirds of patients with angiography-negative SAH. The exact mechanism of perimesencephalic SAH is unknown (51). However, it is thought to be a venous rupture rather than an aneurysmal rupture. There is some evidence that in perimesencephalic SAH, the onset of headache may be more gradual, over minutes as opposed to seconds. However, there is little of the history or physical exam that can reliably decipher a mild aneurysmal hemorrhage from perimesencephalic hemorrhage without additional imaging. Patients with perimesencephalic SAH generally have good outcome compared to aneurysmal SAH as perimesencephalic SAH is not associated with vasospasm development and does not require surgical repair (51).

Other potential causes of SAH include an inflammatory lesions of the brain or spinal cord, arterial dissection, rupture of an arteriovenous malformation (AVM), dural arteriovenous fistula, cavernous angioma rupture, tumor with hemorrhage, and drug use, as mentioned (51). In patients who experience an SAH following drug use, the SAH is rarely related to the drug use alone. Often these patients have an underlying aneurysm or other vascular malformation that is exacerbated by the drug use (50). Cocaine-related SAH as occurs in younger patients has mortality and morbidity rates similar to those of aneurysmal SAH (48).

Mortality

SAH causes death in half of the patients who are afflicted with the disease. SAH causes 6,700 in-hospital deaths annually (50). There is some evidence that mortality associated with SAH is beginning to decline (48). Caucasians have a lower mortality rate than African Americans, Hispanics, American Indians, and Asians in the United States (48).

Of patients who survive the hemorrhage to hospital discharge, approximately 33% remain functionally dependent, and up to 80% of patients who survive the hemorrhage report significant reductions in quality of life 4 months after the hemorrhage. At 18 months after the hemorrhage, 70% of patients who survived their hemorrhage reported some reduction in their quality of life (50).

Factors known to influence mortality include patient factors, aneurysm factors, and institutional factors (48). Related to the patient presentation, severity of initial hemorrhage, advanced age, male sex, increased time to treatment, and medical comorbidities such as atrial fibrillation, hypertension, heart failure, coronary artery disease, and renal disease are associated with higher mortality (48). Larger aneurysm size, location in the posterior circulation, and morphology of the aneurysm are also associated with higher mortality (48). Finally, institutional factors appear to play a role in patient outcome following an SAH. The availability of endovascular management and higher volume of SAH patients treated annually are associated with lower mortality rates (48).

Pathophysiology

As mentioned, the development of aneurysm occurs over years and the presence of an aneurysm does not ensure rupture will occur (48). Size is one of the best predictors of hemorrhage risk, with larger aneurysms posing higher risk for rupture. The exact mechanism behind aneurysmal rupture is unclear. Hypertension and strain likely play a role, as do size and location of the aneurysm. Once the aneurysm ruptures and leaks blood into the subarachnoid space, the concepts of primary and secondary injury in the brain apply to the development of neurologic injury in SAH (48). Primary and secondary injury are discussed elsewhere in this chapter. Another critical stage in the progression of SAH is the development of vasospasm. The exact mechanism causing vasospasm is unknown. Vasospasm is thought to be caused by irritation of vessels that occurs as blood degrades in the subarachnoid space (48).

Clinical Presentation

A patient presenting with an acute headache that they report is the "worst headache of my life" is the quintessential presentation of SAH as reported in the literature. The headache is sudden in onset and unusually severe in nature (50). Some have referred to the headache associated with aneurysm rupture to be a "thunderclap headache." While this is widely taught as the signature presentation of SAH, it is important to note that many patients report symptoms other than headache and certainly may present with an SAH and not report the extreme headache. Other symptoms associated with SAH include a transient or persistent loss of consciousness often associated with a headache, nausea, and/or vomiting that may or may not be associated with a headache and signs of meningeal irritation such as nuchal rigidity or photophobia (50).

Seizure at the time of headache has been reported in 6% to 20% of patients presenting with SAH, but it is currently unclear if it is truly seizure activity or some other symptom related to the acute hemorrhage and not epileptic in origin (48). Thirty percent of patients develop some focal neurologic symptom around the headache onset (50). The focal neurologic symptom is associated with the location of SAH and therefore varies from patient to patient (50). In patients who have had a previous trauma or skull fracture, dural AVM should be investigated as a possible source of hemorrhage. Patients reporting pain between the shoulder blades without radiation (known as coup de poignard or the dagger thrust) should lead to suspicion of a spinal AVM or fistula rupture (50). Sudden unusual head movements immediately preceding headache may indicate a vertebral artery dissection as the source of the subarachnoid blood (50).

Focal neurologic deficits related to aneurysm rupture may reveal suspected location of the aneurysm that ruptured (48). A partial third nerve palsy is more likely to be associated with an inferior/posterior cerebral artery rupture. Monocular blindness may indicate the rupture of an anterior cerebral artery aneurysm. Bilateral sixth nerve palsy in the setting of SAH is generally associated with the development of hydrocephalus, which often arises in the hours after the hemorrhage. Bilateral lower limb weakness may be associated with anterior cerebral artery aneurysm rupture (48). Hemiparesis is rarely associated with SAH but if present is most often related to middle cerebral artery aneurysm rupture (48). Other assessment findings may include retinal hemorrhages, meningismus, and decreased level of consciousness.

There is some evidence that some patients may experience a "sentinel bleed" or "warning leak" where a minor hemorrhage occurs from the aneurysm anywhere from 2 to 8 weeks prior to a larger hemorrhage, resulting in a headache of smaller magnitude and possibly associated symptoms (48). Recognition of the warning leak is very important for those caring for outpatients and patients presenting to the emergency department.

Recognition of a sentinel hemorrhage may help to avoid major rupture if caught early by caregivers (48).

Diagnosis

Based on the SAH incidence rates, a full-time general practitioner will only see one SAH patient every 7 to 8 years (51). Hospitals serving smaller populations also rarely care for SAH patients. Therefore, misdiagnosis is a real concern due to the infrequency with which many caregivers care for an SAH patient. Prior to advanced imaging, misdiagnosis rates were estimated to be as high as 64%. With advanced CT and MRI, misdiagnosis rates remain around 12% and are associated with much higher death and disability at 1 year after hemorrhage. Failure to obtain a head CT is the most common diagnostic error (54), as is failure to follow up with an LP in appropriate patients (52). Most often, SAH is mistaken for migraine and tension headache (49).

Noncontrast CT of the brain is the first line imaging in a patient with suspected SAH (48). Blood will appear hyperdense, generally surrounding the basal cisterns if SAH is aneurysmal in nature. In patients with traumatic SAH hemorrhage, it is less common to see blood in the basal cisterns; this pattern is more characteristic of an aneurysmal cause of hemorrhage. Blood from trauma is more likely to be in the subarachnoid space around the cerebral convexities and often associated with a skull fracture in the area of hemorrhage (50). CT imaging of a patient with a perimesencephalic SAH often shows hemorrhage confined to the basal cisterns and located anterior to the midbrain (51). However, location of blood in the subarachnoid space is confirmatory of SAH and further imaging is generally necessary to confirm origin of hemorrhage. CT is most reliable in detecting subarachnoid blood in the first 12 to 24 hours after a hemorrhage. CT imaging becomes less reliable in detecting smaller amounts of blood in the subarachnoid space after a day has passed. Generalized brain edema may yield a false diagnosis of SAH as the edema causes subarachnoid congestion that can mimic hemorrhage (51). CT scanning is most sensitive in the first 12 to 24 hours after initial hemorrhage, after which time blood begins to break down and may be less visible in cases of smaller hemorrhage.

CTA is a function of CT imaging that may serve as an alternative to angiography or MRA (50). CTA requires less contrast be given compared to an angiogram or MRA and is also minimally invasive (53). This imaging does require special software, scanning procedure, and postprocessing of the images to allow for an angiography-like view. CTA is as sensitive as MRA and has been found in one study to aid in the identification of aneurysms that were missed with conventional angiography. CTA is highly dependent on the skill of the technologists administering the exam and the radiologist, neurologist, and neurosurgeon interpreting the scan but may be increasingly used in place of conventional angiography and MRI (50).

MRI and MRA may be useful in the identification of blood in the subarachnoid space and may provide clues as to the etiology of the SAH by detecting venous malformation or other possible sources of hemorrhage (50). As CT becomes less reliable to detect SAH in the days after hemorrhage, MRI is increasingly useful in detecting blood in the subarachnoid space and may be used in conjunction with an LP to make a diagnosis in a patient where time has elapsed between hemorrhage and imaging or medical care (53). MRA may be used to identify the presence of an aneurysm but can be difficult due to the time it takes to obtain motionless images, and the SAH patient may be agitated or unable to tolerate the exam, requiring sedation or anesthesia. MRA has a sensitivity of 69% to 100% of detecting one aneurysm but is slightly less sensitive in the detection of all aneurysms in the cases of more than one aneurysm. MRA is less invasive than angiography and may be useful in certain patient situations. Currently, angiography remains the gold standard for aneurysm or vascular malformation detection (50).

LP is performed when SAH is suspected but initial CT imaging is negative (50). Preferably 12 hours will have elapsed between hemorrhage and LP to allow enough time for the red blood cells in the CSF to lyse and bilirubin and oxyhemoglobin to form (50). The presence of bilirubin and oxyhemoglobin helps to distinguish between a traumatic LP and the true presence of blood in the subarachnoid space.

Cerebral angiography is currently the gold standard for imaging the cerebral vasculature to determine the etiology of SAH and is the test of choice for initial evaluation of the presence of aneurysm. However, advancements in CTA and MRA may result in practice change over the coming decade (50). Cerebral angiography has a complication rate (transient or permanent) of approximately 0.8% but may vary according to expertise from center to center. Imaging of all the cerebral arteries is necessary when performing cerebral angiography as 15% of patients have multiple aneurysms (50).

Management

Part of what makes the management of a patient with SAH so complex is the multiple phases of disease process. Initial management of the patient with SAH is aimed at airway and hemodynamic stabilization, addressing any hydrocephalus and hypertension, locating the cause of hemorrhage, and securing the aneurysm. Following obliteration of circulation to the bleeding aneurysm, the patient enters a window of surveillance and treatment of vasospasm, which is the major cause of secondary injury in patients with SAH (48).

In the initial hours after an SAH, management is focused on patient stabilization. As many facilities do not currently have the capabilities to treat a patient with SAH, rapid emergency department triage and treatment or transfer to a facility able to treat is necessary (48). Protection of airway with endotracheal intubation may be necessary if the patient declines neurologically and is not able to protect the airway (48). Health care personnel in the emergency department and ICU are encouraged to use an established scale to monitor patients on an hourly or more frequent basis. There is not yet consensus as to which neurologic assessment scale should be used. The Glasgow Coma Scale (GCS), NIHSS, and Hunt and Hess scale for SAH are all options that may be considered (48). Patients with SAH require an ICU level of care for initial monitoring and management (51).

Prevention of Aneurysm Rehemorrhage

In the absence of overt trauma and until vascular imaging is performed, it is assumed the patient has an active vascular lesion such as an aneurysm or AVM that is at risk for rerupture and expansion of hemorrhage side. Until the lesion is detected and secured, initial management is aimed at prevention of rebleeding (48). The risk of rebleeding is highest in the first 24 hours after initial hemorrhage (4% overall risk of rebleeding) and then remains elevated (1% to 2% risk of rebleeding) daily over the next 4 weeks if the aneurysm is not secured (48). Rebleeding of an aneurysm increases the mortality rate for SAH from 50% to 70% (48). Therefore, active interventions must be implemented to minimize the risk of rehemorrhage. Factors associated with increased risk of rebleeding include a longer time from hemorrhage to hospital admission and securing of aneurysm, higher initial blood pressure, and worse neurologic status on admission (48).

Early treatment of the aneurysm has become the mainstay of aneurysm rerupture prevention (48). Bed rest alone will not prevent rebleeding but is often used as part of a care plan to minimize rebleeding risk until the aneurysm is secured (48). Reduced noise and stimulation also may be helpful as part of a comprehensive care plan until the aneurysm is secured, but further research is needed to best determine the appropriate activity and level for patients until their aneurysm is secured (49).

It is recognized that hypertension plays a role in aneurysm rupture and rerupture. There is agreement that hypertension should be controlled until the aneurysm is secured, but there is no current consensus on the ideal blood pressure in this patient population (48). There is some evidence that a systolic blood pressure greater than 150 or 160 mm Hg is associated with aneurysm rerupture. However, studies have been mixed and the true link between the rupture process and the role of blood pressure remains to be defined (48). General practice based on the concern for rebleeding and the association between hypertension and increased rebleeding rate have lead to a practice of decreasing systolic blood pressure to 140 to 160 mm Hg (48, 49). Preferred medication to reduce blood pressure includes nicardipine, labetalol, and esmolol. Sodium nitroprusside should be avoided in patients with SAH as the drug may raise ICP and is associated with toxicity with prolonged infusion (48). Antifibrinolytic therapy (specifically tranexamic acid) has been studied with mixed results on rebleeding rates and ischemic complications. This remains an area of active research. Antifibrinolytic therapy is currently not recommended (48).

Aneurysm Management

Recent developments and research in the area of aneurysm management have greatly advanced the understanding and management of aneurysmal SAH. It has also led to a debate over how aneurysms are best managed. Prior to the 1990s, the mainstay of aneurysm treatment was microsurgical clipping of the aneurysm. The first successful clipping of an aneurysm was completed in 1937. Aneurysm clipping requires extensive neurosurgery and results in a clip being placed on the outside of the aneurysm to occlude blood flow to the aneurysm while attempting to maintain the blood flow within the parent vessel. In the 1970s, a Russian physician, Dr. Fedor Serbinenko, began exploring the possibility of securing an aneurysm from within the vessel instead of the open craniotomy and aneurysm clipping. He initially trialed the use of latex balloons placed within the aneurysm to stop blood flow to the aneurysm. This technique was abandoned because of the frequent growth of the aneurysm and recannulation with blood around the latex balloon. In 1991, Dr. Guido Guglielmi introduced detachable platinum coils that could be placed endovascularly, causing thrombosis of the aneurysm and cessation of blood flow to the aneurysm. Since 1991, coil embolization technique and technology have garnered international attention and research and has become an increasingly popular treatment method (53). The two treatment options have led to increased debate over which method is ideal in the treatment of an aneurysm (53, 54). Further complicating this picture is that surgical clipping is generally offered by a neurosurgeon, whereas endovascular intervention is most often offered by interventional neuroradiologists, leading to competing fields and at times conflicting interests (53).

Research has shown that hospitals that offer endovascular management of aneurysms tend to have improved outcomes (48). To appropriately determine the best option on a patient-by-patient basis, the practitioner must understand the implications of each surgical option and the literature fueling the debate. Coil embolization is generally a neuroendovascular interventional radiology procedure

performed in a biplane angiography suite. The procedure is generally performed under general anesthesia. Diagnostic angiography is performed via the femoral artery in most cases. Other arteries may be accessed if necessary to perform the angiography. Patients are often anticoagulated during the procedure. A guide wire is traced to the neck of the aneurysm, and coils are passed over the catheter into the aneurysm until enough coils are placed inside the aneurysm to induce thrombosis (53). Previously, only aneurysms with a narrow neck (berry aneurysms) could be treated with coils because the narrow neck was necessary to hold the coils in place. However, some centers are now using stents to assist coiling where the stent is placed across the parent artery of the aneurysm and coils are passed through the stent into the aneurysm (53). This technique requires long-term antiplatelet therapy, which can complicate the course of the SAH. This is a rapidly developing field of neurologic intervention, and more research is needed (53).

Coil embolization is minimally invasive and has a lower procedural complication rate (albeit not absent) compared to neurosurgical microclipping (48). In some centers, coil embolization has been associated with improved morbidity and mortality and overall better patient outcomes (48). However, coil embolization may not totally stop blood flow to the aneurysm and may require additional treatments, whereas aneurysm clipping is thought to be definitive treatment of the aneurysm. This is of concern as incomplete treatment of the aneurysm is associated with higher rates of rebleeding. Coil embolization also requires follow-up angiography monitoring, which is associated with some procedural risk to the patient (48). Finally, surgical clipping is the only technique that allows for clot drainage, which has been suggested to decrease complications and speed recovery (55).

Guidelines have suggested that aneurysm morphology and location should dictate preferred treatment method (48). For example, basilar tip and internal carotid aneurysms are generally best treated with coil embolization, whereas middle cerebral artery aneurysms tend to be difficult to coil and may be more amenable to clipping (48). There is little literature available that directly compares clipping to coiling. It has been suggested that the best option for patient care is to be treated at a center that provides both surgical and endovascular treatment. Treatment by a multidisciplinary team is the standard of care proposed in the latest SAH guidelines, and a joint decision should be made between surgical and endovascular team at the time of the initial angiography. The decision regarding which treatment is best should take into consideration aneurysm size, morphology, and location and the skill of surgical and endovascular teams (48).

Obstructive hydrocephalus is a complication of SAH that is generally seen in the hours to days after SAH (53). Acute hydrocephalus is present in 20% to 30% of SAH patients (55), and as many as 67% of patients with SAH will experience either acute or chronic hydrocephalus as a complication of their hemorrhage (55). Progressive obtundation with slower pupillary response to light and sixth nerve palsy is characteristic of the development of hydrocephalus and should prompt the practitioner to evaluate ventricle size and rule out other complications with a follow-up CT scan of the brain (55). Placement of an external ventricular drain is the standard of care for acute hydrocephalus (55).

The calcium channel blocker nimodipine (60 mg every 4 hours oral for 21 days) has been studied in the setting of SAH and resulted in improved outcomes 90 days after hemorrhage (48). The exact mechanism by which nimodipine improves the outcome of SAH patients is unknown. Benefit is suspected to be related to neuroprotection and support of collateral circulation to injured areas of the brain. Administration of nimodipine does not reduce the occurrence or severity of vasospasm but does decrease the incidence of permanent neurologic deficit at 90 days. Administration of nimodipine is currently standard of care (48).

Cardiovascular side effects of SAH include a phenomenon of cardiac stunning that is believed to result from a catecholamine surge that depresses systolic and diastolic heart function (48). This effect appears to be more common in women and in the more severe hemorrhages. Electrocardiographic (ECG) changes may be visible and include T-wave inversion, QT prolongation, and ST-segment elevation. The degree of myocardial injury ranges from a "stunned" effect that is reversible over days to actual infarction and a picture of contraction band necrosis (48). The catecholamine surge reduces left ventricular ejection function and creates a heart failure picture (takotsubo cardiomyopathy, apical and ventrical akinesis). This dysfunction is visible on cardiac echocardiography on 8% to 12% of patients and diastolic dysfunction may be present in as many as 70% of patients. Elevated troponin I is seen in as many as 30% of SAH patients. Cardiac enzymes and an ECG should be obtained on admission and a cardiac echocardiogram should be obtained on anyone with cardiac or pulmonary complications (48). The depressed heart function is usually transient and reverses over days but may lead to significant hemodynamic compromise and pulmonary oxygenation complications in the interim (48). Cardiac catheterization, reduction of blood pressure, and/or anticoagulation should be avoided in patients with cardiac complications of SAH. Gentle use of beta-blockers or inotropic medication may be considered in certain patients. There is some evidence that brain natriuretic peptide (BNP) may be a prognostic indicator of cardiac complications from SAH and may be a useful diagnostic test in certain patients with cardiac complications (54).

Neurogenic pulmonary edema is another complication of SAH that occurs in 8% of patients, generally those with the most severe hemorrhages (48). The mechanism behind the formation of pulmonary edema is thought to be primarily from the cardiac stunning resulting from catecholamine release. However, noncardiac sources such as hypothalamic injury and elevated ICP may result in disruption of alveolar endothelium and capillary endothelium, causing increased pulmonary vascular permeability that results in interstitial and alveolar pulmonary edema. Any SAH patient with impaired oxygenation, with or without abnormal appearing chest radiograph, should receive a thorough work-up and neurogenic pulmonary edema should be included in the differential while evaluating for pneumonia, atelectasis, or another pulmonary cause. SAH patients with neurogenic pulmonary edema have higher morbidity and mortality rates compared to SAH patients without, although this is likely also related to the size and effect of the initial hemorrhage. Regardless, early recognition and treatment of neurogenic pulmonary edema may result in improved patient outcomes.

Additional management considerations in the care of the SAH patient include attention to quality ICU nursing and medical management (51). SAH patients should receive early nutrition orally if the swallow is intact and level of consciousness permits or enteral nutrition if level of consciousness is depressed or the patient has dysphagia. Patients should be started on an aggressive bowel regimen to maintain soft stools and prevent constipation. Straining with stools should be avoided as it may raise ICP. Patients with SAH are at risk for DVT by virtue of being hospitalized and immobile, but risk is also increased by coma and hemiparesis in patients with severe hemorrhage. If the patient is immobile, sequential compression devices should be placed on the patient. Subcutaneous heparin or low-molecular-weight heparin should be added once aneurysm is secured.

Fever in patients with SAH is independently associated with worse outcomes (49). Fever should be aggressively managed according to the literature outlined earlier in this chapter. Hyperglycemia is present in up to 70% of SAH patients and is also independently associated with delayed cerebral ischemia (vasospasm) and overall poor outcomes (49). Debate exists regarding the ideal glucose range for the SAH patient. Most of the ICU literature guiding the current paradigm of aggressive treatment of hyperglycemia was studied in CV and medical/surgical ICU patients. While hyperglycemia has been associated with worse outcomes in all ischemic and hemorrhagic stroke, it is unclear if the aggressive target range of 80 to 110 is ideal in this patient population. A recent study suggested that slight hyperglycemia in the range of 110 to 140 may be beneficial in SAH patients but confirmed that a glucose greater than 140 was associated with worse outcomes (48). This is an area of active investigation, and until further research is available, aggressive glucose control should be the rule.

During the initial management phase, SAH patients should be fluid resuscitated to maintain euvolemia (48). In the initial management of the SAH patient and the subsequent management of vasospasm, there is controversy regarding the role of crystalloid versus colloid fluids. There is currently no evidence that colloids (albumin) improve outcomes.

Seizure prevention with antiepileptic drug (AED) prophylaxis is another area of controversy and interest in the initial management of the SAH patient (48). Traditionally, SAH patients were placed on AEDs upon admission to provide prophylaxis against seizures, and the AED was continued for up to 6 months after hemorrhage. However, recent studies have raised concern regarding the cognitive impact of AEDs and called this traditional practice into question. This concern, combined with thought that the actual seizure rate in SAH is lower than previously suspected, has led to a shortened course of AED prophylaxis or none at all. Current guidelines state short-term prophylaxis in the immediate posthemorrhage period (up to 3 days) may be considered, and long-term use of anticonvulsants is not recommended unless seizure activity is confirmed or another confounding risk is present (48).

There is not sufficient literature about the intraoperative experience of the SAH patient to form clear consensus on intraoperative management. However, periods of hypotension during surgery should generally be avoided (48). The role of induced hypothermia during surgery still is being investigated. Hypothermia may be helpful in individual cases but is not currently recommended for all patients (48).

Vasospasm

Once the aneurysm is secured, the patient enters a period of vasospasm surveillance. This period involves close observation of the patient for the development of vasospasm, a major complication of blood in the subarachnoid space. Cerebral vasospasm is the narrowing of the artery following an SAH, generally occurring in the large vessels of the Circle of Willis and proximal arteries. Vasospasm is thought to be an inflammatory response in the vessel wall in response to the vessel being surrounded by CSF with blood breakdown products in contact with the outside vessel wall (49). While the exact pathophysiology of vasospasm is still unknown, current belief is that both (1) increased vascular wall stress from the ruptured aneurysm and (2) oxyhemoglobin from blood breakdown inhibiting nitric oxide action (a vasodilator) with increased release of vasoconstrictors such as arachidonic acid and endothelin lead to the activation of the smooth muscle layer of the vessel (53, 56). Prolonged contraction of the vessel wall results in morphologic vessel changes and fibrosis of the vessel wall (53). Vasospasm is seen in as many as 70% of SAH patients and results in ischemic events in 36% of patients. Vasospasm generally begins within 3 to 5 days of hemorrhage and resolves over the course of 2 to 3 weeks (56). If left untreated, the narrowed artery will lead to cerebral ischemia, altered cerebral blood flow, and infarction. Vasospasm appears to account for up to 50% of deaths in patients who survive the initial hemorrhage and securing of the aneurysm (48, 56). Severe vasospasm is defined as a decrease in arterial lumen space of more than 50% (56). ICU level of care is generally continued while the patient is monitored during the peak time of vasospasm onset.

Vasospasm diagnosis may occur through several different mechanisms (56). Vasospasm should be suspected in a patient who develops a focal neurologic deficit unexplained by hydrocephalus or rebleeding in the days and weeks following SAH. However, this is reliant on the patient having a neurologic exam to follow. Vasospasm may be silent in patients who are in a coma. Studies have noted that some patients develop increased mean arterial pressures in conjunction with the neurologic deficit as the brain attempts to compensate and improve cerebral perfusion (48, 49). Patient assessment findings in a patient developing vasospasm include the development of focal neurologic deficit, pyrexia, and possibly elevated mean arterial pressure or overall blood pressures (56). The degree of neurologic deficit associated with vasospasm is highly dependent on the location of the affected artery, the amount of vessel narrowing, and the degree of collateral circulation to the area.

TCD monitoring involves using ultrasound to measure velocity flow of large cerebral arteries. Many institutions monitor TCD velocities of cerebral vessels while the patient is in the window of possible vasospasm development (48). Increased vessel velocities and an increased Lindegaard ratio (ratio of the velocity in the brain vessel of choice to the velocity of the ipsilateral extracranial internal carotid artery) may indicate vessel narrowing from vasospasm (48). It is important to monitor velocity trends over time; independent values are generally not as helpful. Studies on TCD find it most reliable in detecting middle cerebral artery vasospasm. When used in conjunction with patient assessment and clinical picture, TCD monitoring may be helpful in the detection of vasospasm and decision on initiating treatment. However, results must be interpreted carefully. Technician proficiency as well as patient factors such as bone windows for ultrasound must be taken into consideration when interpreting results of the study (48).

Angiography continues to be the gold standard diagnostic test to identify vasospasm (48). While angiography is an invasive procedure, it also allows for treatment of the vasospasm at the time of diagnosis. Research regarding the use of CTA, CT perfusion, and MRA in the diagnosis of vasospasm is currently under way, and both imaging modalities could potentially play a role in screening patients for vasospasm formation in the future (54). Timing of angiography is an important point in the diagnosis and management of vasospasm. Routine screening of patients is not generally advised as there is no current consensus on treatment of vasospasm found angiographically in an asymptomatic patient. In general, patients are taken for angiography if initial attempts to correct the vasospasm with "triple H" therapy fail (48).

The management of vasospasm treatment has historically been "triple H" therapy (54), which is a cluster of interventions aimed at providing hypervolemia, hypertension, and hemodilution. The concept of triple H therapy was first introduced in the 1970s and is based on the assumption that the decreased cerebral blood flow through the narrowed vessel is pressure dependent. Theoretically, by increasing the pressure and volume, the spasm of the vessel will be overcome and cerebral blood flow restored. This was adopted quickly into practice in the 1970s and 1980s with no randomized controlled trials to support it. True efficacy of triple H therapy remains unclear (53). Hypervolemia is induced by infusing large volumes of colloids or crystalloid fluids. There is no true standard for how to quantify hypervolemia, nor is there a standard for a specific goal in which to titrate therapy. In general, either CVP or pulmonary artery catheter is used and CVP is increased along with blood pressure while observing patient response (54).

Blood pressure after the aneurysm is secured is generally allowed to rise and hypertension is permitted (48). Hypertension may be induced using vasopressors once vasospasm is suspected or confirmed. Again there is no standard for how elevated the blood pressure should be allowed to rise. Generally, the patient's clinical picture is paired with hypervolemia and hypertension goals. Vasospressor drug choice is made according to the individual's cardiac needs and the titration goal is set on an individual patient basis. Hemodilution occurs as a by-product of increased fluid administration as well as other factors associated with a prolonged ICU stay. However, the role of hemodilution in vasospasm management has fallen under scrutiny. There is evidence that a decreased hemoglobin may impair oxygen delivery and may play a detrimental role in the secondary ischemic injury during vasospasm. Further, initial trials suggest that a higher hemoglobin is associated with improved outcomes in SAH patients. These data suggest that SAH patients may benefit from a lower threshold to transfuse with blood products as the hemoglobin drops. However, concerns exist regarding the side effects associated with transfusions. Ideal hemoglobin goal for the SAH patient is currently being studied in clinical trials (48).

Complications associated with triple H therapy include pulmonary edema, myocardial ischemia, hyponatremia, and cerebral edema (56). Theoretically, triple H therapy works by increasing the circulating blood volume and blood pressure and reducing the blood viscosity, thereby overcoming the vessel narrowing or at least allowing blood to flow more easily through the narrowed vessel, thus maintaining cerebral blood flow. More recent literature on vasospasm has highlighted that the secondary injury that occurs after an SAH is likely multifactorial and not solely related to arterial narrowing with vasospasm. This emphasizes that vasospasm and the resulting ischemic injury are not solely problems of pressure. While reduction in arterial constriction has improved patients' clinical exams and outcomes in some studies, others have shown a reduction in vessel spasm but no real change in long-term outcomes. Recent literature highlights the role that early ischemic damage (immediately following the hemorrhage up to 72 hours post hemorrhage) as well as spreading depression (spreading depolarization that results in spreading ischemia) may be related to poor outcome after SAH. Further, much of the literature to date has focused only on large vessel vasospasm. Smaller cerebral arteries may also play an important role in ischemia and long-term outcome. More research is certainly necessary, but some are calling for a shift in paradigm and movement beyond the traditional understanding of vasospasm and treatment with triple H therapy. Future interventions may be more effective if they are aimed at multiple ischemic pathways (56).

Neuroendovascular interventional radiology also plays a role in the treatment of vasospasm (53). As vessels narrow over an extended period of time, the muscular wall of the vessel undergoes fibrosis that may not be overcome by triple H therapy alone. Intra-arterial therapies such as angioplasty or intra-arterial infusion of vasodilators may be necessary as an adjunct treatment. Transluminal balloon angioplasty may be used alone or in combination with vasodilators to resolve ischemia. Angioplasty works best on large vessels with thick muscular walls. Balloon dilation disrupts the connective tissue and fibrosis in the contracted vessel resulting in sustained vessel dilation. Angioplasty has been shown to be safe and feasible and improves outcomes in patients with vasospasm. However, it is possible to have improved flow angiographically with no improvement in neurologic exam. Reversal of symptoms following successful angioplasty of a vessel in vasospasm has ranged in reports between 31% and 90%.

Intra-arterial pharmacologic intervention with vasodilators such as papaverine, nicardipine, or verapamil has also been investigated (49). Papaverine results in vasodilation but has a short half-life. Therefore, vasospasm often reoccurs in several hours after treatment and repeated treatments may be necessary. Nicardipine also results in vasodilation when applied intra-arterially to a vessel in vasospasm. Nicardipine has a more sustained effect on the vessel in vasospasm, requiring less retreatment than papaverine. There was report of transiently increased ICP immediately following intra-arterial treatment with nicardipine, and this should be considered when choosing an intervention. Finally, verapamil is currently under investigation as another topical intra-arterial vasodilator for use in a vasospasm vessel. Patients who do not improve with triple H therapy should be considered for emergent neurointerventional radiology treatment (49).

It would stand to reason that if vasospasm is related to narrowing of the artery that is pressure dependent and triple H therapy works by increasing pressure and blood flow, then initiating triple H therapy before the patient is symptomatic may be beneficial in preventing vasospasm (56). This notion has been studied in two clinical trials, where it was found that prophylactic triple H therapy did not prevent the formation of vasospasm. Prophylactic triple H therapy places the patient at risk for a multitude of side effects with no effect on vasospasm occurrence and is not supported in the literature (56). During the period of vasospasm surveillance where the patient is at risk for vasospasm but not yet in vasospasm, interventions should be aimed at maintaining euvolemia. Hypovolemia occurs in as many as 30% to 50% of patients and is associated with worse outcomes as it increases risk of vasospasm and ischemia (56). When calculating intravascular fluid needs, fluid lost to third spacing, insensible loss, and blood loss should be taken into consideration.

Hypomagnesemia is found in as many as 40% of SAH patients, particularly with the presence of cisternal or ventricular blood. Low levels of magnesium may increase the risk of vasospasm, and hypomagnesemia should be avoided. Magnesium supplementation is currently being studied for prevention and treatment of vasospasm. Current recommendations are to aggressively replace magnesium to normal levels at a minimum, and some recommend maintaining elevated levels of magnesium, although research regarding the ideal magnesium level to target is under way (48).

High-dose statin therapy is also under investigation as a potential prevention and/or treatment for vasospasm (48). Initial literature suggests that statins confer neuroprotection by enhancing cerebral autoregulation and through their anti-inflammatory properties. Clinical trials are currently ongoing. Aspirin, low-molecular-weight heparin, endothelin antagonists, and antioxidants in vasospasm and ischemic injury after SAH have all been studied in smaller trials and case series. At this time, none are recommended in the guidelines and additional literature is necessary (48).

Other complications of SAH include chronic hydrocephalus, seizures, and hyponatremia (49). As many as 30% of SAH patients may develop chronic obstructive hydrocephalus and ventriculomegaly, requiring permanent ventriculoperitoneal (VP) shunt placement (49, 55). Need for VP shunt placement is associated with older age, early hydrocephalus, intraventricular hemorrhage, poor clinical condition on presentation, and female sex (49).

Hyponatremia is present in 30% of patients and is independently associated with poor outcomes (49). Hyponatremia in SAH is generally due to cerebral salt wasting (CSW), syndrome of inappropriate ADH (SIADH), or possibly a combination of both (49). In SIADH, patients develop hyponatremia, hypervolemia, low serum osmolarity, and elevated urine osmolarity. Treatment includes restriction of free water and possibly diuretics. In CSW, high plasma levels of atrial natriuretic factor (ANF) result in increased urinary sodium losses. Patients exhibit hyponatremia and euvolemia or hypovolemia. Treatment includes fluid resuscitation to euvolemia and salt replacement, with either isotonic saline or hypertonic saline. In a patient with SAH who develops hyponatremia, diagnostic work-up includes assessment of fluid status since admission and serum and urine osmolality (56).

While SAH has been an area of active research in the past decade, many questions remain unanswered. Additional research is under way attempting to address the role of secondary ischemic injury. The role of brain tissue oxygenation, cerebral microdialysis, cerebral blood flow monitoring, and neuroprotection are all areas of active research

Prevention

In patients who have experienced SAH, the risk of forming a new aneurysm is 1% to 2% annually. Patients with multiple aneurysms seem to be more susceptible to forming new aneurysms compared to patients with one or no aneurysms (48). However, little scientific data exists on prevention of aneurysm formation. Controlling known risk factors may decrease the incidence of SAH and/or the severity. Yet improvements in HTN control over the past 20 years do not appear to have made a difference in SAH incidence or prevalence. Regardless, control of hypertension and smoking cessation would be expected to decrease risk of aneurysm formation and rupture (48). Screening of the general population or even high-risk populations has not been adequately studied and is currently not recommended in the literature. Which patients to screen and which imaging modality to use remain matters of debate (48).

Traumatic SAH

Regarding the management of patients with traumatic SAH, there are a few areas where care of the patient with traumatic SAH differs from the care outlined for an aneurysmal SAH (55). Post-traumatic hydrocephalus occurs more often in traumatic SAH compared to aneurysmal SAH and may require a higher percentage of patients to undergo VP shunt placement. Vasospasm does occur in as many as 40% to 60% of traumatic SAH depending on how vasospasm is quantified. However, it is unclear the role vasospasm has on secondary injury and ischemia in this patient population. When vasospasm does occur, it occurs earlier compared to atraumatic SAH but has a similar duration. There is debate over the role of nimodipine in traumatic SAH. Research has shown a modest improvement in mortality in the short term in traumatic SAH patients treated with nimodipine. However, one of the side effects of nimodipine is decreased blood pressure, which should be avoided in trauma patients. Therefore, decision on nimodipine therapy should be made on a case-by-case basis with the risks and benefits weighed in relation to each case (50). In terms of additional management of the patient, please refer to the TBI section.

Unruptured Aneurysm

Patients with unruptured aneurysms are increasingly being treated by either coil embolization or surgical clipping of the aneurysm. The need for treatment versus conservative medical management must be carefully considered in the context of risk of hemorrhage over time. Research has shown that the larger aneurysms are at a higher risk of hemorrhage. Certain comorbid cerebral vascular diseases may also place the patient at higher risk of hemorrhage, such as the presence of an AVM, fibromuscular dysplasia, dissection, and cerebral arteritis. The decision to pursue aggressive surgical or endovascular treatment of an unruptured aneurysm should consider the size of the aneurysm, comorbid cerebrovascular conditions and age of the patient as well as history of SAH, multiple aneurysms, or a strong family history of SAH. Patients should be counseled as to the risks and benefits of conservative medical management, endovascular coil embolization, and surgical treatment (54).

Clinical Nurse Specialist Competencies and Spheres of Influence
Clinical Expert/Direct Care

The CNS acts as an expert clinician as a part of the multidisciplinary team providing care to patient and families. The CNS supports the bedside nurse in advocating for and providing evidence-based interventions. The CNS may also evaluate the patient's care plan and organized care pathways to determine where care needs to be tailored to the individual needs of the patient/family. The CNS provides direct patient care as needed and prescribes pharmacologic and nonpharmacologic interventions, diagnostic measures, nursing therapeutics, and procedures to meet patient needs.

Consultation

The CNS provides consultation to staff at all levels of SAH care. The CNS may develop programs and protocols for the care of the SAH patient based on the evidence and measures the outcomes of programs and protocols for care to guide the health care team toward performance improvement.

Systems Leadership and Collaboration

The CNS may influence the development of a stroke care system, providing systems leadership, using the collaboration competency. The CNS may be responsible for evaluating the patient population and care outcomes across the system to identify opportunities for improvement. The CNS may also coordinate the care of patients as they transfer from the health care system out into the community. By evaluating resource use surrounding the care of the SAH patient, the CNS may identify opportunities for improvement and cost containment. There is increasing literature reporting that hospital characteristics and systems of care play a role in patient outcomes following SAH (48). Hospitals treating higher volumes of SAH appear to have better outcomes. Initial studies report that hospitals caring for fewer than 20 SAH patients annually had higher 30-day mortality. Lower in-hospital mortality has been reported at hospitals who offer endovascular services (4). However, debate remains whether the benefit of being treated at a high-volume center outweighs the risk and cost of transfer. Current consensus is that it is reasonable to transfer patients with SAH or an unruptured aneurysm for care at a high-volume center (48). More research is needed to determine the ideal model of care for SAH patients. The CNS may play a pivotal role in the development of stroke systems of care. In addition, the CNS may apply the collaboration competency through a key role in improving relationships and communication between disciplines and agencies involved in the care of the SAH patient.

Coaching/Teaching/Mentoring

The CNS may provide education and teaching to patients' families, and nurses surrounding the care of the SAH patient. The CNS may be called on to interpret current research to ensure the team is providing evidence-based medical and nursing care or to participate in original nursing and medical research to advance the care of the SAH patient.

Ethical Decision-Making/Moral Agency/Advocacy

The CNS is often called on to guide the health care team in navigating the ethical issues surrounding the care of the SAH patient, including end-of-life issues and futility of care. Participation in local, state, and national committees that guide the care of the SAH patient population strengthens ethics in policy-making decisions.

Intracerebral Hemorrhage
Etiology

ICH is defined as bleeding into brain tissue of parenchyma. ICH accounts for between 10% to 15% of all strokes in the United States. Incidence of ICH is 10 to 30 per 100,000 persons (57). This disease disproportionately affects minority races and ethnicities, with Mexican American, African American, Native American, Japanese, and Chinese having a higher incidence of ICH. Further, hemorrhages in these populations are more often deep in the brain and occur more often in younger and middle age (57). Decreased incidence of ICH over the past several decades is likely related to better hypertension control throughout the nation and access to medical care (57). ICH accounts for 2 million strokes annually worldwide (57). The economic burden associated with ICH is substantial. ICH costs an estimated $125,000 per person per year for a total cost of $6 billion per year in the United States (58).

ICH results in death at 30 days in 35% to 50% of patients afflicted with the disease (59). ICH in-hospital admissions increased by 18% in the past decade but in-hospital mortality rates decreased by only 6% between 1990 and 2000 despite advances in therapies (57). Half of deaths occur in the first 2 days following ICH (59). Mortality rates at 1 year depends on location of hemorrhage with a mortality rate of 51% for deep hemorrhage, 57% for lobar hemorrhage, 42% for cerebellar hemorrhage, and 65% for brainstem hemorrhage. Of patients who survive their hemorrhage, only 20% of patients are functionally independent at 6 months (57). Health-related quality of life (HRQOL) has been studied in ICH patients across several nations, and ICH patients reported substantially lower quality of life than the general public. Deep hemorrhage (as opposed to lobar), higher stroke severity, and stroke volume, as well as worsening clinical status in the first 72 hours after stroke, were associated with worse HRQOL (60).

Causes

ICH is classified as either traumatic or spontaneous. Traumatic ICH will be addressed in the TBI section. Spontaneous ICH can then be further divided into primary ICH resulting from either hypertension or cerebral amyloid angiography (85% of all cases) versus secondary resulting from coagulopathy, tumor hemorrhage, and hemorrhagic conversion of a stroke or vasculitis (58).

ICH is more common in certain areas of the brain. ICH is classified as deep (50% of hemorrhages), lobar (35% of all hemorrhages), cerebellar (10% of all hemorrhage), or brainstem (6% of all hemorrhages) (59). Location of ICH is often related to cause of the hemorrhage (61). Forty percent of ICH cases involve extension of hemorrhage into the ventricles (58).

Primary ICH is caused by hypertension or cerebral amyloid angiopathy and accounts for 85% of all ICH cases. Secondary ICH is caused by coagulopathy, tumor with hemorrhage, stroke with hemorrhagic conversion, trauma, or vasculitis (57).

Risk Factors

Nonmodifiable risk factors for ICH include gender and race. Men are at higher risk for development of ICH, as are those of African American and Hispanic race (59).

Cerebral amyloid angiopathy (CAA) accounts for 20% of ICH cases in patients over the age of 70 (62).

Amyloid angiopathy involves the deposition of beta-amyloid protein in the vessel wall of arteries, arterioles, and capillaries. The deposition of amyloid results in vessel fibrosis (62). CAA is genetically linked, and there is some evidence that it may be more common in people of European and Asian descent (62). CAA should be considered as a cause of ICH in patients over age 55, particularly those who are normotensive and if investigation into other causes of hemorrhage is negative (62). The most common site of hemorrhage associated with CAA is lobar (2). Definitive diagnosis of CAA can only be made post mortem on autopsy. Clinically, CAA is a diagnosis of exclusion and is considered "probable" in a patient over age 55 with history of multiple hemorrhages with no other apparent cause and "possible" in a patient over the age 55 with a single hemorrhage with no other apparent cause (62).

Modifiable risk factors/causes of ICH include hypertension. Hypertension is responsible for nearly 60% of cases of ICH (61). Chronic hypertension results in decreased vessel compliance and microaneurysm formation that causes the vessel to be more susceptible to hemorrhage, particularly when placed under the stress of elevated blood pressure (61). Hypertensive ICH most often affects the vessels at the bifurcation of smaller penetrating arteries. Most common sites for hypertension caused ICH include the thalamus, basal ganglia, cerebellum, and pons (61).

Anticoagulant use is also associated with an increased risk of ICH. Warfarin in particular is a cause of ICH in as many as 25% of ICH cases (61). Warfarin use is particularly a risk in patients who have other risk factors such as hypertension, anticoagulant use plus antiplatelet use, CAA, or the presence of leukoaraiosis (white matter changes seen on CT and MRI, attributed to vascular changes and linked to risk factors such as hypertension and diabetes and thought to be associated with the development of dementia and changes in gait). Warfarin is associated with larger bleeds and increased mortality compared to other causes of ICH (61). An elevated INR of greater than 3 is a risk for hemorrhage, but still a majority of warfarin-related ICHs occur with an INR in a therapeutic range below 3. There is an increased risk of ICH as INR elevates, and once INR is greater than 4.5, the risk of ICH doubles with every increase of 0.5 (61). ICH associated with warfarin use is more likely to occur in the first months after warfarin initiation (63). There has been some concern that the use of antiplatelet medications such as aspirin or clopidogrel may increase the size of ICH and therefore be associated with higher mortality. This has even prompted some centers to routinely transfuse platelets in patients who had a history of recent antiplatelet use. However, reports recently published have yielded conflicting results as to the role of antiplatelet medication on

ICH size, expansion, and mortality. More research is needed as to the role of platelet transfusion in this patient population (61).

Other risk factors or causes of ICH include treatment with thrombolytic medication (59). Similar to patients taking warfarin, hemorrhage after thrombolytic treatment is often associated with large, multifocal hemorrhage and poor patient outcome. Thrombolytic use in acute ischemic stroke associated with ICH in 3% to 9% of patients treated and less than 1% in patients treated with fibrinolytics for other reasons (59). Epidemiologic studies have revealed that populations with low serum LDL cholesterol have higher rates of ICH (58). This trend appears to be more associated with populations who have low LDL as a result of their diets than with people who are treated with medications such as statins to lower their LDL. Heavy alcohol intake is associated with the development of ICH, because heavy alcohol use contributes to the development of hypertension as well as platelet dysfunction, coagulopathy, and vessel wall changes (58). Stimulants such as cocaine and amphetamines are a cause of hemorrhage in a small percentage of ICH patients. However, 40% of patients who experience an ICH surrounding the use of stimulant drugs have an underlying vascular lesion. Therefore, further investigation into additional causes of hemorrhage is necessary and vascular imaging is warranted (64).

Additional causes of ICH include hemorrhage of a primary or metastatic brain tumor. The hemorrhage may be the initial presentation of a tumor, may be a hemorrhage in someone with a known tumor, or may related to treatment of the tumor through surgery or chemoradiotherapy (65). ICH may be the result of an ischemic stroke with hemorrhagic conversion, vascular malformation such as aneurysm, AVM, or fistula that has ruptured or possibly venous thrombosis with associated infarct and hemorrhage (57, 58, 61).

Pathophysiology

Central to the understanding of the effect of the ICH on the brain tissue and structures is the role of primary and secondary injury in the brain. The primary injury results from the damage from initial hemorrhage directly to brain tissue and structures. The secondary injury the brain sustains in the days to weeks following a hemorrhage includes the process of blood breakdown and resolution of the hemotoma, which can include the development of edema and hydrocephalus among other complications. Cerebral edema associated with ICH is a multistage process. Initially, the hemorrhage dissects along white matter (primary injury) and the cell disruption associated with the hemorrhage results in edema formation within several hours. In the next several days, the presence of blood in the brain tissue results in a complex interplay of inflammatory response, coagulation cascades, activation of the complement system, and recruitment of immunomediators. This response results in a cyclic effect of edema as the process disrupts the blood-brain barrier, which in turn contributes to additional edema formation (61). During this stage, there is significant activity in the injured tissue surrounding the hematoma. Studies have shown changes in metabolism and glucose uptake in the perihematomal area and current research is focused on mitigating the damage in this area (66). As red blood cells begin to lyse, they create a period of delayed edema as the by-products of the blood irritate surrounding tissue. Cerebral edema generally increases by 75% within 24 hours of the hemorrhage and peaks between 5 and 6 days but can last upward of 2 to 3 weeks (57). This process is difficult to predict and highly specific to each patient, the size of the hemorrhage, and the location of the hemorrhage. As pressure in and around the hematoma compresses microcirculation around the hemorrhage, ischemic damage may occur in the tissue surrounding the clot (61). Elevated ICP is a result of the combination of the cerebral edema process, mass effect from the hematoma itself, as well as hydrocephalus (59, 61).

Intraventricular hemorrhage (IVH) may be present in patient with ICH (67). The intraventricular blood may be the primary site of hemorrhage. In the case of primary hemorrhage, blood is generally confined to the ventricular system and is ventricular in origin. Causes of primary IVH include ventricular AVM, aneurysm, tumor, hypertension, or coagulopathy. IVH is considered to be secondary if it results from the extension of ICH or SAH.

Hematoma expansion is a concern in patients with ICH (59). A significant number of patients will expand their hemorrhage or have additional bleeding events. Hematoma expansion seems to be correlated to lack of acute blood pressure control and coagulopathy.

Clinical Presentation

Initial presentation of ICH generally includes the sudden onset of focal neurologic deficit. The exact deficit is highly dependent on where in the brain the hemorrhage occurs and the size of the hemorrhage (59). The patient presenting with ICH may report a headache, nausea and/or vomiting, and a decreased level of consciousness (59). It is impossible to differentiate ICH from other stroke syndromes based on assessment alone and brain imaging is immediately necessary (57, 59).

Diagnosis

Diagnosis of ICH is based on clinical history, physical exam, and CT imaging of the brain (59). Differential diagnosis includes ischemic stroke. Differentiation between ischemic and hemorrhagic stroke cannot be made on assessment alone. Confirmation by head CT of the presence or absence of hemorrhage leads to a definitive diagnosis of ICH or ischemic stroke.

A noncontrast CT of the brain is the first line test to identify ICH due to speed in which the test can be obtained and the ability to quickly visualize blood. ICH is hypodense on CT imaging and is immediately apparent. CT imaging is more reliable than MRI in evaluating intraventricular extension and hydrocephalus (59). MRI is useful in imaging ICH as it is as reliable as CT imaging in identifying ICH and may be more sensitive than CT in identifying underlying lesions that may have caused the ICH. MRI may also identify areas of previous hemorrhage, which is particularly useful in making a diagnosis of CAA. However, in the setting of initial diagnosis, it is often more difficult to obtain MRI because of the time it takes to obtain the scan as well as patient factors such as agitation and instability (59). Therefore, MRI may be useful in identifying the underlying cause of the ICH and as an alternative to angiography in some patients. Angiography is useful to identify vascular causes of hemorrhage, particularly in patients with bleeding in unusual locations or suspicion of vascular abnormality or ICH with SAH. Angiography may also be warranted in patients with only IVH (59).

Management
Initial Stabilization

Initial stabilization is aimed at airway management, minimizing the expansion of the hemorrhage through blood pressure management, and correction of coagulopathy, if present, and early ICU management. Endotracheal intubation is necessary in patients who are no longer able to protect their airway (59). Neurologic assessment generally associated with a need for endotracheal intubation is a GCS score less than 8 (59, 68). Care must be given during intubation and stabilization to minimize elevated ICP and effects on blood pressure (59). Rapid sequence intubation with attention to adequate sedation so as not to elevate blood pressure or ICP is recommended.

Blood pressure management in the patient with ICH has been a matter of debate as understanding of ICH pathophysiology has evolved. Many patients with ICH have a history of chronically elevated blood pressure. However, even in the absence of a history of hypertension, blood pressure is often elevated with the acute hemorrhage (61). Prior to the last decade, a mainstay of ICH management was tolerating an elevated blood pressure out of concern that lowering blood pressure would result in increased mass effect and subsequent perihematomal ischemia. However, concerns with this treatment methodology emerged as it was noted that hemorrhages tended to increase in size in the hours after the initial hemorrhage, and elevated blood pressure was thought to promote the hemorrhage extension. Positron emission tomography (PET) imaging studies

were also conducted to challenge the notion that decreasing blood pressure increased perihematomal ischemia and showed that reduction in blood pressure did not result in decreased blood flow or ischemia around the hematoma. However, in the setting of acutely elevated ICP, abruptly decreasing blood pressure may result in globally compromised blood flow. Studies are currently under way to identify ideal blood pressure for ICH patients. ICH guidelines published in 2007 generally recommend reducing blood pressure to less than 160/90 while maintaining a CPP between 60 and 80 mm Hg in patients with elevated ICP. Patients with suspected elevations in their ICP should have their ICP monitored and blood pressure titrated to maximize CPP (59, 61, 69) Medications that may be used to decrease blood pressure include labetalol and hydralazine for intermittent dosing or infusion and nicardipine and esmolol for infusions to maintain lowered blood pressure (59). All patients with ICH should be assessed for elevated ICP. Management of elevated ICP is outlined elsewhere in this chapter.

Of immediate concern is assessment for and correction of any coagulopathy (70). Coagulation studies should be checked on admission and interventions tailored to the cause of hemorrhage. The half-life of warfarin is 36 to 42 hours (70). Therefore, in patients with warfarin-induced ICH, anticoagulation must be counteracted or reversed. Warfarin's mechanism of action is to inhibit the vitamin K pathway, an essential step in the clotting cascade, resulting in clotting factors with reduced activity (70). Therefore, standard anticoagulation reversal treatment includes the administration of vitamin K 10 mg (59, 61). Side effects include hypotension and anaphylaxis. Vitamin K takes a minimum of 6 hours to normalize INR and often requires repeated doses. Consequently, fresh frozen plasma (FFP) must be transfused in order to replace vitamin K–dependent coagulation factors. FFP is generally administered at 15 to 20 mL/kg. However, concentration of coagulation factors may vary considerably from infusion to infusion. In clinical practice, total amount of FFP administered is generally titrated to effect on normalization of INR. Side effects of FFP administration include blood transfusion reactions and allergic reactions. One of the difficulties with the treatment of warfarin-induced coagulopathy with vitamin K and FFP is that it may take hours to normalize the INR and requires a large amount of fluid if multiple transfusions are necessary. Prothrombin complex is another treatment option that requires less volume and reverses INR quickly. Unfortunately, prothrombin complex is associated with ischemic complications and disseminated intravascular coagulation (DIC) and therefore often not used.

Recombinant factor VII (rfVII) is a treatment option to reverse warfarin coagulopathy. rFVII normalizes the

INR within minutes with no associated fluid load (58, 59, 63, 71). Dosage is weight based. rFVII has been through phase II and III trials that showed it was effective in providing rapid reversal of INR as well as decreased hemorrhage expansion. Unfortunately, the phase III trial showed no change in patient outcomes at 90 days despite the decreased hematoma size in patients treated with rFVII. Therefore, rFVII is not currently considered standard of care for all ICH patients. However, it may be an option in patients who would benefit from surgical treatment and need rapid INR reversal, patients who are unable to tolerate the fluid associated with FFP, and patients with a hemorrhage in precarious locations where small increases in hemorrhage volume may mean loss of life (such as the brainstem). While rFVII is not recommended as standard treatment in all patients with warfarin-associated ICH, it may be useful on a case-by-case basis.

Currently, there are unclear data on when and in which cases to restart anticoagulation after an ICH. More studies in this area are needed. Current clinical practice is to wait 7 to 10 days and reinstitute only in patients with a high risk of thromboembolism (59, 61).

As previously mentioned, whether to transfuse platelets in patients with ICH and a history of antiplatelet use has been a matter of recent debate (72). The concern is that loss of platelet function results in larger initial hemorrhage, hemorrhagic extension, and poor patient outcomes. Further, antiplatelet medication inhibits platelet activity for the life of the platelet (10 to 14 days). Therefore, stopping the antiplatelet medication is not sufficient to restore the platelet function. More studies are needed to guide the care of these patients. Data are emerging that while antiplatelet medication is associated with larger strokes and higher mortality, the infusion of platelets does not result in a better outcome (61, 72).

Regarding correction of coagulopathy in ICH related to fibrinolytic agents, these hemorrhages are generally massive and multifocal with a mortality rate that exceeds 60%. Treatment includes rapid infusion of platelets and cryoprecipitate (59).

ICH can be managed either medically or surgically with open craniotomy for clot aspiration or minimally invasive surgery for clot evacuation. The number of ICH patients taken to surgery has decreased over the past decade, likely related to trials that showed overall patients did not have a better outcome if their hemorrhage was removed surgically. However, subgroup analysis showed that patients with lobar hemorrhages that were close to the surface did have improved outcome if their hematoma was surgically removed, suggesting surgery is a suitable option for some patients depending on hematoma location (59, 68). Cerebellar hemorrhage patients generally have a better outcome when the hematoma is surgically removed. This is particularly true if the hemorrhage is

greater than 3 cm. Cerebellar hemorrhages are associated with hydrocephalus because of proximity to the fourth ventricle as well as sensitivity to edema because of proximity to the brainstem. Early surgical treatment is often indicated (59, 68).

For patients who are candidates for surgery, ideal timing of surgery remains a topic of debate. There are little scientific data to guide this decision. There is some suggestion that within 12 hours of initial hemorrhage is the ideal time frame but more research is needed (59). Delayed surgery defined as greater than 96 hours after initial hemorrhage may be more harmful than no surgery at all (59).

In the surgical management of ICH, there may be a role for minimally invasive surgery, clot aspiration, and/or thrombolytic therapy (59). There is some evidence that endoscopic aspiration may improve ICH mortality rates but not quality of life. More research is needed in this area. Endoscopic aspiration may be ideal for supratentorial hemorrhages that are close to the surface of the brain. There are currently several studies under way evaluating the use of thrombolytic agents in ICH. Thrombolytic agents that are administered into the clot in small doses every several hours may facilitate clot breakdown and minimize secondary injury (58, 73). Initial studies look promising and trials are ongoing. Many centers have already adopted intraventricular thrombolytic agents for primary or secondary IVH. At a dosage of 1 mg every 8 hours, tPA is thought to be safe and may decrease mortality and improve the speed of clot clearance within the ventricle (58, 67, 74).

ICU and Acute Care

The most common complications in patients with ICH include extension of the hemorrhage, neurologic deterioration, infection, and thromboembolic events (59, 75). ICU care should be aimed at mitigating these events and managing any situations that may worsen secondary brain injury. Depending on bleed size and location, the patient must be assessed for obstructive hydrocephalus. In the event that hydrocephalus develops, treatment with an external ventricular drain is the standard of care (57).

Fever is common in patients with ICH and independently associated with mortality and morbidity, even at "low-grade" levels of fever. Fever also exacerbates elevated ICP thereby worsening the secondary injury to the brain. Aggressive control should be undertaken using acetaminophen and cooling blankets (58).

Hyperglycemia is also present in many patients with ICH regardless of prestroke diabetes status. Hyperglycemia is independently associated with 30-day mortality in ICH patients (58). Aggressive glucose control is recommended for all ICH patients. There is some debate over the ideal target glucose range for stroke patients as there is some evidence of increased glucose needs in injured brains (58). At this time, all stroke guidelines recommend aggressive control. Glucose should be maintained less than 150, and additional research is needed regarding ideal ranges for stroke patients (58).

Early nutrition is associated with better outcomes in ICH patients (57). Posthemorrhage, patients are in a hypermetabolic state and studies show ICH patients are often undernourished. As with all other stroke patients, the ICH patient must be screened for dysphagia and for need of speech therapy prior to initiating oral nutrition. If oral nutrition is not safe, enteral nutrition should be provided (61). ICH patients are at increased risk for gastric ulceration and hemorrhage. The development of gastrointestinal hemorrhage in an ICH patient is associated with significantly worse outcomes. ICH patients should receive prophylaxis with H2 blockers (57). Respiratory failure as a result of coma or other complication results in the need for long-term ventilation and tracheostomy in approximately 10% of patients with ICH (57).

During the ICU stay, the ICH patient should be fluid resuscitated to a goal of maintaining euvolemia. Only isotonic fluids should be used. ICH patients are at high risk for the development of venous thromboembolism due to immobility and hemiparesis. Sequential compression devices should be placed on all immobile patients upon hospital admission. There is debate over the role of heparinoids in a patient with ICH because of risk of bleeding. A small review of the literature consisting of small trials and case series suggested that the addition of heparinoids 2 to 3 days after the hemorrhage is both safe and efficacious. Patients had less venous thromboembolism and no additional bleeding (59, 76). Some still question the risk, and more data are needed to guide the health care team.

Thirty-day incidence of seizure in ICH is around 8% (77). Presence and likelihood of seizure activity vary according to location of hemorrhage and are more common in lobar hemorrhages than in deep hemorrhages. The presence of subdural blood or an elevated INR increase risk of late-onset seizure (77). When seizure occurs, it is associated with increased cerebral blood flow, elevated ICP, and hematoma expansion. Seizure should be treated emergently if identified. However, there remains debate over the role of seizure prophylaxis in patients with ICH (59, 77). Prophylaxis used to be considered standard of care in all patients with an ICH. New literature has emerged that says seizure prophylaxis is associated with poor cognitive outcome in survivors and may carry more risk than the benefit it confers (59, 77). Current ICH guidelines support a brief period of several days of AED prophylaxis only in patients who have lobar hemorrhages (59, 77).

The role of poststroke depression in stroke patients and its effect on stroke recovery have gained attention in the past decade. Clinical depression affects approximately 20% of ICH survivors and is associated with a decreased quality of life. ICH patients should be screened for and treated for depression (78).

Rehabilitation is often necessary in patients with hemorrhagic stroke to allow them to reach their maximum functional recovery. Most of the literature related to stroke and rehabilitation focuses on the ischemic stroke patient only. Because of secondary injury and prolonged edema, the ideal type of rehabilitation and timing of rehabilitation in ICH patients are areas in need of research.

To prevent the recurrence of ICH, risk factors must be modified. Blood pressure should be controlled and tobacco use, illegal drug use, and heavy alcohol use should be stopped. These risk factor modifications should be a part of the acute management of the patient with ICH and incorporated into their discharge plan (59).

ICH patient management remains an area of active research. Current studies are investigating the role of hypertonic saline and statin therapy. Hypertonic saline to maintain elevated levels of serum sodium may be helpful in decreasing cerebral edema (58). There is also some evidence that statin use prior to ICH may have a protective effect on the patient and some suggestion that statins administered during the acute phase of ICH may improve outcomes. More research is needed regarding these medications (79).

Traumatic Brain and Spinal Cord Injury
Etiology

TBI accounts for over 1 million emergency department visits annually in the United States, resulting in more than 200,000 hospitalizations and 50,000 deaths (80). TBI generally affects more men than women and is most commonly seen during teenage and elderly years (80). Falls, motor vehicle accidents, being struck or hit, and assault are the most common causes of TBI (81). It is estimated that TBI costs the nation over $56 billion a year, and survivors of TBI often manage lifelong disabilities (82). TBI is generally divided into mild and severe. Mild TBI is characterized by a higher GCS, whereas severe TBI is generally defined as neurologic injury from trauma resulting in a GCS score less 8 than (81, 107). Spinal cord trauma (TSCI) most commonly results from motor vehicle crashes, falls, assaults, and sporting injuries (83). TSCI is classified according to spinal location (83). There are approximately 10,000 new spinal cord injuries each year, and this estimate may be low as many patients do not report their injury (83). Advancements in the management of TBI and TSCI have resulted in a drastic decrease in mortality associated with trauma (84). Increased knowledge in supportive management and prevention of secondary injury is thought to account for this decline.

Pathophysiology

As discussed in the section on elevated ICP, the cornerstone of TBI and TSCI pathophysiology is the primary and secondary injury to the brain. The primary injury is the direct neuronal injury caused by the trauma event. Secondary injury is the metabolic processes that occur over minutes, hours, and days after the primary injury. Secondary injury includes the development of cerebral edema, decreased cerebral blood flow, release of excitatory neurotransmitters, and breakdown of the blood-brain barrier that results in elevated ICP, infarction, and hemorrhage (2). Nursing and medical interventions in the time immediately following the trauma and during the disease progression are aimed at mitigating the secondary injury (2).

Clinical Presentation

Mild TBI is characterized by a GCS score greater than 8 to 13 with any period of observed or self-reported transient confusion, disorientation, impaired consciousness, dysfunction of memory, or loss of consciousness lasting less than 30 minutes. The term "concussion" is often used for mild TBI. Concussion is graded according to severity. Grade 1 concussion is characterized by transient confusion lasting less than 15 minutes and no loss of consciousness. Grade 2 concussion is characterized by transient confusion lasting longer than 15 minutes with no loss of consciousness, and Grade 3 concussion is characterized by a loss of consciousness of any duration. TBI is graded as severe once GCS score drops below 8. Collecting a detailed history of events surrounding the trauma and any fluctuations in level of consciousness may reveal important clues to diagnosis and complications to expect following the trauma.

TSCI is classified according to the American Spinal Injury Association (ASIA) scale. The ASIA scale grades the injury according to location, complete or incomplete injury, and motor and sensory function. ASIA criteria result in a score of A to E.

Diagnosis

Diagnosis of TBI is largely based on the history of a traumatic event involving the head and any decrease in level of consciousness or focal neurologic deficit. CT and MRI may reveal intracerebral, subarachnoid, epidural, or subdural hemorrhage as well as contusion and cerebral edema. Diagnosis of TSCI is based on history and neurologic deficit in combination with CT and MRI of the spinal cord to assess structure and stability. Atraumatic SCI should be ruled out as a cause of neurologic deficits.

Management

Guidelines from the Brain Trauma Foundation (BTF) help to set the standard and guide the management of TBI. Evan a single prehospital or intrahospital episode of hypotension or hypoxia is associated with worse outcomes in patients with TBI and should be avoided. Blood pressure should be closely monitored, and systolic blood pressure should be maintained above 90 mm Hg. Oxygenation should also be closely monitored, and oxygen saturation below 90% or PaO_2 below 60 mm Hg should be avoided (81). If ICP is elevated in the setting of TBI, a stepwise approach to the management of elevated ICP should be used as discussed elsewhere in the chapter. TBI evidence supports the use of mannitol therapy if ICP is elevated at doses between 0.25 and 1 g/kg provided hypotension is avoided. Prolonged hyperventilation and steroids should be avoided in TBI patients (81). Studies are ongoing regarding the usefulness of hypertonic saline in TBI with elevated ICP (81). ICP should be monitored in patients with TBI and a GCS score between 3 and 8 and abnormal findings on CT (81). Even with a normal CT scan, ICP monitoring should be considered if the patient is over age 40 or has unilateral or bilateral posturing or hypotension (81). ICP treatment threshold is debated and may be patient specific (81). Studies have shown that patients with ICP maintained at less than 20 mm Hg did better overall than patients with ICP greater than 20 mm Hg (81).

CPP should be monitored and fluid resuscitation and pressor therapy initiated if CPP falls below 50 mm Hg. Maintaining CPP greater than 70 mm Hg is associated with the development of adult respiratory distress syndrome (ARDS) (81). Brain oxygen monitoring may be helpful in patients with TBI. Jugular venous saturation below 50% or brain tissue oxygen level less than 15 mm Hg warrants further investigation as to the cause and consideration for treatment (81). TBI patients who are agitated or in pain may experience higher elevations in ICP, blood pressure, and temperature (81). Barbiturates and analgesics should be provided as needed to minimize pain and agitation (81). High-dose barbiturates or propofol may be considered for patients with elevated ICP that is refractory to other treatment (81).

Several studies have evaluated the usefulness of induced hypothermia in TBI with mixed results. At this time, the induction of induced hypothermia to minimize secondary injury in TBI is not supported by the literature (81). However, mild induced hypothermia may be useful to decrease elevated ICP that is refractory to other treatments (81). DVT is a common complication of immobility associated with TBI, and patients should receive early and ongoing DVT prophylaxis. Intermittent pneumatic compression devices are helpful in preventing DVT formation (100). Low-molecular-weight heparin or low-dose unfractionated heparin should be used in addition to mechanical compression devices (100). There is debate regarding how quickly to start pharmacologic DVT prophylaxis, particularly if the patient has intracranial hemorrhage associated with their TBI (100).

Continuous enteral nutrition begun within the first several days of hospitalization is associated with better outcomes in TBI patients. Maintaining normoglycemia is also associated with better outcomes (81). Patients with a blood glucose greater than 110 mg/dL should be considered for aggressive glucose management provided hypoglycemic episodes are avoided (81). Seizures may increase ICP and have been shown to occur in both the early and late phases of TBI (81). However, there is debate regarding the role of seizure prophylaxis in patients with TBI. Current consensus is that seizure prophylaxis is indicated for the prevention of early TBI-related seizures but should not be continued beyond 7 days unless seizure activity has occurred (81).

Patients with TSCI should be placed in cervical collar immobilization as soon as possible to prevent any additional damage and should remain immobilized until images of the injury are obtained (83). Patients with high cervical spine injury will require mechanical ventilation (83). Additional management of secondary injury should be carried out according to the BTF guidelines. Patients with TSCI may require surgical decompression (83). There is debate over the ideal timing of surgical decompression. Nevertheless, all TSCI patients should be evaluated emergently by a neurosurgical team (83). Studies on the use of corticosteroids in TSCI have yielded mixed results. Currently, the use of methylprednisolone is considered a treatment option in TSCI. If a patient is treated with corticosteroids, careful management of side effects such as hyperglycemia must be considered (83).

The use of hypothermia in TSCI gained national attention when it was used in the high-profile football injury of Kevin Everett in 2007. His dramatic recovery was credited by many to the rapid induction of hypothermia following his injury (83). However, there have been no randomized controlled trials in humans supporting the use of induced hypothermia in TSCI. Current consensus is that there is not enough scientific evidence to encourage standard use of therapeutic hypothermia in this patient population (83).

Autonomic dysreflexia (AD) is a complication often seen in patients with TSCI above the level of T5 (85). AD is characterized by an increase in systolic blood pressure greater than 20 to 30 mm Hg and may be accompanied by tachycardia or bradycardia, flushing, and headache. If left untreated, AD may result in dangerously high blood pressure, intracranial hemorrhage, seizures, and death (85). AD is often triggered by pain, constipation, and an overextended bladder. AD may be minimized by regular catheterization to prevent an overdistended bladder, an aggressive bowel regimen to prevent stool impaction, and prevention of pain. Management of AD includes removing the source of irritation as quickly as possible. If this is not effective in decreasing the blood pressure, calcium channel blockers or nitrates are often used to decrease blood pressure, although randomized trials are lacking in this area (85).

Patients with high cervical cord injury may have episodes of neurogenic shock characterized by hypotension caused by low systemic vascular resistance (83). Episodes of hypotension should be aggressively treated with fluid resuscitation and vasopressors to maintain a systolic blood pressure of 90 mm Hg (83). Dopamine may be helpful as it increases blood pressure and heart rate. A key to preventing neurogenic shock after TSCI is maintaining adequate hydration (83).

Safety Issues

A major patient safety issue surrounding trauma care is the overall availability of care. Trauma care is a highly specialized area requiring investment of hospital resources in maintaining trauma designation and high-quality care. Lack of trauma services results in increased time to treatment and increased mortality for patients experiencing brain or spinal cord trauma. In addition, coordination of the entire care team from the prehospital setting through hospital discharge is associated with better patient outcomes. A study of the emergency medical services showed that no documentation of the prehospital scene was significantly associated with higher mortality (84). This indicates that when critical information is not communicated from the prehospital team to the hospital trauma team, patients suffer the consequences.

Another study related to safely delivering trauma care reviewed the presence of management errors at a major trauma center (86). The study revealed that even in a trauma center with established protocols, order sets, and continuous quality improvement, management errors occurred in 10% of trauma patients. Errors were most common in the emergency department and the operating room during the critical resuscitation phase (86). A similar study yielded similar findings and estimated that between three and five errors occur per trauma patient (87). This patient population is tremendously complex with opportunities for error that have serious impact on patient outcomes (86, 87).

Clinical Nurse Specialist Competencies and Spheres of Influence

Clinical Expert/Direct Care and Consultation

There is evidence that following the BTF guidelines for management of TBI improves patient mortality and morbidity (80). The coordination of care and development of clinical pathways and order sets based on guidelines and consensus statements are key roles of the CNS in many hospital settings. By acting as consultant and expert clinician, the CNS has the opportunity to work with the multidisciplinary team to standardize care and ensure guideline-based care.

Coaching/Teaching/Mentoring

Through the role of educator, the CNS may work to mentor the bedside nurse and lead other advanced practice nurses and colleagues on the multidisciplinary team in guideline-based care of TBI patients. CNSs often develop patient education materials and learning packets for staff.

Disorders of the Neuromuscular Junction

The neuromuscular junction, also known as the motor end plate, is the junction where the efferent neuron innervates the motor nerve fiber, initiating the action potential that results in muscle contraction. The process of muscle contractions occurs through calcium-mediated channels and is dependent on acetylcholine. The neuromuscular junction is beyond the protection of the blood-brain barrier and vulnerable to antibody-mediated attack. Antibodies from an autoimmune-mediated attack against receptors and channels in the neuromuscular junction are responsible for myasthenia gravis and Guillain-Barré syndrome (88).

Neuromuscular diseases encompasses multiple diagnoses including multiple sclerosis, amyotrophic lateral sclerosis (ALS, also sometimes referred to as Lou Gehrig's disease), Guillain-Barré, chronic inflammatory demyelinating polyneuropathy (CIDP), muscular dystrophy, and myasthenia gravis. Because multiple sclerosis, muscular dystrophy, and CIDP are primarily outpatient-managed diseases, they will be covered only briefly in this section.

Guillain-Barré Syndrome
Etiology
Guillain-Barré syndrome was initially described by French Drs. Guillain, Barré, and Strohl in 1916 as they detailed the development and spontaneous recovery of acute paralysis with areflexia. Since then the disease has been called Guillain-Barré (89). In the past, Guillain-Barré was recognized as a single disease entity. However, with increased research and understanding, Guillain-Barré is now recognized as a syndrome composed of multiple subtypes that all likely exist on a continuum of acute neuropathies. Much remains unknown and misunderstood regarding these diseases. For the purposes of this chapter, the Guillain-Barré subtypes will be discussed as they are most often hospitalized with a brief mention of deciphering the Guillain-Barré subtypes from CIDP.

Guillain-Barré is a rare disorder, but the most common cause of acute flaccid paralysis (90). With an incidence of one to three cases per 100,000 persons, Guillain-Barré occurs across all ages, with a slightly higher incidence in young adults and the elderly. Guillain-Barré is often described as having a bimodal onset as the disease increases with age, with a slight rise in young adults as well. Guillain-Barré occurs in men more than in women, and there is a slightly higher incidence in Caucasians in the United States (90). There is an increased risk and incidence in those who are immunocompromised, and there is some evidence that there is an increased risk of Guillain-Barré right after giving birth while the incidence is lower during pregnancy (90). There is no true geographic pattern to Guillain-Barré, although there may be clusters of cases after breakouts of bacterial or viral illness (90).

Causes
Seventy-five percent of patients with Guillain-Barré have a preceding viral or bacterial infection (91). The preceding disease is thought to be a trigger of the autoimmune response, not a direct cause of neuron breakdown (91). *Campylobacter jejuni* is the most common preceding bacterial infection. It is generally associated with bacterial enteritis in the United States, and the number of cases is on the rise. In the United States, *C. jejuni* is now more common than *Salmonella* or *Shigella* as a source of bacterial enteritis. *C. jejuni* is associated with eating raw or undercooked meat (specifically poultry), unpasteurized milk, home-canned foods, and foods that are prepared either in or out of the home. It is also found in contaminated water (91). The second most common bacterial infection associated with the development of Guillain-Barré is *Mycoplasma pneumoniae*, which generally results in an upper respiratory tract illness (91).

Cytomegalovirus (CMV), Epstein-Barr virus (EBV), and human immunodeficiency virus (HIV) are the viral infections most commonly associated with the development of Guillain-Barré (91). CMV is the most common preceding viral infection. However, CMV is often a silent virus so its role may be underappreciated. CMV infection seems to be more common in younger women and is associated with increased Guillain-Barré severity with cranial nerve palsy, severe sensory loss, respiratory complications, and liver disease (91). EBV is suspected to be associated with Guillain-Barré but has not been well studied. HIV is associated with Guillain-Barré most commonly before and during seroconversion (91). Many HIV patients are coinfected with CMV, so the exact role coinfection plays in the development of Guillain-Barré is unknown (91). HIV-associated Guillain-Barré is associated with recurrence of Guillain-Barré and also with the development of chronic IDP. Viruses such as herpes simplex virus (HSV) I and II; *Haemophilus influenzae* A and B; hepatitis A, B, C, and D; and the varicella-zoster viruses (VZV) are less frequent but still associated with the development of Guillain-Barré (91).

One of the more controversial causes of Guillain-Barré is the role of vaccination in the development of the disease (91). The 1992 to 1994 seasons of flu vaccine were particularly implicated in the development of Guillain-Barré. When studied, these flu vaccines were found to have a risk of one to two cases per 1 million vaccines administered. According to the Centers for Disease Control and Prevention, the risk of contracting severe flu is greater than the risk of developing vaccine-related Guillain-Barré (91). The widespread swine flu vaccination in the late 1970s was also associated with 8 or 9 cases of Guillain-Barré per 1 million people vaccinated (91). Overall, when evaluating the role of vaccination in the development of Guillain-Barré, studies have established an overall association but not established a true causation (111). More research is needed regarding the risk/benefit of disease versus the development of Guillain-Barré. Other vaccines have been identified as possible triggers of Guillain-Barré, but more studies are needed to identify association. They include polio, rabies, tetanus, MMR, DTP, hepatitis B, hepatitis A, and meningitis (91).

The role of a genetic link in the development of Guillain-Barré is highly debatable. Some cases of familial Guillain-Barré have been identified, but they are quite rare (91).

Economic Considerations

Guillain-Barré is associated with a high economic impact in the United States related to disability and death (92). The disease costs $1.7 billion annually, with $0.2 billion related to hospital admissions and the remaining $1.5 billion related to indirect costs such as premature death. Per patient, the mean cost of Guillain-Barré is estimated to be $318,966 (92).

Mortality

Between 4% and 15% of patients with Guillain-Barré will die from the disorder (91). This has decreased over the past decades with improved intensive care of complications such as respiratory failure and cardiac rhythm abnormalities (91). Major causes of death include infection, pulmonary embolism, and cardiac rhythm disturbances, and death is seen mostly in mechanically ventilated patients (91, 92). Twenty percent of patients have persistent disability. Advanced age is associated with worse outcomes (92). In immunotherapy studies of patients who were unable to walk, a full 20% remained unable to walk unaided at 6 months (93). The Erasmus Guillain-Barré Syndrome Outcome Score (EGOS) can be used to predict the chance of independent walking at 6 months. This score uses age, symptom severity at peak of disease, and presence or absence of diarrhea to predict chance of independent walking at 6 months (90).

Pathophysiology

Guillain-Barré is an autoimmune disease process, although the exact mechanism by which the autoimmune system is activated is not fully understood. Several theories have been postulated, one being that it is a process of molecular mimicry whereby the immune system mistakes similar proteins in the peripheral nervous system for a recent antigen from an infection and institutes an inflammatory reaction. This has been supported by the isolation of lipo-oligosaccharides of *C. jejuni* that mimic carbohydrates of gangliosides, suggesting a similarity between the carbohydrates that may be mistaken by the immune system (89). Antibodies and activated T cells infiltrate the nerves and activate the immune response. Macrophages invade the Schwann cells and strip the myelin sheath from the axon. Degeneration of the actual axon may occur and motor or sensory nerves may also degenerate (in part explaining the differences in variants of Guillain-Barré) (89, 91).

Guillain-Barré is a syndrome, not a disease. At least three forms of Guillain-Barré have been identified. In the United States, 95% of Guillain-Barré cases are acute demyelinating polyradiculoneuropathy (AIDP), while the other 5% are either acute axonal motor disorder or acute sensory and motor axonal neuropathy (91). The distribution of Guillain-Barré variants varies across continents. AIDP Guillain-Barré may have components of Miller-Fisher syndrome (MFS), which is an inflammatory neuropathy that affects cranial nerves that innervate eye muscles. Conversely, MFS may exist on its own (94). As advances in the understanding of the disease have revealed various subtypes of Guillain-Barré, classification of the disease has varied from source to source. Some classify the subtypes into five distinctly different variants of Guillain-Barré, while others subclassify several subtypes as forms of AIDP (94).

AIDP is an antibody-mediated autoimmune variant of Guillain-Barré generally triggered by infection or vaccination, as already discussed. Inflammatory demyelination of the nerves is present, and remyelination occurs after cessation of immune reaction. Acute motor axonal neuropathy (AMAN) is a subtype of AIDP and is most often associated with *C. jejuni* infection. Neuropathy in AMAN is a pure axonal form. AMAN most often affects children and recovery is rapid. Antiganglioside antibodies are present (94). AMAN may be an extreme case of AIDP, or some argue it may be a separate Guillain-Barré subtype (94). Acute motor sensory axonal neuropathy (AMSAN) is another subtype of AIDP with minimal inflammation and demyelination of myelinated motor and sensory fibers. AMSAN most often affects adults and affects both motor and sensory nerves and roots. Acute panautonomic neuropathy (APN) is the rarest of all AIDP subtypes. Recovery is generally gradual and incomplete. APN involves sympathetic and parasympathetic nerves and may also have cardiac involvement.

MFS is a rare subtype of Guillain-Barré. Demylination and inflammation of cranial nerves III and IV as well as spinal ganglia and peripheral nerves are present. This results in rapid ataxia, areflexia, limb weakness, and ophthalmoplegia. Proprioception may be impaired, but sensory loss is not common. This subtype is most closely associated with antiganglioside antibodies (94). MFS generally resolves in 1 to 3 months.

Subacute inflammatory demyelinating polyneuropathy or CIDP is classified as taking longer than 4 weeks to reach maximum symptoms. CIDP is thought to behave differently than AIDP or other Guillain-Barré variants and thought to be a different, although possibly related, disease process (89). In addition to taking longer than 4 weeks to reach maximal symptoms, CIDP is defined as a clinical course longer than 8 weeks. A subacute disease somewhere between Guillain-Barré and CIDP has been proposed and is sometimes referred to as acute-onset CIDP (A-CIDP). Patients with an initial diagnosis of Guillain-Barré may cross over into this diagnosis if the course of their disease is unusually long or they do not respond to conventional treatment as expected (89). More research is needed in this area to help decipher between Guillain-Barré recurrences, treatment-related fluctuation, and A-CIDP/CIDP (89). These diseases likely lie along a clinical spectrum based on immune reaction (89). More research is also needed to identify the exact inflammatory processes involved with each subtype of Guillain-Barré.

Clinical Presentation

Guillain-Barré encompasses a range of presentations from mild to life-threatening paralysis (91). Presentation is characterized by acute-onset, symmetrical weakness in the arms or legs with or without sensory or cranial nerve involvement that is usually accompanied by hyporeflexia or areflexia. These symptoms occur in the absence of CSF pathology that would explain the development of symptoms (89). Early symptoms include pain, numbness, paresthesia, and/or weakness that then evolves over the course of weeks and peaks in severity within 4 weeks (and most often within 2 weeks) of initial symptoms (89, 90). After the peak severity of symptoms, the symptoms generally plateau and then the patient enters a recovery phase. The progression of weakness, plateau, and recovery varies greatly from patient to patient (95).

Limb weakness from Guillain-Barré involves both proximal and distal nerves. In very mild forms of the disease, patients may have only distal involvement (95). The degree of sensory involvement is variable from patient to patient (95). Reflexes are often lost early in the disease course, with the possible exception of AMAN, where reflexes may be preserved (95). Autonomic dysfunction signs such as tachycardia and other cardiac arrhythmias, hypertension or hypotension, abnormal hemodynamic response to drugs, sweating abnormalities, pupillary abnormalities, and bladder and bowel dysfunction are present in over 60% of Guillain-Barré cases (90, 95). Thirty-three percent of patients will develop respiratory failure. Therefore, monitoring vital capacity is very important as many patients will not develop dyspnea or hypoxia until late in failure (95). Cranial nerve weakness and bulbar palsy may be present (95). The clinical presentation varies from case to case and occasionally may be atypical and present with unilateral weakness or weakness only in the arms. Therefore, Guillain-Barré must be considered as a differential diagnosis in any person who develops acute weakness (95).

Diagnosis

Differential diagnosis for Guillain-Barré includes hypokalemia, polymyositis, transverse myelitis, porphyria, and lead poisoning (90). Nerve conduction tests are abnormal in 85% of patients with Guillain-Barré. Nerve conduction will show conduction block, prolonged distal latencies, and delayed F waves (90). Conduction is usually abnormal early in the disease but should be repeated after 2 weeks in a patient with a normal test but high index of suspicion for Guillain-Barré. Motor conduction velocities are normal early but slow later in the course of the disease.

CSF testing in Guillain-Barré will reveal elevated protein that is specific to the disease but not sensitive as many disease processes other than Guillain-Barré result in elevated CSF protein (95). Protein elevates in the second week of the disease, so CSF levels obtained early may not show any abnormality. In Guillain-Barré, the protein is elevated in the setting of a normal white blood cell count. Further CSF abnormalities warrant additional work-up for a cause other than Guillain-Barré (90). Serum antiganglioside antibodies or antibodies to *C. jejuni* are not routinely performed and probably do not aid in initial diagnosis but may be helpful in specific cases (95).

Management
Immunotherapy

Mildly affected patients, those who are able to walk aided or unaided, and those who have remained stable for 2 weeks or longer will likely remain stable and not progress. These patients are generally managed as outpatients (110). Guillain-Barré patients are admitted to the hospital and often the ICU if the disease is progressing and there is threat of respiratory failure (95). The mainstay of treatment is immunotherapy with either plasma exchange or intravenous immunoglobulin (IVIg). Plasma exchange was first studied in Guillain-Barré in the late 1970s. In the studies, plasma exchange was effective when applied early in the disease course, ideally within the first 2 weeks (95). Plasma exchange is performed five times in 2 weeks, with a total exchange of five plasma volumes (93). IVIg was studied in 1992 and shown to be as effective as plasma exchange (93). IVIg is administered at a dosage of 0.4 g/kg over 5 consecutive days (93). Since the introduction of IVIg, it has slowly become the treatment of choice despite equal efficacy compared to plasma exchange, most likely due to convenience and availability. When comparing the treatments, there is debate over short- and long-term outcomes as well as side effects and complications. IVIg is associated with fewer short- and long-term complications but is more costly in the short term (95). The benefits and risks of each treatment modality should be compared and weighed on an individual basis. Studies have shown there is no significant difference in outcomes between plasma exchange and IVIg, and the combination of plasma exchange and IVIg was not significantly better than either treatment modality alone (93). Looking at practice patterns across the United States, IVIg is overall the preferred treatment modality. However, plasma exchange is still used preferentially in older patients and those with pulmonary or infectious complications (93).

When patients do not respond to the initial treatment choice, a logical question is if the patient would benefit from the other treatment. IVIg following plasma exchange has been studied and not found to improve outcome. However, plasma exchange following IVIg has not been studied and no data exist to guide this treatment choice. Some reason that plasma exchange after IVIg would wash out the IVIg and be of no benefit. For patients who continue to deteriorate despite treatment, one argument for continued deterioration is a prolonged immune attack that, in theory, may benefit from extended immunotherapy. But little is known about why some patients continue to deteriorate and why some respond quickly, and little literature exists to guide their care (114). From 5% to 10% of patients deteriorate after a period of initial stabilization or even improvement of their symptoms. Clinical practice is to give these patients a second course of IVIg, although this has never been studied in a randomized controlled trial. A trial evaluating the role of a second course of IVIg in patients who continue to deteriorate is under way (93).

There is some debate over how to treat patients with "mild" disease, meaning they can walk with or without assistance (93). IVIg has not been tested on patients who were minimally affected by the disease, and only small case studies exist evaluating the benefit of plasma exchange in mild cases. To date, no randomized controlled studies exist to guide the management of these patients. However, those with mild disease often have residual deficits. There may be an indication to treat patients with minimal disease, but literature is lacking.

Most patients with MFS have good outcomes and a full functional recovery. Observational studies have evaluated the effect of IVIg and plasma exchange in MFS and concluded that immunotherapy did not have a significant effect and patients tended to do well overall (93). In patients with MFS overlapping another subtype of Guillain-Barré, treatment may be warranted but no literature exists specific to this patient population (93).

Intravenous and oral steroids, alone or in combination with IVIg, proved to be of no benefit in Guillain-Barré outcomes (93). However, they are the treatment of choice in CIDP. Therefore, it is very important to distinguish between the diseases.

Supportive Care

Guillain-Barré patients are at high risk for the development of venous thromboembolism because of immobility. Sequential compression devices and unfractionated or fractionated heparin are recommended for nonambulating patients (92). All Guillain-Barré patients should be monitored for autonomic insufficiency. Blood pressure and pulse should be frequently monitored in patients until they no longer require ventilatory support and are past the most acute phases of the disease (93). Care should be taken in administering medications with hemodynamic effects as patients may have an exaggerated response. As a

result, hypertension is often tolerated and treated only gently in clinical practice. Bradyarrhythmias and other cardiac arrhythmias must be managed and may require transcutaneous pacemaker and/or atropine (93).

All hospitalized patients should be monitored for respiratory failure (92). Serial vital capacity should be monitored as well as clinical assessment for distress, including tachypnea, diaphoresis, use of accessory respiratory muscles, or respiratory muscle dyssynchrony. Rapid disease progression, bulbar facial palsy, and autonomic dysfunction are associated with respiratory failure and need for intubation and mechanical ventilation. Inability to cough or raise the head off of the bed is also associated with need for mechanical ventilation. A rapid decline in vital capacity or a forced vital capacity of less than 20 mL/kg is concerning for respiratory failure, but more studies are needed to better define clinical parameters associated with respiratory failure. Vital capacity values need to be put in the context of the clinical picture of the patient. Once the patient is intubated and mechanically ventilated, weaning from the ventilator can be guided by patients improving strength as assessed by serial pulmonary function tests (92).

Patients with respiratory failure and continued need for mechanical ventilation should be considered for tracheostomy (92). There is debate over the benefits versus the risks of early tracheostomy. Guillain-Barré is associated with a mean duration of ventilation between 15 and 43 days depending on the study. Current recommendations are to monitor respiratory recovery for 14 days and then pursue tracheostomy if there is no significant improvement in pulmonary function tests.

All Guillain-Barré patients should receive early nutrition (92). Because the disease process can affect bulbar function, patients should be assessed for dysphagia and interventions initiated aimed at prevention of aspiration.

Pain is often reported in patients with Guillain-Barré, and pain management is an important element of supportive care (92). Pain is reported early in the disease course in as many as 71% of patients and throughout the disease course in as many as 89% of patients, with over half of patients reporting the pain as severe. Pain may be different during different courses of the disease and may include parasthesia, dysaethesia, backache, muscle pain, joint pain, and visceral pain (93). Theoretically, pain during the acute phase is nociceptive because of inflammation, which then progresses to non-nociceptive neuropathic pain as the disease advances and nerves degenerate and regenerate (93). Small studies have examined using gabapentin and carbamazepine and found some relief in the neuropathic pain. These may be used in addition to simple analgesia and nonsteroidal anti-inflammatory medications. Care must be taken in patients receiving narcotics as they may aggravate the autonomic instability (92).

Bowel dysfunction, constipation, and ileus are all complications of Guillain-Barré as a result of both immobility as well as autonomic dysfunction. An aggressive bowel plan is necessary. Avoid promotility agents in patients with dysautonomia. Bladder catheterization is often necessary in the acute phase of the disease, and a bladder regimen may be necessary depending on functional recovery (92). As many as 30% of patients may have urinary dysfunction after the acute phase of the disease, with 10% experiencing retention (96).

Rehabilitation is often necessary in Guillain-Barré patients but not at all well studied in this patient population. Rehabilitation requires a complex care plan and must balance the need to maintain or regain strength with the risk of overfatigue of the affected nerves (92). Throughout the hospital stay, active nursing interventions should be implemented to prevent the complications of immobility (92).

Severe fatigue is present in up to 80% of patients even as the motor function is regained. The mechanism behind the prolonged fatigue is not clearly understood. Exercise has proved to be useful in small studies and pharmacologic interventions are currently being studied (92).

Because of the role vaccination may play in the development of Guillain-Barré, there is often a question about immunizations post Guillain-Barré. Current recommendation is that the patient with active Guillain-Barré should avoid immunization during the acute phase of the disease and probably after the disease, although an exact time has not been studied. It has been suggested to avoid vaccination for 1 year after disease and then administer immunization as needed on a case-by-case basis (92).

Myasthenia Gravis
Etiology
Myasthenia gravis has a history that dates back several centuries. The initial description of a myasthenia gravis–like condition was that of Native American Chief "Eagle Plume" Opencancanough, who died in 1664. He was described as experiencing bouts of excessive fatigue. In 1672, English physician Thomas Willis described a fatigable weakness in the limbs and bulbar muscles. In the 1800s, additional case reports shaped what we now know as myasthenia gravis. The name "myasthenia gravis" comes from the Greek (*myasthenia* means "muscle weakness" and *gravis* means "severe"). It was recognized in the 1930s that myasthenia gravis symptoms were similar to those of curare poisoning, which was treated at the time with the cholinesterase inhibitor physostigmine. Physicians experimented with treating myasthenia gravis with physostigmine, and anticholinesterase drugs have been a mainstay of myasthenia gravis treatment since.

The incidence of myasthenia gravis is 3 to 4 million cases per year (98). Incidence is equal between genders in children through puberty. Between puberty and middle-age, women are three times more affected then men. However, after age 50, men are affected more than

women (120). Myasthenia gravis occurs with a prevalence of 20 cases per 100,000 people. This has increased over time and is thought to be due to both improved disease recognition and an overall increase in average life span and survival of myasthenia gravis patients (98). There does appear to be some geographic variation to the disease throughout the world as childhood-onset myasthenia gravis is much more common in Asian countries (98).

Pathophysiology
Myasthenia gravis is an autoimmune disorder that results in destruction of the postsynaptic nicotinic acetylcholine receptor of skeletal muscles (97). In a healthy individual, muscle movement is initiated when an action potential is carried down a motor neuron from the ventral horn of the spinal cord, down the peripheral nerve to the skeletal muscle cell. The action potential results in the release of acetylcholine (ACTH) into the synaptic cleft where ACTH binds with the ACTH receptor, causing the contraction of the muscle fiber and continued spreading of the action potential down the muscle fibers. In a healthy individual, far more ACTH is released than is needed to initiate muscle contraction and the additional ACTH is inactivated by acetylcholinesterase (97). In myasthenia gravis, an autoimmune process targeted at destruction of the postsynaptic ACTH receptors results in less action potential to initiate skeletal muscle movement. Bulbar and extraocular muscles are more susceptible to this process as they have less postsynaptic ACTH receptors to begin with and they fire at a higher frequency than fast-twitch skeletal muscle fibers. Further, extraocular muscles and muscles of bulbar function are more susceptible to the activation of an autoimmune response. As a result, muscles of bulbar function and extraocular muscles are often involved in myasthenia gravis symptomatology (97).

As more is learned about myasthenia gravis, it is clear this is not a homogeneous disease process. Several subtypes of myasthenia gravis have been identified, and the actual autoimmune process is likely very specific to the subtype of myasthenia gravis that the patient portrays. The immune process, the resulting symptoms, age of onset, and antibodies all differ among the subtypes, as does prognosis (98, 99). Early-onset myasthenia gravis has an age of onset less than 40 and is associated with thymic hyperplasia, and patients are positive for ACTH receptor antibodies. In this subtype, the thymus, an immune organ, is implicated in the triggering of the autoimmune process, and these patients generally show abnormal thymus histology.

Late-onset myasthenia gravis occurs at an age greater than 40. In these patients, the thymus is normal. Patients with late-onset myasthenia gravis are positive for the ACTH receptor as well as titin and ryanodine receptor antibodies. Although the thymus generally does not show abnormal histology in this version of myasthenia gravis, it is believed the thymus is still involved as a trigger of the autoimmune process. In these patients, thymus activity may be suppressed, possibly by antitumor autoimmune processes.

Patients with a thymoma as the cause of their myasthenia gravis generally have an age of onset between 40 and 60 (98, 100). These patients exhibit a thymic neoplasia and are positive for the ACTH receptor as well as the titin, ryanodine receptor, and KCNA4 antibodies.

Anti-MUSK myasthenia gravis occurs in patients less than 40 years of age (98, 100). This subtype of myasthenia gravis exhibits normal thymus histology and normal antibodies, with the exception of positive MUSK antibodies. This form is disproportionately found in women and tends to present with selective oropharyngeal, facial, and respiratory weakness. MUSK is a postsynaptic polypeptide involved in the signaling pathway of the neuromuscular junction. Breakdown of the MUSK pathway results in reduced number of functional ACTH receptors.

Seronegative generalized myasthenia gravis has a variable age of onset and thymic hyperplasia in some but negative antibodies. There is some thought that antibodies may be present in these patients, but just at a low enough level that it is not identified on current serology tests. Finally, ocular myasthenia gravis is a subtype that has an adult onset in the United States and Europe and childhood onset in Asia (98, 100). The level of thymic involvement in ocular myasthenia gravis is unknown. ACTH receptor antibodies are positive in 50% of patients.

Clinical Presentation

The hallmark symptom of myasthenia gravis is fatigable weakness, most often involving more susceptible muscle groups such as bulbar functions and facial muscles (97). Presentation depends in part on subtype and severity. Weakness tends to fluctuate from day to day and even hour to hour, is worse with activity, and is improved with rest. Initial presentation most often includes ocular weakness and ptosis, which occur in 85% of patients. Occasionally, myasthenia gravis crisis and respiratory failure of unknown origin are the presenting symptoms, although this is not typical (97).

Neurologic deficit may include ocular symptoms such as ptosis, generally asymmetrical, fatigue with upgaze or diplopia (93, 97, 99). Bulbar symptoms may include dysarthria with a nasal quality to speech, dysphagia (often painless), excessive clearing of throat, recurrent pneumonias, dysphonia (hoarseness), and masticatory weakness (jaw fatigue particularly with jaw closing). Facial symptoms include incomplete eyelid closure (inability to bury eyelashes with forced eye closure) and lower facial weakness with poor cheek puff and/or drooling. Limb muscles may be weak with primarily proximal weakness, which is often symmetrical, with arms more affected than legs. The neck may be weak in both flexion and extension. As mentioned previously, when the respiratory muscles are involved, respiratory symptoms may include exertional dyspnea, orthopnea, tachypnea, and overall respiratory failure. Most patients will reach the maximum severity of their weakness within 2 years. From 10% to 20% will experience a myasthenia gravis crisis, which also generally occurs within the first 2 years as severity of symptoms reach their peak.

Diagnosis

Differential diagnoses include: Lambert-Eaton syndrome, botulism (rapid descending pattern, pupillary and autonomic involvement), motor neuron disease, mitochondrial disorders, AIDP, and thyroid disorder (99).

Several diagnostic tests may be useful in making the diagnosis of myasthenia gravis. Bedside testing includes an edrophonium chloride challenge and the ice pack test. Edrophonium chloride is a short-acting acetylcholinesterase inhibitor that increases the duration of time that ACTH exists in the synaptic cleft. Edrophonium can be administered intravenusly at the bedside and the patient is observed for clinical improvement. This test is not as sensitive in generalized myasthenia gravis disease but may be helpful in patients with ptosis or extraocular weakness. Complications include bradycardia and syncope, so patients should be monitored while the test is conducted. In the ice pack test, an ice pack can be placed over an eye for 2 to 5 minutes and the patient is observed for improvement. This is not well tested and appears to be useful only in patients with ptosis. However, it may be considered in a patient with ocular signs of myasthenia gravis who is unable to tolerate the edrophonium test.

Serologic testing is a standard diagnostic test to detect ACTH receptor antibodies or antibodies against muscle proteins such as actin or striational protein (99). Presence of the ACTH receptor antibody confirms the diagnosis of myasthenia gravis, but its absence does not refute the diagnosis. Depending on the type of myasthenia gravis, detection of ACTH receptor antibodies has differing sensitivity and specificity (99). Patients with generalized myasthenia gravis will have ACTH receptor antibodies 80% of time, whereas ocular myasthenia gravis will only have positive antibodies 50% of the time. Values vary widely throughout the course of the disease, and levels are not used to monitor progression or severity of disease. False-negative results may occur in immunocompromised patients and those who are tested too early in the course of the disease (99). ACTH receptor antibodies should be measured on all patients with myasthenia gravis. In patients who are ACTH receptor antibody negative, they are tested for the presence of several other serum antibodies (99). Forty percent of patients who are ACTH receptor antibody negative will have anti-MUSK antibodies; 5% of patients will be ACTH receptor antibody and anti-MUSK antibody negative (99). Additional antibody testing includes low-affinity anti-AChR, anti-tinin, and anti-ryanodine receptor may be useful in confirming the diagnosis but are limited in availability from site to site (99).

Electrodiagnostic testing should be performed on all patients with suspected myasthenia gravis. Single-fiber electromyography (EMG) will reveal abnormal neuromuscular transmission in 90% to 95% of patients (99). This testing records muscle fiber action potentials and specific guidelines exist to guide the testing and diagnosis of myasthenia gravis. Repetitive nerve stimulation is an additional electrodiagnostic test that is abnormal in 75% of generalized myasthenia gravis patients and 50% of patients with ocular myasthenia gravis (99). If single-fiber EMG is available, it is the electrodiagnostic test of choice (99).

Additional diagnostic work-up should include CT and/or MRI on all patients with suspected myasthenia gravis to exclude thymoma (99). A thyroid panel should be evaluated on all patients as myasthenia gravis often coexists with thyroid disease, and all patients should be screened for tuberculosis as patients will often need immunosuppression as a part of their treatment regimen.

Management

Management is divided into symptomatic relief, short-term immunosuppression, and long-term immunosuppression (99). Symptomatic relief is attempted with pyridostigmine 30 to 90 mg every 4 to 6 hours. Dosage is increased or decreased to maximize symptomatic relief while minimizing side effects, which include gastrointestinal distress and excessive salivation or thickened saliva. This medication may be taken 30 to 60 minutes before meals if bulbar dysfunction is causing swallowing difficulties. This medication does not slow disease progression but provides symptomatic relief and management. Overdose of pyridostigmine mimics myasthenia gravis crisis and overdose should be ruled out in patients with acute worsening of their disease. Overdose signs and symptoms include bradycardia, hypersalivation, lacrimation, and miosis (99).

Short-term immunotherapy for myasthenia gravis includes plasma exchange and IVIg (99). Plasma exchange works by removing circulating antibodies. The treatment regimen consists of an exchange of one to two plasma volumes completed every other day for a total of four to six treatments. Strength improves as treatment takes effect. The side effects of plasma exchange include coagulopathy, thrombocytopenia, electrolyte disturbances, dysrhythmias, and hypotension (99). Close monitoring of bloodwork is essential during treatment with plasma exchange (99).

With short-term immunosuppression with IVIg, improvement is generally seen approximately 5 days after initiating treatment (99). There is less clear evidence of IVIg's role compared to plasma exchange in myasthenia gravis compared to the literature existing in Guillain-Barré. However, the national trend has shown an increased use of IVIg and decreased use of plasma exchange in the treatment of myasthenia gravis. This is likely related to the changing trend in Gullian Barré management (93). Dosages of both 1 g/kg of ideal body weight and 2 g/kg of ideal body weight have been studied, with no change in efficacy between the two doses. Therefore, 1 g/kg is the preferred IVIg dosage (93). IVIg side effects include headache, fever, chills, myalgia, aseptic meningitis, and fluid overload. Rarely, thromboembolic complications lead to acute renal failure, myocardial infarction, DVT, ischemic stroke, and/or pulmonary embolus. Slow infusion of IVIg limits thromboembolic complications (93). Prior to initiating IVIg, check serum immunoglobulins. IgA-deficient patients may have an anaphylactic response to infusion (93). Patients undergoing immunotherapy are certainly at high risk for infection; however, empiric antibiotics are not recommended as antibiotics may interfere with neuromuscular transmission and cause clinical worsening (93).

Long-term immunotherapy may be necessary in the management of myasthenia gravis. Corticosteroids have become a mainstay of myasthenia gravis treatment despite poor research and lack of randomized controlled trials to support their use. Corticosteroids are often used in clinical practice, initially started in high doses and then may be maintained for years in lower doses. Patients often respond well (99). Corticosteroids are often started when patients fail to have symptomatic relief with pyridostigmine. Dosing regimen is generally high dose at 0.75 to 1 mg/kg daily and then tapered over time to as low a dose as provides relief. Some clinicians prefer to begin a lower dose of 10 to 25 mg daily and increase every other day as needed to provide symptomatic relief, then taper over time as tolerated (99). Patients may have a temporary exacerbation for the first 7 to 10 days after starting high-dose steroids, then improvement begins. Corticosteroids are standard treatment in patients with ocular myasthenia gravis and may slow the progression of disease to more generalized myasthenia gravis (99). In ocular myasthenia gravis, a lower dose of steroids is often effective. Start at 20 mg daily and increase every third day by 5 to 10 mg until the patient experiences symptomatic relief. As with any corticosteroid treatment plan, the practitioner must monitor and manage side effects of steroid therapy such as fluid retention, weight gain, electrolyte imbalances, hypertension, hyperglycemia, osteoporosis, anxiety, cataracts, glaucoma, steroid myopathy, and peptic ulcer disease (99). If corticosteroids are necessary, treatment is aimed at adding other drugs to manage the disease with less or no steroids (99).

Azathioprine is a purine antimetabolite that interferes with T- and B-cell proliferation thereby decreasing the inflammatory response (99). Azathioprine is highly effective in treating myasthenia gravis but may take up to 12 months to see a benefit. Dosage is 50 mg daily and increased by 50 mg per week to total dose of 2 to 3 mg/kg. Patients started on azathioprine must be closely monitored for reaction to the medication that generally occurs

10 to 14 days after initiation of medication. Patients will develop a flu-like syndrome that requires the drug to be stopped. If no reaction occurs, continue to titrate the medication to the maximum dose while monitoring for leukopenia and hepatotoxicity. Both leukopenia and hepatotoxicity are reversible if caught early and the dose is decreased. Therefore, patients started on azathioprine therapy must be monitored closely (99). Prior to beginning therapy, check patients for thiopurine methyl transferase deficiency as patients who are deficient do not fully metabolize the medication and will need a lower dose (120). As with any long-term immunosuppression, patients must be monitored for the development of malignancies over the course of treatment (99).

Other long-term immunosuppressive therapies include mycophenolate mofetil, a medication that blocks purine synthesis suppressing T- and B-cell proliferation (99). This medication is started at a dosage of 1,000 mg twice daily and titrated up to a maximum dosage of up to 3,000 mg twice daily if necessary. There is mixed literature as to use of this medication alone or in conjunction with prednisone. Cyclosporine is another treatment choice. Cyclosporine works by inhibiting T-cell proliferation and is used in patients with no response to azathioprine or those who have side effects to azathioprine. Dosage is 4 to 6 mg/kg divided into two doses daily and then tapered to 3 to 4 mg/kg divided into two doses daily. Side effects include hirsutism, tremor, gum hyperplasia, anemia, hypertension, and nephrotoxicity. Hypertension and nephrotoxicity warrant discontinuation of the drug (99). Tacrolimus is another treatment option. Tacrolimus has a mechanism of action similar to that of cyclosporine. There are limited data on its use in myasthenia gravis, but it may be of benefit and is less nephrotoxic than cyclosporine (99). For patients who are refractory to the treatment listed above, high-dose intravenous cyclophosphamide has been shown to be a rescue therapy and rituximab may also have a role (99).

Surgical management options for myasthenia gravis include thymectomy. Thymectomy used to be a mainstay of treatment but its use has decreased in practice some since the publishing of a landmark American Academy of Neurology review that suggested the data for surgical intervention were lacking (101, 102, 103). Thymectomy is likely ideal for younger patients with a thymus pathology such as anti-ACTH receptor patients under the age of 50 and possibly for patients with no anti-ACTH receptor antibodies on a case-by-case basis. Obviously, thymectomy is the treatment of choice for patients with a thymoma. A randomized controlled trial is currently underway to try to clarify the role of thymectomy in nonthymomatous patients (103).

Management of Myasthenia Gravis Exacerbation and Crisis

From 15% to 20% of myasthenia gravis patients will experience a crisis. If a crisis occurs, it generally happens within the first 2 years as the disease reaches peak severity (97). Generally there is a precipitating event, and 60% to 70% of patients have an identifiable trigger. Infection is the most common trigger and is often an upper respiratory tract infection or pneumonia. Initiation of new medication or a change in medication can also trigger a myasthenia gravis crisis (97, 98). Several medications are known for triggering myasthenia gravis crisis. They include antibiotics such as D-penicillamine (contraindicated in myasthenia gravis patients), aminoglycosides, macrolides, fluoroquinolones, and telithromycin. Curare and related drugs, botulinum toxin, quinine, quinidine, procainamide, and interferon-alpha also are known for triggering a crisis. Additional medications that should be used with caution in myasthenia gravis patients include magnesium salts, calcium channel blockers, beta-blockers, lithium, iodine contrast agents, and statins. The role of statins in myasthenia gravis is debated and more research is needed. A true causal relationship has not been established between statins and myasthenia gravis. Statins should be used with caution until more research is available.

Other triggers of myasthenia gravis crisis include the stress of surgery or trauma and the presence of a thymoma. In approximately 30% of patients there is no identifiable trigger, however (97). Occasionally the crisis is the presentation of the disease, although this is unusual (97). The development of myasthenia gravis crisis is a clinical emergency as it is associated with rapid deterioration in muscle strength that often compromises respiratory function. Patients in crisis are at risk for respiratory failure and are often admitted to the ICU (97).

All patients in crisis should be assessed for respiratory failure. Patients may exhibit paradoxical chest movement, decreased neck strength, a wet voice or inability to speak, and stridor if neck muscles are weak. Respiratory insufficiency occurs as bulbar muscles and neck muscles weaken, resulting in the inability to protect the airway and manage oral secretions. Indications for mechanical ventilation include a forced vital capacity of less than 15 mL/kg, negative inspiratory force of less than 20 cm H_2O, peak expiratory flow less than 40, and/or an arterial blood gas revealing hypoxia or hypercapnia (97). Noninvasive mechanical ventilation may be useful in some patients, particularly those with hypercapnia. Many patients require invasive mechanical ventilation (97). Rapid sequence intubation with avoidance of paralytics is preferred. Ventilation settings should initially allow for rest (97).

Pyridostigmine is generally held during the acute crisis as it does not affect recovery from the crisis and may cause increased thick oral secretions (97). After initial stabilization, efforts should turn to a search for a trigger and treat the trigger as necessary. This is particularly true if the trigger is infection (97). All patients should be assessed for the presence of thymoma with CT or MRI (97). Treatment includes the initiation of acute immunotherapy such as plasma exchange or IVIg as discussed above (97). Once through the acute crisis, it is appropriate to reinstitute pyridostigmine and develop a plan to prevent exacerbations in the future (97). The outcomes after myasthenia gravis crisis are much better than in past decades. Seventy-five percent of patients in myasthenia gravis crisis are off of mechanical ventilation within 1 month of the crisis and mortality rates associated with myasthenia gravis crisis are between 4% and 8% (97, 102).

MOVEMENT DISORDERS

Parkinson's Disease
Etiology

Parkinson's disease (PD) is a chronic disease that the health care community has struggled to manage for many years. However, the disease has ancient roots. PD was first described in early ancient Egyptian and Indian texts and also described during biblical times (104). The symptomatology of PD was first linked to pathologic findings on autopsy in the 1700s (105). The seminal paper describing PD as we know it today was published by Dr. James Parkinson in 1817, titled "An Essay on Shaking Palsy." This publication analyzed what had been written before about clinical symptomatology and postmortem findings and synthesized them into the concept of the disease (105). He named the disease "shaking palsy" or "paralysis agitans." Charcot later renamed the disease "Parkinson disease" because not all who have the disease experience a tremor or paralysis (106).

PD is the second most common neurodegenerative disease, with a reported incidence between 5 and 24 per 100,000 (107, 108). There has been no significant change in incidence in the past century, although variant identification and incidence have changed. For example, postencephalopathic Parkinson's is no longer prevalent, whereas drug-induced Parkinson is an emerging phenomenon now recognized. Understanding and identification of variants of PD have evolved over the past century (109). Survival and longevity of patients with PD have increased in the past 20 years. This is largely attributed to the use of levodopa in treatment (109). From 35% to 42% of PD cases are thought to be underdiagnosed at any given time (109). Therefore, prevalence data likely underestimate true cases. In the United States, PD prevalence is 300 per 100,000. Prevalence increases with age and is similar between men and women.

Several risk factors have been associated with the development of PD. There is a possible correlation between a rural upbringing and the development of PD (109, 110). PD is also associated with gardening and industry-based professions (109). There is increased risk of developing PD with occupational exposure to herbicides, insecticides, pesticides, paints, wood preservatives, and fungicides, although no specific chemicals have been implicated (109).

PD does appear to have a genetic link. Development of PD is more likely if there is a positive family history of PD (127). Geneticists have also linked PD to five genes. However, no single environmental or genetic cause has been strongly linked to the development of PD.

Pathophysiology

By the time the initial symptoms of PD appear, 60% to 70% of neurons within the substantia nigra have degenerated (111). In PD, neuronal loss and gliosis are most marked in the substantia nigra. Much of the mechanism of neuronal loss and gliosis in PD remains unclear.

Clinical Presentation

PD is characterized by motor and nonmotor symptoms. Motor symptoms of PD include bradykinesia, resting tremor, and postural instability (111). As the disease progresses, neuronal degeneration outside of the of dopamine system results in nonmotor symptoms of the disease. These include autonomic symptoms such as drenching sweats and sialorrhea, gastrointestinal symptoms such as constipation and bowel problems, genitourinary symptoms, and psychological symptoms including depression, cognitive decline, apathy, anxiety, hallucinations, fatigue, sleep disorders, and pain.

Diagnosis/Differential Diagnosis

The diagnostic criteria for PD are debated and continue to evolve. PD can be difficult to diagnose. It is estimated that 50% of patients are misdiagnosed, especially early in the course of the disease and of those who carry a diagnosis of PD, as many as 20% will reveal a different pathology as the cause of their symptoms at autopsy, such as multiple system atrophy (MSA), progressive supranuclear palsy (PSP), AD-type pathology, and cerebrovascular disease. With strict adherence to the current diagnostic criteria, a diagnosis is still only thought to be 90% confident (112). One theory as to the diagnostic difficulty is there may not be one PD, but rather a collection of parkinsonian diseases. PD has been linked to five separate genes and can have multiple etiologies and different clinical symptoms (113).

The current diagnostic criteria are based on clinical symptoms and includes the presence of bradykinesia, muscular rigidity, resting tremor, and postural instability. The clinician then rules out other diagnoses that may be causing the symptoms such as history of repeated strokes, history of trauma, cerebellar signs, presence of tumor, or failure to respond to large doses of levodopa. The clinician then confirms findings that support a diagnosis of PD such as unilateral onset, resting tremor, progressive nature, persistent asymmetry, and a positive response to levodopa (114).

An older age at onset (over age 60), rigidity or hypokinesia as a presenting symptom, presence of associated comorbidities, and male sex are associated with a more rapid progression of disease. Older age at onset and presenting symptom of rigidity/hypokinesia are associated with earlier cognitive decline and dementia. Tremor as the presenting symptom is associated with slower disease progression and better response to levodopa therapy (112). The average life expectancy from diagnosis to death is 17 years (112).

Diagnosis

Diagnosis of PD is largely based on exclusion of other diagnoses and the confirmation of the presence of PD symptoms. There are no diagnostic tests that specifically diagnose PD. However, during the process of ruling out other disease processes, many patients will undergo CT and MRI of the brain as well as other testing as appropriate (112).

Management

Most patients with PD will be managed on an outpatient basis. Patients who are admitted to the hospital with PD are generally admitted with another diagnosis, and the PD must be managed as a comorbid condition. Some patients may be admitted for surgical treatment of their PD through placement of a deep brain stimulator (111).

The hallmark of PD treatment is pharmacologic therapy to manage the motor symptoms of PD. There is no accepted treatment algorithm for PD, and treatment must be tailored to each patient. Prior to initiating pharmacologic therapy, patients should be assessed for the impact of their symptoms on their quality of life, current age, comorbidities, and life expectancy (111). Levodopa, the gold standard pharmacologic treatment for PD, is less effective over time. Therefore, pharmacologic treatment is often withheld until the health care practitioner and patient agree that the symptoms are sufficiently affecting the patient's quality of life.

Dopaminergic drugs improve bradykinesia and rigidity in patients with PD. The hallmark domaminergic drug is levodopa. Levodopa is the most potent of the dopimenergic drugs but has a shorter half-life, requiring multiple dosing for symptom control. Levodopa's effect also decreases over time, requiring dose adjustments and increases as the disease progresses. There is a low risk of cognitive side effects (111).

This therapy is generally saved to be started as late as possible in the disease due to the decreasing effect of the drug over time (110, 111). As the effect decreases, the daily dose may be increased or daily dosing frequency or delivery system (extended versus immediate release) may be changed to increase the effect of the medication. Catechol O-methyltransferase (COMT) inhibitors may be added to the levodopa regimen. COMTs decrease the gastrointestinal breakdown of levodopa, thereby increasing the amount of levodopa available for absorption. COMTs such as entacapone 200 mg may be given with each levodopa dose up to 8 times daily. Tolcapone is another option but may cause hepatotoxicity. Liver function should be monitored while on this therapy. As a COMT is added, the patient may require an overall levodopa dose reduction. Additional side effects of COMT include discoloration of urine and diarrhea.

Higher daily doses of levodopa are associated with motor complications, specifically dyskinesia. Total daily dose should be limited by using adjuvant medications such as adding a monoamine oxidase B (MAOB) inhibitor (110).

Some have questioned the conventional wisdom of waiting until the disease progresses to add levodopa. Evidence suggests that starting levodopa treatment at the time of diagnosis is associated with better overall health status. There is also some thought that initiation of levodopa at diagnosis may confer a protective effect on dopaminergic neurons and slow disease progression (110). There is currently no standard and pharmacologic therapy is generally tailored to the patient's needs.

Dopamine agonists are also used to treat PD (111). Ropinirole and pramipexole both have long half-lives and may be useful in patients with dyskinesia. These drugs are generally dosed three times a day. Side effects generally include somnolence, peripheral edema, cognitive disturbance, and behavioral changes. However, these drugs are associated with few motor side effects. Dopamine agonists should be avoided in those with cognitive disorders or symptoms of cognitive decline. Ergot-related dopamine agonists are associated with cardiac valve fibrosis. Echocardiogram should be monitored routinely.

MAOB inhibitors are generally used as monotherapy in early disease and adjuvant therapy in more progressed disease (111). Selegiline is the most effective when given early in the disease course. Selegiline is shown to improving motor symptoms and activities of daily living (ADL) scores. This drug is dosed once a day and should be avoided in patients with cognitive decline. Rasagiline is used in the treatment of both early and late PD. This drug is also dosed once a day. Rasagiline is well tolerated and does not have any amphetamine metabolites. The lack of amphetamine metabolites is thought to result in fewer cognitive adverse effects.

Other options in treatment of advanced disease include amantadine, parentral dopaminergic therapy, and surgical therapy (111). Amantadine improves peak-dose dyskinesia. Amantadine is dosed at 200 to 400 mg daily divided into two doses per day. Adverse effects include confusion and livedo reticularis. Parenteral dopaminergic therapy is an alternative for patients who do not qualify for surgery. Subcutaneous apomorphine therapy improves motor control and fluctuations and may be given in a continuous or intermittent infusion. Jejunal levodopa infusion via PEG tube is also an option.

Surgery is an option for certain patients with PD (111). Patients with a well-established diagnosis of PD and have responded well to dopaminergic therapy may benefit from surgical therapy. Surgery appears to be of no benefit for those with atypical parkinsonism. Ideal surgical candidates are cognitively intact and suffer disability related to their motor complications. Patients may also have failed pharmacologic therapy. Surgical options include a pallidotomy or deep brain stimulation (DBS). DBS is generally placed in the subthalamic nucleus or globus pallidus. DBS improves cardinal features of PD and dyskinesia. However, disability still occurs over time as nondopaminergic sites degenerate. DBS may be placed bilaterally and adjustments to the stimulation are made to titrate to the maximum benefit. DBS is associated with a complication rate of 2% to 3%. Common complications include lead malfunction, migration or break, infection, and skin erosion.

Depression, psychosis, and dementia are often associated with the progression of PD (108, 111). Diagnosis and treatment are important to general function and ADLs. All patients with PD should be screened for depression. The Beck Depression Inventory and the Hamilton Depression Rating Scale are two scales that may be useful in screening PD patients for depression (108). Studies on depression in PD suggest treatment with tricyclic antidepressants or serotonin selective reuptake inhibitors (SSRIs) (111). Amitriptyline, nortriptyline, citalopram, fluoxetine, sertraline, pergolide, pramipexole, and nefazodone have been studied specifically in PD. Few studies were powered adequately to show clear benefit of one drug over another. In one study evaluating amitriptyline and fluoxetine in severe depression, those treated with amitriptyline showed significant improvement compared to those treated with fluoxetine. In PD, amitriptyline may be beneficial. The side effect profile of any antidepressant treatment should be considered as PD patients may have a particularly difficult time with cholinergic side effects. This may be especially problematic with the tricyclic antidepressants. All PD patients started on an antidepressant should be closely observed for worsening cognition, orthostatic hypotension, and falls (108).

There are multiple screening tools available to screen for psychosis. One specific to PD has been developed, the Parkinsons Psychosis Rating Scale. This tool demonstrated good interrater reliability and consistency when the scale was applied to patients with known PD (108). Clozapine has been studied for psychosis treatment in patients with PD and shown to improve symptoms of psychosis. In some cases, clozapine improved motor function as well (108, 111, 114). Agranulocytosis is a potential side effect of clozapine and may be fatal. Patients should have their absolute neutrophil count monitored while on this therapy. Quetiapine may also be considered as a treatment

option. Olanzapine was also studied and did not improve psychosis and has the potential to worsen motor function (108). Overall, patients on atypical neuroleptics should be monitored closely as these drugs have been associated with increased mortality in elderly patients treated for dementia. Risk and benefit profiles should be closely monitored.

Several screening tools are available to detect dementia in patients with PD (108). The Mini Mental Status Exam (MMSE) and the Cambridge Cognitive Examination (CCE) have both been tested in PD and are reliable tools for screening for dementia. Rivastigmine has been studied and shown to modestly improve cognitive function in PD patients with dementia. However, this drug may worsen tremor and patients should be monitored closely. Donepezil also may result in a modest improvement in cognitive function (108).

Finally, sleep disorders are common in patients with PD. Insomnia should be carefully investigated to explore potential causes and solutions. In general, the health care provider should work with the patient to improve overall sleep hygiene. If the patient has nocturnal motor symptoms, they may benefit from treatment with oxybutynin, tolterodine, or amitriptyline (111). Modafinil may be helpful for daytime drowsiness.

Clinical Nurse Specialist Competencies and Spheres of Influence

Clinical Expert/ Direct Care and Systems Leadership

The CNS may be helpful in managing the chronic needs of PD patients when they are admitted to the hospital regardless of what diagnosis causes their admission. Issues such as insomnia, dementia, and psychosis may contribute to hospitalization in PD patients and may go undetected by other nursing and medical practitioners. The CNS may work to influence the care of the patient and meet organizational needs by screening patients for common psychological complications of PD.

Coaching/Teaching/Mentoring

CNSs also help play a key role in patient education. A majority of patients report that they received little or no education on their disease at the time of diagnosis (115). CNSs play a critical role in educating the patient and helping to bridge the gap between the knowledge of the health care team and the knowledge of the patient (115).

NEUROINFECTIOUS DISEASES

A rare but often deadly neurologic cause of admission to the hospital is infection of the brain or layers of tissue surrounding the brain. Infectious disease of the central nervous system (CNS) may be classified according to location. Infections affecting the CNS may occur in the meninges surrounding the brain and spinal cord (meningitis), the brain parenchyma (encephalitis), collection of infection as an abscess within or around the brain or spinal cord tissue, or infection within the ventricles or the CSF within the ventricles (ventriculitis) (116, 117). CNS infection may present with a variety of clinical signs and symptoms and can be difficult to recognize. Delay in diagnosis and treatment of only hours may result in a significant increase in morbidity and mortality (116, 117).

Pathophysiology

The brain is a less common site for infection compared to other organs in the body due to anatomic barrier provided by the blood-brain barrier and the blood-CSF barrier (116, 117). Both barriers consist of a tight lining of epithelial cells around the nonfenestrated capillaries within the brain and the ventricles within the brain (118). This structural and biochemical barrier restricts the diffusion of molecules, including bacteria, virus, and drugs, from the bloodstream into brain tissue (118). The blood-CSF barrier is formed by similar nonfenestrated capillaries lining the ventricles and the choroid plexus. The blood-brain and blood-CSF barriers serve as the major barriers to infections within the CSF: Nonfenestrated capillaries with endothelial cells form tight junctions and prevent diffusion of drugs, bacteria, and virus from the endovascular space into the brain tissue (118).

Infection of the CNS is handled by the body's immune response differently than in any other area of the body. There is a decreased response of the immunoglobulin and complement-mediated immune response inside the CNS (118). Therefore, once infectious agents have traversed the blood-brain and/or blood-CSF barrier, there is less of an immune response to the invaders. In addition to damage caused by the invading microbe, secondary injury to the brain results from the activation of the immune and inflammatory systems (116). The blood-brain and blood-CSF barriers also pose a challenge when treating a CNS infection. Permeability of blood-brain barrier to various antimicrobial agents must be taken into account when prescribing treatment. In addition, the permeability of the blood-brain barrier may be altered as a result of injury and inflammation from the infection (118).

Infiltration of bacteria or virus into the CNS is thought to occur via one of several mechanisms. Infectious agents may attach to and cross the epithelium of the nasopharynx, where they are absorbed into the bloodstream. Due to a host of chemical defenses, these bacteria are able to elude the immune system and cross the blood-brain barrier.

Meningitis
Pathophysiology

In meningitis, bacteria generally enters the nasopharynx and cross the nasopharygeal endothelium, where they are absorbed into the bloodstream. Due to a host of chemical defenses such as secreting proteases that prevent their destruction, the bacteria then cross the blood-brain barrier and enter the CSF (116, 118). Bacteria may also enter through parameningeal spreading of other head or neck infection as common as sinusitis or otitis media. Exposure to dental infection or recent dental work or any recent neurosurgical procedure may also be entry points of bacteria into the CSF (117).

As the body begins to react to the invading microbe, the immune system is activated and an inflammatory response results. Inflammatory mediators and proinflammatory cytokines ignite an inflammatory cascade that may result in vasogenic edema, elevated ICP, disruption in cerebral perfusion, development of vasculitis, and seizures. If meningitis is not recognized and rapidly treated, infarct and herniation may result. The infection may spread to include systemic involvement and sepsis may result. Systemic complications seen in meningitis include septic shock, DIC, and pneumonia (116, 117).

Clinical Presentation

Meningitis is divided into septic (confirmed bacterial invasion of the meninges) or aseptic (suspected infectious or inflammatory process with no confirmed bacterial pathogen) (117). Generally, patients presenting with septic meningitis have more severe signs and symptoms and have a higher risk for neurologic sequelae as they recover (117). The classical triad of meningitis (fever, neck stiffness, and altered mental status) has a low sensitivity for the diagnosis of meningitis. Most patients will have at least two of four symptoms, including fever, headache, neck stiffness, and AMS (118). The elderly and immunocompromised are less likely to mount a febrile response (118). Meningococcal meningitis is often associated with a petechial purpural rash (118). Ataxia and labyrinthitis is often associated with *H. influenzae* meningitis, while cough, weight loss, night sweats, and cranial nerve deficits are most often associated with tuberculosis meningitis (118). Seizures are reported in a quarter of patients with meningitis. Seizure is indicative of cortical irritation, and the presence of seizures is an independent predictor of mortality in patients with meningitis (118).

Diagnosis

Because meningitis may present with a variety of signs and symptoms, the advanced practice nurse must keep meningitis in the differential for anyone who presents with altered mental status, particularly in the setting of a fever or other sign of infection. Other CNS infections must be ruled out. In addition, meningitis should be differentiated from ischemic and hemorrhagic stroke as well as seizure.

Diagnostic work-up of suspected meningitis includes CSF analysis, CT, MRI of the brain, and a complete blood cell count. CSF analysis is helpful in differentiating between viral and bacterial meningitis. CSF profile indicative of meningitis includes an increased white blood cell count with increased neutrophils, decreased glucose, and increased protein. A CSF absolute neutrophil count greater than $1000/mm^3$ is indicative of bacterial meningitis. In viral meningitis, the CSF white blood cell count generally increases, but not as dramatically as in bacterial meningitis (116). CSF should also be analyzed for presence of bacteria using culture and Gram stain (116).

If the patient has signs and symptoms of elevated ICP, there is concern that an LP and drainage of CSF could result in herniation. The need for CT of the brain prior to LP is debated (117). There is evidence that obtaining a CT scan prior to LP in all cases of suspected meningitis delays antibiotic administration and worsens patient outcomes. General consensus is that if the patient is showing signs and symptoms of elevated ICP, CT should be obtained prior to LP. However, administration of empiric antibiotics should not be delayed while waiting to obtain CSF (117). CSF analysis and culture should ideally be obtained before the administration of antibiotics. However, delay in antibiotic administration in suspected meningitis increases mortality. Signs and symptoms that would warrant a CT scan prior to LP include evidence of immunosuppression, significant decrease in level of consciousness, focal neurologic deficit, seizure, papilledema, decreased reactivity of pupils, gaze palsy, Cushing's triad, or recent administration of sedatives or paralytics that would alter a complete neurologic exam (117).

CT imaging in meningitis may be unremarkable or may reveal complications associated with meningitis such as cerebral edema, infarction, empyema, hydrocephalus, or subdural effusion (142). MRI with contrast often reveals meningeal enhancement. CTA or MRA may reveal vasculitis or sinus venous thrombosis (142). Complete blood cell count may show an elevated white count with a left shift. However, immunocompromised patients may not mount a febrile response or elevate their white blood cell count. SIADH is often associated with meningitis. Therefore, serum sodium should be obtained at hospital admission and monitored during the course of the disease. Blood samples should also be sent for culture and Gram stain (116).

Management

Management of meningitis includes early administration of antibiotics and recognizing and managing the neurologic and systemic complications of the disease. Evidence shows that delay in antibiotics of only 3 hours after admission to the hospital is associated with significantly increased mortality in bacterial meningitis patient's (119). Broad-spectrum antibiotics should be started after evaluating the patient's recent travel, exposure, and risk factors and then narrowed according to CSF culture

findings. Antibiotics should be dosed for meningitis to allow for crossing of the blood-brain barrier (119). Prior to the *H. influenzae* vaccine, *H. influenzae* accounted for a majority of bacterial meningitis cases. Since the vaccine, a majority of bacterial meningitis cases are caused by *Streptococcus pneumoniae, Nesseria meningitides,* and group B streptococci (119). However, previous exposure to antibiotics and recent hospitalization would warrant consideration for additional microbes and a different antibiotic profile (119). Duration of antibiotic, therapy ranges from 7 to 21 days and is based on suspected pathogen, selected antibiotic, and improvement in patient status.

Patients with acute meningitis should be monitored closely for acute neurologic decompensation as this may indicate the development of complications associated with the disease. Elevated ICP, hydrocephalus, vasculitis resulting in infarction, and sinus venous thrombosis should be recognized early and managed appropriately (116). In addition, patients should be monitored for systemic complications such as pneumonia, septic shock, and DIC.

There is mixed evidence that suggests administration of glucocorticoids such as dexamethasone for patients with acute bacterial meningitis decreases inflammation and improves outcomes. However, the role of glucocorticoids in meningitis has been a source of debate. Current consensus is to administer dexamethasone (0.15 mg/kg every 6 hours for 2 to 4 days) in patients with suspected or known pneumococcal meningitis. At this time, there is no consensus for the role of dexamethasone in meningitis caused by other pathogens (119).

Safety Issues

Antibiotic dosing and administration is a key safety issue in patients with meningitis. Medications must be reconciled and kidney and liver function closely monitored to determine safe dosages and administration of antibiotics (119).

Encephalitis
Etiology

Encephalitis is the acute diffuse inflammation of the brain tissue or parenchyma generally associated with a viral infection (118). The location and degree of neurologic dysfunction are associated with the location and degree of inflammation (120). Viruses most commonly associated with encephalitis include mumps, HSV, CMV (particularly in immunocompromised patients), VZV, enteroviruses, togaviruses (eastern and western equine viruses), lymphocytic choriomeningitis virus (LCM), West Nile virus (recent addition) (WNV), monkey-pox in North America, and chandipura virus (CHPV) in developing countries (120). Encephalitis cases generally peak in the winter and summer when certain viruses peak and history may reveal a prodrome of fever, headache, myalgia, or upper respiratory tract illness followed by change in mental status (117, 118). Despite testing, the etiology of encephalitis often remains unknown.

Pathophysiology

With the exception of HSV, most encephalitis cases result from a viral infection that localizes in the CNS (116). HSV encephalitis most often results from a reactivation of the HSV within the neuron after a period of dormancy (116, 117). CNS damage in encephalitis occurs as a result of nerve destruction from the viral pathogen as well as inflammation and immune-mediated response to the pathogen. Complications such as vasculitis, cerebral edema, and demyelination of axons may occur as the disease progresses (116).

Clinical Presentation

Signs and symptoms associated with encephalitis vary according to pathogen as well as location and degree of inflammation (116). Encephalitis should be considered in any patient with decreased level of consciousness particularly in the setting of recent viral illness, travel, or animal bite. In addition to decreased level of consciousness, personality changes, fever, and focal neurologic deficits, encephalitis patients may also present with focal or generalized seizure (116). HSV encephalitis is often associated with personality changes and psychosis followed by fever and decreased level of consciousness (117). HSV patients may also have a herpetic rash. Patients with brainstem involvement of HSV encephalitis may also have diplopia, dysarthria, and ataxia as presenting signs and symptoms (118).

Diagnosis

The clinician must distinguish between infectious encephalitis, postinfectious encephalitis, postimmunization encephalitis, encephalomyelitis (acute disseminated encephalomyelitis [ADEM]), and other noninfectious causes of disease such as vasculitis, paraneoplastic syndromes, and stroke or seizure (118). Differentiation is most often made by a careful history.

Diagnostic workup of encephalitis includes CSF analysis, CT imaging, and MRI. The CSF profile of a patient with encephalopathy is similar to meningitis with less marked CSF leukocytosis and a normal glucose count (116). Hemorrhage into the CSF is characteristic of HSV encephalitis and CSF analysis may reveal an elevated red blood cells count. CSF should be sent for viral culture and polymerase chain reaction (PCR) for suspected viruses. CSF immune serology may also be helpful in differentiating between viral pathogens (116).

CT imaging in encephalitis may be normal or may reveal complications such as edema, infarction, hemorrhage, or hydrocephalus. In HSV encephalitis, CT may reveal hemorrhage within the frontal and temporal lobes of the brain (116). MR imaging is also useful in HSV encephalitis as it characteristically reveals hyperintensities in the frontal and temporal lobes.

Blood culture may reveal infection in some cases of encephalitis, and CBC may reveal leukocytosis or leukopenia (116). As with meningitis, SIADH is a complication of CNS infections. Serum sodium should be obtained at baseline and monitored as the disease progresses to identify hyponatremia.

Management

Much of the management of encephalitis is supportive. Depending on the suspected virus, antiviral drug therapy may be helpful. Suspected HSV encephalitis should be treated with acyclovir (120). Early treatment of HSV is associated with improved mortality and morbidity. Acyclovir is often started empirically while waiting for CSF study confirmation of the diagnosis. CMV encephalitis is most often seen in patients with severe immunocompromised status from AIDS or status-post organ transplantation. Current consensus is to treat suspected CMV encephalitis with a combination of ganciclovir and foscarnet. Patients must be closely monitored for neurologic and systemic complications of encephalitis and managed appropriately (120).

Brain Abscess
Etiology

Cranial, epidural, and subdural abscesses are rare but potentially fatal forms of CNS infection (121). Abscesses are characterized by a focal collection of purulent infection within the brain tissue or in the epidural or subdural space. Abscesses are most commonly associated with trauma or neurosurgical procedures but may result from bacterial or viral infection or as a complication of meningitis or encephalitis (121). Overall incidence of abscesses has decreased for the general population in the United States (121). However, abscesses incidence has increased in immunocompromised patient populations.

Pathophysiology

Abscess may form as a result of introduction of infection into the CNS as a result of trauma or neurosurgery or as a result of migration of infection elsewhere in the body such as endocarditis or pulmonary infection (121). Untreated sinusitis or otitis media may result in abscess formation (121). Abscess may also form as a complication of meningitis or encephalitis. Formation of abscess can be divided into early and late cerebritis stages and early and late capsule stages. The early cerebritis stage is generally defined as the first several days of infection during which bacterial presence results in local inflammation and edema. Late cerebritis is characterized by the formation of a central necrotic area and occurs between 4 and 9 days after bacterial invasion. Early capsule stage occurs by the 14th day of bacterial invasion and is characterized by the formation of a ring-enhancing capsule. Late capsule stage occurs after the 14th day and is characterized by the presence of a well encapsulated infection.

Unlike other CNS infections, CNS abscesses are generally multimicrobial. Most commonly identified agents include streptococci, staphylococci, and anaerobic bacteria. Infectious agent varies according to location and history of trauma, surgery, or other infection within the body (121).

Clinical Presentation

The clinical presentation of abscess is highly dependent on the location and size of the abscess. Focal neurologic signs and symptoms will correspond with the location of the abscess (116, 121). In addition to focal neurologic deficits, abscess may present with headache, nausea, vomiting, fever, and decreased level of consciousness. Depending on the size of the abscess, elevated ICP may be present (121).

Diagnosis

Differential diagnoses for abscess include mass lesions, hemorrhage, and other CNS infectious processes. Diagnosis of abscess is generally confirmed with radiologic imaging such as CT and MRI. Depending on the stage of abscess formation, contrast-enhanced CT and MRI will reveal edema and inflammation or a ring-enhancing lesion at the site of the abscess (116, 121). LP is generally not indicated unless meningitis or encephalitis is suspected (121). Antibiotic therapy is generally narrowed according to culture of the purulent drainage through aspiration or surgical drainage.

Management

Most abscesses must be removed surgically (121). If the abscess is causing spinal cord compression or elevated ICP, surgical evacuation is emergent. Broad-spectrum empiric antibiotic therapy should be started as soon as possible and narrowed according to culture findings. Antibiotic choice should be guided by history of surgery or hospitalization, history of antibiotic treatment, and presence of infection elsewhere in the body.

Clinical Nurse Specialist Competencies and Spheres of Influence

Systems Leadership and Collaboration

Because the early recognition and treatment of CNS infections have such a large bearing on the morbidity and mortality of the disease, the CNS has a particular role in coordinating care for these patients. Patients may benefit from protocols and order sets aimed at the coordination of care, diagnosis, and timely administration of antibiotics. Similar to the management of a sepsis patient, the CNS may be critical in coordinating care to decrease time to antibiotic administration as well as improving recognition of the common complications associated with meningitis.

Seizure
Etiology

Approximately 150,000 patients will present to the hospital or their primary care provider with a first-time seizure each year in the United States. From 40% to 50% of first-time seizures will develop into recurrent seizures, and those patients in time will receive a diagnosis of epilepsy (122). The annual cost of epilepsy in the United States was last estimated to be in excess of $12.5 billion (122). Misdiagnosis and mismanagement contribute to inappropriate pharmacologic therapy and worse patient outcomes (122).

Pathophysiology

In a healthy individual, there is a balance of excitatory and inhibitory neurotransmitters. Each patient has a threshold commonly referred to as the "seizure threshold." Seizure activity is the abnormal discharge of cerebral electrical impulses (123). A decrease in the seizure threshold or an increase in the excitatory neurotransmitter discharges will result in a seizure. There are many different cases of a seizure (123). Seizures generally last seconds to minutes long and subside without intervention. Some patients report an aura or a prodrome for minutes or hours prior to seizure activity. Common symptoms include emotional changes and a general feeling of malaise.

Seizures are classified as idiopathic, cryptogenic, or symptomatic (123). Ideopathic seizures are related to an identified genetic mechanism that is causing the seizure activity. Cryptogenic seizures are seizures with an unknown etiology not associated with previous CNS injury or other suspected cause. Symptomatic or provoked seizures are associated with CNS injury such as TBI, stroke, or tumor. An acute symptomatic seizure generally occurs within one week of known CNS injury, whereas a remote symptomatic seizure occurs more than 1 week from known CNS injury.

Seizures are classified according to the International Classification of Epileptic Seizures (122). Seizures are classified as partial or general. Partial seizures are classified as having motor signs, having somatosensory or special-sensory symptoms, and having autonomic symptoms or psychotic symptoms. Partial motor seizures are further classified as motor seizure without march, motor seizure with march (Jacksonian), versive, postural, or phonatory. Partial seizures with somatosensory or special-sensory symptoms are further classified as visual, auditory, olfactory, gustatory, or vertiginous. Partial seizure with psychic symptoms include dysphasia, dysmnesic, cognitive, affective, illusions, and/or structured hallucinations.

Complex partial seizures are further subclassified according to level of consciousness and development of seizure (123). Complex partial seizures may start as simple partial seizures and be followed by an impairment of consciousness. These seizures may have simple partial features or automatisms. Complex partial seizures may also have impairment of consciousness at onset or they may be partial seizures evolving to secondarily generalized seizures.

Generalized seizures are further classified into absence, atonic (drop attacks), myocolonic, or tonic-clonic seizure (122). Typical absence seizures include impairment of consciousness only or may have mild clonic or atonic components. Absence seizures may also have automatisms or autonomic components as well.

A patient who experiences multiple seizure episodes that are unprovoked and associated with biochemical, anatomical, or physiologic changes is diagnosed with epilepsy (122). Epilepsy diagnosis is made according to localization. Epilepsy is classified as idiopathic with age-related onset, benign childhood epilepsy with centrotemporal spikes, childhood epilepsy with occipital paroxysms, and symptomatic or mesial temporal lobe sclerosis.

Generalized epilepsy may be classified as idiopathic with age-related onset, benign neonatal familial convulsions, benign neonatal convulsions, benign myoclonic epilepsy of infancy, childhood absence epilepsy (pyknolepsy), juvenile absence epilepsy, juvenile myoclonic epilepsy (JME), epilepsy with grand mal seizures on awakening, idiopathic and/or symptomatic infantile spasms, Lennox-Gastaut syndrome, epilepsy with myoclonic astatic seizures, epilepsy with myoclonic absences, and symptomatic epilepsy (122).

Status epilepticus occurs when a patient experiences multiple seizures without returning to their baseline neurologic function between seizure activity or experiences continuous seizure activity for more than 30 minutes (123). Any patient with any seizure type or epilepsy classification may present with status epilepticus. If seizing continues, patients with status epilepticus will develop cerebral edema, elevated ICP, and other secondary complications. Status epilepticus is considered a medical emergency and should be treated immediately and expeditiously (123).

Diagnosis

Seizures are generally a diagnosis made based on clinical history and physical exam. Seizure activity may be reported by witnesses and is generally followed by a period of decreased responsiveness called the "postictal phase." Epilepsy diagnosis is made when two or more seizures occur more than 24 hours apart that have no immediate identifiable cause (122, 123). Diagnostic tests include laboratory work such as electrolytes and complete blood count to evaluate metabolic and/or infectious causes. Hypoglycemia and hyperglycemia may both contribute to seizure activity as can rapid changes in serum sodium levels. One of the most common causes of seizure activity is failure to take prescribed AEDs. If the patient has a history of taking AEDs, serum levels may be obtained.

CT with and without contrast is generally done to rule out ischemic or hemorrhagic stroke and tumor as possible causes of neurologic changes or causes of seizure activity (122, 123). MRI may also be done to determine the presence of seizure or infection. EEG is ideally performed within 24 hours of event and may be performed under sleep-deprived conditions if appropriate. Hospitalized patients may suffer subclinical seizure activity that could be contributing to the decline in mental status in common

diagnoses such as ischemic and hemorrhagic stroke or trauma. In such patients, continuous EEG monitoring for 24 to 48 hours may be helpful to identify seizure activity. LP may be warranted to identify CNS infection in suspected patients. Seizure activity is of concern in patients with existing neurologic injury such as stroke or trauma as it elevates ICP and contributes to cerebral edema and other causes of secondary injury to the brain (123).

Management

Seizure management and prevention of another seizure are often dependent on identifying and treating the underlying etiology. Not all first-time seizures require treatment. After identification of the classification of the seizure and underlying cause, risk assessment generally dictates the likelihood of treatment. Those at higher risk for recurrent seizures are those under the age of 16, with a history of a remote symptomatic seizure, with seizure occurring in the early morning, with presence of a prior provoked seizure history of a primary relative with seizures, and with a history of an episode of status epilepticus.

Pharmacologic treatment is also largely guided by the suspected underlying cause and if this is a first-time or recurrent seizure. Benzodiazepines are often administered to quiet seizure activity but only offer temporary control. AEDs offer long-term control. There are many AEDs available according to type of presenting seizure (Table 8-1) (124). Patients who are actively seizing

TABLE 8–1 Anti-seizure and Antiepileptic Drugs (AEDs): Choice depends on type of seizure, new onset or chronic condition, individual response, drug interactions, and toxicity

carbamazepine (Tegretol)
phenobarbitol
phenytoin (Dilantin)
primidone (Mysoline)
valproic acid (Depakote)
ethosuximide (Zarontin)
gabapantin (Neurontin)
lamotrigine (Lamictal)
topiramote (Topamax)
levetiracetam (Keppra)
oxycarbazepine ((Trilepfal)
zonisamide (Zonegran)
tiagabine (Gabitril)

should be helped to the bed or floor, and all furniture should be moved to protect their safety (123).

Safety Issues

All patients and family members should be educated regarding epilepsy and the medication regimen expected to control seizure activity. The most common cause of admission to the hospital for seizure is related to noncompliance with medication. Many states have laws regarding the operation of a motor vehicle within several months of having a seizure. Patients should be counseled regarding the local laws and restriction against driving and working (123).

Many common over-the-counter medications, foods, and prescription medications interact with AEDs. Patients should be counseled regarding each medication and the expected side effects and interactions with other medications. In particular, patients on warfarin and AEDs should be counseled regarding potential interactions and effects on the INR. Some AEDs are also associated with birth defects if taken during pregnancy. Women in childbearing years should be closely counseled regarding pregnancy and their medication (123).

Clinical Nurse Specialist Competencies and Spheres of Influence

Clinical Expert/Direct Care

In Europe, the CNS role has taken a primary responsibility in the chronic management of epilepsy patients (125). Epilepsy specialist nurses counsel patients on treatment of epilepsy and frequently titrate medications to minimize side effects while controlling for seizure activity. As they continue to define the role, expansion of prescriptive authority and scope of services is being evaluated at a national level (126). In a national survey of all advanced practice nurses in England working with epilepsy patients, 40% held clinic hours and 40% were responsible for evaluating patients with new seizures not yet seen by anyone else on the medical team (127). The epilepsy advanced practice nurse has been embraced in Europe and may have a role in the United States.

References

1. Zuckerman A, Markham C. Why neuroscience business development? Healthc Fin Manage. Retrieved June 1, 2006, from http://www.allbusiness.com/health-care/medical-practice-oncology/10542141-1.html

2. Rangel-Castillo L, Gopinath S, Robertson R. Management of intracranial hypertension. Neurol Clin 2008;26:521-541.

3. Bershad E, Humphries W, Suarez J. Intracranial hypertension. Semin Neurol 2008;28:690-702.

4. Lescot T, Abdennour L, Boch A, et al. Treatment of intracranial hypertension. Curr Opin Crit Care 2008;14:129-134.

5. Mayer S, Sessler D. Therapeutic Hypothermia. Boca Raton, FL: Taylor and Francis Group; 2005.

6. Polderman K. Induced hypothermia and fever control for prevention and treatment of neurological injuries. Lancet 2008;371:1955-1969.

7. Badjatia N. Fever control in the neuro-ICU: why, who and when? Curr Opin Crit Care 2009;15:79-82.

8. Thompson H, Kirkness C, Mitchell P. Intensive care unit management of fever following traumatic brain injury. Intens Crit Care Nursing 2007;23(2):91-96.

9. Polderman K, Herold I. Therapeutic hypothermia and controlled normothermia in the intensive care unit: practical considerations, side effects and cooling methods. Crit Care Med 2009;37(3):1101-1120.

10. Thompson C, Mitchell P, Webb D. Fever management practices of neuroscience nurses: national and regional perspectives. J Neurosci Nursing 2007;39(3):151-162.

11. Laupland K, Shahpori R, Kirkpatrick A, et al. Occurrence and outcome of fever in critically ill adults. Crit Care Med 2008;36(5):1531-1535.

12. Badjatia N, Bodock M, Guanci M, et al. Rapid infusion of cold saline (4°C) as adjunctive treatment of fever in patients with brain injury. Neurology 2006;66:1739-1741.

13. Badjatia N, Strongili, E, Gordon E, et al. Metabolic impact of shivering during therapeutic temperature modulation: the bedside shivering assessment scale. Stroke 2008;39:3242-3247.

14. Gentile NT, Siren K. Glycemic control and the injured brain. Emerg Med Clin North Am 2009;27:151-169.

15. Wijdicks E. The diagnosis of brain death. N Engl J Med 2001;344(16):1215-1221.

16. American Academy of Neurology. Practice Parameters: Determining Brain Death in Adults. Summary Statement from the Report of the Quality Standards Subcommittee of the American Academy of Neurology. 1994. Retrieved July, 2011, from www.aan.com/professionals/practice/guidelines/pda/Brain_death_adults.pdf

17. Choi E, Fredland V, Zachodni C, et al. Brain death revisited: the case for a national standard. J Law Med Ethics N Engl J Med 2001; 344:1215-1221 April 19, 2001.

18. Manno EM, Wijdicks EFM. The declaration of death and withdrawal of care in the neurological patient. Neurol Clin 2006;24:159-169.

19. Wijdicks EFM, Barelas PN, Gronseth GS, et al. Evidence-based guideline update: determining brain death in adults—report of the quality standards subcommittee of the American Academy of Neurology. Neurology 2010;74:1911-1918.

20. Shafer T, Wagner D, Chessare J, et al. Organ donation breakthrough collaborative: increasing organ donation through system redesign. Crit Care Nurse 2006;26:33-48.

21. Mascia L, Mastromauro I, Viberti S, et al. Management to optimize organ procurement in brain dead donors. Minerva Anesthesiol 2009;75:125-133.

22. Goldstein L, Adams R, Alberts M, et al. Primary prevention of ischemic stroke: a guideline from the American Heart Association/American Stroke Association. Stroke 2006;37:1583-1633.

23. Adams H, del Zoppo G, Alberts M, et al. Guidelines for the early management of adults with ischemic stroke. Stroke 2007;38:1655-1711.

24. Summer D, Leonard A, Wentworth D, et al. Comprehensive overview of nursing and interdisciplinary care of the acute ischemic stroke patient: a scientific statement from the American

Heart Association. Stroke. Retrieved July, 28, 2011, from http://stroke.ahajournals.org/content/40/8/2911.

25. Grysiewicz R, Thomas K, Pandey D. Epidemiology of ischemic and hemorrhagic stroke: incidence, prevalence, mortality and risk factors. Neurol Clin 2008;26:861-895.

26. Amarenco P, Bogousslavsky J, Caplan L, et al. Classification of stroke subtypes. Cerebrovasc Dis 2009;27:493-501.

27. Amarenco P, Bobousslavsky J, Caplan L, et al. New approach to stroke subtyping: the A-S-C-O (phenotypic) classification of stroke. Cerebrovasc Dis 2009;27:502-508.

28. Switzer J, Hess D, Nichols F, et al. Pathophysiology and treatment of stroke in sickle-cell disease: present and future. Lancet Neurol 2006;5:501-512.

29. Gamlimanis A, Mono M, Arnold M, et al. Lifestyle and stroke risk: a review. Curr Opin Neurol 2009;22:60-68.

30. Brown D, Boden-Albala B, Langa K, et al. Projected cost of ischemic stroke in the United States. Neurology 2006;67:1390-1395.

31. Doyle K, Simon R, Stenzel-Poore M. Mechanisms of ischemic brain damage. Neuropharmacology 2008;55:310-318.

32. Emsley H, Smith C, Tyrrell P, et al. Inflammation in acute ischemic stroke and its relevance to stroke critical care. Neurocrit Care 2008;9:125-138.

33. Schwamm L, Audebert H, Amarenco P, et al. Recommendations for the implementation of telemedicine within stroke systems of care: a policy statement from the American Heart Association. Stroke. Retrieved July 28, 2011 from http://stroke.ahajournals.org/content/40/7/2635.short.

34. Meyers P, Schumacher C, Higashida R, et al. Indications for the performance of intracranial endovascular neurointerventional procedures: a scientific statement from the American Heart Association Council on Cardiovascular Radiology and Intervention, Stroke Council, Council on Cardiovascular Surgery and Anesthesia, Interdisciplinary Council on Peripheral Vascular Disease, and Interdisciplinary Council on Quality of Care and Outcomes Research. Circulation 2009;119:2235-2249.

35. Sacco R, Adams R, Albers G, et al. Guidelines for prevention of stroke in patients with ischemic stroke or transient ischemic attack. Stroke 2006;37:577-617.

36. Alberts M, Hademenos G, Latchaw R, et al. Recommendations for the establishment of primary stroke centers. JAMA 2000;283(23):3102-3109.

37. Alberts M, Latchaw R, Selman W, et al. Recommendations for comprehensive stroke centers: a consensus statement from the Brain Attack Coalition. Stroke 2005;36:1597-1618.

38. Schwamm L, Panciolo A, Acker J, et al. Recommendations for the establishment of stroke systems of care: recommendation from the American Stroke Association's Task Force on the Development of Stroke Systems. Circulation 2005;111:1078-1091.

39. Holloway RG, Tuttle D, Baird T, et al. The safety of hospital stroke care. Neurology 2007;68:550-555.

40. Michaels AD, Spinler SA, Leeper B, et al. Medication errors in acute cardiovascular and stroke patients: a scientific statement from the American Heart Association. Circulation 2010;121:1664-1682.

41. Lawson C, Gibbons D. Acute stroke management in emergency departments. Emerg Nurse 2009;17(5);30-34.

42. Fitzpatrick M, Birns J. Thrombolysis for acute ischemic stroke and the role of the nurse. Br J Nurs 2004;13(20):1170-1174.

43. Alexandrov AW, Brethour M, Cudlip F, et al. Postgraduate fellowship education and training for nurses: the NET SMART experience. Crit Care Nurses Clin North Am 2009;21(4):435-449.

44. Oswald SK, Hersch G, Kelley C, et al. Evidence-based educational guidelines for stroke survivors after discharge home. J Neurosci Nursing 2008;40(3):173-191.

45. Ellis G, Rodger J, McAlpine C, et al. The impact of stroke nurse specialist input on risk factor modification: a randomized controlled trial. Age Aging 2005;34(4):389-392.

46. Werner H. The benefits of the dysphagia clinical nurse specialist role. J Neurosci Nursing 2005;37(4):212-215.

47. Easton D, Saver J, Albers G, et al. Definition and evaluation of transient ischemic attack: a scientific statement for health care professionals from the American Heart Association/American Stroke Association Stroke Council. Stroke 2009;40:2276-2293.

48. Bederson JB, Connolly ES, Batjer H, et al. Guidelines for the management of aneurysmal subarachnoid hemorrhage. Stroke 2009; 40:994-1025.

49. Suarez J, Tarr R, Selman W. Aneurysmal subarachnoid hemorrhage. N Engl J Med 2006;354(4);387-396.

50. Van Gijn J, Rinkel G. Subarachnoid hemorrhage: diagnosis, causes and management. Brain 2001;124:249-278.

51. Van Gijn J, Rinkel G. Subarachnoid hemorrhage. Lancet 2007;369:306-318.

52. Edlow J, Caplan L Avoiding pitfalls in the diagnosis of subarachnoid hemorrhage. N Engl J Med 2000;342(1):29-36.

53. Linfante I, Wakhloo AK. Brain aneurysm and arteriovenous malformations: advancements and emerging treatment in endovascular embolization. Stroke 2007;38:1411-1417.

54. Navai N, Stevens R, Mirski M, et al. Controversies in the management of aneurysmal subarachnoid hemorrhage. Crit Care Med 2006;34: 511-524.

55. Varelas P, Helms A, Sinson G, et al. Clipping or coiling of ruptured cerebral aneurysms and shunt-dependent hydrocephalus. Neurocrit Care 2006;4(3):223-228.

56. Cook N. Subarachnoid hemorrhage and vasospasm: using physiological theory to generate nursing interventions. Intens Crit Care Nursing 2004;20:163-173.

57. Qureshi A, Mendelow A, Hanley D. Intracerebral hemorrhage. Lancet Neurol 2009;373:1632-1644.

58. Rincon F, Mayer S. Clinical review: critical care management of spontaneous intracerebral hemorrhage. Crit Care 2008;12:237.

59. Broderick J, Connolly S, Feldman E, et al. Guidelines for the management of spontaneous intracerebral hemorrhage in adults 2007 update. Stroke 2007;38:2001-2023.

60. Christensen M, Mayer S, Ferran J. Quality of life after intracerebral hemorrhag: results of the factor seven for acute hemorrhagic stroke (FAST) trial. Stroke 2009;40:1677-1682.

61. Testai F, Aiyagari V. Acute hemorrhagic stroke pathophysiology and medical interventions: blood pressure control, management of anticoagulant-associated brain hemorrhage and general management principles. Neurol Clin 2008;26:963-985.

62. Pezzini A, Padovani A. Cerebral amyloid angiopathy-related hemorrhages. J Neurol Sci 2008;29:S260-S263.

63. Cavallini A, Fanucchi S, Persico A. Warfarin-associated intracerebral hemorrhage. J Neurol Sci 2008;29:S266-S268.

64. Pozzi M, Roccatagliata D, Sterzi R. Drug abuse and intracranial hemorrhage. J Neurol Sci 2008;29:S269-S270.

65. Salmaggi A, Erbetta A, Silvani A, et al. Intracerebral hemorrhage in primary and metastatic brain tumors. J Neurol Sci 2008; 29:S264-S265.

66. Vespa P. Metabolic pneumbra in intracerebral hemorrhage. Stroke 2009;40:1547-1548.

67. Engelhard H, Andrews C, Slavin K, et al. Current management of intraventricular hemorrhage. Surg Neurol 2003;60:15-22.

68. Mendelow A, Unterberg A. Surgical treatment of intracerebral hemorrhage. Curr Opin Crit Care 2007;13:169-174.

69. Koch S, Forteza A, Rabinstein A. Rapid blood pressure reduction in acute intracerebral hemorrhage: feasibility and safety. Neurocrit Care 2008;8:316-321.

70. Aiyagari V, Testai F. Correction of coagulopathy in warfarin associated cerebral hemorrhage. Curr Opin Crit Care 2009;15:87-92.

71. Torbey M. Intracerebral hemorrhage: what's next? Stroke 2009; 40:1539-1540.

72. Creutzfeldt C, Weinstein J, Longstreth W, et al. Prior antiplatelet therapy, platelet infusion therapy and outcome after intracerebral hemorrhage. J Stroke Cerebrovasc Dis 2009;18(3):221-228.

73. Naval N, Nyquist P, Carhuapoma J. Advances in the management of spontaneous intracerebral hemorrhage. Crit Care Clin 2007;22:607-617.

74. Nyquist P, LeDroux S, Geocadin R. Thrombolytics in intraventricular hemorrhage. Curr Neurol Neurosci Rep 2007;7(6):522-528.

75. Lyden M, Sacco R, Shuaib A, et al. Natural history of complications after intracerebral hemorrhage. Eur J Neurol 2009;16:624-630.

76. Freitas G, Nagayama M. Deep vein thrombosis after intracerebral hemorrhage, gender and ethnicity: a challenge for therapeutic approaches. Cerebrovasc Dis 2009;27:320-321.

77. Garrett M, Komotar R, Starke R, et al. Predictors of seizure onset after intracerebral hemorrhage and the role of long-term antiepileptic therapy. J Crit Care 2009;24(3):335-339.

78. Christensen M, Mayer S, Ferran J, et al. Depressed mood after intracerebral hemorrhage: the FAST trial. Cerebrovasc Dis 2009;27(4):353-360.

79 Tapia-Perez H, Sanchez-Aguilar M, Torres-Corzo J, et al. Use of statins for the treatment of spontaneous intracerebral hemorrhage: results of a pilot study. Cen Eur Neurosurg. 2009;70(1):15-20.

80. Brain Trauma Foundation. Guidelines for the management of severe traumatic brain injury, 3rd ed. J Neurotrauma 2007;24:S1.

81. American Association of Neuroscience Nurses. Nursing management of adults with severe traumatic brain injury. AANN clinical practice guideline series. Retrieved July 28, 2011, from http://www.aann.org/pdf/cpg/aanntraumaticbraininjury.pdf.

82. Centers for Disease Control and Prevention. Injury prevention and control: traumatic brain injury. Retrieved July 28, 2011 from http://www.cdc.gov/TraumaticBrainInjury/.

83. Miko I, Gould R, Wolf S, et al. Acute spinal cord injury. Int Anesthesiol Clin 2009;47(1):37-54.

84. Sugrue M, Caldwell E, D'Amours S, et al. Time for a change in injury and trauma care delivery: a trauma death review analysis. ANZ J Surg 2008;78(11):949-954.

85. Krassioukov A, Warburon DE, Teasell R, et al. A systematic review of the management of autonomic dysreflexia after spinal cord injury. Arch Phys Med Rehabil 2009;90:784-695.

86. Ivatury RR, Guilford K, Malhotra AK, et al. Patient safety in trauma: maximal impact management errors at a Level 1 trauma center. J Trauma 2008;64(2):265-270.

87. Laudermilch DJ, Schiff MA, Nathens AB, et al. Lack of emergency medical services documentation is associated with poor patient outcomes: a validation of audit filters for prehospital trauma care. J Am Coll Surg 2010;210:220-227.

88. Lang B, Vincent A. Autoimmune disorders of the neuromuscular junction. Curr Opin Pharmacol 2009;9 (3) 336-340.

89. Hadden R. Deterioration after Guillain-Barré syndrome: recurrence, treatment-related fluctuation or CIDP? J Neurol Neurosurg Psychiatry 2009;80:3.

90. Mantay, MK, Armeau E, Parish T. Recognizing Guillain-Barré syndrome in the primary care setting. Internet J Allied Health Sci Pract 2007;5(1):1-8).

91. Winer J. Guillain-Barré syndrome. BJM 2008;33:a671.

92. Hughes R, Wijdicks E, Benson E, et al. Supportive care for patients with Guillain-Barré syndrome. Arch Neurol 2005;62:1194-1198.

93. Hughes R, Swan A, Raphael J, et al. Immunotherapy for Guillain-Barré syndrome: a systematic review. Brain 2007;130:2245-2257.

94. Newswanger W. Subtypes of Guillain-Barre syndrome. Am Fam Phys 2004;69(10):4.

95. Van Doom P, Ruts L, Jacobs B. Clinical features, pathologies and treatment of Guillain-Barré syndrome. Lancet Neurol 2008;7:939-950.

96. Sakakibara R, Uchiyama T, Kuwabara S, et al. Prevalence and mechanism of bladder dysfunction in Guillain-Barré syndrome. Neurourol Urodynam 2009;28(5):432-7.

97. Bershad E, Feen E, Suarez J. Myasthenia gravis crisis. South Med J 2008;101(1):63-69.

98. Meriggiolo M, Sanders D. Autoimmune myasthenia gravis; emerging clinical and biological heterogeneity. Lancet Neurol 2009;8:475-490.

99. Lunn M, Willison H. Diagnosis and treatment in inflammatory neuropathies. J Neurol Neurosurg Psychiatry 2009;80:149-158.

100. Conti-Fine B, Milani M, Kaminski H. Myasthenia gravis: past, present, and future. J Clin Investig 2006;116:2843-2854.

101. Gronseth G, Barohn R. Practice parameter: thymectomy for autoimmune myasthenia gravis: an evidence-based review. Neurology 2000;55:7-15.

102. Alshekhlee A, Miles J, Katirji B, et al. Incidence and mortality rates of myasthenia gravis and myasthenic crisis in US hospitals. Neurology 2009;72:1548-1554.

103. Bachmann K, Burkhardt D, Schreiter I, et al. Thymectomy is more effective than conservative treatment for myasthenia gravis regarding outcome and clinical improvement. Surgery 2009;145(4):392-398. Epub 2009 Feb 8.

104. Ruiz G. Prehistory of Parkinson disease. Neurolgia 2004;19(10): 735-737.

105. Kempster P, Hurwitz B, Lees A. A new look at James Parkinson's essay on the shaking palsy. Neurology 2007;69:482-485.

106. Zesiewicz T, Elble R, Louis E, et al. Therapies for essential tremor: report of the Quality Standards Subcommittee of the American Academy of Neurology. Neurology 2005;64: 2008-2020.

107. Klein C, Schlossmacher M. Parkinson disease, 10 years after its genetic revolution: multiple clues to a complex disorder. Neurology 2007;69:2093-2104.

108. Miyasaki J, Shannon K, Voon V, et al. Evaluation and treatment of depression, psychosis and dementia in Parkinson disease (an

evidence based review): report of the Quality Standards Subcommittee of the American Academy of Neurology. Neurology 2006;66:996-1002.

109. Rajput A, Birdi S. Epidemiology of Parkinson disease. Parkinson Relat Disord 1997;3(4):175-186.

110. Marras C, Lang A. Changing concepts in Parkinson disease: moving beyond the decade of the brain. Neurology 2008; 70:1996-2003.

111. Schapira A. Treatment options in the modern management of Parkinson disease. Arch Neurol 2007;64:8 1083-1088.

112. Suchowersky O, Reich S, Perlmutter J, et al. Diagnosis and prognosis of new onset Parkinson disease (an evidence based review): report of the Quality Standards Subcommittee of the American Academy of Neurology. Neurology 2006;66:968-975.

113. Weiner W. There is no Parkinson disease. Arch Neurol 2008;65:6 705-708.

114. Suchowersky O, Gronseth G, Perlmutter J, et al. Neuroprotective strategies and alternative therapies for Parkinson disease (an evidence based review): report of the Quality Standards Subcommittee of the American Academy of Neurology. Neurology 2006;66:976-982.

115. Heisters D. Effective communication in diagnosis Parkinson's. Br J Nursing 2007;16(7):382-383.

116. Ziai W, Lewin J. Update in the diagnosis and management of central nervous system infections. Neurol Clin 2008;26:427-468.

117. Suarez JI. Critical Care Neurology and Neurosurgery. Totowa, NJ: Humana Press; 2004.

118. Ziai W, Lewin J. Advances in the management of central nervous system infections in the ICU. Crit Care Clin 2007;22:661-694.

119. Tunkel A, Hartman B, Kaplan S, et al. Practice guidelines for the management of bacterial meningitis. Clin Infect Dis 2004;39: 1267-1284.

120. Tunkel A, Glaser C, Bloch K, et al. The management of encephalitis: clinical practice guidelines by the Infectious Diseases Society of America. Clin Infect Dis 2008;47:303-327.

121. Greenberg B. Central nervous system infections in the intensive care unit. Semin Neurol 2008;28:682-689.

122. Krumholz A, Wiebe S, Gronseth G, et al. Evaluating an apparent unprovoked first seizure in adults (an evidence based review): report of the Quality Standards Subcommittee of the American Academy of Neurology and the American Epilepsy Society. Neurology 2007;69;1996-2007.

123. AANN Clinical Practice Guideline Series. Care of the patient with seizures: AANN clinical practice guideline series. Retrieved July 28, 2011, from http://www.aann.org/pdf/cpg/aannseizures.pdf.

124. French JA, Kanner AM, Bautista J. Efficacy and tolerability of the new antiepileptic drugs: treatment of new onset epilepsy. Neurology 2004;62:1252-1260.

125. Hosking PG. Prescribing and the epilepsy specialist nurse. Seizure 2003;12:74-76.

126. Hosking PG. Epilepsy and supplementary nurse prescribing. Br Med J 2006;332(7532):2.

127. Goodwin M, Higgins S, Lanfear JH, et al. The role of the CNS in epilepsy: a national survey. Seizure 2004;13(2):87-94.

CHAPTER 9

Cardiovascular Problems

Cathy J. Thompson, PhD, RN, CCNS

INTRODUCTION

Cardiovascular disorders are among the most prevalent acute and chronic conditions in the world. About 30% of the world's population has some type of cardiovascular disease (CVD), and it remains the number one cause of death throughout the world (1). In the United States, over 80 million adults have CVD and over 38 million are 60 years of age or older (2). Over 700,000 deaths are attributed to CVD in the United States each year (2).

CVD includes diseases of the heart and vascular system, including the cerebrovascular system. Chronic conditions such as hypertension, diabetes mellitus, and chronic renal disease are risk factors for CVD—and often precipitate or coexist with CVD. The total health care cost of CVD for 2009 is estimated to be over $475 billion. That figure is over twice the health care dollars estimated for the cost of all malignant and benign cancers in 2008 (2, 3). (See Table 9-1.)

Coronary heart disease (CHD) includes diseases of the structure and function of the heart, including the lining of the heart and the heart valves. Over 16,800,000 adults in the United States have some form of CHD incurring a direct and indirect cost estimated at $165.4 billion (2009 dollars) (2). Over the years, due to risk factor modification and the use of evidence-based interventions, there has been a 50% reduction in the mortality rate from CHD (4); however, the number of people afflicted by CHD is still significant (2).

Coronary artery disease (CAD) is caused by atherosclerosis, the accumulation of lipid-rich plaques in the coronary arteries. Atherosclerosis eventually may cause a temporary decrease in coronary artery blood flow resulting in ischemia or angina pectoris (pain in the chest) or result in coronary atherothrombosis, the development of a clot that partially or fully occludes a coronary artery causing acute coronary syndrome (ACS). Thirteen million Americans have a history of myocardial infarction (MI), angina, or both (5). According to the American Heart Association (AHA), ACS was the single largest cause of death in the United States, accounting for over 500,000 deaths per year (5). Atherothrombosis is the underlying cause of cerebrovascular, coronary, and peripheral vascular diseases.

RISK FACTORS

Risk factors for CVD (shown in Table 9-2) and CHD are well known and include modifiable risk factors (those that are amenable to lifestyle strategies) and nonmodifiable risk factors (variables such as gender, genetic profile, race/ethnicity, family history, and age). Smoking, obesity (body mass index [BMI] >30), physical inactivity, diet, dyslipidemia, high levels of inflammatory markers (C-reactive protein [CRP], fibrinogen, protein C, plasminogen activator inhibitor), hyperhomocysteinemia, stress, depression, anxiety, behavior type, inflammation, hypertension, diabetes, certain infectious agents (e.g., *Helicobacter pylori*,

TABLE 9-1 Elements of Direct and Indirect Cost Measures

Cost Measure	Typical Elements
Direct costs	Cost of primary care visits and visits to other health care professionals (i.e., specialist visits); hospitalization; nursing home/skilled facility/home health care services; medications; treatment costs; disposable and consumable medical supplies/durable medical equipment
Indirect costs	Lost productivity from morbidity and mortality; value of the patient's time

TABLE 9–2 Common Risk Factors for Cardiovascular Disease (CVD)

Risk Factor	Affect on Risk of CVD
Increased age	↑ risk
Adiposity (BMI >30)	↑ risk
Behavior pattern	Inconclusive, but some evidence shows 2× risk with type A personality profile
Cigarette smoking	2-6× the risk; cumulative risk ↑ with the number of cigarettes smoked
	Risk ↓ when smoking stopped
Diabetes mellitus (DM)	2× risk compared to non-DM
Gender	Male > female until 75 years old, then risk equalizes
Heredity	Family history ↑ risk
HTN	2-3× risk
	↑ frequency of MI; ↑ DBP → ↑ risk
Triglycerides, lipoproteins	↑ LDL, ↑ TG = ↑ risk
	↓ HDL = ↑ risk
	↑ HDL = ↓ risk
Oral contraceptive use	↑ risk
Physical inactivity	↑ risk
	May lead to obesity → ↑ risk
Premature menopause	↑ risk

BMI, body mass index; DBP, diastolic blood pressure; HDL, high-density lipoprotein; HTN, hypertension; LDL, low-density lipoprotein; MI, myocardial infarction; TG, triglycerides; ↑, increased; ↓, decreased.

Chlamydia pneumoniae), and cardiometabolic syndrome are risk factors that influence the development of coronary artery and other vascular diseases (1, 2, 6, 7). The use of oral contraceptives and estrogen level changes post menopause are risk factors unique to women. Many of these risk factors may be mediated through the implementation of preventive health strategies to decrease CVD risk.

The risk of CVD increases as the number of risk factors increase. Data from a large randomized trial showed an increase of yearly risk for atherothrombotic events from 5.5% for persons with zero to one risk factor to 22% for those with eight or more risk factors (8). Atherothrombotic disease in one arterial vascular bed (CVD, coronary disease, or peripheral vascular disease) increases the likelihood of atherothrombotic disease in another arterial bed (9). For example, within 6 months of discharge, MI patients have up to 4 times the risk of stroke; patients with severe peripheral arterial disease have 2.2 times the risk of having an MI or stroke (9). Thus, the modifiable risk factors are the focus of major national prevention initiatives to decrease the morbidity and mortality of CVD.

Cigarette smoking is the principal reason for disease and death in the United States and a fitting target for preventive strategies. Though the percentage of Americans who smoke has decreased since the 1960s, data from the 2006 National Health Interview Survey confirm that 21% of Americans currently smoke (10). Consequently, one of the national health goals for the U.S. population is to reduce the prevalence of adult cigarette smoking to less than 12% (National Health Goal Objective 27-1a) (11).

A comparison of prevalence of cigarette smoking by race/ethnicity and gender is found in Table 9-3 (10). The clinical nurse specialist (CNS) can counsel patients to stop smoking and provide referrals to smoking cessation programs.

Of the primary familial dyslipoproteinemias (see Figure 9-1), type IV is the most common, affecting 1 in

TABLE 9–3 Prevalence of Current Smoking (Adults 18 years and older) by Race/Ethnicity and Gender According to 2006 National Health Interview Survey U.S. Data

	Men	Women
NH-American Indian/ Alaskan Native	35.6%	29.0%
NH-Black	27.6%	19.2%
NH-White	24.3%	19.7%
Hispanic	20.1%	10.1%
NH-Asian	16.8%	4.6%
NH: non-Hispanic		

From Centers for Disease Control and Prevention, 2007 (10).

Primary Dyslipoproteinemias

Name	Laboratory Findings	Clinical Features	Therapy
Type I: exogenous hyperlipidemia; fat-induced hypertriglyceridemia	Cholesterol normal Triglycerides increased three times Chylomicrons increased	Abdominal pain Hepatosplenomegaly Skin and retinal lipid deposits Usual onset: childhood	Low-fat diet
Type IIa: hypercholesterolemia	Triglycerides normal LDL increased Cholesterol increased	Premature vascular disease Xanthomas of tendons and bony prominences Common Onset: all ages	Low-saturated-fat and low-cholesterol diet Cholestyramine[a] Cholestipo[b] Lovastatin[c] Nicotinic acid[d] Neomycin[e] Intestinal bypass
Type IIb: combined hyperlipidemia; carbohydrate-induced hyperglyceridemia	LDL, VLDL increased Cholesterol increased Triglycerides increased	Same as IIa	Same as IIa; *plus* carbohydrate restriction Chlofibrate[f] Gemfibrozil[g] Lovastatin
Type III: dysbetalipoproteinemia	LDL or chylomicron remnants increased Cholesterol increased Triglycerides increased	Premature vascular disease Xanthomas of tendons and bony prominences Uncommon Onset: adulthood	Weight control Low-carbohydrate, low-saturated-fat, and low-cholesterol diet Alcohol restriction Chlofibrate Gemfibrozil Lovastatin Nicotinic acid Estrogens[h] Intestinal bypass
Type IV: dysbetalipoproteinemia	Glucose intolerance Hyperuricemia Cholesterol normal or increased VLDL increased Triglycerides increased	Premature vascular disease Skin lipid deposits Obesity Hepatomegaly Common onset: adulthood	Weight control Low-carbohydrate diet Alcohol restriction Chlofibrate Nicotinic acid Intestinal bypass
Type V: mixed hyperlipidemia; carbohydrate and fat-induced hypertriglyceridemia	Glucose intolerance Hyperuricemia Chylomicrons increased VLDL increased LDL increased Cholesterol increased Triglycerides increased three times	Abdominal pain Hepatosplenomegaly Skin lipid deposits Retinal lipid deposits Onset: childhood	Weight control Low-carbohydrate and low-fat diet Chlofibrate Lovastatin Nicotinic acid Progesterone[i] Intestinal bypass

Legend
[a] *Cholestyramine* (Questran), anion exchange resin; bind bile acids; enhances cholesterol excretion.
[b] *Colestipol* (Colestid), same as cholestyramine.
[c] *Lovastatin*, 3-hydroxy-3-methylglutaryl coenzyme a (HMG-CoA) reductase inhibitor; decreases cholesterol synthesis in the liver.
[d] *Nicotinic acid* (niacin), decreases release of free fatty acids from adipose tissue; increases lipogenesis in liver; decreases glucagon release; most effective for type V disorder.
[e] *Neomycin*, experimental medication; questionable mode of action; decreases LDSs.
[f] *Chlofibrate* (Atromid-S), decreases release of free fatty acids from adipose tissue; decreases hepatic secretion of VLDL and increases catabolism of VLDL.
[g] *Gemfibrozil* (Lopid), similar to clofibrate but inceases HDLs more.
[h] *Estrogens*, decrease LDL levels in type III disorders; experimental.
[i] *Progesterone*, decreases plasma triglycerides in type V disorders; experimental.
Adapted from Brashers, VL. Table 30-6 In McCance, KL, Heuther, S (*Pathophysiology: The Biologic Basis for Disease in Adults and Children*, 6th Edition. Mosby, 112009. 30.2.9.1.1.

FIGURE 9–1: Primary dyslipoproteinemias. *(Adapted from Brashers VL, Table 30-6. In: McCance KL, Huether SE, editors. Pathophysiology: The Biological Basis of Disease in Adults and Children, 6th ed. Maryland Heights, MD: Mosby Elsevier; 2010. With permission.)*

every 300 people in the United States. Total cholesterol and total low-density lipoprotein (LDL) cholesterol levels have the most significant effects on atherogenesis. Stress will elevate lipid levels due to the production of glucocorticoids, which then inhibit fat catabolism and promote adiposity and hyperlipidemia. Multiple studies have shown the effects of negative stressors on lipid levels, whereas the effects of positive life events have been shown to reverse elevated lipid profiles (6). The cellular mechanisms of selected atherogenic risk factors are described in Table 9-4 (6, 12, 13). CNSs can help reduce anxiety and stress in patients by providing accurate information and answering questions from patients and family members regarding their disease processes and treatment strategies. Additionally, CNSs can provide referrals for stress management classes and support groups.

Atherosclerotic lesions have been detected in children (14) and young adults (14, 15). Friedman et al. (14) were among the first to study CHD risk factors in young adults. The CARDIA (Coronary Artery Risk Development in Young Adults) study was a longitudinal, prospective cohort study of young African American and Caucasian adults aged 18 to 30 years. The purpose of that study was to evaluate racial differences in the distribution of CHD risk factors in young adults and to prospectively evaluate lifestyle choices, habits, and behaviors that affect the development and progression of modifiable risk factors for CVD. CARDIA participants were evaluated at years 0, 2, 5, 7, 10, and 15.

TABLE 9-4 Cellular Mechanisms for Selected Atherogenic Risk Factors

Atherogenic Risk Factor	Pathophysiology of Cellular Mechanisms
Adiposity (BMI >30)	• Specific cellular mechanisms unknown; however, obesity → risk factors independently associated with CAD: type 2 diabetes, HTN, hypercholesterolemia, hypertriglyceridemia • Accumulation of visceral fat, especially in abdomen → ↑risk (waist-to-hip ratio >0.90 men; >0.85 women; "apple" shape)
Cigarette smoking	• ↑ CO thought to cause cellular hypoxia, platelet aggregation → endothelial damage; • Smoking induces ↑ SVR, ↑ LDL oxidation → endothelial damage
Diabetes mellitus (DM; type I [T1D] and type 2 [T2D])	• Increases probability of concomitant CAD risk factors such as HTN and hyperlipidemia • Induces procoagulant state from interference with the liver's ability to remove LDL, ↑ platelet aggregation, ↑ production of clotting factors • ↑ LDL oxidation • ↑ SMC proliferation, ↑ foam cell development, alterations in vascular tone from hyperinsulinemia (T2D) or insulin boluses (T1D) • Hyperglycemia induces proatherogenic state in vessel walls
Female gender	• Before menopause: Estrogens believed to increase the ability of the liver to produce more LDL receptors thereby increasing LDL removal (protective effect) • After menopause: Protective effect lost and risk equalizes
Male gender	• No protective effect of estrogens on LDL receptors
Heredity	• Variety of genetic mechanisms thought to increase risk, such as congenital defects in LDL receptors
Hyperlipidemia with low HDL	• ↑ LDL cholesterol damages endothelium → accumulation on lining and proliferation of SMC
Hypertension	• ↑ SVR, ↑ shear stress → endothelial damage, ↑ platelet aggregation, ↑ permeability of endothelial lining; • RAAS may cause cellular changes from link with ↑ AT II via stimulation of AT receptor; AT I → ↑ LDL oxidation

AT I, angiotensin I; AT II, angiotensin II; CAD, coronary artery disease; CO, carbon monoxide; LDL, low-density lipoprotein; HDL, high-density lipoprotein; HTN, hypertension; RAAS, renin-angiotensin-aldosterone system; SMC, smooth muscle cells; SVR, systemic vascular resistance; ↑, increased; ↓, decreased; →, leads to/leading to.

From Brashers, 2010 (6); Shapiro, 2002 (91).

Loria et al. (15) used the CARDIA data to evaluate the amount of coronary artery calcium (CAC) deposited in atherosclerotic plaques of the CARDIA participants at year 15. Calcium presence in the coronaries was assessed in relation to modifiable risk factors, and to age, gender, and race. Histologic plaque and area of calcium infiltration are highly correlated (16). Calcium deposits are measured using electron-beam computed tomography. The presence, extent, and severity of coronary artery calcification quantity is measured in Agatston units. Plaque calcification occurs throughout the life span, but seems to accelerate after age 40 (15). Calcium scores of 0 to 10 indicate no evidence of CAD to minimal evidence; scores of 11 to 100 indicate mild disease; scores over 400 signify severe and widespread disease (17). Loria et al. reported that CAC levels in young adulthood were predictive of future CHD events and that modifying habits, behaviors, and other lifestyle factors may decrease calcium deposition and reduce future risk of heart disease.

Middle-aged and older Caucasians have higher levels of CAC than other racial/ethnic groups. Questioning whether differences in CAC deposition exist among racially diverse groups, Bild et al. (16) conducted a comparison of CAC levels among different U.S. ethnic groups in the Multi-Ethnic Study of Atherosclerosis (MESA) study. Results from the MESA study showed that Caucasian men and women have much higher rates of coronary calcification (70% and 45%, respectively; relative risk [RR] 1.0) compared to African Americans (RR 0.78), Hispanics (RR 0.85), and Chinese (RR 0.92) after adjustment for known coronary risk factors (16). That is, compared to Caucasians, African Americans, Hispanics, and Chinese have less risk of calcium deposition (22%, 15%, and 8%, respectively), even after controlling for cardiac risk factors. Bild et al. (16) noted that while coronary risk factors and calcium levels are related, the differences in CAC are not fully explained by ethnic/racial differences and further research in this area is needed. However, knowledge of ethnic variations in CAC levels may aid clinicians in interpreting CAC scores differently and individualizing the plan of care. For example, because these ethnic groups have less risk, determining the range of CAC levels to prompt the practitioner to order additional testing may need to be adjusted for nonwhite patients (16). CAC testing is not yet widely used as a screening test for CAD, and more research is needed to identify how the results can be used to modify risk (17).

ADVANCED PRACTICE IN ACUTE CARE

Patients can benefit from the expert knowledge base of the advanced practice nurse (APN). Preventive health strategies can be taught and encouraged among young adults and people at risk in hopes of having an impact on disease-risk profiles to avoid or delay the onset of CVD in middle and old age (14, 15). In acute care, APNs are called upon to use their clinical expertise to help manage patients with acute presentations of cardiovascular problems and acute exacerbations of chronic disease. Admissions for coronary atherosclerosis account for over 1 million patients a year; over 800,000 people are admitted with a diagnosis of acute MI and almost 300,000 are admitted for management of ischemic heart disease (IHD) (5). The CNS is influential in promoting positive outcomes for these vulnerable patients. Management of acutely and critically ill patients incorporates all of the CNS core competencies and occurs in all three spheres of influence: Patient/Family, Nursing/Other Disciplines, and the System/Organization. This chapter will cover common acute cardiovascular conditions likely to be influenced by CNSs either through direct patient- and family-centered care or indirectly through work behind the scenes with nurses and the organization. CNSs influence the Patient and System/Organization spheres through the preparation and mentoring of the nursing staff, and by translating evidence into practice through a systems focus on evidence-based practice (EBP), quality and safety, effective interprofessional teamwork, and advocacy for the patient and the nurse at the system level. National initiatives and resources for quality improvement and patient safety will be addressed in each section as appropriate.

ACUTE CORONARY SYNDROMES

Etiology

Acute coronary syndrome (ACS) is a term used for a continuum of progressively harmful conditions that stem from the underlying disorder of CAD. ACS is used to identify patients presenting with clinical signs and symptoms consistent with acute myocardial ischemia. The syndromes included in this initial diagnosis consist of (a) unstable angina (UA); (b) MI without Q-wave development or ST-segment elevation (non–ST-segment elevation MI [NSTEMI], also known as non–ST-segment elevation ACS or non-ST ACS); (c) MI as evidenced by Q-wave formation and ST-segment elevation (STEMI); or (d) sudden cardiac death (SCD) (18, 19). This new terminology reflects the understanding that cardiac ischemia and injury can present with or without elevation of the ST segments or development of Q waves, depending on which layers of the myocardium are involved. ACS is the initial working diagnosis for patients presenting with signs and symptoms of ACS but before confirmation of a specific diagnosis of UA, NSTEMI, or STEMI is made.

ACS is caused by formation of a thrombus or a thromboembolism arising from the rupture or erosion of an atherosclerotic plaque. ACS primarily affects males, women after menopause, and African Americans at higher rates than Caucasians or other racial/ethnic groups. In 2004, almost 1.6 million patients were hospitalized for either primary or secondary ACS (20). Over 1 million Americans will suffer from a new or recurrent MI each year (785,000/470,000, respectively) and, of those, almost half will die (2). Even after treatment, complications remain high for ACS patients: in the first 30 days after admission for ACS, there remains a high risk of future adverse cardiac events (19). More than $83 billion is spent each year in the United States for the direct care of ACS patients (21).

ACS may be asymptomatic or present with predictable chest pain progressing to unpredictable chest pain. Myocardial ischemia, MI, and death may follow. However, all patients do not necessarily experience ACS symptoms in a classic manner and SCD can occur at any time. Almost 300,000 people are treated by emergency medical services (EMS) teams for out-of-hospital SCD each year (2).

Angina is chest pain of cardiac origin caused by an imbalance of oxygen supply and demand. This imbalance is temporary and reversible causing no death of cardiac myocytes. Angina affects almost 10 million people in the United States (2). Anginal syndromes include stable angina and Prinzmetal's, or variant, angina and are differentiated in Table 9-5. People with stable angina are at risk of progression of their CAD to UA, which is a change in the clinical presentation or triggers of anginal attacks, as a result of worsening coronary artery blockage. Because the extent and duration of the blockage influence the viability of cardiac tissue, MIs can occur solely in the endocardial or epicardial layers or extend into the myocardium (nontransmural) or can involve all three layers of the heart (transmural). Signs and symptoms and treatment of nontransmural versus transmural infarctions will differ based on the area of the heart affected. MI affects 8 million people annually in the United States (2).

Education is vital for informing the public of the signs and symptoms of ACS so that those affected get to the hospital for prompt treatment and a better survival advantage. Delays in seeking treatment are common among older adults, women, and minorities. One factor related to the rationale for these delays is the fact that women (Table 9-6) and certain ethnic minorities tend to describe their symptoms differently than white males and, as a result, do not necessarily link their discomfort or shortness of breath with the signs of ACS. The AHA (2) reported that women's awareness of heart disease as the principal reason for death among U.S. women has risen steadily since 1997 but is still only at 57%. CNSs can help to close this information gap through one-to-one education with patients and family members, as well as providing group education for religious, athletic, social, civic, and other community-based groups.

People with significant risk factors for CAD who suffer from disease processes that include neuropathies—such as those with diabetes or spinal cord injury—warrant a high degree of clinical suspicion on the part of the advanced clinician. These patients may have considerable CAD, but be asymptomatic due to dysfunction or disruption of the afferent nerve fibers that transmit chest pain, lipid abnormalities related to sedentary lifestyles and increased fat reserves, and decreased physical activity (22-24). For example, in patients with a high cervical or thoracic spinal cord injury (i.e., T6 or higher), chest pain may be absent or present in a more subtle manner such as an episode of autonomic dysreflexia or as tooth or jaw pain (22, 23). Table 9-6 outlines differences in atypical or uncommon signs and symptoms of angina, known as anginal equivalents, as well as common pain locations and possible electrocardiographic (ECG) changes in selected vulnerable populations.

Pathophysiology

ACS can be caused by coronary artery inflammation or spasm or any obstruction to coronary arterial flow that lasts long enough for myocytes to be injured. However, the majority of ACS events are caused by varying degrees of atherothrombosis (18, 19). Table 9-7 outlines common coronary and noncoronary causes of ACS.

Atherogenesis is the formation of atherosclerotic plaque that begins early in life and leads to diseases of the coronaries, carotids, and other arterial vessels. Areas of high turbulence or high shear force are most vulnerable to atherosclerotic plaque formation, and multiple plaque sites are common. Studies have shown that 80% of patients with ACS have two or more active plaques (5). Atherothrombosis is the sudden erosion, rupture, or fissure of the plaque cap allowing the lipid and cellular contents to leak into the vessel lumen, causing the activation of platelets and thrombosis formation (25).

The thrombus may be occlusive or nonocclusive. Occlusive thrombus will cause ischemia and infarction; a nonocclusive thrombus will cause ischemic symptoms during the time the blood flow is obstructed. Plaque is considered "active" because it releases cellular and chemical mediators: vascular cell adhesion molecules (e.g., VCAM-1) to ensnare leukocytes at the plaque site for penetration into the intima; cytokines, such as tumor necrosis factor-alpha (TNF-α), interleukin-1 (IL-1), and other procoagulant factors; and human leukocyte antigen-DR (HLA-DR) (26). Microvascular clots can form and embolize from activated plaque causing distal inflammation and obstruction and possible

TABLE 9-5 Comparison of Anginal Syndromes and Acute Coronary Syndromes

	Precipitating Causes	Quality of Pain (Typical Pain Descriptors)	Radiation of Pain	Associated Signs and Symptoms	Diagnostic Clues	Treatment Measures
Anginal Syndromes						
Stable angina	Known cause • Exercise or exertion • "Heavy" meal • Stress • Emotional upset • Cold weather exposure	Pain lasts <20 min (pressure, heaviness, squeezing, strangling, constricting, bursting, burning, "a band across the chest," "a weight in the center of the chest," "a vise tightening around the chest")	May radiate to upper chest, epigastrium shoulders, neck, jaw, arms, back	Symptom duration usually 2-5 min—5-15 min: SOB, diaphoresis palpitations Anxiety, nausea, or vomiting	Predictable frequency, severity, duration, time of appearance, and therapeutic response; Ear crease is sign of hyperlipidemia; Levine's sign or other diagnostic pain clues (two hands with fingers spread over precordium, or one hand with spread fingers with palm circling chest area)	Rest NTG
Prinzmetal's (variant) angina	Coronary vasospasm with no known trigger; typically wakes patient from sleep at night	Similar to stable angina	Similar to stable angina	Similar to stable angina	ECG only shows ischemic changes if patient is experiencing chest pain at the time of the ECG tracing	Calcium channel blockers prescribed to prevent future episodes
Acute Coronary Syndromes						
Unstable angina (UA)	Atypical triggers unlike what the patient has experienced before: e.g., • Differing amount of exercise now triggers pain episode;	Rest angina; similar to anginal descriptors	To neck, jaw, shoulder blades, left and/or right arms	Symptom duration usually >20 min; occurs at rest (rest angina) or with minimal exertion: SOB, diaphoresis, palpitations, anxiety, nausea or vomiting	Levine's sign or other diagnostic pain clues	Rest or NTG does not relieve pain; Seek emergency treatment; ACS protocols

Continued

TABLE 9-5 Comparison of Anginal Syndromes and Acute Coronary Syndromes—cont'd

	Precipitating Causes	Quality of Pain (Typical Pain Descriptors)	Radiation of Pain	Associated Signs and Symptoms	Diagnostic Clues	Treatment Measures
	• New onset of symptoms (within previous 4-6 weeks); • Symptoms more frequent, severe, or prolonged					
MI	Occlusive thrombus in coronary artery; Prolonged coronary spasm or obstruction	Pain lasts >30 min; Similar to anginal descriptors (Heaviness, crushing squeezing, pressure, like an "elephant sitting on my chest")	Similar to UA	Symptom duration usually >30 min; Diaphoresis Feeling of impending doom, Nausea, vomiting Weakness, dizziness, anxiety, lightheaded Syncope Dysrhythmias	Levine's sign or other diagnostic pain clues	Rest or NTG does not relieve pain; Seek emergency treatment; ACS protocols
STEMI	Transmural MI	May not have chest pain (silent MI); or similar to MI descriptors	Similar to UA	Similar to MI	ST segment elevation and Q waves seen in leads overlying infarcted area; New BBB may obscure diagnosis	Seek emergency treatment; ACS protocols; STEMI SOC
NSTEMI	Nontransmural MI: Subendocardial, subepicardial, or intramural MI alone or in combination	May not have chest pain (silent MI) ; or similar to MI descriptors	Similar to UA	Similar to MI	No ST segment elevation seen; ST segment depression noted in leads overlying infarcted area	Seek emergency treatment; ACS protocols; NSTEMI SOC

ACS, acute coronary syndrome; BBB, bundle branch block; ECG, electrocardiogram; MI, myocardial infarction; NSTEMI: non–ST-segment elevation MI; NTG, nitroglycerin; SOB, shortness of breath; SOC, standard of care; STEMI, ST-segment elevation MI; UA, unstable angina.

TABLE 9–6 Comparison of Ischemic Pain Presentations in Vulnerable Populations

Population	Common Anginal Equivalents	Pain Location	ECG
OLDER ADULTS			
	• Exertional dyspnea (most common complaint) • Fatigue • Syncope • Nausea • Anorexia • Confusion • Dyspnea at rest • Abdominal or epigastric discomfort	May not c/o chest pain; May c/o abdominal or epigastric pain	Less likely to have ST elevation on the first ECG. ECG changes normally found in aging patients may hinder diagnosis
WOMEN			
	• Aching • Tightness • Pressure • Sharpness • Burning • Fullness • Tingling Acute S/S • Shortness of breath • Weakness • Unusual fatigue • Cold sweats • Dizziness • Nausea/vomiting	May not c/o chest pain; May c/o pain in: • Back • Shoulder • Neck • Chest	
DIABETICS			
	• Generalized weakness • Syncope • Light-headedness • Change in mental status	May not c/o chest pain	
SPINAL CORD INJURY (SCI)			
	• Dull or heavy pain • Referred pain • Episode of autonomic dysreflexia (may be refractory to treatment) • Variability in vital signs likely in patients with history of autonomic dysreflexia	C/O pain will vary with level of injury • T4 and above—chest pain may be absent or modified • Referred pain in areas not affected by SCI May c/o pain in: • Tooth/teeth • Jaw	ECG changes normally found in aging patients may hinder diagnosis

c/o, complain of; ECG, electrocardiogram; S/S, signs and symptoms.

Sources: Chen et al., 2005 (54); Mosca, 2007 (49); McSweeney et al., 2010 (55); Thompson and Smith-Love (in press) (68).

TABLE 9-7 Mechanisms of Imbalances in Myocardial Oxygen Supply and Demand

Decreased Myocardial Oxygen Supply	Location
Decreased coronary blood flow due to narrowed coronary arteries or other causes	• Usually occurs on ruptured, thinned, or eroded plaque
• Atherothrombosis (thrombus or thromboembolism) • Total occlusion • Subtotal occlusion (can progress to total occlusion) • Microvascular thromboembolism • Coronary vasospasm (including cocaine-induced spasm) • Restenosis of coronary artery • Post-PCI or CABG • Chronic atherosclerosis • Coronary artery inflammation • Coronary artery dissection (very uncommon)	• Of a major vessel → STEMI; • Of small, downstream collateral vessels → NSTEMI (majority of patients) • Degree of injury r/t extent of collateral vessel development • Usually occurs on top of established plaque • Usually occurs in a distal location due to shedding of a plaque-associated thrombus • Can occur in macrovascular (i.e., epicardial) and/or microvascular vessels, and on top of established plaques;
Selected noncoronary causes of ↓ coronary blood flow	• Any coronary artery
• Hypotension (e.g., shock, maldistribution of blood flow) • Hypoxemia (i.e., ↓ Do$_2$ to heart) • Anemia (i.e., ↓ Do$_2$ to heart) • Compression of coronary arteries (e.g., massive pulmonary embolism, neoplasms, hemopericardium)	
Increased myocardial oxygen demand	
• Anxiety • Fever • Tachycardia • Thyrotoxicosis • Heavy exercise • Pulmonary congestion • Tension pneumothorax • Fluid overload	

CABG, coronary artery bypass graft; Do$_2$, oxygen delivery; NSTEMI, non–ST-segment elevation MI; PCI, percutaneous coronary intervention; STEMI, ST segment elevation MI; UA, unstable angina; ↑, increased; ↓, decreased; →, leads to/leading to.

long-term complications in the heart, brain, and peripheral tissues (26).

From Fatty Streak to Advanced Lesion

Atherogenesis starts as an inflammatory response to damage or injury of the endothelial lining of the blood vessels. Endothelial damage can be caused by high serum cholesterol or triglycerides, shear forces from high blood pressure, or high blood iron levels. Inflammation plays a role in the initiation of the lesion, the progression of the lesion, and the thrombotic complications that result from disruption of the plaque (9). Common agents stimulating an inflammatory response in the endothelial cells are listed in Box 9-1. At an early age, fat molecules (primarily oxidized LDL particles) are deposited in the subendothelium producing a fatty streak, which in early stages does not decrease the diameter of the artery, nor does the fatty streak manifest clinically. Fatty streaks can get smaller or remain dormant (27). However, activation of the fatty streak causes the release of chemical mediators from the inflamed endothelium, promoting coagulation and attracting inflammatory cells (i.e., leukocytes, monocytes, mast cells), which promote the progression of the fatty streak to a fatty plaque and possibly toward an advanced lesion. The release of chemical mediators from endothelium causes alterations in vessel patency and vasodilatory response, affects the ability of endothelium to release antithrombotic cytokines to balance the procoagulant effects, and induces growth factors (e.g., angiotensin II [ATII], fibroblast growth factor [FGF],

---

BOX 9-1 Agents Triggering Inflammatory Reactions in Endothelial Cells

- Dyslipidemia (especially ↑ LDL w/↓HDL)
- DM
- Cigarette smoking
- ↑ Homocysteine levels
- Autoimmune mechanisms
- ↑ Blood viscosity
- Vessel wall shear stress
- Increased C-reactive protein and fibrinogen
- Viral infection of endothelial cells (e.g., CMV, *Chlamydia pneumoniae*, *Helicobacter* pylori)

DM, diabetes mellitus; CMV, cytomegalovirus; LDL, low-density lipoprotein; HDL, high-density lipoprotein; ↑, increased; ↓, decreased.

---

and platelet-derived growth factor [PDGF]) that promote smooth muscle cell (SMC) growth within vessel wall (6).

LDLs increase the permeability of the vessel wall, enter the intimal layer, and become oxidized by free oxygen radicals produced during cellular metabolism and enzymatic reactions (6). Oxidative stress is defined as the imbalance between the production of free oxygen radicals (reactive oxygen species [ROS]) and the body's ability to neutralize ROS. Disease processes, such as hypertension and diabetes, and other factors, such as smoking and high levels of angiotensin II, increase LDL oxidation (6). The oxidation of LDL stimulates the release of VCAM-1 and other adhesion molecules from the endothelium.

VCAM-1 allows leukocytes (e.g., monocytes, T-lymphocytes) to invade the intimal lining of the vessel. This invasion triggers vascular smooth muscle proliferation in the intimal layer, eventually causing protrusion of the growing plaque into the vessel lumen. Monocytes, called to the site by chemoattractant proteins such as monocyte chemoattractant protein-1 (MCP-1), penetrate the endothelium becoming macrophages and phagocytize the oxidized LDL particles, causing their appearance to look "foamy"—hence the term *foam cells* (6, 9). This process also produces free oxygen radicals, which increase damage to the surrounding tissue. Foam cells, stimulated by macrocyte colony-stimulating factor (M-CSF), are able to multiply within the arterial intima thus enlarging the lipid core (9). Multiple studies have shown the proatherogenic affects of MCP-1 and M-CSF (9). Foam cells also express apolipoprotein E (apoE), procoagulant tissue factor, growth mediators, and other cytokines (21). Other immune cells, activated during inflammation, comprise the atherosclerotic lesion: macrophages, T-lymphocytes, and mast cells (9). Quantities of proatherogenic adhesion molecules and

cytokines (e.g., VCAM-1, MCP-1, M-CSF, TNF-α) are found within atherosclerotic plaques.

Over time, intimal smooth muscle proliferation continues and the foam cells within the atheroma die, releasing their contents and forming the lipid core of the atheroma. This vascular remodeling may take years before the "plaque burden" is large enough to occlude half of the vessel lumen and thus affect blood flow to the point that the obstruction can be seen angiographically (28). An extracellular matrix of fibrous strands composed of collagen, elastin, and proteoglycans overlay the plaque cap; collagen is the major component (28). However, continued expression of cytokines from inflammatory cells and the inflammatory process can cause the release of proteolytic enzymes, interferon-gamma (INF-γ), collagenase, matrix metalloproteinases, and other proteinases that degrade collagen and inhibit its production (28). A reduction in the synthesis of collagen and an increase in its degradation lead to weakening or thinning of the fibrous cap resulting in instability and cap disruption (28). INF-γ also induces apoptosis of the foam cells, thus enriching the lipid contents of the atheroma. Activated platelets express CD40 ligand, which increases the secretion of tissue factor in macrophages promoting the conversion of fibrinogen to fibrin and the development of a platelet-fibrin thrombus (9). Advanced lesions continue to have lipids deposited within the plaque and may have cholesterol crystals and calcium deposits embedded in the fibrous cap (8).

Stable and Unstable Plaques

Research studies have demonstrated that the stability of the plaque cap is responsible for the likelihood of thrombotic complications, more so than the plaque protrusion into the vessel lumen (28). Stable plaques have an intact endothelial layer, a thick fibrous cap made up of many smooth muscle cells with few inflammatory cells, and a small lipid core. Unstable plaques have a corroded endothelial layer, a thin fibrous cap that consists of many inflammatory cells and few SMCs, and large lipid core of activated macrophages (Figure 9-2). The lipid core is extremely thrombogenic if exposed to blood due to the presence of tissue factor expressed by the activated macrophages. Mechanical stress, in the form of shear force (from blood pressure) and circumferential stress, acts upon the fibrous cap—the more fragile the cap, the more vulnerable it is to rupture (28). Additionally, the inflammatory process creates an unstable environment where the fibrous cap can erode (commonly at the lesion edges from apoptosis), fissure, or rupture causing an acute thrombotic event. The site of plaque disruption oozes or hemorrhages its contents that will induce platelet activation and adhesion upon contact with the blood. The resulting thrombus may completely obstruct the vessel lumen or only partially obstruct the lumen. Small fissures or minor erosions of the plaque cap can ooze plaque

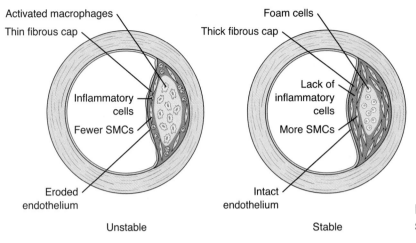

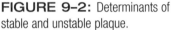

FIGURE 9–2: Determinants of stable and unstable plaque.

contents that temporarily occlude the lumen, leading to transient ischemic episodes—the vessel lumen reopens within 10 to 20 minutes before permanent damage occurs (6). Additionally, platelet thrombi may shed from the disrupted plaque and embolize to the microcirculation (26). The bottom line is a temporary decrease in oxygen delivery to the cardiac myocytes (i.e., ischemia, a reversible dysfunction) or a disruption in blood flow for a long enough time that death of the myocytes occurs (i.e., infarction, irreversible damage).

Patients with UA have soft caps that allow some of the inner core material to leak out of the plaque, causing the change in anginal symptoms. Complete disruption of the cap causes the lipid core to exude, platelet aggregation to occur, the coagulation cascade to become activated, and an obstructive clot to form. Incomplete occlusion of the coronary artery may be clinically silent (i.e., no signs and symptoms), or may cause UA, NSTEMI, or, in some cases, SCD. Complete occlusion of the coronary artery may result in STEMI or SCD. The cardiac myocytes do not have large oxygen or energy stores and therefore within 1 minute of coronary artery occlusion, oxygen tension falls to zero, contraction-relaxation becomes disrupted, energy stores are used up, the lack of oxygen causes lactic acid to be produced from anaerobic metabolism, and ischemia occurs (12).

Time Is Muscle

Obstruction of blood flow to the heart muscle for greater than 20 to 30 minutes results in permanent damage. If the affected site is not reperfused within 40 to 60 minutes, irreversible injury is inflicted and viable tissue surrounding the infarcted site may suffer from myocardial "stunning," injury of heart muscle that may take months for normal function to be restored. The presence of collateral vessels in the ischemic area, continual or intermittent occlusion of the affected artery, myocyte sensitivity to ischemia, preconditioning, and/or myocardial oxygen demand will determine the degree of myocardial compromise and the length of

time to complete myocyte death in the affected area (29). The longer the clot obstructs blood flow to the cardiac myocytes, the more heart muscle is damaged—lending weight to the axiom of "time is muscle" (which is true for any kind of ischemic injury to muscle or tissue—cardiac, skeletal, brain, kidney, etc.). The volume of damaged tissue is determined by the degree of left ventricular (LV) damage: focal necrosis is microscopic damage; necrosis of less than 10% of the LV myocardium is classified as a small MI; a moderate MI denotes 10% to 30% of the LV infarcted; and a large MI is classified as necrosis of greater than 30% of the LV (29). Cardiogenic shock occurs when 40% or more of the cardiac muscle is damaged.

The death of cardiac myocytes keeps the inflammatory system stimulated, and acute MI is recognized histologically by the infiltration of polymorphonuclear leukocytes (PMNs) or neutrophils. As the tissue heals (in about 7 to 28 days), PMNs leave the injured site and mononuclear cells and fibroblasts pervade the area. The presence of necrotic myocytes continues to stimulate the inflammatory process as scavenger cells dispose of the necrotic tissue. Fibrin and collagen replace the damaged myocytes and scar tissue forms, without cellular infiltration. Scar tissue in the heart is recognized as a healed MI and takes about 5 to 6 weeks for the total healing process to be complete (29). Scarred heart muscle is nonfunctional: electrical action potentials will not cross and activate scarred muscle, and the area will not participate in contraction. The larger the area of scar, the more nonfunctional the heart muscle. Echocardiography can identify regional wall motion abnormalities as no contraction (akinesia) or paradoxical contraction or bulging (dyskinesia). Clinically akinesia and dyskinesia have the same consequences and will be manifested as a decreased ejection fraction (EF), cardiac output (CO), and tissue perfusion; dysrhythmias; and heart failure (HF). Additionally, scar tissue is not as strong as muscle and the area can become weakened to the point that an aneurysm forms (most commonly in the LV), further impairing contractility and causing potential clot formation within the aneurysm. LV aneurysmectomy and surgical treatments to remodel scarred muscle (e.g., Dor procedure or Batista procedure) have shown mixed results.

Physiology of Chest Pain

Inflammation, obstruction or restriction, and distention or dilation of the heart or structures surrounding the heart are the etiologic agents of chest pain. Chest pain itself is difficult to diagnose because the afferent nerves in the heart share a common nerve tract with organs in the chest and upper abdomen (Figure 9-3). Pain receptors (nociceptors) are distributed widely, with more nociceptors in the cutaneous tissues and less in the organs. Pain is sensed at the nociceptors and transmitted through the afferent pain fibers through the spinal cord and transverse the cardiac and pulmonary nerves to the dorsal nerve roots. Transmission of pain sensation through rapidly conducting A-delta fibers (medium-sized, lightly mylelinated, found in cutaneous tissue) produces a pain sensation that is sharp and localized (30). Transmission of pain through the C-fibers found in the viscera (small, unmyelinated) is much slower and produces a duller, aching, and poorly localized (diffuse) sensation (30).

Common locations of chest pain radiation include the upper chest, beneath the sternum, the neck, jaw, and/or down the arms (left arm, most commonly), the epigastric area, and the intrascapular regions (Figure 9-4). Recognizing that somatic or visceral pain in the areas sensed by T1-T5 all share a common pain pathway to the brain makes it easier to understand that chest pain may

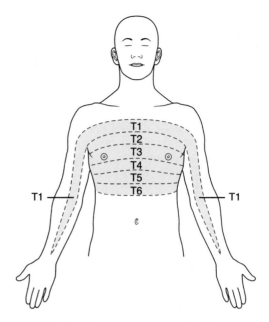

FIGURE 9–3: Common nerve tracts for chest pain sensation.

be of cardiac origin (ischemic or nonischemic etiologies), or from another source. Other causes of "chest" pain include disorders of the pulmonary, gastrointestinal, esophageal, and musculoskeletal systems; mental or somatoform disorders, or from miscellaneous causes (Figure 9-5). Because of the life-threatening nature of MI, all chest pain must initially be considered of cardiac origin until proved otherwise.

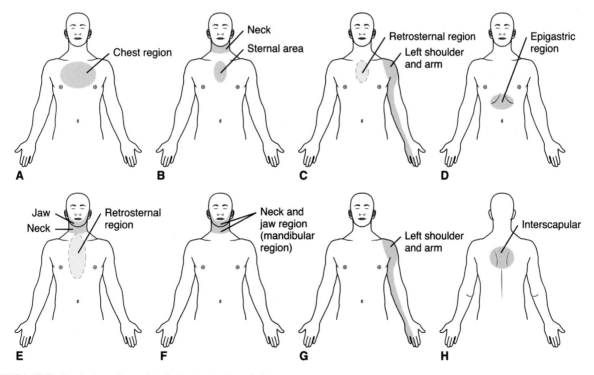

FIGURE 9–4: Locations of typical chest pain radiation.

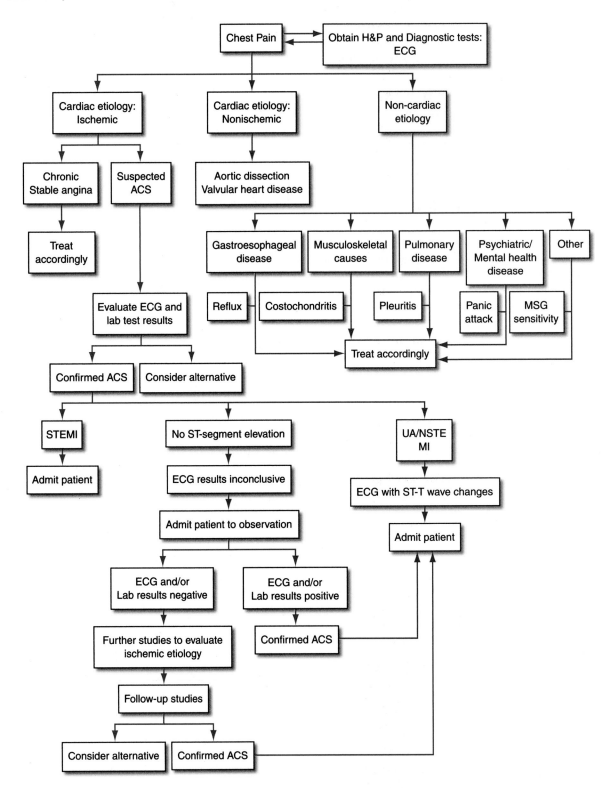

FIGURE 9–5: Algorithm for diagnosis and management of patients with chest pain. *[Sources: Anderson et al., 2007 (18); Fraker et al., 2007 (42); Thygesen et al., 2007 (29).]*

Clinical Presentation

Clinical presentations of ACS are the result of decreased blood flow, and therefore reduced oxygen delivery, to the heart and other tissues. Partial occlusion of the affected vessel may only cause a temporary reduction in flow; reestablishment of blood flow usually occurs upon discontinuance of the activity that caused the transient ischemia, or relaxation of the coronary artery after coronary artery spasm. The more rapidly coronary blood flow is restored, the less heart muscle is permanently damaged. However, studies have shown that many are likely to delay the seeking of emergency care during an ischemic event. The average delay between the onset of prolonged chest pain and treatment seeking is about 2 hours (18).

The classic sign of ischemia is chest pain of varying intensity from discomfort to heavy pressure. Other signs and symptoms of ischemia, which may not be as quickly recognized as chest pain, include pain in the neck, upper jaw, and/or arm (either arm), as well as nonpain indicators of ischemia known as anginal equivalents. Box 9-2 lists signs and symptoms, besides chest pain, observed or reported during ischemic episodes.

Atypical presentations seem to be partially responsible for a delay in early treatment and are common in older adults; those with altered pain perceptions, neuropathies, or sensory dysfunction (e.g., diabetes, spinal cord disease, stroke); and women. Women do not describe pain with the same pain descriptors as men—women's pain tends to be reported primarily in the back, shoulder, neck, and chest—and may delay seeking treatment for MI as a result. Delays in seeking treatment are also seen more frequently in older adults than in younger adults (18). Table 9-6 compares the clinical presentations of ischemia in women, older adults, diabetics, and those with spinal cord injury. This knowledge is helpful in recognizing myocardial ischemia in these vulnerable populations.

Patient gestures may help the clinician differentiate chest pain causes. Levine's sign—the patient signals chest pain as a clenched fist over the precordium (31, 32), an open palm with fingers spread over the precordium (i.e., a flat hand), or the palms of both hands drawn laterally from the sternum across the chest are all gestures typical of patients with ischemic pain (Figure 9-6) (32). The

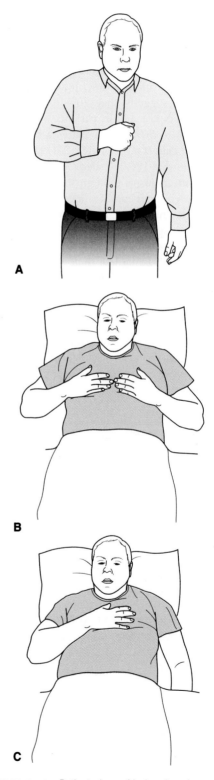

BOX 9–2 Common Anginal Equivalents: Signs and Symptoms of Ischemia in the Absence of Chest Pain/Discomfort

- Generalized weakness
- Fatigue or extreme fatigue
- Dyspnea/Shortness of breath
- Diaphoresis
- Syncope or near syncope
- Palpitations
- Dysrhythmias
- Pain in the abdominal region, back, jaw, arm, or shoulder (may be exercise-induced)
- Disorientation/confusion

FIGURE 9–6: Patient clues of ischemic pain.

ability to point to a specific painful location on the chest wall is more indicative of pleural or musculoskeletal pain. The patient who demonstrates the location of their chest pain by running their fingertips up and down the sides of the sternum are more likely to suffer from esophageal pain than cardiac pain (32). Differential clues for chest pain complaints are listed in Table 9-8. (Refer back to Table 9-5 for a comparison of clinical manifestations of ACS conditions.)

Of note, CNSs should coach their staff that the differentiation of ischemia and infarction cannot be made on the complaints of and descriptions of chest pain alone. Research suggests that 70% to 80% ischemic episodes are asymptomatic in patients with CAD (12) and about 25% to 50% of MI patients have no complaints of chest pain at all (i.e., silent MI) (2, 12, 18). The AHA estimates that 195,000 silent MIs occur each year (2). Biologic mechanisms thought to be responsible for asymptomatic episodes include (a) afferent nerve dysfunction such as that caused by denervation of the heart after transplant, spinal cord injury, or peripheral neuropathy in patients with diabetes; (b) temporary reduction in blood flow lasting less than 30 seconds causing immediate systolic and diastolic dysfunction, but no angina, as angina occurs after 30 seconds of ischemia; and (c) differing individual patient pain thresholds as a result of plasma endorphin differences (12). Patient age may also affect perception of pain and/or physiologic response to pain. For example, older adults commonly present with symptoms other than chest pain when experiencing ACS, such as confusion or shortness of breath; additionally blunted vital sign responses due to normal aging may further confuse the diagnosis. Differential clues in the physical and laboratory assessment and evaluation of ECG findings, with their associated likelihood ratios (LRs) (33, 34), for diagnosing MI are found in Table 9-9. LRs are interpreted as how much more or less a particular sign or symptom is demonstrated in a patient with disease than in a patient without disease (35). For a brief overview of likelihood ratios and how they are used in clinical practice, see Box 9-3 (36).

Diagnosis

The diagnosis of ACS relies on three major findings: (a) the patient's history, (b) the results of the ECG, and (c) the results of cardiac enzyme testing. The ability to differentiate between angina and MI is important, but the diagnosis cannot be made based on signs and symptoms alone. Anginal pain typically does not last as long as that of an MI, the trigger for chest pain is usually known, the pain quality tends to be different, and rest or nitroglycerin usually relieves the pain. However, patients with ACS do not always present in a classic manner, especially older adults. The way people describe the quality of chest pain is variable, and descriptors alone are not reliable in differentiating between the syndromes. Remember that about 25% of MIs are silent—chest pain is not the chief complaint.

Chest pain related to an impending or evolving MI is typically described as squeezing or heaviness radiating to

TABLE 9–8 Differential Clues for Chest Pain

Clinical Sign or Symptom	Pain Origin Most Likely
• Closed fist or open palm on chest with spread fingers	Ischemic
• Fingers of two hands on either side of sternum drawn laterally across the chest	
• Finger-point to pain location	Pleuritic, costochondritis
• Sharp, stabbing	
• Pain increases with inspiration, cough, or position change	Musculoskeletal, pericarditis, pleuritic
• Fingers of two hands running up and down on either side of sternum	GI (including esophagus)
• Pain location primarily in middle or lower abdomen	
• Burning sensation face/chest; feeling of heaviness/fullness	MSG sensitivity
• Sudden in onset	Pulmonary embolism, aortic dissection
• Sharp, stabbing	
• "Tearing" feeling	Aortic dissection
• Severe back pain	
• Affirmative answer to question "Does the chest pain get worse when you smoke?"	Ischemic (R/T effect of nicotine on vasculature)

GI, gastrointestinal; MSG, monosodium glutamate; R/T, related to.

TABLE 9-9 Likelihood Ratios as Diagnostic Clues for Myocardial Infarction in Patients Presenting With Acute Chest Pain

Clinical Symptom or Sign	LR+ (95% Confidence Interval [CI])	LR- (95% CI)
More Likely		
Chest pain radiating to both arms	7.10 (3.6–14.2)	0.67
Hypotension	3.10 (1.8–5.2)	0.96
S$_3$ heart sound	3.20 (1.6–6.5)	0.88
Pulmonary crackles	2.1 (1.4–3.1)	
Diaphoresis	2.00 (1.99–2.20)	0.64
Less Likely		
Pleuritic chest pain	0.2 (0.2–0.3)	1.20
Reproducible chest pain on palpation	0.2–0.4	1.20
Sharp or stabbing chest pain	0.3 (0.2–0.5)	
Positional chest pain	0.3 (0.2–0.4)	
Electrocardiogram (ECG) Finding	**LR+ (95% CI)**	**LR-**
New ST elevation ≥1mm	16.0	0.52
New Q wave	8.7	0.68
New conduction defect	6.3 (2.5–15.7)	0.88
New T-wave inversion	2.5	0.72
Any ST segment elevation	11.2 (7.1–17.8)	0.45
Any ST segment depression	3.2 (2.5–4.1)	
Any Q wave	3.9 (2.7–5.7)	0.60
Any conduction defect	2.7 (1.4–5.4)	0.89
Normal ECG	0.1–0.3	
Cardiac Enzyme Result	**LR+**	**LR-**
Troponin I >1ng per mL (1 mcg/L) at least 6 hours from presentation	18.0	0.10
Troponin T >2ng per mL (2 mcg/L) at least 8 hours from presentation	5.2	0.05

Sources: Caley, 2005 (33); Panju, 1998 (34).

BOX 9-3 What Are Likelihood Ratios and How Are They Used in Clinical Practice?

Likelihood ratios (LRs) are used to help the advanced clinician refine their differential diagnosis by providing information on the "value" of laboratory or diagnostic tests to predict disease. The clinician starts with their clinical suspicion of which disease the patient is likely experiencing (also known as the pretest probability of the disease) based on the patient's chief complaint, history, and physical exam findings. Diagnostic and laboratory testing is then conducted, and the results are used to refine the differential list and therefore decrease the uncertainty of the final diagnosis (thereby determining the posttest probability of disease X). The value of the physical exam findings and test results can be compared using the LRs. LRs are becoming the preferred parameter to help the advanced clinician rule in or rule out a specific diagnosis.

LRs are defined as the odds or chances of a particular sign or symptom occurring in a patient with disease divided by the odds of the same test result, sign, or symptom occurring in a patient without disease. The LR provides an indication of how strongly a test result, sign, or symptom is associated with a particular disease; therefore, LRs can help clinicians decide which tests to order (i.e., the test with the strongest LR+ or LR–). The higher the positive LR (LR+), the more strongly the presence of that sign/symptom/test result is associated with the specific disease you suspect. The lower the negative LR (LR–), the less likely the sign/symptom/test result is associated with the disease you suspect—helping you determine that the patient does NOT have the disease.

Continued

BOX 9–3　What Are Likelihood Ratios and How Are They Used in Clinical Practice?—cont'd

LRs are easily calculated and derived from the sensitivity and specificity of the specific test result, sign, or symptom. An LR can be calculated for every sign/symptom/test result (if you know its sensitivity and specificity); therefore LRs are used to assess the relative worth of a diagnostic test, sign, or symptom and can be compared. LRs are similar to the concept of relative risk. You want to choose a test that will provide you with the best, most accurate result—that is, one that makes the most difference in reducing your uncertainty of the diagnosis—so the tests with the highest or lowest LRs will produce the most change in the probability of disease.

"HOW TO"

Differential diagnosis is the best guess of which disease processes are likely for the patient based on chief complaint, history, and physical exam findings. You have a clinical suspicion of which diseases are more likely and can assign a value to how sure you are the patient has disease X—that's your pretest probability.

When the patient's test result is positive (e.g., an abnormal stress test) or the person demonstrates a particular sign or symptom (e.g., an S_3 is auscultated) the clinician would look up the LR for a positive result (LR+), for that test result/sign/symptom, to assist in determining whether the patient really has the disease or not. You then apply the LR+ to your pretest probability and come up with a posttest probability that the person has or does not have the disease—you increase or decrease diagnostic uncertainty. If the patient has a negative test result or the patient does not exhibit a disease-specific sign or symptom, the clinician would use the negative LR measure (LR–) to figure out the likelihood of disease in that case.

An application to calculate LRs and posttest probability can be downloaded to your SmartPhone or personal digital assistant (PDA). All you need to input is your pretest probability and the LRs of the sign/symptom/test to get the posttest probability. (If you don't know the LRs, you'll need to input the sensitivity and specificity of the particular test/sign/symptom for the LR to be calculated.) The program will apply the LRs to your pretest probability of disease (what you thought the patient had before you started testing) to give you a posttest probability—that is the probability the patient has disease X, now that you have these results. Based on your posttest probability, you make a decision to treat the patient, order more tests because you still cannot be certain of the disease, or consider an alternative diagnosis (and start over!). Positive LRs (LR+) greater than 10 or negative LRs (LR–) less than 0.1 will incur the most change in the posttest probability of disease.

Application to Practice 1: For example, in assessing the electrocardiogram (ECG) of a patient suspected of have a myocardial infarction (MI), new ST elevation of ≥1 mm has a positive LR (LR+) of 16 and a negative LR (LR–) of 0.52.

Interpretation: An ECG finding of new ST elevation of ≥1mm is 16 times more likely to be found in a patient experiencing an MI than in a patient who is not experiencing an MI. The LR+ of 16 is high and will increase your certainty of an MI diagnosis. If you thought the patient had a 25% chance of having an MI, this LR+ of 16 would increase your certainty of diagnosis to 84%. If you started with a 50% pretest probability (a coin toss!) your certainty of the diagnosis would increase to 94%. It is very likely that this patient is having an MI and you would consider beginning treatment.

Application to Practice 2: The patient is suspected of having an MI, but not showing new ST elevation of ≥1 mm is not very likely to be having an MI (LR– 0.52):though there is still a possibility that the patient is experiencing a non–ST-segment elevation MI (NSTEMI).

Interpretation: The odds of a patient having an MI, with no new ST elevation of ≥1 mm, are 0.52. The LR– of 0.52 is not very large and won't change your posttest probability of disease by much. If you thought the patient had a 25% chance of having an MI, this LR– of 0.52 would bring your posttest probability down to 15%. If you started with a 50% pretest probability (a coin toss!), this result would only decrease your diagnostic certainty to 34%. It is unlikely that this patient is having an MI—though there is still a 34% chance! The outcome? You have to do more testing (in this scenario, serial cardiac enzymes) because though the likelihood has decreased, you are still uncertain of the diagnosis: the patient still could be having an MI—or not.

From Thompson, C. J. 2010; Statistical measures used for evidence-based practice. South Fork, CO: CJT Consulting (36). With permission.

the jaw, neck, or arm and lasts for more than 30 minutes despite rest or nitroglycerin (NTG) tablets. Refer to Table 9-5 for distinguishing characteristics of anginal syndromes compared to those of MI. Other clues of ACS in a patient with a history of angina include a description of chest pain as different from what the patient normally experiences, pain lasting longer than 30 minutes, and the presence of one or more risk factors for CAD. The 12-lead ECG, serum biomarkers of myocardial damage, a chest radiograph, diagnostic angiography, and possible cardiac testing with stress testing or nuclear imaging are common diagnostic tests to rule in or rule out ACS.

Intravascular ultrasound may also be considered as it provides an internal look at the patency of the coronary arteries; often lesions that are not apparent on angiography are visualized using this technology (18).

Invasive and Noninvasive Testing

Diagnostic angiography is recommended for patients who meet criteria for a suspected ACS condition, although revascularization is not a viable option for all patients. The decision to refer a high-risk patient (those with multiple risk factors and/or comorbidities, a previous history of cardiac disease or intervention, or positive troponin levels) for angiography or revascularization should be discussed between all parties—the physician, patient, and family member and/or patient advocate (18). Detailed management of the patient post angiography is found in the joint guidelines produced by the AHA and the American College of Cardiology (ACC) (18). Noninvasive stress testing is used to provide diagnostic and prognostic information to determine the need for additional testing and to plan care and is recommended for low-risk and some intermediate-risk patients meeting certain criteria (18). Either treadmill exercise or pharmacologic stress testing (i.e., stress radionuclide ventriculography) can be used to evaluate myocardial function. Stress echocardiography may also be used in the evaluation of ACS patients. Patient performance and response to stress testing are measured and the patient's treadmill score is one data point used to stratify patients according to risk of future coronary events: high risk, intermediate risk, and low risk.

ECG Findings

Dead myocardium is nonfunctional. Necrotic and scarred muscle does not contract nor does it conduct electricity (which is why we can diagnose MIs using the ECG). ECG changes warn of impending injury, allow the determination of the location of the MI and the suspected coronary artery involved, and give an indication of the extent and "age" of the infarction (29).

ST segment monitoring is useful for early recognition of cardiac ischemia. ST elevation is a sign of myocardial injury; ST depression typically a sign of ischemia or reciprocal changes in the leads opposite the infarcted tissue. For example, ST depression noted in V_1 and V_2 are reciprocal changes and instead of indicating ischemic changes actually denote cardiac injury in the posterior wall opposite the lead placement.

Patients with UA may show variable abnormalities on ECG. T-wave inversion is a sign of disruption of electrical conduction in the heart (repolarization abnormalities) and characteristic of MI. Patients suffering from STEMI will show ST elevation in the leads overlooking the area of injury; reciprocal changes may be seen in the leads viewing the heart muscle on the side opposite that of the injured tissue. Additionally, abnormal Q waves will develop overlying infarcted tissue. The development of Q waves signifies a transmural infarction. In patients for whom the injured and infarcted tissue is localized to the epicardial or endocardial layers (and possibly extending into the myocardium), ST segments may not elevate and Q waves may not develop leading to the diagnosis of NSTEMI.

Table 9-10 identifies the ECG findings associated with acute MI (AMI). Findings from ECG testing that have the highest odds of correctly diagnosing AMI are ST-segment elevation, Q-wave development, the presence of a conduction defect, and T-wave inversion; new findings are more diagnostic than those already

TABLE 9–10 Electrocardiogram (ECG) Changes Indicative of Acute Myocardial Infarction (AMI)

	ECG Findings
Early changes	T wave changes
	• Increased hyperacute T-wave elevation with tall, symmetrical T-waves in at least two contiguous leads is an early sign that may be a precursor to the elevation of the ST segment.
	R-wave changes
	• Increased R-wave elevation and width (e.g., large R-wave with shrinking S-wave) usually seen in leads demonstrating ST elevation and tall T-waves due to conduction delay in the ischemic tissue.
	Q-wave changes
	• Transient Q-waves occasionally seen during acute ischemic event; rarely seen during AMI with successful reperfusion.

Continued

TABLE 9–10 Electrocardiogram (ECG) Changes Indicative of Acute Myocardial Infarction (AMI)—cont'd

	ECG Findings
Acute ischemic changes	New ST elevation (measured at J-point) in 2 contiguous leads • Leads V_{2-3}: Men ≥0.2 mV or 2 mm; Women ≥0.15 mV or 1.5 mm and/or • All other leads: ≥0.1 mV or 1 mm New ST depression • Horizontal or down-sloping ST segment depression ≥0.05 mV (0.5 mm) in 2 contiguous leads and/or T-wave inversion • ≥0.1 mV (1 mm) in 2 contiguous leads with prominent R-wave or RS ratio >1

established (33). New ST-segment elevations are diagnostic for MI, and therefore ST-segment monitoring should be instituted if the ECG monitors have this capability. Frequent serial ECG recordings provide data points to compare to baseline recordings. Refer to Table 9-9 to find the LRs of ECG findings in MI.

The diagnosis of MI occurs with permanent damage to one, two, or all three layers of the heart muscle. Members from the European Society of Cardiology (ESC), the ACC, the AHA, and the World Heart Federation organized a global task force to review current evidence and revised an earlier consensus document of the definition of MI (29). The new definition relies heavily on highly sensitive and specific cardiac biomarkers, troponin elevations in particular, for evidence of AMI (Table 9-11).

Cardiac Enzymes
Cardiac enzymes are released from necrotic myocytes at specific time intervals and afford an estimation of the amount of damage incurred via the enzyme types and serum levels (Table 9-12). The earliest enzyme released

TABLE 9–11 Revised Universal Definition of Acute Myocardial Infarction (AMI)

Myocardial infarction is defined as any one of the following criteria:

• Cardiac enzyme changes combined with at least one sign or symptom of myocardial ischemia

• Cardiac troponins (preferred biomarker) rise, fall, or both, with at least one value above the 99th percentile of the upper reference limit (URL)

Plus any of the following:

• Ischemic symptoms
• Development of ECG changes
  • New pathologic Q waves
  • New ST-T changes
  • New left bundle-branch block (LBBB)
• New Imaging evidence
  • Loss of viable myocardium
  • Regional wall motion abnormalities

TABLE 9–11 Revised Universal Definition of Acute Myocardial Infarction (AMI)—cont'd

- Sudden, unexpected cardiac death before ability to draw laboratory samples or before samples are positive for biomarkers

- Percutaneous coronary intervention (PCI)-related MI
  - Defined as an MI occurring during the PCI procedure in patients with baseline troponin levels that are within the normal range
- Coronary artery bypass grafting (CABG)-related MI
  - Defined as an MI occurring during the CABG procedure in patients with baseline troponin levels that are within the normal range

- Pathologic changes of myocardial necrosis

- Cardiac arrest with ischemic symptoms, and new ST-segment elevation or new (LBBB)

and/or

- New thrombus identified at coronary angiography and/or at autopsy
- Elevations >3 times the 99th percentile URL for cardiac enzymes (troponins = preferred biomarker) (AKA PCI-related MI)
- Documented stent thrombosis
- Elevations >5 times the 99th percentile URL

Plus any of the following:

- Development of ECG changes
  - New pathologic Q-waves
  - New LBBB
- Angiographic evidence
  - New graft occlusion
  - Native coronary artery occlusion
- Imaging evidence
  - New loss of viable myocardium
- Pathologic evidence

From Thygesen et al, 2007; Universal definition of myocardial infarction. Circulation 116(22):2634-2653; doi:10.1161/circulationaha.107.187397 (29).

TABLE 9–12 Characteristics of Cardiac Enzymes

	Normal Value	Rise	Approximate Peak	Duration	Comments
Myoglobin	<0.85 ng/mL Males: 17—106 ng/mL * Females: 14—66 ng/mL	1–2 hours	8–10 hours	24 hours	First test to show rise in level, but not specific for cardiac muscle
Cardiac troponins cTpI cTpT	<0.03–0.05 ng/mL 0.05–0.12 = ng/mL minimal cardiac injury ≥0.12 ng/mL = probable MI	3–6 hours (may be detected in blood in 2–4 hours; elevation maybe delayed up to 8–12 h)	18–24 hours	5–14 days	Cardiospecific; Preferred test to R/O MI Noncoronary causes can also raise cTpn levels

Continued

TABLE 9–12 Characteristics of Cardiac Enzymes—cont'd

	Normal Value	Rise	Approximate Peak	Duration	Comments
CPK-MB LDH	<6 ng/mL (6mcg/L) 105–333 IU/L LDH-1 18%–33% LDH-2 28%–40%	4–12 hours 6–12 hours	18–24 hours 24–48 hours	36–72 hours 6–8 days	Measured by mass assay –Flipped LDH pattern: LDH 1 > LHD 2 indicative of MI (normally LDH 2 > LDH 1); –LDH-1 is found primarily in heart muscle and red blood cells –LDH-2 is concentrated in white blood cells –May help "time" MI as high levels early in patient's presentation indicate an infarction that occurred several days before patient presented in the ED

Data from Agruss and Garrett, 2005 (40); Chan and Ng, 2010, (39); Joiss-Bilowich, 2010 (37); Schrieber and Miller, 2009 (38); Thygesen et al, 2007 (29).

ED, emergency department;MI, myocardial infarction; R/O, rule out

by damaged muscle is myoglobin, which rises within 1 to 2 hours of injury (Figure 9-7). Because myoglobin rises so rapidly, it has been used in some emergency departments (EDs) to help diagnose MI early. However, because it is not specific for cardiac muscle damage, myoglobin should not be used as a solitary marker of cardiac damage—a rising myoglobin can be a sign of muscle injury anywhere in the body (37, 38). Additionally, its use is being reconsidered in EDs because of the superiority of the cardiac troponin assays (38).

In contrast, cardiac troponins are very specific to cardiac muscle and are considered the gold standard and preferred biomarker for cardiac enzyme testing and integral to the new definition of MI (18, 29, 37). As little as 1 gram of infarcted cardiac muscle can be detected by cardiac troponin levels; MI is identified as the elevation of troponin levels above the 99th percentile of normal (18). The greater the elevations of troponin above the 99th percentile, the more cardiac muscle is damaged and the greater the mortality rate (18, 29). Both cardiac troponin I (cTpI) and cardiac troponin T (cTpT) are highly sensitive and specific for

cardiac muscle damage. cTpI rises slightly faster than cTpT, within 3 to 6 hours versus 6 to 8 hours. To assist in early diagnosis, the use of an early biomarker (e.g., myoglobin) and a late marker (cTpI or cTpT) together is recommended for patients presenting within 6 hours of ACS symptom onset (class IIb, Level of Evidence [LOE] B recommendation) (18) (Table 9-13).

Creatinine phosphokinase (CPK; CK) is an enzyme also found in a variety of tissues; total CK by itself is no longer a recommended test for initial management of the patient with suspected ACS (18). The CK isoenzyme specific to cardiac muscle (myocardial bands [MB]; CK-MB) is highly specific for myocardial damage. Elevated CK-MB levels are indicative of cardiac injury. Again, because of the superior performance characteristics of the cardiac troponin assays some institutions have stopped the use of CK-MB isoforms (38).

Lactic dehydrogenase (LDH) isoenzyme levels (LHD1 and LDH2) were routinely drawn for suspected MI in the past, although the discovery of the cardiac troponins has caused its use to decline in recent years and it is no longer recommended as a primary test for ACS

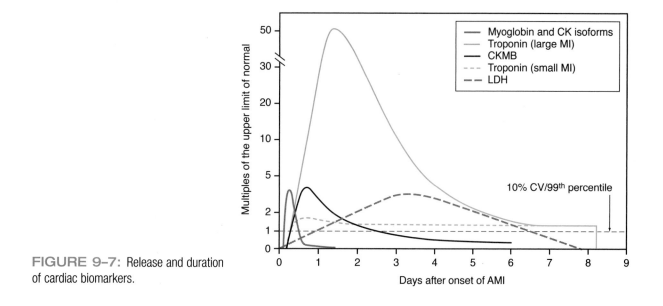

FIGURE 9–7: Release and duration of cardiac biomarkers.

TABLE 9–13 Selected Recommendations for the Immediate and Early Management of Patients at High Risk for UA/NSTEMI

Recommendation

INITIAL EVALUATION AND MANAGEMENT

- Give 162–325 mg of chewable, nonenteric coated aspirin (ASA) unless contraindicated or already taken by patient (e.g., by EMS or self-administered) (LOE C)

(ALL RECOMMENDATIONS ARE CLASS I UNLESS OTHERWISE NOTED)

- 12L ECG within 10 min of ED arrival (LOE B);
  - Nondiagnostic initial ECG:
    - Continue serial ECGs q15–30min → look for development of ST-segment elevation or depression (LOE B)
    - Obtain supplemental ECG leads V_7–V_9 to rule out MI due to left circumflex occlusion (class IIa, LOE B)
- Cardiac biomarkers should be measured in all patients with ACS symptoms (LOE B) q6–8h, 2–3 times or until levels peak (class IIa, LOE B)
  - Cardiac troponins (cTnI/T) preferred test (LOE B)
  - Negative cardiac biomarkers within 6 h of the onset of suspected ACS symptoms should have biomarkers redrawn 8 to 12 h after symptom onset (LOE B)
  - Multimarker method for patients presenting within 6 h of symptom onset: Myoglobin recommended as an early marker of muscle injury combined with late marker (cTnI/T) (class IIb, LOE B)
  - Measurement of BNP or NT-pro-BNP may be considered (class IIb, LOE B)
- Patients with negative results on ECG or biomarkers initially should be observed in monitored unit, with repeat ECGs and biomarkers obtained (LOE B)
- Low risk patients not admitted but referred for outpatient testing should be tested within 72 h and given medications while awaiting test results (LOE C)

Continued

TABLE 9–13 Selected Recommendations for the Immediate and Early Management of Patients at High Risk for UA/NSTEMI—cont'd

Recommendation
(ALL RECOMMENDATIONS ARE CLASS I UNLESS OTHERWISE NOTED)

- Admit patients with definite ACS and ongoing ischemic symptoms, positive cardiac biomarkers, new ST-segment deviations, new deep T-wave inversions, hemodynamic abnormalities, or a positive stress test to a monitored unit (e.g., telemetry). Admission to the critical care unit is recommended for those with active, ongoing ischemia/injury and hemodynamic or electrical instability. (LOE C)
- Patients with definite ACS and ST-segment elevation in leads V_7–V_9 (secondary to left circumflex involvement; i.e., true posterior MI) should be evaluated for immediate reperfusion therapy. (LOE A)

Possible Harm:

- Total CK (without MB), aspartate aminotransferase (AST, SGOT), alanine transaminase, beta-hydroxybutyric dehydrogenase, and/or lactate dehydrogenase should not be utilized as primary tests for ACS patients. (class III, LOE C)

EARLY HOSPITAL CARE

A. ANTI-ISCHEMIC AND ANALGESIC THERAPY

- Bed/chair rest with continuous ECG monitoring (LOE C)
- Administer supplemental oxygen to all patients during the first 6 h after presentation (class IIa, LOE C); and for patients with PaO_2 <90%, respiratory distress, or other signs of hypoxemia. (class I, LOE B)
- Pulse oximetry may be used for continuous measurement of SaO_2. (LOE B)
- Patients with ongoing symptoms of ischemic pain should receive sublingual NTG (0. 4 mg) every 5 min for a total of 3 doses. (LOE C)
- IV NTG is indicated in the first 48 h for treatment of persistent ischemia, heart failure (HF), or hypertension (LOE B); but beta-blockers and ACEI should still be administered if no contraindications. (LOE B)
- Oral beta-blocker therapy should be initiated within the first 24 h for patients without contraindications (e.g., 1) ≥1 of the following: HF signs, 2) low-output state, 3) high risk for cardiogenic shock, or 4) other relative contraindications to beta-blockade (PR interval greater than 0.24 s, second-or third-degree heart block, active asthma, or reactive airway disease). (LOE B)
  - Intolerance to beta-blockers: Give a nondihydropyridine calcium channel blocker (e.g., verapamil or diltiazem), barring contraindications to calcium channel blocker therapy. (LOE B)
- An oral ACE inhibitor should be given within the first 24 h to UA/NSTEMI patients with pulmonary congestion or LV ejection fraction (LVEF) ≤40%, barring low systolic blood pressure or known contraindications to that class of medications. (LOE A)
  - Intolerance to ACE inhibitors: Give an angiotensin receptor blocker if intolerant of ACE inhibitors and have either clinical or radiologic signs of HF or low LVEF. (LOE A)

TABLE 9–13 Selected Recommendations for the Immediate and Early Management of Patients at High Risk for UA/NSTEMI—cont'd

Recommendation	
EARLY HOSPITAL CARE	
	• IV morphine sulfate is reasonable for symptoms not relieved by other methods, even if NTG is being used. (class IIa, LOE B) • Intra-aortic balloon pump counterpulsation is reasonable for patient who could benefit from its use. (class IIa, LOE C) Possible Harm: • Discontinue all nonsteroidal anti-inflammatory drugs (NSAIDs), except for ASA, and do not administer during hospitalization. (class III, LOE C)

B. Antiplatelet/Anticoagulant Therapy
I. ANTIPLATELET THERAPY
II. ANTICOAGULANT THERAPY
	• ASA therapy should be administered on presentation and continued indefinitely (LOE A)
	• Clopidogrel (first line; LOE A) or Prasugrel (second line; LOE B) should be administered at PCI (new recommendation 2009).
	• Clopidogrel (loading dose followed by daily maintenance dose) is an alternative medication for patients who are aspirin sensitive. (LOE A)
	• Anticoagulant therapy should be added to antiplatelet therapy as soon as possible (LOE A), especially if invasive therapy is planned. (LOE A; new recommendation 2009)
	  • Efficacious anticoagulant regimens for patients undergoing invasive strategy include enoxaparin and UFH (LOE A), bivalirudin and fondaparinux. (LOE B)
	  • Efficacious regiments for patients undergoing conservative strategy include enoxaparin or UFH (LOE A) or fondaparinux. (LOE B; preferred for patients with an increased risk of bleeding)
	• Proton-pump inhibitors should be prescribed with ASA and/or clopidogrel therapy concomitantly. (LOE B)
	• Either an IV GP IIb/IIIa inhibitor (eptifibatide or tirofiban; (LOE A) or clopidogrel (loading dose followed by daily maintenance dose; LOE A) should be added to ASA and anticoagulant therapy before diagnostic angiography. (LOE C).
	
	Possible Harm:
	
	• Abciximab should not be administered to patients in whom PCI is not planned. (LOE A)

From Anderson et al. ACC/AHA 2007 guidelines for the management of patients with unstable angina/non–ST-elevation myocardial infarction: a report of the American College of Cardiology/American Heart Association Task Force on Practice Guidelines. J Am Coll Cardiol 2007; 50(7):e1-e157; doi:10.1016/j.jacc.2007.02.013 (18)

ACEI, angiotensin converting enzyme inhibitor; ACS, acute coronary syndrome, BNP, brain natriuretic peptide; ECG, electrocardiogram; EMS, emergency medical services; HF, heart failure; LOE, level of evidence; LVEF, left ventricular ejection fraction; NTG, nitroglycerin; NT-pro-BNP, N-terminal portion of the pro-BNP peptide; PCI, percutaneous coronary intervention; S_aO_2, oxygen saturation; UFH, unfractionated heparin.

(class III, LOE C; 18). LDH1 is found in higher quantities in the cardiac muscle than LDH2, which is found in white blood cells; normally LDH2 is higher than LDH1. A "flipped" pattern (LHD1 > LHD2) is indicative of cardiac damage. LDH isoenzymes may be helpful in establishing the "age" of the MI in patients who may have delayed seeking treatment when the symptoms began, as the LDH levels rise later than cardiac troponins and stay elevated for a longer length of time. Thus, high LDH levels in a patient who presents in the ED may indicate an infarct that occurred several days before the patient sought treatment.

B-type natriuretic peptide (BNP) identifies LV dysfunction and has been used as a prognostic indicator of HF. Its use as a marker of AMI is limited by low specificity, although it may be helpful in identifying residual LV function and prognosis in ACS patients (37-40). Because BNP is rapidly eliminated from the serum, the N-terminal portion of the pro-BNP peptide (NT-pro-BNP) is measured. Other biomarkers being researched for rapid diagnosis of AMI include heart-type fatty acid binding protein (H-FABP), ischemia modified albumin (IMA) (37, 38), high-sensitivity CRP (hs-CRP), pregnancy-associated plasma protein A (PAPP-A), myeloperioxidase (MPO), C-terminal provasopressin (copeptin), and lipoprotein-associated phospholipase A2 (Lp-PLA2) (37-40). In accordance with national guidelines, positive cardiac biomarkers should be drawn every 6 to 9 hours, 2 to 3 times or until peak levels are noted; the higher the level of biomarker in the blood, the more cardiac damage that has occurred (18). Negative serial cardiac biomarker results, drawn through the sixth through the ninth hour after the onset of symptoms, can effectively rule out AMI according to the updated 2007 guidelines (18, 38).

After the diagnosis of acute MI, clinical guidelines call for the evaluation of the patient's LV systolic function (class I) to guide therapeutic decisions (i.e., the prescription of ACEI or ARB, or invasive therapy) and provide prognostic information (LV function is directly related to long-term survival) (41).

Management

Management of ACS will differ based on the final diagnosis of UA or NSTEMI versus STEMI, although many of the initial interventions are the same. The patient presenting with signs and symptoms suggestive of ACS is categorized into four possible diagnoses: (a) a noncardiac diagnosis; (b) chronic stable angina; (c) possible ACS; and (d) definite ACS (ST elevation or non-ST elevation) (5). Almost 80% of patients experiencing an MI will have a non-ST elevation MI (21). Refer to Figure 9-5 for an algorithm to assess and manage patients with suspected ACS. Revised guidelines for chronic stable angina (42) are freely available on the

AHA Web site (www.myamericanheart.org) and will not be discussed in this chapter.

Major professional medical and interdisciplinary organizations have produced evidence-based clinical practice guidelines (CPGs) to assist in the evaluation and management of patients with ACS. As new scientific information becomes available, many guidelines are revised to reflect current best practice; levels of evidence are assigned to research studies to provide an objective measure of the strength of the study, based on quality and scientific criteria. Once the studies are rated, practice recommendations are proposed based on the overall strength of the evidence. Practice recommendations are then assigned a "grade," providing a visual tool of the value of the recommendation for the busy practitioner. Note that there is no universal system of classification for CPGs. Clinicians should not assume that class I evidence or a grade A recommendation is defined the same in all guidelines and should check the document for its explanation of the system used to produce the practice recommendations. The classification system of practice recommendations (class I, II, III, etc.) and study quality, or levels of evidence (LOE) A, B, or C noted in this chapter are provided verbatim from the guidelines cited; detailed descriptions of the system can be found in any of the AHA/ACC guidelines (18, 41-45). The jointly produced American College of Cardiology Foundation (ACCF)/AHA methodology manual provides policies and procedures designed to be "evidence-based, transparent, and systematic" for writing practice guidelines (46, p. 4). This rigor and transparency allow the APN to have confidence in recommendations outlined in the ACC/AHA guidelines. In this chapter, class I and LOE A indicate recommendations with documented benefit that have been shown to consistently produce positive outcomes, and thus should be performed, and are based on studies with the strongest research designs (i.e., multiple randomized clinical trials and/or meta-analyses).

Emphasizing the importance of early recognition and management of ACS, the revised guidelines for the management of patients with UA/NSTEMI (18) and STEMI (43-45) identify new recommendations and update previous recommendations for the clinical assessment, risk stratification, immediate management, and long-term education and care of patients presenting with ACS symptomatology. Table 9-13 outlines the major class I recommendations for acute care of the UA/NSTEMI patient that APNs can use to educate their staff. Not many of the class I recommendations for STEMI management have changed since the last guidelines were published in 2004 (43), so these recommendations are still in effect. However, new and evolving evidence has necessitated the production of focused updates to those guidelines; these were published in 2007 and 2009 (44, 45). Table 9-14 provides new or changed

(Text continued on page 271)

TABLE 9–14 Class I and/or New Recommendations for Acute Care of the STEMI Patient

Recommendation (Class I, unless noted)	Status of 2007 Recommendation	Status of 2009 Recommendation
ANALGESIA		
Use of morphine sulfate for pain management (2–4 mg IV with increments of 2–8 mg IV repeated at 5–15-min intervals) (Level of Evidence (LOE) C)	No change from 2004 recommendation NEW Terminate selective and nonselective NSAID use for chronic users, except for aspirin, at STEMI presentation d/t increased risk of possibly fatal complications. (LOE C) NEW POSSIBLY HARMFUL: Do not administer selective or nonselective NSAIDs, except for aspirin, for STEMI patients while hospitalized d/t increased risk of possibly fatal complications. (Class III; LOE C)	
BETA-BLOCKER USE		
Initiate oral beta-blocker therapy within 24 hours for patients without contraindications to beta-blockade. (LOE B)	Text edited LOE downgraded	
Reevaluation of STEMI patients for beta-blocker therapy, if not started early because of. (LOE C)	No change from 2004 recommendation	
Administer and titrate beta-blocker therapy to patients with moderate or severe LV failure. (LOE B)	No change from 2004 recommendation	
POSSIBLY HARMFUL: Do not administer IV beta-blockers to STEMI patients with any contraindications. (Class III; LOE A)	NEW	

Continued

TABLE 9–14 Class I and/or New Recommendations for Acute Care of the STEMI Patient—cont'd

Recommendation (Class I, unless noted)	Status of 2007 Recommendation	Status of 2009 Recommendation
REPERFUSION THERAPY		
Provision of primary PCI for STEMI patients within 90 min of first medical contact. (LOE A)	Text edited LOE upgraded	
STEMI patients who are candidates for fibrinolytic therapy should be treated within 30 min of hospital presentation if primary PCI capability is not available or the timely ability to transfer patient to a PCI center is not possible. (LOE B)	Text edited LOE downgraded	
It is reasonable to start treatment with glycoprotein IIb/IIIa receptor antagonists abciximab, (LOE A), tirofiban (LOE B), or eptifibatide (LOE B) at the time of primary PCI (with or without stenting) in selected patients with STEMI. (Class IIa, LOE)		Modified recommendation (class of recommendation changed from IIb to IIa for tirofiban and eptifibatide)
IMMEDIATE (OR EMERGENCY) INVASIVE STRATEGY AND RESCUE PCI		
Following fibrinolytic therapy, plan for coronary angiography with intent to perform PCI (or emergency CABG) is recommended for patients with any of the following conditions: a. Cardiogenic shock (<75 years who are candidates for revascularization (LOE B) b. Severe heart failure and/or pulmonary edema (Killip class III) (LOE B) c. Ventricular arrhythmias causing hemodynamic instability (LOE C)	Text edited LOE delineated for each item NEW POSSIBLY HARMFUL: Do not perform coronary angiography with intent to perform PCI (or emergency CABG), for STEMI patients who have received fibrinolytic therapy if additional invasive therapy is not possible or if it is against the patient/designee's wishes. (class III; LOE C)	

TABLE 9–14 Class I and/or New Recommendations for Acute Care of the STEMI Patient—cont'd

Recommendation (Class I, unless noted)	Status of 2007 Recommendation	Status of 2009 Recommendation

ANTICOAGULANTS AS ADJUNCT THERAPY TO REPERFUSION THERAPY

Recommendation (Class I, unless noted)	Status of 2007 Recommendation	Status of 2009 Recommendation

Proven anticoagulant regimens include:
a. UFH (initial IV bolus 60 U per kg [maximum 4,000 U]) followed by an IV infusion of 12 U per kg per hour (maximum 1,000 U per hour); titrate to maintain the activated partial thromboplastin time at 1.5 to 2.0 times control (approximately 50 to 70 seconds) (LOE C).
b. Enoxaparin (in patients with adequate renal function):
• Loading dose:
  • <75 years old: 30 mg IV bolus, followed 15 min later by SC injections of 1.0 mg per kg every 12 hours;
  • ≥75 years old, no loading dose; SC dose is reduced to 0.75 mg per kg every 12 hours.
• Dose is adjusted for creatinine clearance (using the Cockroft-Gault formula).
• Enoxaparin administration should be preferably continued for during hospitalization for up to 8 days. (LOE A)
c. Fondaparinux (in patients with adequate renal function):
• Loading dose 2.5 mg IV; followed by SC injections of 2.5 mg once daily.
	NEW Anticoagulant medications should be administered for at least 48 hours following fibrinolytic therapy (LOE C), preferably continued for during hospitalization for up to 8 days; (Note that UFH treatment >48 h is not recommended because it increases the risk of heparin-induced thrombocytopenia; alternative anticoagulant should be used). (LOE A)
	NEW
	In patients administered anticoagulant therapy before undergoing PCI, specific dosing recommendations for prior treatment with UFH, enoxaparin, or fondaparinux are recommended. (LOE C)
	NEW
	Dual antiplatelet therapy with clopidogrel (75 mg per day PO; caution in patients >75 years old) should be added to aspirin in STEMI patients regardless of reperfusion status (LOE A) and should be continued for at least 14 days. LOE B	

Continued

TABLE 9–14 Class I and/or New Recommendations for Acute Care of the STEMI Patient—cont'd

Recommendation (Class I, unless noted)	Status of 2007 Recommendation	Status of 2009 Recommendation
ANTICOAGULANTS AS ADJUNCT THERAPY TO REPERFUSION THERAPY		
• Fondaparinux administration should be preferably continued during hospitalization for up to 8 days. (LOE B)		
THIENOPYRIDINE THERAPY		
		Loading dose of thienopyridine recommended for STEMI patients for whom PCI is planned. Regimens should be 1 of the following: a. 300 to 600 mg of clopidogrel should be given as early as possible before or at the time of primary or nonprimary PCI. (LOE C) b. Prasugrel 60 mg should be given as soon as possible for primary PCI. (LOE B) c. For STEMI patients undergoing **nonprimary** PCI, the following regimens are recommended: (i) If the patient has received fibrinolytic therapy and has been given clopidogrel, clopidogrel should be continued as the thienopyridine of choice. (LOE C) (ii) If the patient has received fibrinolytic therapy without a thienopyridine, a loading dose of 300 to 600 mg of clopidogrel should be given as the thienopyridine of choice. (LOE C) (iii) If the patient did not receive fibrinolytic therapy, either a loading dose of 300 to 600 mg of clopidogrel should be given or, once the coronary anatomy is known and PCI is planned, a loading dose of 60 mg of prasugrel should be given promptly and no later than 1 hour after the PCI. (LOE B)

TABLE 9–14 Class I and/or New Recommendations for Acute Care of the STEMI Patient—cont'd

Recommendation (Class I, unless noted)	Status of 2007 Recommendation	Status of 2009 Recommendation
THIENOPYRIDINE THERAPY		
Discontinue clopidogrel for 5 days (minimally)–7 days (preferable) in patients for whom surgical revascularization is planned, unless the patient's condition warrants urgent surgical intervention. (LOE B)	No change from 2004 recommendation	The duration of thienopyridine therapy should be as follows: a. In patients receiving a stent (BMS or drug-eluting stent [DES]) during PCI for ACS, clopidogrel 75 mg daily (LOE B) or prasugrel 10 mg daily (LOE B) should be given for at least 12 months. b. If the risk of morbidity due to bleeding > anticipated benefit afforded by thienopyridine therapy, consider earlier discontinuation. (LOE C) Modified recommendation (added prasugrel) In patients taking a thienopyridine in whom CABG is planned and can be delayed, it is recommended that the drug be discontinued to allow for dissipation of the antiplatelet effect. (LOE C) The period of withdrawal should be at least 5 days in patients receiving clopidogrel (LOE B) and at least 7 days in patients receiving prasugrel (LOE C) unless the need for revascularization and/or the net benefit of the thienopyridine > the potential risks of excess bleeding. (LOE C)
ANTIPLATELET THERAPY FOR PATIENTS WITH CHRONIC MUSCULOSKELETAL DISORDERS		
	NEW Before discharge, the STEMI patient should be assessed and managed using a stepped-care approach to pain management. Initial medications should begin with acetaminophen, aspirin, tramadol, short-term narcotics, or nonacetylated salicylates. (LOE C)	

Continued

TABLE 9–14 **Class I and/or New Recommendations for Acute Care of the STEMI Patient—cont'd**

Recommendation (Class I, unless noted)	Status of 2007 Recommendation	Status of 2009 Recommendation
ANTIPLATELET THERAPY FOR PATIENTS WITH CHRONIC MUSCULOSKELETAL DISORDERS		
POSSIBLY HARMFUL: Do not administer COX-2 NSAIDs to STEMI patients with chronic musculoskeletal discomfort when therapy with medications listed above plus nonselective NSAIDs, provide adequate pain relief for the patient. (LOE C)	Text edited	New Each community should develop a STEMI system of care that follows standards at least as stringent as those developed for the AHA's national initiative, Mission: Lifeline, to include the following: Ongoing multidisciplinary team meetings (include EMS, non–PCI-capable hospitals/STEMI referral centers, and PCI-capable hospitals/STEMI receiving centers) to evaluate outcomes and quality improvement data: • Prehospital identification and activation process • Destination protocols for STEMI receiving centers • Transfer protocols for patients who arrive at STEMI referral centers who are primary PCI candidates, are ineligible for fibrinolytic drugs, and/or are in cardiogenic shock (LOE C)
An insulin infusion to normalize blood glucose is recommended for patients with STEMI and complicated courses. (LOE B)		Recommendation is no longer current. It is reasonable to use an insulin-based regimen to achieve and maintain glucose levels less than 180 mg/dL while avoiding hypoglycemia for patients with STEMI with either a complicated or uncomplicated course. (Class IIa, LOE B)

ACE, angiotensin-converting enzyme; BMI, body mass index; CABG, coronary artery bypass graft; COR, class of recommendation; CHF, congestive heart failure; d/t, due to; HDL-C, high-density lipoprotein cholesterol; HF, heart failure; INR, international normalized ratio; IV: intravenous; LDL-C, low-density lipoprotein cholesterol; LOE, level of evidence; LV, left ventricle; LVEF, left ventricular ejection fraction; MI, myocardial infarction; NSAIDs: non-steroidal anti-inflammatory drugs; PCI, percutaneous coronary intervention; STEMI, ST-elevation myocardial infarction; UFH: unfractionated heparin. >: greater than; <: less than; ≥: greater than or equal to; ≤: less than or equal to

From Kushner et al. 2009 focused updates: ACC/AHA guidelines for the management of patients with ST-elevation myocardial infarction (updating the 2004 guideline and 2007 focused update) and ACC/AHA/SCAI Guidelines on percutaneous coronary intervention (updating the 2005 guideline and 2007 focused update): a report of the American College of Cardiology Foundation/American Heart Association Task Force on Practice Guidelines. Circulation 2009; 120,:2271-2306; doi 10.1161/. circulationaha.109.192663 (45).

recommendations from the 2007 and 2009 updated guidelines for the acute care of STEMI patients. New patient education recommendations for secondary prevention of ACS are also outlined in the 2007 focused update for the STEMI guidelines. The major goal of each topic is listed in Table 9-15 (44). The current guidelines can be found, in full, in the publications by Anderson and et al. (18) for UA/NSTEMI and by Antman and et al. (43) for STEMI. Updates to the 2004 STEMI guidelines were published in 2007 (44) and 2009 (45).

TABLE 9–15 Secondary Prevention Topics and Outcome Goals from 2007 STEMI Guideline

Secondary Prevention Topic	2007 Guideline Goal
Smoking	Complete smoking cessation, no exposure to environmental tobacco smoke
Blood pressure (BP) control	BP <140/90 mm Hg or <130/80 (diabetic or chronic kidney disease patients)
Lipid management	LDL-C <100 mg per dL (If triglycerides are ≥200 mg per dL, non–HDL-C should be <130 mg per dL.)
Physical activity	30 min, 7 days per week (minimum 5 days per week)
Weight management	BMI: 18.5–24.9 kg/m2 Waist circumference: Men less than 40 inches (102 cm), women less than 35 inches (89 cm)
Diabetes management	HbA1c <7%
Antiplatelet agents/anticoagulants: aspirin	Unless contraindicated, start and continue long-term aspirin use of 75–162 mg once a day (with some exceptions noted for post-PCI STEMI stented patients in the immediate post-implantation period)
Antiplatelet agents/anticoagulants: clopidogrel	Unless contraindicated, clopidogrel 75 mg daily should be given for at least 12 months for post-PCI (DES) and for a minimum of 1 month and ideally up to 12 months (BMS)
Antiplatelet agents/anticoagulants: warfarin	Unless contraindicated, maintain warfarin levels to an INR equal to 2.0–3.0 for paroxysmal or chronic atrial fibrillation or atrial flutter; post-MI (e.g., atrial fibrillation, left ventricular thrombus)
Renin-angiotensin-aldosterone system blockers: ACE inhibitors	Unless contraindicated, ACE inhibitors should be started and continued indefinitely in all patients recovering from STEMI with poor cardiac function (LVEF ≤40%) and/or hypertension, diabetes, or chronic kidney disease
Renin-angiotensin-aldosterone system blockers: angiotensin receptor blockers	Unless contraindicated, use of angiotensin receptor blockers in selected patients
Renin-angiotensin-aldosterone system blockers: aldosterone blockade	Unless contraindicated, use of aldosterone blockade in selected patients.
Beta-blockers	Unless contraindicated, beta-blocker therapy should be continued indefinitely in all patients who have had MI, ACS, or LV dysfunction with or without HF symptoms
Influenza vaccination	Annual influenza vaccination for all CVD patients

ACE(I), angiotensin-converting enzyme (inhibitor); ACS, acute coronary syndrome; BMI, body mass index; BMS, bare metal stent; DES, drug-eluting stent; HDL-C, high-density lipoprotein cholesterol; HF, heart failure; HbA1C, hemoglobin AIC; INR, international normalized ratio; LDL-C, low-density lipoprotein cholesterol; LV, left ventricle; MI, myocardial infarction; PCI, percutaneous coronary intervention; STEMI, ST-elevation myocardial infarction.

From Antman et al. 2007 focused update of the ACC/AHA 2004 guidelines for the management of patients with ST-elevation myocardial infarction: a report of the American College of Cardiology/American Heart Association Task Force on Practice Guidelines. Circulation 2009;, 117(2):296-329; doi:10.1161/circulationaha.107.188209 (44).

Short-Term Observation

A major change in the guidelines, relevant to all ACS diagnoses, is the recommendation that patients suspected of having ACS, but not showing objective evidence of ischemic changes in their ECG or a rise in cardiac biomarkers during initial testing, should continue to be observed in an area capable of cardiac monitoring and retested at scheduled intervals (5, 18). Short-stay observation units, sometimes called chest pain units, are measures to decrease the number of patients incorrectly diagnosed (e.g., with an alternative diagnosis) or risk-stratified as low-risk and discharged, only to suffer an MI or SCD a short time after discharge (18).

Two percent to 8% of MI diagnoses are missed in the ED (18, 38), depending on the diagnostic algorithm or prognostic scoring tool used. The ability to monitor these patients in a short-stay unit also decreases the number of unnecessary admissions to the hospital, saving money (18) and freeing up beds for patients who can benefit from the admission. Decisions to admit and intervene or discharge and follow-up are facilitated by the use of written, evidence-based protocols. Staff nurses and/or APNs use these specialized protocols and/or critical pathways to monitor these patients and to determine additional testing and length of stay. Stays in these observation units range from 6 to 12 hours (most common) to 24 hours, depending on the specific protocol followed (18). Many times these protocols and policies are written and/or facilitated by the CNS.

Initial Interventions

Barring contraindications to the medications, acute care nurses and CNSs should expect to give chewable aspirin (ASA) upon admission to any patient with ACS symptoms, if the patient has not already received ASA as part of an emergency protocol (18). Guidelines for diagnosis and risk stratification of the UA/NSTEMI and STEMI patient are similar in many regards. Continuous cardiac monitoring, supplemental oxygen to maintain oxygen saturation above 90%, and pulse oximetry are initiated immediately and as needed (class I; 18, 43). A 12-lead ECG within 10 minutes of admission to the emergency department is recommended (18, 43). Cardiac biomarkers are drawn on admission and then every 6 to 8 hours for 2 or 3 times or until the levels peak (see Figure 9-7 and Table 9-12). BNP or NT-pro-BNP may also be drawn. Evaluation of the serial ECGs and cardiac biomarkers, along with the history and physical findings, will help the physician or APN to make a diagnosis. In the case of indeterminate findings, the patient should be observed in a monitored unit, such as a chest pain observation or telemetry unit, where repeat biomarker testing and additional ECGs should be performed (18).

Patients with continued negative or indeterminate results may be scheduled for an exercise or pharmacologic stress test. Patients who have been diagnosed with ACS with continuing symptoms of ischemia, elevated cardiac biomarkers, new ECG changes (e.g., ST-segment deviations, deep T-wave inversions), hemodynamic instability, or a positive stress test should be admitted to the critical care unit or the telemetry unit, depending on the severity of the symptomatology (18). Additionally, new recommendations specific to ischemic changes in

ECG posterior leads V_7-V_9 (true posterior MI leads, left circumflex occlusion) advise the immediate evaluation of the patient for reperfusion therapy (class I, LOE A; 5, 18).

Pharmacologic Interventions

Medications administered to treat symptoms and prevent further problems include anti-ischemic medications, analgesics, anticoagulants, and antiplatelet therapies. Class I anti-ischemic medications include NTG tablets (LOE C) and an intravenous infusion (LOE B) for persistent chest pain; an oral beta-blocker or calcium channel blocker therapy (if beta-blockers are not tolerated) (LOE B); and an ACEI or ARB (LOE A) (18, 43). These medications are recommended to be administered within the first 24 hours after symptom onset. Intravenous morphine is administered as needed for unrelieved pain, anxiety, and/or HF.

ASA, clopidrogrel, and prasugrel are class IA antiplatelet therapy recommendations (18, 45) and PPIs are recommended to decrease gastric upset common with antiplatelet therapies (class I, LOE B; 18). PPI medications include omeprazole, lansoprazole, pantoprazole, rabeprazole, and esomeprazole. There has been some evidence that certain PPIs interfere with the effectiveness of clopidogrel; however, there is not enough evidence to revise the current guideline recommendation at this time (45). Warfarin may be added to long-term antithrombotic medication regimens for patients needing anticoagulation in addition to antiplatelet therapy (class I, LOE A; 18). Other major changes to long-term management of UA/NSTEMI patients include the provision of hydroxymethyl glutaryl-coenzyme A reductase inhibitors (HMG-CoA, also known as statins) to all patients post UA/NSTEMI or post revascularization (class I, LOE A; 18), regardless of their baseline LDL cholesterol levels (5). Statins benefit patients by decreasing inflammation, lowering LDL levels, and raising high-density lipoprotein (HDL) levels (47).

Invasive Therapies

Invasive medical therapies are defined as diagnostic angiography with the intent to perform revascularization if needed (5). Conservative therapy consists of anticoagulant and antiplatelet medications and additional testing. The determination of invasive versus conservative therapy is dependent on the patient's cardiac risk factors and prior history of cardiac disease or cardiac intervention; ACS signs and symptoms, including laboratory and diagnostic testing; presence of dysrhythmias, low EF (<40%), and/or hemodynamic instability; and risk scores (5). Multiple randomized studies have shown the survival and morbidity benefits of early invasive therapy in eligible patients, including positive outcomes for older adults and women (5). New recommendations stated that high-risk women should receive invasive therapies (class I, LOE B; 49) and conservative strategies are appropriate for low-risk women (49).

Anticoagulant Therapy

In both the invasive and conservative therapeutic strategies, anticoagulant therapy is initiated with medications such as low-molecular-weight heparin (LMWH) or unfractionated heparin (UFH), then the patient receives either clopidrogrel and/or an intravenous GPIIb/IIIa inhibitor (e.g., abciximab, eptifibatide, or tirofiban). The clopidogrel and/or GPIIb/IIIA inhibitor is given before angiography according to the invasive strategy protocol. Giving both clopidrogrel and a GPIIb/IIIa inhibitor is indicated for high-risk patients, those whose angiographies have been delayed, and those with repeated bouts of acute ischemic pain (18). Bivalirudin and fondaparinux are two new anticoagulant drugs added to the revised UA/NSTEMI recommendations based on new clinical data (class I, LOE B) (18). Prasugrel is a new thienopyridine that has been shown to have a greater effect on platelet aggregation than clopidogrel and does not seem to be inhibited by PPIs (45). Only patients with acute ST-segment elevation, a true posterior MI, or a presumed new left bundle-branch block (LBBB) are recommended for intravenous fibrinolytic therapy (18, 44).

Management of STEMI Patients

Fibrinolytic and Anticoagulation Therapy

For patients with STEMI, the critical goal is to decrease the time from symptom onset to reperfusion. Reperfusion methods include pharmacologic methods using fibrinolytics (pharmacologic reperfusion) and catheter-based therapies (primary percutaneous coronary interventions [PCIs]) (aka mechanical reperfusion). The quicker the time to reperfusion, the more heart muscle can be saved. Fibrinolytic therapy can be accomplished using the alteplase or tissue plasminogen activator (t-Pa), reteplase (r-PA), tenecteplase (TNKase), anisoylated purified streptokinase activator complex (APSAC), and streptokinase (48). The acute administration of clopidogrel in STEMI patients is recommended based on recent clinical trial evidence, whether or not the patient is undergoing fibrinolytic therapy, and is listed as a Class I recommendation (44). Anticoagulant therapy with UFH should be administered concomitantly with fibrinolytics for a minimum of 48 hours according to the revised STEMI guidelines (44). After 48 hours, the risk of heparin-induced thrombocytopenia (HIT) increases and the anticoagulant medication should be changed from UFH to another anticoagulant, such as enoxaparin or fondaparinux. All three of these anticoagulants are efficacious in this patient population, although all increase the risk of bleeding (44). Recommended dosages and associated comments are noted in Table 9-16.

The following recommendations are found in greater detail in the AHA/ACC guidelines for STEMI patients (43, 44). For hospitals with PCI capability, the time from the first medical contact with the STEMI patient to intervention should be less than 90 minutes

TABLE 9–16 Anticoagulant Dosages for STEMI Patients Undergoing Fibrinolysis

According to the 2009 Update to the STEMI Guidelines: Patients undergoing reperfusion with fibrinolytics should receive anticoagulant therapy for a minimum of 48 hours (Level of Evidence [LOE] C) and preferably for the duration of the initial hospitalization, up to 8 days.

Anticoagulant Regimen	Dosage/Comments
Unfractionated heparin (UFH) (class I, LOE C)	**Bolus:** IV 60 U/kg [maximum 4,000 U]) Followed by: **Intravenous (IV) Infusion:** 12 U/kg/hr (maximum 1,000 U/hr) to start **then titrate** to maintain the activated partial thromboplastin (aPTT) time at 1.5–2.0 times control (approximately 50–70 seconds) • There is no benefit of continuing of the infusion of UFH beyond 48 hours in the absence of ongoing indications for anticoagulation. • Risk of development of heparin-induced thrombocytopenia with prolonged infusions of UFH, therefore alternate regimen recommended after 48 hours.

Continued

TABLE 9-16 Anticoagulant Dosages for STEMI Patients Undergoing Fibrinolysis—cont'd

Anticoagulant Regimen	Dosage/Comments
Enoxaparin (class I, LOE A) Partial renal excretion of drug: Only administered if the serum creatinine <2.5 mg/dL in men and <2.0 mg/dL in women	Patients <75 years of age **Bolus:** IV 30 mg Followed 15 min later by: **Subcutaneous (SC) injection:** 1 mgkg q12h Patients ≥75 years of age: **Bolus:** No IV bolus **SC injection:** 0.75 mg/kg q12h **Titration:** Regardless of age, if the creatinine clearance (using the Cockroft-Gault formula) during the course of treatment is estimated to be <30 mL/min, the subcutaneous regimen is 1 mg/kg every 24 hours. • Maintenance dosing with enoxaparin should be continued for the duration of the index hospitalization, up to 8 days.
c. Fondaparinux (class I, LOE B) Partial renal excretion of drug: Only administered if serum creatinine <3.0 mg/dL	**Bolus:** IV 2.5 mg Followed by: **SC injection:** 2.5 mg qd • Maintenance dosing with fondaparinux should be continued for the duration of the index hospitalization, up to 8 days.

From Antman et al. 2007 Focused update of the ACC/AHA 2004 guidelines for the management of patients with ST-elevation myocardial infarction: a report of the American College of Cardiology/American Heart Association Task Force on Practice Guidelines. Circulation 2008;117(2):296-329. doi:10.1161/circulationaha.107.188209 (44); and from Kushner et al. 2009 Focused updates: ACC/AHA guidelines for the management of patients with ST-elevation myocardial infarction (updating the 2004 guideline and 2007 focused update) and ACC/AHA/SCAI Guidelines on percutaneous coronary intervention (updating the 2005 guideline and 2007 focused update): a report of the American College of Cardiology Foundation/American Heart Association Task Force on Practice Guidelines. Circulation 2009;120:2271-2306; doi:10.1161/circulationaha.109.192663 (45).

(door-to-balloon time) (class I, LOE A). Prehospital fibrinolysis within 30 minutes of EMS arrival is preferred if the EMS providers have been trained in the administration of fibrinolytic therapy and the patient is eligible for treatment (class I, LOE B). Timely reperfusion within 30 minutes of presentation with fibrinolytic therapy (unless contraindicated) is the goal for hospitals without PCI facilities or without the means to transfer the patient to a PCI-capable facility within 90 minutes of first medical contact (class I, LOE B). Improving door-to-balloon time for STEMI patients is a national initiative (44, 50).

Other Medications

STEMI guidelines (43, 44) for pain management specify morphine (2 to 4 mg) to be given IV and repeated every 5 to 15 minutes in increments of 2 to 8 mg, if needed (class I, LOE C). All nonsteroidal anti-inflammatory drugs (NSAIDs), except for ASA, are recommended to be immediately discontinued when the patient presents with STEMI because of evidence showing an increased risk of cardiovascular events (reinfarction, hypertension, HF, and myocardial rupture), shock, and death among patients taking NSAIDs (class I, LOE C; 44). Revised guidelines also recommend oral beta-blockers to be given within 24 hours to STEMI patients who have no contradictions to beta-blockade (class I, LOE B). A new recommendation based on the research stipulates that early administration of beta-blockers should not be given to patients with severe HF or cardiogenic shock, or at high risk for cardiogenic shock, as this intervention has resulted in adverse outcomes (class III, LOE A; 44).

Revascularization Therapies

Revascularization therapies include PCI, coronary artery bypass graft (CABG) surgery, and medical therapy. According to the 2007 guidelines (18), the purpose of revascularization is to "improve prognosis, relieve symptoms, prevent ischemic complications, and improve functional capacity" (p. e84). The choice of revascularization performed is based on the complexity and location of the lesion, the patient's expected benefit, overall cardiac function, the presence of comorbidities, symptom severity, functional ability, and amount of threatened myocardium (18). Indications for coronary revascularization for patients with UA/STEMI and STEMI are found in their respective guidelines (18, 43-45).

Trends in open-heart surgery have stayed level at about 600,000 procedures a year since 1995, while the number of PCI procedures has increased from about 300,000 procedures in 1995 to over 1 million procedures in 2006 (2). In 2006, over 7 million inpatient cardiovascular operations and procedures were performed in the United States (2). Of those operations and procedures, about 1,313,000 were PCI procedures; 1,115,000 were diagnostic cardiac catheterizations; 448,000 were cardiac bypass procedures; 418,000 were pacemaker procedures; and implantable defibrillator placements accounted for about 114,000 procedures (2). A comparison of costs and in-hospital death rates for various cardiovascular operations and procedures is found in Table 9-17.

Basic to all revascularization procedures is the continuation of ASA (class I, LOE A) to decrease the threat of thrombosis and resultant complications. A meta-analysis of 195 clinical trials and over 143,000 high-risk patients noted a 22% decrease in the odds of death, MI, or stroke with antiplatelet therapy, for ASA doses of 75 mg to 1,500 mg daily (5).

Percutaneous Coronary Intervention

As noted, most revascularization procedures are PCIs. PCIs consist of a variety of percutaneous techniques: balloon angioplasty (PTCA), intracoronary stenting, and procedures to remove atherosclerotic tissue, such as atherectomy, thrombectomy, or laser angioplasty. PCI is preferred for patients without significant comorbid conditions or complicated lesions and/or those at high risk for surgical morbidity or mortality (18). Drug-eluting stents (sirolimus-eluting stent or paclitaxel-eluting stent) were the intervention of choice for the majority (70%) of PCI procedures (2) because these drugs have been shown to significantly reduce the restenosis rate after PCI by inhibiting cell growth at the intervention site (18). According to Antman et al. (44), there is no difference in mortality, MI, or stent thrombosis outcomes between bare-metal or drug-eluting stent implantation. Preparation for PCI includes the administration of loading doses of clopidogrel and intravenous GPIIb/IIIa, if they were not already given preangiography (18, 44). Anticoagulant therapy may be discontinued for low-risk cases.

For STEMI patients, rescue PCI is the performance of PCI after failure of full-dose fibrinolytic medications to lyse the clot (44); however, this expression was determined to be misleading and has since been discontinued (45). Clues of reperfusion failure include continued ischemic pain (though the presence or absence of ischemic pain is not reliable by itself) and less than 50% resolution of the most elevated ST segment (from the initial ECG), 90 minutes after the start of the fibrinolytic infusion (44).

Coronary Artery Bypass Graft Surgery

The most invasive therapy, CABG, is reserved for those patients for whom interventional techniques are not appropriate because of the quantity, location, or diffuse nature of the plaques. CABG is recommended in cases with significant left main or left anterior descending artery disease; complicated, multivessel, diffuse lesions; and/or LV dysfunction (18). Preparation for CABG includes discontinuing most of the anticoagulant and antiplatelet medications before surgery. ASA and UFH are continued indefinitely, while clopidogrel should be discontinued 5 days before surgery (LOE B; 45), prasugrel stopped 7 days before surgery (LOE C; 45), and other anticoagulant/antiplatelet medications are stopped 4 to 24 hours before surgery depending on the drug (18).

Care of the CABG patient is focused on vigilant monitoring of hemodynamic and physiologic status, including cardiac rhythm; optimizing the patient's cardiopulmonary and renal function; pain management; and recognition and prevention of postoperative complications. EBP guidelines for the care of the patient after

TABLE 9-17 Mean Charges and In-Hospital Death Rates for Various Cardiovascular Procedures

Procedure	Mean Charges	In-Hospital Death Rate
Valves	$141,120	4.98%
Implantable defibrillator	$104,743	0.64%
Coronary artery bypass graft	$99,743	1.94%
PCI	$48,399	0.71%
Pacemaker	$47,081	0.90%
Diagnostic cardiac catheterization	$28,835	0.77%
Endarterectomy	$25,658	0.38%

From Lloyd-Jones et al. Heart disease and stroke statistics—2010 update: a report from the American Heart Association. Circulation 2010;121(7):e46-e215; doi:10.1161/circulationaha.109.192667 (2).

CABG surgery are available on the ACC Web site at www.cardiosource.org; updated guidelines for CABG are expected to be published in 2011.

Postoperative CABG patients usually stay in the intensive care unit (ICU) for 1-2 days and then transfer to a step-down unit or a general care floor. Selected patients may be eligible for "fast-track" recovery and discharge programs, which have demonstrated positive outcomes (51). Early ambulation to prevent postoperative complications is encouraged for all CABG patients and all suitable patients should be referred to cardiac rehabilitation after discharge (LOE B; 51). ASA therapy is considered the standard of care to prevent saphenous vein graft (SVG) closure after CABG; indefinite ASA therapy is recommended to maintain SVG patency and to prevent future adverse events (LOE A; 51). Acute pain management resources can be found at the American Pain Society, www.ampainsoc.org.

Secondary Prevention

Secondary prevention programs reduce all-cause mortality and the incidence of acute MI (52). After the patient has been discharged from the hospital, modification of known risk factors for CVD should be emphasized as self-care measures and ways for the patient to be an active participant in his or her health care. Preventive measures are important for decreasing disability and death from acute coronary events. For example, post-discharge education on the proper use of NTG tablets, in a sample of UA patients admitted to the ED for chest pain, has been hypothesized as the rationale for a reduction in recurrent acute coronary events (52).

Target areas for modification include smoking cessation, blood pressure control, lipid management, physical activity, weight management, diabetes management, pharmacologic therapies, and prevention of infectious disease (i.e., vaccinations) (44). Patients need to understand that medications to control blood pressure, cholesterol, and/or blood glucose may still need to be prescribed despite the implementation of lifestyle modifications. Nurses should set realistic goals for patient outcomes. Lowering LDL and raising HDL levels decrease CVD risk. The target for lowering LDL cholesterol levels in high-risk patients is to strive for less than 100 mg/dL: this goal is achieved through medication, diet modifications, 30 to 60 minutes of exercise at least 5 days per week, and weight management. Table 9-18 shows the general effect of lifestyle, medications, genetics, and certain disease processes on LDL and HDL levels. Diabetic patients are at high risk for ACS and should be advised to manage their diabetes with a goal of keeping their hemoglobin A1c (HbA1c) level at less than 7%. Finally, resources to help patients quit smoking should be provided. Recommendations for physical activity and cardiac rehabilitation programs for patients with cardiac disease are listed in detail in the 2004 CABG guidelines

TABLE 9–18 The Effects of Different Factors on HDL and LDL

Effects on High-Density Lipoprotein (HDL) Levels		Effects on Low-Density Lipoprotein (LDL) Levels	
Good Effect (Raises Levels)	Bad Effect (Lowers Levels)	Good Effect (Lowers Levels)	Bad Effect (Raises Levels)
Alcohol			
Niacin		Niacin	
Fibrates	Certain drugs	Fibrates	
Statins		Statins	
		Fat reduction	Dietary fats
Smoking cessation	Smoking		
Estrogen	Progesterone	Estrogen	
	Diabetes		Diabetes
Weight Loss	Obesity	Weight loss	Obesity
			Thyroid disease
			Renal disease
			Liver disease
Exercise	No exercise	Resins	Genetics
	High triglycerides	Bile acid sequestrants	

Adapted from Davidson MH, Jacobsen TA. Statins work: The development of cardiovascular disease and its treatment with 3-hydroxy-3-methylglutaryl coenzyme a reductase inhibitors. Retrieved April 29, 2002, from MedscapeCME: http://cme.medscape.com/viewarticle/416521 (47)

(51), 2007 update of the guidelines for prevention of CVD in women (49), and the 2007 STEMI guidelines (44).

Future Trends: Genomics and Cardiovascular Disease

The future of the prevention and treatment of CVD will include more complex genomic research and tailored gene therapies, as an outcome of this new knowledge. CVD clearly has a genetic component—we can see a familial pattern to the predisposition toward various CVD processes, and multiple research studies provide evidence for greater disease risks, and especially the early onset of CVD, among family members (53). In some forms of CVD, Mendelian disorders (e.g., LDL receptor gene or *ApoB* gene mutations) have been identified as the etiologic agents of disease (53). Gene–environment interactions, pharmacogenetics, whole-genome association studies and resequencing studies, and RNA expression profiling are cutting-edge research topics to learn more about the genetic basis of CVD. These studies will hopefully provide information to design individualized interventions to prevent, diagnose, counsel, and effectively manage patients at high risk of CVD. As Arnett and pointed out, current clinical use of these complex techniques and therapies is limited; however, as the science grows and clinical applications become apparent, CNSs with this expertise may well be called upon to administer and measure the outcomes of genetic testing programs and to provide genetic counseling to at-risk patients (53). Determining genetic predisposition will allow for earlier interventions to reduce future risk and disability from all forms CVD.

Clinical Nurse Specialist Competencies and Spheres of Influence

The CNS Core Competencies of Clinical Expert/Direct Care and Consultation; Coaching/Teaching/Mentoring; Research/Evidence-Based Practice and Collaboration; and Systems Leadership are emphasized in the care of the ACS patient. Using these competencies, the CNS influences all three spheres of practice influence.

Clinical Expert/Direct Care and Consultation

The Clinical Expert/Direct Care and Consultation competencies most directly affect the Patient/Family Sphere and the Nursing/Other Disciplines Sphere. In the care of the ACS patient, the CNS applies expert knowledge to facilitate the triage of patients presenting with signs of ACS in the ED. Registration clerks and triage nurses must be aware of the signs and symptoms of ACS, especially in patient populations that may not present with "classic" signs and symptoms—such as women, the elderly, and those with neuropathic disorders. Algorithms are available to triage patients appropriately. In the units, the CNS assists staff to monitor

hemodynamics and cardiac rhythm accurately. Introducing and coaching staff on the importance of evidence-based ECG lead placement and use of ST-segment monitoring will enable the correct diagnosis and management of cardiac dysrhythmias, a common complication of ACS patients. Auditing compliance with unit policies provides the CNS with data on continuing education needs. Vigilance is required when caring for ACS patients to detect any changes in condition and avert potential health crises. Overall, the CNS provides and/or assists in the direct care of ACS patients in the units and on the general-care floors, role modeling effective communication, and authentic presence.

As the clinical expert, the CNS is consulted by the nursing staff to troubleshoot issues related to care management. Additionally, consultation with the bedside nurse is important to facilitate patient transfers from the ICU to the general care floor to free up beds for more acutely ill patients.

Coaching/Teaching/Mentoring

Patient education is extremely important to prevent adverse events. The CNS, working within the Patient/Family Sphere, may design new patient teaching materials or revise existing materials based on new recommendations. The revised guidelines for UA/NSTEMI (18) and STEMI (43-45) provide new recommendations for patient education that the nursing staff may be responsible for conveying to the patient and family. For example, previous education regarding continuing chest pain was to instruct the patient to take up to 3 NTG tablets, 5 minutes apart; this teaching is being replaced with a "one NTG dose" instruction. Patients experiencing anginal discomfort are told to stop the activity or eliminate the stressor causing the angina and to take one dose of sublingual NTG if the discomfort does not subside immediately after the cessation of activity. The new guidelines (18) then teach the patient to quickly access the emergency medical system by calling 911 if the pain continues or worsens 5 minutes after the first NTG dose, and before taking a second dose of NTG. The rationale is to get emergency help to the patient as quickly as possible—teach the patient that "time is muscle" and delaying calling 911 until after three doses of NTG wastes precious minutes and increases the amount of cardiac muscle damage.

Providing teaching about modifiable risk factors is important to give patients the information they need to live healthier lives. In general, lifestyle modifications will assist in lowering blood pressure and lipid levels, regulate insulin levels, and reduce obesity—all risk factors for CVD. Multiple studies have shown the benefits of CVD prevention and nurses have the skill sets needed to administer secondary prevention and chronic disease management programs (52).

Education for vulnerable groups is also important. The CNS can help to raise women's awareness of CVD by providing gender-specific education. For instance, many women do not realize that they are at high risk of experiencing a coronary event because of comorbid conditions or multiple risk factors. Table 9-19 categorizes women into one of three risk groups: high risk, at risk, and optimal risk, based on their history and presence of known risk factors (49). This knowledge may encourage at-risk and high-risk women to implement changes in their lifestyle to decrease their risk profile. Another important avenue of gender-specific education is related to the presentation of ACS in women. Women frequently delay seeking treatment because they do not recognize that they are experiencing ACS because their symptoms may not be what they expect. Multiple research studies have shown that women experience ACS differently than men—they use different words to describe their symptoms than men and so do not always recognize the seriousness of their condition (54-56). Increased awareness of ACS symptomatology specific to women may influence someone to suspect an ACS event and activate emergency services early, thus saving viable heart muscle and perhaps saving a life. Refer to Table 9-6 for a listing of common anginal equivalents in women.

Research/Evidence-Based Practice and Collaboration

The competencies of Research/Evidence-Based Practice and Collaboration are achieved within the Nursing/Other Disciplines and System/Organization spheres of influence. The CNS is the expert clinician and leader responsible for translating evidence into practice. Ensuring that the care provided to patients consists of best practices is hard work. The CNS is expected to identify gaps in practice, find evidence to close the gap, and design and implement plans to change practice. The CNS's knowledge of the organization (e.g., its priorities, bureaucratic structure, culture for change, etc.) and advanced research skills are necessary to successfully implement change. The CNS identifies needed practice change; searches, locates, appraises, and synthesizes the evidence that supports the change; helps facilitate nurse and interprofessional team discussions regarding the practice change; and often leads the team in writing new policies and procedures based on the evidence. The practice change must then be

TABLE 9–19 Stratification of Risk for Women

High Risk	• Established coronary heart disease • Cerebrovascular disease • Peripheral arterial disease • Abdominal aortic aneurysm • End-stage or chronic renal disease • Diabetes mellitus • 10-year Framingham global risk >20% or at high risk from another population-adapted tool used to assess global risk
At Risk *(≥1 major risk factors for CVD)*	• Cigarette smoking • Poor diet • Physical inactivity • Obesity, especially central adiposity • Family history of premature CVD (<55 years of age in male relative and <65 years of age in female relative) • Hypertension • Dyslipidemia • Evidence of subclinical vascular disease (e.g., coronary calcification) • Metabolic syndrome • Poor exercise capacity on treadmill test and/or abnormal heart rate recovery after stopping exercise
Optimal risk	• Framingham global risk <10% and a healthy lifestyle

Adapted from Mosca et al. Evidence-based guidelines for cardiovascular disease prevention in women: 2007 update. J Am Coll Cardiol 2007;9(11):1230-1250; doi:10.1016/j.jacc.2007.02.020 (49).

communicated and the staff persuaded that the change is in the best interest of the patient. Frequently, the CNS is the person who collects data to audit compliance with the policy or protocols.

Searching for the evidence can be time-consuming, but there are many resources available to the CNS. For example, there are multiple evidence-based guidelines, clinical data standards, performance measures, and other evidence-based tool kits available to support the provision of evidence-based care to ACS patients. Many of these resources are freely available on the Web. The AHA (www.myamericanheart.org), ACC (www.cardiosource.org), the Society of Critical Care Medicine (www.sccm.org), the Institute of Health care Improvement (IHI) (www.IHI.org), and the American Association of Critical-Care Nurses (AACN) (www.aacn.org) are just a few of the many professional organizations that have resources available to support the work of CNSs to improve patient care. The AHA's newest campaign, "Mission: Lifeline," is directed toward improving the acute care of patients with STEMI to decrease death and disability from MI (57). CNSs will be vital team members in the success of this program.

With the many resources available, how does the CNS evaluate the quality of those resources? Using their research competency skills, CNSs understand that not all published guidelines are based on a comprehensive and rigorous review of the literature and assumptions of quality cannot be made based just on the national standing of the organization producing the guidelines. The caveat to determine the system the authors used for classifying study strength can be extended to evaluating the quality of CPGs. Be sure to evaluate the organization's process for producing clinical practice guidelines for methodologic rigor and transparency in how the document was produced. Many national professional health care organizations do adhere to a consistent protocol and high standards for producing CPGs, and their standards are usually readily available online on the organization's Web site and/or explained in the introductory material of the published guideline. Once the CNS has established the credibility of the organization or authors producing the CPG, she or he can have more confidence in future publications.

Systems Leadership

The CNS is a systems thinker and therefore a natural leader for a number of quality and safety initiatives aimed at providing best practice to patients suffering from ACS. Resources are available in hard copy and via the Internet for the CNS to use to educate staff and monitor compliance with evidence-based recommendations. For example, the ACC/AHA has produced multiple performance measure tools for tracking system goals for timely treatment of CAD patients with NSTEMI and STEMI, available on their Web site. An outline of the measures evaluated in the ACC/AHA Performance Measures set for 2008 (41) is found in Table 9-20, and these measures are aligned with performance measures previously published by The Joint Commission (TJC) and Centers for Medicare and Medicaid Services (CMS). Details of the performance measures are found in the report by Krumholz et al. (41).

The AHA offers health care providers and their teams a voluntary hospital-based quality improvement (QI) program called "Get With The Guidelines" (GWTG). GWTG–Coronary Artery Disease (GWTG-CAD) offers health care institutions evidence-based guidelines, implementation tips, clinical decision support and QI methodology tools, among other resources, to implement the GWTG program related to CAD. The six key quality measures identified in the GWTG-CAD program are the provision of (a) ASA at discharge; (b) beta-blocker at

TABLE 9-20 2008 Performance Measures and Dimensions of Care for STEMI Patients

Measured on Admission or in Early Management	Measures related to Wait Times or Delays	Test Measures	Measured at Discharge
Aspirin at arrival (T) Evaluation of LVSF (New) (D) Reperfusion therapy (T)	Time to fibrinolytic therapy (T) Time to primary PCI (T) Time from ED arrival at STEMI referral facility to ED discharge from STEMI referral facility in patients transferred for PCI (New) (T)	LDL-C assessment (D) Excessive initial heparin dose (New) (T) Excessive initial enoxaparin dose (New) (T) Excessive initial abciximab dose (New) (T) Excessive initial eptifibatide dose (New) (T)	Aspirin prescribed at discharge (T) Beta-blockers prescribed at discharge (T) Statin at discharge (New) (T) ACEI or ARB for LVSD (T)

Continued

TABLE 9-20 2008 Performance Measures and Dimensions of Care for STEMI Patients—cont'd

Measured on Admission or in Early Management	Measures Related to Wait Times or Delays	Test Measures	Measured at Discharge
	Time from ED arrival at STEMI referral facility to PCI at STEMI receiving facility among transferred patients (New) (T)	Excessive initial tirofiban dose (New) (T) Anticoagulant dosing protocol (structural measure) (New) (T) Anticoagulant error tracking system (structural measure) (New) (T) Clopidogrel at discharge (New) (T)	Adult smoking cessation advice/counseling (PE) Cardiac rehabilitation patient referral from an inpatient setting (PE) Clopidogrel at discharge for medically treated AMI patients (T)

Dimensions of Care: D, Diagnostics; PE, Patient education; T, treatment.

ACEI: angiotensin-converting enzyme inhibitor; AMI, acute myocardial infarction; ARB, angiotensin receptor blocker; ED, emergency department; HDL-C, high-density lipoprotein cholesterol; LDL-C, low-density lipoprotein cholesterol; LVSD, left ventricular systolic dysfunction; LVSF, left ventricular systolic function; PCI, percutaneous coronary intervention; STEMI, ST-elevation myocardial infarction.

From Krumholz et al. ACC/AHA 2008 performance measures for adults with ST-elevation and non-ST-elevation myocardial infarction: a report of the American College of Cardiology/American Heart Association Task Force on Performance Measures (Writing Committee to develop performance measures for ST-elevation and non-ST-elevation myocardial infarction): developed in collaboration with the American Academy of Family Physicians and the American College of Emergency Physicians: Endorsed by the American Association of Cardiovascular and Pulmonary Rehabilitation, Society for Cardiovascular Angiography and Interventions, and Society of Hospital Medicine. Circulation 2008;118(24):2596-2648; doi:10.1161/circulationaha.108.191099 (41).

discharge; (c) ACEI or ARB at discharge for AMI patients; (d) lipid therapy at discharge if LDL is greater than 100 mg/dL; (e) smoking cessation counseling; and (f) ASA within 24 hours of hospital arrival for AMI and angina patients (50).

New 30-day measures are recently released to assist hospitals to track CAD patients after discharge (58). Data collected at 30 days provide data on mortality rates, hospital recidivism, follow-up visits, adherence to medications, patient education, and rehabilitation for analysis. CNSs may be responsible for collecting and submitting quality-of-care and 30-day measurement data to the national GWTG database.

Resource allocation and resource use are other areas the CNS can positively affect a system/organization level. The CNS may want to track patient flow in the unit to ascertain the need for disease-specific education or to design better workflow patterns. One way to find this information is to track disease processes through data mining of the *International Classification of Disease (ICD)* codes common to the unit. Disease processes are assigned an ICD code for billing purposes; these codes can be useful for administrative and research purposes, too. The CNS should be familiar with the *ICD* codes commonly seen on the unit. The *ICD-9-CM (International Classification of Diseases, Clinical Modification, 9th Revision)* and the newer *ICD-10-CM* codes for CVD (minus cerebrovascular disease) are listed in Table 9-21 (2).

HEART FAILURE

Etiology

HF is a complex clinical syndrome marked by the inability of the heart to pump enough blood, because of poor systolic function and/or inadequate ventricular filling or relaxation, to meet the metabolic demands of the body. Structural or functional deficits cause remodeling of the cardiac muscle as a result of neurohormonal interaction. The most common cause of HF is loss of contractile function from coronary disease. MI increases the risk of HF two- to three-fold (59). The resulting pressure and/or volume overload in the heart primarily affects both the cardiac and pulmonary systems.

Aging is a risk factor for the development of HF. HF affects only 1% of the younger population (younger than 50 years), but rises to 10% of the population over 70 years old and to 15% of those 80 and older (60). Besides age, other common risk factors for HF include gender, race/ethnicity, hypertension, and diabetes; the latter risk is higher in women with CAD (2). The lifetime risk of

TABLE 9–21 ICD Codes for Cardiovascular Disease

- Diseases of the Circulatory System—ICD/10 codes (100–199)— included as part of what the American Heart Association calls "Cardiovascular Disease."
- Total Cardiovascular Disease (ICD/9 390–459, 745–747); ICD/10 codes 100–199, Q20–Q28)— includes:
  - Rheumatic Fever/Rheumatic Heart Disease (100–109);
  - Hypertensive Diseases (110–115);
  - Ischemic (Coronary) Heart Disease (120–125);
  - Pulmonary Heart Disease and Diseases of Pulmonary Circulation (126–128);
  - Other Forms of Heart Disease (130–152);
  - Cerebrovascular Disease (Stroke) (160–169);
  - Atherosclerosis (I70);
  - Other Diseases of Arteries, Arterioles and Capillaries (171–179);
  - Diseases of Veins, Lymphatics, and Lymph Nodes not classified elsewhere (180–189);
  - Other and Unspecified Disorders of the Circulatory System (195–199).
  - Congenital Cardiovascular Defects (Q20–Q28).
- Diseases of the Heart—Classification the NCHS uses in compiling the leading causes of death. Includes: ICD/10 codes:
  - Acute Rheumatic Fever/Chronic Rheumatic Heart Diseases (100–109);
  - Hypertensive Heart Disease (111);
  - Hypertensive Heart and Renal Disease (113);
  - Coronary Heart Disease (120–125);
  - Pulmonary Heart Disease and Diseases of Pulmonary Circulation (126–128);
  - Heart Failure (150); (ICD/9 428)
  - Other Forms of Heart Disease (129–149, 150.1–151).
- Coronary heart disease (CHD)

ICD/9 410–414, 429.2;

- 410.00 Anterolateral wall, AMI—episode of care unspecified
- 410.01 Anterolateral wall, AMI—initial episode
- 410.10 Other anterior wall, AMI—episode of care unspecified
- 410.11 Other anterior wall, AMI—initial episode
- 410.20 Inferolateral wall, AMI—episode of care unspecified
- 410.21 Inferolateral wall, AMI—initial episode
- 410.30 Inferoposterior wall, AMI—episode of care unspecified
- 410.31 Inferoposterior wall, AMI—initial episode
- 410.40 Other inferior wall, AMI—episode of care unspecified
- 410.41 Other inferior wall, AMI—initial episode
- 410.50 Other lateral wall, AMI—episode of care unspecified
- 410.51 Other lateral wall, AMI—initial episode
- 410.60 True posterior wall, AMI—episode of care unspecified
- 410.61 True posterior wall, AMI—initial episode
- 410.70 Subendocardial, AMI—episode of care unspecified (NSTEMI)
- 410.71 Subendocardial, AMI—initial episode (NSTEMI)
- 410.80 Other specified sites, AMI—episode of care unspecified
- 410.81 Other specified sites, AMI—initial episode
- 410.90 Unspecified site, AMI—episode of care unspecified
- 410.91 Unspecified site, AMI—initial episode

ICD/10 120–125

- Acute Myocardial Infarction (121–122);
- Other Acute Ischemic (Coronary) Heart Disease (124);
- Angina Pectoris (120); ICD/9 413

Continued

TABLE 9-21 ICD Codes for Cardiovascular Disease—cont'd

- Atherosclerotic Cardiovascular Disease (125.0);
- All other forms of Chronic Ischemic Heart disease (125.1–125.9).
- Acute Coronary Syndrome (ICD/9 Codes 410, 411)

From Lloyd-Jones et al. Heart disease and stroke statistics—2010 update: a report from the American Heart Association. Circulation 2010;121(7):e46-e215; doi:10.1161/circulationaha.109.192667 (2); and from Krumholz et al. ACC/AHA 2008 performance measures for adults with ST-elevation and non-ST-elevation myocardial infarction: a report of the American College of Cardiology/American Heart Association Task Force on Performance Measures (Writing Committee to develop performance measures for ST-elevation and non-ST-elevation myocardial infarction): developed in collaboration with the American Academy of Family Physicians and the American College of Emergency Physicians: Endorsed by the American Association of Cardiovascular and Pulmonary Rehabilitation, Society for Cardiovascular Angiography and Interventions, and Society of Hospital Medicine. Circulation 2008;118(24):2596-2648; doi:10.1161/circulationaha.108.191099 (41).

HF, based on data from the Framingham studies, is roughly equivalent between men and women at about 20%; however, women over 70 tend to have a higher incidence of HF. Racial differences are apparent in the morbidity and mortality of this disease: African Americans are more likely to develop HF, develop HF at an earlier age, and have higher death rates due to HF than either Caucasians or Latinos (60). Over 75% of people with HF have a comorbidity of hypertension (61).

The prevalence of HF in the United States is approaching 6 million people (2) and experts estimate that number to double by 2039 as the population ages (59). Over 1,000 new cases of HF are diagnosed every day accounting for an incidence rate of 550,000 cases a year; over 1 million hospitalizations for HF occur each year (61). HF is the most common cause for hospitalization in people over 65 years of age and 75% of patients admitted for HF exacerbations are between 65 and 75 years old (60).

Although the annual mortality rate has decreased from 20% per year to 8% to 10% per year in the past 30 years (62), the prognosis of a HF diagnosis remains dismal: one in five patients with HF will die. Diagnosis before the age of 65 incurs an 8-year mortality rate of 80% (men) and 70% (women) (2, 60). The 1-year mortality rate of people diagnosed with severe HF is 60%. The relative risk of death is 8 times higher among HF patients suffering from a new MI than in the general population (RR 7.8; 95% confidence interval [CI] 6.9-8.8) (60). Additionally, the risk of SCD in HF patients is 6 to 9 times that of the general population (2). About 300,000 people die from HF each year in the United States (2).

The economic burden of the cost of HF is correspondingly high: the costs of caring for people with HF in 2005 were documented at $27.9 billion; in 2009 direct and indirect costs are estimated at about $38 billion or more than 5% of the total annual health care costs in the United States (2). Of this amount, outpatient care (about

33%) and medications (about 10%) are significant contributors to the total medical costs (59). Recidivism is also a concern for HF patients. Data show that 44% of Medicare patients will be readmitted to the hospital within 6 months of discharge. Of patients with HF, 2% will be readmitted within 2 days and 20% within 1 month, and 50% of patients discharged with HF will be readmitted within 6 months (61).

Acutely decompensated HF (ADHF) presents with acute signs and symptoms of respiratory distress and activity intolerance, along with hemodynamic and neuroendocrine alterations (63), and is seen most often in patients with chronic HF. The distressing nature of the acute symptoms sends these patients to the ED for immediate treatment and/or hospitalization. Only one-fifth of patients present in the ED with a first-time ADHF event (21%); the remaining ADHF patients (79%) have chronic HF (63). CNSs are likely to be consulted by staff to assist in the management of these highly complex patients.

Pathophysiology

The syndrome of HF reflects the inability of the heart muscle either to contract with enough force to propel blood volume forward into the systemic circulation (systolic dysfunction) or to relax enough to adequately fill with blood during diastole (diastolic dysfunction). HF also may manifest as the coexistence of both deficiencies. The end result, regardless of which type of dysfunction is present, is a decrease in stroke volume leading to decreased CO, blood pressure, and decreased tissue perfusion.

Systolic Dysfunction

Poor systolic function is defined as an EF of less than 40% (64, 65). Systolic dysfunction is usually a result of CHD. MI is the most common etiology of systolic HF leading to poor contractility and increased preload and afterload; the outcome is a decrease in EF, stroke volume, CO, and, therefore, tissue perfusion. Other causes of systolic dysfunction include hibernating myocardium, idiopathic dilated cardiomyopathy, congenital heart disease, valvular diseases, obesity, viral infections, long-term alcohol use, peripartum cardiomyopathy, and thyroid dysfunction (60, 65). Alterations in the structure of cardiac muscle and death of cardiac muscle adversely affect its ability to generate and sustain the wall tension needed to open the atrioventricular valves to deliver the stroke volume to the rest of the body. The area(s) of damaged cardiac muscle dilute the power of the overall cardiac contraction, leading to a less than synchronous effort to contract as one muscle and therefore interfering with stroke volume and CO.

Diastolic Dysfunction

Diastolic dysfunction is not as common as systolic dysfunction; at least 20% and up to 60% of HF patients present with normal or near-normal systolic function but have abnormal diastolic function (61, 64, 66). According to the Vasodilator-Heart Failure Trial (VHeFT) studies, the prevalence of diastolic dysfunction increases with age. Thirteen percent of HF patients with an average age of 50 had diastolic dysfunction, while 60% of patients with a mean age of 75 have diastolic dysfunction (61). Abnormal diastolic function can be described in terms of alterations in LV distensibility, filling, or relaxation (64). Stiff or noncompliant ventricles are a result of hypertrophy of the cardiac muscle and increased myocardial collagen deposition; variations in the amount of blood volume, venous tone, and/or arterial compliance can increase diastolic and pulmonary artery pressures causing an acute episode of pulmonary edema (64). Stiff ventricles also prevent the heart from filling normally—so although the EF may be normal at 60%, the stroke volume may still be decreased because the preload volume is lower than normal. In addition, noncompliant ventricles are dependent on atrial filling and any tachydysrhythmia that interferes with ventricular filling during diastole will further compromise end-organ perfusion. Diastolic dysfunction may be caused by normal aging, severe hypertension, ischemic myocardium, restrictive or hypertrophic cardiomyopathy, valvular disorders, atrial myxoma, infective processes, diabetes mellitus, cardiac dysrhythmias, and conditions that increase cardiac workload from increased metabolic demands (60, 61, 63).

Compensatory Mechanisms in Heart Failure

Myocardial Hypertrophy and Chamber Dilation

The heart is able to compensate for changes in metabolic demands, pressure overloads, or volume overloads through stimulation of the central nervous system, hormonal influences, and remodeling or reshaping of the cardiac muscle. Normally an increase in CO is a response to an increase in metabolic or physiologic demands. Compensatory systems kick in when the body is stressed from any cause. In response to pressure overload, such as that resulting from stenotic valves, the enlargement of cardiac myofibrils in the muscle on the affected side (known as concentric ventricular hypertrophy) enables the ventricular wall to generate greater wall tension and therefore a stronger contraction to enable the forward flow of the stroke volume into the systemic circulation. The outcome of concentric hypertrophy is a stiff ventricle that requires high filling pressures to generate an effective contraction. Volume overloads result in an enlargement of the affected cardiac chamber (chamber dilation), producing a thinner muscle layer to accommodate the excess blood volume left over from ineffective contractions. Eccentric hypertrophy is the presence of both cardiac muscle hypertrophy and chamber dilation leading to an increase in end-diastolic volume but maintaining normal filling pressures. Both ventricular hypertrophy and dilation improve the ability of the heart to function normally, for a period of time. However, eventually the sarcomeres become overstretched, decreasing contractile ability; the remodeled cardiac muscle then outgrows its blood supply, and the effectiveness of the compensatory mechanisms declines. Other consequences of ventricular remodeling include sarcomere death and dysfunction, collagen matrix loss, and interstitial fibrosis leading to myocyte and sarcomere slippage, dilation of the heart, scar formation mediated by angiotensin II, and subsequent cardiac dysfunction (61, 63, 64).

Neurohormonal Compensation

Over the years, theories of the causative factors in ventricular remodeling have evolved from a general understanding that hemodynamics drive compensatory changes to a recognition that the interaction of neurohormonal factors are the primary reasons for structural changes occurring in the cardiac muscle. This new understanding is based on the results of many large randomized clinical trials and guides the treatment of HF. The thorough review by Unzek and Francis provides details of the many milestone HF trials that have led to current management (62).

The interaction of neurohormonal and sympathetic nervous system (SNS) activation is now understood to be the underlying cause of LV remodeling and, thus, the progression of HF—and consequently an avenue for new treatments (60, 61). Disproportionate and persistent sympathetic activity and renin-angiotensin-aldosterone system (RAAS) activity stress the heart and perpetuate the remodeling of the cardiac muscle mass. Deficits in cardiac function are immediately recognized by the body, and physiologic systems spring into action to compensate for inadequate CO. Baroreceptors in the aortic arch and carotid sinuses sense a decrease in blood pressure and transmit signals through the sympathetic nerve fibers of the heart to increase heart rate and stimulate beta-adrenergic receptors in the heart to increase contractility. The alpha-adrenergic receptors in the vascular system also are stimulated, causing the blood vessels to vasoconstrict.

Concomitantly, the juxtaglomerular cells in the macula densa of the glomerulus recognize a decrease in blood volume and release renin. Renin cleaves angiotensinogen, a precursor produced by the liver, into angiotensin I. Angiotensin I is converted into angiotensin II (ATII) by ACE found mainly in the lungs. ATII is a potent vasoconstrictor that increases blood pressure and thus increases glomerular filtration rate. Researchers have discovered that ATII directly promotes ventricular remodeling (63). Vasoconstriction increases systemic vascular resistance (SVR) and thus cardiac workload precipitating ventricular hypertrophy. ATII stimulates the adrenal cortex to produce aldosterone to assist in the protection of the body systems. Aldosterone works on the distal convoluting tubule and the collecting ducts of the nephron to reabsorb sodium; water is retained along with the sodium, thus restoring blood volume and blood pressure.

Additionally, aldosterone stimulates antidiuretic hormone (ADH; aka arginine vasopressin [AVP]), which signals the distal tubules and collecting ducts of the kidney to allow water reabsorption—again increasing blood volume to support glomerular filtration. Urine output drops during this time to conserve fluid. Excessive amounts of vasopressin are produced and circulated in chronic HF from activation of the RAAS, causing vascular constriction due to stimulation of the V_1 vasopressin receptors and aquaresis due to V_2 receptor activation (62). Tolvaptan is a selective V_2 receptor antagonist designed to inhibit activation of the V_2 receptor in the distal collecting duct and promote the excretion of mainly free water, decreasing volume overload and improving hyponatremia. Clinical trials are in progress (62).

Enlargement and volume overload cause the atria and the ventricles to stretch, which stimulates the release of atrial natriuretic peptide (ANP), made and stored in the atrial and ventricular granules, and BNP, produced in the ventricles de novo (63). The effects of ANP and BNP counteract the effects of the SNS and RAAS, to some extent. The effect of these cardiac peptides results in decreased levels of aldosterone, ATII, endothelin (a powerful vasoconstrictor), and norepinephrine, decreasing the excess fluid volume through enhanced diuresis and natriuresis and balanced vasodilation (63). BNP also has positive effects on the cardiac muscle: it assists with relaxation of the ventricle for better filling and has antifibrotic and antiremodeling effects (63). BNP levels have been used to risk stratify patients in diagnosis of HF, and an intravenous infusion of BNP (nesiritide) is a treatment strategy for acutely decompensated patients (60, 61).

This complex interaction of nervous system stimulation and endocrine secretion leads to a direct increase in CO and an improvement in patient symptoms; however, the continuous cycle of cardiac stress and its adverse effects eventually cause compensatory mechanisms to fail and pulmonary congestion to ensue, resulting in a compromised heart unable to meet the body's demands. Clinical manifestations of pulmonary congestion are a result of LV failure (LVF); systemic effects, such as jugular venous distention and peripheral edema, result from right ventricular failure (RVF). LVF usually precedes and, ultimately, causes RVF. RVF may also be a result of primary pulmonary hypertension (PPH); *cor pulmonale* is the term used to describe RVF caused by a primary pulmonary process.

Clinical Presentation
Classifications of Heart Failure
Stages of heart failure. Four stages of HF were first proposed by the 2005 Joint Committee of the ACC and AHA and have been updated in the newest revision to the 2005 guidelines (61). The four stages include two asymptomatic stages (stage A and stage B) to identify and proactively treat patients who are at high risk of developing HF. The majority of HF patients fall into stage C, defined as structural heart damage with previous or current clinical manifestations of HF (61). Stage D is the presence of end-stage heart disease requiring specialized medical therapies and/or heart transplantation for survival. The four-stage schema complements the New York Heart Association (NYHA) classification of symptomatic HF that has been used for years. A comparison of the ACC/AHA stages of HF and the NYHA classifications of HF is found in Table 9-22. The most recent guidelines incorporate new clinical trials and other evidence relevant to the diagnosis, management, and prevention of HF (61). The patient with acute decompensated HF may present in a variety of modes, with or without pulmonary edema or cardiogenic shock, or in low- or high-output states (63, 66). Table 9-23 presents management strategies related to the most common hemodynamic and perfusion characteristics seen in ADHF patients (63, 66, 67).

Signs and Symptoms of Right and Left Ventricular (Heart) Failure
In general, HF signs and symptoms are related to the transmission of increased ventricular or systemic pressures into the systemic circulation (from RVF) or into the pulmonary system (from LVF). LVF is usually the result of a large MI or multiple smaller MIs—dead cardiac muscle cannot participate in electrical conduction or cardiac contraction, resulting in dyskinesia or akinesia and thereby reducing the ability of the ventricle to generate enough force to eject its preload. The inability of the

TABLE 9–22 Comparison of ACC/AHA Heart Failure Stages With NYHA Classifications of Heart Failure and Priorities for Treatment

ACC/AHA Stages	NYHA Classification	Treatment Priorities
STAGE A: ASYMPTOMATIC. PRE-HEART FAILURE. High risk of developing HF because of the presence of conditions strongly associated with HF development.No identified structural or functional abnormalities of the pericardium, myocardium, or cardiac valves; no HF signs or symptoms		

	No comparable classification	Reduction of risk factors and patient education:
		
		• Encourage smoking cessation
		• Treat HTN, DM, hyperlipidemia
		• Lifestyle modifications
		  • Encourage physical activity
		  • Diet
		  • Weight loss
		  • Stress reduction
		  • Discourage EtOH, illegal drug use
		
		Pharmacotherapy (unless contraindicated)
		
		• ACEI or
		• ARB (patients with vascular disease, DM)

STAGE B: ASYMPTOMATIC. Latent period. Structural heart disease present and strongly associated with HF development; No HF signs or symptoms		
	Class I: Asymptomatic. Ordinary physical activity does not cause undue fatigue, dyspnea, palpitation; no limitations.	All Stage A interventions Pharmacotherapy (unless contraindicated) • Same as stage A • Beta-blockers for appropriate patients Device therapy as needed: e.g., ICDs
STAGE C: Patients with current or prior symptoms of HF associated with underlying structural heart disease.		
	Class II: Ordinary physical activity causes fatigue, dyspnea, palpitation, or angina; slight limitation. Class III: Comfortable at rest; less than ordinary physical activity causes fatigue, dyspnea, palpitation, or angina; moderate limitations.	All stage A and stage B interventions, plus • Add dietary salt restriction Pharmacotherapy (routine) (unless contraindicated) • Diuretics and • ACEI and • Beta-blockers Pharmacotherapy for selected patients: • Aldosterone antagonist • ARBs • Digitalis • Hydralazine/nitrates Avoid or discontinue use of: • Antiarrhythmic agents • NSAIDs • Most calcium channel blockers

Continued

TABLE 9-22 Comparison of ACC/AHA Heart Failure Stages With NYHA Classifications of Heart Failure and Priorities for Treatment—cont'd

ACC/AHA Stages	NYHA Classification	Treatment Priorities
		Devices in selected patients: • Biventricular pacing • ICD
STAGE D: Advanced structural heart disease and marked symptoms of HF at rest despite maximal medical therapy; require specialized interventions.		

	Class IV: Symptoms at rest; any physical activity increases discomfort; severe limitations.	Stage A, stage B, stage C interventions, plus
		
		• Level of care decisions
		  • Mechanical assist devices
		  • End-of-life care
		• Extraordinary measures
		  • Heart transplantation
		  • Chronic inotropes
		  • Permanent mechanical support
		  • Investigational/experimental surgery or drugs

ACC/AHA, American College of Cardiology/American Heart Association; ACEI, angiotensin-converting enzyme inhibitor; ARB, angiotensin receptor blocker; DM, diabetes mellitus; HF, heart failure; HTN, hypertension; ICD, implantable cardioverter/defibrillator device; NSAIDs, nonsteroidal anti-inflammatory drugs; NYHA, New York Heart Association;

Sources: Hunt et al., 2009 (61), Lamendola, 2008 (59), Neuenschwander and Baliga, 2007 (66), Smith, 2002 (60).

TABLE 9-23 Initial Management Strategies for Common Hemodynamic and Perfusion Profiles of Acute Decompensated Heart Failure (ADHF) Patients

	Congestion at Rest	
	No	**Yes**
Low perfusion at rest No	Warm and dry (HF compensated) (Normal PAOP and CI) Rx: Determine whether S/S are d/t HF	Warm and wet (most common) (high PAOP; normal CI and BP) "Wet" (fluid overload) Rx: IV loop diuretics (furosemide, bumetanide; toresimide) Natriuretic peptides (nesiritide); or vasodilators (nitroprusside, nitroglycerin) added if no/poor response Device Rx: ultrafiltration (UF)
Yes "Cold" (low-output) Rx: inotropic medications: dobutamine, dopamine, milronone Device Rx: IABP, ECMO	Cold and dry (not common most likely d/t over diuresis) (low/normal PAOP; low CI)	Cold and wet (high PAOP; low CI; low BP) Low SVR←→High SVR

Adapted from Neuenschwander JF II, Baliga RR. Acute decompensated heart failure. Crit Care Clin 2007;23(4):737-758; doi:10.1016/j.ccc.2007.08.003 (66).

CI, cardiac index; d/t, due to; PAOP, pulmonary artery occlusion pressure; S/S, signs and symptoms; SVR, systemic vascular resistance.

ventricle to eject its stroke volume means there is extra blood volume and, therefore, extra pressure within the LV. These extra pressures are transmitted backward to the left atrium (LA) and eventually that pressure is transmitted into the pulmonary system, increasing hydrostatic pressure and thereby forcing fluid into the interstitial tissue causing signs and symptoms of pulmonary congestion. Ventricular remodeling occurs to compensate for the extra volume and pressure, forcing the heart to work harder; the ventricular function curve shifts downward. The increased cardiac workload taxes an already compromised cardiac pump and a vicious cycle ensues with a progressive decrease in cardiac function.

LVF also can occur because of stiff ventricles that do not relax enough to fill with blood during diastole (i.e., diastolic HF) or a ventricle that cannot contract and eject sufficient blood into the systemic circulation (i.e., systolic HF). Both types of HF lead to ventricular remodeling. Systolic and diastolic HF can be differentiated, although many times they coexist.

Clinical signs and symptoms of RVF are related to the increase in pulmonary vascular pressure and congestion due to primary pulmonary disorder or to a decrease in LV function (most common). The pressure and/or volume overload in the RV initiates RV hypertrophy and/or dilation because the RV needs to work harder to pump its preload forward against the high pulmonary pressures. The pressure from the RV is transmitted backward into the right atrium (RA). The RA cannot accept all blood from systemic circulation; therefore, blood pools in the RA and RV, increasing pressure and congestion in the vena cava and, ultimately, in the venous circulation. Kussmaul's sign, a significant sign of hypervolemia, is an increase in the jugular venous pressure during inspiration and may be seen in patients with RVF (60, 68). The backed-up blood expands the visceral veins, causing the liver, spleen, and gastrointestinal tract to become distended and enlarged. A hepatojugular reflex producing an increase in the jugular venous pressure greater than 3 mm Hg is considered a positive sign of capillary hydrostatic pressure. As capillary pressure increases, fluid is forced out of the capillaries into interstitial tissues, causing peripheral and dependent pitting edema. A comparison of the clinical signs and symptoms of RVF and LVF is found in Table 9-24.

Signs and Symptoms of ADHF

Decreased exercise tolerance due to dyspnea or fatigue, complaints of leg or abdominal swelling, and acute hypertension are the predominant signs and symptoms of HF (61). Almost 80% of patients have complaints of

TABLE 9-24 Comparison of Clinical Signs and Symptoms of Heart Failure

	Clinical Signs and Symptoms
Right Heart Failure	Signs and symptoms (S/S) of systemic congestion (backward effects)
	• Peripheral and dependent pitting edema
	• Weeping edematous tissues
	• Distended jugular neck veins
	• Anorexia, bloating, nausea
	• Ascites
	• Hepatomegaly
	• Splenomegaly
	• Elevated central venous pressure (CVP)
	• Weight gain
	S/S of inadequate tissue perfusion (forward effects)
	• Low U/O
	• Fatigue
	• Cool, clammy skin
	• Confusion, restlessness
	• Anxiety
	• Faint pulses
	• Tachycardia
	• Tachypnea
	• Hypotension

Continued

TABLE 9-24 Comparison of Clinical Signs and Symptoms of Heart Failure—cont'd

	Clinical Signs and Symptoms
Left Heart Failure	S/S of pulmonary congestion (backward effects)
	• Pulmonary edema
	• Tachypnea
	• Basilar crackles, wheezing
	• Tachycardia, murmur, displaced PMI
	• S_3, S_4
	• Hypoxia
	• PND, orthopnea, DOE
	• Cough w/pink, frothy sputum
	• Dysrhythmias
	• Elevated PA pressures
	• Cyanosis
	S/S of inadequate tissue perfusion (forward effects)
	• Low U/O
	• Fatigue
	• Cool, clammy skin
	• Confusion, restlessness
	• Anxiety
	• Faint pulses
	• Tachycardia
	• Tachypnea
	• Hypotension

DOE, dyspnea on exertion; PA, pulmonary artery; PMI, point of maximal impulse; PND, paroxysmal nocturnal dyspnea; U/O, urine output.

general dyspnea on presentation. Dyspnea on exertion (DOE) is the most sensitive symptom accompanying ADHF (LR– 0.45, 95% CI, 0.35 to 0.67), and the most specific symptom is paroxysmal nocturnal dyspnea (PND) (LR+ 2.6, 95% CI, 1.5 to 4.5) (66). Jugular venous distention (JVD) is a highly accurate (80%) indicator of ADHF and corresponds to pulmonary artery occlusion pressure (PAOP): a JVD greater than 10 cm is equivalent to a PAOP greater than 22 mm Hg (66). Studies reported that patients with JVD are 5 times more likely to have ADHF than patients without JVD and thus JVD is an excellent indicator of ADHF (LR+ 5.1, 95% CI, 3.2 to 7.9); absence of JVD also helps to rule out ADHF (LR– 0.66, 95% CI, 0.57 to 0.77) (66). Radiographic evidence of pulmonary congestion due to ventricular failure is demonstrated in only 75% of ADHF patients (61, 66). Over 30% of ADHF patients have atrial fibrillation (AF), which further complicates HF symptomatology (66).

Some patients may be so decompensated that they present with signs of shock or a combination of shock and fluid overload. In some cases, patients are asymptomatic and cardiomegaly or HF is a serendipitous finding during the evaluation of another physiologic complaint (61). Because many the signs and symptoms of HF are nonspecific, differential diagnoses include acute MI, HF, pneumonia, pulmonary embolism, asthma, chronic obstructive pulmonary disease (COPD) exacerbation, cardiac tamponade, infection, volume overload, and anxiety (66). Table 9-23 depicts a 2 × 2 table, which is useful to classify HF patients and to select appropriate therapeutic options (66). This table identifies therapies specific to the patient with or without congestive symptoms coupled with their perfusion status. The majority of patients have hemodynamic signs marking them in the "warm and wet" or "cold and wet" categories.

Diagnosis

According to the updated guidelines (61), class I interventions for the diagnosis and management of patients presenting in the ED or hospitalized with HF signs and symptoms include posterior-anterior and lateral chest radiographs, a 12-lead ECG, and two-dimensional (2D) Doppler echocardiography (class I, LOE C); coronary angiography may be appropriate for patients suspected of having an acute coronary event causing new-onset or worsening HF signs. Up to 25% of patients have no classic signs of HF on the chest radiograph and changes may not be apparent until at least 6 hours after symptom onset (66). If present, radiographic findings of LVF include enlarged hilar vessels, upper lobe vessels, and pulmonary arteries; enlarged cardiac silhouette; interstitial edema (the presence of which correlates with an increased LA pressure of at least 25 mm Hg); pleural effusion; alveolar edema; engorged superior vena cava, and Kerley B lines (66). A 12-lead ECG may help in differentiating the underlying cause of the HF symptoms: AMI, myocardial ischemia, LV hypertrophy, heart block, dysrhythmias, and/or pacemaker malfunction (66). Echocardiography can determine LVEF and structural dimensions, abnormalities of wall motion and valvular function, and the existence of endocarditis (61, 66). Evaluation of LV function in HF patients is a core measure identified in multiple professional guidelines and recommended by TJC (69).

Additionally, laboratory testing should initially include a complete blood count; urinalysis, basic metabolic panel (serum electrolytes, especially potassium, calcium, and magnesium), blood urea nitrogen (BUN), serum creatinine, fasting blood glucose, lipid panel, liver function tests, and thyroid-stimulating hormone (class I, LOE C; 61). A fasting transferrin saturation also may be considered to assess for hemachromatosis (class IIa, LOE C). High serum BUN (>43 mg/dL), high serum creatinine (Cr >2.75 mg/dL), hyponatremia, low hemoglobin level, and a high red-cell distribution width (RDW) are all associated with poor outcomes (66). Cardiac biomarkers may be evaluated to rule out acute coronary events. Lactate levels may also be ordered (66).

BNP or NT-pro-BNP is released from the overstretched ventricle, and detection of blood levels is available through point-of-care technology. BNP levels are recommended to be drawn in hospitalized patients presenting with the symptom of dyspnea, even though BNP is not an independent predictor of HF and must be evaluated in the context of the other laboratory and diagnostic studies (class I, LOE A; 61). In the hospitalized patient, assessment of natriuretic peptides may be used for confirmation of an uncertain HF diagnosis or to assist with risk stratification (class IIa, LOE A, 61). Normal values of BNP are less than 100 pg/mL and have a sensitivity of 90%, a specificity of 76%, and a negative predictive value (NPV) of 89% (95% CI, 87% to 91%) (66, 70). Patients with previous HF admissions or clinically suspected of an HF diagnosis, with BNP levels between 100 and 500 pg/mL, have a 90% chance of having HF; BNP levels greater than 500 pg/mL make the diagnosis of HF very likely (95%) (66).

Invasive hemodynamic monitoring using a pulmonary artery catheter is controversial but may be used in institutions specializing in HF management. Hemodynamic parameters of interest in ADHF management include CO, pulmonary artery occlusion pressure, systemic arterial pressure, heart rate, and systemic vascular resistance. Noninvasive hemodynamic monitoring such as the use of tissue Doppler or cardiothoracic bioimpedance may also be implemented.

Management

The treatment goals for the ADHF patient are to urgently relieve the patient's symptoms, optimize medical therapy, and lessen the hemodynamic and neuroendocrine effects of compensation to prevent morbidity, reduce adverse effects, decrease length of stay, prevent the need for invasive mechanical therapies, and reduce mortality (61, 66). The addition of interventions specific to the hospitalized HF patient is new to the ACC/AHA HF guidelines (61), as studies for the acute management of ADHF are few. The best evidence, including consensus expert opinion (identified as LOE C), was used to formulate the recommendations for care of the hospitalized HF patient. Class I interventions point to the importance of early assessment of the patient's volume status, systemic perfusion, and LV function, as well as identification of HF as a new occurrence or an acute exacerbation of chronic HF (61); all of the interventions recommended by Hunt et al. (61) and, identified here, have an LOE rating of C, unless otherwise noted.

Oxygen should be started on all patients with hypoxic symptoms; occasionally patients may need to be mechanically ventilated to support respiratory function in acute-onset cardiogenic pulmonary edema. Noninvasive positive pressure ventilation (NIPPV) using biphasic positive airway pressure (BiPAP) and continuous positive airway pressure (CPAP) are alternatives to mechanical ventilation and have been shown to be beneficial to HF patients (66, 71). The use of pulse oximetry is routine in hospitalized patients.

Patients with fluid overload are immediately treated with IV loop diuretics, titrated for the relief of dyspnea and other symptoms of excess fluid volume (class I, LOE B; 61). Furosemide may be started at 40 mg IV push (IVP) in furosemide-naïve patients. Patients already taking furosemide may be given their usual oral dosage or bumetanide may be substituted (1 mg bumetanide is equal to 40 mg of furosemide) (66). Higher dosages of furosemide, a continuous infusion of a loop diuretic, the administration of synergistic diuretic medications, or ultrafiltration may be considered if inadequate diuresis is observed. Ultrafiltration is very effective at removing excess fluid and improving symptoms and has been the focus of a recent clinical study, The Ultrafiltration versus Intravenous Diuretics for Patients

Hospitalized for Acute Decompensated Congestive Heart Failure (UNLOAD) trial (62). Patients in the ultrafiltration group did show a significant decrease in hospital readmission rates, but other outcomes were equivocal (62).

Use caution when administering diuretics to patients with diastolic HF as the ventricular function curve is shifted downward and large volume losses will significantly raise LV diastolic pressure, resulting in decreased CO (64). Diastolic HF patients who develop AF suffer a loss in ventricular filling and may develop severe hypotension; the increase in LV diastolic pressure may be transmitted to the lungs and cause pulmonary edema. In these cases, immediate cardioversion is indicated (64).

Vasodilators are a mainstay of therapy and used to counteract the effects of the RAAS. Intravenous vasodilator therapy (NTG, sodium nitroprusside [SNP], or nesiritide [human BNP]) is frequently implemented for patients who are unresponsive to diuretics or other HF medications. NTG and SNP are effective medications with very short half-lives used to reduce preload and afterload in the heart. NTG is a venodilator that also dilates the coronary arteries at higher dosages. It may be given as an oral or sublingual dose (0.4 mg) or as a continuous IV infusion starting at 0.2 mcg/kg/min (66). As the patient becomes tolerant of the medication, the critical care nurse must constantly titrate the drug upward until dosages of 160 mcg/kg/min or greater are achieved. An SNP infusion, not used as often in current practice, may be instituted at doses of 0.3 mg/kg/min and titrated every 5 to 10 minutes according to the patient's blood pressure. Thiocyanate levels should be drawn for any patient on SNP for a significant amount of time, to check for cyanide toxicity. Nesiritide is an expensive manufactured form of human-BNP, approved by the Food and Drug Administration (FDA) for use in the United States. It is prescribed for patients with acute HF to vasodilate arteries and veins, increase the excretion of sodium and water, and possibly increase blood flow through the coronary arteries (66). The half-life of nesiritide is relatively long compared to SNP and NTG at 18 minutes (61, 62). Adverse effects include potential renal dysfunction, so renal function must be evaluated during nesiritide therapy (61). Morphine sulfate may also be administered at 2 to 5 mg provided the patient has no contraindications (low blood pressure, altered mental status, weak or diminished respiratory drive). Morphine reduces preload through venodilatation, reducing pulmonary pressures and lessening pulmonary edema, as well as patient anxiety. As with all vasodilator use, acute and prolonged hypotension may occur if the patient is volume depleted (61).

To maintain perfusion to the tissues and organ systems, intravenous infusions of positive inotropes may be added to the treatment regimen. Dobutamine is a catecholamine usually given for ADHF patients with low CO, hypoperfusion, and pulmonary congestion. Milrinone is a phosphodiesterase inhibitor causing both a positive inotropic and pulmonary vasodilator effect. The newest inotropic agent, levosimendan, is a calcium sensitizer that works by "binding to the calcium saturated N-terminal domain of cardiac troponin C, thus stabilizing and prolonging the life span of the molecule without impairment in filament relaxation" (62, p. 566). Benefits of levosimendan include positive inotropy without a concomitant increase in myocardial oxygen consumption, peripheral and coronary vasodilation, and anti-ischemic effects (62). Clinical trials in Europe have shown promising effects of levosimendan, although it is not yet approved in the United States. Vasopressors are started in the event of shock but are not beneficial by themselves in the care of ADHF. HF caused by AMI should be treated according to the AMI guidelines, with pharmacologic and revascularization therapies, as indicated.

Continuous cardiac monitoring, serial laboratory assessments of serum electrolytes (especially potassium) and renal function, and documentation of vital signs and fluid status (e.g., daily weight, intake and output, and signs of pulmonary congestion) are essential to assess the patient's response to treatment and guide the need for adjustment of the therapeutic regimen. Invasive hemodynamic monitoring is not routinely recommended but is essential for patients demonstrating signs of low output states, significant hypotension, and/or sustained clinical signs and symptoms despite optimized therapy, as well as for those on vasopressor therapy, with mechanical assist devices, and/or in cardiogenic shock (61). Anticoagulant therapy should be started to decrease the risk of thrombosis. Discharge instructions that include information on diet (including sodium restrictions), medication purposes and potential side effects, activity level, follow-up appointments, importance of daily weights, and recognition of symptoms of HF exacerbation should be provided to the patient.

Long-Term Medical Therapy

Long-term medical therapy for patients with chronic HF is based on the recognition of neurohormonal involvement in the gradual progression of HF and on the results of many large, randomized clinical trials (62). ACEIs, ARBs if ACEIs are not tolerated well by the patient, and beta-adrenergic blockers (once the patient is stabilized and eligible for beta-blocker therapy [LOE B]) are first line therapies to block the LV remodeling effects of excessive sympathetic activity, stress hormone release, and the renin-angiotensin-aldosterone cycle (61, 66). ARB with spironolactone has shown to benefit HF patients without renal dysfunction (66). These drugs, along with diuretic therapy, have been shown to improve patient quality of life and survival outcomes (62). Digoxin may also be used to control the ventricular rate in patients with AF. Organizational performance measures for state-of-the-art HF care are tracked and documented (69). The administration of these evidenced-based medications, either on admission or by discharge, is documented and considered important information for disease-specific and general quality performance ratings.

Cardiac Resynchronization Therapy and Internal Cardiac Defibrillator Therapy

Newer technologies such as cardiac resynchronization therapy (CRT) and implantable cardioverter-defibrillators (ICDs) have significantly improved chronic HF patient survival and quality of life (62, 72). LV hypertrophy leads to impairment in the conduction system and to normally synchronized cardiac contractions. About one-third of patients with systolic HF have interventricular conduction delays (IVCD), as evidenced by prolonged QRS duration of longer than 120 msec. The IVCD causes a paradoxical movement of the septal wall, interfering with contractile force and ventricular filling time and increasing the length of mitral regurgitation (72). Prolonged QRS duration increases mortality risks by 46% to 70% in chronic HF patients (72).

CRT requires the implantation of three pacing leads: one each in the RA and RV, and an LV lead inserted into the coronary sinus to access a lateral coronary vein (72). The purpose of CRT is to induce 100% biventricular pacing to reinstate cardiac synchrony and improve CO. The implementation of CRT has been shown to reverse LV remodeling (62).

CRT is designed for patients in moderate to severe HF (ACC Stage C or D; NYHA III or IV) who are refractory to optimal pharmacologic therapy. Other indications for CRT include EF less than 35%, QRS interval of more than 120 msec, medically refractory patients, LV end-diastolic diameter of 55 mm or more, and evidence of cardiac dysynchrony on echocardiogram (62, 72). CRTs are frequently implanted along with an ICD to treat lethal dysrhythmias. Coordination between the HF team, including the CNS/APN and nursing staff, and the electrophysiology staff is important to optimal management (72). CRT is a life-saving therapy and clinically efficient: implantation of CRT saves one life and prevents three hospitalizations for every nine devices implanted (number needed-to-treat [NNT] = 9) (62).

Mechanical Assistive Therapies

In ADHF patients with cardiogenic shock and in patients with end-stage HF, when pharmacologic therapies become ineffective, mechanical assistive therapy may be indicated. The use of the intra-aortic balloon pump (IABP), extracorporeal membrane oxygenation (ECMO), ventricular assist devices (VADs), and the Tandem Heart (a percutaneously inserted LA–to–femoral arterial bypass system driven via a centrifugal pump) have been reported

in the literature as case reports for use in selected ADHF patients (71). Clinical trials are in progress to test the Impella Recover by Abiomed, a percutaneous ventricular assist device, and the Orqis continuous aortic flow augmentation system (71). Mechanical assistive devices are currently used as rescue therapies and as a bridge to more definitive therapies. The only definitive therapy for end-stage HF is cardiac transplantation. When patients no longer respond to available pharmacologic, medical, and technical treatment strategies, a discussion of palliative and end-of-life care is appropriate. Palliative care strategies may be implemented in any unit of the hospital, including the critical care unit.

Palliative Care

Palliative care is the provision of therapies "to prevent and relieve suffering and support the best-possible quality of life for patients and their families, regardless of the stage of the disease or the need for other therapies" (73, p. 1507). Because the morbidity and mortality of HF are significant and the risk of SCD is substantial, Goodlin (74) suggested that the patient's prognosis be addressed and palliative care planning integrated early, as part of evidence-based guidelines for HF care. Recommendations for end-of-life care are part of the updated guidelines for care of the HF patient (61). Other authors have provided guidance for palliative and end-of-life care of the HF patient (e.g., 74, 75, 77). Goodlin presents a conceptual map of comprehensive care for HF patients that ranges from initial diagnosis to end-of-life (74). Besides evidence-based care interventions, interventions are outlined for decision-making and supportive care (consisting of communication, education, psychosocial and spiritual issues, and symptom management) specific to the stages of the HF trajectory. This matrix would provide helpful guidance for CNSs and HF teams planning a critical pathway for HF management.

The World Health Organization (WHO) defined *palliative care* as that which provides symptom relief and thereby enhances the patient's quality of life, affirms life and validates the natural process of dying without intent to accelerate or delay death, incorporates spiritual and psychological elements of care, supports the patient and family, uses a team approach to patient care, may influence the illness trajectory, and "is applicable early in the course of illness, in conjunction with other therapies that are intended to prolong life" (76). Palliative care strategies are designed to manage the patient's symptoms and increase comfort and involve frank discussions that should include the patient's goals for therapy. Pain or discomfort, dyspnea, fatigue, sleep-disordered breathing, depression, and anxiety are common symptoms that end-stage HF patients may suffer at the end of life, and strategies to relieve these symptoms have been identified (74, 75, 77). Effective end-of-life discussions involve a level of trust between the patient, family, and the caregivers. Excellent communication skills are important to present information effectively and in a caring manner.

The health care team should meet with the patient and family and any other invested health care providers (e.g., primary care provider, nurse practitioner) to discuss the patient's current condition, the patient's desired goals of care, and realistic hopes for recovery or relief of suffering or peaceful death (77). Decisions to withhold or withdraw certain therapies are difficult and may be instituted quickly or after trial periods to give the patient and family time to absorb the reality of the situation. Many therapeutic strategies for advanced HF are continued because they offer palliation of symptoms. Advanced directives should be encouraged to be completed, if not already documented. It is important for the patient and family to understand that "care" itself will not be withdrawn or withheld from the patient at any time, but that the health care team will continue to care for the patient with compassion and respect. Goodlin (74) advised that:

> *Physicians and nurses should be prepared to discuss dying and prognosis whenever they arise. Answers about prognosis, should be honest, and uncertainty should be acknowledged. Discussions with HF patients about length of life should give a range of time, and should acknowledge the possibility for error at either end (p. 392).*

Goals for end-of-life care are to achieve a "good death"—one in which the patient is as comfortable as possible and the family feels supported and cared for throughout the dying process (77). A synopsis of nursing interventions for end-of-life care is found in Table 9-25. CNSs, especially the palliative care CNS, may be the ones to help the family through the dying process. Knowledge of institutional resources, such as a chapel on site and pastoral care or bereavement specialists, may be appreciated by the family, and resources to help staff through the grieving process, such as critical incident debriefing or staff bereavement groups, may also be beneficial (77). Multiple resources from local and national initiatives (books, guidelines, workshops, etc.) are available to assist the nurse with caring for the patient at the end of life. Preprinted materials regarding the goals and benefits of palliative care services may be helpful in these discussions.

Targeted therapy has decreased morbidity and mortality of HF in the past few decades and continues to be a work in progress. Unzek and Francis (62) outlined four prospects for future therapies: (1) pharmacogenomics geared at responders and nonresponders; (2) designer drugs; (3) gene therapy aimed at controlling proteins known to positively affect the progression of HF; and (4) stem cell therapy to stabilize or perhaps reverse structural and functional changes of HF. The CNS will need to stay current with the literature as new therapies are tested and approved for use in this patient population.

Clinical Nurse Specialist Competencies and Spheres of Influence

Many of the CNS core competencies have already been discussed throughout this section. Primary core competencies in the care of ADHF patients include

TABLE 9–25 Nursing Interventions for End-of-Life Care

Topic/Time	Action/Intervention
Treatment Plan Modifications	Ask questions about patient/family's goals and make sure they are available to caregivers.
	Get details about wishes for life-sustaining therapies.
	Develop plans to manage implanted cardiac devices (e.g., pacemakers, implantable cardioverter defibrillators, ventricular assist devices, etc.).
	Review pharmacotherapy regimens and consider medications that could be stopped if they are not having an impact on symptoms.
	Trial changes to give patient/family time to consider impact of treatment decisions and a timeframe for withdrawal of certain therapies.
Good Communication	Begin to develop rapport with patient/family as early in the admission as possible
	Plan discussions early.
	Keep communication open by providing information, including patient/ family in all discussions about care, and using good therapeutic techniques to elicit information.
	Empathize with patient/family
	Advocate for the patient/family
	Individualize care to this patient/family.

TABLE 9–25 Nursing Interventions for End-of-Life Care—cont'd

Topic/Time	Action/Intervention
End-of-Life Decision-Making	Advance care planning needed to be completed, if not already done. • Durable power of attorney for health care of proxy • CPR/defibrillator preferences • Find out level of symptom relief • Site of care delivery (home, hospital, hospice, other) and desired caregiver (hospice, health care provider) • Decisions related to the "plan" if status worsens or changes Plan how to deliver "bad news" beforehand: use Ask-Tell-Ask format (Goodlin, 2009) • Ask patient/family understanding of information before you talk; correct any misinterpretations or false information • Tell patient/family bad news in simple terms • Ask if they have questions, explain any unclear points. Plan family meetings within 3 days of intensive care unit admission. Follow-up.
Treatment Decisions	Involve patient/family in all discussions. Refer to advance directives completed by patient/family to advocate for their wishes. Provide information on procedures for withdrawing or withholding therapies so patient/family knows what to expect about dying, including sounds, feelings, physical changes, patient's ability to participate at different stages of dying.
Symptom Management	Treat symptoms/evidence-based protocols • Discomfort and pain: analgesics, opioids, and sedatives (particularly for withdrawal of life-sustaining therapies) • Congestion: diuretics, morphine • Anxiety: anxiolytics • Dyspnea: oxygen, position for comfort, circulate air on patient with fans • Paroxysmal nocturnal dyspnea: nitroglycerin at bedtime • Loud, wet respirations: anticholinergics • Fatigue: stimulants; lower extremity range-of-motion exercises • Sleep-disordered breathing: continuous positive airway pressure (CPAP) machine, oxygen • Depression: stimulant Keep patient euvolemic
Bereavement	Provide postdeath bereavement resources to family, including pastoral care Staff who knew and care for the patient should also consider attending bereavement support groups

Adapted from Wingate and Wiegand (2008) (77); Goodlin (2009) (74); Wiegand and Williams, (2009) (73).

Consultation, Collaboration, and Ethical Decision Making/Moral Agency/Advocacy, as well as Systems Leadership competency. These CNS competencies primarily involve the Patient/Family and the System/Organization spheres of influence.

Consultation, Collaboration, and Ethical Decision Making/Moral Agency/Advocacy

The complexity of care surrounding the patient with ADHF warrants a team approach to care. Staff will consult the CNS to manage this highly complex care and to plan effective interventions to prevent complications and recidivism. The CNS collaborates with the nursing staff and the rest of the health care team to ensure that the patient is receiving care that is evidence-based and compassionate. Discussions about palliative and end-of-life care should take place with the patient, family, and the interprofessional team. Good interpersonal and communication skills are imperative to engage the patient and family to elicit questions and provide information to assist the patient and family in making decisions about ongoing care. The CNS makes sure that the patient's voice is heard in interprofessional team discussions and decisions. Review the management section for details regarding the CNS's operationalization of these competencies.

Systems Leadership

Multiple performance measures exist for the management of patients with HF. A joint collaboration between the ACC and the AHA has produced several data collection forms for physician inpatient and outpatient clinical performance improvement for adults with HF. CNSs may be asked to help collect data for these, or other organizational performance measures, and can use or adapt these measures for the tracking of institutional performance in the areas of diagnostics, patient education, treatment, self-management, and HF disease monitoring. For example, the AHA's Get With the Guidelines–Heart Failure (GWTG-HF) Program aims to improve the quality of HF care (69). Measures of LV function, medications administered on admission and at discharge, discharge instructions, and smoking cessation counseling are among the 30-day measures tracked that are amenable to CNS influence.

The CNS can be extremely influential in decreasing readmission rates of HF patients by implementing population-focused, evidence-based care. National quality initiatives have begun to focus on reducing the hospital readmission rate. According to a Medicare advisory commission, readmissions accounted for almost 18% of all Medicare hospital admissions and cost about $15 billion each year (78). The commission asserts that of that $15 billion cost, 80% could be saved due to potentially preventable incidents. The 30-day readmission rates for chronic HF patients are higher than the average at 20%

to 24% (78) and 6-month readmission rates are documented at 50% (61). Factors most commonly associated with hospital admission for HF patients are multifactorial and found in Box 9-4. Noncompliance with the medical or lifestyle regimen, due to socioeconomic or other factors, is responsible for 30% to 50% of recurrent episodes of HF (66).

The Institute for Healthcare Improvement's (IHI) new time-limited program titled Reducing Readmissions by Improving Transitions in Care Collaborative, aims to develop solutions to improve coordination of care and therefore the quality of the patient and family experience with the transition from hospital to home (78). The ultimate goal is to decrease the 30-day readmission rate by 30%. The proposed interventions are perfectly aligned with the team skills and system competencies of the CNS, including "enhanced assessment of post-discharge needs, enhanced teaching and learning, enhanced communication at discharge, and timely postacute follow up" (www.ihi.org/IHI/Programs/Collaboratives).

The CNS can assist the multidisciplinary team and guide the nursing staff to provide teaching and information to patients and their families to smooth the transition to outpatient care, improve the patient's quality of life, assist patients to identify and self-manage situations likely to result in an acute exacerbation of their HF, and reduce distressing, and expensive, hospital readmissions. A systematic review of multidisciplinary interventions validated that patient morbidity is decreased and survival

---

BOX 9–4 Common Factors Precipitating Hospital Admission for Heart Failure

- Noncompliance/nonadherence/inappropriate discontinuation of the medical regimen, sodium and/or fluid restriction
- Acute myocardial ischemia
- Uncontrolled or uncorrected high blood pressure
- Atrial fibrillation and other dysrhythmias
- Recent addition of negative inotropic drugs (e.g., verapamil, nifedipine, diltiazem, beta-blockers)
- Pulmonary embolus
- Nonsteroidal anti-inflammatory drugs
- Anemia
- Renal insufficiency
- Excessive alcohol or illicit drug use
- Endocrine abnormalities (e.g., diabetes mellitus, hyperthyroidism, hypothyroidism)
- Concurrent infections (e.g., pneumonia, viral illnesses)
- Excess intake of salty foods

Sources: Hunt et al., 2009 (61); Aurigemma and Gaasch, 2004 (64).

is increased when multidisciplinary interventions for clinic and home care are applied: all-cause admissions were reduced by 13%, mortality rates were reduced by 20%, and hospital admissions for HF were reduced by 30% (79). APNs frequently work in or manage HF clinics. Nurse-led HF clinics have been shown to improve patient outcomes and to reduce overall health care costs, including those associated with hospital recidivism (63, 79).

PERICARDIAL DISEASE

Etiology

Pericardial disease consists of any pathology affecting the pericardial sac covering the heart. Pericardial disease can take many forms—as an acute disorder, frequently occurring after an MI, or as a chronic disorder requiring surgical intervention. Pericardial syndromes consist of a congenital absence of a section or the entire pericardial layer (very rare); acute, chronic, recurrent, or constrictive pericarditis; or pericardial cysts (80). As many as 20% of HIV-positive/AIDS patients manifest with some type of pericardial disease (81). Pericarditis is common in adults aged 20 to 50 years old and is more common among men than among women (82).

Pericardial disease is commonly classified into two major etiologies, infectious or noninfectious, but is caused by a variety of mechanisms. It can occur (a) as a physiologic response as part of the inflammatory or immune process (e.g., deposition of toxins due to renal disease or an autoimmune reaction) or from a viral, bacterial, or fungal agent from an infectious source (e.g., infection of any structure adjoining the heart) (80, 83) (Table 9-26); (b) from the buildup of scar tissue (adhesions) and fibrosis from certain medications or repeated bouts of pericardial disease; (c) as a result of exudation from damaged myocardium (e.g., after an MI); (d) from pericardial trauma; (e) from malignancies; or (f) from iatrogenic sources (e.g., radiation therapy, surgical procedures, surgical complications, and medications) (80). The most common form of pericardial disease in the United States is acute idiopathic pericarditis (90%). Acute and chronic pericarditis will be the pericardial diseases most frequently encountered by CNSs and are the focus of the rest of this section.

Pathophysiology

The pericardial sac comprises two layers: one layer is a thin transparent mesothelial membrane that adheres to the heart and great vessels (visceral layer) connected to the second layer made up of relatively inelastic, strong elastin fibers, and collagen bundles that serve to protect the heart (parietal layer) (84). Attachments to the pericardial sac under the sternum, to the vertebral bodies, and to the diaphragm help to keep the heart positioned within the mediastinal space; the sac also helps protect the heart from overdistention due to excess volume (84). The pericardial fluid is an ultrafiltrate of the plasma and serves to lubricate the sac, decrease friction, and allows for the visceral and parietal layers to smoothly glide over each other during systole (84, 85). The amount of fluid in the pericardial sac normally ranges from 20 to 50 mL (84, 85).

TABLE 9–26 Infectious Agents Causing Pericardial Disease

Viral Agents (30% to 50% incidence)	Bacterial Agents (5% to 10% incidence)	Fungal/Parasitic Agents (rare)
Enteroviruses (seasonal following epidemics of coxsackievirus A+B and echoviruses)	*Mycobacterium tuberculosis*	*Histoplasma*
Echoviruses	*Staphylococcus*	*Coccidioides*
Adenoviruses	*Streptococcus*	*Candida*
Cytomegaloviruses (CMVs)	*Pneumococcus*	*Aspergillus*
Ebstein-Barr virus	Diphtheria	*Blastomyces*
Herpes simplex	*Gonococcus*	*Nocardia*
Influenzaviruses	Gram-negative bacilli	*Actinomyces*
Parvovirus B19	*Escherichia coli, Salmonella*	Toxoplasma
Hepatitis C		Amebiasis
Human immunodeficiency virus (HIV)		
Mononucleosis		
Mumps		
Rubella		
Rubeola		

Sources: Maisch and Ristic, 2005 (80); Maisch et al., 2004 (83).

The fundamental mechanism of action in acute and chronic pericarditis is the inflammatory process. The etiologic agent (e.g., uremic toxins, bacterial or viral infections, radiation damage, certain medications, etc.) causes an inflammatory response. The inflammatory cascades are triggered causing the release of cytokines that regulate and stimulate the inflammatory response. There is an increase in vascularity and the pericardial sac becomes infiltrated with neutrophils (PMNs, the primary immune defense cells). The resulting exudate causes an increase in the amount of pericardial fluid normally present in the pericardial sac, leading to a potential for cardiac constriction and tamponade (discussed later in this chapter). In addition, fibrin deposits on the pericardial layers support the development of adhesions and the pericardial walls become roughened causing irritation, which sustains the inflammatory process.

The pain of pericarditis is theorized to come from mechanical stretch-receptors located in the pericardium and from the end-products of inflammation and ischemia (e.g., bradykinin, proteolytic enzymes, lactic acid) causing chemical damage to the pericardial surfaces and stimulating the many pain fibers in the parietal pleura (85, 86). Additionally, inflammation of the parietal pericardium may spread to the epicardium, parietal peritoneum, or the lung pleura (86). Pericardial pain is able to be localized because parietal pain is directly transmitted into the local spinal nerves (86)—thus the patient can frequently point to the painful region—a differential clue that may help in the determination of the diagnosis.

Two types of pericarditis may occur after MI (postinfarction pericarditis). Pericarditis epistenocardica is the early, although less commonly recognized form seen in 5% to 20% of patients with transmural MIs and exudative damage (80). The second type, Dressler's syndrome, can occur after any kind of MI and has a delayed onset of about 1 week to a few months after MI (80); although the mechanism of action is not fully known, it is believed that self-antigens to the myocardial tissue stimulate an autoimmune reaction (82). The incidence of Dressler's syndrome is small at only 0.5% to 5% and is even less in patients who received thrombolytic therapy (80). However, patients with Dressler's syndrome may suffer from hemopericardium and greater than 50% experience cardiac tamponade and/or rupture of the ventricular free wall (80).

Pericarditis as a consequence of renal disease is caused by the inflammatory effect of uremic toxins on the pericardium. The patient in chronic renal failure is not able to eliminate nitrogenous and other wastes; the concentration of urea can increase up to 10-fold (86). An elevated BUN signifies nitrogenous waste buildup and patients with uremic pericarditis usually have a BUN of greater than 60 mg/dL (84). The toxins irritate the pericardial sac, thereby increasing the production of fluid within the sac. This inflammation can affect adjoining structures such as the epicardium and extend into the myocardium, causing a myocarditis and decreased ventricular function (86). Three forms of pericarditis can manifest in patients with end-stage renal disease. Common etiologies, incidence rates, and treatments of pericarditis frequently found in end-stage renal disease patients are listed in Table 9-27 (87).

Viral agents are the most common infections causing pericardial disease as the presence of the virus or viral fragments stimulate the immune response producing both T and B cells to eliminate the viral antigens. Sometimes the immune responses are targeted against the cardiac tissue itself, causing an autoimmune reaction. The viruses identified in causing pericarditis are listed in Table 9-26. Viral agents are identified through polymerase chain reaction (PCR) or in situ hybridization techniques (80). Immunoglobin treatments for cytomegalovirus (CMV) pericarditis and adenovirus and parvovirus B19 perimyocarditis, as well as interferon treatment for coxsackievirus B pericarditis, are being studied. Acute or chronic myocarditis may occur as a complication of viral pericarditis. Viral pericarditis is usually self-limited, producing small amounts of serous effusion fluid (81).

Bacterial pericarditis usually results from infections in adjoining structures or in the bloodstream. Patients who are immunocompromised or otherwise debilitated are at greatest risk, and mortality rates are high, regardless of treatment. Purulent pericarditis, as well as pericarditis resulting from neoplastic or tuberculous sources, produces large amounts of pericardial fluid. The characteristics of this fluid are indicative of inflammation with high protein levels, blood, and large numbers of white blood cells (81).

Drugs known to cause pericarditis include dantrolene (Dantrium), doxorubicin (Adriamycin), hydralazine

TABLE 9–27 Forms of Pericarditis in Patients With ESRD

Form of Pericarditis	Etiology (Incidence)	Treatment
Uremic pericarditis	Uremia (40% to 50%)	Dialysis
Dialysis-associated pericarditis	Infection/multiple factors (20% to 30%)	Intense dialysis
		Anti-inflammatory drugs
Chronic constrictive pericarditis	Chronic inflammation (4%)	Pericardiectomy

ESRD, end-stage renal disease.

Source: Berg J. Assessing for pericarditis in the end-stage renal disease patient. Dimens Crit Care Nursing 1990;9(5):266-271 (87).

(Apresoline), isoniazid (INH), mesalamine (Rowasa), methysergide, penicillin, phenytoin (Dilantin), procainamide (Procanbid), and rifampin (Rifadin) (81). The signs and symptoms and treatment regimens are similar for other types of pericarditis. The offending medication should be discontinued.

Acute pericarditis in the early stages is typically more of a dry irritation; in the late stages the exudate can be serous and hemorrhagic. In chronic pericarditis, the incessant irritation of the pericardial sac causes a continual inflammatory response and the buildup of fibrin deposition and adhesions. This response may cause the pericardial sac to become thickened and therefore stiff and rigid. The inflexibility of the pericardial sac causes a constrictive and compressive effect on the heart leading to signs of RVF and LVF from compromised ventricular filling and forward flow, as well as chronic pain.

Chronic pericarditis is defined as pericarditis lasting longer than 3 months. There are several types of chronic pericarditis manifesting as effusive, adhesive, or constrictive. Chronic effusive pericarditis is caused by agents that incite a continual inflammatory response or from a complication of HF called hydropericardium (80). Adhesive or constrictive forms of chronic pericarditis may be the result of repeated pericardial insults, myxedema, or renal or autoimmune diseases (80); scarring and adhesion

formation cause the pericardium to contract and adhere to the heart (84). Chronic pericarditis is a common complication of tuberculosis, radiation therapy, pericardial trauma, renal failure, and metastatic cancer. Table 9-28 provides the definition, etiologies, and complications of pericardial syndromes (80, 83).

Clinical Presentation

Diagnosis of pericarditis is based on the patient's presentation (signs and symptoms), especially the presence of precordial pain and a pericardial friction rub, along with ECG changes and detection of a pericardial effusion (85). The most common sign of acute pericarditis is the patient's complaint of chest pain. Precordial chest pain in pericarditis is usually described as a sharp, stabbing pain (i.e., pleuritic pain) but may also be described in terms similar to ischemic pain. The chest pain may radiate to the back and epigastric areas and frequently to the left side, especially to the left neck and shoulder regions (trapezius ridge). A differential clue of pericardial disease–related chest pain is chest pain that is worsened by deep breathing on inspiration, coughing, the supine position, or body movement—thus the patient compensates for these aggravators by limiting body movement and breathing very shallowly. Patients with pericardial pain are frequently seen leaning forward over the bedside table; this maneuver relieves

TABLE 9–28 Definition, Etiologies, and Complications of Pericardial Syndromes

Disorder	Definition	Etiologies	Complications
CONGENITAL PERICARDIAL DEFECTS			
	Partial or total absence of the pericardium • Partial left absence—70% • Partial right absence—17% • Bilateral—rare	Congenital defect	Increased risk of traumatic injury Cardiac herniation and strangulation (due to partial left absence) • Treatment (Tx): Immediate surgical pericardioplasty
ACUTE PERICARDITIS			
	Acute inflammation of the pericardial sac Classifications: dry, fibrinous, or effusive	Multiple	Pleural effusion Cardiac tamponade
CHRONIC PERICARDITIS			
	Chronic disease of the pericardial sac • Effusive • Adhesive • Constrictive	Inflammation Heart failure Infection Autoimmune Systemic diseases	Cardiac tamponade

Continued

TABLE 9–28 Definition, Etiologies, and Complications of Pericardial Syndromes—cont'd

Disorder	Definition	Etiologies	Complications
RECURRENT PERICARDITIS			
	Inflammation of pericardial sac that presents either sporadically with symptom-free periods or continually if medication is stopped	Inflammation Heart failure Infection Autoimmune Systemic diseases	Cardiac tamponade
CONSTRICTIVE PERICARDITIS			
	Result of chronic inflammation causing increase in thickness of the pericardium (sometimes)	Chronic inflammation Tuberculosis Radiation therapy Previous surgical interventions	Decreased left ventricular function Cardiac tamponade Venous congestion Hepatomegaly Ascites Pleural effusions • Tx: Pericardiectomy • Mortality rate 6% to 12% • Surgical complications: acute cardiac insufficiency; ventricular wall rupture
PERICARDIAL CYSTS			
	Unilocular or multilocular growths consisting of encapsulated pleural effusions from a variety of etiologies	Congenital (rare) Inflammation Rheumatic pericarditis Bacterial infection Trauma Cardiac surgery	
NEOPLASTIC PERICARDITIS			

	Primary (rare) or secondary tumor formation (from primary lung or breast cancer, malignant melanoma, lymphoma, leukemia) on the pericardium	Primary neoplasia
		Metastatic disease
			Cardiac tamponade
			Constrictive pericarditis
			Large recurrent pericardial effusions
			
			• Tx:
			  • Neoplastic pericarditis without cardiac tamponade: systemic antineoplastic therapy
			  • Pericardiocentesis and/or radiotherapy to treat/prevent recurrent effusions
			  • Instillation of sclerosing, cytotoxic agents, or immunomodulators into pericardial sac to prevent reoccurrences

From Maisch B, Ristic AD. Pericardial diseases. In MP Fink, E Abraham, V Jean-Louis, and PM Kockanek, editors. Textbook of Critical Care. 5th edition. Philadelphia: Saunders; 2005:851-860 (80).

parietal pain to some extent by moving the heart away from inflamed diaphragmatic lung pleura.

Dyspnea is a common finding, along with a low-grade fever due to inflammatory cytokines, malaise, and myalgia. Heart rate may be normal or rapid, and regular. A paradoxical pulse is a result of the accumulation of fluid in the pericardium (pericardial effusion); it is also a sign of cardiac tamponade and must be treated emergently. Blood pressure may be labile due to a reduction in LV stroke volume. A narrowing pulse pressure may also indicate cardiac tamponade. Any suspicion of cardiac tamponade must be validated and aggressive maneuvers to decrease cardiac compression enacted immediately.

A hallmark, but possibly transient, sign of pericarditis is a pericardial friction rub, a grating sound caused by the rubbing together of the inflamed layers of the pericardial sac. The diagnostic accuracy of a pericardial friction rub shows a high specificity of almost 100% but a low sensitivity (81). Auscultation should be repeated frequently to identify a transient friction rub. A pericardial friction rub is heard best using the diaphragm of the stethoscope at the left lower sternal border (at intercostal space 4-5) with the patient sitting up (high Fowler's) and leaning forward. Asking the patient to exhale while you auscultate will move the heart and pericardium nearer to the chest wall (82). The pericardial rub may be classified as monophasic, biphasic, or triphasic (80) and may be heard during all phases of cardiac contraction and relaxation. The sounds of a triphasic rub correlate to the heart's movement during atrial contraction, ventricular contraction, and ventricular relaxation (81). Differentiating a pericardial friction rub from a pleural friction rub is accomplished by asking the patient to hold his or her breath—if you still hear the rub, it is a pericardial rub. Of course, if the inflammation has spread to the pleura, a pleural friction rub may also be evident once the patient starts breathing again. A pericardial friction rub is not present in about half of all patients with pericarditis (88).

Atypical presentations of pericardial disease may be seen in elderly patients or patients with neuropathic pain syndromes. For example, elderly patients may not present with a fever because of normal decreases in immune responses with age.

Infectious Pericarditis

Patients with a viral or bacterial etiology may have additional signs or symptoms. Bacterial pericarditis presents acutely with severe symptoms of a short duration. Bacterial infections may produce purulent exudate and the infection can become life-threatening if not treated promptly. Tuberculous pericarditis also has a mortality rate of 85% if left untreated and results in constrictive pericarditis in 30% to 50% of patients (80). The presence of a temperature over 38.5°C, night sweats, loss of weight, elevated serum globulin levels, and a normal total white blood cell count is diagnostic of tuberculous pericarditis (81). Fungal infection of the pericardium is rare and, like bacterial and tubercular forms of pericarditis, primarily occurs in immunocompromised patients. Refer to Table 9-26 for viral, bacterial, and fungal agents causing pericardial disease.

Constrictive Pericarditis

Signs and symptoms of constrictive pericarditis are similar to those of HF and related to the compressive effects of pericardial scar tissue: fatigue, exercise intolerance, dyspnea, orthopnea, peripheral edema, and ascites (84). Distended neck veins during inspiration, known as Kussmaul's sign, is observed in 30% to 40% of patients with constrictive pericarditis (89). A pericardial "knock" may be apparent during auscultation of the heart. A pericardial knock is a loud sound occurring early in diastole (after S_2 and slightly before an S_3 would be heard) during rapid diastolic filling (89). The cadence of a pericardial knock is similar to: "Lub, dub, thock . . . lub, dub, thock."

Clinical manifestations of chronic pericarditis are dependent on the degree of cardiac compromise from the inflamed pericardium and the amount of pressure applied to the cardiac muscle from the constrictive sac. Precordial pain, palpitations, and fatigue may be reported. Chronic pain and AF are also common.

Diagnosis

Laboratory data may show the results of the inflammatory process. Expect to see an elevated total white blood cell count and neutrophil count, as well as elevations in the erythrocyte sedimentation rate (ESR), CRP, and LDH levels. The anti–streptolysin O (ASO) titer may also be elevated with autoimmune diseases and the patient may have a positive purified protein derivative (PPD) test, if tuberculosis is the etiology. An elevated BUN and creatinine may occur if the cause of the pericarditis is renal in nature. Gram staining, acid-fast staining, fungal staining, and PCR testing of pericardial fluid; blood cultures; and a culture of the pericardial fluid or tissue may be performed for suspicions of an infectious process. cTnI and CPK-MB enzymes may be elevated due to inflammation of the epicardium or myocardial damage, but large elevations in cTnI, greater than 1.5 ng, are not common (80). One study reported that when cTnI was elevated, the patients, mostly young males, presented with ST elevation and pericardial effusion (80).

Echocardiography is the recommended procedure for evaluating the patient with pericarditis (90). Echocardiography is easily performed at the bedside and provides immediate and accurate information about ventricular function and the presence of pericardial fluid (91).

Changes in the ECG are helpful in diagnosing pericarditis but may also be deceiving depending on when the ECG is performed. Comparison of the current 12-lead with previous ECGs will aid in the diagnosis. Four characteristic stages of ECG changes in a patient with acute pericarditis have been identified. In general, ECG changes due to pericarditis show global changes in the

ST segments and T waves with decreased QRS voltage. The decreased QRS voltage is related to the accumulation of fluid in the pericardium (86). These changes are unique to pericarditis and can help the clinician to differentiate pericarditis from the typical ECG changes for MI. In addition, the patient with pericarditis will not demonstrate reciprocal or mirror ECG changes, nor will Q waves develop (81).

A quick way to remember the stages of ECG change is to remember that the changes are widespread across the ECG and can be simply identified as "all up," signifying concave ST-segment elevation in most leads in the first stage; "normal," as the ST segments come back down to baseline; "all down," reflecting widespread T-wave inversion in the third stage; and "normal," as the waveforms resume their prepericarditis morphology. Table 9-29 lists the ECG changes typical of acute pericarditis (80, 83, 85). If the ECG is initially documented during the third stage when T-wave inversions are seen throughout the recording, differentiating pericarditis from other myocardial damage, such as myocardial stunning, myocarditis, or biventricular strain will be difficult (80). Dysrhythmias, such as supraventricular tachycardia (SVT), may be seen (80).

A chest radiograph may be performed to ascertain involvement of the pulmonary system or pathologies of the adjoining structures. The cardiac silhouette may be completely normal or present in a classic "water bottle" shape (82). A widened mediastinum may or may not be appreciated. Other diagnostic tests that may be used to confirm the diagnosis are an echocardiogram, computed tomography (CT) scan, or magnetic resonance imaging (MRI) to identify pericardial effusions and pathologies of the pericardium and epicardium, or pericardiocentesis, pericardial/epicardial biopsy, or pericardioscopy to classify the etiologic agent (66).

Management
Acute Pericarditis

Collaborative interventions for the care of the patient with acute pericarditis include pain assessment and management, oxygen therapy to relieve the dyspnea, vigilant monitoring of vital signs, administration of anti-inflammatory medications and antibiotics if indicated by culture and sensitivity testing, and the prevention and recognition of complications.

Whether the pericarditis is acute or chronic, frequent pain assessment is essential. Of particular importance is the ability of the nurse to recognize the chest pain as that of ischemic origin rather than inflammatory. The possibility that the patient's pain is from an ischemic source versus a pericardial source should be seriously considered. The CNS as the clinical expert should be able to differentiate normal versus abnormal heart sounds (i.e., clicks, rubs, extra sounds, murmurs) to aid in the diagnosis and reevaluation of the patient.

Pericardial pain is managed with anti-inflammatory medications. NSAIDs are the foundation of pericarditis treatment. ASA (325 to 650 mg PO every 4 to 6 hours) or ibuprofen (300 to 800 mg every 6 to 8 hours) is commonly prescribed (85). Indomethacin is used cautiously in the elderly and in patients with CAD because it can decrease coronary artery perfusion (80). Colchicine, an older drug that has waxed and waned in popularity for treatment of acute pericarditis, is back in favor due to the positive outcomes of several clinical trials and may be used to treat pericarditis if NSAID therapy is ineffective by itself. Colchicine can be administered either in combination with an NSAID or as monotherapy at a dose of 0.5 mg twice daily/1 mg daily (81). The COPE trial (COlchicine for acute PEricarditis) demonstrated significant beneficial effects of colchicine on the reoccurrence rate of acute pericarditis (relative risk reduction [RRR] 66% with an NNT = 5) and symptom relief (RRR 66%; NNT = 3) (92).

Steroids administered orally, intravenously, or intrapericardially usually are reserved for pericarditis and recurrent pericardial effusions unresponsive to other drug therapy or from pericarditis resulting from connective tissue disorders or uremic toxins. Systemic effects of high-dose steroid therapy (1 to 1.5 mg/kg/day) include gastrointestinal upset, osteoporosis, and aseptic necrosis of the femoral head (93); intrapericardial application causes few to no systemic side effects (80, 94). Complications of acute pericarditis include pericardial effusion; if significant effusion exists cardiac filling is decreased and myocardial function

---

TABLE 9–29 ECG Changes Typical of Patients With Acute Pericarditis

	Electrocardiogram (ECG) Change
Stage I ("All Up")	ST segment elevation in the inferior (II, III, AVF) and anterior (I, AVL, V_3–V_6) leads ST segment always depressed in AVR, possibly in V_1 and/or V_2 PR segment opposite in polarity to P wave
Stage II ("Normal")	Early: ST segments return to baseline; PR segments remain deviated Late: Flattening and inversion of T waves
Stage III ("All Down")	Global T wave inversions in all leads (usually)
Stage IV ("Normal")	Return of ECG waveforms to patient's normal state

Sources: Maisch et al., 2004 (83); Maisch and Ristic, 2005 (80).

can be compromised leading to cardiac tamponade and possible death. Up to 24% of patients who have had acute pericarditis will have a return of pericardial symptoms within a few weeks after their initial illness (81).

Chronic, Constrictive, or Recurrent Pericarditis

In addition to pain management, the treatment of chronic, constrictive, and recurrent pericarditis is symptomatic. Steroids are considered for those cases for which traditional therapies are unsuccessful, leading to frequent reoccurrences. Maisch and Ristic (80) noted that too frequently providers prescribe an ineffective dose or taper the drug too quickly. A month's worth of prednisone (1 to 1.5 mg/kg) should initially be prescribed and gradually tapered over a 3-month period. Other immunosuppressive drugs are added to the regimen if the prednisone alone is ineffective: azathioprine (75 to 100 mg once daily) or cyclophosphamide may be administered in combination with the prednisone. Anti-inflammatory drugs such as an NSAID or colchicine (0.5 mg twice or three times daily) should be started near the end of the tapering period and continued for 3 to 6 months (80).

Treatment for Pericardial Effusions

For large or recurrent pericardial effusions, pericardiocentesis should be performed. The CNS should continually observe the patient for signs of cardiac distress and the patient's ECG for changes indicating contact of the heart with the pericardiocentesis needle during the procedure. Emergency equipment should be nearby in case of cardiac arrest. Interventional techniques such as balloon pericardiotomy or surgical interventions such as creation of a pericardial window or pericardiectomy are usually reserved for patients with severe recurrent and chronic pericardial disease. The goal of balloon pericardiotomy or a surgical pericardial window is to prevent reaccumulation of pericardial fluid by draining the fluid through the created hole or window. The drained fluid flows into either the pleural or mediastinal space (91), where it is eventually reabsorbed. The injection of sclerosing agents into the pericardial space, such as talc powder or bleomycin, is another treatment for recurrent effusions, especially those from a malignant source (85, 91). If pericardiectomy is planned, steroids need to be discontinued several weeks before surgery. Mortality rates of up to 40% have been documented for pericardiectomy procedures in patients with severe constrictive pericarditis (85); the percentage of patients who obtain complete relief and return of normal cardiac function from this procedure is only 60% (80).

Patient education should include information related to an increase in physical activity as the pain and fever subside and to proper administration and side effects of medications. For patients with chronic pericarditis, signs of decreased CO and cardiac tamponade should be emphasized and the patient should be instructed to seek immediate treatment.

Clinical Nurse Specialist Competencies and Spheres of Influence
Clinical Expert/Direct Care and Coaching/Teaching/Mentoring

The CNS is a clinical expert in the care and management of patients with pericarditis. The CNS may influence the Patient/Family Sphere by directly role modeling evidence-based care for these patients, but most likely will be called upon to perform in a supervisory role and for expert advice (Nursing/Other Disciplines Sphere). Clinical expertise in cardiac auscultation is critical in caring for cardiovascular patients. The patient with pericarditis presents a unique challenge to the clinician in that a pericardial rub is not always heard; and if it is heard, the sound is usually transient. The CNS can bolster the confidence of the staff nurse by sharing this knowledge and assessing the patient with the nurse. The CNS may be called upon to assist the physician or nurse practitioner (NP) in performing pericardiocentesis to relieve a pericardial effusion. The CNS assures and prepares the patient, helps to explain the procedure, and monitors the patient's response. Failure to rescue can be avoided by vigilant monitoring of the patient with pericarditis for signs of ischemic pain and signs of cardiac tamponade. The CNS can coach the staff as to the signs and symptoms of cardiac tamponade and encourage staff to seek rapid consultation with the attending physician or hospitalist for suspicion of tamponade.

In the Patient/Family Sphere, the CNS also uses his or her competency in coaching/teaching/mentoring by providing education to patients regarding medication side effects, steps toward progressive physical activity, and the signs of pericardial effusions and cardiac tamponade to patients with chronic disorders. In the Nursing/Other Disciplines Sphere, the CNS mentors the staff's familiarity with best practices by translating the evidence into a form that makes sense for the staff.

CARDIAC TAMPONADE

Etiology

Cardiac tamponade is a life-threatening condition that causes a decrease to total absence of cardiac pumping ability as a result of compression of the heart within the pericardial sac. Cardiac tamponade may occur after any surgical or traumatic injury to the chest or heart, bleeding after cardiac surgery, massive pulmonary embolism, aortic dissection, acute pericarditis, iatrogenic injury, or malignant diseases (80, 95, 96). About 15% to 20% of patients with acute pericarditis experience a pericardial effusion large enough to cause cardiac tamponade (80). The mortality rate is high if signs of cardiac tamponade are not recognized and treated promptly.

Pathophysiology

Cardiac compression is due to the accumulation of extra fluid (serous, sanguineous, or chylous [very rare]) in the pericardial sac or outside of the pericardial sac. As noted in the previous section, the pericardial sac is fairly stiff and typically holds about 20 to 50 mL of serous fluid. In an acute situation, the accumulation of blood will quickly increase the volume of fluid in the pericardial sac and thereby increase the pressure within the sac. This elevated pressure will compress the myocardium, ultimately affecting its ability to pump—to the point at which CO will decline precipitously and the patient goes into cardiac arrest. Cardiac compression can also occur from external forces of excess pressure in the chest, impeding the ability of the heart to pump. Tension pneumothorax, pulmonary embolism, or dissecting aortic aneurysm can acutely increase intrathoracic pressure.

Determinants of intrapericardial pressure are the absolute fluid volume, the rate of fluid accumulation, and the distensibility of the pericardial sac (96). Figure 9-8 shows the relationship of intrapericardial volume and pressure—just small changes in volume in the pericardial sac can cause a large change in pressure. Since the pericardial sac has the ability to stretch to accommodate its volume, the rate at which the fluid accumulates is of more significance than the ultimate volume (80, 95, 96). Rapid accumulation of fluid up to 250 mL over a short time period (e.g., minutes to hours) will cause more rapid deterioration in the patient than a slower accumulation of a much larger fluid amount (e.g., >1000 mL). The reason lies in the fact that while the pericardial sac is relatively noncompliant, the slower accumulation gives the sac time to stretch and accommodate the extra fluid (84, 96). For example, a patient recovering from cardiac bypass surgery may deteriorate very quickly with obvious signs of tamponade, due to a rapid bleed into the pericardial sac from a missed, unligated arterial feeder vessel. In another scenario, a patient recovering from cardiac bypass surgery may not show signs of cardiac tamponade from a slowly leaking vessel anastomosis until after they are transferred out of the ICU or possibly even discharged to home. Eventually the extra fluid in the sac will create enough pressure on the heart to compromise its function and signs and symptoms will be manifested.

Clinical Presentation

Classic signs of cardiac compression include the observation of Beck's triad (increased central venous pressure [CVP], muffled heart sounds [quiet precordium], and hypotension), narrowed pulse pressure, JVD, pulsus paradoxus, tachycardia, tachypnea, and signs of decreased CO (e.g., change in mentation; decreased urine output; weak pulses; pale, cool, moist skin). Hepatomegaly and peripheral edema may also be evident. Ewart's sign is a classic finding of large pericardial effusions and is considered positive when there is dullness to percussion and increased tactile fremitus, increased bronchial breath sounds, and a blowing sound between the vertebral column, just below the left scapular area (95, 97). Patients with purulent pericarditis may show signs of severe illness with fever, chills, and increasing temperature (88).

Major hemodynamic findings consist of elevation and equalization of all intracardiac pressures (±5 mm Hg), which can be seen during right heart catheterization and/or pulmonary artery pressure monitoring (95). Pulsus paradoxus, an exaggerated fall in arterial pressure during inspiration (greater than 10 mm Hg), occurs due to the inability of the RV to expand outward to accommodate venous return during inspiration due to high pressure in pericardial space. Normal intrapericardial pressure of 1 to 5 mm Hg can increase to over 30 mm Hg in tamponade (93). This increased ventricular effort causes the interventricular septum to shift and bulge into the LV, which decreases the size of the LV chamber, decreases

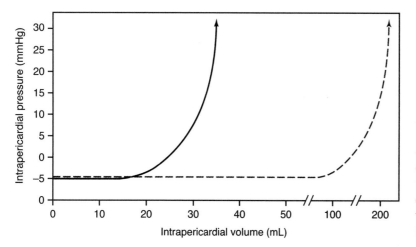

FIGURE 9–8: Relationship between intrapericardial volume and pressure. In acute situations, small changes in volume in the pericardial sac can cause a large change in intrapericardial pressure. In chronic situations, with a slow change in intrapericardial volume the pericardial sac can distend to accommodate the extra fluid without dramatically increasing the intrapericardial pressure, up to a point.

LV filling and stroke volume, and therefore decreases CO and arterial blood pressure. Additionally, an RV "dip and plateau" or "square root sign" can be seen. This phenomenon is related to a rapid rise in RV diastolic pressure followed by a flat plateau of pressure indicating no further diastolic filling can occur due to high pericardial pressure. Sinus tachycardia, SVT, atrial flutter, or AF may be seen (80, 95).

Permanent distention of the pericardial sac can occur in patients who have experienced multiple bouts of recurrent pericarditis and in patients with cardiomegaly from end-stage heart disease. Signs of cardiac tamponade may take longer to become apparent in these patients because the enlarged pericardial sac would require a larger amount of fluid to accumulate before cardiac compression would occur.

Diagnosis

The gold standard for diagnosis of pericardial effusion is echocardiography (83, 90), which is identified as a class I intervention in the latest ACC/AHA clinical practice guidelines for echocardiography (90). Signs of cardiac tamponade may be first identified on the echocardiogram before clinical signs are apparent (90). Echocardiographic criteria for confirming the diagnosis of tamponade include identification of the "swinging heart" sign, right-heart chamber collapse, reduction in heart chamber volume with respiration, and RA invagination (91). Collapse of RV chamber in diastole and the RA chamber in systole are signs of decreased CO; RA chamber collapse is sensitive to high pressure within the pericardial space and RV collapse in diastole is specific for cardiac tamponade (90). The collapse of the ventricular and atrial chambers is a compensatory mechanism and equalization of pressures within the chambers is a consequence. As the volume in the pericardial space rapidly increases against a noncompliant pericardium, the intrapericardial pressure also rises. To accommodate the increased volume and pressure in the pericardial space, the heart chambers must decrease in size, equalizing the diastolic compliance of all heart chambers (84). Confirmation of pericardial effusion also may be made with CT or MRI to identify pericardial thickness, the location and amount of effusion, and the presence of pericardial cysts or masses.

A routine chest radiograph (CXR) is not very sensitive or specific for the diagnosis of pericardial effusion. A CXR may show the lack of pulmonary edema or congestion and it may be helpful in identifying a widened mediastinum or enlarged, globular heart silhouette, but differentiation of pericardial effusion in a hypertrophied heart, or small or retropericardial effusions may not be appreciated (96). An ECG may provide additional evidence showing a global decrease in QRS voltage, diffuse ST and T-wave changes, electrical alternans (i.e., a "swinging heart" associated with huge effusions greater than 500 mL [96]), and pulsus paradoxus.

Management

For patients with rapid onset of signs of tamponade, until definitive management can be instituted, treat decreased CO with fluids and possibly inotropic medications. Collaborative management includes continuous cardiac and vital sign monitoring, alleviation of patient anxiety, and assisting with or performing therapeutic invasive procedures. In the immediate postoperative period after cardiac surgery, patients are vulnerable for the development of cardiac tamponade. These postoperative patients should be monitored for signs of diminishing chest tube output, decreased CO (such as tachycardia, hypotension, narrowed pulse pressure, increasing CVP, decreased urine output), and ECG changes and/or dysrhythmias. Postinfarction patients should be monitored for complaints of chest pain and questions to differentiate the chest pain from pericardial pain (e.g., is the pain positional or worse with inspiration?) should be used.

Removal of the accumulated fluid via pericardiocentesis is paramount to restoring the patient to optimal health. Patients who are post cardiac surgery may require reopening of their chest incision to alleviate the pressure on the heart and remove accumulated blood clots. Surgical intervention may be necessary to find the cause of the tamponade. Assisting the physician or specially trained APN in performing a pericardiocentesis is an important responsibility for the clinician. The patient and family are prepared for the procedure by providing information about the rationale and a description of what to expect; informed consent is obtained (98). The patient is positioned, skin is prepared for needle insertion, and intravenous sedation may be administered to make the patient more comfortable. A combination of a sedative with an amnesic is a common approach. Morphine (0.1 mg/kg) or merperidine (1 mg/kg) and midazolam (3 to 5 mg) is a common combination (85).

Using a subxiphoid approach (most common), pericardiocentesis is performed by inserting a 16- to 18-gauge needle, 3-inch pericardial needle or catheter over the needle into the pericardial space (98). The pericardial needle is guided into the pericardial space, under constant suction from the attached syringe, either by ECG (by attaching an alligator clip lead wire to the proximal end of the needle and monitoring on a V lead), echocardiography, or fluoroscopy. In the ECG-guided approach, the needle is advanced until it contacts the epicardium. This needle-to-muscle contact is seen as ST-segment elevation on the cardiac monitor. The needle is withdrawn until the ST segment returns to baseline and then pericardial fluid is slowly withdrawn through the needle or via a catheter placed in the pericardial space.

Pericardial fluid may be sent to the laboratory for determination of the cause of the effusion. Typically, a post-procedure CXR is obtained immediately to evaluate for iatrogenically induced pneumothorax or hemothorax. To assess for recurrent or residual pleural effusion, a 2D echocardiogram should be performed within a few hours of the conclusion of the procedure (98).

The pericardial catheter may remain in the pericardial space up to 4 days if further drainage or interventional treatments are expected (85, 98). Care of the patient after pericardiocentesis includes continued monitoring of vital signs, assessing the pericardiocentesis site for signs of bleeding or infection, and observing the patient's condition, with special attention for signs of recurrent effusion or tamponade. Drainage of the pericardial space should be performed every 8 hours and the catheter should be maintained with 5 mL of a heparinized flush (100 U/mL) solution (96). Because the patient is at risk for infection, the site is kept clean and a sterile occlusive dressing is applied. The pericardial catheter should be removed as soon as possible.

Clinical Nurse Specialist Competencies and Spheres of Influence

The CNS competencies of Clinical Expert/Direct Care and Collaboration are vital to the care of the patient in cardiac tamponade. The Spheres of Influence include the Patient/Family and System/Organization spheres.

Clinical Expert/Direct Care and Collaboration

The emergent nature of caring for a patient with cardiac tamponade requires the characteristics of clinical judgment, clinical expertise, and teamwork. Cardiac tamponade can occur from a variety of causes and the astute nurse recognizes the importance of being attentive to, sometimes subtle, signs and symptoms that warn of an impending crisis. The patient in cardiac tamponade does not have time on his or her side—measures to decrease the pressure surrounding the heart must be undertaken immediately or the patient may die. The CNS lends expert skill to conduct a rapid assessment of the general situation and of the patient. Maintaining a calm atmosphere in the midst of the chaos of a crashing patient is important. "Thinking aloud" by the CNS while performing clinical tasks may help new nurses make sense of the experience. Emergency protocols are enacted and the CNS assists the team to manage the patient, pitching in where needed and providing expert advice. The CNS may assist the physician or APN to perform a pericardiocentesis to relieve the pressure around the heart. There are evidence-based guidelines available on care of the patient with pericardial disease. The CNS is responsible to make sure that the current guidelines are being reflected in the unit policies and procedures and the standards of care (SOC) for this vulnerable patient population.

VALVULAR DISORDERS

Etiology

Valvular heart disease (VHD) affects over 5 million Americans and consists of congenital and acquired disorders affecting all four heart valves (2). Congenital defects include conditions such as bicuspid mitral and bicuspid aortic valves. Rheumatic heart disease is the most common cause of valve disease in adults (99). In addition, MI, thoracic trauma, inflammatory conditions, or certain medications may cause acquired VHD (99). For example, the diet medication phentermine (Fen-Phen) may cause heart valve disease as well as primary pulmonary hypertension and cardiac fibrosis. Structural alterations in valve fit can occur from deposition of calcium deposits on valve leaflets and the annulus or from ventricular dilation from HF or aortic dissection.

There are three main abnormalities that affect valve function: (a) stenosis prevents the valve from opening completely, (b) regurgitation or insufficiency prevents the valve from closing completely, or (c) mixed lesions that have elements of both stenosis and regurgitation. The most common valve disorders affect the left side of the heart because that is where the heart is most stressed from muscle mass and workload. Mitral stenosis, mitral regurgitation, mitral valve prolapse, aortic stenosis, and aortic regurgitation are the most common disorders observed; tricuspid valve disorders are common in intravenous drug abusers and patients with infective endocarditis (99).

Pathophysiology

Heart valves consist of an opening or annulus with two or three leaflets, which are attached to the papillary muscles by the chordae tendineae. When closed, the valve leaflets are approximated and no leakage of blood into the adjacent chamber occurs. The AV valves (tricuspid and mitral) open due to the pressure of the blood volume as it collects in the RA and LA. This pressure on the proximal side of the valve pops open the valve, allowing the atrial contents to empty into the respective ventricles. The semilunar valves (pulmonic and aortic) open due to the buildup of wall tension within the ventricle, also a function of blood volume and blood pressure, for muscle contraction leading to ejection of the stroke volume into the pulmonary artery or the aorta (86).

Stenotic valves do not open completely. The valve leaflets and chordae tendineae may become fused and thickened due to inflammatory conditions or calcium deposits. The fused leaflets cannot open, thus obstructing forward blood flow into the RV (tricuspid stenosis), pulmonary artery (pulmonic stenosis), LV (mitral stenosis), or aorta (aortic stenosis). Obstructed blood flow translates into decreased blood volume delivered, resulting in decreased stroke volume and CO. The obstruction to flow causes the chamber behind the stenotic valve to work harder (by increasing the wall tension or pressure) to deliver its blood volume—this pressure overload causes the heart muscle to compensate by increasing its muscle mass (myocyte hypertrophy). Hypertrophy of the cardiac muscle in the affected chamber may be evident on a CXR and/or ECG.

Regurgitant valves, also known as insufficient or incompetent valves, do not close completely. Again, the valve leaflets may be damaged by infection, inflammation, or dilation of the annulus from HF or another condition. Because the leaflets are not sealing tight, a quantity of blood volume will leak back into the chamber that delivered it during systole: from the RV into the RA (tricuspid regurgitation), pulmonary artery into the RV (pulmonic regurgitation), LV into the LA (mitral regurgitation), and aorta into the LV (aortic regurgitation). The addition of this extra blood volume to the volume collecting in the chamber for the next contraction results in a volume overload. The heart muscle compensates for the extra blood volume through chamber dilation. The chamber walls stretch and thin to accommodate the extra volume.

Mixed lesions—those that cause both obstruction to forward flow and regurgitation—are common, causing hypertrophied cardiac muscle and dilated chambers at the same time. Hypertrophy and dilation work well as compensatory responses to pressure and volume overloads, respectively, but only for a short time as eventually the muscle will be unable to compensate further and HF will be the result. The damaged valve will need surgical repair and/or replacement.

Mitral valve prolapse is a syndrome that normally affects young women aged 20 to 40 years old. It is typically a benign condition but can cause disturbing signs and symptoms. Table 9-30 outlines the etiology, epidemiology, pathophysiology, clinical manifestations, and diagnostic testing for the most common valvular heart disorders.

Clinical Presentation

The clinical signs and symptoms of VHD are those of RVF or LVF. Damaged right-sided heart valves will cause the RV and/or RA to hypertrophy and/or dilate. Signs of RVF affect the venous circulation: JVD, hepatosplenomegaly, peripheral edema, and elevated CVP may be seen. LVF signs and symptoms are dyspnea, cough, paroxysmal nocturnal dyspnea (PND), orthopnea, and pulmonary edema, and elevated pulmonary and LA pressures are manifestations of cardiac and pulmonary compromise. Additionally, aortic stenosis may cause LV hypertrophy, syncopal episodes due to inadequate flow to the brain via the right internal carotid artery from which the middle cerebral artery branches, and angina due to

TABLE 9–30 Etiology, Epidemiology, Pathophysiology, Clinical Manifestations, and Diagnostic Testing for Left-Sided Valvular Heart Disorders

VHD	Major Etiology	Epidemiology	Pathophysiology	Clinical Manifestations (S/S [signs and symptoms])	Diagnostic Tests
MITRAL STENOSIS					
	RHD	Women 60% to 75% 66% <45 years	Thickened fibrotic leaflets Shortened contracted chordae tendineae → obstructed forward flow = LV gets ↓ preload = ↓ SV, CO, BP = ↑ LAP = dilated, hypertrophied = ↑ PAP → pulmonary congestion → RVH → RVF	Mild MS: asymptomatic S/S pulmonary congestion first S/S RVF = late signs Afib common (notify MD if new)	CXR: LAE, prominent PA, RVH ECG: LAE, RVH

Continued

TABLE 9–30 Etiology, Epidemiology, Pathophysiology, Clinical Manifestations, and Diagnostic Testing for Left-Sided Valvular Heart Disorders—cont'd

VHD	Major Etiology	Epidemiology	Pathophysiology	Clinical Manifestations (S/S [signs and symptoms])	Diagnostic Tests
MITRAL REGURGITATION					
	RHD Papillary muscle dysfunction/ rupture IE Congenital	RHD W > M PMR: M > W	Backflow blood into LA during systole = increased LV preload during diastole LA and LV → dilate, hypertrophy → LVF = pulmonary congestion → RVF	Gradual progression, no S/S until LVF S/S LVF and ↓CO Anxiety Chest pain Palpitations Prominent S₃ S/S RVF = late signs Afib common in 75% of patients	CXR: cardiomegaly (LVH, LAE)
MITRAL VALVE PROLAPSE					
	Varied causes, usually benign but can progress to MR Marfan syndrome Congenital	5% to 10% of population Women 20–40 years	Enlarged valvular leaflets balloon into LA during systole	Most asymptomatic HR/BP usually WNL Exercise intolerance Atypical chest pain (sharp, left-sided) Ventricular or atrial dysrhythmias: dizziness, syncope, palpitations Late systolic murmur, mid-systolic click louder on inspiration.	
AORTIC STENOSIS					
	Congenital Atherosclerosis/calcifications >70 years RHD	80% male Biscupid aortic valve (<30 years) 50% patients 30–70 years	Forward flow obstructed into aorta = ↑ resistance to ejection = ↑ afterload = ↓ SV, CO	Signs of ↓ CO DOE, angina, syncope on exertion, narrowed pulse pressure, Prominent S₄	CXR: LVH, pulmonary congestion

TABLE 9-30 Etiology, Epidemiology, Pathophysiology, Clinical Manifestations, and Diagnostic Testing for Left-Sided Valvular Heart Disorders—cont'd

VHD	Major Etiology	Epidemiology	Pathophysiology	Clinical Manifestations (S/S [signs and symptoms])	Diagnostic Tests
AORTIC STENOSIS					
			↑ pressure = LVH → LVF, ↑ LAP → LAE →↑ PAP = pulmonary congestion → RVH and RVF	Late signs: marked fatigue, debilitation, peripheral cyanosis	
AORTIC REGURGITATION					
	IE Congenital HTN Marfan syndrome	75% men	Incomplete closure during diastole, dilated or deformed annulus → backflow into LV = ↑ preload to LV = LVH, LAE = LVF, pulmonary congestion → RVF	Asymptomatic for years S/S pulmonary congestion first DOE, PND, orthopnea, palpitations, nocturnal angina with diaphoresis Bounding pulse ("water hammer") Wide pulse pressure S/S RVF = late signs	CXR: LAE, LV dilation, pulmonary congestion

Afib, atrial fibrillation; BP, blood pressure; CO, cardiac output; CXR, chest x-ray; DOE, dyspnea on exertion; ECG, electrocardiogram; HR, heart rate; HTN, hypertension; LA, left atrial/atrium; LAE, left atrial enlargement; LAP, left atrial pressure; LV, left ventricle; LVF, left ventricular failure; M, men; MD, medical doctor; MS, mitral stenosis; PA, pulmonary artery; PAP, pulmonary artery pressure; PMR, papillary muscle rupture; PND, paroxysmal nocturnal dyspnea; RHD, rheumatic heart disease; RVF, right ventricular failure; RVH, right ventricular hypertrophy; SV, stroke volume; VHD, valvular heart disease; W, women; WNL, within normal limits.

From Shapiro S. Cardiac problems in critical care. In F. S. Bongard, and D. Y. Sue, Current Critical Care: Diagnosis and Treatment (2nd ed, pp. 503-534). New York: Lange Medical Books/McGraw-Hill; 2002 (91).

From Wiegand et al. 2008; Care of patients with acquired valvular disease. In D. K. Moser and B. Riegel (Eds.), Cardiac Nursing: A Companion to Braunwald's heart disease (pp. 1030-1051). St Louis, MO: Saunders. (99)

compromised blood flow to the coronary arteries during diastolic filling.

Heart murmurs are diagnostic indicators of turbulent blood flow through narrowed, obstructed, or abnormally functioning valves. Table 9-31 outlines the different murmurs of the valvular heart disorders and their diagnostic indications. Differentiation of heart murmurs is an advanced skill—but there are many resources available on the Internet and worldwide Web to assist clinicians in learning the sometimes subtle sounds of heart and valvular abnormalities.

Diagnosis

A CXR may show an enlarged heart silhouette or enlarged heart chambers from the hypertrophy and/or dilation, along with pulmonary edema (if left-sided valves

TABLE 9–31 Differentiation of Systolic and Diastolic Murmurs

Source and Type	Etiologies	Auscultation Site/Timing/ Stethoscope Bell or Diaphragm	Sounds and Pitch	Radiation
Systolic Murmurs **AORTIC STENOSIS**				
	Rheumatic fever Calcification Congenital valve malformation	Aortic area (2nd ICS, RSB) Midsystole Diaphragm	Medium pitch, harsh, grating sound; louder if patient lying flat, or squatting, crescendo-decrescendo	Neck, sternal border, upper back, right carotid
PULMONIC STENOSIS				
	Congenital valve malformation	Pulmonic area (2nd–3rd ICS, LSB) Midsystole Diaphragm	Medium pitch, harsh louder with patient supine	Left side of neck, shoulder
MITRAL REGURGITATION				
	Chronic rheumatic fever ABE MI or ischemia Papillary muscle rupture Annular dilation secondary to dilated LV MVP	Mitral area (5th ICS, LMCL) Holosystolic Diaphragm	High pitch, blowing, worse during expiration, and with patient supine or on left side	Left axilla, back
TRICUSPID REGURGITATION				
	Annular dilation 2nd to dilated RV IE (rare) IVDA	Tricuspid area (3rd (ICS, LSB) Holosystolic Diaphragm	Medium-high pitch, blowing, louder on inspiration and with patient supine	Right sternal border
Diastolic Murmurs **AORTIC REGURGITATION**				
	Rheumatic fever Congenital valve malformation IE Trauma Marfan syndrome Aortic stenosis (may be concurrent)	Aortic area (2nd-3rd ICS, RSB) Diaphragm	High pitch, blowing, louder with patient leaning forward and holding breath, decrescendo	Left or right sternal border, apex

TABLE 9-31 Differentiation of Systolic and Diastolic Murmurs—cont'd

Source and Type	Etiologies	Auscultation Site/Timing/ Stethoscope Bell or Diaphragm	Sounds and Pitch	Radiation
PULMONIC REGURGITATION				
	Congenital valve malformation PHTN IE (rare)	Pulmonic area (2nd ICS, LSB) Diaphragm	High pitch, blowing, louder with inspiration	Left lower sternal border, Apex
MITRAL STENOSIS				
	Rheumatic fever Congenital valve malformation (rare)	Mitral area (5th ICS, LMCL, apex) Bell	Murmur rare Low pitch, rumbling, increases with exercise, inspiration, and left lateral position Opening snap (early diastole, sharp, high pitch) best at apex Loud S_1	Usually does not radiate; may radiate to axilla
TRICUSPID STENOSIS				
	Rheumatic fever IVDA	Tricuspid area (4th ICS, LSB) Bell	Low pitch, rumbling, increases with inspiration Opening snap (early diastole, sharp, high pitch)	Apex, xiphoid

ABE, acute bacterial endocarditis; ICS, intercostal space; IE, infective endocarditis; IVDA, intravenous drug abuse; LMCL, left midclavicular line; LSB, left sternal border; LV, left ventricle; MI, myocardial infarction; MVP, mitral valve prolapse; PHTN, pulmonary hypertension; RSB, right sternal border; RV, right ventricle.

Sources: Wiegand et al. Care of patients with acquired valvular disease. In Moser DK, Riegel B, editors. Cardiac Nursing: A Companion to Braunwald's Heart Disease. St Louis, MO: Saunders; 2008:1030-1051 (99); Brashers VL. Alterations of cardiovascular function. In McCance KL, Huether SE, editors. Pathophysiology: The Biological Basis of Disease in Adults and Children. 6th edition. Maryland Heights, MD: Mosby; 2010:1142-1208; Guyton AC, Hall JE. Textbook of Medical Physiology. 11th edition. Philadelphia: Saunders; 2006.

involved). Insertion of a pulmonary artery catheter or cardiac catheterization will show increased pulmonary pressures. Echocardiography (2D/3D echo or transesophageal echocardiography [TEE]) is a standard method of evaluation of VHD. Echocardiography will be able to demonstrate abnormalities of the valve leaflets and cusps, degree of calcification and/or vegetation growth, dyskinesia, wall thickness, and cardiac pressures and function. Cardiac catheterization and coronary angiography may be performed as an adjunct.

Management

The APN will most likely see the patient with VHD hospitalized for exacerbations of pulmonary congestion or after valve interventional procedures or surgery. Interventional procedures are increasing in number and range from percutaneous balloon valvuloplasty (PTV) to open stenotic mitral and aortic valves. Surgical intervention for VHD includes valvuloplasty, annuloplasty, or valve replacement. It is preferable to repair the valve, if possible, rather than to replace it (100) as repair prevents the need for extensive surgery and lifetime medications with anticoagulants, and decreases complications. Newer minimally invasive approaches to valve replacement are being tested and offer alternatives to patients who might not be able to tolerate surgery. Transcatheter pulmonary and aortic valve replacement has been available since 2000 and 2002, respectively (101). The minimally invasive transapical approach can be used if femoral or iliac grafting is not an option. Clinical trials are under way with both of these new methods; early outcomes have been promising.

Care after Valve Surgery

Care of patients after valvular surgery is much like the care for a patient after any type of major cardiac surgery. One of the differences in VHD surgery from other cardiac surgeries is the patient's need for higher filling pressures postoperatively. The patient with VHD is used to higher volumes and pressures for cardiac contraction, so the patient's fluid status, monitored using the CVP or the pulmonary artery readings, is generally kept on the high side of normal. Continuous cardiac and blood pressure monitoring, as well as routine documentation of pulmonary artery pressure, mixed venous oxygen demand, and/or CO readings, can be used to assess the patient's response to surgery and collaborative interventions and to manage the postoperative medical regimen. Focused assessments of the cardiac and pulmonary systems are the standard of care. Regular neurologic checks are very important to assess for embolic complications from calcium or vegetative emboli that may have been dislodged by valvuloplasty (e.g., separation or excision of the fused leaflets). Strategies to decrease oxygen demand and increase oxygen supply will help the patient recover faster. Antibiotic therapy will be continued after the procedure.

Pharmacologic Therapy

Cardiac glycosides, diuretics, and prophylactic antibiotic coverage are part of ordinary care. Nitrates are used cautiously with aortic stenosis as this medication can further decrease preload and therefore CO. Vasodilators, such as nifedipine, are indicated for aortic stenosis and mitral stenosis because they decrease the regurgitant blood flow through, the stenotic opening. New-onset AF should be treated, and attempts to convert the rhythm back to sinus rhythm (SR) are encouraged. Patients with chronic AF, very common in mitral regurgitation in particular, should be on an anticoagulant to prevent clot formation and embolization. Complications from valvular interventional or surgical interventions include cardiac tamponade and hemorrhage.

Clinical Nurse Specialist Competencies and Spheres of Influence
Coaching/Teaching/Mentoring

The competency of Coaching/Teaching/Mentoring occurs in the Patient/Family Sphere, as well as in the Nursing/Other Disciplines Sphere. The patient with VHD needs a lot of teaching and support. Patient and family teaching is essential before and after invasive procedures. Preoperative teaching includes systematically describing the events the patient and family should expect before and after the procedure. Preoperative

routines, the actual surgery or procedure, equipment used, and all tubes placed should be explained. Exercises to prevent pneumonia and deep vein thrombosis should be taught and the patient should return the demonstration. These exercises include the use of an incentive spirometer for deep breathing and coughing every hour; regular turning, and/or early ambulation.

Nurses caring for VHD patients should be able to identify murmurs. CNSs should coach their staff to actively listen for murmurs and extra sounds during their assessments, noting the medical adage—"you only hear what you listen for" (89). Differentiating murmurs takes practice and there are many resources available, especially on the Internet, to hone one's listening and discerning skills.

PERIPHERAL VASCULAR DISEASE

Etiology

Peripheral vascular disease (PVD) is a collection of cardiovascular disorders that consist of diseases of the arterial and venous system, with the exception of the heart and brain. New terminology for arterial vascular diseases has been proposed because of the nonspecificity of current nomenclature (102). The label "peripheral vascular disease" is criticized as too vague as its meaning refers to diseases of the arteries, veins, and lymphatics, as well as vasospastic diseases (102). Peripheral venous diseases includes acute venous thrombosis (i.e., venous thromboembolism [VTE]) and chronic venous insufficiency (CVI). CVI resulting in leg ulcers and varicose veins is a chronic condition that is usually managed on an outpatient basis, although the patient with CVI may need to be hospitalized for surgical management of leg ulcers or amputation. While the same assessment parameters are used for peripheral artery disease (PAD) and CVI, the patient presentations will be different. Table 9-32 compares the findings for both PAD and peripheral venous disease. This section will cover PAD, as defined by Creager et al. (102) and Hirsh et al. (103), as well as selected peripheral venous diseases; aortic disease and VTE are covered in future sections of this chapter.

PERIPHERAL ARTERY DISEASE

"Peripheral artery disease (PAD) is recommended to describe disease that affects the lower- or upper-extremity arteries" (103, p. 2812). PAD is sometimes referred to as peripheral artery occlusive disease (PAOD); however PAOD does not include vasoreactive or aneurysmal disorders (103). The most common cause of PAD is atherosclerosis. As a primarily atherosclerotic process, the presence of PAD suggests other concomitant

TABLE 9–32 Comparison of Clinical Manifestations of Arterial and Venous Peripheral Vascular Disease

Assessment Parameter	Arterial Disease	Venous Disease
PAIN		
	Acute, sudden, severe	Acute: little or no pain, tenderness along inflamed vein Chronic: heaviness, fullness, muscle fatigue
PALLOR (SKIN COLOR)		
	Pallor or reactive hyperemia, dependent rubor	Reddish-brown (brawny), cyanotic when dependent, mottled skin
PULSES		
Intensity recorded: 0, absent; 1, diminished; 2, normal; 3, bounding	Diminished, weak, absent	Normal
POIKILOTHERMIA		
(Skin temperature = environment temperature)	Cool	Warm
SENSATION		
	Paresthesia, paralysis (poor prognostic sign) (denotes irreversible ischemia)	Normal
SKIN TEXTURE		
	Thick, shiny, dry	Stasis dermatitis, varicose or visible veins
SKIN BREAKDOWN (i.e., ULCER FORMATION)		
	Severely painful, ulcers form between toes, on upper foot over metatarsal heads, on bony prominences Ulcer appearance: "punched-out," well-demarcated edges, pale gray or necrotic base	Mildly painful—usually ankle area, pain relieved with elevation of leg
EDEMA		
	None or mild; usually unilateral	Unilateral or bilateral, usually foot to calf
BLOOD FLOW		
	Possibly bruit, blood pressure lower below the stenosis	Normal

Continued

TABLE 9–32 Comparison of Clinical Manifestations of Arterial and Venous Peripheral Vascular Disease

Assessment Parameter	Arterial Disease	Venous Disease
HAIR		
	Hair loss distal to occlusion	No hair loss
NAILS		
	Thick, brittle, opaque	Normal
SKELETAL MUSCLE		
	Possibly atrophy, restricted limb movement	Normal
IMPOTENCE		
	Possibly with aortofemoral occlusion	No association

Sources: Guyton and Hall, 2006 (86); Hirsch et al., 2006 (103); Kuznar, 2004 (104); Khan et al., 2006 (106); Norgren et al., 2007 (107).

atherosclerotic diseases and increases with age: PAD is present in 12% to 20% of persons older than 65 to 70 years (2, 104).

It is estimated that PAD affects 8 to 12 million people in the United States, although that number is considered to be low as it is believed that PAD is under-diagnosed because its signs and symptoms may not be immediately obvious and are often falsely identified as other disease processes (105). Patients with PAD have a 5-times greater risk of MI and 2- to 3-times the risk of stroke, but only about 20% of people with PAD are diagnosed and only 25% are receiving targeted treatment (2, 105).

Risk factors for PAD are analogous to those for CAD: smoking (smokers are 2 to 3 times more likely to develop PAD than CAD), presence of diabetes or impaired glucose tolerance (diabetics have a 4-fold increase in risk for the development of PAD), hypertension, obesity, sedentary lifestyle, dyslipidemia [including elevated lipoprotein(a)], elevated homocysteine and CRP, and age, male gender, postmenopausal women, and genetic predisposition (103, 104). The existence of these risk factors increases the risk of the development of PAD and subsequent complications by at least 2-fold; some factors increase the risk up to 10-fold, depending on gender, predisposition, and/or dose or degree (103). Recognized as a worldwide health problem, the costs associated with PAD extract a personal, social, and economic toll in the United States, Europe, South America, and Asia (103). Preventive strategies are foremost in the clinician's arsenal to decrease the complications associated with PAD.

Pathophysiology

The pathophysiology of PAD is systemic, includes a variety of pathophysiologic processes (atherosclerosis, degenerative diseases, dysplastic disorders, vascular inflammation [arteritis], thrombosis, and thromboembolism), and usually results in alterations of the structure and function of the vessel wall and obstruction to blood flow (103). The most common pathology is the process of atherosclerosis. Atherosclerotic plaques build up in the arteries, causing stenotic walls and occlusive lesions that block blood flow and deprive tissue of necessary nutrients. Plaques tend to form at the junctions or bifurcations of the arteries. When the velocity of blood flow increases across a stenotic lesion, claudication occurs. The rate of blood flow, degree of stenosis in the lesion, and number of obstructive lesions are the mechanisms responsible for the manifestations that present in PAD (106). The number one risk factor for PAD is also a risk factor for CAD: smoking. Smoking causes endothelial damage stimulating the inflammatory system and promoting coagulation. Plus, the nicotine in cigarette smoke is a vasoconstrictor, further decreasing blood flow in stenotic or atherosclerotic tissues.

Many patients with PAD are asymptomatic but still have occult disease. For example, patients who are normally sedentary may experience claudication during times of physical stress and activity—the sudden demand for blood flow to the lower extremities and the occlusive lesion blocking that blood flow leave the tissues starved for oxygen and ischemia occurs. Leg pain at rest is a PAD symptom that requires no physical exertion. Severe stenotic and occlusive disease of the lower extremities that results in little to no blood flow is labeled critical limb ischemia (CLI).

Clinical Presentation

Clinical signs and symptoms of PAD are a result of decreased blood flow and tissue perfusion to the muscles of the legs. Most people have symptoms, but 30% to 50% of people with PAD are asymptomatic (103). Significant problems with mobility and exertional discomfort that can severely affect the patient's quality of life are associated with PAD. Signs and symptoms include walking impairment, unilateral or bilateral intermittent claudication, ischemic rest pain, thin, shiny skin on legs and feet, hair loss on legs, dependent rubor, skin pallor with legs elevated, thickened toenails, cool skin, prolonged capillary refill, arterial ulcerations, nonhealing wounds, and decreased peripheral pulses. Pain may be reported in the buttock, thigh, calf, or foot. Hip, buttock, thigh pain, and even calf pain can be a result of occlusive disease in the iliac artery. The most likely cause of calf pain is due to disease in the femoral and popliteal arteries. Calf pain and foot pain and numbness may be signs of tibial artery occlusive disease, as well (103). Keep in mind that pain, including rest pain, may not be perceived by patients with peripheral neuropathies. PAD is classified according to stages or grades of severity. The most common systems, the Fontaine or Rutherford staging systems, are compared with the patient's clinical status in Table 9-33.

Intermittent Claudication

Vague leg symptoms are reported by 40% to 50% of patients (102, 103). Intermittent claudication, a sign of ischemic muscle, is the classic symptom, although not present in all persons with PAD. Roughly, 10% to 35% of patients report classic claudication symptoms (102, 103). Intermittent claudication refers to leg discomfort during activity that results from inadequate oxygen delivery to working muscles, as well as from the effects from the skeletal muscle (e.g., metabolic), neurologic, and inflammatory systems (103). As with angina (a similar pathophysiology), the leg pain and discomfort may subside with rest. Diabetics have an increased risk of claudication: 3.5 times the risk in men and 8.6 times the risk for women (48). Quality descriptors of claudication are described as aching, burning, heaviness, pain, cramping, and muscle fatigue. Box 9-5 provides differential diagnosis considerations for the symptoms of intermittent claudication. Clinical signs and symptoms with the greatest diagnostic accuracy per the LRs are listed in Table 9-34.

Critical Limb Ischemia

CLI presents in 1% to 2% of PAD patients and is an extensive, sometimes complete, obstruction of the leg arteries that result in little to no blood flow to the affected area. CLI is described as extremely painful, can cause ulcers or gangrenous lesions, and can lead to limb amputation due to tissue infarction (103-106). The pain profile of CLI is foot pain at rest, typically over the dorsum of the foot or in the toes, which may be relieved by placing the feet in a dependent position (106). Ischemic rest pain usually occurs at night when the patient is supine. The horizontal position naturally decreases blood pressure to the legs, causing decreased blood flow and inadequate tissue perfusion (103). Standing up increases blood flow to the feet via gravity and thus decreases the pain.

TABLE 9–33 Classification of Peripheral Arterial Disease: Comparison of Fontaine's Stages and Rutherford's Categories

Fontaine Stage	Rutherford Grade—Category	Clinical Status
I	0–0	Asymptomatic
IIa	I–1	Mild claudication
IIb		Moderate-severe claudication
	I–2	Moderate claudication
	I–3	Severe claudication
III	II–4	Ischemic rest pain
IV		Ulceration or gangrene
	III–5	Minor tissue loss
	IV–6	Ulceration or gangrene

Adapted from Hirsch et al. ACC/AHA 2005 practice guidelines for the management of patients with peripheral arterial disease (lower extremity, renal, mesenteric, and abdominal aortic): a collaborative report from the American Association for Vascular Surgery/Society for Vascular Surgery, Society for Cardiovascular Angiography and Interventions, Society for Vascular Medicine and Biology, Society of Interventional Radiology, and the ACC/AHA Task Force on Practice Guidelines (Writing Committee to Develop Guidelines for the Management of Patients With Peripheral Arterial Disease). Circulation 2006;113(11):e463-e654. doi:10.1161/circulationaha.106.174526 (103).

BOX 9–5 Differential Diagnosis of Intermittent Claudication

- Intermittent claudication: calf, thigh and buttock, foot
- Nerve root compression
- Spinal stenosis
- Inflammatory process
- Foot/ankle arthritis
- Hip arthritis
- Baker's cyst
- Venous claudication
- Chronic compartment syndrome

From Hirsch et al., 2006 (103).

Treatment options for CLI are revascularization, medical therapy, or limb amputation (107). Morbidity and mortality are significant with this complication—30% to 40% of patients will have a limb amputation within the year and 20% to 25% will die (105, 109).

Differential diagnoses to consider include vascular, neurologic, musculoskeletal, and inflammatory conditions such as deep venous thrombosis (DVT), phlebitic syndrome, sciatica, myositis, lumbar intervertebral disc disorder, peripheral neuropathy, restless leg syndrome, muscle/ligament/tendon strain, lumbar spinal stenosis, osteoarthritis, arteritis, thromboangitis obliterans (Buerger disease), and connective tissue disease (104, 106).

Diagnosis

Testing for PAD begins with a comprehensive medical history and physical exam. Diagnostic tests to confirm the diagnosis consist of the ankle-brachial index (ABI), duplex ultrasound, X-ray angiography, and megnetic resonance angiography (MRA). Figure 9-9 provides an algorithm for the diagnosis of PAD (103, 104, 107).

Ankle-Brachial Index

The gold standard for diagnosing PAD and evaluating the severity of the disease is the ABI, also known as the ankle-arm index (AAI), which is a simple, accurate (sensitivity 95%; specificity 99%), noninvasive tool to assess the presence of decreased blood flow. The ABI is calculated from the blood pressure measurements of the arms (brachial artery) and ankles (both posterior tibial and dorsalis pedis arteries are assessed). Brachial blood pressure may be measured using any method (auscultation with a stethoscope, oscillometric, or a hand-held Doppler ultrasound probe), but the same method should be used by all caregivers for consistency and comparability between the measurements (106). Vascular laboratories normally use the Doppler method to record all values. Besides use as a screening measurement, ABIs are also documented as part of routine postoperative care monitoring after peripheral bypass procedures (aortofemoral, aortoiliac, femoropopliteal, femorotibial, etc.) to assess graft patency.

In an unobstructed system, blood pressure is expected to be the same, if not slightly higher, in the feet than in the arms. The highest systolic blood pressure in the ankle arteries is divided by the highest systolic blood pressure of the arms. Each side is a separate measurement. The results are documented. Normal values range from 0.91 to 1.30. Values below 0.90 indicate decreased blood flow and PAD. An ABI between 0.71 and 0.90 is reflective of mild PAD; 0.41 to 0.70 is moderate PAD, and values below 0.40 indicate severe PAD. Rest pain is seen at ABIs of less than 0.50, and ischemia and gangrene at ABIs of less than 0.20 (108). Patients with questionable or borderline results may be asked to perform a treadmill test (or exercise ABI) to try to

---

TABLE 9–34 Positive Likelihood Ratios of Common Signs of Peripheral Artery Disease (PAD)

PAD Signs	Positive Likelihood Ratio (LR+) (95% Confidence Interval)
Claudication	LR, 3.30 (2.30–4.80)
Femoral bruit	LR, 4.80 (95% CI, 2.40–9.50)
Any pulse abnormality	LR, 3.10 (95% CI, 1.40–6.60)
Cool skin	LR, 5.90 (95% CI, 4.10–8.60)
At least 1 bruit	LR, 5.60 (95% CI, 4.70–6.70)
Any palpable pulse abnormality	LR, 4.70 (95% CI, 2.20–9.90)
Absence of any bruits (iliac, femoral, or popliteal)	LR, 0.39 (95% CI, 0.34–0.45)
Pulse abnormality	LR, 0.38 (95% CI, 0.23–0.64)

From Khan et al. Does the clinical examination predict lower extremity peripheral arterial disease? JAMA 2006;295(5):536-546 (106).

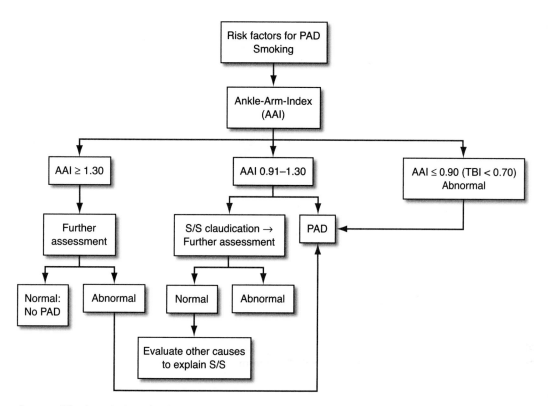

Sources: Hirsch et al., 2006 (103); Kuznar, 2004 (104); Norgren et al., 2007 (107)

FIGURE 9–9: Algorithm for the diagnosis of peripheral arterial disease.

provoke symptoms of claudication and get a better idea of the severity of the disease. Figure 9-10 presents the ABI procedure.

ABIs over 130 are found in diabetic patients, patients with chronic renal failure, and the very old. High values for the ABI indicate arteries that may be calcified and therefore noncompressible leading to falsely high systolic pressures (106). ABI results are not reliable in these patient populations, and alternative measures should be used (103, 105). A toe-brachial index (TBI) (using special toe cuffs), segmental limb pressure measurements, segmental plethysmography (pulse volume recording), waveform analysis, or selected imaging procedures are alternatives to ABI.

Other Diagnostic Testing

Arteries in the toes will reflect a truer blood pressure in high-risk patient populations (very old, chronic renal failure patients, diabetics) because calcification is not likely in those distal vessels (109). A normal toe pressure is 30 mm Hg less than the pressure in the ankle; therefore an abnormal TBI is less than 0.70 (107). Segmental limb pressures (SLPs) are valuable to detect arterial lesions and to identify the location of the lesions. The approximate site of the arterial lesion is identified by the differences in blood pressure below

the level of the lesion (107). Blood pressure gradients of 20 mm Hg or more indicate an arterial lesion (109). Segmental plethysmography produces a pulse volume recording (PVR) that can detect blood volume changes in the limbs. The combined use of SLP and PVR measurements increases diagnostic accuracy to 95% (107).

Doppler velocity waveform analysis evaluates the contours of the arterial waveform. In PAD, the normal triphasic waveform progressively disappears and the initial wave becomes flat (109). Thus in patients with PAD, the triphasic pattern is altered to a biphasic pattern and, finally, to a monophasic form as the disease progresses (107).

Imaging procedures are performed to assist with diagnosis but also to identify the location and extent of the lesion(s) for revascularization. Imaging and revascularization are routine for patients with CLI who are candidates for interventional or surgical procedures. Angiography is the current reference standard but is invasive and expensive and incurs a high risk of complications. Multidetector CT angiography (CTA) is considered to have a moderate risk for complications. This machine presents rapid imaging and "3D" pictures from the axial images. MRA of PAD patients is becoming the "preferred" imaging procedure (107). Rapid 3D high-resolution imaging, less artifact, and

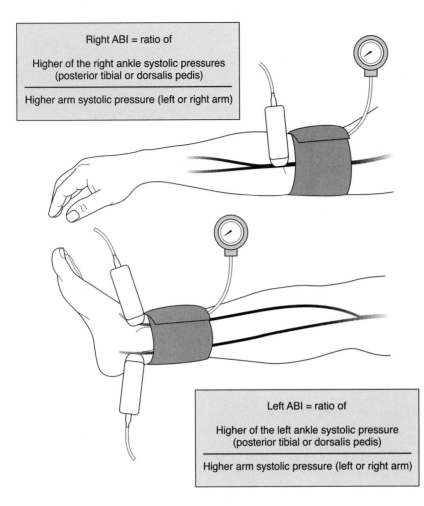

Right ABI = ratio of

Higher of the right ankle systolic pressures
(posterior tibial or dorsalis pedis)

Higher arm systolic pressure (left or right arm)

Left ABI = ratio of

Higher of the left ankle systolic pressure
(posterior tibial or dorsalis pedis)

Higher arm systolic pressure (left or right arm)

FIGURE 9-10: Procedure for obtaining an ankle-brachial index.

its safety profile are among the advantages of this technique; the high-magnetic field produced during the procedure is a contraindication for many patients with implanted metal clips and devices. Contrast-enhanced MRA has a sensitivity and specificity of greater than 93% in the diagnosis of PAD (107); the range of sensitivity and specificity for the multidetector CTA for PAD is calculated at 89% to 99% and 83% to 100%, respectively (102). Duplex ultrasonography assists the provider to evaluate the integrity of the arterial vessels and the quality of blood flow noninvasively and at a much lower cost than the other modalities (107).

Management
Assessment and Risk Stratification
Patient goals for PAD include symptom relief, prevention of complications, risk factor modification, and maintenance or improvement of functional capacity (105). Initial management of patients with PAD begins with good assessment skills. The "6Ps" mnemonic is useful to remember signs of acute limb ischemia, in order of increasing disease severity: leg or foot **P**ain, extremity **P**allor, **P**ulselessness, **P**oikilothermia (cool, cold skin), **P**aresthesia, and **P**aralysis. Assess the color, movement, sensation, and temperature of

the extremity—are the findings normal or abnormal? Bilateral or unilateral? The lack of hair, atrophic skin changes, and thickened nails are common signs of the lack of arterial blood flow. Check the pulses in the extremities—Are they palpable or do you need a Doppler to locate them? For upper extremity PAD, check the patency of the palmar arch with the Allen test. What is the ABI of each leg?

Pallor on elevation and dependent rubor can be assessed by changing the position of the legs. With the patient in a supine position, elevate the limb 30 to 40 degrees above the bed—the ischemic limb will become pale. To assess for dependent rubor, let the patient's legs dangle over the bed and observe for a reddish-blue-purplish color to the ischemic limb. Stenotic lesions create blood turbulence, so assess for bruits over the major arteries. Poor capillary refill is not a strong diagnostic sign in PAD (LR, 1.90; 95% CI, 1.20 to 3.20) (106). Be sure to document all findings. Refer to Table 9-32 for assessment parameters for PAD.

Risk Factor Modification
A variety of tools exist for the stratification of risk and documentation of clinical manifestations (110). The Walking Impairment Questionnaire is an easy-to-administer,

validated tool to assess functional disability in patients with PAD. The domains assessed on the tool are walking distance, walking speed, and stair climbing, with additional questions related to PAD and other causes of walking impairment. The San Diego Claudication questionnaire (SDCQ) and the Rose Claudication questionnaires are also used in PAD research and clinical practice. These tools assess leg symptoms in people suspected of having PAD. For example, the SDCQ classifies PAD patients as having (a) no leg symptoms, (b) atypical leg symptoms, or (c) typical symptoms of intermittent claudication (110).

People diagnosed with PAD are treated with interventions to reduce the progression of atherosclerosis. Risk factor modification can have dramatic effects on patient well-being and possibly reverse the progression of the disease. Lifestyle modifications, medications, or combinations of both are recommended interventions for PAD and identified as class I (considered beneficial, useful, and effective) in the most current PAD clinical guidelines (103). Counseling for changes to one's lifestyle includes smoking cessation, increasing physical activity, control of diabetes and blood pressure, and diet modifications (low saturated fat, low cholesterol). If lifestyle modifications are not sufficient to manage and reduce symptoms, interventional therapies, such as angioplasty or surgical interventions, may be necessary (111).

Smoking causes inflammation of the arteries, damaging endothelium from the chronic inflammatory process, thus promoting plaque formation and the development of occlusive lesions. Smokers have 3 times to as much as 8 times the risk of PAD than do nonsmokers. Therefore, a plan for smoking cessation has the highest priority in the hierarchy of lifestyle management strategies (103).

Increasing physical exercise has beneficial effects on weight loss, body image, blood pressure, cholesterol levels, diabetes, claudication symptoms, and mood. Exercise, such as walking, can be initiated and then gradually increased in duration and difficulty as the patient tolerates longer exercise periods without symptoms. Evidence-based exercise guidelines for patients with claudication include 5 to 10 minutes for warm-up and cool-down exercises and a treadmill or track walking regimen of 3 to 5 times per week at an intensity to induce symptoms of claudication within 3 to 5 minutes; resting briefly between symptom bouts; and repeating the process (112). Patients should be encouraged to begin with 35 minutes of exercise and gradually increase exercise duration to 50 minutes per workout (112). A formal referral to a claudication exercise rehabilitation program and follow-up are recommended (103). In addition to exercise, nutrition counseling with a registered dietitian is important for tailoring a food plan low in saturated fat, cholesterol, and sodium acceptable to the patient.

Pharmacologic Therapy

Drug therapy includes antiplatelet medications to reduce the risk of clot formation from impaired blood flow or occlusive disease, and drugs like cilostazol (100 to 200 mg twice daily) and pentoxifylline (400 mg three times daily) are used to improve symptoms and increase walking distance (103), as well as cholesterol-lowering agents (i.e., statins). The TASC II group (Trans-Atlantic Inter-Society Consensus Document on Management of Peripheral Arterial Disease) recommended antiplatelet drugs be started before revascularization, maintained as therapy post interventional or surgical procedures, and continued for an indefinite period (Recommendation 41) (107). ASA (81 to 325 mg per day) and thienopyridines (ticlopidine, clopidogrel) may be prescribed; combinations of ASA and a thienopyridine are more effective than ASA therapy alone. The dosage of ticlodipine is 250 mg twice daily and clopidogrel dosage is 75 mg once a day (109).

Cilostazol, a phosphodiesterase III inhibitor, improves symptoms because of its vasodilator, metabolic, and antiplatelet effects. Headache, diarrhea, and palpitations are listed as side effects. A meta-analysis demonstrated the positive effects of cilostazol over pentoxifylline in terms of peak treadmill performance, quality of life, and safety (107). Naftidrofuryl (not available in the United States) and L-carnitine and propionyl-L-carnitine have been shown to improve walking distances, decrease symptoms, and improve quality of life in patients with PAD. Pentoxifylline decreases blood viscosity and, although still widely used, has not been shown to have any significant clinical utility (107). Additionally, antithrombotic agents, vasodilators, and prostaglandins, among others, have not shown clinical efficacy in the treatment of intermittent claudication and in some cases showed harm. New drug treatments with angiogenic growth factors, such as vascular endothelial growth factor (VEGF) and basic fibroblast growth factor (bFGF), are being studied for the treatment of claudication (107).

Management of Comorbidities

Control of chronic diseases such as diabetes, dyslipidemia, and hypertension is obtained with medications and provider follow-up, along with the lifestyle interventions already discussed. The coexistence of diabetes, hypertension, and dyslipidemia increases the risk of PAD 6 times. Keeping glycosylated hemoglobin level (HgA1c) below 7% is recommended in diabetic patients, controlling blood pressure to below hypertensive parameters, and monitoring and treating high lipid levels also are important. For diabetics, the risk of PAD increases with rises in the HgA1c level: for every 1% rise in HgA1c, the risk for PAD increases by 28% (113). Hypertension alone increases the PAD risk in men 2½ times; the PAD risk in women is almost 4 times higher than in women without hypertension. Glucose modulators, HMG-coreductase inhibitors (statins), fibrates, beta- and calcium channel blockers, and other drugs are used to manage these three chronic disease states.

Interventional and Surgical Therapies

In patients with disseminated or complex disease, invasive measures may be undertaken. Angiography, angioplasty, and atherectomy assist with the diagnosis and management of PAD. Percutaneous transluminal angioplasty (PTA) and vascular stenting are used to open blocked arteries with localized, discrete lesions. The patient is given a mild sedative, the procedure is conducted and completed, and in many cases, the patient is brought to the PACU and assessed for discharge after recovery from the procedure. If interventional techniques are not possible due to location of the lesion, diffuse disease, or patient contraindications, surgical interventions are considered. Peripheral artery or vascular bypass with or without graft placement or ischemic ulcer repair or amputation, if the tissue is gangrenous, may save the patient's life. New surgical procedures are focused on developing minimally invasive surgery, such as minimally invasive arterial reconstructions (107). Average economic costs of the various procedures was calculated as PTA, $10,000 ($20,000 if the procedure fails initially or later), peripheral bypass grafting, $20,000 ($40,000 if revision is required), and limb amputation, $40,000. The addition of rehabilitation for postprocedure care usually doubles the costs (107).

Postoperative care of the patient after surgical intervention includes monitoring vital signs and neurovascular status, including sensation, movement, and perfusion of the feet; assessing the operative site and dressings for bleeding; checking and documenting peripheral pulses and an ABI on the operative site; administering anticoagulants; managing pain; encouraging early ambulation; and providing education for the patient and family. Once the surgical bandage is removed, evaluate the incision for redness, swelling, or drainage. A small amount of numbness surrounding the incision site is normal and results from the ligation of multiple small nerves in the skin. Pain medications are usually needed within the first 48 to 72 hours after surgery. A patient-controlled analgesia (PCA) pump and narcotics are typical pain management orders.

Clinical Nurse Specialist Competencies and Spheres of Influence

The ACC/AHA 2005 practice guidelines for the management of patients with peripheral arterial disease are available on the AHA Web site (www.myamericanheart.org) (103). This and other helpful resources (e.g., 100, 107, 112) provide the CNS with the evidence for translation into practice.

Coaching/Teaching/Mentoring and Research/Evidence-Based Practice

Facilitating the learning of patients (Patient/Family Sphere) and staff (Nursing/Other Disciplines Sphere) are at the heart of the core competencies for CNSs caring for PAD patients. CNSs providing preventive health teaching, either one-on-one or in the community, can provide evidence-based information for patients to manage their PAD symptoms and decrease their health risks for the development of other atherosclerotic disease processes. The CNS has the skills to translate evidence into manageable pieces of information that patients can understand. Resources for the CNS include materials available from The Peripheral Artery Disease Coalition. A series of patient education materials are readily accessible and will be helpful to the busy clinician. Other resources include patient management guidelines, slide sets, clinical tools, and professional education resources (www.padcoalition.org).

ABI testing after peripheral vascular surgery is easy to perform and supplies important information about the patency of the vascular graft. CNSs teach staff how to perform ABI testing, identify critical values related to graft patency, and audit future performance for accuracy and consistency.

Collaboration

Another competency applicable to care of the PAD patient is collaboration and is mainly accomplished through the System/Organization Sphere of Influence. The CNS communicates important information and collaborates with the interprofessional team to provide safe, evidence-based care. The CNS formally refers patients to a claudication exercise rehabilitation program that may be managed by APNs and/or physical therapists and encourages follow-up as needed.

VENOUS THROMBOEMBOLIC EVENTS

Etiology

VTE is a collective term for DVT and pulmonary embolism (PE), events that are very common in the acute and critical care setting. Ninety percent of pulmonary emboli originate from DVT. VTE is a preventable event in most circumstances; trauma and critical-care patients are at particular risk of developing VTE because of multiple risk factors and should be screened upon admission to assess their risk. Staff nurses and CNSs have a responsibility to keep the number of venous thromboembolic events to a minimum through identification of patients at risk, institution of preventive interventions, constant vigilance in monitoring for early event onset, and aggressive collaborative treatment when the event occurs.

According to the literature, first time VTE rates range from 71 to 117 cases per 100,000, with 75% of VTE cases occurring in medical patients (114). Each year over 250,000 patients are diagnosed and treated for VTE, but the majority of cases are diagnosed on autopsy (115). About 50,000 to 200,000 people die from VTE each year in the United States (116) and the treatment cost is estimated at $1.5 billion (21). The incidence of VTE in general is 0.1 to 0.2 per 100 person-years; this incidence is increased in the presence of strong hereditary risk factors coupled with additional thrombophilic deficiencies or defects to 2.64 per 100 person-years (117). One-quarter to almost one-half of all people with VTE have at least one inherited risk factor (116). The most common inherited coagulation disorders are AT deficiency, protein C and protein S deficiencies, factor V Leiden mutation, hyperhomocyteinemia, prothrombin gene mutation, and elevated factor VIII (116).

Deep Vein Thrombosis

DVT occurs frequently in hospitalized patients and is considered a hazard of immobility, age greater than 60 years, acute illness, and venipunctures (114). Over 2 million people will develop a DVT each year. It is estimated that patients hospitalized for general surgery and acute or chronic medical conditions have a risk of DVT of 10% to 40%; orthopedic surgery incurs a higher risk of 40% to 60%; major trauma and spinal cord injury patients have an absolute risk ranging from 40% to 80%; and critical care patients have an absolute risk of 10% to 80% (118). The exact incidence of DVT is unknown because the signs and symptoms are usually nonspecific and therefore pinpointing the diagnosis can be difficult. Elderly patients double their risk of DVT with each decade of life; 80-year-olds have a 100-fold risk of developing DVT compared with patients younger than 40 years (114). As with most predictive factors, patients with multiple risk factors are at higher risk of developing DVT than those with just one risk factor.

Pulmonary Embolism

PE is caused by a thrombus or thrombi that dislodge from their point of origin, travel through the bloodstream (i.e., embolize), and settle in the pulmonary artery or its segmental branches. Emboli can travel from other parts of the body and frequently come from the deep veins of the pelvis or lower extremities (DVT). Blood clots may also form and travel from upper extremity veins, from blood pooling in the RA or RV, or from a central venous catheter end tip (119). A saddle embolus is a large embolus that obstructs the main pulmonary artery at the bifurcation of the right and left pulmonary artery trunks. PE not caused by blood clots may form from air, fat, or amniotic fluid. The rate of fatal PE is 26% to 30% (115, 120).

The risk factors related to VTE include genetic predisposition (including inherited coagulation disorders), inflammation or infection, and acquired or exogenous causes. The majority of hospitalized patients have one or more risk factors for VTE—and there is a direct relationship between the number of risk factors and the rate of VTE (118). PE accounts for 10% of all hospital deaths (118). Trauma patients are especially vulnerable to the development of VTE and possibly fatal PE. Studies have

shown that spinal cord injury, lower extremity or pelvic fracture, the need for a surgical procedure, increasing age, femoral venous line insertion or major venous repair, prolonged immobility, and longer duration of hospital stay are independent risk factors for VTE (118). A table of factors that predispose to VTE is found in Table 9-35.

Strong hereditary risk factors are deficiencies of protein S, protein C, or AT factor, but the occurrence of these deficiencies is rare (117). Other hereditary risk factors have a milder effect on risk, independently and include the presence of factor V Leiden or the prothrombin *G20210A* mutation or high levels of coagulant factors VIII, IX, and XI; hyperhomocysteinemia; and antiphospholipid antibodies (117). People with type I hereditary AT deficiency (HD) have a high risk of VTE, probably prompted by events or procedures that are already considered high risk for VTE, such as pregnancy, surgery, immobilization, etc. Half of HD type I patients between 10 and 35 years of age will suffer at least one thrombotic episode (121).

Brouwer et al. conducted a retrospective family cohort study (N = 468) and demonstrated that the risk for VTE increases with the number of thrombophilic hereditary defects and the number of exogenous risks (117). Relatives of family members who had had a venous thromboembolic event, and who had deficiencies of protein S, protein C, or AT, were tested to determine the presence of thrombophilic deficiencies or defects. Those individuals with protein S and protein C deficiencies were 16 times more likely to develop a VTE (protein S: RR 16.2, 95% CI, 6.1 to 43.4; protein C: RR 16.2, 95% CI, 6.4 to 41.2) and persons with AT deficiency were 18 times more likely to develop a VTE than persons without these inherited deficiencies (RR 18.4, CI, 6.7 to 50.1) (117). As the number of deficiencies increased and/or the combination of deficiencies included these stronger risk factors, the risk for VTE increased as well. Individuals with two or more additional deficiencies or thrombophilic defects (without concurrent protein S, protein C, or AT deficiencies) had a relative risk of 10.4 (95% CI, 1.1 to 99.1); individuals who had protein S or C or AT deficiency plus two or more additional thrombophilic disorders had a relative risk of almost 103 (95% CI, 12.5 to 843.4) (117). Because there was not a large number of adverse events in this study, the confidence intervals are extremely wide, as would be expected.

Pathophysiology

Thrombosis is the process of clot formation, and an embolus is a blood clot that travels from its site of origin. The most frequent site of clot formation is in the deep veins of the legs. DVT from thrombosis in the upper extremities also has been diagnosed. Risk factors include the presence of central venous catheters, thrombophilic states, and previous leg DVT. Thirty-six percent of patients with upper extremity thrombosis are diagnosed with PE (122). About

TABLE 9–35 Predisposing Factors for Venous Thromboembolism (VTE)

Risk Factors	*Disease Factors*
• Age (>60 years) • Cigarette smoking (including passive smoke inhalation) • Family history of VTE • Use of estrogens (treatment for menopausal symptoms, contraception [highest risk among women >35 or who smoke], or use of estrogen receptor modulators) • Immobility • Paralysis • Decreased mobility • Prolonged bedrest or illnesses that lead to decreased activity • Prolonged surgery • Phlebotomy • Recent trauma • Major surgery within the past 3 months • Chemotherapy or other IV irritating substances • Pregnancy or the period after delivery • Varicose veins • Airplane travel • IV drug abuse	• Acute medical illness • Sickle cell disease • Blood clotting disorder/hypercoagulable state • Hyperviscosity • Obesity (controversial) • Trauma/injury to the pelvis, hip, or leg • Indwelling peripheral and central venous catheters • Heart failure • Nephrotic syndrome • Sickle cell anemia • Myeloproliferative disease (e.g., polycythemia vera or essential thrombocytosis) • COPD • Stroke • Inflammation • Infection • Cancer • Diabetes • Hypertension • Atrial fibrillation • Heparin-induced thrombocytopenia • Antiphospholipid antibody syndrome • Previous deep vein thrombosis or pulmonary embolism

80% of symptomatic patients with confirmed DVT have DVT in the popliteal, femoral, or iliac proximal veins; 20% have DVT restricted to the calf veins (distal DVT) (123). The differentiation of proximal versus calf vein DVT is important because proximal DVT is associated with a higher occurrence of PE (and therefore should be treated immediately), while PEs are rarely seen in conjunction with isolated calf vein thrombosis (123). However, extension of thrombi into the proximal veins occurs with 10% to 20% of calf vein thrombi (118). Chronic DVT (longer than 2 weeks) is less likely to embolize because the thrombi have adhered to the vessel wall in that timeframe (122). A complication of distal vein DVT in particular, the thrombus adhering to the vessel wall can cause permanent impairment of blood flow and may result in limb pain and discomfort, dermatitis, leg ulcers, and chronic leg edema for the rest of the patient's life, a condition labeled postthrombotic syndrome (124). Postthrombotic syndrome is costly both in terms of its effects on quality of life and the direct and indirect expenses of this chronic medical problem. A DVT reoccurrence rate of 20% has been observed in these patients (124).

Risk Factors for VTE

The development of VTE is a function of impaired venous blood flow (venous stasis), loss of integrity or damage of the endothelial vessel wall (venous injury), and an imbalance of blood components toward a procoagulant state. The presence of any of these three components can cause a thrombus to form and embolize. The combination of these three components is known as Virchow's triad, and any or all of these mechanisms are common in hospitalized patients.

Patients who are immobile, paralyzed, or confined to bedrest or who stay in bed voluntarily (due to pain, intravenous equipment, drainage tubes, etc.) are at risk for blood pooling in the vessels causing venous blood flow to decrease or stop; blood that pools is likely to clot. The problem lies with a foot and calf-muscle pump that cannot function properly as a result of activity restrictions. The foot pump and the calf-muscle pump allow for the propelling of blood in the lower extremities to the inferior vena cava and then on to the right side of the heart. This delivery of blood volume occurs by the mechanical action of pressure on the plantar arch (i.e., weight-bearing or stretching), thus flattening the plantar artery, forcing venous blood into the saphenous veins, and emptying the venous sinuses. The venous system of the entire foot is emptied when pressure is placed on the heel of the foot and the metatarsal heads (125). Immobility or sitting for long periods of time, especially in confined spaces such as during international air flights, may predispose to venous compression and sluggish blood flow.

Air Travel as a Risk Factor

Up to one-quarter of patients presenting with signs and symptoms of VTE have a history of recent air travel (118). Studies comparing the relationship of air travel with VTE events have reported mixed results, although prolonged flights lasting 6 to 10 hours or longer have been associated with an increased risk of VTE (118). Causative factors for VTE during air travel may be related to the effects of immobilization or due to dehydration and the maintenance of high-altitude cabin pressures (118). Preventing venous compression by wearing loose clothing, performing simple leg exercises to stretch the calf muscles, and suggestions to "get up and move about the cabin" periodically may help to decrease travel-related VTE risk.

The WRIGHT Project (**WHO** **R**esearch **I**nto **G**lobal **H**azards of **T**ravel), sponsored by the World Health Organization, was started in 2001 to review epidemiologic, clinical, and physiologic evidence on the relationship between air travel and VTE and to conduct research in this area (126). The evidence from the phase one summary supported the relationship between "prolonged seat immobility" and a risk of VTE twice that of normal for flights longer than 4 hours in duration. "The risk increases with the duration of the travel and with multiple flights within a short period . . . [and] in the presence of other known risk factors of VTE. The risk factors identified as contributors to the increased risk of travel-related VTE were obesity, extremes of height, use of oral contraceptives and the presence of prothrombotic blood abnormalities" (126, p. 1).

VESSEL WALL INJURY

Vessel wall injury stimulates the inflammatory system to dispatch immune cells to repair the injury, causing a variety of proinflammatory cytokines to be expressed. The coagulation cascade is activated during inflammation, and thus clots are formed to protect the injured area. Vessel injury can occur due to intravenous catheter insertion, intravenous therapy solutions, surgery, or routine venipunctures (e.g., phlebotomy) (117). Cigarette smoking also causes chronic inflammatory damage to the vessels.

Hypercoagulable States

Hypercoagulable states are caused by physiologic, pathophysiologic, acquired, and genetic factors. Pregnancy is a risk because there is a physiologic increase in coagulation factors and a concomitant decrease in fibrinolytic activity (121). Dehydration causes the blood to become concentrated. Pathophysiologic causes are related to disturbances in clotting functions secondary to inflammatory or infectious causes. Acquired or environmental/exogenous causes are related to traumatic or iatrogenic vein injury, obesity, cigarette smoking, and air travel ("economy-class syndrome") (118). Acquired thrombophilic disorders result from surgery or disease processes that increase blood coagulation. Genetic predisposition leads to hypercoagulable conditions.

Inherited Disorders

Inheritance of thrombophilic disorders such as those listed above affect the clotting system by either stimulating or supporting coagulation or inhibiting fibrinolysis. A brief discussion of the hereditary defects known to be strong risk factors of VTE: proteins S and C and AT, follows, as well as an overview of some inherited coagulation defects that have a fairly high incidence in VTE.

Protein C, protein S, and AT are natural anticoagulants. Protein C and protein S are vitamin K–dependent glycoproteins that either degrade (protein C) or inactivate (protein S) coagulation factors. Protein S works together with protein C to inhibit thrombosis. The inability of these proteins to function appropriately results in an accumulation of coagulation factors and therefore increased thrombosis. Both protein C and S deficiencies are autosomal dominant traits and carriers of homozygous genes resulting in a higher risk of VTE. Protein C and S deficiencies are rare with general population risks ranging from 0.2% to 0.3% for protein C and 1% to 2% for protein S (116). Multiple types of protein C and S deficiencies have been identified.

Antithrombin (AT) is a serine protease inhibitor (serpin) with a wide range of inhibitory activity and, as such, is major factor in blood coagulation (121). Antithrombin is also known as AT III (ATIII). Anticoagulation is accomplished when AT attaches to thrombin, inactivating it, as well as inactivating factors IXa, Xa, XIa, XIIa, and VIIa bound to tissue factor (116). In general, AT deficiency results in an increase in the risk of thrombosis 20 times higher than that of the general population (116).

HD is expressed in an autosomal dominant inheritance pattern and affected people usually are heterozygous for this gene. There are several types of HD: type I denotes a quantitative deficiency—there are low circulating levels of AT and AT antigen to about 50% of normal (prevalence 0.04% to 0.05%), and type II shows a decrease in functional AT, but AT antigen levels are normal—a qualitative deficiency; a variant protein supplies half of AT (121). Type III shows normal AT function and AT antigen; however, the interface between AT and heparin is impaired. Type II HD is more common but carries less risk of VTE; people with homozygous genes for type III HD are at very high risk for thrombosis (116). Type I HD patients have a high prevalence of spontaneous thromboembolic events (42%) and a risk 50-times greater than non-HD patients for the development of VTE associated with surgery, pregnancy, delivery, trauma, and/or use of oral contraceptives (121).

Factor V Leiden mutation (FVLM) is associated with resistance to activated protein C and is the inherited coagulation defect most frequently associated with VTE (116). FVLM is seen in about 5% of the population, with Caucasians the most affected race; FVLM is not common in African or Asian populations (116). People with homozygous FVLM genes are the most susceptible to VTE, especially in the presence of triggering events, often experiencing their first venous thromboembolic event before 40 years of age; they carry a lifetime risk of VTE 80 times the risk of the unaffected population (116).

Homocysteine

High levels of homocysteine (greater than 15 mmol/L) are known to be risk factors for CAD, stroke, and PVD (127). Homocysteine is a protein and, when present in high levels, is postulated to damage the endothelial lining of the blood vessel. Diet and genetic factors are strongly associated with high homocysteine levels. Diets deficient in folate and vitamins B_6 and B_{12} will lead to abnormally high homocysteine levels because these components break down homocysteine. Other factors that affect homocysteine levels are renal insufficiency, diabetes, hypothyroidism, anemia, inflammatory bowel disease, cancer, or a gene mutation for methylenetetrahydrofolate reducatase (116). In the general population, about 5% of people have high levels of homocysteine; hyperhomocysteinemia increases to 10% in people with VTE. The presence of hyperhomocysteinemia triples the risk of VTE. A mutation in the prothrombin *G20210A* gene causes an increase in the thrombin precursor, prothrombin. This mutation is considered the second most common inherited coagulation defect associated with VTE. Factor VIII is the coagulation factor that is deficient or absent in hemophiliacs. In VTE, factor VIII is abnormally elevated in one-quarter of the people affected and is present in 11% of the general population. Elevation of factor VIII above 150 IU/dL indicates a risk of VTE 5 times that of the normal population (116).

Clinical Presentation

The clinical manifestations of DVT and PE may range in intensity from clinically silent to severe and dramatic. Clinical correlates of DVT are nonspecific in nature—pain, leg tenderness, edema, and erythema—can be caused by, and coexist with, other processes such as leg trauma, cellulitis, obstructive lymphadenopathy, superficial venous thrombosis, postphlebitic syndrome, or Baker cysts (123) and are, therefore, as independent predictors

not reliable. For example, Homan's sign, pain upon passive dorsiflexion of the foot, is often cited as a sign of DVT, but it is not a reliable clinical marker with sensitivity ranging from 10% to 54% and specificity varies from 39% to 89% (122, 128). As a clinical exam, this combination of signs and symptoms pointing to DVT has low validity and reliability.

The clinical signs of pain, tenderness, edema, Homan's sign, swelling, and erythema have sensitivities of 60% to 88% and specificities of 30% to 72% in well-designed studies, using venography as the reference standard. Studies of Homan's sign suggest it is positive in from 8% to 56% of people with proven DVT but also positive in more than 50% of symptomatic people without DVT (129, p. 181)

A clinical prediction rule can help with the diagnosis of DVT. Clinical prediction rules (CPRs) contain clusters of components that when combined are helpful, predictive tools in the risk assessment, diagnosis, and management of disease; for many disease processes, individual clinical manifestations are not reliable in the prediction of disease (129). CPRs that are most useful in practice incorporate easily obtained patient data from the history, physical exam, and laboratory or diagnostic test results and have been validated in more than one patient population. The Wells clinical prediction rules for DVT and PE are widely used in the determination of pretest probability of DVT and PE and therefore used for decision-making regarding additional testing (124, 130). The Wells clinical prediction rule is a validated tool that can be used to determine the pretest probability of DVT (128, 130). Table 9-36 outlines the Wells clinical prediction rule for DVT (131). McGee suggested that clinicians continue to use compression ultrasonography as their first line test to diagnose DVT and reserve the use of the Wells criteria to determine the need for additional testing (128).

Symptom presentation in patients with PE is variable and therefore can be difficult to diagnose. Many of the signs and symptoms of PE are nonspecific and competing disease processes, such as pneumonia, pneumothorax, pleuritis, rib fracture, COPD exacerbation, congestive HF, or lung cancer, must be ruled out before a definitive diagnosis can be made. The severity of the symptoms is associated with the extent of thrombosis, the existence and quality of collateral vessels, the degree of inflammation, and the size of the embolism relative to the presence of concommitant disease processes (115).

The most common but nonspecific symptom of PE is acute-onset dyspnea and/or wheezing. Other manifestations are tachycardia, cough, hemoptysis, fever, hypotension, syncope, and anxiety. Wells also has tested a clinical prediction rule that can help with the diagnosis of PE; this rule can be found in Table 9-37 (132). Ventilation-perfusion (V/Q) mismatch, bronchoconstriction, and pulmonary vasoconstriction (a

TABLE 9–36 Wells Clinical Prediction Rule for Pretest Probability of Deep Vein Thrombosis (DVT)

Clinical Sign or Symptom/Risk Factor	Criterion Score
Risk Factor	
Cancer (active treatment ongoing, within last 6 months, or palliative)	1
Confined to bed >3 days (recent) or major surgery within last 12 weeks requiring anesthesia	1
Lower extremity involvement*	
Lower extremity immobilization (paralysis, paresis, recent plaster cast)	1
Localized tenderness of lower leg venous system	1
Entire leg swollen	1
Unilateral calf swelling 3 cm larger than asymptomatic leg†	1
Pitting edema on symptomatic leg	1
Collateral nonvaricose superficial veins	1
Alternative Diagnosis Possible	
Alternative diagnosis at least as likely as DVT	–2

*If symptoms occurring in both legs, use the more symptomatic leg for score
†Measured 10 cm below the tibial tuberosity
Score: ≤0 = low clinical probability (low risk, 3%; 95% CI, 2%–6%)
      1–2 = intermediate clinical probability (moderate risk, 17%; 95% CI, 12%–23%)
      ≥3 = high clinical probability (high risk, 75%; 95% CI, 63%–84%)

Adapted from Ebell MH Evaluation of the patient with suspected deep vein thrombosis. Fam Pract 2001; 50(2). Retrieved from JFPOnline: http://www.jfponline.com/Pages.asp?AID=2143#bib8 (131)
From Ebell MH Evidence-Based Diagnosis. New York: Springer; 2001 (130)

TABLE 9–37 Wells Clinical Prediction Rule for Pretest Probability of Pulmonary Embolism (PE)

Clinical Sign/Risk Factor	Criterion Score
Risk Factor	
Previous history of pulmonary embolism or deep vein thrombosis	+1.5
Recent surgery or immobilization	+1.5
Cancer	+1.0
Clinical Signs	
Tachycardia (HR >100 bpm)	+1.5
Hemoptysis	+1.0
Signs of deep vein thrombosis	+3.0
Alternative Diagnosis Not Possible	
Alternative diagnosis less likely than PE	+3.0

Score: 0–1 = low clinical probability (low risk of PE, 1.3%)
      2–6 = intermediate clinical probability (moderate risk, 16.2%)
      ≥7 = high clinical probability (high risk, 40.6%)
Score <4 = less likely
Score >4 = likely

Adapted from Ebell MH 2004;69:367-369. Suspected pulmonary embolism. Part I. Evidence-based clinical assessment. Amn Fam Physician, (132)
From Ebell MH Evidence-Based Diagnosis. New York: Springer; 2001 (130)

compensatory mechanism to combat V/Q imbalance) lead to decreased oxygenation, hypoxemia, tachypnea, and hyperventilation in compensation (115). Sudden onset of pleuritic chest pain is seen in many patients, but a large number may be completely asymptomatic. Syncope and circulatory collapse (i.e., shock states) are signs of a massive PE. The presence of shock increases the risk of death 5 times that of a patient with PE without shock (115). Signs and symptoms of DVT and PE, along with associated diagnostic parameters, are provided in Table 9-38.

Diagnosis

Diagnostic testing for a diagnosis of DVT includes compression ultrasonography, venography, D-dimer assay, or impedance plethysmography. Compression Doppler ultrasonography (DUSG) is a very sensitive and specific test for detecting proximal DVT in symptomatic patients (sensitivity 89% to 96%, specificity 94% to 99%;) and 73% to 93% in distal calf veins (120) and is often the first test used to confirm DVT; however, in asymptomatic patients, the sensitivity and specificity parameters are not as helpful to guide decision-making (sensitivity and specificity 68%) (115).

Contrast venography is an invasive test that uses a small amount of radioactive dye injected into a leg vein to evaluate venous patency. Venography is extremely accurate in the diagnosis of proximal and calf vein DVT (123) and is still considered the authoritative test to rule-out DVT (120), although because of multiple limitations in the use and availability of this test, the DUSG is the most widely used test for DVT diagnosis (102). Impedance plethysmography can be performed at the bedside and measures changes in blood volume and therefore

TABLE 9–38 Signs and Symptoms of Venous Thromboembolism: Comparing DVT and PE

Deep Vein Thrombosis (DVT)			Pulmonary Embolism (PE)		
	Sensitivity (Sn) and Specificity (Sp)	LR+ LR–		Sensitivity and Specificity	LR+ LR–
Unilateral (usually) swelling of the calf, ankle or foot	Sn = 35% to 97%; Sp = 8% to 88%*		Sharp Chest pain (worse during deep breathing)		
			Chest wall tenderness (11%)		
Calf asymmetry ≥2.0 cm**	Sn: 61% Sp: 71%	LR+ 2.1 LR– 0.6	Tachypnea (48%) (RR >25/min) JVD (3%)	Sn: 75% Sp: 55%	LR+ 1.7 LR– 0.5
Thigh swelling**	Sn: 50% Sp: 80%	LR+ 2.5 LR– 0.6			
Palpable cord	Sn: 15% to 30% Sp: 73% to 85%	LR+ NS LR– NS	Pleural friction rub (4% to 18%)	Sn: 14% Sp: 91%	LR+ NS LR– NS
Asymmetric skin coolness**	Sn: 42% Sp: 63%	LR+ NS LR– NS	Rales or wheezing		
Tenderness or pain in the calf or upper leg (Sensitivity of calf pain for acute DVT = 66% to 91%; specificity = 3% to 87%)*	Sn: 42% to 85% Sp: 10% to 65%	LR+ NS LR– NS	Dyspnea and/or hyperventilation		
Purple or blue discoloration of the skin on the leg			Hemoptysis		

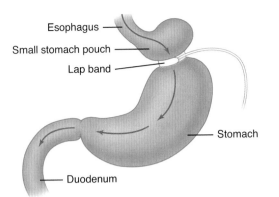

Esophagus

Small stomach pouch

Lap band

Stomach

Duodenum

LAP-BAND ADJUSTABLE GASTRIC BANDING SYSTEM

The Lap-Band, made by BioEnterics Corporation, is a hollow silicone band that is placed around the upper portion of the stomach, creating a small pouch that holds a limited amount of food. The band is inflated with saline through an access port placed under the skin, which is connected to the band by tubing. The degree of inflation can be adjusted, with a more inflated band leading to a narrower opening and therefore slower passage of food between the pouch and the rest of the stomach. The Lap-Band is inserted via laparoscopy. The Lap-Band offers some benefits over traditional gastric bypass surgery but may not be as effective.

http://win.niddk.nih.gov/notes/winter01notes/fda.htm.

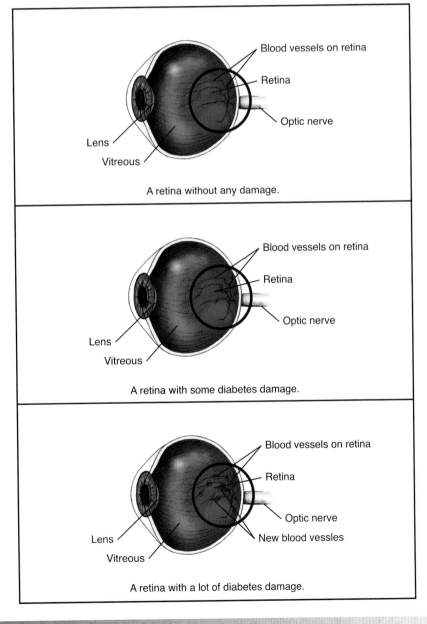

Blood vessels on retina

Retina

Optic nerve

Lens

Vitreous

A retina without any damage.

Blood vessels on retina

Retina

Optic nerve

Lens

Vitreous

A retina with some diabetes damage.

Blood vessels on retina

Retina

Optic nerve

New blood vessels

Lens

Vitreous

A retina with a lot of diabetes damage.

DIABETES RETINAL CHANGES FROM NORMAL TO SEVERE

http://www.catalog.niddk.nih.gov/ImageLibrary/searchresults.cfm?type=recordtype&recordtype=1

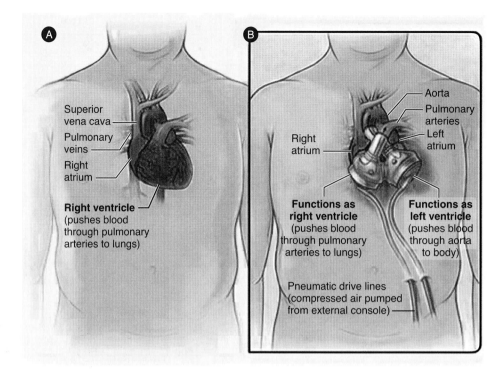

NORMAL HEART AND CARDIOWEST TOTAL ARTIFICIAL HEART

The CardioWest has tubes that, through holes in the abdomen, run from inside the chest to an outside power source. http://www.nhlbi.nih.gov/health/dci/Diseases/tah/tah_what.html.

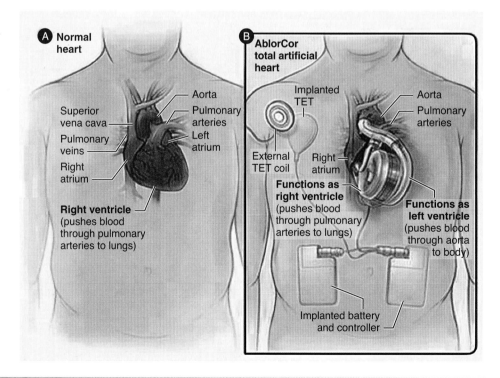

NORMAL HEART AND ABIOCOR TOTAL ARTIFICIAL HEART

The AbioCor Total Artificial Heart (TAH) is completely contained inside the chest. A battery powers this TAH. The battery is charged through the skin with a special magnetic charger. http://www.nhlbi.nih.gov/health/dci/Diseases/tah/tah_what.html.

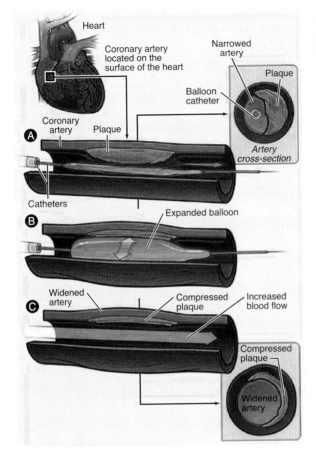

Heart

Coronary artery located on the surface of the heart

Narrowed artery

Plaque

Balloon catheter

Artery cross-section

A Coronary artery Plaque

Catheters

B Expanded balloon

C Widened artery Compressed plaque Increased blood flow

Compressed plaque

Widened artery

CORONARY BALLOON ANGIOPLASTY

During angiography, a small catheter is inserted in an artery, usually the femoral. The catheter is threaded to the coronary arteries. Dye, which can be seen on x-ray, is injected through the catheter. X-ray pictures are taken as the dye flows through the coronary arteries. This outlines blockages, if any are present, and indicates the location and extent of the blockages.

For the angioplasty procedure, a balloon catheter is inserted in the coronary artery and positioned in the blockage. The balloon is then expanded. This pushes the plaque against the artery wall, relieving the blockage and improving blood flow.

http://www.nhlbi.nih.gov/health/dci/Diseases/ Angioplasty/Angioplasty_howdone.html.

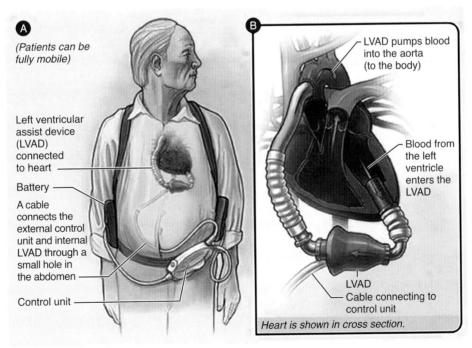

A (Patients can be fully mobile)

Left ventricular assist device (LVAD) connected to heart

Battery

A cable connects the external control unit and internal LVAD through a small hole in the abdomen

Control unit

B LVAD pumps blood into the aorta (to the body)

Blood from the left ventricle enters the LVAD

LVAD Cable connecting to control unit

Heart is shown in cross section.

VENTRICULAR ASSIST DEVICE

The device takes blood from the ventricle of the heart and helps pump it to the body and vital organs.
http://www.nhlbi.nih.gov/health/dci/Diseases/vad/vad_what.html.

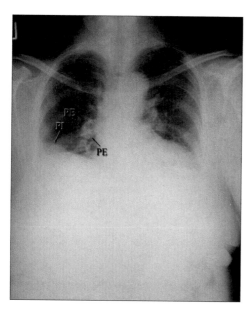

PULMONARY EMBOLISM

This anterioposterior (AP) chest x-ray revealed a right pulmonary arterial embolism (PE) and a pulmonary infarct (PI) distal to the blockage.

Note the radiolucency produced by the moredense pulmonary embolism, and just distal, i.e. further to the left, note the infarct located in the right lung base, representing ischemic lung tissue due to the blockage.

Courtesy of CDC/Dr. Thomas Hooten, 2011.

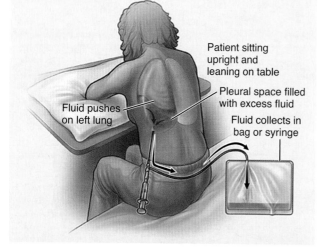

THORACENTESIS

The patient sits upright and leans on a table.

http://www.nhlbi.nih.gov/health/dci/Diseases/thor/thor_all.html.

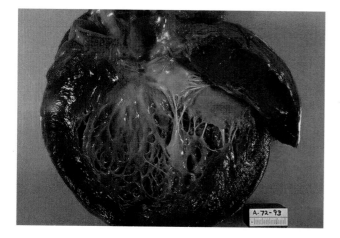

CARDIOMYOPATHY

Gross pathology of idiopathic cardiomyopathy. Opened left ventricle of heart shows a thickened, dilated left ventricle with subendocardial fibrosis manifested as increased whiteness of endocardium.

Courtesy of CDC/ Dr. Edwin P. Ewing, Jr.

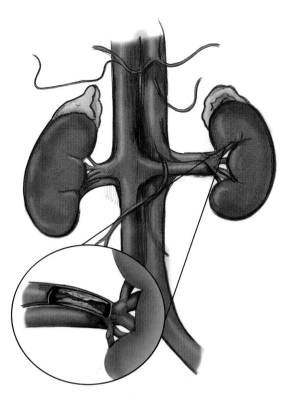

RENAL ARTERY STENOSIS

In renal artery stenosis, plaque builds up on the inner wall of the artery that supplies blood to the kidney.

http://www.catalog.niddk.nih.gov/ImageLibrary/searchresults.cfm?type=recordtype&recordtype=1.

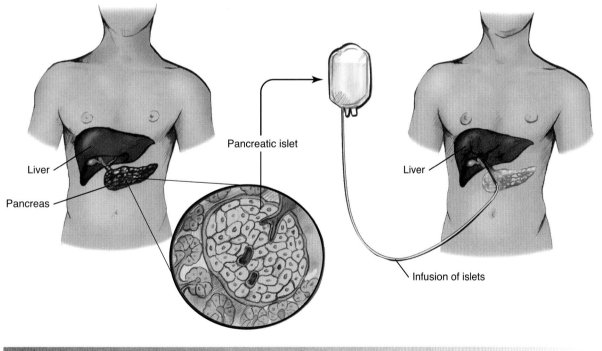

Liver

Pancreas

Pancreatic islet

Liver

Infusion of islets

PANCREATIC ISLET CELL TRANSPLANT

Islets extracted from a donor pancreas are infused into the liver. Once implanted, the beta cells in the islets begin to make and release insulin.

http://www.catalog.niddk.nih.gov/ImageLibrary/searchresults.cfm?type=recordtype&recordtype=1.

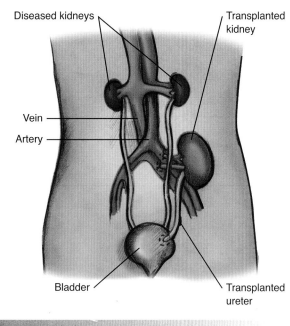

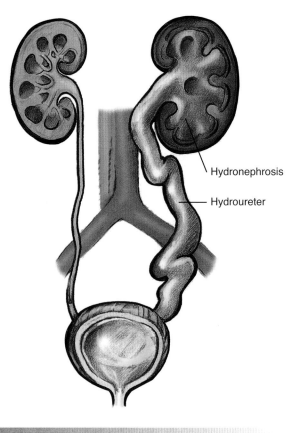

TRANSPLANTED KIDNEY

Anatomical diagram of a female figure with a transplanted kidney. The two diseased kidneys are still in place on either side of the spine, just below the rib cage. The transplanted kidney is located on the left side, just above the bladder. A transplanted ureter connects the new kidney to the bladder.

http://www.catalog.niddk.nih.gov/ImageLibrary/searchresults.cfm?type=recordtype&recordtype=1.

HYDROURETER AND HYDRONEPHROSIS

http://www.catalog.niddk.nih.gov/ImageLibrary/searchresults.cfm?type=recordtype&recordtype=1

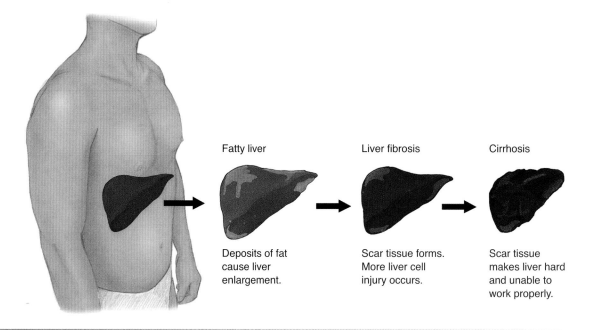

LIVER DISEASE

Stages of liver damage: Normal liver, fatty liver (where deposits of fat cause liver enlargement), liver fibrosis (where scar tissue forms and more liver cell injury occurs), and cirrhosis (where scar tissue makes the liver hard).

http://www.catalog.niddk.nih.gov/ImageLibrary/searchresults.cfm?type=recordtype&recordtype=1.

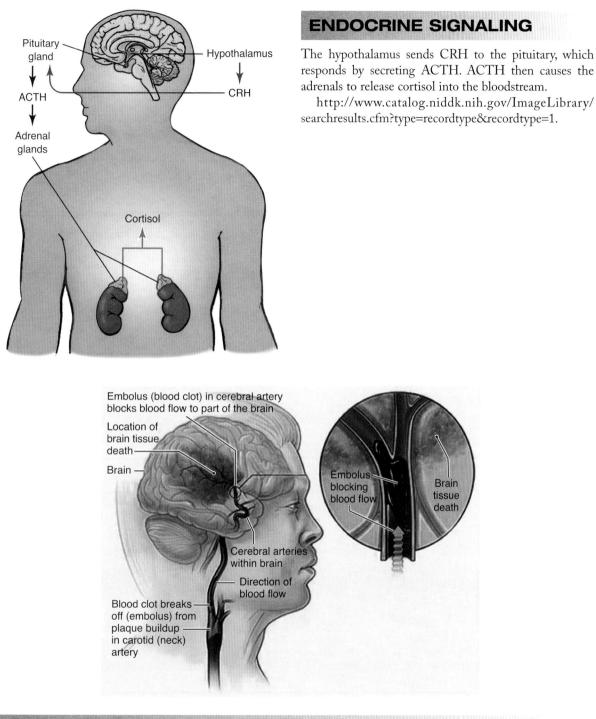

ENDOCRINE SIGNALING

The hypothalamus sends CRH to the pituitary, which responds by secreting ACTH. ACTH then causes the adrenals to release cortisol into the bloodstream.

http://www.catalog.niddk.nih.gov/ImageLibrary/searchresults.cfm?type=recordtype&recordtype=1.

ISCHEMIC STROKE

The two types of ischemic stroke are thrombotic and embolic. In a thrombotic stroke, a thrombus forms in an artery that supplies blood to the brain.

In an embolic stroke, a blood clot or other substance (such as plaque, a fatty material, or septic emboli) travels through the bloodstream to an artery in the brain.

http://www.nhlbi.nih.gov/health/dci/Diseases/stroke/stroke_types.html.

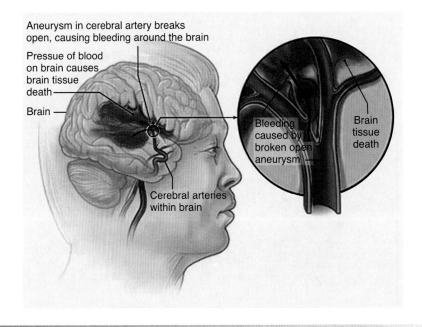

HEMORRHAGIC STROKE

The two types of hemorrhagic stroke are intracerebral and subarachnoid. In an intracerebral hemorrhage, a blood vessel inside the brain leaks blood or ruptures.

In a subarachnoid hemorrhage, a blood vessel on the surface of the brain leaks blood or ruptures. When this happens, bleeding occurs between the inner and middle layers of the membranes that cover the brain.

In both types of hemorrhagic stroke, the leaked blood causes swelling of the brain and increased pressure in the skull. The swelling and pressure damage cells and tissues in the brain.

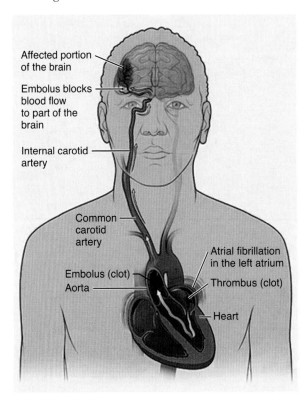

ATRIAL FIBRILLATION AND STROKE

During atrial fibrillation, the atria fail to pump all of their blood to the ventricles. Some blood pools in the atria. When this happens, a thrombus can form. If the clot breaks off and travels to the brain, it can cause a stroke.

http://www.nhlbi.nih.gov/health/dci/Diseases/af/af_all.html.

TABLE 9–38 Signs and Symptoms of Venous Thromboembolism: Comparing DVT and PE—cont'd

Deep Vein Thrombosis (DVT)			Pulmonary Embolism (PE)		
Increased warmth of the leg	Sn: 29% to 71% Sp: 51% to 77%	LR+ 1.4 LR– NS	Tachycardia (81%) Loud P$_2$ (split S$_2$) (19% to 57%)	Sn: 81% Sp: 55% Sn: 19% Sp: 84%	LR+ 1.8 LR– 0.3 LR+ NS LR– NS
			S$_3$ or S$_4$ (6% to 34%) Increase in HR ≥20 bpm	Sn: 41% Sp: 84%	LR+ 2.5 LR– NS
Erythema	Sn: 16% to 48% Sp: 61% to 87%	LR+ NS LR– NS	Syncope (20% to 80% of patients with massive PE)**	Sn: 29% to 71% Sp: 51% to 77%	LR+ 1.4 LR– NS
Pitting edema			Diaphoresis (11%-36%)		
Dilated superficial veins	Sn: 29% to 33% Sp: 82% to 85%	LR+ 1.9 LR– NS	Fever (7%)		
Tenderness in the calf or upper leg (calf tenderness, sensitivity = 56% to 82%; specificity = 26% to 74%)*			Cyanosis (3% to 19%)		
			Cough (more common in pulmonary infarction)		
Homans sign	Sn: 13% to 48%* Sp: 39%-84%	LR+ NS** LR– NS	Crackles (58%)		
Calf swelling with history of Active cancer**	Sn: 20% to 39% Sp: 90% to 92%	LR+ 3.2	Accessory muscle use (17%)		
Recent immobilization**	Sn: 24% to 41% Sp: 82% to 90%	LR+ 2.3	Tender or swollen calf (15% to 52%)	Sn: 52% Sp: 80%	LR+ 2.6 LR– 0.6
			Calf asymmetry of ≥1.5 cm (16%)	Sn: 13% to 48%* Sp: 39% to 84%	LR+ NS** LR– NS
			Hypoxemia (74% to 81%) (PaO_2 <80 mm Hg)	Sn: 74% to 81% Sp: 24% to 29%	LR+ NS LR– NS
			Hypocapnia (51% to 70%)	Sn: 92% to 99% Sp: 12% to 15%	LR+ NS LR– NS
			Increased A-a gradient		
			Known cancer	Sn: 22% to 26% Sp: 94% to 95%	LR+ 4.1 LR– 0.8

A-a, Alveolar-arterial; JVD, jugular venous distention; NS, not significant; PaO_2, partial pressure of arterial oxygen dissolved in the blood; RR, respiratory rate.

Data from American Thoracic Society, 1999 (122); Anand et al, 1998, (123); Cardin and Marinelli, 2004 (115); McGee, 2007 (128)

* Data from American Thoracic Society (122); **data from McGee (128).

identifies blood vessel occlusion in the affected extremity. Impedance plethysmography has a sensitivity of about 70%—it is more sensitive in detecting proximal occlusive DVT but has a lower sensitivity for the diagnosis of nonocclusive proximal or distal DVT (123). D-dimers are protein fragments of a degraded blood clot via fibrinolysis. Increased levels of D-dimers are found in almost all patients with VTE.

The clinical approach to the patient with suspected PE is to combine the data obtained from a history and physical examination together with a CXR, ECG, and arterial blood gas (ABG) analysis to make a decision as to the need for further testing. ECG changes in PE are nonspecific and include T-wave changes, ST-segment abnormalities, and left- or right-axis deviation. One-quarter to one-third of patients with massive or submassive PE may demonstrate ECG changes consistent with acute cor pulmonale: an S_1 Q3 T3 pattern, new RBBB, P-wave pulmonale, or right-axis deviation (122). ABG analysis will indicate hypoxemia and respiratory alkalosis in the early period. Age affects the demonstration of hypoxemia—younger people with PE tend to have higher PaO_2 levels (greater than 80 mm Hg). One distinction between PE and preexisting pulmonary disease is a large elevation in the alveolar-arterial (A-a) gradient of more than 20 mm Hg (122).

Chest radiography is an adjunct but nonspecific test for the diagnosis of PE and helpful in ruling-out alternative diagnoses. The majority of CXRs in PE will be abnormal; frequent findings include atelectasis (68%), pleural effusion (48%), pulmonary infiltrates, and hemidiaphragm elevation. Hampton's hump or Westermark's sign (indicating decreased vascularity) is a classic sign of pulmonary infarction but rarely observed (122). A strong constellation of findings indicative of PE is a patient presenting with severe dyspnea, hypoxemia, no evidence of bronchospasm or anatomic cardiac shunt, and a normal chest radiograph (122).

Pulmonary embolism can be confirmed by V/Q lung scanning, spiral CT scanning, or pulmonary angiography. A V/Q scan identifies areas in the lung that are ventilated and perfused. This test uses inhaled and injected radioactive isotopes to ascertain areas of the lungs that are not receiving adequate ventilation from a presumed PE in a pulmonary artery or branch. PE is more difficult to detect in patients with preexisting cardiovascular or lung diseases (115). The Prospective Investigation of Pulmonary Embolism Diagnosis (PIOPED) study helped establish the diagnostic accuracy of the V/Q scan in the diagnosis of PE (122). Even though a high-probability V/Q scan is indicative of PE 96% of the time, more testing is usually conducted (122). A normal V/Q scan rules out PE (99). The addition of clinical data to the V/Q scan results increases the certainty of PE diagnosis: 96% of patients with high probability scans and a high clinical suspicion of PE are correctly diagnosed; low probability coupled with a low suspicion based on clinical findings accurately rules out PE 90% of the time (115).

A helical (spiral) CT scan also uses an injected dye bolus to allow for direct visualization of the cardiac and pulmonary vasculature. The CT rotates quickly around the body (i.e., in a spiral) to obtain a 3D view of the blood supply to the heart and lungs. The sensitivity and specificity of the spiral CT in the diagnosis of PE have shown some variability. The American Thoracic Society reported the sensitivity and specificity as greater than 95% (122); Qaseem et al. (120) reported sensitivities ranging from 66% to 93% and specificities from 89% to 98%. The newest helical CT scanner is a multidetector model that may have diagnostic accuracy characteristics closer to the range of 90% to 95% (120).

Pulmonary angiography is the gold standard for diagnosing PE, as it is the most accurate. A catheter is inserted into a vein, usually in the groin, and the catheter is positioned into a blood vessel that leads to the lungs. Once positioned, a contrast dye is injected and radiographs are obtained of the pulmonary vasculature. The pulmonary vascular tree fills with the contrast dye and areas that are nonperfused due to an embolus or emboli appear dark.

Laboratory Testing

Blood testing includes an evaluation of D-dimer levels and identification of thrombophilic disorders. D-dimers are fragments of fibrin clots broken down naturally by the fibrinolytic system. Small amounts of D-dimers are found in healthy people, but levels are increased in certain disease and stress states: cancer, infection, HF, renal failure, and VTE, as well as with aging, hospitalization, and in surgery (115). Diagnostic accuracy of D-dimer varies—levels have been reported to be eight times normal in VTE with a negative predictive value of 97% (115). Recent research showed that high-sensitivity D-dimer assays (sensitivity 96-100%) may be helpful for diagnosis of PE; values of less than 500 ng/mL can help to rule out pulmonary embolism (NPV = 95%) (122, 133).

Plasma BNP levels may be adjunctive tests for diagnosing PE. Possible new biomarkers for PE testing in the emergency department include BNP testing (115), CRP, and myeloperoxidase (134). BNP is released from the ventricles in response to increased wall tension. An increase in RV wall tension from pulmonary emboli could cause BNP to rise, but the sensitivity and specificity of BNP for PE diagnosis have not been definitively established. Sensitivity and specificity are limited because BNP levels are elevated in patients with preexisting cardiac illness and patients have died of PE but showed normal BNP levels on autopsy (115). More research is indicated in this area.

The presence of hereditary or acquired thrombophilic defects can be confirmed by a variety of blood assays including factor V Leiden mutation (activated protein C resistance), prothrombin and prothrombin time, prothrombin gene mutation (*G20210A*), AT level and activity, protein C activity, protein S activity, free (active) and total protein S antigen levels, factor VIII level, fasting plasma homocysteine levels, methylenetetrahydrofoloate reducatase mutation, anticardiolipin antibodies and lupus anticoagulants (part of the antiphospholipid antibody syndrome), and heparin antibodies (116, 135).

As noted earlier, validated clinical prediction rules are available to assist in the diagnosis of both DVT and PE (refer to Tables 9-36 and 9-37). Work-up options can be evaluated, using the risk scores from the Wells criteria for prediction of DVT and include the use of ultrasound and venogram; an abnormal venogram is diagnostic of DVT. Recommendations from national guidelines for diagnostic testing are further delineated in Table 9-39 (120).

Management

Nurses and CNSs play important roles in the diagnosis and management of VTE. A high index of suspicion is necessary, especially for patients predisposed to the development of VTE. Nurses need to be aware of the risk factors for VTE and perform a risk assessment on patients on admission and throughout their hospital stay. Identification of these at-risk patients will raise the awareness and vigilance of the nursing staff. Close monitoring, early recognition of signs of trouble, and rapid initiation of aggressive treatment are imperative. Massive PE is usually sudden with no warning signs. In addition, two-thirds of patients who develop a massive PE will die within 1 to 2 hours of symptom onset (115, 136). Early recognition of PE is not always possible as patients present differently and some of the signs are nonspecific—some patients may not complain of pain or show signs of hemodynamic compromise until a large portion of the pulmonary vasculature is blocked and CO is affected. In some patients, fatal PE may be the first indication of a VTE disorder (118).

Various risk assessment tools and evidence-based clinical practice guidelines are available for DVT and PE (120, 122, 124, 130, 133). Geerts et al. (118) and the American College of Chest Physicians (ACCP) guidelines offer rationale for the implementation of preventive interventions in hospitalized patients (137) (Table 9-40). Clinical practice guidelines offer recommendations for VTE risk assessment, diagnosis, prophylaxis, and management (118, 120, 124). Recommendations for acute care management are found in Table 9-41 (137).

Patient care goals for the patient with DVT are to relieve symptoms, prevent progression or recurrence of VTE, and reduce the risk of complications from anticoagulation therapy. Anticoagulants are the foundation of therapy. Patients with folic acid deficiencies causing a thrombophilia should be prescribed a folic acid supplement. Mechanical prophylaxis is used as a solo strategy for low-risk patients or as an adjunct therapy in combination with medications. Interventional radiology techniques also may be used to treat the clot through direct fibrinolysis. Surgical alternatives also are available.

Anticoagulation Therapy

Anticoagulation is standard therapy in the treatment of VTE, including direct thrombin inhibitors, and antiplatelet therapies (21). The major risk of anticoagulation therapy is bleeding (21). However, prophylactic doses of low-dose unfractionated heparin (LDUH), (LMWH) or a vitamin K antagonist have been shown to have little to no effect on the rates of clinically important bleeding; in fact, when thromboprophylaxis is used appropriately the risk/benefit ratio is maximized and overall costs are reduced (118).

The choice of using LDUH, LMWH, warfarin, fondaparinux (a factor X inhibitor), platelet inhibitors, direct thrombin inhibitors, or GIIb/IIIa inhibitors is based on the patient's history, risk factors, and current condition. For example, in patients with symptomatic HD or known HD in situations likely to trigger clot formation, such as surgery, prophylactic anticoagulants (warfarin or heparin) are usually administered. In the Prevention of Recurrent

---

TABLE 9–39 Recommendations for Diagnosis of VTE

Recommendation 1

Validated clinical prediction rules should be used to estimate pretest probability of venous thromboembolism (VTE), both deep venous thrombosis (DVT) and pulmonary embolism, and for the basis of interpretation of subsequent tests.

Recommendation 2

In appropriately selected patients with low pretest probability of DVT or pulmonary embolism, obtaining a high-sensitivity D-dimer is a reasonable option, and if negative, indicates a low likelihood of VTE.

Recommendation 3

Ultrasound is recommended for patients with intermediate to high pretest probability of DVT in the lower extremities.

Recommendation 4

Patients with intermediate or high pretest probability of pulmonary embolism require diagnostic imaging studies.

Adapted from Qaseem et al. Current diagnosis of venous thromboembolism in primary care: a clinical practice guideline from the American Academy of Family Physicians and the American College of Physicians. Ann Fam Medi 2007; 5(1):57-62. (120)

TABLE 9–40 Preventive Interventions for VTE Prevention Based on Patient Risk

Risk Stratification	Clinical Criteria	Management
LOW RISK		
	• Patient under age 40 • Minor surgery, no additional risk factors	• Aggressive and early mobilization • Leg exercises while in bed
MODERATE RISK		
	• Patient age 40–60, no additional risk factors • Minor surgery, with additional risk factors • Major surgery in patients younger than 40 years who have no additional risk factors	• Prophylaxis with low-dose unfractionated heparin (LDUH) (5,000 U bid) or low-molecular-weight heparin (LMWH) ([<3,400 U once daily]) • Graduated compression stockings • Pneumatic compression stockings • Thromboprophylaxis with LDUH (5,000 U tid) or LMWH (>3,400 U daily)
HIGH RISK		
	• Patient over age 60 • Patient age 40–60 with ≥1 additional risk factor (prior VTE, cancer, molecular hypercoagulability)	• Graduated compression stockings and/or • Pneumatic compression stockings
HIGHEST RISK		
	• Patient with multiple risk factors • Hip or knee arthroplasty • Hip fracture • Major trauma • Spinal cord injury	• Combination of pharmacologic methods (LDUH three times daily or LMWH, >3,400 U daily), fondaparinux, oral VKAs (INR, 2–3): with the use of • Graduated compression stockings and/or • Intermittent pneumatic compression devices

INR, International normalized ratio; VKA, vitamin K antidote.
From Geerts et al. (2004) (118); Hiatt, 2007 (113); Kearon et al. (2008) (137).

Venous Thromboembolism (PREVENT) study, warfarin was titrated to achieve a serum international normalized ratio (INR) of 1.5 to 2, instead of the conventional target of 2.0 to 3.0, and compared to placebo. Low-dose warfarin was shown to reduce the risk of recurrent VTE by 64%, but increase minor bleeding episodes by 92% (hazard ratio [HR] 1.92; 95% CI, 1.26 to 2.93) compared to placebo (138). While it seems to make sense that low-dose warfarin would decrease bleeding risk, conventional warfarin therapy targets have still been shown to be more effective in decreasing recurrent VTE greater than the low-dose regimen (139). The Extended Low-Intensity Anticoagulation for Thrombo-Embolism (ELATE) trial, a double-blind, randomized clinical trial, did not demonstrate a protective effect of low-dose warfarin. In fact, the incidence of recurrent VTE for the low-dose experimental group was almost 3 times that of conventional-dose control group (HR 2.8, 95% CI, 1.1 to 7.0) and death rates were twice that of the conventional dose (HR 2.1, 95% CI, 0.9 to 4.8) (139).

The use of LDUH is well established in VTE prophylaxis. A loading dose of 5000 U of LDUH may be given

TABLE 9–41 Recommendations for Acute Care Management of VTE: 2004 American College of Chest Physicians Guidelines

Recommendation	Grade of Recommendation
• Low-molecular-weight heparin or low-dose unfractionated heparin is recommended for acutely ill medical patients who are:	1A
• Admitted to the hospital with congestive heart failure or severe respiratory disease	
• Confined to bed and have at least one additional risk factor	
• Upon admission to a critical care unit, all patients should be assessed for their risk for DVT	1A
• Accordingly, most should receive thromboprophylaxis	
• Mechanical methods of prophylaxis should be used primarily in patients who are at high risk for bleeding or as an adjunct to anticoagulant-based prophylaxis	1C+
	2A

Grade 1 recommendations are strong and indicate that the benefits do, or do not, outweigh risks, burden, and costs; Grade 2 suggests that individual patients' values may lead to different choices.

From Kearon et al. Antithrombotic therapy for venous thromboembolic disease: American College of Chest Physicians Evidence-Based Clinical Practice Guidelines. 8th edition. Chest 2008; 133:(6 [suppl])454S-545S.

intravenously and then a continuous infusion is initiated of 30,000 U/24 hr. Weight-based protocols are used to manage the heparin dose titrated to the partial thromboplastin time (PTT). Side effects of heparin therapy may be significant and include heparin resistance and heparin-induced thrombocytopenia (HIT). Heparin is the drug of choice for pregnant women because it does not cross the placenta. Heparin resistance may occur when administered to AT-deficient patients (121). Antithrombin concentrates from human donors are available for transfusion for HD patients undergoing surgery or during childbirth.

LWMH (i.e., enoxaparin in medical patients; dalteparin and tinzaparin in orthopedic surgery patients) has become the drug of choice for most patients with VTE as research studies have shown its effectiveness and low-risk profile over LDUH (118). Administer LWMH subcutaneously twice a day (every 12 hours) at 1 mg/kg or 1.5 mg/kg once a day. LMWH does not require coagulation studies to monitor effectiveness.

Oral vitamin K antagonists (VKAs) are introduced into the therapy regimen to transition the patient from intravenous to oral therapy. Warfarin (starting dose 2 to 5 mg/day) is started about a day after the patient has been started on the intravenous LDUH or LMWH infusion. Monitoring INRs are important to maintain a therapeutic range of warfarin (a range of 2 to 3 for VTE patients or 4 to 5 for patients with concomitant prosthetic valves) is warranted. Intravenous heparin may be discontinued once the INR has reached the target range. The delayed onset of warfarin of 2 to 3 days is beneficial to achieve surgical hemostasis; however, its burden of

follow-up monitoring and potential drug interactions has caused it to fall out of favor in the European community as a mainstay VKA for total hip replacement. Warfarin remains widely used in North America post total hip replacement (118).

Fondaparinux is a synthetic pentasaccharide (114) and a factor Xa inhibitor. It is administered subcutaneously once a day and eliminated through the kidneys, so it is prohibited in patients with renal failure. Antiplatelet therapies (e.g., ASA, clopidogrel, and GP IIb/IIIa inhibitors) are used but not as monotherapy (118). ASA is effective to decrease platelet aggregation; however, it cannot prevent VTE because venous thrombi are not composed of platelets but rather of fibrin and red blood cells (114).

Mechanical Interventions

Mechanical interventions to prevent VTE work because they increase venous circulation and therefore decrease clot formation; an added benefit is that they do not increase bleeding risk. Clearly, patients who have active bleeding or bleeding disorders should not be started on anticoagulants—patients with bleeding that is temporary and reversible (e.g., from trauma) may be started on anticoagulants after the cause of the bleeding is identified and treated (140). Mechanical interventions are safe and effective strategies in the prevention of venous stasis and DVT (118).

Graduated compression stockings (GCS), intermittent pneumatic compression (IPC) devices, the venous foot pump, and range-of-motion and leg exercises are all designed to stimulate venous muscles to contract and move blood back up to the heart, thereby preventing VTE formation. Evidence for the long-term effect of GCS is particularly compelling: the incidence of postthrombotic syndrome was reduced over 50% in patients wearing over-the-counter or custom-fit compression stockings (124); however, GCS should not be used in patients with compromised arterial blood flow (118). Proper fitting and application of GCS is extremely important and usually the responsibility of the bedside nurse; proper fit can make the difference in patient compliance with this therapy. GCS should be worn most of the day, only removed for a short time per protocol (usually 30 minutes per shift), and then reapplied. Intermittent pneumatic compression machines can be used independently or with GCS. Air pressure of about 45 mm Hg applied to the legs, either sequentially or longitudinally, decreases venous blood pooling and therefore improves blood flow to the heart. The venous foot pump (e.g., the A-V Impulse System), applies pressure to the plantar arch to flatten it and thereby empty the venous sinuses in the feet.

The easiest mechanical interventions to apply are foot and ankle exercises to promote venous return through plantar flexion and dorsiflexion of the foot and ankle (114). These exercises are easily taught to patients and can be performed any time. Range-of-motion exercises provide the same benefits and may be performed by family members or health care professionals if the patient is unable to perform these alone. Preventive measures may be needed for patients vulnerable to friction on the heels; patients with bone injuries should not be taught these exercises (114).

Interventional Techniques

Interventional techniques to treat in situ or graft thromboses include catheter-directed thrombolysis to directly dissolve the clot with thrombolytic agents, percutaneous mechanical thrombectomy to remove the thrombosis, and a new technique, ultrasound accelerated thrombolysis (USAT) (141). USAT joins low-power, high-frequency ultrasound with catheter-directed thrombolysis; this combination speeds up the process of clot lysis (141). A special multilumen catheter capable of delivering both ultrasound and the thrombolytic infusion is inserted in the interventional radiology department, the ultrasound component and the infusion is started, and the patient is transferred to the ICU for continued postprocedure monitoring of the catheter site, peripheral pulses, and patient's response to therapy. Lytic checks are performed at scheduled intervals after the procedure to assess the extent of clot dissolution and recannulation of the artery and to assess the need for additional interventional procedures. Early use of this therapy for a patient with an occluded right femoral–tibial peroneal bypass graft has shown this new technology to be extremely promising (141).

Surgical Interventions

Vena caval filters (VCF) may be placed in the inferior vena cava or femoral vein to snare emboli traveling from the lower extremities and prevent the ascent into the pulmonary system. Filters may be placed in the internal jugular vein also for upper extremity emboli (140). VCFs are considered good alternatives for patients who are not able to tolerate anticoagulant therapy; however, results are mixed: one study showed that the incidence of recurrent DVT seems to be significantly higher in patients who receive a VCF versus anticoagulant therapy alone (124). Complications from VCF placement include migration of the filter from its original position, filter occlusion, and thrombosis of the insertion site and the access vein (140). New retrievable VCFs are used for short-term protection and therefore decrease the risk of long-term complications (140). The evidence as to the efficacy of VCF is currently inadequate to make definitive practice recommendations (140). Surgical intervention to remove the embolus may be necessary.

Clinical Nurse Specialist Competencies and Spheres of Influence

The CNS Core Competencies of Coaching/Teaching/Mentoring, Research/Evidence-Based Practice, and Systems Leadership are the primary competencies required of CNSs practicing in this area of expertise. The performance of these competencies requires skill in all three Spheres of Influence.

Coaching/Teaching/Mentoring

Keeping the staff informed of changes in the standard of care and hands-on practice with new devices is important to safe and quality care. Ensure that the staff can recognize early signs and symptoms of adverse events and impending crises. CNSs should design and implement annual staff competency testing for patient care devices that decrease DVT risk (Nursing/Other Disciplines Sphere).

Patient and family education about short- and long-term complications of VTE and its therapy are important (Patient/Family Sphere of Influence). Ensure that the patient is educated on the risks of VTE and encourage the patient's adherence to the treatment regimen to prevent increased risk of DVT and PE—especially to self-care interventions that can be continued at home such as limiting time in bed and in stationary positions, and performing leg exercises on a regular basis. Geerts et al. (118) noted that a large number of symptomatic VTE associated with hospitalization occur after the patient has been discharged from the hospital.

Patient education regarding anticoagulant medications is imperative to prevent patient harm. Make sure your patient knows the signs and symptoms of adverse effects from anticoagulant and antiplatelet therapies; discourage the use of medications that contain ASA or other NSAIDs, or vitamin and herbal supplements that may potentiate or preclude the desired effects of the anticoagulants. Instruction in foods that are high in vitamin

K is important for patients on warfarin, as vitamin K will interfere with warfarin's anticoagulant effect.

Examples of resources to use for patient, family, and staff education include tools from the American Medical Directors Association's Web site (www.amda.com), which provides resources for use by the CNS and organization related to DVT and PE. For example, a DVT Inpatient Evaluation form (http://www.amda.com/tools/clinical/dvt/US%20NMH%2007%2009%20014%20Evaluation.pdf), a DVT risk assessment form http://www.amda.com/tools/clinical/dvt/US%20NMH%2007%2009%20027%20Assess%20DVT.pdf), an outpatient treatment algorithm (http://www.amda.com/tools/clinical/dvt/US%20NMH%2007%2009%20019%20Algorithm.pdf) and patient education materials, among others, are available for free. A sample documentation form for DVT risk may be found at http://www.amda.com/tools/clinical/DVT/dvtform.doc (140).

Research/Evidence-Based Practice

There are many EBP guidelines for VTE available: guidelines produced by the Institute for Clinical Systems Improvement were originally published in 2000 and are updated annually are available on their Web site (www.icsi.org) (133). Other guidelines for VTE can be found on the National Guidelines Clearinghouse Web site, the Eighth ACCP Conference on Antithrombotic and Thrombolytic Therapy: Evidence-based Practice Guidelines (137), and joint guidelines developed by the American Academy of Family Physicians and the American College of Physicians (120, 124) are also available. Guidelines by the American College of Chest Physicians (137) recommended VTE treatment based on the assessment of patient risk (see Table 9-40). The CNS may lead efforts to make sure that prophylaxis recommendations are included in preprinted or computerized admission and transfer orders. Preprinted order sets and computerized reminders along with a written policy have been shown to increase compliance (118).

Translating research and evidence into practice is a major role function of the CNS. Vigilance and knowledge are key factors related to rescuing patients from harm. Both DVT and PE are preventable incidents that could, and frequently do, cost the patient his life. The Agency for Healthcare Research and Quality (AHRQ) report on patient safety practices, by the University of California at San Francisco-Stanford University Evidence-based Practice Center (142), was a systematic review that identified 79 patient safety interventions from the literature and summarized the evidence supporting the interventions. Eleven patient safety interventions were ranked as the ones that had the highest quality and quantity of evidence support and were recommended for "widespread implementation" (142, Clear Opportunities for Safety Improvement paragraph). The most highly rated safety practice, as both cost-effective and significant for reducing adverse patient outcomes, was the "appropriate use of prophylaxis to prevent venous thromboembolism in patients at risk" (142, Clear Opportunities for Safety Improvement paragraph). The CNS stays current with the newest guidelines and recommendations and ensures that staff is aware of the latest evidence surrounding preventive measures.

Systems Leadership

Multiple quality initiatives are related to VTE prevention and prophylaxis. DVT and PE are considered hospital-acquired conditions (HACs) and therefore are on the list of the Centers for Medicare & Medicaid Services (CMS) "Never-Events" (143). The consequence of a patient developing DVT or PE that was not present on admission is largely economic—neither Medicare nor patients will pay to treat these HACs (144). DVT prophylaxis is recommended as part of quality measures in patient care from the National Quality Forum (145) Safe Practices 28 and 29, TJC 2008 National Safety Goal 3E (146), and the Surgical Care Improvement Project measures to prevent postoperative complications (147). The Surgical Care Improvement Project noted that in patients undergoing major surgical procedures who do not receive anticoagulation prophylaxis, 25% will develop a DVT and 7% will develop a PE (147). CNSs work with the hospital system to ascertain that EBP guidelines are communicated, instituted, and updated, as new evidence is published that may change practice.

There are national registries for patients confirmed with a diagnosis of DVT. Patients are entered into the registries for audit, quality documentation, and research purposes. Some early findings from the Deep Vein Thrombosis Free (DVT FREE) national database indicated that 50% of general medical and surgical patients developed DVT while in the hospital and that the majority of these patients received no DVT prophylaxis (148). VTE prevention and quality patient management are one of the 16 areas for quality improvement as identified by TJC. "The purpose of The Joint Commission's National Patient Safety Goals is to promote specific improvements in patient safety. The goals highlight problematic areas in health care and describe evidence and expert-based consensus to solutions to these problems" (146, p. 1).

Anticoagulation therapy is requirement 3E in the National Patient Safety Goals document. In addition, the National Consensus Standards for the Prevention and Care of VTE is a collaborative effort between TJC and the National Quality Forum. Six core VTE measures, three on prevention and three on treatment, can be viewed on the TJC Web site (http://www.jointcommission.org/PerformanceMeasurement/PerformanceMeasurement/VTE.htm) or in the related document (149).

CNSs should monitor unit compliance with established VTE policies and procedures, collect data on incidence rates, and submit data on VTE prevention and treatment. These data will help guide the design and implementation of quality improvement initiatives.

There are venous thromboembolism measures available from the National Quality Measures Clearinghouse (www.qualitymeasures.ahrq.gov) to assist the CNS with documentation of the incidence and diagnosis of VTE and the use of therapeutic measures (e.g., GCS and LMWH).

The Medicare Quality Improvement Community (MedQIC) Web site (www.qualitynet.org) and the Institute for Clinical Systems Improvement (www.icsi.org) are two Web sites that offer shared tools and resources to promote quality patient care. A Venous Thrombolembolism Diagnosis and Treatment guideline, including algorithms, clinical prediction rules, and order sets, is available at http://www.icsi.org/venous_thromboembolism/venous_thromboembolism_4.html. In addition, Table 9-42 shows other resources available to the CNS.

The CNS documents outcomes in recoverable formats for audit and quality analysis. The addition of a DVT prophylaxis reminder on documentation forms for interdisciplinary rounds or daily patient goal sheets also demonstrated improved communication among the staff and reduced the length of stay by 1 day (150). The FASTHUG mnemonic is an interdisciplinary approach to daily care of the critically ill patient (151). Seven components of evidence-based care for the critically ill (**F**eeding, **A**nalgesia, **S**edation, **T**hromboembolic prophylaxis, **H**ead-of-bed elevation, stress **U**lcer prevention, and **G**lucose control) are reminders of questions to ask and strategies to implement to prevent common complications in critical care and can be incorporated in verbal or written reports and interdisciplinary rounds. Strategies to successfully implement CPGs include designing systems to monitor implementation, safety, and compliance in areas where the guideline will be used; developing systems to provide patient education and risk awareness; and developing protocols and policies for organizational education (e.g., to nursing staff, physicians, and other staff) (133).

Professional nursing organizations have resources to assist in the translation of research into practice. The American Association of Critical-Care Nurses (AACN) produces Practice Alerts, which provide the evidence-base for common conditions seen in acute and critically ill patients in a concise format for easy reference (www.aacn.org). The Practice Alerts are standardized to provide information on expected practice, the scope and impact of the problem, supporting evidence with references, and nursing actions. For some Practice Alerts, there may be an audit tool available to measure compliance with expected

TABLE 9–42 Resources Available for APRNs With Permission

Resources Available

*	Author/ Organization	Title/Description	Audience	Web Sites/ Order Information
	American Venous Forum/Venous Educational Institute of America (VEIN)	Provides a general overview of the condition, a clinical discussion group, referral center, and links to other resources.	Health Care Professionals; Patient and Families	http://www.dvt.info.com
	Health Information Translation or Ohio State University Medical Center, Ohio Health, Mount Carmel Foundation, Nationwide Children's Hospital	Site contains downloadable print education materials on cardiovascular and other topics in a wide range of languages.	Health Care Professionals; Patient and Families	http:www.healthinfotranslations.com
*	Institute for Clinical Systems Improvement	Development of Anticoagulation Programs at Seven Medical Organizations (#29, 12/04)	Health Care Professionals	http://www.icsi.org
*	Institute for Clinical Systems Improvement	Family Health Systems Minnesota Improvement Case Report on Anticoagulation Therapy (#12, 11/99)	Health Care Professionals	http://www.icsi.org

TABLE 9–42 Resources Available for APRNs With Permission—cont'd

Resources Available

*	Author/ Organization	Title/Description	Audience	Web Sites/ Order Information
	Mayo Clinic	Overview of deep vein thrombosis.	Patients and Families	http://www. mayoclinic.com (Select D under Diseases and Conditions)
	National Alliance for Thrombosis and Thrombophilia ("NATT")	A patient-led advocacy organization that includes many of the nation's foremost experts on blood clots and blood clotting disorders.	Patients and Families	http://stoptheclot.org/
	National Heart, Lung, and Blood Institute	Overview of heart, lung and blood disorders. Provides educational resources and information of on-going research.	Health Care Professionals	http://www.nhlbi.nih. gov
	National Library of Medicine-Medline Plus	Overview of varicose veins and related conditions, diagnosis, causes and treatment. Connects to additional DVT resources.	Patient and Families	http://www.nlm.nih. gov/medlineplus/ ency/article/ 001109.htm
*	Park Nicollet Health Services	Deep Vein Thrombosis: brochure	Patient and Families	http://www.icsi.org
	Vascular Disease Foundation	A nonprofit educational organization dedicated to increasing awareness of prevention, diagnosis and management of vascular diseases.	Health Care Professionals	http://www.vdf.org
	Vascular Disease Foundation (VDF)	This Web site is dedicated to reducing death and disability from vascular diseases and improving vascular health.	Health Care Professionals	http://www.vdf.org

*Available to ICSI members only. www.icsi.org

Copyright 2010 by Institute for Clinical Systems Improvement. Used with permission.

practice. For CNSs, especially new CNSs, these tools are valuable resources to plan dissemination, education, and performance audits of new innovations. A Practice Alert on VTE prevention covers expected practice along with the supporting evidence and nursing actions to ensure that patients are protected from this preventable incident and provides additional materials to assist in the collection and documentation of data (150).

THORACIC AND ABDOMINAL AORTIC ANEURYSMS

Etiology

Every year about 45,000 Americans die from diseases of the aorta and its branches (152). The average survival rate at 5 years is around 60% (153). The normal aorta is about 1 inch (2.5 cm) in diameter; women typically have slightly smaller aortas (154). The older-adult aorta grows slowly at a rate of about 0.07 cm per year and at a rate of about 0.19 cm per year in the descending and thoracoabdominal aorta (152). Aortic growth rate is a function of aortic diameter—the larger the diameter, the faster is the growth rate. In aortic dissection, the aorta grows almost 2 to 4 times the normal rate (152).

Aortic aneurysm is defined as a widening of the aortic wall 50% greater than the average aortic diameter; less than 5.5 cm for the average person (152). Aneurysms are created by a weakening of the inner layers of an arterial blood vessel due to damage to elastin and collagen fibers because of increased blood pressure or blood glucose, atherosclerotic plaque accumulation, vessel dilation, or attenuation of the aortic wall and can be found in any vessel (155, 156). As the aneurysm gets bigger, the wall tension also increases, causing a vicious cycle to occur. Of abdominal aortic aneurysms (AAAs), 90% are located below the renal arteries (infrarenal). Each year about 200,000 people are diagnosed with AAA (157). When the weakened wall begins to peel away from its other layers, it forms a false pocket that diverts blood flow; the condition is termed a dissecting aortic aneurysm (DAA). Half of all people with an aortic rupture from a DAA will die before they reach the hospital. DAA is discussed later in the chapter.

Aneurysms may develop anywhere along the aorta or the arterial vessels. Sixty percent of aneurysms occur in the thoracic ascending aorta, 30% occur in the thoracic descending aorta or the abdominal aorta, and 10% of aortic aneurysms are located in the aortic arch (Figure 9-11). Abdominal aneurysms are more common than thoracic aneurysms by a rate of 4:1. Men have a 5- to 7-fold increase in the incidence of AAA compared with women (158). Aneurysms in the lower arterial system are associated with abdominal aneurysms. Patients with popliteal aneurysms have a 62% chance that they also have an AAA; the probability rises to 85% for patients with femoral artery aneurysms. The converse is also true; about 14% of AAA patients will also have a femoral or popliteal artery aneurysm (154).

Aneurysm formation increases with age and is rare in persons under 50 years of age (158). For persons over 65 years of age, the incidence of AAA in men is 13% and is 6% in women. Upchurch and Schaub (154) noted 1-year incidence rates of aortic rupture at 9% for aneurysms 5.5 to 6.0 cm in diameter, 10% for aneurysms 6.0 to 6.9 cm, and 33% for aneurysms with diameters of 7.0 cm or more. The mortality rate from ruptured aortic aneurysm is about 80% and accounts for 15,000 deaths a year in the United States (156). The underlying mechanism of action for "why, in some people the aorta 'pops' and in others, the aorta dissects" is unknown (153).

Smoking is a major cause of aneurysm development and increases the incidence of aneurysm formation by 3- to 5-fold in former smokers (159) and 7-fold in current smokers (160) and has been shown to promote aortic wall inflammation and enlargement. Other causative factors include high blood pressure, atherosclerosis, collagen-vascular defects (e.g., Marfan syndrome, Ehlers-Danlos syndrome), tertiary syphilis (causes medial degeneration of ascending aorta and arch), poststenotic dilation (seen in aortic stenosis or mixed aortic stenosis and regurgitation), vessel injury/trauma, inflammation, infection, aging (decreased production of functional elastin), excessive protease activity (breaks down elastin), male gender (60 years or older), and genetics (154, 158). A family history of aortic disease is a major risk factor. First-degree relatives (primarily men) of persons with an

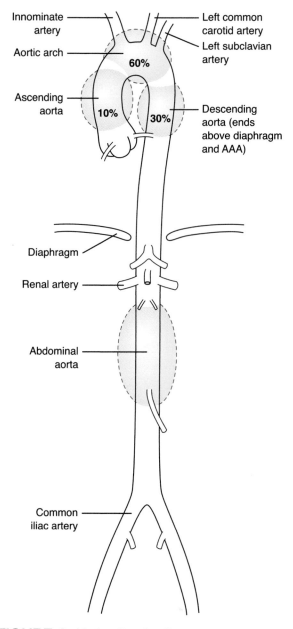

FIGURE 9–11: Location of aortic aneurysms.

AAA have a 12% to 19% chance of also developing an aneurysm (154).

The location and size of the aneurysm will dictate the levels at which medical or surgical therapies are prescribed. These cut points or "hinge points" denote the thresholds at which the aneurysm is vulnerable to rupture or dissection. For example, in the ascending aorta there is a 34% risk of rupture or dissection for aneurysm growth to 6 cm. An aneurysm of 7 cm in the descending aorta has a 43% risk of rupture or dissection (152). Because people have different physiologic structures and genetic tendencies, criteria for surgical intervention are appropriately conservative with the goal to prevent aortic ruptures and dissections. Patients with an aortic diameter of 5.5 cm for the ascending aorta and 6.5 cm for the descending aorta are referred for surgical management. For patients with a history of connective tissue disorders (e.g., Marfan syndrome, bicuspid aortic valve, Ehlers-Danlos syndrome), with chronic aortic dissection, or with a positive family history for aortic disease, especially aortic rupture or dissection, smaller size criteria (e.g., aortic diameter less than 5 cm) may be considered for surgical intervention (152). Svensson et al. advocated that symptomatic patients need to be treated regardless of the size of the aneurysm because the presence of signs and symptoms often indicate impending rupture (152).

Pathophysiology

Arterial vessels have three major layers: the tunica intima (endothelial lining of the vessel), tunica media (thick smooth muscle layer), and the tunica adventitia (outer fibrous layer). The aorta and its major branches and the pulmonary trunk are arteries that contain more elastic fibers in the tunica media than smooth muscle fibers to allow for arterial stretch and recoil. Researchers have found that at the cellular level, there is more elastic tissue in the ascending aorta and collagen fibers are dominant in the abdominal aorta (153). Weakening of the aortic wall occurs due to excess shear forces from high blood pressure and/or the deposition of atherosclerotic plaque between the intimal and medial layers. These forces lead to decreased elasticity and dilation and thinning of the vessel walls. The increased wall stress also causes a compensatory hypertrophy of the aortic wall (153). This compensatory effect does have a physiologic limit. The medial fibers break down and the weakened wall eventually protrudes, increasing the diameter of the vessel wall. This increased aortic circumference places pressure on surrounding vessels and tissues, causing impaired blood flow distal to the aneurysm and, as the aneurysm enlarges, may dissect and/or rupture.

Aneurysm morphology may vary. True aneurysms involve all three layers of the arterial wall. Pseudoaneurysms or false aneurysms do not involve all three layers and may result from traumatic aortic injury. Fusiform aneurysms are the most common and cause a uniform enlargement of the aortic wall circumference. Saccular aneurysms are weakened areas in only a small area of the aortic wall causing a distention or ballooning of the wall, like a bubble. A synchronous aneurysm is one that is proximal and distal to a previous graft (154).

Clinical Presentation

The patient with a thoracic aneurysm or an abdominal aneurysm is most often asymptomatic until the aneurysm enlarges, and then signs are usually related to compression of surrounding structures or the aneurysm starts to dissect or ruptures.

Thoracic Aneurysms

Signs of a thoracic aortic aneurysm (TAA) may be manifested as impaired blood flow distal to the aneurysm location, such as decreased pulses and pain in the right or left arm (from an ascending or arch aneurysm obstructing the innominate artery or left subclavian artery, respectively) or a stroke. Twenty-five percent of patients with a TAA complain of neck, chest, or back pain; other symptoms are shortness of breath, difficulty swallowing, hoarse cough, or signs of superior vena cava compression (congestion of head, neck, and upper extremities) (161). However, most commonly, signs of a thoracic aneurysm are those of dissection or rupture.

Abdominal Aneurysms

Frequently, the AAA is discovered by chance during a routine physical examination. The advanced clinician may note a prominent abdominal pulsating mass and a bruit may be auscultated just above the umbilicus. The patient may complain of tenderness in the area. Abdominal or back pain is a sign of AAA in some patients, as is general epigastric distress/discomfort. Presence of an AAA can affect the celiac artery, superior and inferior mesenteric arteries, renal arteries, and lumbar artery.

Mortality rates for elective AAA surgery average about 5% to 7% (162). Steyerberg et al. constructed a clinical prediction rule to estimate mortality of elective AAA surgery for an individual patient (162). This validated clinical prediction rule used both individual patient data collected in one institution and data from published studies. The resulting tool is clinician-friendly as it incorporates patient data that are readily available (HF and cardiac ischemia on the ECG, renal impairment, history of MI, pulmonary impairment, and female gender) and is easy to calculate and find the corresponding risk estimate, specific to institutional surgical mortality rates (162). See the article by Steyerberg et al. for more details (162).

Aneurysms Due to Trauma

Patients suffering from aortic aneurysms due to trauma (e.g., frontal impact of motor vehicle accident, direct high force chest injury) may have no initial symptoms of a pseudoaneurysm or subsequent aortic rupture in the ED or may offer general complaints of backache, intrascapular soreness, chest pain, hoarseness, dysphasia, and/or cough (163). However, "the index of suspicion must be high in all possible rapid deceleration events" (163, p. 52). A helical CT is the diagnostic test of choice. A CXR may show a widened mediastinum or fractures of the first and second ribs; a CT scan may reveal the pseudoaneurysm. According to research, three factors predicted death from sudden free intrapleural aortic rupture within 30 minutes of hospital arrival in a patient with blunt thoracic aortic trauma: a grossly widened mediastinum, left hemothorax, and transient hypotension (164). The positive predictive value (PPV) of this constellation of findings is 92% and the NPV is 100%. Emergency surgery is clearly indicated in patients presenting with these signs (164); the choice of an open thoracotomy approach or endovascular graft repair is based on multiple factors: the location of the aortic injury and availability of practitioners credentialed in the techniques being paramount (164). See Table 9-43 for a comparison of the two approaches.

AAA rupture may be immediately fatal if the bleed is in the abdomen. Large blood loss will cause hemorrhagic shock and circulatory collapse. Signs of shock ensue and ecchymosis of the umbilical area and/or abdominal flanks may be present. A retroperitoneal bleed may buy the patient some time as those bleeds do not have room to expand and therefore keep blood loss to a minimum and the growing blood volume may actually work to help tamponade the bleed (162).

Diagnosis

Abdominal ultrasonography is the procedure of choice. The circumference of the aorta is normally about 2.5 cm. Because the sensitivity and specificity of abdominal ultrasound in the detection of AAA is almost 100%, the U.S. Preventive Services Task Force (USPSTF) published screening recommendations (165). The USPSTF acknowledges that male patients aged 65 years and older, who have ever smoked at least 100 cigarettes, benefit the most from AAA screening. These men are urged to undergo a one-time ultrasound screening for AAA (154); Medicare has added this screening to its benefits. Other tests that may be ordered are an abdominal CT scan, MRI, or an aortogram.

Because atherosclerosis is a causative factor in the development of arterial disease, patients may be subjected to a battery of tests to establish baseline blood levels and vascular patency. Laboratory studies may include a CBC, chemistry panels, lipid panel, and coagulation profile. Cardiac stress testing may be ordered to detect atherosclerosis and guide further cardiac testing. Carotid artery assessment with carotid duplex ultrasonography, cardiac catheterization, and vascular studies of the distal vessels in the legs may provide information about the extent of atherosclerotic plaque formation (154, 155, 158).

A CXR to evaluate the heart and pulmonary system may be ordered, as well as a 12-lead ECG to assess for previous MI, signs of ischemia, LV hypertrophy, and dysrhythmias. Blood work will show elevated inflammatory cytokines: interleukin (IL)-1β, IL-6, CRP, and TNF-α.

Management

For most patients with AAA aneurysms smaller than 2 inches in diameter (5 to 5.5 cm), the aortic circumference is monitored every 6 to 12 months with CT or

TABLE 9–43 A Comparison of Endovascular Versus Open Repair Methods for Aortic Aneurysm

	Open Thoracotomy Approach	**Endovascular Approach**
Anatomical location of approach	Site ascends above left subclavian artery	Site at isthmus, size of aorta matche commerically available grafts
Hemodynamic stability	Sign/symptoms usually related to urgent rupture	Decreased procedure time, blood loss, decreased hemodynamic stress
Morbidity and mortality	3.8% inhospital mortality 1.1% to 2.7% 30-day mortality	1.2% inhospital mortality 0% to 1.7% 30-day mortality
Pros	Direct access of aneursym, definitive repair—no follow-up x-rays needed, low incidence of graft-related complications (0.4% to 2.3%)	Small incisions over femoral vessels; decrease in abdominal aortic aneursym size over time decreases rupture risk, hospital length of stay 1–3 days
Cons/risks	Aortic clamping, long midline abdominal incision, renal failure, spinal cord ischemia, systemic anticoagulation, transfusion consequences, 4–6 hours of anesthesia, longer healing time; hospital length of stay 5–10 days	Mechanical breakdown stent, retrograde dissection, false aneurysms at ends of endograft, aortobronchial fistula, graft life span unknown; need CT scan at 1 month, 6 months, 12 months and then annually; may still need open repair

From Collins and Dinsmore (2007) (163); Jones et al. (2000) (156); Upchurch and Schaub (2006) (154).

ultrasound and the patient may be treated with medications if appropriate (e.g., for hypertension). Patients with rapidly growing aneurysms that grow more than 1 cm in 6 months should be monitored every 6 months (166). Patients with AAAs greater than 5 cm should be referred for surgical treatment as soon as possible as the larger the aneurysm grows, the more likely it is to rupture. The probability of aneurysms greater than 6 cm to rupture causing massive hemorrhagic shock is 50% (156). AAAs smaller than 5 cm are usually treated medically and with lifestyle interventions (smoking cessation, control of type 2 diabetes and hypertension, diet changes).

For patients undergoing elective surgery, routine preoperative testing such as blood work and a CXR will be performed. To optimize their medical conditions, expect the patient with coronary artery disease to be on a beta-blocker for a week before surgery, the smoker to be encouraged to quit (pulmonary morbidity is decreased in patients who quit smoking at least 2 months before surgery), and to optimize renal function in the patient with impairment of renal function—the mortality rate in elective AAA repair is 7 times higher in patients with impaired renal function than in those with normal function (154). Antibiotics are usually given prophylactically before surgery, during surgery, and then continued postoperatively to prevent infection. Patient education about the procedure and postoperative care is important. Use of the incentive spirometer, coughing and deep breathing exercises, a splint pillow, early ambulation, and the PCA pump should be explained. Teaching should be reinforced in the postoperative period. The patient will be in pain after the procedure, so providing the rationale for why these interventions, which may cause pain, are necessary is important to obtaining patient cooperation and commitment to this regimen. These evidence-based interventions help to prevent complications of bedrest, including pneumonia and that could complicate recovery and further extend the patient's hospitalization.

Surgical Repair

Surgical intervention entails the use of a multifaceted procedure to incise and repair the aneurysm site without damaging surrounding tissue or the use of a minimally invasive endovascular graft. For the open surgical procedure, a midline incision is made and the abdominal aorta is cross-clamped proximal and distal to the aneurysm. Most AAAs are infrarenal and therefore the proximal cross-clamp would be placed below the renal arteries, maintaining renal artery perfusion. Suprarenal AAAs would require the vascular clamp to be placed above the renal arteries, thus depriving the kidney of blood flow. In this case, the clamp would need to be removed within an hour to avoid kidney damage. The surgeons and anesthesiologist keep a close eye on ischemic time to avoid postoperative complications of tissues that have been deprived of blood flow during the aneurysm repair. Postoperatively, nursing interventions will focus on identifying complications of prolonged ischemic time—frequent evaluations of urine output, peripheral sensation, and limb and toe movement are the norm.

Surgical intervention of the aneurysm entails slicing open the aneurysm, removing any thrombotic debris, and suturing a prosthetic graft in place; the aneurysmal sac is then sutured around the graft (155, 156). Heparin is administered in the operating room and in the ICU to prevent clotting of the graft. Expected recovery time after AAA surgery includes 1 day in the ICU and 4 to 7 days on a general floor or unit (157). In-hospital mortality rates average 3.8% (154).

Endovascular Repair

Endovascular aneurysm repair (EVAR), also known as aortic aneurysm stenting, is a minimally invasive procedure, approved by the FDA in 1999, where an endovascular stent graft carried on a balloon catheter is delivered via cutdowns in both femoral arteries and placed across the aneurysm site (155, 156). The patient is usually sedated. A percutaneous technique with local anesthesia has also been performed (166). The inferior mesenteric artery is occluded with this procedure to stop blood flow into the aneurysm. Preoperative testing includes an angiogram to make certain that the inferior mesenteric artery is not needed for intestinal perfusion and that the internal iliac artery is patent (156). Once positioned, the stent is deployed and small hooks or barbs on the graft allow it to be affixed to the aortic wall. An arteriogram is obtained to confirm the position of the endovascular stent graft via gold radiopaque markers and the catheter is removed. A bifurcated graft, consisting of a tube graft divided distally into two limbs positioned in the iliac arteries, is the most popular graft form, used in 25% to 40% of AAA repairs (156) (Figure 9-12). Anesthesia is reversed, and the patient usually is extubated in the operating room. Then the patient is transferred to the postanesthesia care unit and, once recovered, transferred to the floor. Operative time averages 2 to 3 hours with minimal blood loss of less than 600 mL; operative and in-hospital mortality rates are low (1% to 2%) (155, 156). An excellent clinical pathway and care plan for patient care following endovascular grafting can be found in the article by Jones et al. (156).

Complications of the EVAR procedure, from the most prevalent to the least, include leaks around the endovascular graft, graft dysfunction, femoral or iliac artery injury, hemorrhage, procedural complications, stent fracturing, infection at the incision sites, renal artery occlusion from displaced or migrated grafts, graft-limb thrombosis, and hematoma formation (156).

The EVAR procedure has many benefits for the patient and the institution by avoiding an abdominal incision and the resultant pain and postoperative complications

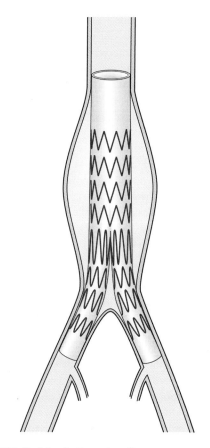

FIGURE 9–12: Aortic endograft.

that accompany a major invasive procedure, speeding up recovery time from up to 3 months to 1 to 2 weeks, and reducing costs by decreasing the length of stay from around 7 days (including an ICU stay) for an open repair to about 2 to 3 days on the floor (156, 157, 160). Endograft insertion via the percutaneous technique typically requires only an overnight stay for observation (166). However, EVAR does require scheduled follow-up CT scans at 1, 6, and 12 months, and then yearly to establish that the graft is functioning without any complications (154). In cases where endovascular grafting is not successful, the operation may be converted to a traditional AAA repair at the time of the initial procedure or in later weeks (156). Recent studies from the Endovascular Aneurysm Repair (EVAR) 1 and 2 trials have documented no difference in outcomes between EVAR and open repairs or between EVAR and "watchful waiting" (154).

At this time, for descending thoracic aorta repairs, evidence from randomized clinical trials regarding the benefit of medical versus surgical therapy is lacking, as is high-level evidence related to the outcomes of open surgical procedures weighed against those of endovascular stent-graft procedures (152). This lack of evidence to guide practice spurred a group of expert cardiothoracic, cardiovascular, and vascular specialists to develop a consensus document for the care of patients with endovascular grafts (152).

Postoperative Care

Postoperative care requires good clinical judgment and vigilance on the part of the nursing staff and the CNS (Clinical Expert/Direct Care Competency: Nursing/ Other Disciplines Sphere). Assessing neurologic status often assists the nurse to monitor the patient's recovery from anesthesia and identifies potentially devastating complications of the surgery—stroke, acute renal failure, or spinal cord injury.

Abdominal surgery creates a potential for massive fluid shifting and blood loss. Hemodynamic assessments are frequently performed and the CNS may be consulted to interpret hemodynamic data, collaborate with the inter-professional team to identify problems related to blood loss or third-space fluid shifting, and to evaluate the patient's response to interventions. The patient is continuously monitored for changes in vital signs or hemodynamic parameters (e.g., CO, systemic vascular resistance, and systemic venous oxygen saturation). The CNS may assist the staff to provide aggressive fluid resuscitation with crystalloid, colloids, and blood products.

Assessment of distal pulses and pulse quality every 15 minutes for the first hour and hourly after that, or per protocol, plus the ability to wiggle toes, is essential to recognizing ischemic damage or graft complications. Assessment and documentation of the incision site are performed. Pain is assessed according to protocol and is managed using a PCA pump with a combination opioid and analgesic administered through an epidural catheter, and additional pain medications, as needed. Routine postoperative interventions to prevent complications are initiated. Potential complications after AAA repair to be aware of are noted in Box 9-6.

Depending on the institution's policies, once stable and extubated, the patient will be transferred to a step-down unit or the floor. As the patient recovers, the epidural catheter will be removed and the PCA infusion will be changed to deliver pain medications through a central line. Eventually, the intravenous pain medications will be replaced with oral forms. Progressions of patient activities of daily living are monitored. Hospital stays of 4 to 7 days are the norm for AAA surgery. Complete recovery ranges from 6 weeks to 3 months. The success rate for open AAA surgical repairs is 90% (157).

Dissecting Aortic Aneurysm
Etiology

A DAA is a life-threatening event and one that acute and critical care nurses should be prepared to manage. The literature notes a wide range for the incidence of acute aortic dissection in the United States of 5 to 30 per 1 million people, or about 2,000 new cases per year (155). The majority of DAAs occur in the thoracic aorta (95%) (thoracic

BOX 9–6 Postoperative Complications of AAA Surgery

- MI
- Heart failure
- Dysrhythmias
- Shock (hemorrhagic, hypovolemic, or septic)
- Graft failure/occlusion/thrombosis
- Perigraph/incisional bleeding
- Hematoma
- Graft infection
- Atelectasis
- Pneumonia
- ARDS
- Acute renal failure
- Spinal cord ischemia/paralysis/neuropathies
- Ischemic colitis
- Prolonged ileus
- Aortoenteric fistula
- Thromboembolism
- Erectile dysfunction
- Pain

ARDS, acute respiratory distress syndrome; MI, myocardial infarction.
Sources: Jones et al., 2000 (154); Upchurch and Schaub, 2006 (156).

Pathophysiology

An aneurysm forms as noted in the previous section on TAAs and AAAs. Dissection occurs as the bulging aortic wall enlarges and the intimal lining pulls away from the medial layer, creating a false lumen; thus, the intimal wall dissects from the medial wall. As blood begins to fill this false pocket, the pressure from the excess volume causes the lumen to dissect further, creating a larger false lumen. As blood fills this false lumen, less blood is delivered to the tissues, causing signs of tissue ischemia leading to nerve damage, stroke, MI, shock, and death. Multiple causes of aortic dissection are reported; 66% of aortic dissections are caused by hypertension. The most common cause among younger people (younger than 40 years old) is a bicuspid aortic valve, prior surgery on the aorta, or some type of connective tissue disorder such as Marfan syndrome (155). Pregnancy is another risk factor: over 50% of aortic dissections occur in young women in their last trimester. Risk factors for aortic dissections are listed in Box 9-7.

Either the location of the aortic tear or the location of the dissection is used to categorize dissecting aneurysms. There are three types of dissections outlined in the DeBakey classification system (types I, II, and III) and there are two types of dissections that characterize the Stanford classification system (type A, proximal; Type B, distal). Table 9-44 and Figure 9-13 compare the two systems.

Clinical Presentation

Signs and symptoms of an acute aortic dissection include sudden chest pain and signs of impaired blood flow to

ascending aneurysms, 65%; thoracic descending aneurysm, 20%; aortic arch aneurysm, 10%) and 5% occur in the abdominal aorta (155).

The risk of DAA increases with gender, race, and age. African American men over the age of 40 are more likely to suffer DAA than Caucasians; Asians have the lowest rates. Individuals between 40 and 70 years of age are the most vulnerable, with the peak incidence occurring from ages 50 to 65 (155).

Aortic rupture is an often fatal complication of DAA—about 80% to 90% of patients will die from exsanguination before they get to the hospital (154); of those who make it to the hospital alive, only 50% will survive. Hospitals performing more than 30 elective AAA repairs a year (defined as high-volume hospitals) have better outcomes in terms of lower mortality rates and fewer postoperative complications than hospitals that have low rates of AAA repairs (154). Rupture of the proximal ascending aorta can cause cardiac tamponade. Other complications involve stenosis, occlusion, or dissection of branch vessels near the expanding false lumen, causing impaired blood flow to the heart, brain, mesentery, liver, spinal cord, or extremities. The aortic valve is also extremely vulnerable if the dissection is located in the ascending aorta and displaces the aortic valve leaflets, causing valve prolapse and aortic regurgitation.

BOX 9–7 Risk Factors for Aortic Dissection

- Hypertension (66% cases)
- Dyslipidemia
- Inherited connective tissue disease: e.g., Marfan syndrome, Ehlers-Danlos syndrome
- Existing disease of the aortic valve or vessels: previous aortic dissection, previous aortic surgery, coarctation of the aorta, congenital bicuspid aortic valve
- Iatrogenic causes: equipment-based intervention (e.g., catheter), aortic surgery
- Inflammatory causes: giant cell arteritis, syphilitic aortitis
- Deceleration trauma: MVA, substantial fall
- Chromosomal abnormalities: Turner's syndrome, Noonan's syndrome
- Pregnancy
- Smoking
- Cocaine use

MVA, motor vehicle accident. From Coughlin, 2008 (155).

TABLE 9–44 Comparison of DeBakey and Stanford Aortic Classification Systems and Clinical Presentation

DeBakey System	Stanford System	Clinical Presentation
Type I: Ascending aorta, aortic arch, descending aorta • Etiologies: Hypertension, atherosclerosis Type II: Confined to ascending aorta • Marfan syndrome, Ehlers-Danlos syndrome	Type A: ascending aorta; proximal tear • See etiologies for DeBakey types I, II • Usually requires emergency surgery	• Acute aortic regurgitation (AEB diastolic murmur) • >50% of patients will develop • Acute myocardial ischemia or MI (if coronary blood flow is obstructed) AEB ECG changes • Chest pain (w/ascending aortic dissection) radiating to neck, throat, or jaw (w/aortic arch dissection); • Retrosternal or midscapular sharp, tearing pain that radiates down back as dissection progresses • Anginal pain (if coronary blood flow is compromised) • Cardiac tamponade or SCD • Hemothorax • Hypotension • Neurologic deficits (stroke, altered consciousness, syncope, visual changes, hemiplegia) • Pericardial effusion • Pulse deficits (carotid, brachial, or femoral); absent upper extremity pulses or blood pressure differential • Vocal cord paralysis, hoarseness (from pressure on left recurrent laryngeal nerve) • Dyspnea, dysphagia (from tracheal pressure) • Stridor, wheezing (from tracheal compression)
Type III: Only descending aorta distal to LSC IIIa: descending aorta to diaphragm IIIb: descending aorta to below diaphragm • Hypertension, atherosclerosis	Type B: descending aorta; distal tear • Hypertension, atherosclerosis Medical treatment Surgical required only if certain patient conditions exist. For example, "Impending rupture," increasing aortic diameter or hematoma size; or vascular compromise	• Diaphoresis • Hypertension • Interscapular pain (tearing or ripping) radiating to lower back or abdomen • Lower extremity ischemia, limb paresthesia or paralysis • Motor or sensory deficit of one limb • Absent lower extremity pulses • Abdominal pain, metabolic acidosis, N/V, melena (due to mesenteric ischemia or infarction) • Oliguria, anuria, rising BUN and SCr (due to renal ischemia) • Paraplegia (due to spinal cord ischemia)

AEB, as evidenced by; BUN, blood urea nitrogen; ECG, electrocardiogram; MI, myocardial infarction; N/V, nausea and vomiting; SCD, sudden cardiac death; SCr, serum creatinine.

Adapted from Coughlin RM. Recognizing aortic dissection: a race against time. Am Nurse Today 2008; 3(4):31-35 (155).

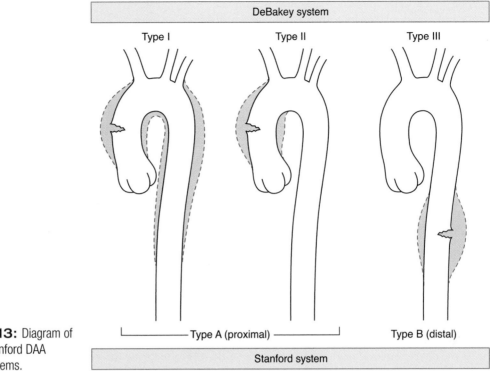

FIGURE 9–13: Diagram of DeBakey and Stanford DAA classification systems.

affected organs. Patients may describe the pain as "tearing" or "ripping" that usually radiates to the back, neck, or jaw. Excruciating back pain is a sign of dissection. Similar to MI, a small percentage of patients (10%) with neuropathic disorders or Marfan syndrome may have no chest pain during an aortic dissection. Suspicion of aortic dissection needs to be considered in patients who present with chest pain similar to that of acute MI, but have no ECG changes typical of an MI; in this case the dissection may be located at the aortic arch or at the aortic root (174). Aortic root dissection may involve one or both coronary ostia causing cardiac ischemia. The right coronary artery is most often affected leading to an inferior wall MI (174). Besides cardiac ischemia, aortic root dissections also can result in aortic regurgitation.

Impaired blood flow causes decreased tissue perfusion and organ dysfunction. Alterations in mental status may range from confusion to coma. Syncope is common and may be a sign of impending cardiac tamponade, decreased cerebral blood flow, or reflex stimulation of cerebral baroreceptors (174). Numbness and tingling of the extremities indicates decreased blood flow to the peripheral nerves. Hoarseness, coughing, or vocal problems may be a result of laryngeal nerve compression. Dyspnea may be a result of HF caused by cardiac strain and/or increased intrathoracic pressure from compression of the trachea, bronchi, or lungs from the growing mass.

Blood pressure may be elevated or depressed depending on the type of dissection. High blood pressure is seen most frequently with Stanford type B dissections, while hypotension is associated more with type A dissections. However, patients who extend their dissections may initially present with signs and symptoms indicative of a type A dissection and then show signs of a type B dissection (155). Hypotension is a consequence of cardiac tamponade. Blood pressure differences greater than 20 mm Hg between the right and left arms are indicative of aortic dissection.

Diagnosis

Astute clinicians need to demonstrate vigilance to recognize the signs of acute aortic dissection and then to begin aggressive treatment to increase the patient's chance of survival. Patients with a DAA presentation should quickly receive a 12-lead ECG, CXR, and blood testing to rule out MI, pulmonary embolism, or other plausible diagnoses. The presence of chest pain warrants the 12-lead ECG. In aortic dissection, the ECG may show some nonspecific ST-segment or T-wave changes or be completely normal. One factor that will hamper the diagnosis is aortic root dissection affecting blood flow to the right coronary artery and therefore to the inferior wall of the heart. Then the clinician would expect to see classic ST-segment changes of ischemia or injury in the inferior leads on the ECG. A CXR may not be definitive, but should be obtained to assess the cardiac size, look for mediastinal widening (an increase in the aortic diameter) and cardiac tamponade, and evaluate the pulmonary vasculature.

Patients with aortic dissection also may demonstrate cardiomegaly, tracheal deviation to the right, pericardial effusion, pleural effusions, or pulmonary edema. Calcifications of the aneurysm may be observed. About 10% of CXRs in acute aortic dissection are normal. Severe aortic regurgitation, a result of displaced aortic valves from the dissection can cause HF. Other imaging studies such as CT scan, MRI, transesophageal or transthoracic echocardiography (TEE or TTE), or aortography can evaluate aneurismal size, lumen diameter and aortic wall thickness, presence of mural thrombi or pericardial effusion, origin and extent of dissection, and valve involvement; these studies may be needed to confirm the diagnosis. Choice of studies will depend on the availability of the equipment, technical competence, and the patient's condition (155).

Blood testing may also be deceptive in aortic dissection. Cardiac enzymes are released and elevated during aortic dissection when the dissection affects the coronary arteries. Aortic dissection in the descending aorta can impair blood flow to the renal arteries, causing acute renal failure and causing an elevation in BUN and creatinine. If the dissection leaks or ruptures, expect the CBC to show a low hemoglobin and hematocrit.

New research indicated that the use of D-dimer levels can increase the confidence of the diagnosis of acute aortic dissection in patients presenting within 24 hours of the beginning of symptoms. Suzuki et al. (167) assessed the D-dimer results in 220 patients admitted for suspected acute aortic dissection. A cutoff value of 500 ng/mL was used to identify patients with aortic dissection and effectively rule out other disease processes (sensitivity 96.6%; specificity 46.6%; LR– 0.07; NPV >90%), with the exception of pulmonary embolism. A specificity of only 20% was documented when evaluating aortic dissection and pulmonary embolism patients. D-dimer levels were 5- to 10-fold higher than control patients within the first 6 hours of symptom onset; a cutoff value of 1600 ng/mL identified patients with a high probability of aortic dissection. These researchers found that D-dimer levels for patients with type A or B dissections were statistically significantly higher than alternative diagnoses (167).

Management

Immediate and aggressive treatment is in order for the patient admitted to the ICU with an acute aortic dissection. Major goals are to manage pain and blood pressure to stabilize the patients and prepare them for urgent and emergent interventions. Providing information about the management plan and maintaining a calm atmosphere will help decrease the patient's and family's anxiety. Emergency procedures include continuous cardiac monitoring and blood pressure monitoring via an arterial line; type and cross for anticipated potential blood transfusions; fluid/blood replacement (two large-bore intravenous lines

should be inserted as soon as possible); providing oxygen or assisting with intubation and mechanical ventilation; recording vital signs per protocol; assessing for neurologic deficits and urine output, administering medications to treat hypertension, myocardial ejection, and anxiety; restricting patient activity; and providing information and comfort to the patient and family (155). The use of pulmonary artery catheters remains controversial, but provide important information if interpreted appropriately.

High blood pressure must be treated to reduce further stress on the aorta and prevent further extension of the dissection. Beta-blockers are given to decrease heart rate, contractility and myocardial ejection velocity, and blood pressure. Calcium channel blockers (e.g., nicardipine, verapamil) may be prescribed for patients who cannot tolerate beta-blockers. Medications are titrated to a systolic blood pressure of 100 to 120 mm Hg or a mean arterial pressure (MAP) of 60 to 65 mm Hg to maintain perfusion to the vital organs. A sodium nitroprusside drip may be started if the BP is not maintained on beta-blockers alone. Nitroprusside is a vasodilator with effects on both the arterial and venous system, depending on the dose given. Its use can cause a reflex tachycardia and should be preceded by beta-blocker therapy. Maintain a calm atmosphere and keep the patient and family informed to reduce their anxiety levels and enable them to participate in the patient's care, if desired. Hypotension may herald ominous events such as cardiac tamponade, aortic rupture, or acute MI. Immediate surgery is indicated for cardiac tamponade or aortic rupture. Fluid or blood replacement is used to maintain blood pressure; alpha agonists such as norepinephrine or phenylephrine may be administered for persistent hypotension. These vasopressors have minimal effects on shear force (155) and therefore are the vasopressors of choice in acute aortic dissection.

If the dissection is leaking, the clinician may be transfusing blood products to maintain the patient's blood volume and prevent shock. If the dissection is a Stanford type A or has ruptured, expect immediate surgical intervention. Mortality rates for acute aortic dissection are 1% to 2% for each hour prior to surgical intervention (155). Type B dissections may be managed medically or surgically depending on the rate of dissection, aortic diameter, proximity of the dissection to major aortic branches, impending rupture, blood leakage into the pleural space, or persistant symptoms despite therapy (155).

Surgical Interventions

Surgical interventions include minimally invasive techniques or multistaged procedures for extensive aneurysms (e.g., ascending and descending aortic involvement). For simple aneurysms, an endovascular graft may be considered. Once deployed, the stent protects the aneurysmal wall from shear forces and intraluminal blood pressure (156). In time, the aneurysm will contract over the graft. This procedure is recommended for high-risk patients who may not be able to tolerate more extensive surgery.

A multistaged procedure known as the elephant trunk procedure (ETP) is performed for extensive aneurysms (168, 169) and involves replacing the ascending aorta and aortic arch with a synthetic graft extending into the descending aorta during the first phase of this surgery (168). The descending aorta is then replaced 4 weeks to 6 months after the initial surgery (168, 169). Early mortality rates after first stage repair range from 8% to 20% and up to 9% after the second stage repair (168); however, in a study by Svensson et al. (169), survival rates for the first stage ETP were 98%, and 92% for the second stage procedure. Complications of stroke and vocal cord paralysis in the first stage ETP were 5.3% each; spinal cord injury occurred in 4.3% of patients undergoing the second stage ETP (169). Other studies have shown a risk of aortic rupture early after the first procedure; although extensive aneurysms may be repaired in one complex operation, the mortality rate is high at about 17% (169). LeMaire et al. (168) conducted a retrospective review of 205 patients with extensive aneurysms who were hospitalized over almost a 16-year period; 148 underwent the ETP. The operative mortality after the first stage of the ETP was 12%, and 4% after the second stage of the procedure in this report (168). Advances in surgical techniques have decreased the mortality and morbidity rates for aortic surgeries to less than 1% for aortic root repairs, aortic valve reimplantations, ascending aortic surgery, bicuspid valve plus ascending aorta repairs, Marfan syndrome surgery, and a 2% mortality rate for complex aortic arch surgery, including ETPs. Likewise, for descending aortic repairs, including endovascular stent grafting, a less than 2% to 3% mortality rate can be expected, and the dreaded complication of leg paralysis for descending or thoracoabdominal aneurysm has been reduced to 3.1% in a most recent analysis of 285 such repairs. Similar results have been achieved in a series of 480 thoracic endovascular grafts (153, p. 1082).

For patients with aortic root dissections—the pressure of the dissection causes the aortic valve to leak blood back into the ventricle during diastole causing severe aortic regurgitation and eventual HF. Replacing the aortic root and the aortic valve is a complicated procedure. A David's and modified David's reimplantation procedure allows the aortic root aneurysm to be repaired without damaging or needing to replace the patient's native aortic valve (170). When the aortic valve does not have to be replaced, the patient has less of a risk of stroke or bacterial endocarditis and is not required to be on long-term anticoagulation therapy. If aortic valve repair is not possible, the aortic valve can be replaced with a prosthetic valve during the aneurysm surgery.

Postoperative Care

Postoperative care of the patient with a DAA continues with many of the interventions initiated before surgery: recording of continuous cardiac and blood pressure monitoring and vital and neurologic signs per protocol; medication administration to maintain heart rate and blood pressure within a target range and decrease pain; monitoring and preventing postoperative complications, such as providing wound care; and providing patient and family education. To prevent stress on the suture lines, elevate the head of the bed no higher than 45 degrees and raise the patient's legs 20 to 30 degrees. Medications administered in the postoperative period include morphine sulfate to control pain; beta-blockers and vasodilators to manage heart rate and blood pressure by decreasing stress on the aorta and maintaining blood flow through the graft; and norepinephrine as the vasopressor of choice to increase blood pressure in the case of hypotension.

Look for signs of postoperative complications. Abdominal distention, hypovolemia, MI, dysrhythmias, cardiac tamponade, sudden cardiac death, thromboembolism, pneumonia, cerebral and spinal cord ischemia, and stroke are potential complications. Postoperative monitoring should include hourly observation of chest tube drainage and other drains, presence of peripheral pulses, urine output, and routine labs. Check the CBC for hemoglobin and hematocrit values—low values indicate bleeding. Low urine output and elevations of BUN and creatinine point to renal damage. Early ambulation and correct and regular use of the incentive spirometer are proven measures to decrease the incidence of pneumonia and atelectasis in postoperative patients.

A collaborative plan should be developed with the patient and family to encourage participation in decision-making and care. Prognosis is very good with 5-year survival rates at 80% and 10-year survival rates at 50%. Predisposing factors for aneurysm formation and follow-up care are managed in the outpatient setting. Patient education should cover signs and symptoms of infection and dissection and emphasize lifestyle interventions that reduce the risk of predisposing factors for aortic dissection: smoking cessation, weight loss, low-fat/low-sodium diet, and increased physical activity.

Clinical Nurse Specialist Competencies and Spheres of Influence
Clinical Expert/Direct Care

The CNS characteristic of clinical expertise is essential to the Direct Care Competency for patients with aneurysms and dissecting aneurysms. Many interventions have already been noted in the management sections on this topic and CNSs play a role in making sure the staff is competent to provide care to these patients before and after medical and/or surgical therapies (Nursing/Other Disciplines Sphere).

Influencing the Patient/Family Sphere, aside from assisting the staff to manage these critically ill patients, the CNS may use their expert knowledge and advanced assessment skills to play a role in AAA detection before the patient needs the ICU! The physician or the APN in primary care is likely to find an AAA during a routine physical exam of the abdomen. In the acute care setting it is possible that a CNS may detect an AAA when examining a hospitalized patient admitted for a completely unrelated reason. Suspicion of an AAA should include palpation of the aorta and deep manipulation to elicit pain on aortic palpation. Almost 30% of the time, an AAA with a diameter ranging from 3 to 3.9 cm is palpable and AAAs with diameters of 5 cm or more are palpable 76% of the time (154).

Coaching/Teaching/Mentoring

With all the different health care plans, helping patients navigate the health care system is a skill with which the CNS must become proficient. Educating patients and their families of the importance of screening tools can help identify problems before they become major crises (Patient/Family Sphere). Screening for AAA has been shown to be cost-effective (165). Medicare now offers a free screening to new members within the first 12 months of enrollment in Medicare. Those eligible for the screening are men who have smoked at least 100 cigarettes during their lifetime, and men and women with a family history of AAA (157).

DYSRHYTHMIAS

Etiology

Cardiac dysrhythmias are defined as deviations in the timing and/or electrical depolarization of the cardiac tissue (171); over 780,000 people are admitted to the hospital each year for treatment of dysrhythmias (172). Dysrhythmia denotes a dysfunction of cardiac rhythm; arrhythmia denotes the absence of cardiac rhythm. Although "dysrhythmia" is the more correct term, "arrhythmia" and "dysrhythmia" continue to be used interchangeably in the literature.

Dysrhythmias may be physiologic or pathologic, benign or malignant. SVTs, heart blocks, BBBs, and sustained ventricular dysrhythmias are cardiac dysrhythmias that may present in an acute state, as an exacerbation of a chronic problem, or as the underlying cause of SCD. One of the ways CNSs influence dysrhythmia management practice is by translating evidence and technical information regarding new treatments or technologies into practical application at the bedside. Though discussion of every dysrhythmia is beyond the scope of this section, overviews of many types of dysrhythmias are incorporated throughout this chapter. AF, differentiation of SVT and ventricular tachycardia (VT), and dysrhythmias underlying SCD will be discussed.

The most common sustained acute and chronic dysrhythmia noted in practice is AF (173). Henry and Ad (174) reported that over 2.3 million people in the United States have AF. Age, gender, and race are risk factors: the prevalence of AF increases with age, male gender, and Caucasian race. Because of the aging of the population, by 2050, AF will affect almost 6 million people—many older than 65 years. Currently, 9% of the population over 80 years old has AF (174). The major complications from AF consist of decreased CO from the loss of atrial kick volume contribution and embolic stroke. People with AF are 5 times more likely to suffer a stroke than people without AF (174). APNs in acute care settings are likely to care for patients admitted to the hospital with acute presentations of AF as evidenced by hypotension, cardiac compromise, and dizziness. Additionally, AF is a complication of physiologic stressors, certain disease states, and therapeutic interventions. For example, the development of acute-onset AF, although usually transient, is common after cardiac surgery, as well as manifesting in those with long-standing AF (175, 176).

Almost 600,000 people in the United States have paroxysmal SVT and about 90,000 new cases are diagnosed each year (175). SVT with aberrancy is a dysrhythmia that may be difficult to differentiate from VT. Many clinicians mistakenly believe that SVT with aberrancy is a frequent occurrence; however, in reality, it is not (175). VT is much more common, and misdiagnosis can lead to erroneous treatment leading to adverse consequences and even death. CNSs can coach their staff on the subtleties of these dysrhythmias so that the dysrhythmias are recognized and treated promptly and appropriately.

SCD accounts for more than 60% of adult deaths in the United States (177). SCD occurs most frequently as a result of a ventricular dysrhythmia—VT or ventricular fibrillation (VF). Pulseless electrical activity (PEA) and asystole are other causes. Inherited electrophysiologic disorders can also cause SCD—long QT syndrome and Brugada syndrome are two briefly discussed in this section.

Pathophysiology
Brief Overview of Cardiac Electrophysiology

Discussion of the principles of electrophysiology and the details of normal cardiac conduction can be found in introductory texts. A brief overview of cardiac electrophysiology is presented here. The process of cardiac contraction starts with electrical stimulation of the heart. Automaticity is the ability of the pacemaker cells to initiate an impulse spontaneously. Cardiac contraction is the result of activation and opening of protein channels (ion channels) allowing the rapid movement of sodium, potassium, chloride, and calcium ions across the cell membrane, creating an action potential. Activation or deactivation of the ion channels occurs as a result of electrical stimulation (voltage-gated sodium and potassium channels), the influence of ligand substances (neurotransmitters, intracellular calcium, and adenosine triphosphate [ATP]), or physical stimulation of volume and stretch receptors (receptor-activated chloride channels) (178). The cardiac action potential relies mainly on voltage-gated channels found in sodium and potassium channels (178). Activation or deactivation of the ion channels affects the action potential and may be manipulated, for example, through medication administration such as the use of class III antiarrhythmics, which block potassium channels, or calcium-channel blockers (class IV).

The electrical property of automaticity is present in pacemaker cells found throughout the heart. Automaticity is the ability of the cardiac myocyte to spontaneously fire an electrical impulse. The property of excitability refers to the ability of the cardiac cell to be stimulated. The action potential results in depolarization of the cell or a change in the electrical membrane potential of the cell from negative to positive (the inside of the cell becomes less negative than the outside). The ability of cardiac cells to spread an action potential from one cell to another is the property of conduction. The mechanical response to these three electrical events is muscle contraction. PEA is the presence of electrical activity, but no mechanical activity, and therefore no cardiac muscle contraction.

The propagation of the action potential moves from the depolarized cells throughout the heart to stimulate adjacent polarized cells—the wave of depolarization moves through the RA to the LA through the three intra-atrial pathways and then on to the AV node. The AV node is located in front of the opening of the coronary sinus on the right side of the heart in an area known as the triangle of Koch (178). Conduction through the AV node slows down due to changes in ion currents, causing a delay in cellular depolarization. This slower impulse transmission, represented in the proximal portion of the PR interval, provides for the mechanics of atrial contraction and contribution of atrial blood volume (i.e., atrial kick) before the AV valves close during systole (178). Conduction speeds up again through the His bundle, which then divides into the right and left bundle branches. The left bundle subdivides into the anterior and posterior fascicles. The bundle branches terminate as the Purkinje fibers within the ventricles. The latter portion of the PR interval indicates His-Purkinje system activation (178). Ventricular depolarization is depicted by the QRS complex on the ECG. A synchronized cardiac contraction occurs as the electrical wavefront continues to move across the ventricles as a coordinated whole; the progression moves from the left to the right septum, then apex to base, and endocardium to epicardium. The normal action potential of the atrial tissue

lasts between 100 to 200 msec; the larger mass of the ventricles increases the duration of the ventricular action potential to about 250 to 300 msec (178). Prolongation of the action potential puts the individual at risk for potentially lethal dysrhythmias and is a consequence of hypertrophic disease states, such as HF.

All pacemaker cells have the electrical property of automaticity, although the dominant pacemaker (generally the sinoatrial [SA] node) usually overrides spontaneous firings of secondary pacemaker cells. Pacemaker tissue throughout the heart acts as a failsafe mechanism for the heart. When the dominant pacemaker slows or fails because of disease or exogenous influences, the next fastest pacemaker site takes over to stimulate the cardiac conduction. Pacemaker rate decreases as one gets further down the conduction pathway. The sinus or SA node pacemaker is located at the junction of the lateral border of the superior vena cava and RA in the sulcus terminalis and fires at a rate of 60 to 100 beats per minute (bpm). The normal rate of the AV node is 40 to 60 bpm, and the rate of the ventricular pacemaker sites ranges from 15 to 40 bpm. Any of the pacemaker sites may be stimulated by other factors to produce an accelerated rate outside of their normal range.

Classification of Dysrhythmias

Dysrhythmias can be classified in many ways. One way to classify dysrhythmias is to group the dysrhythmias according to heart rate: as tachydysrhythmias (those with heart rates greater than 100 bpm) and bradydysrhythmias (those with heart rates less than 60 bpm). Dysrhythmias may also be classified as sinus, atrial, junctional, or ventricular. Dysrhythmias grouped using this taxonomy reflect the location of the dominant cardiac pacemaker.

Sinus rhythms (SR) indicate cardiac conduction that was initiated in the sinus node. Normal sinus rhythm (NSR) (with a pulse) indicates that the cardiac conduction system is performing normally: heart rate is between 60 and 100 bpm and atrial and ventricular depolarization has occurred in the expected manner. Atrial rhythms are initiated by spontaneous firing of one or multiple pacemaker tissue sites within the atria. Atrial rhythms predominate when the atria pacemaker rate(s) overrides that of the sinus node. Junctional dysrhythmias are initiated from the vicinity of the junction of the atria and the ventricles, including the AV node, and therefore the atria are not always stimulated. For atrial contraction to occur the junctional impulse must travel backward up through the atria (retrograde conduction). Junctional rhythms are usually regular, but the atrial contribution to ventricular preload volume may be lost because of the desynchronization of atrial contraction with an open AV valve. Therefore, the loss of atrial kick is a consequence of any dysrhythmia that affects the synchrony of atrial and ventricular contractions. Ventricular dysrhythmias originate in the pacemaker tissue of the ventricles.

Disorders of Impulse Formation

Dysrhythmias may also be described as disorders of impulse formation due to either triggered or spontaneous activity or to a reentrant mechanism. Abnormal impulse formation due to triggered activity can be a result of early electrical activity (early afterdepolarization [EAD]) or late electrical activity (delayed afterdepolarization [DAD]) of the membrane potential (171); however, dysrhythmias due to triggered activity are rare (178). Additionally, the normal conduction pathway from the AV node to the ventricles may be circumvented by the existence of accessory pathways: the Kent bundle, James fiber, Brechenmacher fiber, and Mahaim fiber are accessory pathways, or shortcuts, that excite the cardiac tissue prematurely, resulting in tachydysrhythmias that may compromise CO and tissue perfusion. A slurred wave prior to the QRS complex, known as a delta wave, is a hallmark of preexcitation (178).

Reentry refers to an electrical impulse that reactivates the same portion of tissue over and over again. This restimulation of the same tissue is possible if a conduction block exists (i.e., an impulse that can only travel in one direction), along with a portion of slow conducting tissue and an area of depolarized or nonexcitable cells (179). Reentrant dysrhythmias result from three different mechanisms—reflection, circus movement reentry, or phase 2 reentry (178). These mechanisms cause either a functional block (meaning no physical obstruction) or an anatomical obstruction. Functional blocks manifest as wavefront patterns, and their labels are descriptive of their pathways: leading circle, figure-of-eight, and spiral wave (178). The conduction block stops the impulse from moving through a portion of the tissue normally, so the impulse takes an alternative route through the cardiac tissue. As the impulse moves through the rest of the tissue it eventually reaches the tissue on the other side of the conduction block. The impulse is able to enter and depolarize this tissue in a retrograde manner. If conduction is slow enough through this portion of tissue, the cells that were depolarized first are now repolarized and ready for restimulation from the original impulse moving through the reentrant circuit. This cycle will continue until the refractory period lengthens or the conduction speed increases eventually causing the impulse to die out (179). See Figure 9-14 for a diagram of a reentry mechanism.

The mechanism of AF is a reentrant circuit. Multiple, constantly changing, reentrant wavelets stimulate and restimulate the atria, creating a local circuit of intraatrial reentry (175). There are three types of intraatrial reentry mechanisms identified in AF. Conover (175) described these reentry mechanisms as (a) type I, common to 40% of patients and resulting in activation of the RA via regularly conducted wavelets transmitting quickly down the conducting pathways and resulting in paroxsymal AF; (b) type II AF, occurring in just over one-third of patients and consisting of one or two irregular wavefronts with significant conduction delay and intraatrial blocks; and (c) type III, producing sustained AF by activating the RA by multiple, chaotic wavefronts with significant functional conduction blocks and observed in 28% of patients (175).

Atrial remodeling consists of structural changes in myocardial cell structure and atrial wall and chamber size (i.e., atrial hypertrophy and dilation) and of electrical

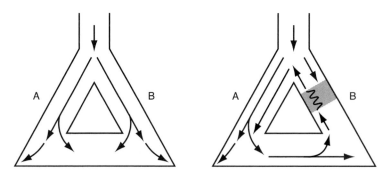

FIGURE 9–14: Diagram of a reentry circuit. Normal cardiac conduction is depicted in the figure on the *left*. All segments are depolarized in the normal manner. Reentry is depicted on the *right*. The impulse comes down the conducting pathways normally, but gets stopped at the area of the block. The impulse traveling down segment A travels normally, but once it moves across the membrane at B it hits muscle cells that have not been depolarized yet. The impulse thus depolarizes segment B in a retrograde fashion and then conducts slowly through the block. The impulse gets to the beginning of the circuit and if the myocytes have been repolarized, they will be activated again—allowing the same impulse to depolarize those cells again (circus movement). The reentrant circuit can continue a long time. When it hits refractory tissue, the cycle will end. *[Sources: Conover, 2003 (175); Calkins, 2008 (178); Wellens and Conover, 2006 (182).]*

remodeling of the conduction system due to AF. Structural changes in cardiac myocytes are progressive in chronic AF and affect almost half (40%) of the atrial myocytes by 8 weeks; remodeling of the LA appendage are also apparent (175). Structural and functional changes to the ventricles may occur because of the rapid ventricular rate in uncontrolled AF leading to tachycardia-related cardiomyopathy. Reductions in LVEF result in volume overloads evidenced by increased end-systolic and end-diastolic blood volumes and increased pulmonary artery pressures.

AF produces changes in intracellular calcium levels and potassium currents affecting repolarization, and increases ATII levels, all of which influence the electrophysiology of the heart and promote, and potentially sustain, AF. Calcium overload adversely affects mitochondrial function because of rapid atrial stimulation; potassium currents are reduced affecting membrane potentials and shortening the duration of the action potential, thereby potentially allowing the recurrent propagation of AF episodes in vulnerable patients; and ATII shortens the atrial effective refractory period, increasing the tendency to promote and sustain AF (175).

Clinical Presentation

Signs and symptoms of dysrhythmias are a result of alterations in CO due to variations in chamber filling, EF, and decreased contractile force. Decreased CO can occur because of cardiac asynchrony decreasing the contribution of atrial volume during atrial kick, shortened diastolic filling time because of a tachydysrhythmias, or ineffective pumping due to rhythm disturbances. Signs of decreased CO include lightheadedness, dizziness, mental status changes, chest pain, palpitations, dyspnea, pallor, fatigue, decreased urine output, tachycardia, and syncope.

Gender Differences and Dysrhythmias

It is well-documented that there are sex-specific differences in the presentation and incidence of cardiac disease. Physiologic gender differences related to hormones and normal life phases may be factors in electrophysiologic status and the response to alterations. For example, men have slower heart rates and shorter corrected QT intervals, on average, than women (173). Women have an average heart rate of 3 to 5 bpm faster than men, and longer corrected QT intervals correspond to an increase in the potential for ectopic beats, torsades de pointes, and antiarrhythmic medication side effects. From a therapeutic standpoint, women tend to recover more rapidly from overdrive pacing because their sinus node recovers faster than that of men (173, 180).

The mechanisms for these gender differences are not completely known, but they influence not only basic electrophysiology but also the predisposition toward and response to certain dysrhythmias. Women are more likely to suffer from inappropriate sinus tachycardia,

atrioventricular nodal reentrant tachycardia, and congenital and acquired long QT syndrome. The cause of SCD in women is most likely to result from asystole and PEA than from ventricular dysrhythmias. Increased prevalence of SVT has been documented in women during menstruation, pregnancy, and in the postpartum period. These findings suggest a possible hormonal link to the dysrhythmias and may warrant consideration of the timing of diagnostic procedures and treatment (173).

Men are twice as likely to develop SCD as women. The cause of the SCD in males is most often due to ventricular dysrhythmias (VT and VF) while asystole and PEA are the most common causes for women (173). Men have a 50% increase in the risk of AF over women and are more likely to develop AF after cardiothoracic surgery. However, the prevalence of AF in women is much higher than in men, women have more symptoms, and women tend to suffer more complications related to AF compared to men (173). Men are twice as likely to have preexcitation from accessory pathways (odds ratio [OR], 1.96 to 1.99) and more dysrhythmias with preexcitation syndromes such as Wolff-Parkinson-White syndrome (WPW) (173). Long QT syndrome affects more women than men, but men have a higher risk for fatal outcomes from first-time cardiac events.

There has been documentation of gender differences in the use of diagnostic procedures and treatments—for example, multiple studies have documented that women tend to be treated more conservatively than men complaining of the same cardiac symptoms (173). The use of ICDs in men is significantly higher compared to women (hazard ratio [HR] 3.15; 95% CI, 2.86 to 3.47 [men]; HR, 2.44; 95% CI, 2.30 to 2.59 [women]) (173). However, it appears that the response to dysrhythmia treatment is equal among men and women. Both men and women benefit from the use of radiofrequency catheter ablation for AF, ICDs, and cardiac resynchronization therapy (CRT) for HF (173).

Atrial Fibrillation and Atrial Flutter

AF, the most common supraventricular dysrhythmia seen in acute and primary care settings, is observed as chaotic atrial activation of multiple sites, producing an atrial rate of 300-600 bpm and causing the atria to lose synchronized contractions and quiver or fibrillate. The quivering of the atria impedes the regular emptying of the atrial chambers causing blood to collect and, thereby, promotes the formation of blood clots—a potentially fatal complication of AF leading to cardiac emboli and stroke. The ventricular response in AF is irregularly irregular, due to random blockage of atrial impulses through the AV node, and usually is rapid (100 to 160 bpm) (175). Ventricular filling is compromised because atrial contractions are not synchronized with AV valve opening so loss of atrial contribution (i.e., loss of atrial kick) to diastolic volume occurs, thus decreasing total CO by about 20% to 30%.

Hemodynamic symptoms can be variable depending on many factors, including the patient's hydration status and the presence of other comorbidities; hypertension, mitral stenosis, cardiomyopathy, and diastolic dysfunction also can increase the severity of the symptoms.

AF may be paroxysmal (sudden start and termination), persistent (requiring conversion back to SR), or permanent (refractory to cardioversion) (175). Premature atrial complexes (PACs) trigger the majority (95%) of episodes of paroxysmal AF; paroxysmal SVT and autonomic nervous system dysfunction inducing vagal stimulation are other known triggers (175). Causes of AF are found in Box 9-8 and include normal aging; acute and chronic disorders; disease states, or conditions that cause the atria to stretch (e.g., HF, pulmonary embolism, fluid volume excess), and post cardiac surgery (174, 175, 181). Studies of cardiac surgery patients have shown cardiopulmonary bypass with cardioplegic arrest to be the primary mechanism

---

BOX 9–8 Causes of Atrial Fibrillation

Normal aging process (increased fibrotic tissue deposition after age 30)
Acute and chronic disorders

- Cardiovascular
  - Hypertension
  - Coronary artery disease
  - Valvular disorders
  - Myocardial infarction and ischemia
  - Myocarditis
  - Heart failure
  - Myocardial irritation (intracardiac catheters, pericarditis)
  - Left atrial enlargement
- Respiratory
  - Pulmonary embolus
  - Bronchopneumonia
  - Bronchial carcinoma
  - Chronic airflow limitation
- Endocrine
  - Hyperthyroidism or thyrotoxicosis
  - Pheochromocytoma
- Metabolic
  - Electrolyte imbalance
- Neurologic
  - Increased sympathetic tone (acute illness, fever)
  - Increased parasympathetic tone (vagal stimulation)
- Other
  - Alcohol intake (acute/chronic, moderate/heavy)
  - "Recreational" drug use
  - Postoperative cardiac or thoracic surgery
  - Sleep disorders (sleep-disordered breathing; obstructive sleep apnea)
  - Obesity

---

predicting postoperative AF: 25% to 30% of patients undergoing CABG and 60% of patients undergoing valve surgery develop AF, usually 48 to 72 hours after the procedure (175). AF that occurs in the absence of a recognized physiologic cause is labeled "lone" AF; these patients are at risk of developing tachycardia-mediated cardiomyopathy.

Patients with paroxysmal AF are usually symptomatic; those with chronic or permanent AF may have adjusted to their symptoms and only speak about generalized complaints or be completely asymptomatic (known as silent AF). Hemodynamic comprise, exacerbated by certain comorbid disease processes, manifests as tachycardia, hypotension, lightheadedness, dizziness, and/or syncope. Other clinical manifestations may include severe dyspnea, palpitations, fatigue, and chest pain. Polyuria may be noted by patients, particularly after termination of the AF event; atrial stimulation releases ANP, which causes the kidney to excrete sodium and water (175, 179). The polyuria may be significant and warrant aggressive fluid resuscitation (175).

ECG findings of AF typically consist of an irregularly irregular ventricular rhythm and rate with indiscernible p waves (fibrillatory waves), because of the rapid atrial rate. Morphology of the QRS complex will vary due to the presence of underlying BBBs or accessory pathways. AF can coexist with a number of other atrial and ventricular dysrhythmias. For example, ventricular rates greater than 200 bpm may indicate an underlying ventricular tachycardia or accessory pathway conduction (176). Very rapid ventricular rates (280 to 300 bpm or greater) with wide QRS complexes are likely due to accessory pathway conduction of WPW syndrome (175).

The rhythm of AF is not always irregularly irregular—and thus can confound the diagnosis. One study of patients with AF noted that episodes of heart rate regularity occurred about 30% of the time and pulse volume regularity was noted more than 50% of the time (129). Additionally, extremely rapid ventricular rates, digoxin toxicity, complete AV block, or conversion to a fixed-conduction atrial flutter may cause AF to appear to be regular (175). Atrial flutter is usually easily differentiated from AF: *P* waves are discernible and resemble the teeth on a handsaw (flutter waves), the atrial rate is about 300 bpm with a range of about 240 to 320, and atrial flutter has a consistent atrial to ventricular block—commonly 2:1, 3:1, or 4:1. Atrial flutter may also have a variable block noted by a consistent pattern of group beating; for example, 2:1, 3:1, 4:1, 2:1, 3:1, 4:1 etc. The best leads in which to observe atrial flutter are II, III, AVF, and V_1. Untreated, atrial flutter may deteriorate into AF; AF may also transform into atrial flutter (176).

SVT and SVT With Aberrancy

SVT is a broad term indicating a narrow-QRS based tachydysrhythmia (greater than 100 bpm) that originates above the ventricles (*supra* = "above"). The mechanism is either an AV nodal reentry tachycardia, circus movement tachycardia, or atrial tachycardia (182). SVT can be paroxysmal or sustained. P waves may not be visible as the rapid rate "hides" the P wave within the QRS complex. In SVT, all of the QRS complexes look alike and the atrial and ventricular rates are in the range of 150 to 250 bpm. The patient complains of his heart "racing" and may be symptomatic.

Paroxysmal SVT with aberrancy is a regular rhythm with a rate of 150 to 250 bpm with a monomorphic wide-based QRS, causing it to look very much like VT. Differentiation of VT from SVT with aberrancy is important because the treatments differ and misdiagnosis can lead to death (175). Conover noted that many clinicians believe that SVT with aberrancy just as likely to occur as VT; however, VT is 4 times more common than SVT with aberrancy (183).

Treatment of SVT with aberrancy begins with vagal stimulation (such as coughing, carotid massage, Valsalva maneuver, facial ice water immersion) in an attempt to lengthen the AV node refractory period and "break" the reentry circuit. If vagal stimulation is not successful, give adenosine 6 mg rapid IVP, which may be repeated at double the initial dose in 3 minutes. Verapamil may be given if adenosine is not available (5 mg [for patients on beta-blockers or hypotensive] to 10 mg IVP over 5 to 10 minutes). If adenosine or verapamil is not effective, administer 10 mg/kg of intravenous procainamide slowly over 5 minutes. Cardioversion is a last step if all other measures are ineffective.

Pharmacologic treatment of VT begins with a 10 mg/kg dose of intravenous procainamide given slowly over 5 minutes instead of adenosine or verapamil (182). If myocardial ischemia is the suspected cause of the VT, lidocaine is recommended. Again, cardioversion is the procedure of choice if drug therapies are unsuccessful.

Wellens and Conover recommend calm in the face of an unsure diagnosis (182). If the patient is hemodynamically unstable, the advanced clinician should cardiovert immediately, regardless of the rhythm. Additionally, administering procainamide over verapamil is a better choice if uncertain of the diagnosis because procainamide works to convert both VT and SVT (182). Giving verapamil to a patient with VT can cause circulatory collapse and cause the dysrhythmia to become refractory to cardioversion (182). There are evidence-based clues to help the advanced clinician distinguish SVT with aberrancy from VT. Diagnostic and morphologic clues to differentiate SVT with aberrancy from VT are found in Table 9-45 (182,183).

VENTRICULAR DYSRHYTHMIAS, SUDDEN CARDIAC DEATH, AND BRUGADA SYNDROME

As noted earlier, SCD is the cause of death for almost 500,000 Americans each year. VT causes more than 70% of SCD episodes; VF, asystole, and PEA are other

TABLE 9-45 Diagnostic Clues Differentiating Supraventricular Tachycardia (SVT) With Aberrancy From Ventricular Tachycardia (VT)

Favors VT	Favors SVT With Aberrancy
General Indicators	***V₁ mainly Positive:***
Patients with a cardiac history	Triphasic RBBB pattern in lead V_1 (rSR´)
AV dissociation	Triphasic RBBB pattern in lead V_6 (qRs) ONLY if
Retrograde conduction to the atria	V_1 is positive
Ventricular fusion or capture beats	QRS <0.14 sec
Negative precordial concordance (diagnostic)	
Positive precordial concordance (strong indicator)	
Northwest axis	
Circulatory collapse	
V₁ mainly Positive:	***V₁ mainly Negative:***
Monophasic R in V_1	Narrow initial r wave in V_1 or V_2
Biphasic complex in V_1	Slick, quick S downstroke in V_1 or V_2
QRS with taller left peak in lead V_1 (Rr´)	Early S nadir in V_1 or V_2
QRS >0.14 sec with RBBB pattern	No Q in V_6
R:S ratio in V_6 <1 when QRS axis is left	

Continued

TABLE 9–45 Diagnostic Clues Differentiating Supraventricular Tachycardia (SVT) With Aberrancy From Ventricular Tachycardia (VT)—cont'd

Favors VT	Favors SVT With Aberrancy
V₁ mainly Negative: Broad R (>0.03 sec V_1 or V_2) (36% sensitivity; 100% specificity; 100% predictive accuracy for VT) Slurred S downstroke (V_1 or V_2) (36% sensitivity; 96% specificity; 96% predictive accuracy for VT) Delayed S nadir (>0.06 sec V_1 or V_2) (63% sensitivity; 96% specificity; 98% predictive accuracy) Any Q in V_6 in V_6 Right axis deviation QRS >0.16 sec with LBBB pattern Combination of broad R, slurred S, delayed S nadir, and Q in V_6 present = 100% sensitivity; 89% specificity; 96% predictive accuracy	

Data from Conover, 2003 (175); Wellens and Conover, 2006 (181).

causes. VT is triggered by a variety of cardiac and metabolic conditions, as well as proarrhythmic medications. Cardiac conditions include CAD, MI, cardiomyopathy, and VHD. Metabolic triggers are hypoglycemia, metabolic acidosis, hypoxemia, and electrolyte abnormalities (hyperkalemia/hypokalemia, hypomagnesemia). Proarrhythmic medications include class I and class III drugs; caffeine, digoxin, theophylline, antipsychotics, tricyclic antidepressants, and cocaine also can induce VT (183). VT is defined as three or more ventricular-initiated beats in a row at a rate between 110 and 250 bpm. The QRS complexes are greater than 0.12 second and often characterized as wide and bizarre. Nonsustained VT terminates within 30 seconds; sustained VT lasts for longer than 30 seconds. The morphology of VT may be monomorphic, all beats look alike and arise from one ectopic ventricular site, or polymorphic with complexes of multiple shapes, sizes, and directions signifying multiple ectopic pacemakers. Torsades de pointes, a complication of congenital and acquired long QT syndrome, is a polymorphic VT.

The rhythm of VF is chaotic and indicates the firing of erratic electrical impulses that cause the ventricles to fibrillate. The fibrillation is a purposeless movement in that no ventricular contraction occurs and therefore no blood is pumped from the ventricle into the systemic circulation. Cardiac arrest occurs and resuscitation measures and defibrillation should be initiated. Correction of reversible causes is the primary treatment for nonsustained VT; class I or class III antiarrhythmic medications may also be prescribed. Pulseless VT and

VF need to be treated immediately with CPR and defibrillation according to the ACLS Pulseless Arrest algorithm (184). IV or intraosseous (IO) access should be obtained. Epinephrine or vasopressin is administered IV/IO in between shocks. Amiodarone is the preferred antiarrhythmic at an initial dose of 300 mg IV/IO or lidocaine 1 to 1.5 mg/kg initially may be administered. One to 2 grams of magnesium sulfate is given for torsades de pointes. For patients refractory to medication, implantation of a cardiac defibrillator is recommended.

Long QT syndrome and Brugada syndrome are inherited disorders that can result in SCD. Long QT syndrome has been mentioned several times in this chapter. Brugada syndrome is a rare, autosomal dominant genetic disorder, which presents as ventricular tachydysrhythmias often leading to SCD in young, seemingly healthy people. In fact, of those presenting with SCD, about half are suspected to have Brugada syndrome (185). People of Southeast Asian ancestry have a higher incidence of this disorder. Within 2 to 3 years following the diagnosis of Brugada syndrome, almost one-third will develop VT or SCD (185). Sodium ion channel dysfunction is the cause for the tendency of ventricular dysrhythmias, and the use of class IA antidysrhythmic drugs in the electrophysiology laboratory can help to expose this syndrome (185).

In 1992, Brugada identified the ECG findings of the syndrome as those (a) similar to a RBBB pattern with a fixed or variable Type I ST segment in leads V_1–V_3; (b) a structurally normal heart; (c) an increased tendency for the development of sustained and nonsustained ventricular tachydysrhythmias provoking syncope (nonsustained), or SCD (sustained); and (d) a positive family history in a number of cases (185). Only the type I ST segment variant is diagnostic of Brugada syndrome and presents as in a coved or saddleback shape: the peak elevation of the J-point or ST segment is greater than 2 mm, followed by a negative T wave (185). Brugada sign is the presence of ventricular dysrhythmias characteristic of Brugada syndrome but without symptoms or a history of cardiac dysrhythmias or SCD. Expert knowledge of the characteristics of Brugada syndrome can help identify these patients in the ED or in other settings. At this time, an implantable ICD is the only treatment that offers short- and long-term effectiveness, although drug trials are in progress (185).

Diagnosis

Diagnosis of heart rhythm disturbances is made by a thorough review of the patient's history, clinical manifestations, and the results of electrophysiologic testing. The 12-lead ECG is usually the first diagnostic test performed when a patient is suspected of having cardiac dysrhythmias. Examination of the rhythm strip may be straightforward or scrutiny of the waveforms may be needed to provide diagnostic clues. Gender differences in the description of clinical signs and symptoms and the meaning of those manifestations have been reported in the literature (173, 180). Ambulatory ECG (commonly known as a Holter monitor) is performed to assess dysrhythmias that may be transient in nature. The patient typically wears the monitor for a 24- to 48-hour period. Long-term Holter monitoring lasting 4 to 6 weeks is used to assess the conversion and maintenance of NSR after cardioversion or surgical intervention. The recording monitor is attached to electrodes placed on the chest and is battery-powered and pocket-sized. The monitor records the heart's electrical activity throughout the day and night and the activity is downloaded and evaluated. The patient keeps a log or diary of any symptoms during the monitoring period: the log and heart rhythms are used together to aid in the diagnosis.

Cardiac mapping is a procedure that may be performed in the electrophysiology laboratory or in surgery. The purpose of mapping is to isolate the source of ectopic activity by stimulating the heart and then recording where the electrical impulses are generated. Ectopic sites may then be isolated or ablated to terminate the ability of the ectopic focus to conduct its impulse. Zak described different mapping techniques to locate and treat the ectopic foci; for details on the actual mapping techniques, see Zak (186). Radiofrequency ablation produces focused lesions using alternating, low-voltage current and is used in the treatment of supraventricular and ventricular dysrhythmias (186). Cardiac scar tissue from MI or surgery can foster the development of reentry circuits by forming areas of slow conduction and blockages in the conducting pathways. Monomorphic VT is a result of such reentrant circuits (186). Radiofrequency lesions are produced by the ablation catheter and placed in critical areas around and in the scar tissue to cut off the reentrant pathways. Moderate sedation with midazolam and fentanyl citrate is used and sedation response is monitored, as well as vital signs. Heparin is used for systemic anticoagulation and activated clotting times are monitored during the procedure. The ablation procedure takes about 3 to 4 hours and patients may be discharged home after a period in the recovery room or short-stay unit. High-risk patients may be kept overnight for observation. Complications include hypotension due to sedation, a vagal response to sheath removal, hypovolemia, bleeding at the groin puncture site, hematoma formation, or possible pericardial tamponade (186). Additional diagnostic testing may include a CBC, basic metabolic panel, thyroid panel, hepatic panel, and renal function tests.

Management

Because AF is the most common supraventricular dysrhythmia seen in both acute and primary care settings, a detailed discussion of management strategies follows. Management of patients with AF includes nonpharmacologic and pharmacologic efforts to control ventricular response, to decrease blood viscosity and platelet adhesion to reduce the risk of thromboembolic events, and to restore and maintain SR (175). In new-onset AF, the goal is to return the patient to NSR as soon as possible.

Preventing thromboembolic events is paramount for patients with AF. Anticoagulation with warfarin or ASA is dependent on the patient's stroke risk or CHADS$_2$ score (181). CHADS$_2$ is a stroke risk predictor tool and a mnemonic for **C**ardiac failure, **H**ypertension history, **A**ge ≥75 years old, and **D**iabetes mellitus (176). Patients are scored 1 point for each risk factor present and given an extra 2 points if the patient has experienced a **S**troke or transient ischemic attack in the past. Low risk is a score of 0: treatment is anticoagulant therapy consisting of low-dose ASA (162 to 325 mg/day is recommended). Moderate risk is a score of 1 and treatment is with either ASA or warfarin to an INR range of 2.0 to 3.0. High risk for stroke is considered 2 or more points, and warfarin is the drug of choice as it reduces the risk of stroke by 70% (181). Obvious contraindications to anticoagulation preclude the use of these medications.

Antiarrhythmic Therapy

The priority of controlling ventricular rate versus restoring SR continues to be studied. Antiarrhythmics are used to both control heart rate and to convert and maintain NSR. To control ventricular rate, stable patients may be administered beta-blockers or calcium channel blockers (class I, LOE B; 176). These drugs work quickly, within 3 to 7 minutes, to reduce heart rate by 25% (175). Digoxin may be also given, although its use has been questioned (175). Antiarrhythmic agents work by prolonging the atrial refractory period or by slowing impulse conduction, but many have proarrhythmic effects as well.

Acute control of ventricular rate is accomplished using Class I and class III antiarrhythmic drugs. Caution should be exercised when administering antiarrhythmics: women and patients with hypertrophied hearts are more likely to develop a prolonged QT interval and torsades de pointes with the use of quinidine, procainamide, and disopyramide (type IA antiarrhythmic medications); as well as with sotalol, dofetilide, ibutilide, and amiodarone (type III) (173). In women, other drugs that can have the same electrophysiologic effect are erythromycin and probucol (173). Table 9-46 outlines commonly used

TABLE 9–46 Electrophysiologic Effects of Commonly Used Antiarrhythmic Agents

Agents (Vaughn Williams Classification)	Electrophysiologic Effect
CLASS I	
• Class IA: quinidine, procainamide, disopyramide, amiodarone, imipramine	• Moderate sodium channel blockade • ↓ conduction velocity • Prolongs repolarization • ECG: prolonged QT interval; widened QRS
• Class IB: lidocaine, mexiletine, tocainide, phenytoin	• Mild sodium channel blockade • ↓ conduction velocity • Shorten repolarization • ECG: shortened QT interval
• Class IC: flecainide, encainide, propafenone, moricizine	• Marked sodium channel blockade • ↓ conduction velocity • ECG: prolonged QT interval; widened QRS
CLASS II	
• Nonselective β_1 β_2: nadolol, sotalol, propranolol, timolol • Selective β_1: esmolol, atenolol, metoprolol, labetalol • Amiodarone	• Beta-adrenergic blockade • ECG: prolonged PR interval, slows sinus rate, bradycardia
CLASS III	
• Bretylium, sotalol, amiodarone, ibutilide, dofetilide, dronedarone	• Potassium channel blockade • Prolongs repolarization • ECG: prolonged PR interval, prolonged QT interval
CLASS IV	
• Dihydropyridines: amlodipine, felodipine, isradipine, nicardipine, nifedipine, nimodipine • Nondihydropyridines: verapamil, diltiazem, amiodarone	• Calcium channel blockade • ECG: heart block, slows sinus rate, slows AV conduction, prolonged PR interval
MISCELLANEOUS	
• Adenosine	• Opens potassium channels decreasing heart rate, ↓ conduction velocity
• Magnesium and potassium salts • Digitalis • Atropine	• Electrolyte replacement • Cardiac glycoside • Muscarinic receptor antagonist

AV, atrioventricular; ECG, electrocardiogram.

antiarrhythmic and miscellaneous agents according to their Vaughn Williams classifications and their general electrophysiologic effects.

Synchronized Cardioversion

Even short episodes of AF can cause structural, functional, and electrical damage to the atria; therefore, the faster AF is converted to NSR, the better. Conversely, the more entrenched AF is (longer than 1 year), the harder it is to convert to NSR, and the more likely AF is to reoccur, if successfully converted (175, 176). Conversion of AF is accomplished through pharmacologic and nonpharmacologic approaches and may be delivered electively or emergently. Patients with hemodynamic compromise should be immediately cardioverted using direct current. Synchronized cardioversion is more effective than pharmacologic conversion, but necessitates the use of conscious sedation or anesthesia (176). An initial shock of 200 joules is recommended for monophasic or biphasic cardioversion of AF, although biphasic shocks have demonstrated better patient outcomes (175, 176). Prophylactic anticoagulation is recommended both before and after cardioversion to reduce the incidence of postprocedure thromboembolism (176). Antiarrhythmic medications are usually administered prior to cardioversion or after discharge to increase the probability of successful maintainence of NSR (176). Class I recommendations for care of the patient in AF are found in Table 9-47.

Carotid sinus massage stimulates vagal tone to prolong the atrial refractory period and can be used as a clinical maneuver to convert AF to NSR. Other interventional procedures with documented effectiveness include transcutaneous catheter methods such as radiofrequency ablation and surgical interventions such as the maze procedure. Catheter ablation involves mapping the atria to detect the location of the wavelet activation. Specific local firing sites

TABLE 9-47 Class I Recommendations for the Management of the Patient With Atrial Fibrillation

Recommendation	Rationale
PHARMACOLOGIC RATE CONTROL DURING ATRIAL FIBRILLATION (AF)	
	Measurement of the heart rate at rest and control of the rate using pharmacologic agents are recommended persistent or permanent AF. (Level of Evidence [LOE]: B)
	In the absence of preexcitation, intravenous (IV) administration of beta-blockers (esmolol, metoprolol, or propranolol) or nondihydropyridine calcium channel antagonists (verapamil, diltiazem) is recommended to slow and control the ventricular response to AF in the acute setting, exercising caution in patients with hypotension or heart failure (HF). (LOE: B)
	IV administration of digoxin or amiodarone is recommended to control the heart rate in patients with AF and HF who do not have an accessory pathway. (LOE: B)
	In patients who experience symptoms related to AF during activity, the adequacy of heart rate control should be assessed during exercise, adjusting pharmacologic treatment as necessary to keep the rate in the physiologic range. (LOE: C)
	Digoxin is effective following oral administration to control the heart rate at rest in patients with AF and is indicated for patients with HF, left ventricular (LV) dysfunction, or for sedentary individuals. (LOE: C)
PREVENTING THROMBOEMBOLISM	
	Antithrombotic therapy is recommended for all patients with AF, except those with lone AF or contraindications. (LOE: A)
	The selection of the antithrombotic agent should be based upon the absolute risks of stroke and bleeding and the relative risk and benefit for a given patient. (LOE: A)

Continued

TABLE 9–47 Class I Recommendations for the Management of the Patient With Atrial Fibrillation—cont'd

Recommendation	Rationale

PREVENTING THROMBOEMBOLISM

For patients at high risk of stroke, without mechanical heart valves, chronic oral anticoagulant therapy with a vitamin K antagonist (VKA) is recommended in a dose adjusted to achieve the target intensity international normalized ratio (INR) of 2.0 to 3.0, unless contraindicated. Two major factors associated with highest risk for stroke in patients with AF are prior thromboembolism (stroke, transient ischemic attack [TIA], or systemic embolism) and rheumatic mitral stenosis. (LOE: A)

Anticoagulation with a VKA is recommended for patients with more than 1 moderate risk factor (e.g., age 75 years or greater, hypertension, Heart Failure, impaired left ventricular (LV) systolic function (ejection fraction 35% or less or fractional shortening less than 25%), and diabetes mellitus. (LOE: A)

INR should be determined at least weekly during initiation of therapy and monthly when anticoagulation is stable. (LOE: A)

Aspirin, 81–325 mg daily, is recommended as an alternative to vitamin K antagonists in low-risk patients or in those with contraindications to oral anticoagulation. (LOE: A)

For patients with AF who have mechanical heart valves, the target intensity of anticoagulation should be based on the type of prosthesis, maintaining an INR of at least 2.5. (LOE: B)

Antithrombotic therapy is recommended for patients with atrial flutter as for those with AF. (LOE: C)

CARDIOVERSION OF ATRIAL FIBRILLATION

a. Pharmacologic Cardioversion

b. Direct-Current Cardioversion

Administration of flecainide, dofetilide, propafenone, or ibutilide is recommended for pharmacologic cardioversion of AF. (LOE: A)

When a rapid ventricular response does not respond promptly to pharmacologic measures for patients with AF with ongoing myocardial ischemia, symptomatic hypotension, angina, or HF, immediate R-wave synchronized direct-current cardioversion is recommended. (LOE: C)

Immediate direct-current cardioversion is recommended for patients with AF involving preexcitation when very rapid tachycardia or hemodynamic instability occurs. (LOE: B)

Cardioversion is recommended in patients without hemodynamic instability when symptoms of AF are unacceptable to the patient. In patients with early relapse of AF after cardioversion, repeated direct-current cardioversion attempts may be made following administration of antiarrhythmic medication. (LOE: C)

For patients with AF of 48-h duration or longer, or when the duration of AF is unknown, anticoagulation (INR 2.0 to 3.0) is recommended for at least 3 wk prior to and 4 wk after cardioversion, regardless of the method (electrical or pharmacological) used to restore sinus rhythm. (LOE: B)

TABLE 9–47 Class I Recommendations for the Management of the Patient With Atrial Fibrillation—cont'd

Recommendation	Rationale
CARDIOVERSION OF ATRIAL FIBRILLATION	
	Administer IV heparin concurrently (unless contraindicated) in patients with AF of >48-h duration requiring immediate cardioversion because of hemodynamic instability, by an initial intravenous bolus injection followed by a continuous infusion in a dose adjusted to prolong the activated partial thromboplastin time to 1.5 to 2 times the reference control value. Thereafter, oral anticoagulation (INR 2.0 to 3.0) should be provided for at least 4 wk, as for patients undergoing elective cardioversion. Limited data support subcutaneous administration of low-molecular-weight heparin in this indication. (LOE: C)
c. Prevention of Thromboembolism in Patients With Atrial 77 Undergoing Cardioversion	For patients with AF of less than 48-h duration associated with hemodynamic instability (angina pectoris, myocardial infarction [MI], shock, or pulmonary edema), cardioversion should be performed immediately without delay for prior initiation of anticoagulation. (LOE: C)
d. Maintenance of Sinus Rhythm	Before initiating antiarrhythmic drug therapy, treatment of precipitating or reversible causes of AF is recommended. (LOE: C)
POSTOPERATIVE ATRIAL FIBRILLATION	
	Treatment with an oral beta-blocker to prevent postoperative AF is recommended for patients undergoing cardiac surgery; unless contraindicated. (LOE: A)
	Administration of AV nodal blocking agents is recommended to achieve rate control (LOE: B)
ACUTE MYOCARDIAL INFARCTION	
	Direct-current cardioversion is recommended for patients with severe hemodynamic compromise or intractable ischemia, or when adequate rate control cannot be achieved with pharmacologic agents in patients with acute MI and AF. (LOE: C)
	Intravenous administration of amiodarone is recommended to slow a rapid ventricular response to AF and improve LV function in patients with acute MI. (LOE: C)
	Intravenous beta-blockers and nondihydropyridine calcium antagonists are recommended to slow a rapid ventricular response to AF in patients with acute MI who do not display clinical LV dysfunction, bronchospasm, or AV block. (LOE: C)
	For patients with AF and acute MI, administration of unfractionated heparin by either continuous intravenous infusion or intermittent subcutaneous injection is recommended in a dose sufficient to prolong the activated partial thromboplastin time to 1.5 to 2 times the control value, unless contraindications to anticoagulation exist. (LOE: C)
MANAGEMENT OF ATRIAL FIBRILLATION ASSOCIATED WITH THE WOLFF-ARKINSON-WHITE (WPW) PREEXCITATION SYNDROME	
	Catheter ablation of the accessory pathway is recommended in symptomatic patients with AF who have WPW syndrome, particularly those with syncope due to rapid heart rate or those with a short bypass tract refractory period. (LOE: B)

Continued

TABLE 9–47 Class I Recommendations for the Management of the Patient With Atrial Fibrillation—cont'd

Recommendation	Rationale

MANAGEMENT OF ATRIAL FIBRILLATION ASSOCIATED WITH THE WOLFF-ARKINSON-WHITE (WPW) PREEXCITATION SYNDROME

Immediate direct-current cardioversion is recommended to prevent ventricular fibrillation in patients with a short anterograde bypass tract refractory period in whom AF occurs with a rapid ventricular response associated with hemodynamic instability. (LOE: B)

Intravenous procainamide or ibutilide is recommended to restore sinus rhythm in patients with WPW in whom AF occurs without hemodynamic instability in association with a wide QRS complex on the electrocardiogram (ECG) (greater than or equal to 120-ms duration) or with a rapid preexcited ventricular response. (LOE: C)

HYPERTHYROIDISM

Beta-blockers are recommended to control the rate of ventricular response in patients with AF complicating thyrotoxicosis, unless contraindicated. (LOE: B)

If a beta-blocker cannot be used, administration of a nondihydropyridine calcium channel antagonist (diltiazem or verapamil) is recommended to control the ventricular rate in patients with AF and thyrotoxicosis. (LOE: B)

In patients with AF associated with thyrotoxicosis, oral anticoagulation (INR 2.0 to 3.0) is recommended to prevent thromboembolism, as recommended for AF patients with other risk factors for stroke. (LOE: C)

Once a euthyroid state is restored, recommendations for antithrombotic prophylaxis are the same as for patients without hyperthyroidism. (LOE: C)

MANAGEMENT OF ATRIAL FIBRILLATION DURING PREGNANCY

Digoxin, a beta-blocker, or a nondihydropyridine calcium channel antagonist is recommended to control the rate of ventricular response in pregnant patients with AF. (LOE: C)

Direct-current cardioversion is recommended in pregnant patients who become hemodynamically unstable due to AF. (LOE: C)

Protection against thromboembolism is recommended throughout pregnancy for all patients with AF (except those with lone AF and/or low thromboembolic risk). Therapy (anticoagulant or aspirin) should be chosen according to the stage of pregnancy. (LOE: C)

MANAGEMENT OF ATRIAL FIBRILLATION IN PATIENTS WITH HYPERTROPHIC CARDIOMYOPATHY (HCM)

Oral anticoagulation (INR 2.0 to 3.0) is recommended in patients with HCM who develop AF, as for other patients at high risk of thromboembolism. (LOE: B)

MANAGEMENT OF ATRIAL FIBRILLATION IN PATIENTS WITH PULMONARY DISEASE

Correction of hypoxemia and acidosis is the recommended primary therapeutic measure for patients who develop AF during an acute pulmonary illness or exacerbation of chronic pulmonary disease. (LOE: C)

TABLE 9-47 Class I Recommendations for the Management of the Patient With Atrial Fibrillation—cont'd

Recommendation	Rationale

MANAGEMENT OF ATRIAL FIBRILLATION IN PATIENTS WITH PULMONARY DISEASE

A nondihydropyridine calcium channel antagonist (diltiazem or verapamil) is recommended to control the ventricular rate in patients with obstructive pulmonary disease who develop AF. (LOE: C)

Direct-current cardioversion should be attempted in patients with pulmonary disease who become hemodynamically unstable as a consequence of AF. (LOE: C)

Adapted from Fuster et al. ACC/AHA/ESC 2006 guidelines for the management of patients with atrial fibrillation-executive summary: a report of the American College of Cardiology/American Heart Association Task Force on Practice Guidelines and the European Society of Cardiology Committee for Practice Guidelines (Writing Committee to Revise the 2001 Guidelines for the Management of Patients with Atrial Fibrillation). Circulation 2006;114(6):700-752 (176).

may be ablated or involvement of the entire atrium may be detected and lesions formed to circumvent the reentrant circuits (181). In some cases of refractory AF, ablation of the AV node may be performed to eliminate electrical conduction between the atria and the ventricles; a pacemaker will need to be implanted to electrically stimulate the heart, if needed (181). Postprocedure monitoring will include frequent assessments of vital signs, distal pulses, and cardiac rhythm; evaluation of incisions for integrity and signs of infection; and observation of complications such as hematoma formation or bleeding at the groin puncture site (181).

Surgical Therapy: The Maze Procedure

The maze procedure attempts to redirect the aberrant atrial impulses by ablating the ectopic pathways and creating a surgical surface route (or maze) for the electrical charge to follow. The surgical scar prohibits the transmission of electrical impulses across the suture line. The LA appendage is oversewn or removed to decrease the incidence of thromboembolic events. The maze procedure has undergone revisions in the years since it was first introduced in 1987 and is now known as the maze IV procedure and has been associated with positive patient outcomes (174). Benefits of the maze IV procedure are that the intervention is a shorter operation performed using a minimally invasive approach versus a median sternotomy and results in fewer complications (174).

Henry and Ad (174) presented detailed care of the patient following the maze procedure; these guidelines include antiarrhythmic therapy to prevent and treat postoperative AF (amiodarone is the drug of choice); maintenance of potassium levels greater than 4 and magnesium greater than 2; aggressive diuretic therapy with furosemide

and aldactone; and anticoagulant therapy (warfarin [Coumadin] is the drug of choice). The full-text version of evidence-based guidelines for the management of patients with AF was produced by the American College of Cardiology (ACC), the American Heart Association (AHA), and the European Society of Cardiology (ESC). The guidelines are available on the AHA Web site (www.myamericanheart.org) and in print (176).

Following the maze procedure, the patient is returned to ICU and cared for according to evidence-based protocols and guidelines. Temporary pacing wires are inserted during surgery, in case the patient requires an external pacemaker and allow for daily atrial ECGs to be obtained. Spironolactone and furosemide are administered to reduce fluid excess and prevent pulmonary edema and pleural effusions. Fluid volume excess ranks as the most frequent complication affecting almost half of all patients after the maze procedure (174). Spironolactone and furosemide are continued for about a month after discharge from the hospital. Follow-up testing of electrolytes is vital. Although a class IIa recommendation for the prevention of AF in cardiac surgery patients in the current guidelines (176), recent studies have shown that amiodarone and amiodarone plus metoprolol have been shown to prevent postoperative AF after cardiac surgery, as well as reduce the incidence of ventricular tachyarrhythmias, stroke, and increased length of stay (174). Long-term treatment with warfarin has been a common intervention to prevent clot formation—although the need of long-term anticoagulation after the maze procedure is being questioned (174). The expected outcome of the maze procedure is a return to NSR. Patients who do not convert to NSR may need to be electrically cardioverted.

Clinical Nurse Specialist Competencies and Spheres of Influence

Clinicians need the expertise of the CNS to translate research and evidence into practice (Nursing/Other Disciplines Sphere of Influence). The CNS characteristics of clinical judgment and caring practices are embodied in the core competency of Clinical Expert/Direct Care and in the Patient/Family Sphere. Clearly, disorders that are potentially life-threatening require expert clinical judgment and vigilance on the part of the nurse. Patients with dysrhythmias that disrupt their activities of daily living and/or are potentially lethal are often anxious and need nursing staff who understand how the dysrhythmia affects their quality of life. Caring practices are considered the soul of nursing care. Facilitation of learning takes place in the Patient/Family and Nursing/Other Disciplines Spheres of Influence and is the characteristic mainly reflected in the core competency of Coaching/Teaching/Mentoring.

Research/Evidence-Based Practice

Accurate diagnosis of dysrhythmias relies on accurate ECG monitoring. Much research has been conducted in the area of ECG, including the best monitoring leads for dysrhythmia identification. CNSs can influence practice by ensuring that policies and procedures for cardiac monitoring reflect best practices. Staff education and competency measures can be developed from the evidence and performance can be monitored to assess understanding of the standards and to ensure safe and effective patient monitoring. Assessment of accurate lead placement is essential because misplaced leads can result in misdiagnosis and potentially erroneous treatment (187). CNSs may need to schedule formal orientation sessions, brief inservices, or continuing education to educate the staff on the use of new monitoring equipment, the setting of alarm parameters, appropriate documentation of dysrhythmias, or management of patients undergoing specialized procedures. Hands-on training helps build confidence, and annual competency testing should be implemented (187). Resources are available to assist the CNS in establishing best practice. AACN has produced a "Practice Alert" on dysrhythmia monitoring available on its Web site (www.aacn.org) (188).

Practice standards for ECG monitoring (187) have been published. The ECG practice standards define patients who would benefit from ECG monitoring and provide expert consensus on recommendations for cardiac monitoring of adults and children (187). QT-interval and ST-segment monitoring are discussed in these practice standards.

QT-interval monitoring to detect prolonged QT intervals is not a universal standard but strongly recommended for (a) patients receiving antiarrhythmic medications that are known to be proarrhythmic, (b) patients who have overdosed on medications that may cause dysrhythmias, and (c) patients with new-onset Bradydysrhythmias (187). ST-segment monitoring is a class I intervention, per expert consensus, to detect myocardial ischemia for patients in early stages of acute coronary syndrome, patients presenting to the ED with chest pain or anginal equivalent symptoms, patients post nonurgent coronary interventional procedures, and patients with possible variant angina from coronary artery spasm, yet ST-segment monitoring also is not universally implemented (187). CNSs can help improve practice in this area by translating the evidence on the efficacy of ST-segment monitoring for their staff and administrators. Resources are available to assist the CNS to communicate the research and measure performance. For example, AACN also has a Practice Alert on ST-segment monitoring (189).

Credible, regularly updated, evidence-based guidelines exist for the management of patients with cardiac rhythm abnormalities (176, 190). The AHA Web site (www.myamericanheart.org) maintains a database of current guidelines produced by the AHA, and in collaboration with other professional organizations, dedicated to cardiovascular health.

Clinical Expert/Direct Care

Identifying patients at high risk for developing lethal dysrhythmias is a first step in providing excellent care and heading off potential crises. The paroxysmal nature of many dysrhythmias renders the characteristic of vigilance all the more important. The expert clinical knowledge of the CNS assists the nurses to recognize and interpret signs of impending events and to respond quickly in critical situations. Potential antiarrhythmic drug interactions and toxicities should be identified early and nurses should remain observant for common complications after therapeutic procedures and medication administration. For example, nursing implications of amiodarone therapy include continuous cardiac monitoring and vigilance for the development of ventricular dysrhythmias due to QRS widening and a prolongation of the QT interval. Amiodarone's long half-life (weeks to months) translates into continual drug effects long after the drug is discontinued. Pulmonary toxicity is a major adverse effect of amiodarone therapy, and signs and symptoms of respiratory distress or failure must be quickly treated. Obtaining routine CXRs can help to identify signs of pulmonary toxicity; laboratory testing of liver, thyroid, metabolic, and coagulation function is important to monitor function after long-term amiodarone therapy (191).

Patients who have experienced the acute onset of dysrhythmias, or especially SCD, may be anxious, fearing another dysrhythmic episode or death. CNSs can provide reassurance and emotional support for patients and their family members, role modeling caring practice.

Coaching/Teaching/Mentoring

CNS expertise in the Coaching/Teaching/Mentoring core competency is very important for patients with dysrhythmias (Patient/Family Sphere) and the nurses who care for them (Nursing/Other Disciplines Sphere). Patients and interested family members should be taught about their particular disease process and/or dysrhythmia, along with information on medications, lifestyle modifications to reduce risk factors that may predispose them to recurrent dysrhythmias, the use of implantable devices, side effects and symptoms to report, exercise recommendations, any physical or social restrictions. Emergency measures, including how to perform cardiopulmonary resuscitation (CPR), the use of an automatic external defibrillator (AED), and calling 911 in an emergency are important skills that family members should be taught to care for their family member with acute-onset dysrhythmias (183).

CNSs should ensure that the nursing staff is educated as to the complex care management of the patient with dysrhythmias. Informal bedside nursing rounds are opportunities for the CNS to assess the skill level and knowledge of the staff nurse. This interaction with the nursing staff presents many chances for teachable moments. Inservices and hands-on demonstrations of the software to monitor ST segments will increase the nurses' confidence in using these new systems. Staff may need education and practice sessions regarding ECG interpretation. Recognizing changes on the ECG and monitoring for potentially lethal dysrhythmias is vital to the safe recovery of the patient.

CARDIOMETABOLIC SYNDROME

Etiology

Cardiometabolic syndrome is a group of endocrine, metabolic, and cardiovascular risk factors (hypertension, insulin resistance, abdominal obesity, and dyslipidemia) known to predispose to type 2 diabetes mellitus (and subsequent cardiovascular diseases (192). The cluster of risk factors for this diagnosis was first identified in the 1920s, and the android type of body obesity was first associated with metabolic syndrome in 1947 (193). Grouping the risk factors into a "syndrome" diagnosis increases the predictive power for identifying subjects at risk for subsequent type 2 diabetes and/or coronary heart disease, better than any individual risk factor (194). However, not all health care professionals agree that metabolic syndrome should be considered as a diagnostic category (195, 196).

A variety of names have been associated with this syndrome: cardiometabolic syndrome, metabolic syndrome, dysmetabolic syndrome, syndrome X, insulin resistance syndrome, plurimetabolic syndrome, and "the deadly quartet" (192, 197, 198). Although insulin resistance is a significant feature that precedes the other characteristics (193), metabolic syndrome is not caused by insulin resistance alone nor can insulin resistance explain all of the manifestations of the syndrome. Additionally, people without insulin resistance also may have metabolic syndrome. In patients with normal glucose tolerance, metabolic syndrome has been identified in 10% of women and 15% of men; in patients with impaired fasting glucose, 42% of women and 64% of men have metabolic syndrome; and the statistics are highest in those with type 2 diabetes: 78% of women and 84% of men (199). Eighty percent of people over 60 years old with type 2 diabetes are estimated to have metabolic syndrome (192). Thus, the term metabolic syndrome was adopted by the WHO to acknowledge the abnormalities of carbohydrate and lipid metabolism in this diagnosis (194).

Health care professionals agree that cardiometabolic syndrome is a huge public health problem in westernized countries because the risk factors, individually and collectively, lead to the number one cause of death in the world—cardiovascular disease (192, 194, 198). In 2000, over 55 million Americans had metabolic syndrome (200) and one-quarter of the world's adult population is affected (201). The overall prevalence of metabolic syndrome in the United States is 22% to 25% depending on which diagnostic criteria are used (192, 198); that risk may be over 50% in the elderly (198). The increase in the prevalence of cardiometabolic syndrome is related to the increasing frequency of obesity and diabetes in the United States and across the world (193). In a national study done in the United States (the third National Health and Nutrition Examination Survey [NHANES]), 58% of obese men had metabolic syndrome (192). The risk of stroke in obese persons with metabolic syndrome is 3 times greater than in persons without the syndrome (202).

The risk of metabolic syndrome is high in certain patient populations and ethnic groups due to higher incidences of diseases that are in the constellation of signs of metabolic syndrome. For example, HIV-positive patients, Filipina women, and Native Americans (particularly Pima Indians) have a high incidence of metabolic syndrome (200). Hispanics, especially Mexicans, have a higher risk than African Americans or Caucasians, because they have a higher incidence of type 2 diabetes than other ethnic groups. African Americans have a higher incidence of hypertension in the United States (22% prevalence), adding to their increased risk for metabolic syndrome.

In the United States, Mississippi has the highest CVD mortality. Researchers conducting the Jackson Heart Study studied over 5,000 African American subjects in Mississippi for risk factors of CVD. Of these subjects over 37% met National Cholesterol Education Program's Adult Treatment Panel III (NCEP: ATP III), diagnostic criteria for metabolic syndrome with incidence rates of 15.9% (34 years or younger), 39.4% (45 to 64 years old), and almost 50% for subjects 65 and older (199). Women had a higher prevalence than men (41.2% to 30.1%) and central obesity and hypertension were present in over 60% of the population. The prevalence rate for metabolic syndrome in Hispanics is 32%; however, it is believed that this group may be underdiagnosed for metabolic syndrome in the United States (202). South Asians from the Indian subcontinent and Southeast Asians (e.g., Polynesian, Japanese) are also a higher risk (199), although the prevalence rates vary by the diagnostic criteria used to diagnose the condition.

Gender plays in role in risk stratification also: African American women are at higher risk than Caucasian women and Caucasian men are at higher risk for metabolic syndrome than African American men (198). In the San Antonio Heart Study (203), a cohort of almost 3,000 people was studied to determine the risk of CVD, using both the NCEP: ATP III criteria and the WHO criteria for metabolic syndrome. After adjusting for age and ethnicity, using the NCEP: ATP III definition, women with metabolic syndrome were almost 5 times more likely to die of CVD than are women who did not have metabolic syndrome (HR 4.65; 95% CI, 2.35 to 9.21); the hazard ratio showed almost 3 times the risk of dying from CVD in women, using the WHO criteria (HR 2.83; 95% CI, 1.55 to 5.17) (203).

HRs for men with metabolic syndrome were 1.82 (95% CI, 1.14 to 2.91; NCEP: ATP III criteria) and 1.15 (95% CI, 0.72 to 1.86; WHO criteria). There was a significant interaction effect between gender and cardiovascular mortality showing the NCEP: ATP III and WHO criteria were significantly more predictive of cardiovascular mortality in women than in men (p = 0.03 and p = 0.02, respectively) (203). Results from the Prospective Cardiovascular Münster (PROCAM) study demonstrated that middle-aged men (40 to 65 years old) with type 2 diabetes or hypertension have a 2.5% increase in the risk of MI; that risk increases to 8 times the risk if both disease processes are present and to 19 times the risk of MI if type 2 diabetes, hypertension, and dyslipidemia are all present (199).

Comparing reports of the prevalence of metabolic syndrome can be difficult because there is no universal definition and the definitions used incorporate different diagnostic criteria (193). These definitions or conceptual frameworks can be classified based on three major causes of metabolic syndrome: (a) environmental causes (e.g., NCEP: ATP III framework); (b) insulin resistance (e.g., WHO framework); or (c) inflammation (195). Currently there are seven definitions of *cardiometabolic syndrome* proposed from the American Heart Association/National Heart, Lung, and Blood Institute (AHA/NHLBI), WHO, the National Cholesterol Education Program's Adult Treatment Panel III (NCEP: ATP III), the

European Group for the Study of Insulin Resistance (EGIR), the American Diabetes Association (ADA), The International Diabetes Foundation (IDF), and the American College of Endocrinology/American Association of Clinical Endocrinologists (ACE/AACE). The WHO definition is considered more relevant for research and used more commonly in Europe, whereas the NCEP: ATP III definition is more accepted and used in the United States and considered more practical for clinical practice (193, 203). Table 9-48 compares these definitions (193, 198, 204).

The central characteristics of metabolic syndrome are defined by the majority of definitions and include dyslipidemia, abnormal glucose metabolism, hypertension, and central obesity; however, insulin resistance, found in the majority of patients with metabolic syndrome, is not a mandatory criterion in three of the six definitions (NCEP: ATP III; AHA/NHLBI; or IDF) of *metabolic syndrome*. According to published research, obesity does not have as strong an influence on insulin resistance as does race (202). *Insulin resistance* is defined as a fasting blood glucose greater than 110 mg/dL. Most of the definitions use this criterion; however, the ACE/AACE and AHA/NHLBI definitions use the lower limit of 100 mg/dL for their definition of insulin resistance. In addition, proinflammatory and prothrombotic states have been identified as associated with insulin resistance and metabolic syndrome, and multiple authors have discussed the addition of specific cytokines to the criteria for diagnosis (193, 195). These definitions should continue to be revised as new markers (i.e., inflammatory cytokines) are found and tested. For example, the addition of highly sensitive CRP (hsCRP) greater than 3 mg/L has been proposed to be added to the current definition of metabolic syndrome (201). Table 9-48 compares the different definitions and diagnostic criteria of the major definitions. The NCEP: ATP III definition is the one most widely used in clinical practice.

There is a lot of disagreement as to the diagnostic criteria that define metabolic syndrome, as well as the underlying mechanisms of action (195, 196, 201). Kahn et al. (196) stated that:

> *While there is no question that certain CVD risk factors are prone to cluster, we found that the metabolic syndrome has been imprecisely defined, there is a lack of certainty regarding its pathogenesis, and there is considerable doubt regarding its value as a CVD risk marker. Our analysis indicates that too much critically important information is missing to warrant its designation as a "syndrome." Until much needed research is completed, clinicians should evaluate and treat all CVD risk factors without regard to whether a patient meets the criteria for diagnosis of the "metabolic syndrome" (p. 2289) . . . [instead of] drawing attention to and labeling millions of people with a presumed disease that does not stand on firm ground (p. 2299).*

TABLE 9-48 Comparison of International and National Definitions of Cardiometabolic Syndrome

	ACE/AACE, 2002	ADA, 1998	AHA/NHLBI, 2005	ERIG, 1999	IDF, 2004	NCEP: ATP III, 2001	WHO, 1999
DIAGNOSIS INCLUDES:							
	2 hr post 75 g glucose challenge >140 mg/dL or fasting glucose 110–125 mg/dL, plus any 2 of the following	Insulin resistance	3 or more of the following:	Insulin resistance, plus 2 or more of the following:	Central obesity with waist circumference r/t ethnicity, plus any 2 of the following:	3 or more of the following:	Type 2 diabetes or impaired fasting glycemia or impaired glucose tolerance or insulin resistance by $HOMA_{IR}$, plus 2 or more of the following:
BMI							
	≥25				>23–24 Asians >25 Caucasians		>30
WAIST CIRCUMFERENCE							
		Central obesity	40″ men (>102 cm) 35″ women (>88 cm)	≥94 cm men ≥80 cm women	>90 (Asian men) >94 cm men >80 cm women	40″ men 35″ women Or if genetically at risk for DM: 37–39″ men 31–35″ women	Waist-hip ratio >0.90 (men) >0.85 (women)

Continued

TABLE 9-48 Comparison of International and National Definitions of Cardiometabolic Syndrome—cont'd

	ACE/AACE, 2002	ADA, 1998	AHA/NHLBI, 2005	ERIG, 1999	IDF, 2004	NCEP: ATP III, 2001	WHO, 1999
HDL CHOLESTEROL	<40 mg/dL men <50 mg/dL women	Low HDL	<40 mg/dL men <50 mg/dL women Or on medications for ↓ HDL-C	<1.0 mmol/L	<40 mg/dL men <50 mg/dL women	<40 mg/dL men <50 mg/dL women Or on medications for ↓ HDL-C	<35 mg/dL men (<1.0 mmol/L) <40 mg/dL women (<1.3 mmol/L)
LDL CHOLESTEROL		Small dense LDL					
TRIGLYCERIDES (TG)	≥150 mg/dL	High TG	≥150 mg/dL Or on medications for ↑ TG	>2.0 mmol/L	≥150 mg/dL	≥150 mg/dL Or on medications for ↑ TG	≥150 mg/dL (≥1.7 mmol/L)
BLOOD PRESSURE	≥130/85 mm Hg	HTN	≥130 mm Hg systolic Or ≥85 mm Hg diastolic Or on medications for HTN (w/Hx of HTN)	≥140/90 mm Hg Or on medications for HTN	≥130/85 mm Hg	≥130/85 mm Hg Or on medications for HTN	≥140/90 mm Hg on medications for HTN OR ≥160/90 mm Hg untreated
FASTING BLOOD GLUCOSE (BG)	≥100 mg/dL Or on medications for ↑ BG		≥100 mg/dL Or on medications for ↑ BG	≥110 mg/dL (≥6.1 mmol/L)	≥100 mg/dL (≥5.6 mmol/L)	≥110 mg/dL Or on medications for ↑ BG	

363 Cardiovascular Problems

OTHER RISK FACTORS

OTHER RISK FACTORS
Family Hx of type 2 diabetes, HTN, CVD; polycystic ovary syndrome; prior gestational diabetes; sedentary lifestyle; advancing age; ethnic group susceptible to type 2 diabetes or CVD
Increased prothrombotic and antifibrinolytic factors Increased atherosclerotic disease
Microalbuminemia ≥ 20 mcg/min Albumin/creatinine ratio >20 mg/g

Data from Eckel et al. 2005 (193); Grundy et al. (2005) (204); Miranda et al. (2005) (198).

International/National Organizations: ACE/AACE, American College of Endocrinology/American Association of Clinical Endocrinologists; ADA, American Diabetes Association; AHA/NHLBI, American Heart Association/National Heart, Lung, and Blood Institute; EGIR, European Group for the Study of Insulin Resistance; NCEP: ATP III, National Cholesterol Education Program's Adult Treatment Panel III; IDF, International Diabetes Foundation; WHO, World Health Organization.

BMI, body mass index; CVD, cardiovascular disease; Dx, diagnosis; HDL, high density lipoprotein; HOMA$_{IR}$, homeostatic model assessment of insulin resistance; HTN, hypertension; Hx, history; LDL, low-density lipoprotein; w/, with.

Patients with metabolic syndrome have a 3-fold increase in the probability of developing cardio/cerebrovascular disease (OR, 2.96), and exhibit an increase in overall mortality rates compared to patients without metabolic syndrome (197).

Pathophysiology

Because metabolic syndrome is a syndrome of related risk factors, the pathophysiology is complex and the four diseases/risk factors intertwined. One hypothesis is that an early underlying pathology of metabolic syndrome is oxidative stress. Oxidative stress contributes to insulin resistance and is a component in the pathogenesis of atherosclerosis, hypertension, and type 2 diabetes (192). Reactive oxygen species (ROS) or free oxygen radicals are a result of normal cellular energy metabolism. Antioxidants scavenge free radicals. *Oxidative stress* is defined as a surplus of ROS to antioxidants. Oxidative stress can occur because of an excess production of ROS overwhelming antioxidant capacity in the body or as a decrease in the production or quantity of antioxidants to inactivate ROS (192).

The pathophysiology of metabolic syndrome has been described as a "two-hit model" consisting of obesity and a metabolic predisposition (201, para. 5). Many researchers believe that obesity is the starting point that eventually leads to the major components identified as metabolic syndrome. Genetics influences the metabolic predisposition to insulin resistance, hypertension, dyslipidemia, etc. Insulin–regulated metabolic pathways are responsible for the production of "coagulation factors, sex hormones, and apolipoproteins . . . thus liver, muscle, endothelium, and adipose tissue are the main affected organs" causing a decrease in the transport and storage of glucose (194, p. 224).

Insulin Resistance

Insulin resistance has also been identified as an underlying pathology (195) or as a "mediating factor" (198) and it should be noted that metabolic syndrome, while linked to insulin resistance, is not solely caused by insulin resistance nor is it caused as a direct result of a deficiency in insulin action (198). Insulin resistance is considered a result of obesity in the two-hit model (201) and leads to the other pathologies of high blood pressure, abnormalities in lipid metabolism, abnormal coagulation, and inflammation (201).

Insulin resistance is defined as a defect in the ability of insulin to maintain normal blood glucose levels. The physiologic effects of insulin include the metabolism of carbohydrate, lipid, protein, and minerals. Insulin increases blood flow in the arterial vessels; promotes the synthesis of fatty acids, glycogen, triglycerides, and glucose; decreases the breakdown of proteins and lipoproteins; and promotes the uptake of glucose, amino acids, and potassium. Multiple factors contribute to insulin resistance: circulating free fatty acids resulting from lipolysis

of adipose tissue and lipoproteins, problems with defects in insulin receptors and mitochondrial energy production, as well as chemical changes in insulin-mediated signalling pathways that impact normal insulin function (193). Normally, insulin inhibits lipolysis from occurring, but changes in the availability and function of insulin receptors cause a resistance to the effects of insulin and therefore abnormally high concentrations of triglycerides and other lipid molecules due to uninhibited lipolysis and hyperglycemia. The discussion of insulin resistance is found in greater detail in Chapter 11.

Atherogenic Dyslipidemia

Atherogenic dyslipidemia presents with elevated triglyceride levels (or very low density lipoprotein [VLDL]) and small dense LDL (sdLDL) particles and low levels of HDL (199). This triad of signs has been labeled atherogenic lipoprotein phenotype and has been shown to increase cardiac risk to the same extent as high LDL levels (198). "Although all LDLs are atherogenic, small dense LDL are more atherogenic, perhaps due to increased penetration of the arterial intima, decreased antioxidant capacity, or other properties" (198, p. 41). Also increased are chylomicrons and glycated LDL particles, which move surplus triglycerides and apolipoprotein B into the circulation. Circulating free fatty acids are oxidized and synthesized back into triglyceride through reesterification. Ineffective oxidation and/or increased transport of free fatty acids to the liver cause the buildup of excess triglyceride in the skeletal muscle cells (198).

Adipose tissue is known to be metabolically active. Cytokine release by adipocytes found in metabolically active adipose tissue is the basis for obesity as a manifestation of metabolic syndrome. Adipokines include leptin, TNF-α, IL-6, resistin, and adiponectin. Increased secretion of angiotensinogen (associated with hypertension and type 2 diabetes), TNF-α, resistin, leptin, and plasminogen activator inhibitor (PAI-1) are linked with large amounts of adipose tissue (198). TNF-α and resistin are associated with insulin resistance in human and animal models, respectively. Leptin is linked with obesity and PAI-1 related to clotting. Reduced levels of adiponectin are found in obesity and type 2 diabetes and seem to be a factor in the development of atherosclerosis and insulin resistance (198).

Adipocytes store energy as triglycerides, preferentially in the peripheral adipocytes, and break down the triglycerides into fatty acids to circulating blood, which are then used for energy production. When the capacity for triglyceride storage is surpassed in the peripheral adipocytes, the extra triglyceride "overflows" and is stored in hepatocytes (pathologically demonstrated as hepatic steatosis or fatty liver), skeletal myocytes, and visceral adipocytes (198). A disruption or dysfunction in the process of triglyceride storage within the peripheral adipocytes (lipodystrophy syndromes) can cause extremely high triglyceride levels, insulin resistance, fatty liver, and diabetes mellitus (198). Manifestations of lipodystrophy syndrome include the development of central obesity and fat pads at the base of the neck with an obvious loss of subcutaneous body fat (198). Dysfunctional energy storage proposes to be the process responsible for the development of insulin resistance (198). Dysfunctional energy storage is an abnormality "in the processing and storage of fatty acids and triglycerides ... [causing] the presence of too much triglyceride, or body fat ... [which] may lead to the development of hepatic and muscular resistance to insulin" (198, p. 38). The breakdown of adipose tissues (lipolysis) increases the quantity of circulating free fatty acids, which get converted into triglycerides, stored, and ultimately, increase VLDL levels (199).

Hypertension

Hypertension is another element attributed to metabolic syndrome—but again, is an independent risk factor that is associated with other elements of metabolic syndrome. Hypertension is correlated with increased weight, is present in many diabetic patients, and is inversely correlated with insulin sensitivity; about 50% of people with insulin resistance have hypertension (198). Mechanisms of action postulated for the increased incidence of hypertension due to insulin resistance include a decrease in nitric oxide–mediated vasodilation, increased sensitivity to salt, or an increase in blood volume (198). It is thought that in patients with insulin-resistance, these same mechanisms may be responsible for a limited response to antihypertensive medications (198).

As noted earlier, large amounts of adipose tissue increase the production of angiotensinogen, the precursor of angiotensin I and II; adipocytes are also responsible for the production of ACE. The conversion of angiotensinogen to angiotensin II can be inhibited by ACEIs.

Other Factors Related to Risk

Other factors are also postulated to be responsible for the risk factor patterns seen in metabolic syndrome. Of these, cellular, hormonal, genetic, and environmental factors play a role in vascular alterations seen in metabolic syndrome. Dysfunction of the endothelial cell lining, systemic inflammation, aberrations of the sympathoadrenal system, and genetic and environmental factors are considered specifically for the alterations in risk factors of a vascular nature (197). Endothelial dysfunction causes a reduction in nitric oxide synthesis resulting in vasoconstriction, as well as induces a proinflammatory and procoagulant condition (199). Elevated levels of inflammatory markers such as hs-CRP are found in patients with insulin resistance before the development of diabetes or metabolic syndrome (195).

Inflammation stimulates the production and release of acute phase reactants from the liver (CRP, fibrinogen, haptoglobulin, serum amyloid A, complement components, coagulation components, protease inhibitors, alpha-1 antitrypsin), which cause systemic changes leading to a procoagulant and chronic inflammatory condition. Thrombosis is stimulated as a result of the trigger of protein cascades during inflammation. The production of PAI-1 and fibrinogen increases clotting potential. High levels of inflammatory markers are associated with higher risks of CAD and type 2 diabetes (195, 198), and some medical professionals advocate for adding inflammatory markers to revised definitions of *metabolic syndrome* (195). Haffner (195) reported on multiple studies that show the association of high hs-CRP levels with the development of metabolic syndrome, new-onset diabetes, and CAD. In one study, patients with hs-CRP levels of 3 mg/L or greater, without metabolic syndrome, had a higher risk of CAD and new-onset diabetes than patients with hs-CRP levels less than 3 mg/L. Patients with the highest risk of coronary events and new-onset diabetes were those with both hs-CRP levels of 3 mg/L or greater plus metabolic syndrome (195). In the Insulin Resistance Atherosclerosis Study, baseline inflammatory markers (CRP, fibrinogen, and PAI-1) of nondiabetic participants showed a statistically significant association with the onset of diabetes (205), showing again the role of chronic inflammation in the development of disease. Genetic and environmental factors play a role in the expression of disease. Gene variants alter responses to metabolic processes and therapeutic interventions.

Microalbuminuria is a sign of renal endothelial damage and has been recognized as a risk factor for metabolic syndrome; in diabetic patients, it also can identify risk for CAD and renal disease (198). The correlation of microalbuminuria and metabolic syndrome was confirmed in a study of over 5,600 people in the United States for the NHANES III study conducted between 1988 and 1994 (206). Palaniappan et al. demonstrated a significant odds ratio between microalbuminuria and both high glucose levels and high blood pressure, for both men and women (206). Men with microalbuminuria were 2½ times as likely to have high blood glucose and hypertension (OR, 2.51; 95% CI, 1.54 to 4.10; and OR, 2.51; 95% CI, 1.63 to 3.86, respectively); women were 2¼ times as likely to have high blood glucose (OR, 2.24, 95% CI, 1.25 to 4.0) and almost 3½ times as likely to have hypertension (OR, 3.34, 95% CI, 2.45 to 4.55) (206).

Clinical Presentation

People with metabolic syndrome are usually asymptomatic of the "syndrome" per se, but demonstrate a variety of signs and symptoms specific to the individual components of the syndrome. Patients may have type 2 diabetes or insulin resistance alone, so high insulin levels and hyperglycemia are common traits. Abnormal lipid profiles, arterial hypertension, adiposity, microalbuminuria, and hyperuricemia are also noted. Laboratory evidence of increased platelet aggregation, decreased fibrinolysis, inflammation, endothelial dysfunction, and hepatic steatosis are other manifestions. Acanthosis nigricans is a discoloration of the skin due to stimulation of insulin receptors, usually seen on the neck and in body folds and low sex hormone binding globulin are both results of extremely high insulin levels (194).

Diagnosis

Diagnosis of metabolic syndrome is dependent on clinical judgment and the presence of risk factors identified in the criteria. Measuring height and weight to calculate a body mass index (BMI) and waist and hip circumference will assist the APN to calculate a waist-to-hip ratio. It is important to determine the waist circumference to avoid missed diagnoses for patients whose BMIs are normal but whose waist circumference may meet the diagnostic criteria (202). The waist measurement is an excellent predictive screening tool and an accurate and simple way to determine the amount of visceral adipose tissue (197). Waist measurement is performed at the level of the umbilicus (the highest point of the iliac crest) and the hip measurement is taken at the widest point. Measurements are rounded to the nearest 0.1 cm. BMI and waist circumference are not necessarily correlated. APNs must remember that even patients with a BMI within the normal range may have a waist measurement that meets the NCEP: ATP III criteria for metabolic syndrome (202) and should have a high index of suspicion for ethnic patients who meet some of the criteria, but not waist circumference or BMI criteria. In several studies, larger waist size is correlated with increased incidence of high blood pressure, high insulin levels, and high lipid levels, regardless of race or ethnicity (202).

Laboratory testing would include fasting blood glucose, glucose tolerance testing, hs-CRP level, and lipid panel (triglyceride and cholesterol levels). The homeostatic model assessment of insulin resistance ($HOMA_{IR}$) is calculated by multiplying the fasting insulin (mU/L) by the fasting glucose (mmol/L) and dividing by a constant of 22.5, which serves to normalize the value to 1.0 in normal persons (198). A urinary albumin excretion rate or albumin/creatinine ratio can be measured from a urine sample. Table 9-49 outlines laboratory and diagnostic tests consistent with metabolic syndrome.

Management

Management of patients with metabolic syndrome includes multiple interventions in a multidisciplinary collaboration. Patient management is also guided by which conceptual framework one perceives to be the most correct. Interventions to manage environmental causes would include weight loss, diet modifications, and increased physical activity to reduce obesity; drug therapy for insulin resistance would be added to lifestyle modifications for those who believe that insulin resistance is the primary causative factor; and the addition of drugs to reduce an elevated CRP (e.g., statins, ACEI, or ARBs mentioned earlier in the chapter) would be added if inflammation is thought to be the major culprit (195). Though there is no universal

TABLE 9–49 Laboratory and Diagnostic Testing for Metabolic Syndrome

Laboratory/Diagnostic Test	Findings
Insulin resistance	Fasting insulin >75th percentile
	Homeostasis model (HOMA-IR) >75th percentile
Hyperglycemia	Fasting plasma glucose >100 mg/dL (>5.6 mmol/L)
	Fasting plasma glucose >110 mg/dL
	Impaired GTT
Dyslipidemia	Fasting triglycerides >150 mg/dL
	HDL cholesterol <35–40 mg/dL men; <40–50 mg/dL women (smaller subclasses predominant)
	Increased concentration of small dense LDLs or apolipoprotein B
Arterial hypertension	Systolic BP >130 or >140 mm Hg
	Diastolic BP >85 or >90 mm Hg
Adiposity	BMI >23–24 kg/m² in Asians, >25 kg/m² Caucasians or >30 kg/m²
	Waist circumference >90–102 cm men
	>80–88 cm women
	Waist-to-hip ratio >0.90
Microalbuminuria	Urinary average excretion rate ≥20 mcg/min
	Albumin/Creatinine ratio >20 mg/g
Uric acid	Hyperuricemia

TABLE 9–49 Laboratory and Diagnostic Testing for Metabolic Syndrome—cont'd

Laboratory/Diagnostic Test	Findings
Hemostatic factors	Elevated plasminogen activator inhibitor-1 (PAI-1) and fibrinogen Increased platelet aggregation Decreased fibrinolysis
Inflammation	Elevated levels of high sensitivity C-reactive protein (hs-CRP), leukocytes, interleukin 6, TNF-α
Endothelial dysfunction	Elevated levels of homocysteine, asymmetrical dimethylarginine, endolthelial-dependent vasodilation, cellular adhesion molecules
Hepatic steatosis	Elevated serum aminotransferases Decreased antioxidant protection: Low vitamin C and α-tocopherol levels
Oxidative stress	Decreased superoxide dismutase activity Increased lipid peroxidation malondialdehyde levels, protein carbonyls, xanthine oxidase activity
Other	Acanthosis nigricans Low sex hormone-binding globulin

BMI, body mass index; CVD, cardiovascular disease; Dx, diagnosis; GTT, glucose tolerance test; HDL, high density lipoprotein; HOMA$_{IR}$, homeostatic model assessment of insulin resistance; HTN, hypertension; LDL, low-density lipoprotein.

Sources: Aguilar-Salinas et al. (2005) (194); Fuster et al, 2006 (176); Haffner, (2006) (195); Roberts and Sindhu, 2009 (192).

standard of care, management of this patient population requires management of each individual modifiable risk factor. An individualized plan of care that is realistic and achievable is desirable.

Diet

Weight control is a key factor in modifying future risk from metabolic syndrome. Weight, height, and waist circumference will have been assessed before therapy begins and sould be monitored periodically throughout therapeutic intervention. A reduced calorie (achieved by decreasing calorie intake of about 500 to 1,000 kcal/day), low fat, low trans-fat, low cholesterol, and high-complex carbohydrate diet is recommended to manage dyslipidemia. Added soluble fiber content (3 to 10 g/day) is recommended to further decrease cholesterol and lipoprotein levels as well as to reduce the risk of other disease processes (197). Obese patients may modify this diet to limit carbohydrates.

Besides decreasing metabolic syndrome risk, weight loss will have other beneficial effects by lowering serum cholesterol, lipoprotein, and triglyceride levels, PAI-1, and blood pressure. Increased glucose tolerance and sensitivity to insulin is a result of weight loss and HDL cholesterol levels are raised (197).

Physical Activity

Multiple studies have been conducted to describe the benefits of physical activity on risk reduction, including a reduction in inflammation, for CVD. Educate the patient on the benefits of regular physical activity to reduce risks of future disease (coronary heart disease, insulin resistance, diabetes, and obesity) and promote well-being. Patients should be encouraged to increase their physical activity to at least 30 minutes of brisk walking every day; alternative exercises may be substituted for patients for which this is not feasible. Remind patients to start any exercise program slowly, with reasonable goals. Patients may be referred to rehabilitation programs, physical therapists, and specialists to tailor an individualized exercise plan that is safe and effective (197).

Managing Risk Factors

Advanced practice nurses may prescribe medications to prevent and/or treat various components of metabolic syndrome. Drug therapy includes medications to reduce the other risk factors in the cluster: high cholesterol/triglycerides, low HDL cholesterol, high levels of inflammatory markers (e.g., CRP), high blood pressure, and high blood glucose/diabetes.

The guidelines recommend the LDL levels be maintained at less than 129 mg/dL. Patients who are at high risk for cardiovascular disease are treated to keep their LDL levels below 100 mg/dL. The National Cholesterol Education Program Adult Treatment Panel III (NCEP-III) guidelines recommend the use of HMG reductase inhibitors (statins) as first line therapy for lowering LDL levels (207). In addition to statins, drug therapy for dyslipidemia includes fibrates (fenofibrate, gemfibrozil) and nicotinic acid (niacin). Statin therapy not only reduces lipid levels, but has been shown to lower CRP levels and thereby dramatically reduce the risk of future cardiovascular events.

Hypertension is treated with a variety of medications, and many studies have shown their effectiveness in reducing morbidity and mortality from cardiovascular (MI, stroke, aneurysm rupture) and ischemic cerebrovascular disease. There are no specific guidelines for antihypertensive drug therapy in metabolic syndrome per se; therefore, the clinician would follow national guidelines for blood pressure control. Common antihypertensive drugs include diuretics, ACEIs, beta-blockers, and calcium channel blockers. The use of ACEIs has been shown to decrease inflammation and make dramatic decreases in cardiovascular and cerebrovascular disease mortality. ARBs may also be used to lower blood pressure and are frequently substituted for patients who cannot tolerate ACEIs. Drug trials have showed the ability of losartan to prevent diabetes (198). Losartan prevents free fatty acid–induced endothelial dysfunction and oxidative stress (208).

Glucose control is recommended to keep blood glucose levels between 60 and 100 mg/mL in patients with diabetes. Other medications may be prescribed to control other CV risk factors. Anticoagulation and antiplatelet agents may be part of the regimen to counteract inflammation. Patients with AF are usually prescribed warfarin, ASA, clopidogrel, dipyridamole, or combination therapy. Daily ASA therapy is recommended (204).

Directions regarding how each medication works, how to take the medications, the side effects, and possible consequences should be discussed with the patient and family. Medication compliance is vital.

Clinical Nurse Specialist Competencies and Spheres of Influence
Clinical Expert/Direct Care, Collaboration, and Research/Evidence-Based Practice

Health promotion and disease prevention are vital areas for APN involvement, especially with patients with, or at risk for, cardiometabolic syndrome (Patient/Family Sphere). Early interventions may prevent or delay the onset of metabolic syndrome or one of its components. Screening for metabolic syndrome is important for early education and treatment to prevent further disease (202, 209). CNSs, in collaboration with their physician and allied health colleagues (dietitian, physical therapist, and/or rehabilitation specialist) and other APNs, have a critical role in educating their patients at risk for metabolic syndrome, or already diagnosed with metabolic syndrome, to make modifications to their lifestyles, and therefore significantly influence their current and future risk of disease. Weight management and increasing physical activity are key interventions. The CNS's sensitivity to the patient's preferences and cultural norms or traditions regarding food may warrant slight modification of the goals or strategies to achieve the goals. Support groups and stress management activities can help the patient feel emotionally supported and provide tips on how to manage multiple demands. Barriers to the patient's full participation in preventive care may come from insurance companies limiting payment for preventive strategies (197). The CNS can help the patient and family brainstorm ways to overcome these barriers.

Systems Leadership

There are validated and reliable practice guidelines available on the care of the patient with dyslipidemia and hypertension. In the Nursing/Other Disciplines Sphere of Influence, the CNS is responsible to make sure the staff is aware of the criteria for the definition of metabolic syndrome and of the steps required for operationalizing EBP guidelines. CNSs can have an impact on policy formulation for the addition of screening for metabolic syndrome at the institutional level (System/Organization Sphere). Unit- or service-based protocols can be written to guide the staff in making decisions about additional lab draws and referrals. Modification of the guidelines, policies, and procedures for metabolic syndrome, regarding waist measurements in particular, may be needed to acknowledge differences in ethnic groups or patient populations at risk. There is some literature to suggest that there are differences in visceral fat stores between African Americans and Caucasians (202). CNS has a role in developing policy and procedures specific to ethnic and patient populations to make staff more aware for screening and risk identification purposes (202).

SHOCK STATES

Etiology

Shock is a life-threatening state of inadequate tissue perfusion of oxygenated blood at the cellular level, resulting in cellular dysfunction, cell death, and organ failure. Shock is not a disease, but a syndrome of interacting systems. Three components are responsible for failure to perfuse the tissues: the pump (problem with the cardiac system), the pipes (problem with the blood vessels), and the fluid or perfusate (problems with blood volume). There are various ways in which these components can be compromised and thus affect the distribution of blood flow. One way many authors have classified the different types of shock is to identify the etiologies are "failures" of normal processes—(a) failure to pump/eject (equal to pump failure or cardiogenic shock); (b) failure to fill (such as from obstructive shock or distributive shock); (c) failure to perfuse (fluid failure or hypovolemic shock); and (d) failure to vasoconstrict (signifies pipe failure or distributive shock). With these etiologies in mind, there are three main classifications of shock: (a) hypovolemic, (b) cardiogenic, and (c) distributive or vasogenic (i.e., anaphylactic, neurogenic, or septic). Some systems will add burn shock and obstructive shock as separate classifications and further delineate hypovolemic shock as hemorrhagic or traumatic shock (210). Table 9-50 defines the different

TABLE 9–50 Manifestations, Body Response, and Outcomes of Shock Stages

Shock Stage	Manifestations	Body Response	Outcome
SUBCLINICAL (INITIAL)			
	No obvious S/S Elevated lactate levels		Progresses to compensatory stage if oxygen delivery not restored
COMPENSATORY			
(Nonprogressive Stage)	Decreases in: ↓ CO ↓ BP ↓ U/O ↑ SVR ↑ Acid ↑ K+ ↑ RR and depth ↑ pH Restless, confusion, lethargy, stupor	Compensatory mechanisms restore CO and tissue perfusion Neural, hormonal, chemical compensation interact	Reversible stage if treatment is initiated in time Ventilatory support; fluid resuscitation Inotropic and vasoactive medications initiated as needed ↑ CO → ↑ BP and ↑tissue perfusion Vasoconstriction • Blood shunted from nonvital organs/organs with "luxury" perfusion (skin, kidneys, GIT, lungs) • ↓ Peristalsis • Skin cool, clammy, pale, mottled Protective oliguria • ↓ U/O • ↑ SG • ↑ Osmolality • ↑ Urine K (= ↓ serum K) Stress response • ↑ HR, contractility • ↑ RR, depth • Respiratory alkalosis • Dilated pupils • Dilated skeletal and coronary arteries • Na/H_2O retention • ↑ Cortisol = ↑ BG
PROGRESSIVE (DECOMPENSATED)			
	↓ CO ↓ BP ↓ $PaCO_2$ ↓ SPO_2 ↓ pH (respiratory and metabolic acidosis) ↓ No U/O Mottled, cold skin Diminished pulses	Compensatory mechanisms fail—ineffective to maintain CO and tissue oxygenation Cellular death occurs in vital organs	Decreased LOC→ coma Respiratory acidosis Metabolic acidosis Circulatory collapse Anuria Leads to MODS High-dose vasopressor and inotropic support Mechanical ventilation

Continued

TABLE 9–50 Manifestations, Body Response, and Outcomes of Shock Stages—cont'd

Shock Stage	Manifestations	Body Response	Outcome
PROGRESSIVE (DECOMPENSATED)			
	↓ LOC ↑ HR Dysrhythmias ↑ P_ACO_2 ↑ K ↑ SVR ↑ PAP		
REFRACTORY			
	No hemodynamic response to therapy Metabolic and respiratory acidosis ↓↓ CO ↓↓ BP Anuria	All systems failing	Irreversible stage leads to MOF and death

BG, blood glucose; BP, blood pressure; CO, cardiac output; CVP, central venous pressure; HR, heart rate; H_2O, water; K, potassium; LOC, level of consciousness; RR, respiratory rate; MODS, multiple organ dysfunction syndrome; MOF, multiple organ failure; Na, sodium; PAP, pulmonary artery pressure; P_ACO_2, partial pressure of carbon dioxide dissolved in the arterial blood; PAOP, pulmonary artery occlusion pressure; SG, specific gravity; SPO_2, saturation of hemoglobin with oxygen; SVR, systemic vascular resistance; U/O, urine output.

types of shock, their etiologies and pathophysiology, clinical presentation, and management.

Shock is a major cause of death worldwide and ranks as the 11th leading cause of death in the United States (211). It is estimated that over 750,000 cases of severe sepsis occur each year (211). Of the different types of shock, septic shock is the most deadly.

Pathophysiology

The basic pathology of shock states result in a reduction in CO (except for distributive shock) and therefore decreased tissue perfusion. The observed mechanism of distributive types of shock is a normal or increased CO; however, the maldistribution of the CO into extravascular spaces still results in poor tissue perfusion. Novel technologies to observe the microcirculation have provided greater clarification of the cellular mechanisms of distributive shock and have found that the problem lies within the microcirculation at the mitochondrial level (213). Elbers and Ince described the pathophysiology as "microcirculatory and mitochondrial distress syndrome" (p. 221).

Apart from transporting nutrients and removing waste products, oxygen delivery is the prime function of [the microcirculation]. The microcirculation is a complex network of resistance and exchange vessels, where perfusion is dependent on numerous factors. These include arterial oxygen saturation, oxygen consumption, blood viscosity, red and white blood cell deformability and flow, shunting of vessels, vasodilatation, vasoconstriction or stasis in arterioles and capillaries, diffusion constants of gasses and nutrients and distances from cells to the nearest blood vessel (213, p. 222).

Regional dysoxia (impaired oxygen extraction) occurs due to shunting of hypoxemic microcirculatory units and/or a defect in the ability of the tissues to use the delivered oxygen for oxidative phosphorylation (known as cytopathic hypoxia): this is seen clinically as elevated mixed venous oxygen saturation (SVO_2). The endothelium is highly involved in the regulation of oxygen delivery and decreased oxygen supply to these cells disrupts normal function. The result is increased capillary membrane permeability, massive nitric oxide production leading to vasodilation, a procoagulant state giving rise to sluggish microvascular blood flow and microthrombi formation, and the production of lactate and tissue acidosis (213). Elbers and Ince noted that therapies that improve systemic variables (e.g., CO, blood pressure) do not necessarily also improve microcirculatory flow and function (213). The use of vasodilatory agents, inotropes, fluids, and activated protein C have been shown to reverse microcirculatory flow stasis and improve microvascular diffusion defects (213).

Ongoing research in this area may lead to new or adjunct therapies to improve microcirculatory flow.

Hypoxia and Cell Death

Cells require oxygen to function. When blood flow is impaired the delivery of oxygen is diminished. Without oxygen, pyruvate is not taken up by acetyl-CoA and directed through the Krebs cycle to produce energy. Instead, pyruvate is converted to lactic acid as a part of anaerobic metabolism (or anaerobic respiration) and the net production of ATP is only 2 moles (from the glycolysis step) versus the 38 moles of ATP that oxidative phosphorylation and the electron transport chain produce via aerobic metabolism/respiration. Without oxygen, cellular metabolism is hindered, lactic acid builds up, and the sodium-potassium (Na^{2+}, K^+) pump is damaged. The nonfunctional Na^{2+}, K^+ pump is not able to remove Na^{2+} from inside the cell, therefore, Na^{2+} builds up within the cell. Water follows Na^{2+} into the cell and the cell swells to the point that the lysosomal membrane breaks open and the cell dies. The cell spills all of its internal components (e.g., enzymes, electrolytes, proteins) into the capillary beds.

With infectious sources, free radicals (ROS as well as reactive nitrogen species) are produced by leukocytes to fight pathologic organisms. Free radical production is a natural consequence of the inflammatory cascades but increase in production in infection and sepsis. The large amounts produced can overwhelm the body's antioxidant defenses and cause tissue damage by stimulating apoptosis.

Shock Stages

There is one subclinical stage in shock and three major stages: compensatory, progressive, and refractory.

Subclinical Stage

The initial stage is cellular and described in the pathophysiology section. The decrease in blood flow to the tissues causes a reduction in the delivery of oxygen and nutrients to the cells. Anaerobic metabolism takes over and produces lactic acid. Energy production is reduced. This subclinical state does not produce obvious signs and symptoms; however the rise in lactic acid would be detected if lactate levels were drawn during the subclinical phase. Because rising lactate levels are an early sign of decreased tissue perfusion, knowledge of blood lactate levels for patients with septic signs and symptoms presenting in the ED one of the first interventions noted in the Sepsis Resuscitation bundle. The goal is to identify sepsis and start aggressive therapy as soon as possible (211).

Compensatory Stage

The compensatory stage of shock is a reversible stage and occurs at the expense of "nonvital" organs, for example, the gastrointestinal tract and skin; and organs with "luxury" perfusion, defined as those receiving more blood than needed for cellular function: the kidneys and the lungs. Intervention at this stage will prevent further deterioration of tissue metabolism and allow a return to homeostasis. In this stage, compensatory neural, hormonal, and chemical mechanisms are activated to restore CO and tissue perfusion. Each compensatory system has independent components but work together to reestablish homeostasis. There is a redundancy or overlap in the effects from each system. Figure 9-15 shows the individual components and the complex interrelationships between the compensatory systems (211-215).

Neural compensation occurs when baroreceptors in the aorta and carotid bodies sense a decrease in blood pressure. The sympathetic nervous system (SNS) is activated via the vasomotor center in the medulla; direct stimulation of the heart occurs and causes the heart to beat faster and with more force. The purpose is to increase stroke volume and therefore CO and blood pressure. The coronary arteries dilate in response to SNS stimulation to feed the heart with oxygen for this increased work. The SNS also causes blood flow to be shunted from the nonvital and luxury perfusion organs to the brain, heart, and skeletal muscles. Vasoconstriction directly increases blood pressure and increases venous return to the RV, thereby increasing stroke volume and therefore blood pressure and tissue perfusion. Additionally, the lungs are stimulated to increase respiratory rate and depth. SNS stimulation also causes the pupils to dilate, skeletal blood flow to increase via vasodilation, and the sweat glands to become activated resulting in cool, clammy skin (diaphoresis).

Hormonal compensation involves the hypothalamus-pituitary-adrenal axis (HPA; triggers the stress response). The SNS is triggered by the low blood pressure state. Low blood pressure is sensed by the juxtaglomerular cells of the macula densa in the glomerulus and cause renin to be secreted. The RAAS is a powerful compensatory mechanism as it influences blood volume and therefore blood pressure. Renin cleaves angiotensinogen, a precursor molecule made in the liver, and produces angiotensin I (AT-I). Angiotensin I is converted in the lungs by ACE to angiotensin II (AT-II). AT-II is one of the most potent vasoconstrictors in the body. Additionally, AT-II induces the production of aldosterone. Aldosterone, a mineralocorticoid, is secreted from the adrenal cortex and works by increasing the retention of sodium in the distal tubules and collecting ducts. The end result is the retention of water as the water follows the sodium molecules. Water retention increases the blood volume, increasing venous return to the heart and therefore CO. Antidiuretic hormone (i.e., ADH) is stimulated by high serum osmolality (from low blood volume) and by aldosterone secretion. ADH works on the aquaporin receptors in the distal tubules of the kidney. The aquaporin receptors stimulate the vasopressin receptors, which increase water retention, lowering urine output, and thereby

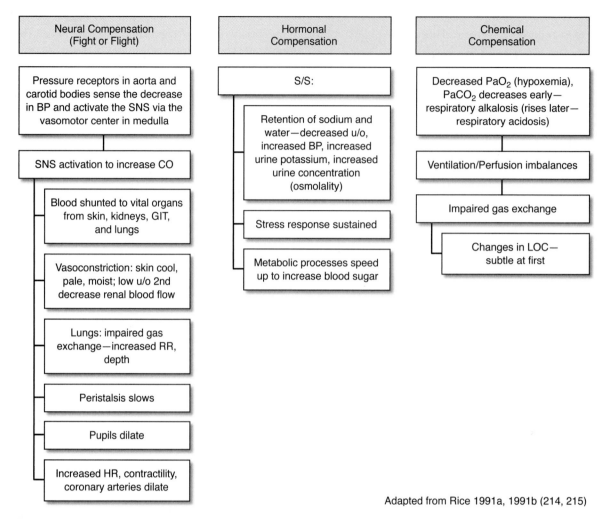

Adapted from Rice 1991a, 1991b (214, 215)

FIGURE 9–15: Interrelationship of neural, hormonal, and chemical compensation in shock.

increasing blood volume. While both aldosterone and ADH have an end result of increased blood volume, the mechanisms are different. Remember that aldosterone retains sodium, which draws water to it; ADH retains water only. The effect of the RAAS has been called "protective oliguria" because the main goal is to protect the kidney from low volume states and possible renal failure.

Stimulation of the SNS triggers the production of epinephrine and norepinephrine from the adrenal medulla. These catecholamines stimulate the beta-receptors of the heart causing the heart to beat faster and harder and, also, stimulate the alpha-receptors on the blood vessels and cause vasoconstriction. The result is a potentiation of the SNS response initiated by through neural compensation. SNS activation also stimulates the anterior pituitary and causes adrenocorticotropin hormone (ACTH) to be released. ACTH stimulates the adrenal cortex to release cortisol, which stimulates the liver to increase glycogenolysis and therefore increase blood glucose levels.

Chemical compensation entails pulmonary compensatory mechanisms that work to restore effective gas exchange. In anaerobic metabolism, there is a decrease in oxygen delivery resulting in hypoxemia and an increase in dead space, which causes a V/Q mismatch. The amount of blood carbon dioxide (CO_2) increases and competes for hemoglobin binding sites with oxygen. The chemoreceptors in the aortic arch and carotid bodies sense the change in oxygen tension (manifesting as a low partial pressure of arterial oxygen or PaO_2) and in blood pH, an acidotic state or low pH resulting from the excess CO_2 levels. They then transmit a message to the medulla to increase the SNS response (already triggered through the neural mechanism) and increase the rate and depth of breathing. The result of this action is to rid the body of the excess CO_2; eventually a respiratory alkalosis develops. Low PaO_2 and low CO_2 levels in the brain cause vasoconstriction of the cerebral blood vessels and cerebral ischemia. Changes in level of consciousness from mild to severe: restlessness, confusion, excitation, lethargy, or coma may occur.

Progressive Stage

Eventually the body's compensatory mechanisms are not able to sustain the patient in a homeostatic state and the compensatory mechanisms begin to fail. The progressive stage is also known as the stage of decompensation. Cardiac output and tissue perfusion are decreased, which lead to cellular dysfunction and eventual cell death. The patient presents with signs and symptoms of major organ dysfunction. The first major system that usually fails is the renal system, followed by pulmonary, heart, and then gastrointestinal tract. With each additional failing organ system the risk of death increases by 20% (216). So there is about a 20% mortality rate with one organ failure, 40% with two organ failures, 60% with three, and so on. Aggressive efforts at this stage can still reverse the shock process.

Refractory Stage

In the refractory stage, the patient does not respond to conventional therapy and death ensues. In this stage, the patient continues to get worse as the tissue perfusion decreases, acidosis increases, and organs fail. Even high doses of vasoactive medications cannot support the patient in this stage. The health care team continues to provide interventions, the patient usually goes into cardiac or respiratory arrest, and ultimately the patient dies. The frustration of the refractory stage is that there is no clear line of demarcation (i.e., definitive signs) that alerts the health care team that the patient has entered this stage from the progressive stage. Therefore, the team continues to provide aggressive therapy, but the patient does not recover. This may be one reason for the prolongation of what seems to be aggressive therapy to some of the staff, but the reality may be that neither the physician nor team fully realize the futility of their efforts, because the team never knows at what point in the resuscitation effort the patient progressed to this final stage. This can be very frustrating for all staff. The CNS may be the person to point out futile efforts during team discussions of patient care.

Clinical Presentation

Signs and symptoms of shock are manifestations of the stages of shock. A decrease in CO and therefore tissue perfusion may present in subtle ways. For example, a patient who has been previously oriented becomes confused or restless—these are signs of decreased tissue perfusion to the brain. Heart rate may be increasing for no apparent reason, blood pressure is decreasing, and urine output is starting to fall. The astute nurse is aware of the complication of shock and looks for these early signs, knowing that prompt intervention may prevent the patient from progressing into a more dangerous and possibly fatal stage.

In the compensatory stage, the signs and symptoms are related to the effect of the different compensatory components—stimulation of neural, hormonal, and chemical mechanisms produce the signs of the stress response—or the flight-or-fight response. Heart rate and force of cardiac contraction increase to deliver more blood and respiratory rate and depth increase to facilitate gas exchange and acid-base balance, nonvital vessels vasoconstrict, catecholamines are released, the RAA system is activated—these processes all serve to increase CO, blood pressure, and therefore, tissue perfusion. HPA axis hormones are released to increase blood glucose to supply energy to the organs and heart, brain, and skeletal vessels dilate to bring oxygenated blood to the working muscles. Skin is cool and may be diaphoretic. These are all effects of compensation. Presentations in this stage are classic and once recognized, require immediate treatment. Aggressive treatment at this stage assists the patient to return to a state of normalcy.

In the progressive stage, the compensatory mechanisms are failing. They are no longer able to maintain the CO and blood pressure and signs of a worsening state manifest. Heart rate continues to climb but contractility decreases and stroke volume is reduced; blood pressure is low; pulses are weak; skin becomes cool, clammy, and pale, capillary refill is prolonged; and only small amounts of concentrated urine are produced. The blood vessels (arterial and venous) become vasoconstricted in an attempt to increase perfusion; microemboli form. SVR increases, but that adds resistance to LV ejection, increasing cardiac workload and further compromising the heart. The lungs and respiratory muscles are not able to maintain the rapid rate and depth of breathing, so breathing becomes shallow—though the rate may remain elevated. Alveolar hypoventilation causes CO_2 to be retained and the respiratory alkalosis that is characteristic of the early stages of shock now has shifted to a respiratory acidosis. Metabolic acidosis also begins to manifest as the insufficient process of anaerobic metabolism produces more lactic acid in the face of decreased oxygen. Increased partial pressure of carbon dioxide in the arterial blood ($PaCO_2$) cause cerebral vessels to dilate increasing intracranial pressure; that and decreased oxygen account for the decrease in level of consciousness seen at this stage. Aggressive efforts at this stage can still assist recovery for the patient. As the progressive stage continues, signs of multiple organ dysfunction occur. As each organ fails the mortality rate increases by about 20% (216).

The signs of the refractory stage are a culmination of multiple organ failure and the inability of the body and aggressive therapies to combat the progressive decline to death. The patient is severely acidotic from multiple causes; mechanically ventilated for pulmonary failure; anuric and uremic from renal failure; demonstrates a decreased level of consciousness; is tachycardic and hypotensive from HF; and unresponsive to conventional therapies. The final outcome is death.

Diagnosis

Hemodynamic monitoring and laboratory testing are primarily used to diagnose the different shocks. While the use of hemodynamic measurements such as CVP and PAOP are routinely used to guide fluid management, it is known that neither of these measurements accurately estimates RV or LV filling pressures or cardiac performance in the face of fluid challenge (217). End-diastolic volume (EDV) is an accurate indicator of fluid volume, but central venous access is required for measurement. Trends should be monitored. Table 9-51 compares the hemodynamic effects of the different types of shock.

To guide fluid therapy decisions, the use of base excess/base deficit (BE/BD) has been proposed as a practical and more accurate indicator of fluid status than using CVP or PAOP measurements (218, 219). Normal BE/BD is −2 to +2 and the results will correlate with the pH label. Some labs will report the BE and others the BD—there is not a standard for which label to use. BE/BD is a difficult concept in that there one must think in opposites to correctly interpret the results. So a BE value of +6 is intuitive—there is a lot of base available; however, a BE of −6 shows a deficit of base (the base excess is negative). The good news is that regardless of the label used, the results are interpreted the same. If a positive number for the BE or BD is reported, the patient has extra base and therefore not enough acid—the pH should be alkalotic (assuming a pure acid-base disturbance); a negative result for the BE or BD means the patient has too little base available (therefore more acid) and the pH should be acidotic. A negative BD value signifies more acid. Fluid therapies are discussed below.

Basic chemical panels, including serum electrolyte levels, blood glucose, BUN, and creatinine are important indicators of organ function. A CBC, including a white blood cell differential, and a coagulation panel, will help to assess the patients hematologic, immune, and coagulation status. Elevation of white blood cells and platelet counts are seen in inflammation and infection. Anemia is possible. In severe, persistent sepsis, a fall in the platelet count and WBCs may occur as the immune cells fighting the infection are overwhelmed and "used up" in the inflammatory process. ABG analysis will provide information on the ability of the lungs to regulate gas exchange and provide a picture of acid-base status. Serum lactate levels are obtained on admission and then regularly to ascertain the patient's current state and response to therapy. Lactate levels over 4 mmol/L signal reduced tissue perfusion and the shift from aerobic to anaerobic metabolism. Cultures of bodily fluids (blood, sputum, urine, cerebrospinal fluid, wound drainage, or respiratory secretions) and gram staining are important to help identify the pathologic microorganism.

Other diagnostic measures include right heart catheterization, echocardiography, ECG, and an FAST (focused assessment with sonography for trauma) examination. FAST can detect pericardial fluid of cardiac tamponade as the cause for cardiogenic shock and can detect intraperitoneal fluid in the abdomen, a possible cause for hypovolemic shock.

Management

One of the most important things a nurse can do is to identify patients at risk for complications and to be vigilant in their monitoring of those patients so complications are caught early and those patients are treated as soon as possible. Mortality rates for cardiogenic and septic shock are high, despite therapy; left untreated or undetected, most patients in shock will die (220).

TABLE 9–51 Hemodynamic Effects of Shock

Type of Shock	CO/CI	BP	HR	SVR	PAP	PAOP	CVP	Svo$_2$
Hypovolemic	↓	↓	↑	↑	↑	↓	↓	↓
Cardiogenic	↓	↓	↑	↑	↑	↓	↓	↓
Distributive: septic								
Early stage	↑	↓	↑	↓	↓	↓	↓	↑
Late stage	↓	↓	↑	↑	↑	↓	↓	↓
Distributive: Neurogenic	↓	↓	↑	↓	↑	↓	↓	↓
Distributive: anaphylactic	↓	↓	↑	↓	↑	↓	↓	↓

BP, blood pressure; CO/CI, cardiac output/cardiac index; CVP, central venous pressure; HR, heart rate; PAP, pulmonary artery pressure; PAOP, pulmonary artery occlusion pressure; Svo$_2$, mixed venous oxygen saturation; SVR, systemic vascular resistance.

Assessment of fluid status is a routine intervention. Daily weights are extremely important measurements as weight is one of the most sensitive indicators of fluid gain or loss. Intake and outputs are recorded as per protocol. Simple hemodynamic parameters such as heart rate and blood pressure and peripheral oxygen saturation (SpO_2) are monitored. Note that the degree of tachycardia is usually correlated to the amount of bleeding—the faster the heart rate, the more bleeding is occurring. Also, be aware that patients may be on medications that may mask the early warning sign of tachycardia. Beta-blockers or calcium channel blockers are the most common agents with this effect.

Assessment of skin color and temperature provides valuable information. Assessments of capillary refill or skin turgor do not have strong diagnostic profiles. Prolonged capillary refill only has a sensitivity of 25% to 28%, so it is not a test that is very good at identifying abnormal tissue perfusion; its specificity is better at 85% (129), but that still means 15% of people with poor tissue perfusion will be misdiagnosed as normal. Sublingual tissue CO_2 is a good indicator of tissue perfusion, is easy to use and interpret, and should be used more (221). Hemodynamic parameters are monitored.

Clearly the goals of shock therapy are to identify those patients at high risk and attempt to prevent shock from occurring. However, once a shock stage is identified, the goal is to locate and correct the underlying cause or causes and start treatment immediately. The specific therapy will vary with the type of shock. In the ED, temporary measures may be used to stabilize the patient before transfer to the ICU. In all shocks, regardless of etiology, fluid resuscitation is vital.

Fluid Resuscitation

Rapid fluid resuscitation is paramount and based on the type of fluid lost. Cardiac output cannot increase without fluid, and fluid that is not in the vascular space (e.g., edema fluid or third-spaced fluid) is not immediately available—so regardless of how "overloaded" a patient looks because of peripheral edema, they may be hypovolemic. Crystalloid infusion alone may be adequate for patients with class I or class II blood loss. For patients with severe blood loss, resuscitation should include blood products to increase the oxygen-carrying capacity and allow for increased oxygen extraction from the tissues. Blood transfusions are indicated for hemoglobin levels less than 7 g/dL or for less than 10 g/dL for patients with cardiovascular or cerebrovascular disease (222). Cardiogenic shock is one type of shock for which large amounts of fluid are usually not indicated.

The controversy over type of replacement fluid (crystalloid or colloid), how much to administer, when to administer, and when to stop is ongoing in the trauma literature (218, 219, 223). Isotonic crystalloids are recommended as the first fluids infused to help "fill up the tank" or the intravascular space. The estimated amount of initial fluid resuscitation is 1 to 2 liters of lactated Ringer's (LR), followed by packed red blood cell transfusion, according to Advanced Trauma Life Support (ATLS) guidelines (223). However, all fluid types do not act the same with the body compartments. One liter of NS will stay in the extracellular fluid space, with 10% to 25% distributed to the intravascular space and 75% to 90% into the interstitial spaces, so this fluid is helpful in hypovolemic patients. Because of this known distribution of crystalloid, ATLS guidelines recommend that for every 1 mL of blood lost, 3 mL of replacement crystalloid be used (210). This concept is known as the "3 for 1" rule. Lactated ringers solution causes less acidosis and thus is preferred as a resuscitation fluid. Caution is used with LR infusions because it does contain calcium, which can cause drug interactions and precipitate blood clotting in the transfused blood. Ensuring that the amount of transfused blood is twice that of infused LR should prevent these reactions (222). Hypotonic solutions are not appropriate for fluid resuscitation.

Although isotonic crystalloids are inexpensive and easy to administer, research studies have shown detrimental effects from the administration of LR or isotonic solutions. Consequences of fluid resuscitation with LR have been documented to affect acid-base balance, cellular function, and the immune system and inflammatory response: increased apoptosis and ROS production, and neutrophil and immune system activation. Increased production of ROS and nitrogen reactive species from increases in neutrophil activation and neutrophilic oxidative (respiratory) burst (210, 223), hyperchloremic acidosis from NS solutions (210, 218), and hemodilution and coagulopathies have also been noted (219). Hyperchloremic acidosis is a concern and can occur with LR or hetastarch administration but not to the same extent as with NS infusions. Additionally, hyperchloremic acidosis has been associated with impairment of renal function, metabolic acidosis, abdominal discomfort, and mental status changes (218, 219). Warming large amounts of replacement fluids is suggested to help decrease the potential for acidosis by preventing hypothermia. Adverse reactions to fluid replacement after hemorrhagic shock, in particular, are labeled resuscitation injury (223).

Hypertonic crystalloids include 3% hypertonic saline (HTS), 5% HTS, and 7.5% HTS. Because of the higher osmotic content, HTS is an effective choice for fluid replacement. Smaller volumes of HTS can be used, as most of this volume stays in the intravascular space and it pulls additional fluid from the extravascular spaces into the blood vessels. Research studies on fluid resuscitation have shown that HTS has the opposite effect on immune function than LR. HTS inhibits neutrophil oxidative burst activity, reduces adhesion molecule "stickiness," and thus reduces the amount of cellular injury (223). Research using HTS and HTS combined with other products, such as Dextran, are in progress (223).

Research studies have provided mixed reviews on the use of colloids in hemorrhagic shock (210, 224). Colloids are nonsynthetic proteins or synthetic proteinS/Starches that because of their high molecular content stay in the intravascular space—so colloids increase blood volume by staying completely in the intravascular compartment and by recruiting fluid from the interstitial spaces because of the pull of the increased oncotic pressure. Therefore, smaller amounts of colloids can be given because they replace fluid at more than a 1:1 ratio.

Albumin reduces the immune effects of increased cellular adhesion and neutrophilic oxidative burst seen with crystalloid infusions; reduces pulmonary, cerebral, and intestinal edema; and enhances urine output (225). Both the macro- (systemic) and micro-circulatory systems are improved with colloid infusion (218). Examples of colloids are 5% and 25% albumin, 6% hydroxyethyl starch (HES), gelatins, and 3% dextran-60 and 6% dextran-70. The disadvantage of colloid replacement is cost, availability, and potential harm in patients with increased capillary membrane permeability—the colloid proteins can leak into the interstitial spaces and pull fluid out of the intravascular space. Colloid administration also has risks that include anaphylactoid reactions, organ damage, and infection (225); impairment of platelet function and coagulation (for volumes of Dextran and HES greater than 1.5 L); considerable neutrophil activation; renal impairment; and hyperchloremic acidosis (210, 222-225). According to a Cochrane review, at this time there is no definitive evidence that one colloid is better than another (224).

Blood products are transfused when the amount of blood loss threatens oxygenation. Although whole blood would be the preferred replacement fluid, it is difficult to store and safely maintain. Therefore, typed and cross-matched packed red blood cells (RBCs) are commonly transfused. One to two units of type O Rh-negative blood may be transfused in emergency situations (222). When multiple units of blood are transfused, they should be administered warmed (37°C), and for patients needing large amounts of blood (8 to 10 units or more), fresh frozen plasma, cryoprecipitate, and platelet transfusions should be considered to replace lost clotting factors (222). There are cautions against overly aggressive fluid resuscitation for patients with hemorrhagic shock from internal hemorrhage as bleeding may be increased (222, 225); a resuscitation endpoint of an MAP between 60 and 80 mm Hg is encouraged to stabilize the patient with internal hemorrhage until surgical correction of the blood loss can be achieved (222). Hematocrit (Hct) values are followed to ascertain the need for more blood. Cardiovascular and cerebrovascular patients needed higher Hct values and are transfused to keep the Hct at or above 30; other patients can usually tolerate an Hct of 23 to 28 mm Hg (200). In hemorrhagic shock, 5 to 10 mL/kg of colloid or packed RBCs is the recommended infusion dose (200).

Blood substitutes can be hemoglobin-based or perfluorocarbons, each carry large amounts of oxygen, do not need to be cross-matched, and can be stored for long periods. There has been ongoing research to find an effective blood substitute, but results have not been conclusive as to safety or outcomes (210, 222). With any fluid resuscitation, it is essential to be sure to continuously assess your patient for signs of fluid overload, such as pulmonary edema.

Management (Pharmacologic)

The following medications are typically used in the management of shock: inotropic agents, vasodilators, vasopressors, beta-blockers, phosphodiesterase inhibitors, catecholamines, alpha agonists, steroids, antihistamines, and anticoagulants. Table 9-52 includes general information about the shock states, including the typical drugs used to manage each type of shock.

Shock Endpoints

The endpoint of shock resuscitation is adequate tissue perfusion. A urine output of greater than 0.5 to 1 mL/kg/hr is a good indicator of organ perfusion. The typical measurements of heart rate, level of consciousness, and capillary refill can vary due to many factors (e.g., is the parameter change due to compensation or true resuscitation?) and therefore are not robust indicators of tissue perfusion. Global indicators of tissue perfusion include serum lactate and base excess or base deficit levels as these are relatively unaffected by other parameters (219). Serum lactate levels should decrease by half after resuscitation measures, but may continue to be elevated for several hours after resuscitation (222). Sublingual CO_2 measurements are very accurate and can rapidly identify changes (221, 222). Base deficit has been studied in trauma situations and found to be a reliable marker of fluid resuscitation. Base deficit responds so quickly to changes in blood pH and blood volume that it may show a change before the blood pressure or urine output. According to some trauma researchers, an indicator of resuscitation success is a corrected lactate and BD levels and a normal platelet count (219).

General Management of Specific Shock States

Hypovolemic Shock

General management of hypovolemic shock includes rapid fluid resuscitation and locating the cause of the hypovolemia for treatment. An overview of hypovolemic shock management is found in Table 9-52.

(Text continued on page 383)

TABLE 9-52 Etiologies, Pathophysiology, Clinical Manifestation, and General Management of Different Types of Shock

Etiology	Pathophysiology/Mechanisms of Action	Clinical Manifestations	General Management Overview
HYPOVOLEMIC: FLUID FAILURE: RESULTS FROM DECREASED INTRAVASCULAR VOLUME MAY BE DELINEATED AS:			
• Hemorrhagic (traumatic) shock • Burn shock			
External fluid losses (most common) • Loss of large amounts of any body fluid • Trauma • Suctioning • Vomiting • Diarrhea • Diuretics • Surgery • Diabetes Insipidus • Hyperglycemia • Bleeding disorders • GI bleeding • Inadequate fluid replacement Internal fluid shifting • Intravascular to intracellular/interstitial space	Loss of intravascular volume results in decreased cardiac output, stroke volume, and blood pressure. Compensatory mechanisms are activated. In hemorrhagic shock, blood vessels spasm to protect the body from blood loss, but the size and extent of the vessels injured overwhelms the body's ability to stem the flow of blood. The clotting cascade is activated. In burn shock, large amounts of plasma proteins are lost in the burned tissue, causing internal fluid shifting to occur.	The amount of blood loss will dictate the clinical signs and symptoms. Class I: up to 15% of total blood volume lost: few S/S as body compensates for loss Class II: 15-30% volume loss: BP may be stable; tachycardia, tachypnea Class III: 30% to 40% total volume loss: worsening tachycardia (HR >120 bpm) and falling BP; AMS; oliguria Class IV: >40% loss is life-threatening; significant tachycardia (HR >140 bpm) General S/S: Tachycardia, hypotension, Narrowed pulse pressure ΔLOC Piloerection then cold, clammy skin Respiratory alkalosis, hypoxemia U/O <30 mL/hr Mottled skin Cyanosis (late) Hemodynamic S/S: decreased CO, CVP, MAP; increased SVR	• Locate cause and correct • Return to surgery for surgical cause • Direct pressure for trauma cause • Antiemetics antidiarrheals, for severe dehydration from vomiting or diarrhea • Provide O_2 • Obtain IV access (at least 2 large-bore IVs recommended) • Fluid resuscitation with crystalloids and/or colloids • Warmed fluids if possible • Transfusion with whole blood or packed red blood cells for blood loss; FFP and/or cryoprecipitate for plasma loss • Hemodynamic monitoring, cardiac monitoring • Hemorrhagic shock: Monitor Hand, platelet counts, and bleeding times; serum lactate & base deficit/excess

Continued

TABLE 9-52 Etiologies, Pathophysiology, Clinical Manifestation, and General Management of Different Types of Shock—cont'd

Etiology	Pathophysiology/Mechanisms of Action	Clinical Manifestations	General Management Overview
HYPOVOLEMIC: FLUID FAILURE: RESULTS FROM DECREASED INTRAVASCULAR VOLUME MAY BE DELINEATED AS:			
• Hemorrhagic (traumatic) shock • Burn shock			
• Increased capillary membrane permeability (edema, third spacing) • Burns • Liver disease • Renal disease • Fluid overload • Surgery		Labs: increased Na, K, serum lactate; BUN/Cr normal; negative BD; low pH Hemorrhagic shock: check H&H	
CARDIOGENIC SHOCK: Pump Failure: results from a cumulative loss of cardiac muscle ≥40% causing impaired ability to deliver blood forward in the systemic circulation. Noncoronary causes of cardiogenic shock may be described as obstructive shock.			
Coronary causes: • AWMI (15% to 20% develop cardiogenic shock) • Highest risk: AWMI with complications: papillary muscle rupture; interventricular septum rupture; ventricular free wall rupture • HF • CMP • LV aneurysm • VHD • Myocardial depression (from septic shock)	Blood volume is adequate however heart can't pump blood in the systemic circulation. Coronary causes: damaged cardiac muscle is nonfunctional—it cannot contract or contract well and therefore cannot move preload forward into the aorta or coronary ostia reducing coronary artery perfusion leading to more ischemia and a vicious cycle	General S/S of hypovolemic shock plus: • Dysrhythmias • ↑ JVD • Dependent edema • ↑ WOB • Low-grade temperature • Angina pain • Gallop rhythm Hemodynamic S/S: • ↑ HR • ↑ CVP • ↑ PAOP • ↑ SVR • ↓ CO/CI • ↓ BP	• MI patients: decrease or minimize infarct size by reducing O_2 demands • Calm, reassuring attitude • Supplemental O_2 • Rest • Pain relief • Combat shivering with thorazine or meperidine • Hemodynamic and cardiac monitoring • Mechanical ventilation • Strict I&O • Fluid resuscitation with caution not to overload the weakened ventricle • Improve heart function • Positive inotropes • Dopamine 400 mg/250 D5W or NS (1,600 mg/mL) at 5–10 mcg/kg/min OR

Noncoronary causes:

- No cardiac muscle damage
- Cardiac tamponade
- Pulmonary HTN
- Pulmonary embolism
- Restrictive pericarditis
- Tension pneumothorax

Noncoronary causes:

- Any disease process or pathology that reduces heart filling will reduce the amount of preload and therefore the CO.
- Any disease process or pathology that reduces the pumping ability of the heart will reduce the amount of blood able to be ejected from the heart in systole, reduce stroke volume, and therefore CO.

Labs:

- Leukocytosis
- ↑ cardiac enzymes
- ↑ C-reactive protein

Diagnostics:

- ECG changes indicative of MI
- CXR
- Spiral CT

- Dobutamine 500 mg in 250 D5W or NS (2,000 mcg/mL) at 2–20 mcg/kg/hr
  - ≤5mcg/kg/min—renal
  - 5 mcg–10 mcg/kg/min—cardiac
  - ≥20 mcg/kg/min—blood vessels
- Vasodilators
- Nitroprusside 50 mg/500 mL D5W (100 mg/mL) start at 10 mg/min (6 mL/hr); increase by 10 mg/min q5–10min
- Nitroglycerin 25 mg/250 mL (100 mg/mL) start at 10 mg/min (6 mL/hr); increase by 10 mg/min q5–10min
- Antiarrhythmics
- Phosphodiesterase enzyme

Inhibitors

- Ventricular assist devices if needed (IABP, VAD)
- Heart transplantation
- Diuretics
- Natriuretic peptides (ANP, BNP)
- Norepinephrine 4 mg/250 D5W or NS (16 mg/mL) at 2–12 mcg/min or 0.05–1 mcg/kg/min
- Ongoing assessments

Continued

TABLE 9-52 Etiologies, Pathophysiology, Clinical Manifestation, and General Management of Different Types of Shock—cont'd

Etiology	Pathophysiology/ Mechanisms of Action	Clinical Manifestations	General Management Overview
CARDIOGENIC SHOCK: Pump Failure: results from a cumulative loss of cardiac muscle ≥40% causing impaired ability to deliver blood forward in the systemic circulation.			
	Noncoronary causes of cardiogenic shock may be described as obstructive shock.		Noncoronary patient: Treat the underlying cause: remove the obstruction to filling or ejection • Relieve the tamponade through pericardiocentesis or surgical intervention • Relieve the constriction of the pericardial sac • Treat PHTN • Thrombectomy for PE • Emergency treatment of tension pneumothorax = 18-gauge needle in 2nd to 3rd ICS; chest tube placement
DISTRIBUTIVE OR VASOGENIC SHOCK: *Pipe Failure:* describes shock states resulting from maldistribution of blood flow and/or to an abnormality of the vascular system			
Three types of vasogenic shock: • Neurogenic shock • Septic shock • Anaphylactic shock			
Neurogenic shock: high spinal cord injury (midthoracic level above T5) that blocks or impairs sympathetic outflow: • Pain • Emotional stress • Drug overdose	Total blood volume is adequate; however the blood volume is not in the intravascular space or the blood vessels are so vasodilated that there is no vascular tone and therefore no ability to increase venous return.	General S/S: systemic: • Hypotension • Warm, dry skin • Hypothermia • Bradycardia • No sweating below level of injury	• Proper stabilization to minimize spinal cord trauma • Proper positioning after spinal anesthesia • Administer pain medications • Maintain patent airway and ventilation • Assess for paralytic ileus, urinary retention • Assess for DVT risk • Avoid fluid volume excess to prevent cord edema

- High spinal anesthesia
- Spinal cord damage

Occurs immediately after injury lasting about 1–6 weeks, may last for months; recovery is gradual
Prevention is possible:
- Careful, early immobilization of SCI patients during transport or procedures
- HOB 15–20 degrees after spinal anesthesia

Septic shock: documented infection unresponsive to conventional therapy with at least one organ failure

Gram-positive and gram-negative organisms
Fungal organisms
Viral organisms

Anaphylactic Shock: a systemic response to an antigen

Neurogenic shock: massive vasodilation of the vasculature due to a loss of sympathetic vasomotor tone below the level of injury. Loss of sympathetic tone means unopposed parasympathetic activity. Sympathetic outflow is blocked or impaired.
Venous pooling
Peripheral vasodilation

Massive vasodilation of the vasculature, increased capillary-membrane permeability, and blood pooling in capillaries due to the presence of microorganisms that triggered the inflammatory response and the immune system. Endotoxin (lipopolysaccharide [LPS]) from gram-negative organisims is the primary agent that stimulates immune cells to release histamines and bradykinins causing the inflammatory effects

Immune-mediated hypersensitivity reaction to a substance the body considers foreign; IgE- covered mast cells are triggered by the antigen; antigen-antibody coupling occurs resulting in the eruption of the mast cell releasing histamine, serotonin, platelet aggregating factor

---

Early stage:
- Warm, dry, flushed skin
- Normal to high-normal BP
- Tachycardia
- Tachypnea
- High cardiac output
- Increased U/O
- Acid-base balance
- Low SVR
- High $Svo_2/Scvo_2$
- Fever with chills
- Confusion

Late stage:
- Classic shock: see hypovolemia S/S

- Vasoactive medications to increase BP
- IV methylprednisolone?
- Atropine
- Anticoagulants
- Antianxiety medications
- Antacids, H2 blockers
- Emotional support
- Relieve anxiety and stress

- O_2 therapy: Keep SaO_2 >95%
- Early IV fluid resuscitation
  - Crystalloids 1–2 L in first 1–2 hours
  - Blood transfusion as needed
  - Colloids mb
- Keep U/O >0.05–1 mL/kg/hr
- Dopamine 400 mg/250 D5W or NS (1,600 mg/mL) at 5–10 mcg/kg/min OR
- Dobutamine 500 mg in 250 D5W or NS (2,000 mcg/mL) at 2–20 mcg/kg/hr
- Norepinephrine 4 mg/250 D5W or NS (16 mg/mL) at 2–12 mcg/min or 0.051 mcg/kg/min
- Phenylephrine 60 mg/250 mL D5W or NS (240 mcg/mL) at 5–10 mcg/kg/min
- Digitalis
- IV epinephrine 1:1,000
  - 0.3–0.5 mL SC may repeat q10–15min ×3
- Unstable/hypotensive: 0.1 mg or more IVP or 1–4 mcg/min infusion

Continued

TABLE 9-52 Etiologies, Pathophysiology, Clinical Manifestation, and General Management of Different Types of Shock—cont'd

Etiology	Pathophysiology/Mechanisms of Action	Clinical Manifestations	General Management Overview

DISTRIBUTIVE OR VASOGENIC SHOCK: *Pipe Failure:* describes shock states resulting from maldistribution of blood flow and/or to an abnormality of the vascular system Three types of vasogenic shock:
• Neurogenic shock
• Septic shock
• Anaphylactic shock
	Causes massive vasodilation, increased capillary-membrane permeability (leaky membrane), and		• Inhaled β-agonists
			• HHN
			• Antihistamines: H1 and H2 blockers should be used together
			• H1 blocker:
			  • Mild reaction: Diphendydramine 25–50 mg PO
			  • Serious reaction: Diphenhydramine up to 2 mg/kg SIVP
			• H2 blocker cimeditine 300 mg IV or ranitidine 50 mg IV
			• Continue for 72 hr: diphenhydramine or hydroxyzine 25–50 mg PO q6h and cimeditine 300 mg q6h or ranitidine 150 mg PO bid
			• Corticosteroids
			  • Hydrocortisone 100–300 mg IV OR
			  • Methylprednisolone 60–125 mg IV OR
			  • Prednisone 40 mg PO
			  • Prednisone 40 mg QD x5–7 days to reduce itching and urticaria

AMS, altered mental status; AWMI, anterior wall myocardial infarction; BG, blood glucose; BP, blood pressure; BUN, blood urea nitrogen; CO/CI, cardiac output/cardiac index; CMP, cardiomyopathy; Cr, creatinine; CT, computed tomography scan; CVP, central venous pressure; CXR, chest x-ray; DVT, deep vein thrombosis; FFP, fresh frozen plasma; H&H, hemoglobin and hematocrit; HF, heart failure; HR, heart rate; HTN, hypertension; IABP, intra-aortic balloon pump; I&O, intake and output; IV, intravenous; JVD, jugular venous distention; K, potassium; delta LOC, change in level of consciousness; LV, left ventricle; MAP, mean arterial pressure; MODS, multiple organ dysfunction syndrome; Na, sodium; O₂, oxygen; PAP, pulmonary artery pressure; PaCO₂, partial pressure of carbon dioxide dissolved in the arterial blood; PAOP, pulmonary artery occlusion pressure; PHTN, pulmonary hypertension; SG, specific gravity; RR, respiratory rate; Spo₂, saturation of hemoglobin with oxygen; Svo₂, mixed venous oxygen saturation; SVR, systemic vascular resistance; U/O, urine output; VAD, ventricular assist device;

Cardiogenic Shock

Cardiogenic shock is pump failure or an inability of the heart muscle to fill and/or move blood forward; it occurs when 40% or more of the cardiac muscle is damaged (coronary cause) or whenever the filling and/or ejection from the heart is restricted from a cause other than cardiac muscle damage (noncoronary cause). Cardiogenic shock due to a coronary cause is type of shock that can occur because of systolic and/or diastolic dysfunction—the most common causes are anterior wall MI (AWMI) and AWMI with complications (papillary muscle rupture, interventricular septum rupture, and ventricular wall free rupture).

As with any MI, damaged heart muscle is nonfunctional and therefore does not contract with the rest of the heart muscle. This area of nonfunctional tissue is a dead zone and creates a desynchronized contraction, which impairs ejection. Right ventricular infarction would decrease preload delivery to the left heart, thus decreasing stroke volume and CO (68). In the case of AWMI, the anterior wall of the LV, the powerhouse of the heart, is the muscle damaged. Damaged cardiac muscle in this location will severely impact cardiac contraction ability. About 15% to 20% of patients with an AWMI suffer from cardiogenic shock with a mortality rate of 80%. The prime point in time for this shock complication to arise is about 2 to 3 days after the AWMI onset. Knowing that cardiogenic shock is a potential consequence for AWMI patients, vigilant nurses should be the ones to pick up the first subtle signs of decreased tissue perfusion and alert their physician or advanced practice colleagues to begin treatment.

Patients can suffer from cardiogenic shock even though their heart is completely normal, without any muscle damage. Noncoronary causes of cardiogenic shock include anything that can restrict the heart from filling or from emptying properly. Classic examples of restricted filling and restricted pumping are cardiac tamponade or restrictive pericarditis. The outside pressure building up in the pericardial sac eventually puts pressure on the heart, from all sides restricting filling capacity and pumping ability. Eventually the heart stops and cardiac arrest occurs. A massive pulmonary embolism, pulmonary hypertension, aortic stenosis, and tension pneumothorax are also examples of noncoronary causes of cardiogenic shock. In some of the literature, the restriction of cardiac filling and forward flow is described as either a subtype of cardiogenic shock or as a separate entity termed obstructive shock.

In both types of pathology, the compensatory responses of tachycardia, vasoconstriction, and fluid retention further exacerbate the problem by presenting a compromised heart with higher resistance pressures and higher volumes thus furthering cardiac dysfunction.

See Table 9-52 for management of cardiogenic shock.

Distributive or Vasogenic Shock

The problem with distributive shocks is the massive vasodilation that occurs and causes fluid to third-space. The goal of therapy is this case is to restore vascular tone. See Table 9-52 for general management of distributive shocks.

Neurogenic Shock

Neurogenic shock is a type of distributive shock because injury to the spinal cord causes a disconnect between the sympathetic nervous system and the nerves below the level of injury. Loss of sympathetic tone below the level of the injury means that the parasympathetic nervous system is unopposed. Therefore, a massive vasodilatory effect occurs in neurogenic shock. Neurogenic shock is sometimes confused with spinal shock—these processes are NOT the same! Spinal shock is immediately seen after injury and is due to the loss of motor and sensory function below the injury level.

The typical picture of neurogenic shock is hypotension without the compensatory tachycardia or the vasoconstriction. Neither the heart nor blood vessels are triggered to compensate for the low blood pressure in the lower extremities. Bradycardia is the common response of the heart. The patient does not sweat below the injury. Neurogenic shock is managed through preventive strategies. Neck stabilization in trauma patients is essential! Proper positioning after spinal anesthesia with the head-of-the-bed (HOB) raised 15 to 20 degrees will allow the patient to recover without reinfusing anesthetic into the spinal cord. Positive inotropes (dobutamine, dopamine) and vasopressors may be used to correct the vasodilation.

Anaphylactic Shock

Anaphylaxis is an IgE-mediated, hyperresponsive, systemic reaction to an antigen; it is considered a type I hypersensitivity reaction. Certain foods, insect venom, and medications (commonly ASA and penicillin) can trigger an allergic reaction. In the acute care setting, commonly used materials for diagnostic procedures and therapies can stimulate a hypersensitive immune response. It is estimated that 5% of the population is allergic to radiocontrast materials. Blood transfusions are responsible for a small percent of anaphylactic reactions occurring about once in every 20,000 to 400,000 units transfused and mainly among IgA-deficient individuals (226). Anaphylactic shock is characterized by massive vasodilation, increased capillary membrane permeability, and possible syncope and circulatory collapse. About 1% to 3% of people suffering from anaphylactic shock die.

The pathophysiology of a type I hypersensitivity reaction includes the introduction of a protein or foreign material that then overstimulates the immune system. The antigen triggers the immune response and the IgE-covered mast cell couples with the antigen. This linkage causes the mast cell to erupt, and multiple cytokines are released from the cell's interior. Histamine is released and causes increased capillary membrane permeability, vasodilation, and bronchoconstriction. Bradykinin is also released and potentiates the effects of histamine. In the normal immune response, these immunologic steps are responsible for eliminating the antigen at a local level. Anaphylaxis is an exaggeration of the immune response and the effects are seen systemically instead of locally. Anaphylactic shock could consist of total circulatory collapse refractory to treatment.

Signs and symptoms are specifically associated with the route of the anaphylactic agent, but then become systemic. Antigens that are inhaled have nasal and upper and lower airway signs: congestion, itchy eyes, angioedema of the lips and mucous membranes, dyspnea, cough, and/or wheezing. Antigens that have a topical effect with present as itching, redness, and urticaria (hives) in the region where the antigenic protein touched the skin or mucous membranes. Antigens that are ingested will primarily manifest as gastrointestinal tract symptoms: dysphagia, nausea, vomiting, and abdominal cramping. Injected antigens typically are the most rapidly lethal. The more rapidly the signs and symptoms of anaphylaxis develop, the sicker the patient. Total circulatory collapse may occur requiring life support measures.

Management of anaphylactic shock is similar to that of any distributive shock—fluid resuscitation and the administration of vasopressor agents to manage blood pressure and tissue perfusion. However, first, identification and removal of the antigen source is critical to stopping the anaphylactic reaction. If the antigen is being infused (e.g., blood transfusion or medication), immediately stop the infusion and maintain the intravenous line with NS to keep the vein open for possible fluid resuscitation and emergency medication administration. Reverse the effect of the proinflammatory cytokines by administering intravenous or subcutaneous epinephrine, antihistamines (both histamine-1 [H1] and histamine-2 [H2] blockers), and inhaled beta-agonists or corticosteroids. (See Table 9-52 for detailed management.)

Nursing care entails getting a detailed history of allergies and any prior allergic events. Extra vigilant monitoring in the first hour of new medications or blood transfusions is paramount to identifying adverse reactions early and instituting emergency treatment. Nurses must also be alert to the possibility of late stage symptoms—anaphylaxis can return due to the late-phase reactants, released during the inflammatory stage, that are still present in the bloodstream.

Septic Shock

Septic shock is part of a continuum that depicts the progressive nature of the pathogenesis of infection to sepsis to severe sepsis to septic shock, multiple organ dysfunction syndrome (MODS), and death. Sepsis is the leading cause of death in ICUs, with 28-day mortality rates ranging from 28% to 50% (211). Every year about 750,000 people in the United States suffer from severe sepsis, 215,000 Americans die from sepsis every year, and it is estimated that sepsis kills 1400 people a day throughout the world (www.survivingsepsis.org). Risk factors include extremes of age (the very old and very young are the most vulnerable) and anything that can compromise the immune system: malnutrition, chronic disease, invasive procedures or devices, traumatic wounds, thermal injury, medications, and general debilitation. Elderly patients have a higher risk of sepsis or septic shock and a higher mortality rate from these as well (216). The growing elderly population, increased use of invasive procedures, and increased number of patients vulnerable to infection in America will increase the annual number of severe sepsis cases to 1 million by 2020; 28% to 50% of patients with a severe sepsis diagnosis die within the first month (212).

Septic shock is near the end of the continuum and is the most common form of distributive shock, affecting over 200,000 patients each year—the mortality rate of septic shock in the ICUs is 40% to 60%. A consensus document on the definitions of systemic inflammatory response system (SIRS), sepsis, and septic shock was outlined by the American College of Chest Physicians and the Society of Critical Care Medicine in 1991 in an effort to create universal definitions so that practitioners would be clear on the delineation between the terms and that the results of research studies could be more easily compared. Definitions of the sepsis continuum terms are found in Table 9-53 (211).

The annual cost of sepsis and sepsis syndrome is estimated at $17 billion a year in the United States (216). The complexity of patient care, need for specialized staff and equipment, and time spent on individual patient care accounts for about 40% of total ICU costs (www.survivingsepsis.org). The burden of costs on the patient, including physical, emotional, social, and psychological, are immense and for some sepsis survivors, long-standing. Sepsis research has been ongoing for over 20 years and scientists recently unlocked key parts of the mechanism of action. A result of this research has been the testing of new interventions that show promise in the treatment of severe sepsis and septic shock (211, 212).

TABLE 9–53 Definitions of Continuum of Sepsis Terms

	Definition	Characteristics or Criteria
SIRS		
	A systemic response to inflammation or clinical insults	Dx: Presence of 2 or more: • Body temperature >38°C or <36°C • Heart rate >90 beats/min (bpm) • Respiratory rate >20 breaths/min AND • White blood cell count >12,000/mm^3 or <4,000/mm^3 or with >10% bands
SEPTICEMIA		
	Acute invasion of bloodstream by microorganisms	Fever Chills Tachycardia Tachypnea Altered mentation
SEPSIS		
	Complex syndrome characterized by an overwhelming systemic response to infection	Documented infection 2 or more of SIRS criteria Heart rate >120 bpm; Partial pressure of arterial carbon dioxide (P$_A$CO$_2$) <32 mm Hg Nausea/vomiting/diarrhea Confusion Fever Shaking chills
SEVERE SEPSIS		
	Sepsis plus sepsis-induced organ dysfunction or decreased tissue perfusion	Lactic acidosis Oliguria Change in mental status Signs of organ dysfunction
SEPTIC SHOCK		
	Sepsis with hypotension refractory to therapy	BP <90 mm Hg or drop of 40 mm Hg from baseline value in absence of other causes Elevated lactate Oliguria

Source: www.survivingsepsis.org; www.lilly.com/pdf/sepsis_overview.pdf

Gram-negative and gram-positive bacteria are the main etiologic agents of septic shock. Over half of infecting organisms in septic shock are gram-negative species (60% to 70%) such as *Pseudomonas*, *Escherichia coli*, *Klebsiella*, *Enterobacter*, and *Serratia*. Gram-positive organisms such as staphylococci and streptococci are seen mainly as community-acquired organisms or from indwelling intravenous catheters in 20% to 30% of sepsis cases. Less frequent organisms to cause septic shock are fungal organisms (*Candida*, *Aspergillus*), which are more common in immunosuppressed patients and postoperative patients needing long-term intravenous access and antibiotics, and viruses such as CMV, herpes simplex, and respiratory syncytial virus (RSV).

The effects of endotoxin or lipopolysaccharide (LPS) released by gram-negative organisms and exotoxin from gram-positive organisms cause a generalized inflammatory response and alterations in the peripheral circulation resulting in massive vasodilation, maldistribution of blood volume due to shunted blood flow, and increased capillary-membrane permeability causing fluid shifting into the interstium and third-spaces. These alterations in the circulation reduce the amount of preload presented to the RV and LV. The heart is affected by endotoxin and the expression of TNF in inflammation. These myocardial depressant factors decrease the contractile force of the myocardium. The outcome of reduced preload and decreased cardiac function is decreased CO. The end result is a decrease in oxygen delivery to cells and cellular dysoxia—an inability of the cells to extract and/or use the oxygen that is delivered. Cellular dysfunction and cell death occur followed by organ dysfunction and failure.

The clinical presentation of septic shock is usually sudden in onset with signs that are easily recognized, and manifests in two stages. The early stage of septic shock used to be labeled warm shock because the patient's skin is warm, dry, and flushed from the massive vasodilation—not the common picture of a "shock patient." Temperature is increased and shaking chills are common; tachypnea and respiratory alkalosis is present; blood pressure may be normal to the high normal; tachycardia is present, as is a hyperdynamic myocardium unique to this shock state; finally, restlessness and a feeling of impending doom signified decreased perfusion to the brain. Classic signs of early stage septic shock are high CO (from the hyperdynamic myocardium), low SVR (from the massive vasodilation), and high mixed venous oxygen saturation (Svo_2) (from the dysoxia).

The late stage of septic shock is more typical of "classic shock" as the patient's compensatory mechanisms fail and organ dysfunction sets in. The patient is severely ill; hypotensive with worsening tachycardia and tachypnea; decreased level of consciousness (LOC); skin is cool to cold, clammy, and pale; the fever and chills continue; urine output drops; the respiratory alkalosis changes to respiratory acidosis as the patient tires of fast and deep breathing; and coagulation abnormalities are present.

Atypical presentations or a gradual onset of the signs and symptoms are common in the elderly. For example, the elderly patient in septic shock may be hypothermic (temperature less than 36.5°C) rather than hyperthermic. Nausea, vomiting, diarrhea, or an ileus may hinder the diagnosis of sepsis; however, the presence of other signs and symptoms may give clues as to the etiology of the infecting organism. If a rash is present, the vesicles or pustules may be cultured to help identify the organism (bacterial or fungal). Petechiae are indicative of meningococcus. *Pseudomonas* can cause ecthyma gangrenosum, necrotizing or bullous skin lesions characterized by erythema encircling a necrotic center, an effect of hemorrhagic infarctions from the invading organism.

Global indicators of oxygen supply and demand are at the center of sepsis diagnosis and consist of Svo_2 or central venous oxygenation ($Scvo_2$), arterial lactate concentration, base deficit, and pH. These global indicators provide important information about sepsis in the face of, possibly, normal vital signs (216).

Diagnostic testing for septic shock includes a CBC and a peripheral smear to look for signs of infection (i.e., leukocytosis with a "left shift") or overwhelming infection (leukopenia), thrombocytopenia (from chronic inflammation/infection and/or beginning of DIC), anemia (from inflammation), and abnormal RBC morphology seen in DIC (microangiopathic hemolytic anemia).

Blood cultures and cultures from other potential sources of infection including the sputum, skin lesions, urine, cerebrospinal fluid (CSF), and intravenous catheters and invasive lines should be obtained. A urinalysis may help identify the infectious cause (urinary tract infection [UTI] is a common source of sepsis in the elderly) and signs of early renal problems. Acute tubular necrosis (ATN) can develop secondary to shock; mild proteinuria is an early sign of ATN. Electrolytes, glucose, and liver function are also assessed.

A CXR is obtained. Abdominal radiographs are obtained if a gastrointestinal source of infection is possible because of perforation, ischemic bowel, or inflammation (e.g., cholecystitis, diverticulitis); a lumbar puncture may be performed if the signs indicate a neurologic source for the infection.

Clearly the goals of therapy for septic shock include identifying the source of the infection through cultures of tissue and fluid and in eliminating the identified source by removing invasive devices (Foley catheter, IV catheters), draining infected secretions, and debriding necrotic tissue. Once cultures are obtained, administer antibiotics immediately—broad-spectrum antibiotics are usually given first, changing once the specific organism has been identified and drug therapy can be individualized for that organism. Aminoglycosides, such as gentamycin and tobramycin, are commonly prescribed for gram-negative organisms; third generation cephalosporins such as cefotaxime or ceftazidime may be given for gram-positive and gram-negative organisms. Penicillins such as nafcillin sodium are effective against gram-positive organisms. Chloramphenicol is given for anaerobic bacteria and amphotericin B or fluconazole are effective against fungal agents.

Collaborative therapy is dependent on the team working together. New protocols for the treatment of the septic syndrome and suspected sepsis have been tested in multiple institutions and have been shown to decrease morbidity and mortality of septic shock. A Sepsis Resuscitation Bundle and Sepsis Management Bundle are available through many organizations and are based on the work of Dr. Emmanuel Rivers (216) and the concept of early goal-directed therapy.

Early goal-directed therapy (EGDT) is the strategy to rapidly identify and treat patients with sepsis or suspected sepsis to prevent them from progressing to severe sepsis and septic shock. Rapid treatment consists of early identification, early administration of antibiotics, rapid fluid resuscitation with crystalloid, and manipulation of hemodynamic variables (CVP, MAP, SvO_2) (216). Early administration of antibiotics and aggressive fluid resuscitation are essential in eradicating the causative agent and in supporting the macro- and microcirculation. It is now known that delaying fluid resuscitation causes the release of proinflammatory cytokines and the inhibition of anti-inflammatory cytokines such as IL-10 (227). Review the discussion under fluid resuscitation, if needed. Of note, microvascular resuscitation is perhaps more important than macrovascular resuscitation because it is at this level that oxygen is truly delivered to the tissues (213). Elbers and Ince suggested that microvascular resuscitation be added as a goal to EGDT (213).

Rivers et al. randomly assigned 263 patients with sepsis, septic shock, or sepsis syndrome to standard therapy or early goal-directed therapy in the emergency room (216). An algorithm for patient management was employed that concentrated on the provision of mechanical ventilation and/or sedation, initiation of central venous access for continuous monitoring of CVP and oxygenation (ScVO2), the administration of fluid boluses to maintain a CVP of greater than 8 mm Hg, vasoactive support for MAP less than 65 mm Hg or greater than 90 mm Hg, blood transfusion to a Hct of 30%, and the use of inotropic support after optimization of the hemodynamic variables. The study results were significant and showed that EGDT treatment protocols reduced mortality rates by 30% for severely septic patients and by 50% for patients with only beginning signs of sepsis (216). Multiple other researchers across the world have instituted the concepts of EGDT with great success.

Guidelines for what has become known as the Surviving Sepsis Campaign were first written in 2004 and were updated in 2008 (211). Key management recommendations are found in Box 9-9. Complications of septic shock include DIC, hyperglycemia followed by hypoglycemia, and the inability of the cells to use protein, glucose, or fat substrate for energy production.

Clinical Nurse Specialist Competencies and Spheres of Influence
Clinical Expert/Direct Care and Collaboration

All spheres of influence are affected when dealing with a patient in shock. The major characteristics required of the nurse in caring for the patient in shock are clinical judgment and caring practices, in which vigilance is a main component. The patient in shock is critically ill and may die if the warning signs of shock are not recognized and/or if the treatment of the shock is not implemented promptly. The CNS facilitates the recognition of these patients by synthesizing and interpreting multiple, and sometimes inconsistent, information sources. The CNS may think aloud to give the staff the benefit of hearing the CNS work through process to diagnose actual or potential patient problems. The CNS applies evidence-based guidelines to provide the highest quality care to this vulnerable population of patients. As the expert clinician, the CNS sees the patient's situation as fluid and knows that the complexity of the patient's problems require intraprofessional and interprofessional collaboration and consultation to promote the best possible outcomes.

The family of the shock patient is understandably anxious about what is happening to their loved one and fearful of potentially bad outcomes. Caring practices are demonstrated when the CNS anticipates the family's need for information, providing status updates on the patient's condition and answering questions honestly. The CNS designs strategies or provides resources or referrals according to the family's needs and requests.

The health care microenvironment surrounding the care of the shock patient is extremely stressful, and at times chaotic. The patient's vulnerability in shock and unpredictability of the outcome despite aggressive therapies can be discouraging to the health care team caring for the patient. The CNS creates a healthy environment for the patient by maintaining a calm atmosphere amidst the stress and promoting healthy staff relationships to facilitate communication and promote patient safety.

AACN has been the leader in developing guidelines to assess, create, and maintain healthy work environments for the benefit of the patients, staff, and institution, as a whole. AACN's Standards for Establishing and Sustaining Healthy Work Environments are an excellent resource for the CNS as these outline the components

BOX 9–9 Key Evidence-Based Recommendations from the International Guidelines for the Management of Sepsis and Septic Shock

INITIAL SIX HOURS, DIAGNOSIS, ANTIBIOTIC THERAPY

1. Early goal-directed resuscitation of the septic patient during the first 6 hr after recognition of sign/symptoms (grade 1, Quality C);
2. Blood cultures prior to antibiotic therapy if therapy is not delayed (1C);
3. Imaging studies performed quickly to confirm potential source of infection (1C);
4. Administration of broad-spectrum antibiotic therapy within 1 hr of diagnosis of septic shock (1B) and severe sepsis without septic shock (1D);
5. Daily reassessment of antibiotic therapy with microbiology and clinical data to narrow coverage, when appropriate (1C);
6. A usual 7-10 days of antibiotic therapy guided by clinical response (1D);
7. Source identified within first 6 hours of presentation (1D); control source recognizing pros and cons of therapy chosen (1C);

FLUID RESUSCITATION THERAPY, PHARMACOLOGIC THERAPIES

8. Administration of either crystalloid or colloid fluid resuscitation (1B); Aim for CVP $\geq$8 mm Hg (or 12-15 mm Hg in mechanically ventilated patients) (1C)
9. Fluid challenge to restore cardiac filling pressures and hemodynamic stability; volume and rate dependent on degree of hypoperfusion and clinical response (1D);
10. Reduce fluid administration rate for rising cardiac filling pressures with no improvement in tissue perfusion (1D);
11. Vasopressor preference for norepinephrine or dopamine to target keep mean arterial pressure $\geq$65 mm Hg (1C);
12. Dobutamine inotropic therapy for low cardiac output refractory to fluid resuscitation and combined inotropic/vasopressor therapy (1C); Keep CI within normal limits (1B)
13. Stress-dose steroid therapy given only in septic shock after blood pressure is identified to be poorly responsive to fluid and vasopressor therapy (2C);
14. Hydrocortisone is drug of choice over dexamethasone (2B); Keep hydrocortisone to $\leq$300 mg/day (1A)
15. rhAPC in patients with severe sepsis and clinical assessment of high risk for death (2B except 2C for postoperative patients); do not administer in low risk patients (APACHE II $\leq$20 or one organ failure)
16. Protocols for weaning and sedation/analgesia should be used (1B);
17. Use of intermittent bolus sedation or continuous infusion sedation with daily wake-up (1B);
18. Neuromuscular blockers should be avoided, if at all possible (1B);

OTHER THERAPEUTIC INTERVENTIONS

19. In the absence of tissue hypoperfusion, coronary artery disease, or acute hemorrhage, target a hemoglobin of 7-9 g/dL (1B); a low tidal volume of 6 mL/kg (1B); inspiratory plateau pressure strategy $\leq$30 mm Hg (1C) for ALI/ARDS patients
20. Application of at least a minimal amount of PEEP (1C)
21. Use weaning protocols to guide discontinuation of mechanical ventilation (1A)
22. Head of bed 30° (1B) or 30-45° (2C) in mechanically ventilated patients unless contraindicated
23. Avoiding routine use of pulmonary artery catheters in ALI/ARDS (1A);
24. To decrease days of mechanical ventilation and ICU length of stay, a conservative fluid strategy for patients with established ALI/ARDS who are not in shock (1C);
25. Institution of glycemic control protocols (1B) targeting a blood glucose <150 mg/dL after initial stabilization (2C);
26. Renal replacement therapy with either continuous veno-veno hemofiltration (CVVH) or intermittent hemodialysis is equally effective (2B);
27. Prophylaxis for deep vein thrombosis (1A);
28. Prophylaxis for stress ulcers using H2 blockers (1A) or PPIs (1B);
29. Communicate with patients and families; Advance care planning is recommended where appropriate (1D).

Grade 1, strong recommendation; Grade 2, weak recommendation; Quality of evidence: A, high; B, moderate; C, low; D, very low.

ALI, acute lung injury; APACHE, Acute Physiology and Chronic Health Evaluation; ARDS, acute respiratory distress syndrome; CVP, central venous pressure; CVVH, continuous veno-veno hemofiltration; ICU, intensive care unit; PEEP, positive end-expiratory pressure; PPI, proton pump inhibitors; rhAPC, recombinant human activated protein C.

From Dellinger et al., 2008 (211).

required to assess and establish work environments that respect the knowledge, skills, and talents of the members of the health care team (228). The premise of AACN's Healthy Work Environment standards is that nurses can only make their optimal contribution to patient care in a healthy work environment. The components of a healthy work environment entail skilled communication, true collaboration, effective decision making, appropriate staffing, meaningful recognition, and authentic leadership (228). An explanation of these components, along with a host of resources to implement a healthy work environment, is available from the AACN Web site, www.aacn.org.

Research/Evidence-Based Practice

The CNS's efforts to integrate evidence-based guidelines into the care of the shock patient is facilitated by the many professional organizations that produce tools and quality improvement processes for the purpose of improving care of specific patient populations. The CNS is the person who evaluates current practice and acquires the knowledge needed to change practice. For example, there has been a concerted effort in recent years to tackle the problem of sepsis in hospitalized patients. The Surviving Sepsis Campaign (SSC), an international effort to "improve the management, diagnosis, and treatment of sepsis," ended its collaboration with its founding groups in December 2008. One of the outcome goals of this initiative was to decrease mortality from sepsis by 25% in 5 years (www.survivingsepsis.org). This collaborative was truly unique in that it relied on volunteers to participate and work together in the pursuit of the campaign's goals. By the end of its last phase, over 250 sites in 18 countries in 3 continents had participated (229). The SSC produced excellent materials to educate health care providers on the basics of sepsis and the management of this complex series of disease processes (from SIRS to septic shock). International evidence-based guidelines were produced to standardize the recognition, diagnosis, and management of severe sepsis and septic shock (211). Benchmarking databases were instituted to document and compare institutional efforts using the evidence-based guidelines.

There were two sepsis bundles created to assist the clinician with the management of septic patients. The Sepsis Resuscitation bundle included the protocol and algorithm for managing patients within the first 6 hours of admission to the emergency department. The Sepsis Management bundle continued the treatment of the septic patient through the first 24 hours. The sepsis bundles are available on the Institute of Health Care Improvement (IHI) Web site (www.ihi.org), which also include quality improvement and measurement tools

for CNSs to implement these practice changes. Other organizations and professional organizations have produced materials to implement, monitor, and track progress of institutional goals to reduce sepsis and septic shock; www.survivingsepsis.org and SCCM (www.sccm.org) are two examples. Implementation of the sepsis bundles is an interprofessional endeavor as many disciplines need to buy in to the need for these tools and then collaborate in the implementation and auditing of the protocols. The SSC developed the **LEADER** anagram to identify steps in the adoption and implementation of the SSC guidelines (though these steps work for any quality initiative): **L**earn about sepsis and the quality improvement initiatives; **E**stablish baseline data on sepsis patients in your unit; **A**sk for buy-in from the key stakeholders (e.g., administrative, department, and unit leaders, QI personnel, nursing staff). Form an interdisciplinary team and get input for the plan, publicize efforts to raise awareness of the issues/initiative; **D**evelop a protocol specific to your institution, seek feedback and refine; **E**ducate all stakeholders to familiarize the staff with the protocols; **R**ecount successes and failures every month (www.survivingsepsis.org).

Systems Leadership

The care of severely ill patients includes the administration of fluids, blood products, and vasoactive medications that could spell disaster for the patient if not administered correctly or if the patient is not monitored appropriately. Safety measures for the administration of medications and blood products are part of the policies in every hospital and a renewed effort to decrease medication errors has been initiated by the National Quality Forum and other agencies. The CNS creates a culture of safety in the unit and brings an awareness of national initiatives to the institution so they can be instituted on a local level.

The Institute of Medicine (IOM) noted that many problems with patient safety are directly related to poor communication between providers (230, 231). National initiatives include strategies to improve "handoff" communication when transferring the patient from one service or care environment to another. The SBAR (Situation-Background-Assessment-Recommendation) technique was developed in Colorado and now is used nationally, in response to this patient safety issue (www.ihi.org). TeamSTEPPS™ is a program collaboratively developed by the Department of Defense and the Agency for Health care Research and Quality (232). This program provides "an evidence-based teamwork system to improve communication and teamwork skills among health care professionals . . . to improve patient safety" (232, Homepage). TeamSTEPPS includes training modules, tools, and other materials to implement and sustain this program. The IOM published a book titled: Keeping Patients Safe: Transforming the Work Environment of Nurses in 2004 that offered strategies to improve patient safety through improving the work environment (233). This text, as well as others from the IOM Web site, is available for purchase in hard copy, can be downloaded in pdf format, or read online for free (www.iom.edu).

References

1. World Health Organization. Cardiovascular Diseases: Fact Sheet No. 317. February 2007. Retrieved June 1, 2009, from World Health Organization: http://www.who.int/cardiovascular_diseases/en/

2. Lloyd-Jones D, Adams RJ, Brown TM, et al. Heart disease and stroke statistics—2010 update: a report from the American Heart Association. Circulation 2010;121(7):e46-e215. doi:10.1161/circulationaha.109.192667

3. National Heart, Lung, and Blood Institute. Fact Book—Fiscal Year 2007. Washington, DC: National Institutes of Health; 2008.

4. Ford ES, Ajani UA, Croft JB, et al. Explaining the decrease in US deaths from coronary disease, 1980–2000. N Engl J Med 2007;356(23):2388-2398.

5. Committee on Post-Graduate Education, Council on Clinical Cardiology, American Heart Association. Non-ST-Segment Elevation Acute Coronary Syndrome (NSTE-ACS): Pathophysiology, Epidemiology, Risk Stratification, Evaluation, and Management. [Slide Presentation]. June 29, 2004. Retrieved July 27, 2009, from American Heart Association: http://american-heart.org/presenter.jhtml?identifier=3024822

6. Brashers VL. Alterations of cardiovascular function. In McCance KL, Huether SE, Brashers VL, Rote NS, editors. Pathophysiology: The Biological Basis for Disease in Adults and Children (6th edition. pp. 1142-1208). St. Louis MO: Mosby; 2010.

7. Zebrack JS, Anderson JL. The role of infection in the pathogenesis of cardiovascular disease. Progr Cardiovasc Nursing 2003;18(1):42-49.

8. Reduction of Atherothrombosis for Continued Health. Long-term Management of Patients at Risk of Atherothrombosis. Section 1: Pathogenesis of Atherothrombosis: Long-term Outcome in Patients at Risk. Retrieved July 27, 2009, from Theheart.org: http://www.theheart.org/documents/nonMenuItems/823207/ppt/section1.ppt

9. Libby P. Inflammation and the Pathogenesis of Atherothrombotic Disease. Baylor College of Medicine. Retrieved July 27, 2009, from www.Lipidsonline.org: http://www.lipidsonline.org/ppt_dir/client_zips/592623.zip

10. Centers for Disease Control and Prevention. Cigarette Smoking Among Adults—United States, 2006. MMWR Morb Mortal Wkly Rep 2007;56(44):1157-1161.

11. US Department of Health and Human Services. Objective 27: Tobacco Use. Healthy People 2010: Understanding and Improving Health (2nd ed.). Vol. II. Washington, DC: US Government Printing Office.November 2000. Retrieved from http://www.healthypeople.g.ov/Document/HTML/Volume2/27Tobacco.htm#_Toc489766222

12. Kusumoto F. 2003; Cardiovascular disorders: Heart disease. In McPhee SJ, Lingappa VR, Ganong WF, editors. Pathophysiology of Disease: An Introduction to Clinical Medicine. 4th edition. New York: Lange Medical Books/McGraw-Hill; 2003: 260-300.

13. Ganong WF. Cardiovascular disorders: Vascular disease. In McPhee SJ, Lingappa VR, Ganong WF, editors. Pathophysiology of Disease: An Introduction to Clinical Medicine. 4th edition. New York: Lange Medical Books/McGraw-Hill; 2003:301-327.

14. Friedman GD, Cutter GR, Donahue RP, et al. CARDIA: Study design, recruitment, and some characteristics of the examined subjects. J Clin Epidemiol 1988;41(11):1105-1116. doi:10.1016/0895-4356(88)90080-7

15. Loria CM, Liu K, Lewis CE, et al. Early adult risk factor levels and subsequent coronary artery calcification: the CARDIA study. J Am Coll Cardiol 2007;9(20):2013-2020. doi:10.1016/j.jacc.2007.03.009

16. Bild DE, Detrano R, Peterson D, et al. Ethnic differences in coronary calcification: the Multi-Ethnic Study of Atherosclerosis (MESA). Circulation 2005;111(10):1313-1320. doi:10.1161/01.cir.0000157730.94423.4b

17. Radiological Society of North America. Cardiac CT for Calcium Scoring. Retrieved September 3, 2009, from http://www.radiologyinfo.org/en/info.cfm?pg=ct_calscoring

18. Anderson JL, Adams CD, Antman EM, et al. ACC/AHA 2007 guidelines for the management of patients with unstable angina/non–ST-elevation myocardial infarction: a report of the American College of Cardiology/American Heart Association Task Force on Practice Guidelines. J Am Coll Cardiol 2007;50(7):e1-e157. doi:10.1016/j.jacc.2007.02.013

19. Moustapha A, Anderson HV. Contemporary view of the acute coronary syndromes. J Invas Cardiol 2003;15(2):71-79.

20. Rosamond W, Flegal K, Friday G, et al. Heart disease and stroke statistics—2007 update: a report from the American Heart Association Statistics Committee and Stroke Statistics Subcommittee. Circulation 2007;115(5):e69-e171. doi:10.1161/circulationaha.106.179918

21. Haines SY. Challenges in managing venous thromboembolism and acute coronary syndrome: case studies of the use of antithrombotic and antiplatelet therapies. Am J Health-System Pharmacy 2008;65(15 suppl 7):S3-S4.

22. Lee C-S, Lu Y-H, Lee S-T, et al. Evaluating the prevalence of silent coronary artery disease in asymptomatic patients with spinal cord injury. Int Heart J 2006;47(3):325-330. doi:10.1536/ihj.47.325. Retrieved August 17, 2010, from http://www.jstage.jst.go.jp/article/ihj/47/3/325/_pdf

23. Ho CP, Krassioukov AV. Autonomic Dysreflexia and Myocardial Ischemia [Abstract]. Spinal Cord, doi:10.1038/sc.2010.2 Retrieved August 17, 2010, from http://www.nature.com/sc/journal/vaop/ncurrent/full/sc20102a.html

24. Groah SL, Menter RR. Long-term cardiac ischemia leading to coronary artery bypass grafting in a tetraplegic patient. Arch Phys Med Rehabil 1998;79(9):1129-1132. Retrieved August 17, 2010, from http://www.archives-pmr.org/article/S0003-9993(98)90183-6/abstract

25. Drouet L. Atherothrombosis as a systemic disease. Cerebrovasc Dis 13 2002;(suppl 1):1-6. doi:10.1159/000047782

26. Libby P. Atheroma: More than mush. Lancet 1996;348 (suppl 1):S4-S7. doi:10.1016/S0140-6736(96)98002-2

27. Reduction of Atherothrombosis for Continued Health (REACH). The Burden of Atherothrombosis: Chapter 1: An introduction to atherothrombosis. Retrieved July 27, 2009, from Theheart.org:

http://www.theheart.org/documents/nonMenuItems/823207/ppt/Burden_ch1.ppt

28. Libby P. Molecular bases of the acute coronary syndromes. Circulation 1995;91:2844-2850.

29. Thygesen K, Alpert JS, White HD, Joint ESC/ACCF/AHA/WHF Task Force for the Redefinition of Myocardial Infarction, et al. Universal definition of myocardial infarction. Circulation 2007;116(22):2634-2653. doi:10.1161/circulationaha.107.187397

30. Huether SE. Pain, temperature regulation, sleep, and sensory function. In McCance KL, Huether SE, editors. Pathophysiology: The Biological Basis of Disease in Adults and Children. 6th edition. St. Louis, MO: Mosby; 2010:481-524.

31. Alpert JS, Thygesen K, Antman E, et al. Myocardial infarction redefined: a consensus document of The Joint European Society of Cardiology/American College of Cardiology Committee for the Redefinition of Myocardial Infarction. J Am Coll Cardiol 2000;36(3):959-969.

32. Edmondstone WM. Cardiac chest pain: does body language help the diagnosis? Br Med J 1995;311(7021):1660-1661.

33. Caley WE Jr. Diagnosing the cause of chest pain. Am Fam Phys 2005;72(10):2012-2021.

34. Panju AA, Hemmelgarn BR, Guyatt GH, et al. The rational clinical examination. Is this patient having a myocardial infarction? JAMA 1998;280(14):1256-1263.

35. Greenhalgh T. How to Read a Paper: The Basics of Evidence Based Medicine. 3rd edition. London: Blackwell Publishing; 2006.

36. Thompson CJ. Statistical Measures Used for Evidence-Based Practice. South Fork, CO: CJT Consulting; 2010.

37. Joiss-Bilowich PR. Cardiac biomarkers: how to use them wisely. Emerg Med Rep 2010;31:25.

38. Schreiber D, Miller SM. Use of Cardiac Markers in the Emergency Department. Retrieved August 4, 2009, from emedicine.medscape.com: http://emedicine.medscape.com/article/811905-print

39. Chan D, Ng LL. Biomarkers in acute myocardial infarction. BMC Med 2010;8:34-45. doi:10.1186/1741-7015-8-34

40. Agruss JC, Garrett K. New markers for CVD. Nurse Pract 2005;30(11):26-31.

41. Krumholz HM, Anderson JL, Bachelder BL, et al. ACC/AHA 2008 performance measures for adults with ST-elevation and non-ST-elevation myocardial infarction: a report of the American College of Cardiology/American Heart Association Task Force on Performance Measures (Writing Committee to Develop Performance Measures for ST-Elevation and Non-ST-Elevation Myocardial Infarction—Developed in collaboration with the American Academy of Family Physicians and the American College of Emergency Physicians: Endorsed by the American Association of Cardiovascular and Pulmonary Rehabilitation, Society for Cardiovascular Angiography and Interventions, and Society of Hospital Medicine. Circulation 2008;118(24):2596-2648. doi:10.1161/circulationaha.108.191099

42. Fraker TD Jr, Fihn SD, Gibbons RJ, et al. 2007 chronic angina focused update of the ACC/AHA 2002 guidelines for the management of patients with chronic stable angina: a report of the American College of Cardiology/American Heart Association Task Force on Practice Guidelines Writing Group to Develop the Focused Update of the 2002 Guidelines for the Management of Patients With Chronic Stable Angina. Circulation 2007;116(23):2762-2772. doi:10.1161/circulationaha.107.187930

43. Antman EM, Anbe DT, Armstrong PW, et al. ACC/AHA guidelines for the management of patients with ST-elevation myocardial infarction: a report of the American College of Cardiology/American Heart Association Task Force on Practice Guidelines (Committee to Revise the 1999 Guidelines for the Management of Patients With Acute Myocardial Infarction). Circulation 2004;110:e82-e293. doi:10.1161/01.cir.0000134791.68010.fa

44. Antman EM, Hand M, Armstrong PW, et al. 2007 focused update of the ACC/AHA 2004 guidelines for the management of patients with ST-elevation myocardial infarction: a report of the American College of Cardiology/American Heart Association Task Force on Practice Guidelines. Circulation 2008;117(2):296-329. doi:10.1161/circulationaha.107.188209

45. Kushner FG, Hand M, Smith SC Jr, et al. 2009 focused updates: ACC/AHA guidelines for the management of patients with ST-elevation myocardial infarction (updating the 2004 guideline and 2007 focused update) and ACC/AHA/SCAI Guidelines on percutaneous coronary intervention (updating the 2005 guideline and 2007 focused update): a report of the American College of Cardiology Foundation/American Heart Association Task Force on Practice Guidelines. Circulation 2009;120:2271–2306. doi 10.1161/circulationaha.109.192663

46. ACCF/AHA Task Force on Practice Guidelines. Methodology Manual and Policies from the ACCF/AHA Task Force on Practice Guidelines. Retrieved October 4, 2010, from http://assets.cardiosource.com/Methodology_Manual_for_ACC_AHA_Writing_Committees.pdf

47. Davidson MH, Jacobsen TA. Statins work: The Development of Cardiovascular Disease and Its Treatment With 3-Hydroxy-3-methylglutaryl Coenzyme A Reductase Inhibitors. Retrieved April 29, 2002, from MedscapeCME: http://cme.medscape.com/viewarticle/416521

48. Rivera-Bou WL, Cabanas JG, Villanueva SE. Thrombolytic Therapy. Retrieved September 4, 2009, from http://emedicine.medscape.com/article/811234-overview

49. Mosca L, Banka CL, Benjamin EJ, et al. Evidence-based guidelines for cardiovascular disease prevention in women: 2007 update. J Am Coll Cardiol 2007;9(11),1230-1250. doi:10.1016/j.jacc.2007.02.020

50. American Heart Association American Stroke Association. Coronary Artery Disease Fact Sheet. Retrieved May 26, 2009, from http://www.americanheart.org/downloadable/heart/1247859527251sfactsheet1-CAD-web.pdf

51. Eagle KA, Guyton RA, Davidoff R, et al. ACC/AHA 2004 guideline update for coronary artery bypass graft surgery: a report of the American College of Cardiology/American Heart Association Task Force on Practice Guidelines (Committee to Update the 1999 Guidelinesfor Coronary Artery Bypass Graft Surgery). J Am Coll Cardiol 2004;4:e213-e310. doi:10.1016/j.jacc.2004.08.002

52. Berra K, Miller NH, Fair JM. Cardiovascular disease prevention and disease management: a critical role for nursing. J Cardiopulm Rehabil 2006;26(4):197-206.

53. Arnett DK, Baird AE, Barkley RA, et al. Relevance of genetics and genomics for prevention and treatment of cardiovascular disease: a scientific statement from the American Heart Association Council on Epidemiology and Prevention, the Stroke Council, and the Functional Genomics and Translational Biology Interdisciplinary Working Group. Circulation 2007;115(22):2878-2901. doi:10.1161/circulationaha.107.183679

54. Chen W, Woods SL, Puntillo KA. Gender differences in symptoms associated with acute myocardial infarction: a review of the research. Heart Lung 2005;34(4):240-247.

55. McSweeney JC, O'Sullivan P, Cleves MA, et al. Racial differences in women's prodromal and acute symptoms of myocardial infarction. Am J Crit Care 2010;19(1):63-73. doi:10.4037/ajcc 2010372

56. King KM, Khan NA, Quan H. Ethnic variation in acute myocardial infarction presentation and access to care. Am J Cardiol 2009;103(10):1368-1373. doi:10.1016/j.amjcard.2009.01.344

57. Jones DW, Peterson ED, Bonow RO, et al. Translating research into practice for health care providers: the American Heart Association's strategy for building healthier lives, free of cardiovascular diseases and stroke. Circulation 2008;118(6):687-696. doi:10.1161/circulationaha.108.189934

58. American Heart Association, American Stroke Association. Heart Failure/Coronary Artery Disease Fact Sheet: 30-Day Measures. Retrieved August 4, 2009, from http://www.americanheart.org/downloadable/heart/1248113023270factsheet-HFCAD-4.pdf

59. Lamendola C. Reducing the Risk of Heart Failure. Retrieved August 5, 2009, from http://cme.medscape.com/viewarticle/576929

60. Smith AL. Emerging Concepts in the Assessment and Treatment of Systolic and Diastolic Dysfunction: A "State-Of-The-Heart" Review. Retrieved March 10, 2008, from http://cme.medscape.com/viewprogram/2165

61. Hunt SA, Abraham WT, Chin MH, et al. 2009 Focused update incorporated into the ACC/AHA 2005 guidelines for the diagnosis and management of heart failure in adults: a report of the American College of Cardiology Foundation/American Heart Association Task Force on Practice Guidelines. Circulation 2009;119(14):e391-e479. doi:10.1161/circulationaha.109.192065

62. Unzek S, Francis GS. Management of heart failure: a brief review and selected update. Cardiol Clin 2008;26(4):561-571. doi 10.1016/j.ccl.2008.06.001

63. Lowery SL, Massaro R, Yancy CW Jr. Advances in the management of acute and chronic decompensated heart failure. Lippincotts Case Manage 2004;9(1):4-20.

64. Aurigemma GP, Gaasch WH. Diastolic heart failure. N Engl J Med 2004;351(11):1097-1105.

65. Colucci WS. Predicators of Survival in Heart Failure Due to Systolic Dysfunction. Retrieved April 19, 2005, from http://www.uptodateonline.com/applicatio...=hrt_fail/17977&type=A&selctedTitle=2~2

66. Neuenschwander JF II, Baliga RR. Acute decompensated heart failure. Crit Care Clin 2007;23(4):737-758. doi:10.1016/j.ccc.2007.08.003

67. Nieminen MS, Bohm M, Cowie MR, et al. Executive summary of the guidelines on the diagnosis and treatment of acute heart failure: the Task Force Acute Heart Failure of the European Society of Cardiology. Eur Heart J 2005;26(4):384-416. doi:10.1093/eurheartj/ehi044

68. Thompson, CJ, Smith-Love, J. (2011). Right versus left ventricular infarctions. NurseWeek & Nursing Spectrum Online CE offering. Retrieved August 8, 2011 http://ce.nurse.com/60173/Right-Versus-Left-Ventricular-Infarctions/

69. American Stroke Association. Heart Failure Fact Sheet: 30-Day Measures. Retrieved August 4, 2009, from http://americanheart.org/downloadable/heart/1248113502577factsheet-HF-4.pdf

70. Bhalla V, Maisel AS. B-Type Natriuretic Peptide: Role of BNP in the Emergency-Care Setting. Retrieved October 7, 2010, from http://www.medscape.com/viewarticle/480601_print

71. Kale P, Fang JC. Devices in acute heart failure. Crit Care Med 2008;36(suppl):S121-S128. doi:10.1097/01.ccm.0000297318.39219.2d

72. Trupp RJ. Cardiac resynchronization therapy: optimizing the device, optimizing the patient. J Cardiovasc Nursing 2004;19(4):223-233.

73. Wiegand DL-M, Williams LD. End-of-life care. In Carlson KK, editor. AACN Advanced Critical Care Nursing. St Louis, MO: Saunders; 2009:1507-1525.

74. Goodlin SJ. Palliative care in congestive heart failure. J Am Coll Cardiol 2009;54(5):386-396. doi:10.1016/j.jacc.2009.02.078

75. Medina J, Puntillo K; American Association of Critical-Care Nurses, editors. AACN Protocols for Practice: Palliative Care and End-of-life Issues in Critical Care. Sudbury, MA: Jones and Bartlett; 2006.

76. World Health Organization. WHO Definition of Palliative Care. Retrieved August 20, 2009, from http://www.who.int/cancer/palliative/definition/en/

77. Wingate S, Wiegand DL-M. End-of-life care in the critical care unit for patients with heart failure. Crit Care Nurse 2008;28(2):84-96.

78. Institute for Health Care Improvement. Reducing Readmissions by Improving Transitions in Care. Retrieved June 25, 2009, from http://www.ihi.org/IHI/Programs/Collaboratives/IHICollaborativeIReducingReadmissionsbyImprovingTransitionsinCare.htm

79. Holland R, Battersby J, Harvey I, et al. Systematic review of multidisciplinary interventions in heart failure. Heart 2005;91(7):899-906. doi:10.1136/hrt.2004.048389

80. Maisch B, Ristic AD. Pericardial diseases. In Fink MP, Abraham E, Jean-Louis V, Kockanek PM, editors. Textbook of Critical Care. 5th edition. Philadelphia: Saunders; 2005:851-860.

81. Tingle LE, Molina D, Calvert CW. Acute pericarditis. Am Fam Phys 2007;76(10):1509-1514.

82. Carter T, Riegel B. Care of patients with pericardial diseases. In Moser DK, Riegel B, editors. Cardiac Nursing: A Companion to Braunwald's Heart Disease. St Louis, MO: Saunders; 2008:1159-1166.

83. Maisch B, Seferović PM, Ristić AD, et al. Guidelines on the diagnosis and management of pericardial diseases executive summary: the Task Force on the Diagnosis and Management of Pericardial Diseases of the European Society of Cardiology. Eur Heart J 2004;25(7):587-610. doi:10.1016/j.ehj.2004.02.002

84. Mangi AA, Torchiana DF. Pericardial disease. In Cohn LH, editor. Cardiac Surgery in the Adult. 3rd edition. New York: McGraw-Hill; 2008:1465-1478.

85. Holt BD. Pericarditis. Retrieved June 10, 2009, from http://www.merck.com/mmpe/sec07/ch078/ch078a.html

86. Guyton AC, Hall JE. Textbook of Medical Physiology. 11th edition. Philadelphia: Saunders; 2006.

87. Berg J. Assessing for pericarditis in the end-stage renal disease patient. Dimens Crit Care Nursing 1990;9(5):266-271.

88. Valley VT, Fly CA. Pericarditis and Cardiac Tamponade. Retrieved June 10, 2009, from http://emedicine.medscape.com/article/759642-overview

89. Wilson JM. Heart Sounds Auscultation. Retrieved June 16, 2009, from http://texasheart.org/Education/CME/explore/events/eventdetail_5056-presentation.cfm

90. Cheitlin MD, Aurigemma GP, Beller GA, et al. ACC/AHA/ASE 2003 Guideline Update for the Clinical Application of Echocardiography: A Report of the American College of Cardiology/American Heart Association Task Force on Practice Guidelines (ACC/AHA/ASE Committee to Update the 1997 Guidelines for the Clinical Application of Echocardiography). Retrieved May 1, 2009, from http://www.herzdoktor.ch/de/pdf/Guidelines/Echocardiography.pdf

91. Shapiro S. Cardiac problems in critical care. In Bongard FS, Sue DY, editors. Current Critical Care: Diagnosis and Treatment. 2nd edition. New York: Lange Medical Books/McGraw-Hill; 2002:503-534.

92. Imazio M, Bobbio M, Cecchi E, et al. Colchicine in addition to conventional therapy for acute pericarditis: results of the COlchicine for acute PEricarditis (COPE) trial. Circulation 2005;112(13):2012-2016.

93. Shabetai R. Recurrent pericarditis: recent advances and remaining questions. Circulation 2005;112(13):1921-1923.

94. Maisch B, Karatolios K. Neue Möglichkeiten der Diagnostik und Therapie der Perikarditis [New possibilities of diagnostics and therapy of pericarditis] [abstract]. Der Internis Numerest 2008;49(1):17-26.

95. Clark VL. Pericardial tamponade. In Kruse JA, Fink MP, Carlson RW, editors. Saunders Manual of Critical Care. Philadelphia: Saunders; 2003:100-101.

96. Palacios IF. Pericardiocentesis for pericardial effusion and tamponade. In Parrillo JE, Dellinger RP, editors. Critical Care Medicine: Principles of Diagnosis and Management in the Adult. 2nd edition. St Louis, MO: Mosby; 2002:82-90.

97. Ewart's Sign. Retrieved June 10, 2009, from http://www.whonamedit.com/synd.cfm/2346.html

98. Becker DE. Pericardiocentesis (perform). In Wiegand DJ-M, Carlson KK, editors. AACN Procedure Manual for Critical Care. 5th edition. St Louis, MO: Saunders; 2005:281-288.

99. Wiegand DL-M, Pruess T, Hambach C. Care of patients with acquired valvular disease. In: Moser DK, Riegel B, editors. Cardiac Nursing: A Companion to Braunwald's Heart Disease. St Louis, MO: Saunders; 2008:1030-1051.

100. Hill KM. Mitral valve repair: A new choice. Am Nurse Today 2009;4(5):8-10.

101. McRae ME, Rodger M, Bailey BA. Transcatheter and transapical aortic valve replacement. Crit Care Nurse 2009;29(1):22-37.

102. Creager MA, White C, Hiatt WR, et al. Atherosclerotic Peripheral Vascular Disease Symposium., II:. Executive summary. Circulation 2008;118(25):2811-2825.

103. Hirsch AT, Haskal ZJ, Hertzer N, et al. ACC/AHA 2005 practice guidelines for the management of patients with peripheral arterial disease (lower extremity, renal, mesenteric, and abdominal aortic): a collaborative report from the American Association for Vascular Surgery/Society for Vascular Surgery, Society for Cardiovascular Angiography and Interventions, Society for Vascular Medicine and Biology, Society of Interventional Radiology, and the ACC/AHA Task Force on Practice Guidelines (Writing Committee to Develop Guidelines for the Management of Patients With Peripheral Arterial Disease). Circulation 2006;113(11):e463-e654. doi:10.1161./circulationaha.106.174526

104. Kuznar KA. Peripheral arterial occlusive disease: Evaluation and management in the primary care setting. Adv Nurse Pract 2004; 12(2):36-44.

105. Johnson C. Peril on the periphery. Am Nurse Today 2009;4(6): 28-30.

106. Khan NA, Rahim SA, Anand SS, et al. Does the clinical examination predict lower extremity peripheral arterial disease? JAMA 2006;295(5):536-546.

107. Norgren L, Hiatt WR, Dormandy JA, et al. Inter-Society consensus for the management of peripheral arterial disease (TASC II). Eur J Vasc Endovasc Surg 2007;33(suppl 1): S1-S70.

108. Sacks D, Bakal CW, Beatty P.T. Position statement on the use of the ankle-brachial index in the evaluation of patients with peripheral vascular disease: A consensus statement developed by the standards division of the Society of Cardiovascular and Interventional Radiology. J Vasc Interv Radiol 2002;13:353.

109. Sieggreen M. A contemporary approach to peripheral artery disease. Nurse Pract 2006;31(7):14-25.

110. Schiano V, Brevetti G, Sirico G, et al. Functional status measured by walking impairment questionnaire and cardiovascular risk prediction in peripheral arterial disease:. Results of the Peripheral Arteriopathy and Cardiovascular Events (PACE) study. Vasc Med 2006;11:147-154.

111. American Heart Association. Peripheral Vascular Disease. Retrieved July 1, 2009, from http://www.americanheart.org/presenter.jhtml?.identifier=4692

112. Stewart KJ, Hiatt WR, Regensteiner JG, et al. Medical progress: Exercise training for claudication. N Engl J Med 2002;347: 1941-1951.

113. Hiatt WR. Atherosclerotic peripheral arterial disease. In Goldman: Cecil Medicine. 28th edition. Philadelphia: Saunders; 2007.

114. Kehl-Pruett W. Deep vein thrombosis in hospitalized patients: a review of evidence-based guidelines for prevention. Dimens Crit Care Nursing 2006;25(2):53-60.

115. Cardin T, Marinelli A. Pulmonary embolism. Crit Care Nursing Q 2004;27(4):310-322.

116. Mayden KD. Heading off VTE. Adv Nurse Pract 2007; October:85-87.

117. Brouwer J-LP, Veeger NJ, Kluin-Nelemans HC, et al. The pathogenesis of venous thromboembolism: Evidence for multiple interrelated causes. Ann Intern Med 2006;145(11): 807-815.

118. Geerts WH, Pineo GF, Heit JA, et al. Prevention of venous thromboembolism: the Seventh ACCP Conference on Antithrombotic and Thrombolytic Therapy. Chest 2004;124 (3 suppl):338S-400S.

119. Mayo Clinic. Pulmonary Embolism. Retrieved May 27, 2009, from http://www.mayoclinic.com/health/pulmonary-embolism/DS00429

120. Qaseem A, Snow V, Barry P, et al. Current diagnosis of venous thromboembolism in primary care: a clinical practice guideline from the American Academy of Family Physicians and the American College of Physicians. Ann Fam Med 2007;5(1):57-62.

121. GTC-Biotherapeutics. What Is Hereditary Antithrombin Deficiency? Retrieved May 26, 2009, from http://www.atiii.com/overview_intro.htm

122. American Thoracic Society. The diagnostic approach to acute venous thromboembolism: clinical practice guideline. Am J Respir Crit Care Med 1999;160:1043-1066.

123. Anand SS, Wells PS, Hunt D, et al. Does this patient have deep vein thrombosis? JAMA 1998;279(14):1094-1099.

124. Snow V, Qaseem A, Barry P, et al. Management of venous thromboembolism in primary care: a clinical practice guideline from the American College of Physicians and the American Academy of Family Physicians. Ann Intern Med 2007;146(3):204-210.

125. Lindsay ET, Hampton S. Short-Stretch Compression Bandages and the Foot Pump. Retrieved July 1, 2009, from http://www.nursingtimes.net/nursing-practice-clinical-research/short-stretch-compression-bandages-and-the-foot-pump/205367.article

126. World Health Organization. WHO Research Into Global Hazards of Travel (WRIGHT) Project: Final Report of Phase I. Retrieved July 1, 2009, from http://www.who.int/cardiovascular_diseases/wright_project/phase1_report/en/index.html

127. American Heart Association. What Is Homocysteine? Retrieved May 28, 2009, from http://www.americanheart.org/presenter.jhtml?identifier=535

128. McGee S. Evidence-Based Physical Diagnosis. 2nd Edition. St Louis, MO: Saunders Elsevier; 2007.

129. Joshua AM, Celermajer DS, Stockler MR. Beauty is in the eye of the examiner: reaching agreement about physical signs and their value. Intern Med J 2005;35:178-187.

130. Ebell MH. Evidence-Based Diagnosis. New York: Springer; 2001.

131. Ebell MH. Evaluation of the Patient With Suspected Deep Vein Thrombosis. J Fam Pract 2001;50(2). Retrieved from http://www.jfponline.com/Pages.asp?AID=2143#bib8

132. Ebell MH. Suspected pulmonary embolism:. Part I. Evidence-based clinical assessment. Am Fam Phys 2004;69:367-369.

133. Institute for Clinical Systems Improvement (ICSI). Health Care Guideline: Venous Thromboembolism Diagnosis and Treatment. 10th Edition. Retrieved July 28, 2010, from http://www.icsi.org/venous_thromboembolism/venous_thromboembolism_4.html

134. Nordenholz KE, Mitchell AM, Kline JA. Direct comparison of the diagnostic accuracy of fifty protein biological markers of pulmonary embolism for use in the emergency department. Acad Emerg Med 2008;15(9):795-799.

135. Cleveland Clinic. What You Need to Know About Hypercoagulable States (Blood Clotting Disorders). Retrieved May 28, 2009, from http://my.clevelandclinic.org/heart/disorders/vascular/hypercoagstate.aspx

136. Newman, JH. Pulmonary Embolism. Retrieved May 27, 2009, from http://www.merck.com/mmhe/sec04/ch046/ch046a.html#sec04-ch046-ch046a-433d

137. Kearon C, Kahn SR, Agnelli G, et al. Antithrombotic therapy for venous thromboembolic disease: American College of Chest Physicians Evidence-Based Clinical Practice Guidelines (8th Edition). Chest 2008;133(6 suppl):454S-545S.

138. Ridker PM. Long-term, low-intensity warfarin therapy for the prevention of recurrent venous thromboembolism. N Engl J Med 2003;348(15):1425-1434.

139. Kearon C, Ginsberg JS, Kovacs MJ, et al. Comparison of low-intensity warfarin therapy with conventional-intensity warfarin therapy for long-term prevention of recurrent venous thromboembolism. N Engl J Med 2003;349(7):631-639.

140. Bartley MK. Keep venous thromboembolism at bay. Nursing 2006;36(10):36-42.

141. Crouch SD, Hill D, Bridwell D. New technology for the treatment of peripheral arterial and venous occlusions: ultrasound accelerated thrombolysis. J Radiol Nursing 2008 27(1):14-21.

142. University of California at San Francisco (UCSF)-Stanford University Evidence-based Practice Center. Making Health Care Safer: A Critical Analysis of Patient Safety Practices [Evidence Report/Technology Assessment, No. 43]. Retrieved July 1, 2009, from http://archive.ahrq.gov/clinic/ptsafety/summary.htm

143. CMS: Centers for Medicare and Medicaid Services. CMS Improves Patient Safety for Medicare and Medicaid by Addressing Never Events. Retrieved May 30, 2009, from http://www.cms.hhs.gov/apps/media/press/factsheet.asp?Counter=3224&intNumPerPage=10&checkDate=&checkKey=2&srchType=2&numDays=0&srchOpt=0&srchData=never+events&keywordType=All&chkNewsType=6&intPage=&showAll=1&pYear=&year=0&desc=&cboOrder=date

144. CMS: Centers for Medicare and Medicaid Services. Hospital-Acquired Conditions (HAC) and Present On Admission (POA) Indicator Reporting. Retrieved May 30, 2009, from http://www.cms.hhs.gov/HospitalAcqCond/Downloads/HACFactsheet.pdf

145. The National Quality Forum (NQF). Safe Practices for Better Health Care, 2006 Update: A Consensus Report. Washington, DC: National Quality Forum; 2006.

146. The Joint Commission. 2008 National Patient Safety Goals. Retrieved May 28, 2009, from http://www.jointcommission.org/NR/rdonlyres/0B4EB2A3-0AD5-4B9B-B891-D2BCE33D8D49/0/08_CAH_NPSGs_Master.pdf

147. Surgical Care Improvement Project. MedQIC Medical Quality Improvement Community website. Retrieved June 27, 2009, from http://www.qualitynet.org/dcs/ContentServer?c=MQParents&pagename=Medqic%2FContent%2FParentShellTemplate&cid=1137448680860&parentName=Topic

148. Goldhaber SZ, Tapson VF, for the DVT Free Steering Committee. A prospective registry of 5,451 patients with ultrasound confirmed deep vein thrombosis. Am J Cardiol 2004;93:259-262.

149. The Joint Commission. APPROVED: more options for hospital core measures. Jt Comm Perspect 2009;29(4):406.

150. American Association of Critical-Care Nurses. AACN Practice Alerts: Deep Vein Thrombosis Prevention. Retrieved August 2006, from http://www.aacn.org/WD/Practice/Docs/DVT_Prevention_12-2005.pdf

151. Vincent J-L. Give your patient a fast hug (at least) once a day. Crit Care Med 2005;33(6):1225-1229.

152. Svensson LG, Kouchoukos NT, Miller DC, et al. Expert consensus document on the treatment of descending thoracic aortic disease using endovascular stent-grafts. Ann Thorac Surg 2008;85(1 suppl):S1-S41.

153. Svensson LG, Rodriguez ER. Aortic organ disease epidemic, and why do balloons pop? Circulation 2005;112(8):1082-1084.

154. Upchurch GR Jr, Schaub TA. Abdominal aortic aneurysm. Am Fam Phys 2006;73(7):1198-1204, 1205-1206.

155. Coughlin RM. Recognizing aortic dissection: a race against time. Am Nurse Today 2008;3(4):31-35.

156. Jones M, Hoffman LA, Makaroun MS. Endovascular grafting for repair of abdominal aortic aneursym. Crit Care Nurse 2000;20(4):38-51.

157. Abdominal Aortic Aneurysm. Retrieved June 25, 2009, from http://www.vascularweb.org/

158. Phillips JK. (1998). Abdominal aortic aneurysm. Nursing 98, (5):35-39.

159. Carmona RH. The Health Consequences of Smoking: A Report of the Surgeon General. Retrieved June 25, 2009, from http://www.surgeongeneral.gov/library/smokingconsequences/index.html

160. Cook Medical. Learn the Facts About Abdominal Aortic Aneurysms (AAA) [PowerPoint Presentation]. Retrieved June 12, 2009, from http://www.cookmedical.com/ai/content/mmedia/AAA_PPT_Hetrick.1.ppt

161. Cook Medical. Learn the Facts About Thoracic Aortic Aneurysms (TAA) [PowerPoint Presentation]: Aortic intervention: PowerPoint Library. Retrieved June 27, 2009, from http://www.cookmedical.com/ai/content/mmedia/TAA_PPT_Hetrick.2.ppt

162. Steyerberg EW, Kievit J, de Mol Van Otterloo JC, et al. Perioperative mortality of elective abdominal aortic aneurysm surgery: a clinical prediction rule based on literature and individual patient data. Arch Intern Med 1995;155(18):1998-2004.

163. Collins AS, Dinsmore D. Caring for patients with traumatic injuries of the thoracic aorta. Dimens Crit Care Nursing 2007;26(2):51-56.

164. Simon BJ, Leslie C. Factors predicting early in-hospital death in blunt thoracic aortic injury. J Trauma 2001;51(5):906-911.

165. US Preventive Services Task Force. Screening for abdominal aortic aneurysm: recommendation statement. Ann Intern Med 2005;142(3):198-202.

166. Watson K. The ABC's of AAA. Retrieved June 18, 2009, from http://www.sleh.com/sleh/downloads/innov/03spring_thi.pdf

167. Suzuki T, Distante A, Zizza A, et al. Diagnosis of acute aortic dissection by D-dimer: the International Registry of Acute Aortic Dissection Substudy on Biomarkers (IRAD-Bio) experience. Circulation 2009;119(20):2702-2707.

168. LeMaire SA, Carter SA, Coselli JS. The elephant trunk technique for staged repair of complex aneurysms of the entire thoracic aorta. Ann Thorac Surg 2006;81(5):1561-1569.

169. Svensson LG, Kim K-H, Blackstone EH, et al. Elephant trunk procedure: newer indications and uses. Ann Thorac Surg 2004;78(1):109-116.

170. Cleveland Clinic. Modified David's Reimplantation Procedure. Retrieved June 27, 2009, from http://my.clevelandclinic.org/heart/disorders/aorta_marfan/davidreimplantation.aspx

171. Calkins H, Brugada J, Packer DL, et al. HRS/EHRA/ECAS expert consensus statement on catheter and surgical ablation of atrial fibrillation: recommendations for personnel, policy, procedures and follow–up. A report of the Heart Rhythm Society (HRS) Task Force on Catheter and Surgical Ablation of Atrial Fibrillation developed in partnership with the European Heart Rhythm Association (EHRA) and the European Cardiac Arrhythmia Society (ECAS); in collaboration with the American College of Cardiology (ACC), American Heart Association (AHA), and the Society of Thoracic Surgeons (STS). Endorsed and approved by the governing bodies of the American College of Cardiology, the American Heart Association, the European Cardiac Arrhythmia Society, the European Heart Rhythm Association, the Society of Thoracic Surgeons, and the Heart Rhythm Society. Heart Rhythm 2007;4(6):816-861. doi:10.1016/j.hrthm.2007.04.005

172. American Heart Association. What Is an Arrhythmia? Retrieved from http://www.americanheart.org/downloadable/heart/110063301052708%20WhatIsanArrhyt.pdf

173. Yarnoz MJ, Curtis AB. More reasons why men and women are not the same (gender differences in electrophysiology and arrhythmias). Am J Cardiol 2008;101(9):1291-1296.

174. Henry L, Ad N. The maze procedure: a surgical intervention for ablation of atrial fibrillation. Heart Lung 2008;37(6):432-439. doi:10.1016/j.hrtlng.2008.02.004

175. Conover MB. Understanding Electrocardiography. 8th edition. St Louis, MO: Mosby; 2003.

176. Fuster V, Rydén LE, Cannom D S, et al. ACC/AHA/ESC 2006 guidelines for the management of patients with atrial fibrillation-executive summary: a report of the American College of Cardiology/American Heart Association Task Force on Practice Guidelines and the European Society of Cardiology Committee for Practice Guidelines (Writing Committee to Revise the 2001 Guidelines for the Management of Patients with Atrial Fibrillation). Circulation 2006;114(6):700-752.

177. Zheng ZJ, Croft JB, Giles WH, et al. Sudden cardiac death in the United States, 1989 to 1998. Circulation 2001;104:2158-2163.

178. Calkins H. Principles of electrophysiology. In Goldman L, Ausiello D, editors. Cecil Textbook of Medicine. 23rd edition. Philadelphia: WB Saunders; 2007.

179. Peterson KJ. Advanced dysrhythmias. In Carlson KK, editor. AACN Advanced Critical Care Nursing. St Louis, MO: Saunders; 2009:173-206.

180. Cottrell DB, Jones MM. Women with dysrhythmia: a clinical challenge. Crit Care Nursing Clin North Am 2008;20(3):311-314.

181. Prudente LA. Quelling atrial chaos: current approaches to managing atrial fibrillation. Am Nurse Today 2008;3(8):21-25.

182. Wellens HJ, Conover M. The ECG in Emergency Decision Making. 2nd edition. St Louis, MO: Saunders; 2006.

183. Coughlin RM. Recognizing ventricular arrhythmias and preventing sudden cardiac death. Am Nurse Today 2007;2(5):38-43.

184. American Heart Association. Handbook of Emergency Cardiovascular Care. Dallas, TX: Author; 2004.

185. Gallahue FE, Uzgiris R, Burke R, et al. Brugada syndrome presenting as an "acute myocardial infarction." J Emerg Med 2009;37(1):15-20.

186. Zak J. Mapping ventricular tachycardia. Crit Care Nurse 2006;26(5):13-20.

187. Drew BJ, Califf RM, Funk et al. AHA scientific statement: practice standards for electrocardiographic monitoring in hospital settings: an American Heart Association Scientific Statement from the Councils on Cardiovascular Nursing Clinical Cardiology, and Cardiovascular Disease in the Young: endorsed by the International Society of Computerized electrocardiology and the American Association of Critical-Care Nurses. J Cardiovasc Nursing 2005;20(2):76-106.

188. American Association of Critical-Care Nurses. AACN Practice Alert: Dysrhythmia Monitoring. Retrieved September 2009, from http://www.aacn.org/WD/Practice/Docs/Dysrhythmia_Monitoring_04-2008.pdf

189. American Association of Critical-Care Nurses. AACN Practice Alerts: ST-Segment Monitoring. Retrieved September 2009, from http://www.aacn.org/WD/Practice/Docs/ST_Segment_Monitoring_05-2009.pdf

190. Zipes DP, Camm AJ, Borggrefe M, et al. ACC/AHA/ESC 2006 guidelines for management of patients with ventricular arrhythmias and the prevention of sudden cardiac death: a report

of the American College of Cardiology/American Heart Association Task Force and the European Society of Cardiology Committee to Develop Guidelines for Management of Patients With Ventricular Arrhythmias and the Prevention of Sudden Cardiac Death): Developed in Collaboration With the European Heart Rhythm Association and the Heart Rhythm Society. Circulation 2006;114(10):e385-e484. doi:10.1161/circulationaha.106.178233

191. Brantman L, Howie J. Use of amiodarone to prevent atrial fibrillation after cardiac surgery. Crit Care Nurse 2006;26(1): 48-58.

192. Roberts CK, Sindhu KK. Oxidative stress and metabolic syndrome. Life Sci 2009;84(21-22):705-712.

193. Eckel RH, Grundy SM, Zimmet PZ. The metabolic syndrome. Lancet 2005;365(9468):1415-1428.

194. Aguilar-Salinas CA, Rojas R, Gomez-Perez FJ, et al. The metabolic syndrome: a concept hard to define. Arch Med Res 2005;36(3):223-231.

195. Haffner SM. The metabolic syndrome: inflammation, diabetes mellitus, and cardiovascular disease. Am J Cardiol 2006;97 (2, suppl 1):3-11.

196. Kahn R, Buse J, Ferrannini E, et al. The metabolic syndrome: time for a critical appraisal: joint statement from the American Diabetes Association and the European Association for the Study of Diabetes. Diab Care 2005;28:2289-2304.

197. Fowler SB, Moussouttas M, Mancini B. Metabolic syndrome: contributing factors and treatment strategies. J Neurosci Nursing 2005;37(4):220-223.

198. Miranda PJ, DeFronzo RA, Califf RM, et al. Metabolic syndrome: definition, pathophysiology, and mechanisms. Am Heart J 2005;149(1):33-45.

199. Grundy SM. Metabolic Syndrome: A Growing Clinical Challenge. Retrieved November 2007, from http://cme.medscape.com/ viewarticle/484166

200. Ford ES, Giles WH, Mokdad AH. Increasing prevalence of the metabolic syndrome among US adults. Reprinted from Diabetes Care 2004;27(10). Retrieved November 2007, from http://www. medscape.com/viewarticle/490660

201. Dall T. The Metabolic Syndrome: To Be or Not to Be? Retrieved June 16, 2009, from http://cme.medscape.com/viewarticle/ 566293_print

202. Prussian KH, Barksdale-Brown DJ, Dieckmann J. Racial and ethnic differences in the presentation of metabolic syndrome [electronic version]. J Nurse Pract 2007;3(4):229-239.

203. Hunt KJ, Resendez RG, Williams K, et al. National Cholesterol Education Program Versus World Health Organization metabolic syndrome in relation to all-cause and cardiovascular mortality in the San Antonio Heart Study. Circulation 2004;110(10): 1251-1257.

204. Grundy SM, Cleeman JI, Daniels SR, et al. Diagnosis and management of the metabolic syndrome: an American Heart Association/National Heart, Lung, and Blood Institute scientific statement. Circulation 2005;112(17):2735-2752.

205. Festa A, D'Agostino R Jr, Tracy RP, et al. Elevated levels of acute-phase proteins and plasminogen activator inhibitor-1 predict the development of type 2 diabetes: the insulin resistance atherosclerosis study. Diabetes 2002;51(4):1131-1137.

206. Palaniappan L, Carnethon M, Fortmann SP. Association between microalbuminuria and the metabolic syndrome: NHANES III. Am J Hypertens 2003;16:952-958.

207. Expert Panel on Detection, Evaluation, and Treatment of High Blood Cholesterol in Adults. Executive summary of the third report of The National Cholesterol Education Program (NCEP) Expert Panel on Detection, Evaluation, and Treatment of High Blood Cholesterol in Adults (Adult Treatment Panel III). JAMA 2001;285:2486-2497.

208. Watanabe S, Tagawa T, Yamakawa K, et al. Inhibition of the renin-angiotensin system prevents free fatty acid–induced acute endothelial dysfunction in humans. Arterioscler Thromb Vasc Biol 2005;25(11):2376-2380.

209. Palmer DM, Luther B. Screening for metabolic syndrome. Orthop Nursing 2007;26(5):293-295.

210. Spaniol JR, Knight AR, Zebley JL, et al. Fluid resuscitation therapy for hemorrhagic shock. J Trauma Nursing 2007;14(3): 152-160.

211. Dellinger RP, Levy MM, et al. Surviving Sepsis Campaign: International guidelines for management of severe sepsis and septic shock: 2008. Intens Care Med 2008;34(1):17-60.

212. Filbin MR. Septic Shock. Retrieved September 4, 2009, from http://emedicine.medscape.com/article/786058-overview

213. Elbers PW, Ince C. Bench-to-bedside review: mechanisms of critical illness—: classifying microcirculatory flow abnormalities in distributive shock. Crit Care 2006;10(4):221-228.

214. Rice V. Shock, a clinical syndrome: an update. Part 1. An overview of shock. Crit Care Nurse 1991;11(4):20-24, 26-27.

215. Rice V. Shock, a clinical syndrome: an update. Part 2. The stages of shock. Crit Care Nurse 1991;11(5):74, 76, 78-79, passim.

216. Rivers E, Nguyen B, Havstad S, et al. Early goal-directed therapy in the treatment of severe sepsis and septic shock. N Engl J Med 2001;345(19):1368–1377.

217. Parker MM. Goals for fluid resuscitation: a real challenge. Crit Care Med 2007;35(1):295-296.

218. Boldt J. The balanced concept of fluid resuscitation. Br J Anaesth 2007;99(3):312-315.

219. Moore KM. Controversies in fluid resuscitation. J Trauma Nursing 2006;13(4):168-172.

220. Weil MH. Shock. Retrieved July 8, 2009, from http://www. merck.com/mmpe/sec06/ch067/ch067b.html

221. Ahrens TS. Monitoring carbon dioxide in critical care: the newest vital sign? Crit Care Nursing Clin North Am 2004;16 (3):445-451.

222. Weil MH. Intravenous Fluid Resuscitation. Retrieved July 8, 2009, from http://www.merck.com/mmpe/sec06/ch067/ch067c.html

223. Alam HB, Rhee P. New developments in fluid resuscitation. Surg Clin North Am 2007;87(1):55-72.

224. Bunn F, Trivedi D, Ashraf S. Colloid Solutions for Fluid Resuscitation. Cochrane Database Syst Rev 2008(1): CD001319. Retrieved July 8, 2009, doi:10.1002/14651858. cd001319.pub2

225. American Thoracic Society. Evidence-based colloid use in the critically ill: American Thoracic Society consensus statement. Am J Respir Crit Care Med 2004;170(11):1247-1259.

226. Taylor C, Navarrete C, Contreras M. Immunological Complications of Blood Transfusion: Allergic and Anaphylactic Reactions. Retrieved July 22, 2010, from http://www.medscape.com/ viewarticle/583195

227. Lee C-C, Chang I-J, Yen Z-S, et al. Delayed fluid resuscitation in hemorrhagic shock induces proinflammatory cytokine response. Ann Emerg Med 2007;49(1):37-44.

228. American Association of Critical-Care Nurses. AACN Standards for Establishing and Sustaining Healthy Work Environments: A Journey to Excellence. Available at http://www.aacn.org/WD/HWE/Docs/HWEStandards.pdf.

229. Levy MM, Dellinger RP, Ramsey G. Success Yields Success: The Surviving Sepsis Campaign Past, Present, and Future. Campaign Update, p. 2. Retrieved from http://www.survivingsepsis.org/CampaignUpdate/Pages/default.aspx

230. Institute of Medicine. To Err Is Human: Building a Safer Health System. Washington, DC: National Academies Press; 1999. Available at http://iom.edu/Reports/1999/To-Err-is-Human-Building-A-Safer-Health-System.aspx

231. Institute of Medicine. Crossing the Quality Chasm: A New Health System for the 21st Century. Washington, DC: National Academies Press; 2001. Available at http://iom.edu/Reports/2001/Crossing-the-Quality-Chasm-A-New-Health-System-for-the-21st-Century.aspx

232. Agency for Health care Quality and Research. TeamSTEPPs: National Implementation. 2006. Available at http://teamstepps.ahrq.gov/index.htm

233. Institute of Medicine. Keeping Patients Safe: Transforming the Work Environment of Nurses. Washington, DC: National Academies Press; 2004. Available at http://www.iom.edu/Reports/2003/Keeping-Patients-Safe-Transforming-the-Work-Environment-of-Nurses.aspx

10

Pulmonary Problems

Deborah L. Weatherspoon, RN, CRNA, MSN, and
Christopher A. Weatherspoon, RN, MS, FNP-BC

INTRODUCTION

Pulmonary problems are one of the most common reasons for hospitalization in the adult population. Patients may suffer an exacerbation of a chronic disease or experience an episodic acute illness. Additionally, problems may arise from iatrogenesis. All can be costly problems in terms of health care resource consumption, hospital stay, and patient time off work. Chronic diseases addressed in this chapter include chronic obstructive pulmonary disease, asthma, obstructive sleep apnea, and pulmonary hypertension. Lung cancer is included, which can be a chronic disease, depending on the cell type, treatment modality and response, and the nature of complications that may occur. Community-acquired pneumonia (CAP) can be deadly for certain population segments such as the elderly, immune suppressed, and people with comorbidity. Hospital-acquired pneumonia, (HAP), a serious iatrogenic complication, particularly in intubated critically ill patients supported with mechanical ventilation, has been the subject of recent widespread efforts toward prevention, using evidence-based approaches. Pulmonary edema and respiratory failure are potentially deadly complications of many diseases; this chapter will address cardiac, renal, and neurologic in addition to primary pulmonary etiology. Chest trauma requires prompt recognition and intervention. All of the conditions carry high morbidity and mortality rates.

Clinical nurse specialists (CNSs) integrate all of the competencies required of advanced practice nurses across three spheres of influence for patients with pulmonary problems, whether acute or chronic in nature. CNSs play a pivotal role in management of the acute crises, as well as coordination of multiple disciplines for meticulous planning as patients recover and transition to varying levels of care. Patients and families rely on interactive teaching and educational materials provided by CNSs that assist in the long-term management of their disease. Finally, CNSs provide consultation to front line caregivers, using their expert knowledge to facilitate safe, evidence-based practice that yields the best outcomes for patients.

PNEUMONIA

Etiology

Pneumonia is inflammation of the lungs resulting in consolidation. It is an obstruction in gas exchange on the alveolar level and is most often categorized by the causative agent. Pneumonia is currently the eighth leading cause of death in the United States with an age-adjusted death rate of 16.3 per 100,000 population. The cost of pneumonia has been historically reported as high as $8.4 billion, and approximately 92% of this amount has been spent on hospital care. In addition, HAP has been shown to increase total hospital charges by 75%. Pneumonia may present as either an acute or chronic manifestation depending on onset of symptoms. It is typically broken down into two classifications: CAP and HAP. HAP is synonymous with long-term care facility and nosocomial pneumonias. Causative agents for pneumonia may include bacterial, fungal, viral, and chemical inhalation. The *ICD-10* classification includes influenza and pneumonia with codes from J09 to J18 (1-4).

Pathophysiology

The lungs are typically inoculated with a pathogen through aspiration, droplet inhalation, or blood-borne pathogens. Aspiration is the most common cause and may occur in individuals who currently have an oropharyngeal infection such as *Streptococcus pneumoniae*. It may also occur in individuals with decreased gag reflex, depressed consciousness, or excessive gastroesophageal reflux. Aspirated material may result in a large number of anaerobic bacteria present in the lower respiratory tract.

Droplet inhalation is the second most frequent cause of pneumonia, resulting from exposure to aerosolized droplets that are 0.5 to 1 micron in size. This mechanism of infection is limited to organisms such as *Mycobacteria tuberculosis, Legionella pneumoniae, Yersinia pestis, Bacillus anthracis,* and some viral infections. Blood-borne pathogens may also result in pneumonia; however, this is less common. It is typically seen with staphylococcal sepsis or right-sided endocarditis, and gram-negative bacteremias particularly in immunocompromised patients. In addition, inoculation may occur from penetrating chest trauma or local infected organisms such as amoebic liver abscess (4, 5).

After inoculation, the pathogen results in an immune response causing protein-rich fluid to move into the alveoli from supporting capillary structures. This process is further complicated with pustulant production by the organism. The result is a decrease in alveolar surface area. Consequently, oxygen and carbon dioxide diffusion is hindered resulting in elevation of PCO_2 and a decrease in PO_2 levels. As the disease progresses, consolidation may be seen. Consolidation will typically occur in a lobar fashion; however, it is also seen with multiple consolidations often referred to as bronchial pneumonia. Bronchial pneumonia has been typically associated with HAP; the most common specific organisms are *Staphylococcus aureus, Klebsiella, Escherichia coli,* and *Pseudomonas* (4, 6, 7).

Community-Acquired Pneumonia

CAP refers to pneumonia in persons living within the community, and specifically those not receiving medical treatment within a health care facility. This also includes patients who have been hospitalized for less than 48 hours and develop respiratory symptoms. Table 10-1 shows specific pathogens associated with pneumonia and underlying risk factors. Bacterial organisms that are typically found with CAP include *S. pneumoniae, H. influenzae,* and *Moraxella catarrhalis.* Other atypical bacteria may include *Mycobacterium tuberculosis, Legionella, Chlamydia pneumoniae,* and *Mycoplasma pneumoniae.* In addition to bacterial organisms, viral organisms, such as influenza, respiratory syncytial virus (RSV), and fungi, may be encountered (3, 8).

TABLE 10–1 Underlying Risk Factors and Specific Pathogens Resulting in Pneumonia

Active smoking/chronic obstructive lung disease	*Streptococcus pneumoniae, Haemophilus influenzae, Legionella pneumophila*
Long-term care residents	*S. pneumoniae,* gram-negative bacilli, *H. influenzae, Staphylococcus aureus, Chlamydia pneumoniae,* anaerobes, tuberculosis
Alcohol abuse	*S. pneumoniae* (including drug-resistant strains), gram-negative bacilli, anaerobes, tuberculosis
Traveled to southwestern United States	*Coccidioides immitis*
Exposure to bats	*Histoplasma capsulatum*
Exposure to birds	*Cryptococcus neoformans, Chlamydia psittaci, H. capsulatum*
Exposure to rabbits	*Francisella tularensis*
Exposure to farm animals	*Coxiella burnetti* (Q fever)
Viral influenza	Influenza, *S. aureus, S. pneumoniae, H. influenzae*
Anatomical abnormality of the lung parenchyma (e.g., bronchiectasis, cystic fibrosis)	*Pseudomonas aeruginosa, Pseudomonas capacia, S. aureus, Aspergillus* spp., *Mycobacterium avium*
Intravenous drug use	*S. aureus,* anaerobes, tuberculosis, *Pneumocystis jiroveci*
Endobronchial obstruction	Anaerobes
Recent antibiotic therapy	Drug-resistant *S. pneumoniae, P. aeruginosa*
Incarceration	*Mycobacterium tuberculosis*
Neutropenia	*Aspergillus* spp., *Zygomycetes*
Asplenia	*S. pneumoniae, H. influenza*

Adapted from the American Thoracic Society guidelines for management of adult with community-acquired pneumonia: diagnosis, assessment of severity, initial antimicrobial therapy, and prevention. Am J Respir Crit Care Med 2001:163:1730-1754; Mandell LA, Bartlett JG, Dowell SF, et al. Update practice guidelines for the management of community acquired pneumonia and immunocompetent adults. Clin Infect Dis 2003;37:1405-1433.

Clinical Presentation

People with CAP typically present with a cough, fever, chills, dyspnea, fatigue, and /or pleuritic chest pain. Cough may be dry or productive depending on the pathogen. The presentation of symptoms is typically acute; however, an insidious onset may be seen in immunocompromised individuals. Medical history is essential to identify comorbid conditions and risk factors. Common pathogens and their occurrence rates are shown in Table 10-2.

Tachypnea or central cyanosis due to poor gas exchange may be observed during initial inspection. Typically the patient is febrile, with temperature exceeding 38°C (100.4°F). Cough with or without sputum production may be present, sometimes with hemoptysis. Percussion may reveal dullness over consolidated areas or increased tactile fremitus with palpation. Crackles, rhonchi, wheezing, or egophony may be heard during auscultation. Atypical organisms such as *Mycoplasma*, *Chlamydophila*, and viruses can manifest constitutional symptoms, no fever, nonproductive cough, and absent or diffuse adventitious findings on auscultation.

Diagnosis

Laboratory testing to diagnose pneumonia should include leukocyte count and basic metabolic profile to assist with assessment of fluid status and organ function to avoid toxicity when selecting antimicrobials. Routine blood cultures and sputum Gram stains generally yield low positive culture rates; production of adequate sputum quantity for culture occurs in only about 50% of patients with CAP. However, these tests may be beneficial in determining treatment for more severe cases such as atypical or resistant organisms (3, 4).

Standard posterior/anterior and lateral chest radiographs are absolutely necessary for diagnosis of pneumonia. Radiographic testing may reveal the severity of disease and other underlying differential diagnoses that are present. Use of computed tomography (CT) scanning is not routinely advised; however, this may be utilized if anthrax is suspected. Common radiographic patterns associated with pneumonia are shown in Table 10-3.

Bronchoscopy may be performed to provide sampling of secretions for culture. This is typically reserved for immunocompromised individuals and patients who have not responded and/or are progressively worsening with empiric therapy.

Risk stratification is critical in determining severity of the disease process and requirement for hospitalization. The Pneumonia Severity Index may be useful for classification of severity. Class I and II candidates are considered at low risk for mortality and may respond well to outpatient therapy. Patients in risk class III may be considered for hospital admission, and those in risk class IV or V should be admitted to the hospital. Diagnosis for CAP is shown in Table 10-4.

TABLE 10-2 Pathogens Associated With Community-Acquired Pneumonia

Pathogen	Cases (%)
Streptococcus pneumoniae	20–60
Haemophilus influenzae	3–10
Staphylococcus aureus	3–5
Gram-negative bacilli	3–10
Legionella sp	2–8
Mycoplasma pneumoniae	1–6
Chlamydia pneumoniae	4–6
Viruses	2–15
Aspiration	6–10
Others	3–5

Adapted from Mandell LA, Bartlett JG, Dowell SF, et al. Update practice guidelines for the management of community acquired pneumonia and immunocompetent adults. Clin Infect Dis 2003;37:1405-1433.

TABLE 10-3 Common Radiographic Patterns With Different Sources of Pneumonia

Chest Xray Pattern	Source of Pneumonia
Focal, large pleural effusion	Bacteria
Cavitary	Bacterial abscess, fungi, acid-fast bacilli
Miliary	Acid-fast bacilli, fungi
Rapid progression/multifocal	Legionella, pneumococci, staphylococci
Interstitial	Viruses, *Pneumocystis jiroveci*, *Mycoplasma*, *Chlamydia psittaci*
Mediastinal widening without infiltrate	Inhalation anthrax

TABLE 10–4 Diagnosis for Community-Acquired Pneumonia

Clinical Setting	Test
All patients with suspected pneumonia PORT risk classes II to V	Chest radiography
	Sputum Gram stain and culture (optional)
	Complete blood count
	Complete metabolic profile
	Blood gases or pulse oximetry
All inpatients	Sputum Gram stain and culture
	Blood cultures: two sets for antibiotics
In patients with appropriate history or physical findings	HIV serology
	Legionella serology, urinary antigen, direct fluorescent antibody testing
	Mycoplasma serology
	Chlamydia serology
	Fungal serology
	SARS-associated coronavirus serology or PCR
	Stains are cultures for fungi, *Mycobacterium, Pneumocystis jiroveci*
	Analysis are cultures of pleural or cerebrospinal fluid
	Nasopharyngeal swab for viral direct fluorescent antibody or other rapid technique
	Tuberculin skin testing
Deteriorating patient without definitive diagnosis of cause	Bronchoscopy
	Thoracoscopic or open lung biopsy
	Radiographically guided transthoracic aspirate
	Legionella, Chlamydia, Mycoplasma serology
	Fungal serology
	Evaluation for congestive heart failure, pulmonary embolus, neoplasm, connective tissue disease

Adapted from Mandell LA, Bartlett JG, Dowell SF, et al. Update practice guidelines for the management of community acquired pneumonia and immunocompetent adults. Clin Infect Dis 2003;37:1405-1433.

Management

Antimicrobial therapy is the standard of care for treatment of pneumonia. Many experts believe the pathogen should be identified so antimicrobial therapy can be tailored to the individual and therefore limit concerns associated with antimicrobial overuse and increasing bacterial resistance. However, testing may be time-consuming and therefore empiric therapy should be initiated based on history and presenting symptomatology. Viral agents may also be used if viral infection is suspected. However, early initiation of zanamivir and oseltamivir is necessary within 48 hours of onset to be effective. In CAP, *S. pneumoniae* and *H. influenzae* are the most common pathogens; however, atypical pathogens such as in M. *pneumoniae, C. pneumoniae,* and *Legionella* can be the primary or coinfecting agents in up to 40% of cases. Treatment should be tailored to specific region and based on risk stratification of pneumonia in outpatient or inpatient settings (4, 5). Pathogen-specific antibiotic therapy for CAP is shown in Table 10-5.

Symptom management is an important factor in maintaining quality of life during treatment. Oxygenation should be used to maintain a saturation of greater than 91%. Antipyretics, cough suppressants, and expectorants should be provided to alleviate symptoms. Bronchodilators may also be beneficial if other comorbid conditions exist. Maintaining adequate and proper nutrition should be addressed in the treatment plan. In addition, emphasis should be made on avoiding primary and second-hand smoke as it further impedes the healing process.

Hospital-Acquired Pneumonia

HAP refers to pneumonia in persons who have received care in a health care institution such as recent hospital admission or long-term care facility for at least 2 days in the last 90 days prior to the infection. This also includes patients contracting pneumonia within 48 hours of endotracheal intubation and is commonly referred to as ventilator-associated pneumonia (VAP). Health

TABLE 10–5 Pathogen-Specific Antibiotic Therapy for Community-Acquired Pneumonia in Adults

Organism	Primary Therapy
Streptococcus pneumoniae	
Penicillin susceptible	Penicillin G, amoxicillin
Penicillin resistant	Cefotaxime, ceftriaxone, fluoroquinolone, vancomycin, others dependent on susceptibility studies
Haemophilus influenzae	Secondary third generation cephalosporin, doxycycline, beta-lactam or beta-lactamase inhibitor, and azithromycin, trimethoprim-sulfamethoxazole
Moraxella catarrhalis	Second or third generation cephalosporin, trimethoprim-sulfamethoxazole, macrolide, beta-lactam or beta-lactamase inhibitor
Legionella	Macrolide with rifampin, fluoroquinolone
Mycoplasma pneumoniae	Doxycycline, macrolide
Chlamydia pneumoniae	Doxycycline, macrolide
Anaerobes	Beta-lactam or beta-lactamase inhibitor, clindamycin
Enteric gram-negative bacilli	Third generation cephalosporin aminoglycoside; carbapenem
Pseudomonas aeruginosa	Aminoglycoside + ticarcillin, mezlocillin, ceftazidime, cefepime, aztreonam, carbapenem
Staphylococcus aureus	
Methicillin susceptible	Nafcillin or oxacillin, rifampin and or gentamicin
Methicillin resistant	Vancomycin, rifampin, or gentamicin
Bacillus anthracis	Ciprofloxacin or doxycycline + two of the following: rifampin, vancomycin, penicillin, ampicillin, chloramphenicol, imipenem, clindamycin, clarithromycin
Influenza A, within 48 hours of symptom onset or immunocompromised host	Amantadine, rimantadine, oseltimivir, zanamivir
Influenza B, within 48 hours of symptom onset or immunocompromised host	Oseltamivir, zanamivir

Adapted from Mandell LA, Bartlett JG, Dowell SF, et al. Update practice guidelines for the management of community acquired pneumonia and immunocompetent adults. Clin Infect Dis 2003;37:1405-1433.

care–associated pneumonia includes infections contracted in any health care facility such as dialysis centers, long-term care facilities, and nursing homes. HAP may be referred to as nosocomial pneumonia and represents the second most common nosocomial infection. Pathogens that commonly cause HAP are listed in Table 10-6. HAP is associated with a 25% to 50% risk of mortality and occurs most often in the elderly. VAP occurs in patients with endotracheal intubation for a period greater than 48 hours and is found in approximately 28% of patients receiving mechanical ventilation. The incidence of VAP increases at a rate of 3% for the first 5 days and 1% for every day after 10 days. Mortality rate with VAP is 27% to 76%. Common differential diagnoses for VAP include acute decompensated heart failure, pulmonary embolism or infarction, acute respiratory distress syndrome (ARDS), collagen-vascular diseases, and pulmonary drug reactions (7, 10, 11).

Clinical Presentation

The clinical presentation of HAP and diagnosis are similar to those of CAP with the exception that the organisms tend to be more virulent and difficult to treat. Additionally, patients in institutional settings tend to be of a higher acuity level and therefore require more intense treatment with greater attention to comorbidities and complications. Common symptoms may include dry or productive cough, increased respiratory rate, and shortness of breath. Comorbid factors such as history of respiratory disorders should also be considered to identify likely underlying pathogens.

TABLE 10–6 Common Organisms Involved in Hospital-Acquired Pneumonia

Pathogens in HAP	Comment
COMMONLY ASSOCIATED	
Pseudomonas aeruginosa	
Klebsiella spp.	
Escherichia coli	
Acinetobacter spp.	Intensive care unit setting
Staphylococcus aureus	Specifically methicillin-resistant *S. aureus* (MRSA)
Streptococcus pneumoniae	Should be considered an early-onset HAP; causes up to 9% of pneumonias in elderly patients in nursing home settings
Haemophilus influenzae	Should be considered an early-onset HAP
LESS COMMONLY ASSOCIATED	
Serratia spp.	
Legionella spp.	
Influenza A virus	
Respiratory syncytial virus	
Parainfluenza virus	
Adenovirus	
EXTREMELY RARELY ASSOCIATED	
Enterobacter spp.	
Stenotrophomonas maltophila	Formerly *Pseudomonas maltophila*
Burkholderia cepacia	Formerly *Pseudomonas cepacia*
Candida spp.	

Adapted from American Thoracic Society and the Infectious Diseases Society of America. Guidelines for the management of adults with hospital-acquired, ventilator-associated, and healthcare-associated pneumonia. Am J Respir Crit Care Med 2005;171(4):388-416.

Symptoms are similar to CAP including tachypnea, cyanotic changes, and fever greater than 38°C (100.4°F). Symptom onset will likely be acute but may present insidiously. Patients with a history of immunocompromise may not show typical signs. Crackles, rhonchi, wheezing, and/ or egophony may be heard with auscultation and increased tactile fremitus may be detected during palpation. Since atypical organisms are the most likely cause, lack of fever, nonproductive cough, and absent or diffuse adventitious findings on auscultation may occur. Pulse oximetry or blood gas evaluation should be performed in all patients diagnosed with or suspected of HAP (4, 7).

Diagnosis

Laboratory testing should include leukocyte count and a basic metabolic profile. Blood cultures and sputum gram stains should be performed to identify the organism for proper selection of antimicrobial. Although treatment may begin empirically, it is important in such cases that resistant organisms be identified and antibiotic therapy appropriately adjusted.

Standard posterior/anterior and lateral radiographs should be performed. Severity of the disease and identification of underlying comorbid conditions may be evident on the films. Bronchoscopy may be necessary to obtain sputum samples for culture and is often used therapeutically in patients with copious secretions and higher acuity level. Common differential diagnoses for patients with infiltrates on chest radiography include acute decompensated heart failure, pulmonary embolism or infarct, ARDS, pulmonary drug reactions, and collagen-vascular diseases.

Management

The first line treatment is antibiotic therapy based on laboratory cultures. Due to the seriousness of infection, empiric antimicrobials should be given prior to the availability of cultures. Basic treatment should include intravenous antibiotics and fluids, oxygen supplementation, proper nutrition, and management of comorbid conditions. The patient may require ventilator support and/or admission to the intensive care unit due to high acuity level.

The following points should be remembered while treating HAP: (a) sdministration of antibiotics should not be delayed for a definitive diagnosis; (b) empiric antibiotic choice should be based on patient's relative risk for a specific pathogen; (c) combination antimicrobial therapy is preferred in patients at risk for resistant pathogens; (d) local antibiograms should be reviewed when selecting empiric therapy; (e) if the patient has recently received antibiotics, then an antibiotic from a different class should be used; (f) the duration of antibiotic therapy should be limited to absolute need to decrease the risk of resistance; and (g) false-negative cultures may occur in patients who have received antibiotics in the last 24 to 72 hours.

HAP empiric monotherapy may be initiated in early onset with ceftriaxone, ertapenem, levofloxacin, or moxifloxacin. Ciprofloxacin, cefazidime, or imipenem should not be used since they are likely to result in resistance. Late-onset HAP and VAP require combination therapy using a broad-spectrum cephalosporin with gram-negative activity, beta-lactam, carbapenem, anti-pseudomonal fluoroquinolone, aminoglycoside, linezolid, or vancomycin in various combinations. Table 10-7 provides guidelines for antibiotic treatment for HAP and VAP.

Consultation with infectious disease specialists should be considered to address complex issues such as multiple or resistant organisms, drug toxicity, and comorbid conditions in the treatment plan. Pulmonologist consultation

TABLE 10–7 Antibiotic Treatment of Hospital- and Ventilator-Acquired Pneumonia

Antibiotic, Generic (Brand)	Description	Dosage
Cefepime (Maxipime)	Fourth generation cephalosporin with good gram-negative coverage	2 g IV q12h
Meropenem (Merrem)	Not a beta-lactam antibiotic, effective against most gram-positive and gram-negative bacteria	1 g IV q8h
Pipercillin (Pipracil)	Antipseudomonal penicillin used in combination with other antibiotics	4 g IV q8h
Aztreonam (Azactam)	Activity against gram-negative bacilli	2 g IV q8h
Amikacin (Amikin)	Used for gram-negative bacterial coverage of infections resistant to gentamicin and tobramycin	7.5 mg/kg q 12 hours or 5 mg/kg q 8 hours not to exceed 15 mg/kg/day
Levofloxacin (Levaquin)	Second-generation quinolone	750 mg PO/IV q24h
Pipercillin and tazobactam sodium (Zosyn)	Antipseudomonal penicillin plus beta-lactamase inhibitor	4.5 g IV q6h
Doripenem (Doribax)	Carbapenem antibiotic	500 mg IV q8h and use over 1 h (Adjust dosage to creatinine clearance.)
Ceftriaxone (Rocephin)	Third generation cephalosporin with gram-negative activity	1–2 g IV daily or divided bid (Not to exceed 4 g/day.)
Imipenem and cilastatin (Primaxin)	Carbapenem antibiotic	500 mg IV q6h (Not to exceed 4 g/day; adjust for creatinine clearance.)
Linezolid (Zyvox)	Use as alternative if the patient is allergic to vancomycin and to treat vancomycin-resistant enterococci	600 mg PO/IV q12h for 10–14 days

Adapted from Global Initiative for Chronic Obstructive Lung Disease (GOLD). Global strategy for the diagnosis, management, and prevention of chronic obstructive pulmonary disease. Bethesda, MD: Global Initiative for Chronic Obstructive Lung Disease (GOLD); 2008:94.

should also be considered if mechanical ventilation is required. Underlying comorbid conditions and differential diagnoses requiring consultation include rheumatology, cardiology, and oncology.

Clinical Nurse Specialist Competencies and Spheres of Influence
Research/Evidence-Based Practice, Coaching/Teaching/Mentoring, and Systems Leadership

For patients in the intensive care unit who require intubation and mechanical ventilator support, there is research support for bundled interventions that effectively prevent VAP. The Practice Alert for Ventilator Associated Pneumonia (12) and the Practice Alert for Oral Care for Patients at Risk for Ventilator Associated Pneumonia (13), both published by the American Association of Critical Care Nurses, are available at no cost for download and distribution to bedside nurses, respiratory therapists, educators, novice nurses, and others who may benefit from this information. Head of bed elevation, use of an endotracheal tube that facilitates continuous suctioning of tracheal secretions, and frequent oral care with a toothbrush, when all implemented (or bundled), reduce the risk of VAP (12, 13). Hospitals rely on CNSs to access such resources, educate caregivers, and provide leadership for development and implementation of order sets that reflect state of the science information.

CHRONIC LUNG DISEASE

Etiology

Chronic obstructive pulmonary disease (COPD) is a group of conditions characterized by airflow limitation that is not fully reversible, usually progressive, and associated with inflammation of the lungs. The World Health Organization (WHO) reports that the term COPD includes emphysema, chronic bronchitis, and small airway disease. Emphysema is characterized by anatomical structural change via destruction and enlargement of the alveoli. Chronic bronchitis is associated with chronic cough and increased mucous production that causes chronic airflow restriction. Small airway disease refers to a generalized narrowing of the bronchioles and may include asthma. All of these conditions create the symptoms of COPD (14-17).

COPD is the fourth leading cause of death and continues to increase in prevalence. According to WHO and the U.S. Centers for Disease Control and Prevention (CDC), 210 million people currently have COPD. More than 3 million people died of COPD in 2005 (the latest figures at the time of this publication), which corresponds to 5% of all deaths globally (16). In 2002, WHO projected a 30% increase in the reported occurrence rate of COPD over the next 10 years. This increase will elevate the mortality rate of COPD to be the third leading cause of death worldwide by 2030. The Global Initiative for Chronic Obstructive Lung Disease (GOLD), an organization working to improve the prevention and treatment of COPD, projects an even more grim prediction that COPD will be the third leading cause of death by 2020. Smoking tobacco is highly correlated with the occurrence of COPD and an increase in smoking and an aging population is cited as reasons for the increased occurrence and mortality (14, 15, 18).

COPD presents a significant economic and social burden. The National Heart, Lung, and Blood Institute (NHLBI) reported the direct costs of COPD in the United States for 2005 as $21.8 billion and the indirect costs totaled $17.0 billion. In the United States, per-patient direct costs related to COPD were estimated in the range of $2,700 to $5,900 annually. An even higher cost was attributed in the Medicare population with an average of $6,300 per COPD patient (19-21).

The most important risk factors for COPD are tobacco smoking, indoor air pollution (such as biomass fuel used for cooking and heating), outdoor air pollution, and occupational dusts and chemicals. Other factors are gender, socioeconomic status, and genetics (15, 18). Historically, males have had a higher incidence of COPD; however, as the number of females who smoke has increased, the gender gap has diminished. Lower socioeconomic status is associated with increased occurrence of COPD. The reason is unclear, but crowding, poor nutrition, and exposure to indoor and outdoor air pollutants are possible contributors.

Cigarette smoking was first recognized as a major risk factor in 1964 and continues to be a major contributing source of COPD. Cigarette smokers show an increasing decline in forced expiratory volume over 1 second (FEV_1) compared to nonsmokers; studies of nonsmoking men demonstrate a decline in FEV_1 of approximately 30 mL per year after age 30, whereas average smokers' declines at approximately 60 mL per year, leading to disability from dyspnea late in life. Approximately 15% to 20% of smokers decline as much as 100 mL per year and may develop dyspnea in middle life. The number of cigarettes smoked, generally measured in pack-years (packs per day multiplied by number of years of smoking), correlates positively with loss of pulmonary function and accounts for the higher prevalence rates for COPD with increasing age. To a lesser degree, other forms of smoking, such as pipe, cigar, or even passive smoke inhalation, increase morbidity rates. Children exposed in utero to maternal smoking demonstrate significantly reduced lung growth and reduction in postnatal pulmonary function (14, 15).

Occupational exposure to dust or chemical agents and fumes is suspected to increase the risk of COPD. For example, coal mining, gold mining, and working with cotton textile dust have been identified as risk factors for chronic airflow obstruction. Researchers have shown some reduction in FEV_1 in workers in these occupations, but the evidence is nonconclusive. Cadmium exposure, a metal commonly found in industrial workplaces, particularly where any ore is processed or smelted, is another risk factor for airflow obstruction and emphysema. Cadmium is especially dangerous as it emits a relatively nonirritating fume when heated that does not alarm the exposed individual. Workers should be aware that cadmium is also found in some industrial paints and batteries (22).

Air pollution in urban areas may increase respiratory symptoms, though this has not been conclusively studied. There is some evidence linking prolonged exposure to smoke produced by biomass combustion with development of COPD. This is seen especially in countries where biomass fuels are used indoors for cooking (17, 18).

Genetics play a role in the development of COPD. For instance, it is well documented that a severe hereditary deficiency of alpha-1 antitrypsin increases one's susceptibility for small airway disease. Most common in persons of northern European origin, this recessive trait occurs in approximately 1% to 2% of individuals with COPD. In the United States, it is estimated that 1 in 3,000 individuals are alpha-1 antitrypsin deficient; however, few have been tested to establish the genetic disorder. Screening for alpha-1 antitrypsin deficiency in suspected individuals, which involves a simple serum analysis, may be beneficial in counseling people about smoking and toxic chemical exposure (14, 15). Other genetic deficiencies may be associated with the development of COPD. For example, airflow obstruction has been found in relatives of individuals with a confirmed diagnosis COPD (15).

Pathophysiology

Changes in the pulmonary structure include both large and small airways, alveolar spaces, and pulmonary vasculature. Exaggerated inflammatory responses to chronic irritants, such as cigarette smoke, lead to chronic bronchitis and emphysema (14, 16-18).

Chronic bronchitis is characterized by inflammation, hypersecretion of mucus, and a chronic productive cough. Inspired irritants increase the size and number of mucous glands and goblet cells in the airway epithelium. The mucus is thicker and more tenacious, making clearance more difficult and increasing the risk for colonization of bacteria. As infection and injury increase mucus production, the bronchial walls become inflamed and swollen. Bronchial smooth muscle becomes hypertrophied. Chronic inflammation narrows the airways and leads to bronchospasm, which, in turn, narrows them further. Generally, damage begins in the larger airways and eventually extends to the smaller airways. Air trapping occurs as the airway opens during inspiration followed by collapse of the distal portions of the airways early during expiration (Figure 10-1). This results in retained carbon dioxide and impaired oxygen diffusion. Eventually, gas exchange is so severe that ventilation-perfusion (V/Q) mismatch occurs, resulting in hypercapnia and hypoxemia (23).

Emphysema is a permanent structural change in the anatomy of the lung. Bronchioles and alveoli are enlarged due to damage in the extracellular matrix of the lung. Inflammatory cytokines are released, which increase protease activity resulting in breakdown of elastin in the alveolar septa. Septal destruction eliminates portions of the pulmonary capillary bed, increases air volume in the acinus (small airway sacs), and hyperinflates the

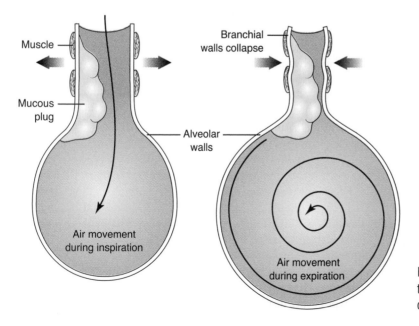

FIGURE 10–1: Mechanisms of air trapping in chronic obstructive pulmonary disease.

alveoli. Significant reduction in alveolar surface area diminishes gas exchange and eventual respiratory failure may result (23).

Clinical Presentation

COPD progresses insidiously over many years, and the individual does not usually seek medical care until symptoms of dyspnea occur. The three most common indicators of COPD are cough, sputum production, and exertional dyspnea, which typically does not occur until the FEV_1 is approximately 50% of normal. Often, people experience dyspnea initially during episodes of acute bronchitis, with increasing frequency over 10 to 15 years until they have exertional dyspnea in the absence of acute bronchitis. Eventually, they have dyspnea even at rest, along with wheezing. A productive cough is usually worse in the morning (14, 17, 18). Periodic exacerbations of severe dyspnea, coughing, wheezing, and excessive mucus production necessitate hospitalization. Yellow or green sputum is usually indicative of bacterial infection. Systemic manifestations of COPD include impaired skeletal muscle function, osteoporosis, anemia, depression, pulmonary hypertension, and cor pulmonale (17). Advanced disease may cause weight loss and skeletal muscle atrophy, which are ominous prognostic signs.

When conducting the history and physical exam, the clinician should determine the degree of acute distress by comparing with the usual baseline activity tolerance. For example, activities that allow the patient to brace his or her arms and use accessory breathing muscles may be better tolerated than those that involve significant arm work, particularly at or above shoulder level. Severe dyspnea often interferes with routine activities of daily living. Tachycardia, tachypnea, use of accessory muscles, perioral or peripheral (nailbed) cyanosis, the ability to speak in complete sentences, and the patient's mental status should be assessed. A prolonged expiratory phase and expiratory wheezing usually indicate advanced disease. Increased anterior-posterior diameter of the chest (barrel chest) indicates hyperinflation. The examiner should observe the patient in sitting position; leaning forward on his or her arms facilitates use of accessory muscles for respiration (sternocleidomastoid, scalene, and intercostals). Advanced disease may lead to secondary pulmonary hypertension and right heart failure known as cor pulmonale. Signs of cor pulmonale include a prominent pulmonic component of the S_2 heart sound, jugular venous distention, hepatic congestion, and ankle edema.

Diagnosis

The diagnostic plan consists of a thorough history and physical exam, pulmonary function tests (PFTs), laboratory tests, and radiographs. Progressive worsening of persistent dyspnea is usually the chief complaint and a key element of COPD diagnosis. A chronic, productive cough and history of exposure to tobacco or other types of smoke or occupational dusts and chemicals raise the index of suspicion (18).

With positive findings in the history and physical exam, the patient should then undergo PFTs. Airflow is assessed with spirometry, which measures the FEV_1 and forced vital capacity (FVC). A reduction in FEV_1, FVC, and FEV_1/FVC ratio favors a diagnosis of COPD. As the disease progresses, total lung capacity, functional residual capacity, and residual volume increase. Dynamic hyperinflation during exercise, measured by the FEV_1, is thought to be a greater contributor to the sensation of dyspnea than airflow obstruction alone (17). Classification of severity and stages of COPD are based on the degree of airflow obstruction defined in the GOLD disease classification (http://www.who.int/respiratory/copd/GOLD_WR_06.pdf).

Laboratory tests should include arterial blood gases (ABGs), complete blood count (CBC), and a basic metabolic profile. ABG analysis reveals mild-to-moderate hypoxemia without hypercapnia in the early stages of disease. As lung injury progresses, hypoxemia worsens and hypercapnia begins, which occurs when the FEV_1 falls below 30% of the predicted value (17). Pulmonary mechanics and gas exchange deteriorate during acute exacerbations. Classification of ventilatory failure, defined as PCO_2 greater than 45 mm Hg, may be determined as acute or chronic by monitoring changes in pH in the ABG analysis. A more acidotic pH in relation to the PCO_2 indicates an acute change in ventilatory status, whereas in chronic ventilator failure, the pH is less acidotic due to renal compensation with secretion of bicarbonate.

The neutrophil count may be elevated, indicative of bacterial infection. An elevated hematocrit may result as a compensatory mechanism for chronic hypoxemia. Renal and hepatic function should be evaluated for appropriate selection of medications to minimize the risk of toxicity. Radiographic studies may show increased lung volumes and flattening of the diaphragm, which suggest the presence of emphysema and right ventricular (RV) hypertrophy. CT scan is more sensitive and therefore more accurate than radiographic studies. High-resolution CT scanning demonstrates bullae that are not always seen on the radiograph; it is also helpful in determining the various forms of COPD (14, 16, 17).

A questionnaire or self-report of exercise tolerance may be used to assess a patient's functional capacity (24). Typical questions includes the number of stairs the patient can climb or how far they can walk before stopping to rest; the findings can provide a broad basis of activity tolerance or indications for further diagnostic studies. A more standardized approach to measuring functional capacity and mortality predictability associated with COPD is the 6-minute walking test. Specific guidelines are available; however, basically the test evaluates the distance the patient can walk in 6 minutes (17).

Management

The GOLD guidelines for routinely managing COPD focus on reduction of risk factors, bronchodilator and inhaled glucocorticoid use, and cardiopulmonary rehabilitation. The goal of treatment is to improve quality of life by preventing exacerbations. Management begins with educating the patient about his or her disease and encouraging the patient to participate in gaining control of their symptoms. If the patient smokes, cessation assistance can be the most important intervention. The U.S. Preventive Services Task Force has issued guidelines for health care providers regarding the use of tobacco products and cessation (Table 10-08). The recommendations advise brief behavioral counseling and offer of pharmacotherapy. If the patient generally smokes a cigarette within 30 minutes of awakening, the patient is most likely highly addicted to nicotine and will likely benefit from replacement therapy. Transdermal nicotine patches or nicotine Polacrilex chewing gum both have a better success rate than placebo; long-term success rates are 22% to 42% compared to 2% to 25% placebo (17). Antidepressant therapy, such as bupropion, may be used to counter the enhanced central nervous system nonadrenergic function. A more recent drug approved for smoking cessation is varenicline. Although a promising and effective medications for smoking cessation, the U.S. Food and Drug Administration requires manufacturers to include a Black Box Warning in the prescribing information highlighting the risk of serious mental health events such as changes in behavior, depressed mood, hostility, and suicidal thoughts when taking bupropion and varenicline (25).

Pulmonary medications for COPD target bronchial smooth muscle contraction, bronchial mucosal congestion and edema, airway inflammation, and increased airway secretions (14, 16-18). Inhaled bronchodilators improve symptoms related to bronchoconstriction. Anticholinergic agents, such as ipratropium bromide, improve FEV_1 and reduce exacerbations. Beta-agonists provide symptomatic benefit but have uncomfortable side effects of tremor and tachycardia. Long-acting inhaled beta agonists, such as salmeterol, have benefits comparable to ipratropium bromide and are more convenient than

TABLE 10–8 U.S. Preventive Services Task Force (USPSTF) Guidelines

Ask about tobacco use.
Advise to quit through personalized messages.
Assess willingness to quit.
Assist with quitting.
Arrange follow-up care and support.

short-acting agents. During an acute exacerbation nebulized therapy should be initiated. After stabilization, inhaled metered dose is equally effective in smooth muscle relaxation. Although numerous factors may cause acute exacerbation of the disease, one of the most common is infection of the tracheobronchial tree. Antibiotics specific to the cultured organism should be prescribed whenever possible and otherwise are empirically prescribed for acute infections. Antibiotics are not recommended for prophylactic treatment due to the risk of resistant organisms.

Decisions of when to hospitalize and when to admit to the intensive care unit (ICU) are defined in the GOLD Report (18). Indications include severe underlying COPD with a sudden increase in dyspnea at rest. Signs of peripheral edema or cyanosis, cardiac arrhythmias, and some comorbidities are indications for hospitalization and possibly the ICU, depending on the hospital's available nursing and respiratory care services. Failure to respond to rescue inhalers, older age, and insufficient home support are all factors to consider when the patient presents with an acute exacerbation (18). Changes in mental status and worsening hypoxemia (PaO_2 less than 40 mm Hg) or severe hypercapnia ($PaCO_2$ greater than 60 mm Hg) likely necessitate mechanical ventilation, and unstable hemodynamics is an indication for aggressive support (18).

Glucocorticoids are effective in the treatment of an acute exacerbation. Studies show that glucocorticoids reduce the length of stay, hasten recovery, and reduce the chance of subsequent exacerbation or relapse for a period of up to 6 months. The GOLD guidelines recommend 30 to 40 mg of oral prednisolone or its equivalent for a period of 10 to 14 days. Patients should be monitored for hyperglycemia especially if the patient has a history of diabetes mellitus (14, 15, 18). Chronic use of oral glucocorticoids for treatment of COPD is not recommended because of an unfavorable benefit/risk ratio. Significant side effects include osteoporosis, cataracts, glucose intolerance, and increased risk of infection. Inhaled glucocorticoids may reduce exacerbations and mortality by approximately 25%. Side effects for which to educate patients and monitor include oropharyngeal candidiasis and increased rate of bone density loss. Client education regarding rinsing the mouth after administration and good oral hygiene is important (14, 15).

Theophylline is effective for moderate to severe COPD and may be used as an adjunct treatment. Mild to moderate improvements in expiratory flow rates, vital capacity, and arterial oxygen and carbon dioxide levels have been established with theophylline treatment. Common side effects include nausea, tachycardia, and tremors (14, 15, 17).

Oxygen is the only pharmacologic therapy shown to decrease mortality in patients with COPD. Patients with resting O_2 saturation less than 90%, signs of pulmonary hypertension, or right heart failure should be on continual oxygen supplementation as home therapy. The goal of supplemental O_2 is to maintain arterial saturations at or above 90%. Loss of hypoxic respiratory drive in the COPD patient may result in modest increases in arterial P_{CO_2}; however, researchers have demonstrated that in patients with both acute and chronic hypercapnia, the administration of supplemental O_2 does not reduce minute ventilation; hence, there is no substantial increase in carbon dioxide. Clinicians should administer oxygen to correct hypoxemia in patients experiencing an acute exacerbation of COPD.

Additional GOLD guidelines advise that patients with COPD receive the influenza vaccine annually and the polyvalent pneumococcal vaccine as recommended. Also, a rehabilitation program that incorporates education and cardiovascular conditioning is recommended and has been shown to improve quality of life and reduce rates of hospitalization.

Exacerbations are frequently associated with a respiratory infection, and it is often difficult to positively identify the microorganism responsible for a particular clinical event. Commonly occurring pathogens include *S. pneumoniae*, *H. influenzae*, and *M. catarrhalis* (Table 10-9) (18). *Pseudomonas aeruginosa* may be seen in patients with severe disease. Recent hospitalization and four or more courses of antibiotics in a year are risk factors for *P. aeruginosa* (18). The choice of antibiotic should be based on susceptibility of the above pathogens as well as the patient's clinical condition. Generally, it is accepted practice to treat patients with moderate or severe exacerbations with antibiotics, even prior to identification of a specific pathogen. Table 10-10 lists the most commonly indicated antibiotics (18).

Mechanical Ventilatory Support

Noninvasive positive pressure ventilation (NPPV) is effective for many patients with respiratory failure and replaces the need for intubation. NPPV decreases complications of therapy, and is associated with a decreased hospital length of stay. Contraindications for NPPV are shown in Table 10-11.

Mechanical ventilation via endotracheal intubation is indicated for patients with severe respiratory distress. Some indications are tachypnea greater than 25, hypercapnia

TABLE 10–10 Antibiotics Recommended for Exacerbations of Chronic Obstructive Pulmonary Disease

Penicillin	Tetracyclines
Ampicillin/amoxicillin	Sulfamethoxaole
Azithromycin	Levofloxin
Clarithromycin	Moxifloxacin
Cephalosporins	

High-dose fluorquinolones (ciprofloxacin and levofloxacin) are indicated for pseudomonal infections.

TABLE 10–11 Contraindications to Noninvasive Positive Pressure Ventilation

Cardiovascular instability	Significant burns
Impaired mental status	Craniofacial abnormalities or trauma precluding effective fitting of mask
Inability to cooperate	
Copious secretions or inability to clear secretions	Extreme obesity

National Heart, Blood and Lung Institute. National Institutes of Health.
Expert Panel Report 3 (EPR-3): Guidelines for the Diagnosis and Management of Asthma - Summary Report 2007. Retrieved August 8, 2011 from http://www.nhlbi.nih.gov/guidelines/asthma/asthsumm.htm.

(Pa_{CO_2} greater than 45), severe acidosis (pH less than 7.25), respiratory arrest, shock, and impaired mental status. Ventilatory settings should provide sufficient expiratory time in patients with severe airflow obstruction and adjustment of positive end-expiratory pressure

TABLE 10-9 Respiratory Pathogens Frequently Colonized in Patients With Chronic Oobstructive Pulmonary Disease

Most Frequently Occurring Pathogens	In 5% to 10% of Exacerbations
Streptococcus pneumoniae, Haemophilus influenzae, Moraxella catarrhalis	*Mycoplasma pneumonia, Chlamydia pneumoniae*

(PEEP). Although beneficial for most patients with severe respiratory distress, mechanical ventilation does not always help those with end-stage disease and other conditions. The overall mortality rate for patients with COPD who require intubation is 17% to 30% during the hospitalization, which is even higher in patients older than 65 (16). (Better predictive models are needed to aid in decision-making about who can benefit from intubation and mechanical ventilator support.)

COPD is the single leading indication for lung transplantation. The current recommendations for lung transplantation are age less than 65 years, severe disability despite maximal medical therapy, and absence of comorbid conditions such as liver, renal, or cardiac disease (16).

Clinical Nurse Specialist Competencies and Spheres of Influence
Coaching/Teaching/Mentoring

Ongoing evaluation, education, and support for people with COPD are fundamental to physical and psychological well-being, with an overriding goal of requiring fewer hospitalizations. The CNS monitors for correct use of inhalers and adverse effects of bronchodilators. Teaching includes relaxation exercises to reduce stress, tension, and anxiety to optimize oxygen utilization. Suggestions for energy conservation and positioning for comfort to decrease dyspnea should be provided. Breathing exercises should be observed to ensure correct pursed lip breathing for control of rate and depth of respiration and to improve respiratory muscle coordination.

Education and assistance in identifying and eliminating all pulmonary irritants, particularly cigarette smoke, helps reduce acute exacerbations. The CNS provides self-help resources and referrals for smoking cessation and prescribes nicotine substitutes and other medications to quell withdrawal symptoms. For example, CNS-initiated smoking cessation educational programs using television and written materials, with enrollees selecting the method of nicotine cessation, have been successful in achieving significant abstinence rates (26). Suggestions that assist in keeping the patient's home as dust-free as possible also help control exacerbations. Patients should be instructed to avoid extremely hot or cold weather and offered a high-efficiency particulate mask to be worn when extreme temperatures are unavoidable. Patients should be advised to avoid persons with respiratory illness, maintain annual influenza and pneumonia vaccination, and taught the signs and symptoms of respiratory infection. Other guidance should include meeting nutritional and hydration needs; monitoring oxygen saturation at rest and during activity; and administering continuous oxygen if needed.

Systems Leadership, Collaboration, and Research/Evidence-Based Practice

CNS-led interdisciplinary teams providing pulmonary rehabilitation using evidence-based practice guidelines have been successful in achieving improved quality of life, improved functional status, greater participation in physical activity, and reduced resource utilization for people with COPD (27). Programs like this potentiate patients' sense of well-being and help curb hospitalizations, which reduces expenditures for an otherwise costly disease. When hospitalization and mechanical ventilation are required, many hospitals place these patients in CNS-run, protocol-driven units, which is successful in reducing ventilator days and length of stay.

ASTHMA

Etiology

Asthma is a clinical syndrome of unknown etiology characterized by spontaneous variations in airflow obstruction. Recurrent episodes of an exaggerated bronchoconstrictor response to stimuli lead to wheezing, varying degrees of airway obstruction, and dyspnea. An underlying inflammation in the airways responds to a wide range of triggers known as airway hyperresponsiveness. Narrowing of the airways is usually reversible, but in some patients with chronic asthma there may be an element of irreversible airflow obstruction (28-30).

The WHO estimates that 300 million people suffer from asthma, with 255,000 deaths occurring in 2009 (the latest figures at the time of this writing) (31). Although mortality is primarily related to lung dysfunction, mortality has also been linked to asthma management failure, especially in young persons. Other factors that impact mortality include age older than 40 years, cigarette smoking more than 20 pack-years, blood eosinophilia, FEV_1 of 40% to 69% predicted, and greater reversibility (32). The high prevalence rate and severity of disease consume a disproportionate amount of health care spending. In the United States in 2009 the asthma prevalence was 8.2%, affecting 24.6 million people. In 2006 in the United States, 3,163 people died from asthma. Estimates of direct and indirect costs of asthma care exceed $8 billion per year in the United States alone (28). Asthma occurs in all races; however, in the United States, morbidity and mortality are higher in blacks than whites. Asthma is the most common chronic disease in childhood, affecting an estimated 6 million children (15%) and a common cause of hospitalization for children in the United States (29-31). The prevalence of asthma is increasing in children, with 8.9% in the United States aged 2 to 17 years affected. The number is rising in developing countries as well, which appears to be associated with increased urbanization. In childhood, twice as many males as females are affected, but by adulthood the occurrence is equal. Asthma may present in childhood, become asymptomatic during adolescence, and then return during adult life and is attributed to airway responsiveness and lower levels of lung function (33).

Approximately half of all children diagnosed with asthma have a decrease or disappearance of symptoms by early adulthood (34).

The National Asthma Education and Prevention Program Expert Panel from the U.S. National Institutes of Health issued a definition, guidelines for the diagnosis, and recommendations for the management of asthma. The most recent report defines asthma as a common chronic disorder of the airways that is complex and characterized by variable and recurring symptoms, airflow obstruction, bronchial hyperresponsiveness, and an underlying inflammation. The interaction of these features of asthma determines the clinical manifestations and severity of asthma and the response to treatment. Asthma management decisions now focus on categorization of asthma severity and, subsequently, on assessment of asthma control (35).

The etiology of asthma includes both genetic and environmental factors. Different genes may contribute to asthma specifically, and there is increasing evidence that the severity of asthma is also genetically determined (30). Genetic screens with classical linkage analysis indicate that asthma is polygenic and suggests that the interaction of many genes is important. There is increasing evidence for a complex interaction between genetic polymorphisms and environmental factors.

Genetic predisposition, atopic syndrome, airway hyperresponsiveness, gender, and possibly ethnicity are endogenous links to asthma. The prevalence of atopic syndrome and other allergic diseases associated with asthma suggests a systemic response rather than one local to the lungs. A genetic tendency toward allergic diseases is known as atopic syndrome (or atopy) and is recognized as a major risk factor for asthma (29, 30). In the atopic individual, a genetically determined IgE antibody is produced in response to environmental proteins or triggers. Often viewed as a type of eczema, atopy is characterized by itching, skin rashes, allergic rhinitis, and asthma. Atopy may be found in 40% to 50% of the population, and although only a proportion of atopic individuals develop asthma, it is a major risk factor. The most consistent genetic findings involve chromosome 5q, including the T helper 2 (TH2) cells interleukin (IL)-4, IL-5, IL-9, and IL-13, which are associated with atopy (30). Other environmental factors or allergens lead to sensitization and include proteins that have protease activity (30).

Environmental risk factors include indoor and outdoor allergens, pollution, passive smoking, and early respiratory infections (Table 10-12). Other known triggers include exercise and hyperventilation, cold air, sulfur dioxide, stress, and irritants such as paint fumes or aerosol sprays (Table 10-13). Common allergens include house dust mites, cat and dog fur, cockroaches, and grass and tree pollens (36). Multiple environmental triggers have been identified; however, the house dust mite *Dermatophagoides*

TABLE 10–12 Risk Factors for Asthma

Endogenous Factors	Environmental Factors
Genetic predisposition	Indoor allergens
Atopy	Outdoor allergens
Airway hyperresponsiveness	Occupational
Gender	Passive smoking
Ethnicity	Respiratory infections
	Obesity
	Early viral infections

pteronyssinus is the most common environmental allergen (28, 29).

Numerous inhaled allergens act as triggers of allergic sensitization and asthma symptoms. Exposure to house dust mites in early childhood is a risk factor for allergic sensitization and asthma. In affluent countries where houses have carpeting, central heat, and poor ventilation, the higher incidence of house dust mites is implicated in the increasing prevalence of asthma for this population. Other perennial allergens are from domestic pets and cockroaches. Domestic pets, particularly cats, have also been associated with allergic sensitization, but early exposure to cats in the home may be protective through the induction of tolerance (30). Seasonal allergens include grass pollen, ragweed, tree pollen, and fungal spores. Pollens usually cause allergic rhinitis rather than asthma but can trigger severe asthma exacerbations (30). Of the environmental factors, allergic reactions remain the most important trigger.

Air pollutants, such as sulfur dioxide, ozone, and diesel particulates, may trigger asthma symptoms. Indoor air pollution may be more important with exposure to nitrogen oxides from cooking stoves and exposure to passive cigarette smoke. Chronic contact with allergens may occur due to occupational exposure and may affect up to 10% of young adults. Over 200 sensitizing agents have been identified, and examples include chemicals, small animal allergens, and fungal amylase in wheat flour (30, 36).

The role of dietary factors is uncertain, although diets low in antioxidants or high in sodium are associated with an increased risk of asthma. Studies involving nutrition as an intervention have not supported diet as a contributing factor. Obesity is recognized as an independent risk factor for asthma, but the mechanism is not known.

Viral infections of the respiratory tract are common triggers of acute exacerbations of asthma. Rhinovirus, RSV, and coronavirus have been implicated, though the mechanism of action is not completely understood. An

TABLE 10–13 Triggers Involved in Asthma

Exercise and hyperventilation
Cold air
Sulfur dioxide
Drugs (beta-blockers, aspirin)
Stress
Irritants (household sprays, paint fumes)
House dust mites, animal allergens (especially cat and dog), cockroach allergens, and fungi are most
   commonly reported

Environmental Allergens	House dust mites, animal allergens (especially cat and dog), cockroach allergens, and fungi are most commonly reported. Environmental pollutants, tobacco smoke
Upper Respiratory Tract Viral Infections	Chronic sinusitis or rhinitis
Exercise	Hyperventilation Exposure to cold or dry air Duration and intensity of exercise Allergen exposure in atopic individuals Coexisting respiratory infection
Pharmacologic Agents	Aspirin or nonsteroidal anti-inflammatory drug (NSAID) hypersensitivity, sulfite sensitivity Use of beta-adrenergic receptor blockers (including ophthalmic preparations)
Obesity	Based on a prospective cohort study of 86,000 patients, those with an elevated body mass index are more likely to have asthma.
Occupational Exposure	Irritants (dust or sprays, paint fumes)
Perinatal Factors	Prematurity and increased maternal age increase the risk for asthma. Both maternal smoking and prenatal exposure to tobacco smoke also increase the risk of developing asthma.

increase in airway inflammation with increased numbers of eosinophils and neutrophils is one connection. There is evidence to show that production of type I interferons by epithelial cells of people with asthma results in an increased susceptibility to these viral infections and a greater inflammatory response (30). There is some association between RSV infection in infancy and the development of asthma. RSV infects the lungs and breathing passages, usually with no further sequelae after 1 to 2 weeks. However, infection can be severe and is the most common cause of bronchiolitis and pneumonia in children under 1 year of age in the United States. In addition, RSV is more often recognized as an important cause of

respiratory illness in older adults (30). Recent research findings show a key and expanding role for viral respiratory infections in the pathology of asthma (35).

Some pharmacologic agents may trigger asthma. Beta-adrenergic blockers mediate an increased cholinergic bronchoconstriction and may be fatal. Recommendations include avoiding all beta blockers including selective beta-2 blockers. Angiotensin-converting enzyme (ACE) inhibitors may reduce breakdown of kinins, which are bronchoconstrictors and theoretically should be avoided (30). Aspirin and some cyclooxygenase (COX) inhibitors may worsen asthma in approximately 1% of asthma patients. Referred to as aspirin-sensitive asthma, this phenomenon is more common in individuals with severe asthma. A genetic predisposition to increased production of cysteinyl-leukotrienes with functional polymorphism of cys-leukotriene synthase produces rhinorrhea, conjunctival irritation, facial flushing, and wheezing in response to aspirin and nonselective COX inhibitors. Selective COX-2 inhibitors may be administered when an anti-inflammatory analgesic is needed. Although antileukotrienes should be effective in these patients, they are no more effective than in allergic asthma and usual therapy with inhaled corticosteroids should be effective.

Exercise-induced asthma is common, especially in children. The overall prevalence rate of exercise-induced bronchospasm is 3% to 10% of the general population and 12% to 15% of the general population if patients with underlying asthma are included. The rate of exercise-induced symptoms in persons with asthma has been reported to vary from 40% to 90% (37). The pathogenesis of exercise-induced bronchospasm is controversial. The mechanism may be due to water loss from the airway, heat loss from the airway, or a combination of both (29, 30). The upper airway is designed to keep inspired air at 100% humidity and body temperature at 37°C (98.6°F). Hyperventilation, especially when mouth breathing occurs, interferes with this normal mechanism. Increased osmolality in airway lining fluids and temperature changes triggers mast cell mediator release, resulting in bronchoconstriction. Dry, cold weather exacerbates the effects, which usually begin after the exercise has ended and lasts about 30 minutes. The most effective treatment includes regular administration of inhaled glucocorticoids, which reduce the population of surface mast cells. Administration of beta-2 agonists and antileukotrienes may also be beneficial (30, 31).

Changes in weather, strong smells, perfumes, and hyperventilation, including laughter, have been reported as asthma triggers. However, the mechanisms are not clearly understood. Many patients believe that their symptoms are triggered by particular food, and although some foods may induce severe anaphylactic reactions, no connection to asthma has been established. Some food additives, however, may trigger asthma. An example is metabisulfite, which is used as a food preservative and may trigger asthma through the release of sulfur dioxide gas in the stomach (31).

Exposures to air pollution containing sulfur dioxide, ozone, and nitrogen oxides are associated with an increase in asthma symptoms. These sensitizing agents may also be contacted in the workplace, resulting in occupational exposure. Recognition and identification of the trigger are necessary to prevent long-term airway damage. Symptoms that typically worsen at work and diminish over the weekend or a long holiday may indicate an occupational exposure.

Other factors include hormonal imbalance, gastroesophageal reflux, and stress. Hormonal imbalance may precipitate asthma. Both thyrotoxicosis and hypothyroidism have been linked to a worsening of asthma, although the mechanisms are not certain. A premenstrual fall in progesterone may act as a trigger as well. Gastroesophageal reflux has been linked to asthma and is a trigger to bronchoconstriction. Antireflux medication is often prescribed but typically does not reduce asthma symptoms. Stress can induce bronchoconstriction through cholinergic reflex pathways.

Pathophysiology

Asthma is a disease of chronic inflammation of the mucosa of the lower airways characterized by acute exacerbations that limit airflow. The major components of asthma are airway inflammation, intermittent airflow obstruction, and bronchial hyperresponsiveness. Three characteristics are (a) constriction of airway smooth muscle, (b) thickening of the airway epithelium (airway edema), and (c) the presence of liquids or mucus in the airway lumen (28-30). This results in a reduction in FEV_1, FEV_1/FVC ratio, and peak expiratory flow (PEF) and an increase in airway resistance. Air trapping occurs due to early closure of peripheral airways in lung hyperinflation and increased residual volume. In more severe asthma, reduced ventilation and increased pulmonary blood flow result in mismatching of ventilation and perfusion and in bronchial hyperemia. In patients with severe asthma, the arterial $PaCO_2$ tends to be low due to increased ventilation.

The presence of airway hyperresponsiveness or bronchial hyperreactivity in asthma is an exaggerated response to numerous exogenous and endogenous stimuli. Both direct stimulation of airway smooth muscle and indirect stimulation by pharmacologically active substances from mediator-secreting cells such as mast cells or non-myelinated sensory neurons are identified as mechanisms of action. The degree of airway hyperresponsiveness generally correlates with the clinical severity of asthma (28-30).

Airway hyperresponsiveness describes the excessive bronchoconstrictor response to multiple inhaled triggers that would not affect a normal airway. It is the characteristic physiologic abnormality of asthma and is linked to the frequency of asthma symptoms. Both direct and indirect stimuli affect the airway smooth muscle; however, most triggers for asthma symptoms appear to act indirectly.

Several endogenous mediators are identified that stimulate the symptoms of wheezing and dyspnea during an asthma attack. Acetylcholine released from the intrapulmonary motor nerves causes constriction of airway smooth muscle through direct stimulation of muscarinic receptors of the M3 subtype. Mast cells are prominent in the airway tissues and release histamine, a known potent bronchoactive agent. Bradykinin, a plasma precursor of the enzymes known as kallikreins, is also released from mast cells and is a potent bronchoconstrictor. Cysteinyl-leukotreines are produced by mast cells, eosinophils, and alveolar macrophages and are potent contractile agonists on airway smooth muscle. Other mediators include neuropeptides, nitric oxide, and platelet-activating factor.

Varying degrees of mononuclear cell and eosinophil infiltration, mucus hypersecretion, desquamation of the epithelium, smooth muscle hyperplasia, and airway remodeling are present in the patient with asthma (29). Bronchoscopic and biopsy studies show hyperemia, edema, and airway mucosa infiltrated with activated Th2 phenotype lymphocytes, mast cells, and eosinophils. T-lymphocytes play an important role in the regulation of airway inflammation through the release of numerous cytokines. The lymphocytes produce IL-3, IL-4, and IL-5, which promote the synthesis of an important allergic effector molecule: immunoglobulin E (IgE). Chemokines produced by the epithelial and inflammatory cells amplify and perpetuate the inflammatory events within the airway (29, 30).

Bronchographic findings show uneven narrowing of the airways consistent with a patchy involvement of the airways. Eosinophils release fibrogenic factors and the airway wall itself may be thickened and edematous. In severe chronic asthma, there is hypertrophy and hyperplasia of airway glands and secretory cells, as well as hyperplasia of smooth muscle. Subepithelial collagen deposition leads to thickening of the basement membrane and frequently presents as a chronic cough and inflammation in the airway. Vasodilatation and increased numbers of blood vessels (angiogenesis) lead to narrowed, reddened, edematous airways. Mucus glycoproteins secreted from goblet cells, clusters of shed airway epithelial cells, and plasma proteins from leaky bronchial vessels may create a mucus plug and occlude the airway. Occlusion of the airway lumen by a mucus plug is a common finding in fatal asthma (28, 30). The cartilaginous airways of the bronchi are primarily affected with inflammation of the respiratory mucosa. Variable airflow due to airway hyperresponsiveness may be attributed to local IgE production. Although asthma is often viewed as an acute inflammatory change, it is a chronic condition.

Diagnosis

The diagnosis begins with a detailed assessment of the medical history. The initial consideration is whether the symptoms are attributable to asthma or another cause. Determining family history may be helpful in highlighting a genetic tendency. If asthma is suspected or confirmed the asthma severity and the identification of possible precipitating factors should be determined (29). The profile of a typical asthma exacerbation should be obtained and include the number of emergency department visits, hospitalizations, ICU admissions, or need for ventilatory support. Determine how many days of work or school were missed or if the patient limited activity due to difficulty breathing.

The hallmark symptom of asthma is wheezing, and although it is noted that all asthmatics wheeze, all wheezing is not asthma. Wheezing is generally louder on expiration but audible on inspiration and described as polyphonic. Adventitious sounds may include crackles and the expiratory phase is prolonged relative to the inspiratory phase. The patient may report a cough that is worse at night (39), chest tightness or shortness of breath, decreased exercise tolerance, and sputum production (28-30). Symptoms may vary seasonally or at night or early mornings. Asthma symptoms may be continual or episodic and vary in duration, severity, and frequency. Sputum color may be clear or opaque with a greenish or yellow tinge. This is not necessarily an indication of infection but may be due to the presence of eosinophils, which may affect color. Determining the presence of infection requires a Gram stain or Wright-stained smear.

Hyperinflation and increased ventilation including use of accessory muscles may also be noted. Symptoms include dyspnea, shortness of breath, and coughing that may be worse at night. Some variants of asthma cause hoarseness or an inability to sleep through the night. Prodromal symptoms may precede an attack, with itching under the chin, discomfort between the scapulae, or an inexplicable fear of impending doom.

Vital signs during an acute attack include tachypnea (25 to 40 breaths per minute), tachycardia, and an exaggerated inspiratory decrease in the systolic pressure known as pulsus paradoxus. Pulse oximetry typically is 90% on room air. Use of accessory muscles of respiration may be noted. Electrocardiographic (ECG) findings may show right-axis deviation, right bundle-branch block, or even ST-T wave abnormalities during an acute attack (30). Physical exam usually reveals an end-expiratory wheeze, although an inspiratory wheeze may also be heard. Diminished breath sounds and chest hyperinflation (especially in children) may be observed during acute asthma exacerbations. The presence of inspiratory wheezing or stridor may prompt an evaluation for an upper airway obstruction such as vocal cord dysfunction, vocal cord paralysis, thyroid enlargement, or a soft tissue mass (e.g., malignant tumor). The upper airway should be assessed for erythematous turbinates or polyps from sinusitis, allergic rhinitis, or upper respiratory tract infection. The skin should be observed for the presence of atopic dermatitis, eczema, or other allergic skin conditions (28-30).

The diagnosis of asthma is usually apparent from the symptoms but should be confirmed by objective measurements of lung function. A decrease in airflow rates throughout the vital capacity is the cardinal pulmonary function abnormality during an asthma attack (30). Spirometry assessments should be obtained as the primary test to establish the asthma diagnosis. Ideally, spirometry should be performed prior to initiating treatment in order to establish the presence and determine the severity of baseline airway obstruction (29, 39). Optimally, the initial spirometry should also include measurements before and after inhalation of a short-acting bronchodilator in all patients in whom the diagnosis of asthma is considered. Simple spirometry confirms a reduced FEV_1, FEV_1/FVC ratio, and PEF. Reversibility is demonstrated by a greater than 12% and 200 mL increase in FEV_1 at 15 minutes after an inhaled short-acting beta-2 agonist (SABA) or by a 2- to 4-week trial of oral glucocorticoids (28, 29).

Peak-flow monitoring is ideal for ongoing monitoring of patients with asthma. The test is simple to perform and the results are a quantitative and reproducible measure of airflow obstruction. It can be used for short-term monitoring, exacerbation management, and daily long-term monitoring; however, it is not reliable to establish the initial diagnosis of asthma. Results can be used to determine the severity of an exacerbation and to help guide therapeutic decisions as part of an asthma action plan, including guidelines for the use of peak-flow meters for asthma (29).

Hematologic tests and ABGs are not usually helpful. Many asthmatics are atopic; therefore, eosinophilia is common. Blood eosinophilia greater than 4% or 300 to 400/μL supports the diagnosis of asthma, but an absence of this finding is not exclusionary. Eosinophil counts greater than 8% may be observed in patients with concomitant atopic dermatitis (29). Except during severe asthma attacks, blood gas analysis is not necessary. If ABGs are measured, expect respiratory alkalemia at the onset of the attack. If the attack is prolonged the pH normalizes by a compensatory metabolic academia. A normal $PaCO_2$ in a patient with severe airflow obstruction may indicate that the ventilator load is greater than can be sustained and herald impending ventilatory failure (30).

The chest radiograph is usually normal but may show hyperinflated lungs in more severe disease. In mild to moderate asthma without adventitious sounds other than wheezing, a chest radiograph is not necessary. However, if symptoms are more severe, it is recommended. It may also be useful to rule out other causes. During exacerbations, there may be evidence of a pneumothorax. The presence of lung shadowing usually indicates pneumonia or eosinophilic infiltrates. High-resolution CT may show areas of bronchiectasis in patients with severe asthma, and there may be thickening of the bronchial walls, but these changes are not diagnostic of asthma (28, 30).

Allergy skin tests to common allergens are frequently positive in allergic asthma but negative in intrinsic asthma; therefore, they are not helpful in diagnosis. Obtaining radioallergosorbent (RAST) testing may be useful for teaching certain allergens to avoid but are generally not indicated as part of the treatment plan for asthma. Two methods are available to test for allergic sensitivity to specific allergens in the environment: allergy skin tests and blood tests (RAST). Allergy immunotherapy may be beneficial in controlling allergic rhinitis and asthma symptoms for some patients (28-30). In patients with asthma and symptoms of gastroesophageal reflux disease (GERD), 24-hour pH monitoring can help determine if GERD is a contributing factor.

Differential Diagnoses

It is usually not difficult to differentiate asthma from other conditions that cause wheezing and dyspnea in patients without comorbid conditions. A history of exacerbating and remitting airway obstruction accompanied by blood eosinophilia that responds quickly to bronchodilator treatment is usually conclusive. Challenge testing in which subjects are exposed to inhaled bronchoconstrictor agonists measure airway hyperresponsiveness. A positive hyperresponsive airway suggests asthma, while wheezing and a negative test indicate a need for further testing (30).

Common diagnoses that present with similar symptoms as asthma include acute bronchiolitis, aspiration of a foreign body, bronchial stenosis, cardiac failure, chronic bronchitis, cystic fibrosis, and eosinophilic pneumonia. Less common diagnoses include upper airway obstruction due to a tumor or mass. This may include external compression from central thoracic tumors, superior vena caval syndrome, or a substernal thyroid mass. Left ventricular (LV) failure may mimic the wheezing of asthma but basilar crackles are present in contrast to asthma. COPD may be differentiated from asthma as symptoms never completely remit and do not respond well to bronchodilators. Approximately 10% of people with COPD have asthma concomitantly as evidenced by increased sputum eosinophils and a response to oral corticosteroids (37).

Management

The treatment plan is directed at the chronic long-term nature of asthma and the severity of acute exacerbations. The aims of therapy are to reduce airway obstruction and inflammation. Goals for successful assessment and management of asthma are outlined in the 2010 Global Initiative for Asthma (GINA) publication "Global Strategy for Asthma Management and Prevention" and include the following: (a) achieve and maintain control of asthma symptoms, (b) maintain normal activity levels, including exercise, (c) maintain pulmonary function as close to normal as possible, (d) prevent asthma exacerbations, (e) avoid adverse effects from asthma medications, and (f) prevent asthma mortality (40).

Management of asthma is based on severity of disease. Essentially there are two types of drugs for asthma: bronchodilators, which give rapid relief of symptoms mainly through relaxation of airway smooth muscle, and controllers, which inhibit the underlying inflammatory process. Treatment options are based on classification of asthma severity (41). A six-step approach to asthma treatment is outlined in Table 10-14.

Bronchodilator Therapy

The first line of treatment during an acute attack is often referred to as a rescue agent, and its purpose is an immediate bronchodilation. Acting primarily on airway smooth muscle, bronchoconstriction is reversed. Three classes of

TABLE 10–14 A Six-Step Approach to Asthma Therapy

Step 1: Intermittent asthma is present. Intermittent symptoms occurring less than once a week Brief exacerbations Nocturnal symptoms occurring less than twice a month Asymptomatic with normal lung function between exacerbations FEV_1 or PEF rate greater than 80%, with less than 20% variability	A controller medication is not indicated.	The reliever medication is a short-acting beta-agonist (SABA) as needed for symptoms.
Step 2: Mild persistent asthma is present. Symptoms occurring more than once a week but less than once a day Exacerbations affect activity and sleep Nocturnal symptoms occurring more than twice a month FEV_1 or PEF rate greater than 80% predicted, with variability of 20% to 30%	The preferred controller medication is a low-dose inhaled corticosteroid (ICS).	Alternatives include cromolyn sodium, nedocromil sodium, or a leukotriene receptor antagonist (LTRA) (40)
Step 3: Moderate persistent asthma is present. Daily symptoms Exacerbations affect activity and sleep Nocturnal symptoms occurring more than once a week FEV_1 or PEF rate 60-80% of predicted, with variability greater than 30%	The preferred controller medication is either a low-dose ICS plus a long-acting beta-agonist (LABA) (combination medication preferred choice to improve compliance) (41) or a medium-dose ICS.	Alternatives include a low-dose ICS plus either an LTRA, theophylline, or zileuton.
Step 4: Moderate-to-severe persistent asthma is present. Continuous symptoms Frequent exacerbations Frequent nocturnal asthma symptoms Physical activities limited by asthma symptoms FEV_1 or PEF rate less than 60%, with variability greater than 30%	The preferred controller medication is a medium-dose ICS plus an LTRA (combination therapy).	Alternatives include a medium-dose ICS plus either an LTRA, theophylline, or zileuton.

TABLE 10–14 A Six-Step Approach to Asthma Therapy—cont'd

Step 5: Severe persistent asthma is present.	The preferred controller medication is a high-dose ICS plus an LTRA.	Consider omalizumab for patients who have allergies.
Step 6: Severe persistent asthma is present.	The preferred controller medication is a high-dose ICS plus an LTRA plus an oral corticosteroid	Consider omalizumab for patients who have allergies.

Adapted from McCance K, Huether S. Pathophysiology: The Biologic Basis for Disease in Adults and Children. 6th edition. St Louis, MO: Elsevier Mosby; 2010.

bronchodilator include beta-2 adrenergic agonists, anticholinergics, and theophylline.

Beta-2 agonists are by far the most effective and most widely used. The mechanism of action is activation of beta-2 adrenergic receptors. Beta-2 receptors are coupled through a stimulatory G protein to adenylyl cyclase, resulting in increased intracellular cyclic AMP, which relaxes smooth muscle cells and inhibits certain inflammatory cells (28-30). The generalized action of the beta-2 agonists reverses and prevents contraction of all airway smooth muscle cells and effectively promotes bronchodilation. Additional therapeutic benefits are inhibition of mast cell mediator release, reduction in plasma exudation, and inhibition of sensory nerve activation.

SABAs, such as albuterol and terbutaline, provide rapid onset of bronchodilation and last 3 to 6 hours. SABAs are administered by nebulizer or via a metered dose inhaler with a spacer. The treatment usually consists of two puffs from an inhaler administered 3 to 5 minutes apart. The first puff dilates narrowed airways, allowing the second puff better access to lower affected airways. Aerosol spacers are recommended to enhance deposition and reduce oral impaction of the medication. SABAs should be used primarily for rescue; however, they are useful in preventing exercise induced asthma if taken prior to exercise. Frequent or escalating use of SABAs indicates that asthma is not controlled and signals a need to reevaluate the treatment plan.

Long-acting beta-2 agonists (LABAs) have replaced the regular use of SABAs. Examples of LABAs are salmeterol and formoterol; both have duration of action of greater than 12 hours and are administered twice daily. Despite their longer action, LABAs should not be prescribed without including inhaled corticosteroids (ICSs). While an effective bronchodilator, neither SABAs nor LABAs treat the underlying airway inflammation associated with asthma. Ideally, combination therapy that includes ICS and LABAs allows a lower dose of corticosteroid and improves control. Fixed combination inhalers that contain a corticosteroid and an LABA have proved to be highly effective in the control of asthma (29, 30).

The most common adverse effects of beta-2 agonists when given via inhalation are muscle tremor and palpitations, which are seen more commonly in elderly patients. There is a small fall in plasma potassium due to increased uptake by skeletal muscle cells, but this effect does not usually cause a clinical problem. Tolerance to agonists may develop when used chronically. Mast cells are rapidly affected; however, this may be prevented by concomitant administration of ICSs (30).

Anticholinergics such as atropine inhibit the effects of acetylcholine released from the intrapulmonary motor nerves that run in the vagus and innervate airway smooth muscle. Adverse central nervous system effects limits their usefulness until the development of ipratropium bromide. A muscarinic receptor antagonist, ipratropium bromide prevents cholinergic nerve–induced bronchoconstriction and mucus secretion. The mechanism of action is inhibition of the cholinergic reflex component of bronchoconstriction. They are less effective and have a slower onset than beta-2 agonists and should be used only as an adjunct bronchodilator for asthma not controlled on other inhaled medications. There is little or no systemic absorption and the most common side effect is dry mouth; in elderly patients, urinary retention and glaucoma may also be observed (30).

The bronchodilator effect of theophylline is due to inhibition of phosphodiesterases in airway smooth muscle cells. Once widely used as an oral bronchodilator, inhaled beta-2 agonists have replaced their role in bronchodilation. Although theophylline is inexpensive, the beta-2 agonists are more effective and have fewer side effects. There is increasing evidence that theophylline at lower doses has anti-inflammatory effects and, used in low doses, is well tolerated.

Therapeutic plasma concentrations of 10 to 20 mg/L are required for severe asthma, although these concentrations are often associated with side effects and reserved for refractory situations. Low-dose therapeutic levels of theophylline (5 to 10 mg/L plasma concentration) have additive effects to ICSs. Oral theophylline administered as a slow-release preparation once or twice daily gives stable plasma concentrations. Abrupt withdrawal of theophylline may precipitate an acute asthma attack.

Oral theophylline is well absorbed and is largely inactivated in the liver. The most common side effects are related to plasma concentration greater than 10 mg/L and include nausea, vomiting, and headaches. Diuresis and palpitations may also occur, and at high concentrations cardiac arrhythmias, epileptic seizures, and death may occur due to adenosine receptor antagonism; measurement of plasma theophylline may be useful in determining the correct dose (30). Theophylline is metabolized by CYP450 in the liver, and thus plasma concentrations may be elevated by drugs that block CYP450, such as erythromycin and allopurinol. Other drugs may also reduce clearance by other mechanisms leading to increased plasma concentrations.

Intravenous aminophylline (a soluble salt of theophylline) has now been largely replaced by inhaled SABAs, which are more effective and have fewer side effects. Aminophylline is occasionally used (via slow intravenous infusion) in patients with severe exacerbations that are refractory to high-dose SABAs (30).

Systemic corticosteroids are effective for the treatment of moderate to severe persistent asthma and for exacerbations of mild asthma. Treatment usually consists of prednisone 40 to 60 mg/day tapered down to zero over 7 to 14 days. Intravenous methylprednisolone 125 mg every 6 hours may be used in extreme life-threatening situations. ICSs provide a therapeutic effect with fewer side effects than systemic steroids and have been clearly shown to be effective for the treatment of asthma. Numerous products are available and considered effective treatment. The major disadvantage is the potential for systemic effects including growth retardation in children, loss of bone mineralization, cataracts, and glaucoma. Oral thrush and hoarseness of voice (from myopathy of the laryngeal muscles) are common adverse effects that can be minimized by using aerosol spacers and good oropharyngeal hygiene.

An exacerbation of asthma may flare suddenly and lead to life-threatening situations. Typical presentation begins with increasing chest tightness, wheezing, and dyspnea that is not relieved with rescue inhalers. In severe cases the patient may be breathless and unable to complete a sentence or may be cyanotic. Signs of increased ventilation, hyperinflation, and tachycardia are typical, while pulsus paradoxus may be present. Spirometry measures are decreased and oxygen saturation is usually less than 90%. ABGs on room air show hypoxia due to airway constriction and hypocapnia due to hyperventilation. A normal or rising $PaCO_2$ is an indication of impending respiratory failure and requires immediate monitoring and therapy. A chest roentgenogram is not usually informative but may show pneumonia or pneumothorax (30).

Emergency treatment begins with a functional assessment of airway obstruction with a measurement of the FEV_1 or PEF initially to assess the patient's response to treatment. Assess arterial oxygen saturation and obtain a brief history including asthma symptoms, onset of exacerbation, medications, prior emergency department visits, and hospitalizations (including endotracheal intubations). Perform a physical examination of the overall patient status, including other diseases. Laboratory studies should be considered based on the status of the patient. These and other studies may include ABG measurement, CBC, serum theophylline level (if indicated), chest radiography to assess for complications, and ECG in patients older than 50 years (29).

Following the initial assessment, begin treatment by administering a high concentration of oxygen to achieve saturation of greater than 90%. High doses of inhaled SABAs are administered either with a nebulizer or metered dose inhaler. Initially, three treatments every 20 to 30 minutes are given. In extreme cases an inhaled anticholinergic may be added if there is not a satisfactory response to beta-2 agonists alone. Systemic corticosteroids should be given early if there is an incomplete response to beta-agonists. Corticosteroids speed the resolution of airway obstruction. Oral administration is equivalent in efficacy to intravenous administration.

Infusion of aminophylline may be effective, but it is important to monitor blood levels. Prophylactic intubation may be indicated for impending respiratory failure, when the $PaCO_2$ is normal or rises. Sedatives should never be given as they may depress ventilation.

Approximately 5% of asthmatics are difficult to control despite maximal inhaled therapy. It is important to identify triggers for the asthma and correct any that may be aggravating asthma. Noncompliance with medication is the most common cause of refractory asthma. ICSs do not provide an immediate benefit and patients may not recognize the therapeutic effects. A combination of LABA and ICS may enhance compliance. Other factors to consider are high levels of allergens and upper respiratory disease. Some patients may have chronic infection with *Mycoplasma pneumoniae* or *Chlamydophila pneumoniae* and benefit from treatment with a macrolide antibiotic (29). Some COX inhibitors, beta-adrenergic blockers, and aspirin may worsen asthma. A premenstrual worsening of asthma may occur and requires treatment with progesterone or gonadotropin-releasing factors. Gastroesophageal reflux may occur due to bronchodilator therapy; however, treatment for reflux does not improve the asthma. Excess or insufficient thyroid function may increase asthma and should be evaluated. Refractory asthma is difficult to control and requires a careful examination of correct use of inhalers, minimizing triggers, and frequently a maintenance dose of oral corticosteroids.

Clinical Nurse Specialist Competencies and Spheres of Influence
Clinical Expert/Direct Care, Coaching/Teaching/Mentoring, and Consultation

Management of patients with asthma begins with clinical expertise. CNSs must provide skillful physical examination and recognize signs of increasing distress, with implementation of appropriate treatment steps. Spirometry evaluation, chest radiography interpretation, and blood gas analysis for detection of impending respiratory failure are key aspects of expert care. Patient education materials and programs for self-management are commonly developed by CNSs. Consultation requests by frontline nurses in the acute care setting occurs when patients show increasing respiratory distress; CNSs are able to assess the patient and rally other team members in preparation for possible intubation, mechanical ventilator setup, and transfer to a higher level of care.

SLEEP APNEA

Etiology

Sleep apnea may be divided into the two broad categories of central sleep apnea (CSA) and obstructive sleep apnea (OSA). CSAs are respiratory pauses caused by lack of respiratory effort. Although these pauses may occur normally during rapid eye movement (REM) sleep or sleep onset, they are more frequently associated with cardiac failure or neurologic disease, especially stroke. Defects in the ventilatory drive may be related to hypercapnia or hypocapnia. Patients may present with symptoms of daytime sleepiness. OSA is a sleep disorder that involves cessation or significant decrease in airflow in the presence of breathing effort (42, 43). OSA occurs more frequently and is a major cause of morbidity and mortality throughout the world. OSA is the most common medical cause of daytime sleepiness and is defined as having five or more obstructed breathing events per hour of sleep. Apnea is defined as breathing pauses lasting 10 seconds or longer, while hypopnea is a 50% or more decrease in ventilation.

In severe OSA, sleep apnea may occur hundreds of times per night lasting 1 to 2 minutes each time. Recurrent sleep arousals, recurrent precipitous oxygen desaturation, and wide swings in heart rate occur in OSA. Electroencephalogram (EEG) arousals occur simultaneously with stertorous breathing sounds as a bolus of air is exhaled when the airway reopens (43).

OSA is strongly associated with many debilitating medical conditions, including hypertension, cardiovascular disease, coronary artery disease, insulin-resistance diabetes, depression, and sleepiness-related accidents. Irregular breathing during sleep occurs in approximately one-fourth of the middle-aged male population. However, for most patients, daytime sleepiness does not occur and these individuals are asymptomatic. OSA is an increasingly prevalent condition in both adults and children in modern society. Approximately 24% of men and 9% of women have OSA, with and without excessive daytime sleepiness (44). Predisposing factors are obesity, a short mandible, male gender, age 40 to 65 years, myotonic dystrophy, and smoking. Untreated OSA patients are typically heavy users of health care seeking help for the symptoms without treatment of the root problem.

The National Commission on Sleep Disorders Research has estimated that 7 to 18 million people in the United States have some degree of sleep disturbance and 1.8 to 4 million people with relatively severe cases (44). The prevalence increases with age. It is less common but also occurs in children; enlarged tonsils or adenoids is usually the cause. A 2007 study suggests that approximately 6% of adolescents have weekly sleep-related disordered breathing (45). According to the American Academy of Sleep Medicine (AASM), OSA is characterized by repetitive episodes of complete (apnea) or partial (hypopnea) upper airway obstruction occurring during sleep (46). The definition of apneic and hypopneic is an event lasting a minimum of 10 seconds. At least five apnea events must occur per hour of sleep time in association with clinical symptoms, or at least 15 apnea events must occur per hour of sleep time with or without clinical symptoms (43).

Pathophysiology

During sleep, pharyngeal muscles relax and the airway collapses on inspiration. Sleep apnea occurs not only due to these muscles relaxing but due to a narrow upper airway. While the patient is awake, the airway dilating muscles ensure airway patency; however, during sleep, striated muscles relax and the airway narrows. Transmural pressure is the difference between intraluminal pressure and the surrounding tissue pressure. As transmural pressure decreases, the cross-sectional area of the pharynx narrows and may progress to pharyngeal closure. As the airway partially occludes, snoring may occur. Progression of the occlusion results in apnea. Arousal returns the upper airway muscle tone and restores airway patency (42, 43).

Clinical Presentation

Three cardinal symptoms of OSA include snoring, sleepiness, and significant-other report of sleep apnea episodes (43). The patient's spouse or someone close to him or her should be included in taking a sleep history because the sleeper is often unaware of the symptoms. The patient may report that they have no problem sleeping and can doze off easily. Excessive daytime sleepiness (EDS) may account for motor vehicle accidents and other hazards and is one of the greatest potentially morbid consequences of sleep apnea. Patients with OSA do not perform as well as healthy control subjects during driving simulation tests, but their performance may return to normal after treatment. Moreover, the profound and repetitive hypoxia that occurs during apnea can affect end organ systems (43).

Dynamic factors of OSA include nasal and pharyngeal airway resistance. The typical physical presentation includes any anatomic feature that decreases the size of the pharynx. Retrognathia, a condition in which either or both jaws recede with respect to the frontal plane of the forehead, is recognized as a risk factor. This condition is known as Pierre Robin syndrome and may be treated with a mandibular-advancement device (43).

Obese individuals, particularly those with fat deposition in the neck, are most likely to have OSA. Neck circumference may correlate with OSA better than body mass index (BMI). Approximately 30% of patients with a BMI greater than 30 kg/m^2 have OSA, and 50% of patients with a BMI greater than 40 kg/m^2 have OSA. This is of particular concern in the United States as 20% of men and 25% of women have a BMI greater than 30 kg/m^2. Patients with obesity hypoventilation syndrome and some patients with OSA may have evidence of pulmonary hypertension and right-sided heart failure. Due to the volume of the soft tissue, including the tongue, lateral pharyngeal walls, soft palate, and parapharyngeal fat pads, the cross-sectional area of the airway is smaller than that of people without OSA (43, 47). Weight loss in patients with OSA decreases occurrence of apneic episodes. Position also affects OSA and, for most patients, worsens in the supine sleeping position.

Risk factors include race as African Americans appear to be more predisposed to sleep disorders than white persons (43). Gender shows a 3:1 prevalence rate in males compared to females. Interestingly, postmenopausal women are three times more likely to have moderate-to-severe OSA compared with premenopausal women (43). Women who were taking hormone replacement therapy were half as likely to have OSA compared with postmenopausal women who were not on hormone replacement therapy (48). Age is also a factor, and persons 65 and older are 2 to 3 times more likely to have OSA compared with individuals aged 30 to 64 years (43).

Patients with sleep disturbances have a 2- to 4-fold increased risk of nocturnal complex arrhythmia. Bradyarrhythmias occurs in approximately 10% of OSA patients, especially in the REM sleep state and when greater than 4% drop in oxygen saturation occurs. Additionally, atrioventricular block, asystole, and premature ventricular contractions are more common. People with OSA have double the prevalence of coronary artery disease. OSA apparently affects the timing of sudden cardiac death because research shows that greater than 50% of sudden cardiac deaths that occur in OSA patients do so between 10 PM and 6 AM; the more common time for sudden cardiac death is between 6 and 11 AM (49). The Sleep Heart Health Study showed the strongest relationship was between OSA and stroke versus any other cardiovascular disease (50).

Patients may present complaining of EDS, decreased memory and concentration, or decreased motor coordination. Impaired vigilance, decreased cognitive performance, depression, waking up tired, nocturnal choking, nocturia, decreased libido, and hypertension are all associated with OSA (44). These symptoms relate to sleep fragmentation and hypoxemia during apneic episodes. Treatment is not usually needed unless symptoms interfere with activities of daily living (42). Daytime sleepiness may range from mild to severe and may result in inability to work effectively. The chronic sleepiness is dangerous when driving, with a 3- to 6-fold risk in accidents on the road or when operating machinery.

Diagnosis

Diagnosis may be suspected but should be confirmed by a specialist. OSA is a condition requiring long-term treatment and the diagnosis needs to be accurate. A thorough sleep history from the patient and partner using a screening tool such as the Epworth Sleepiness Score (Figure 10-2) establishes a baseline. Physical examination must include assessment of obesity, jaw structure, the upper airway, blood pressure, and possible predisposing causes, including hypothyroidism and acromegaly. Valuable information may be obtained from partners including a history of loud snoring punctuated by the silence of apneas. Researchers have found support for the notion of a sleep-related disordered breathing (SRDB) continuum (50). The SRDB continuum illustrates that snoring is the initial presenting symptom, and it increases in severity over time. Comorbid medical disorders, such as obesity, exacerbate the disorder. As the disease progresses SRBD patients begin to develop increased upper airway resistance that results in sleepiness. Sleepiness is caused by increased arousals from sleep.

Routine laboratory tests usually are not helpful in obstructive sleep apnea except to rule out or identify comorbid conditions. A thyrotropin hormone level should be considered, especially in the elderly population. An ABG analysis should be obtained if hypoventilation is suspected. Imaging studies may be used to identify sites of upper airway obstruction, although their usefulness is not confirmed.

Numerous conditions may present with symptoms similar to OSA and should be considered as a differential diagnosis. A careful history may indicate many possibilities such as insufficient sleep. Shift work, rotating shifts, or night shift work can cause chronic sleepiness; this is especially apparent in age 40 and older. Depression is a

Epworth Sleepiness Scale

Name: _____ Today's date: _____

Your age (Yrs): _____ Your sex (Male = M, Female = F): _____

How likely are you to doze off or fall asleep in the following situations, in contrast to feeling just tired?

This refers to your usual way of life in recent times.

Even if you haven't done some of these things recently try to work out how they would have affected you.

Use the following scale to choose the **most appropriate number** for each situation:

> 0 = would **never** doze
> 1 = **slight chance** of dozing
> 2 = **moderate chance** of dozing
> 3 = **high chance** to dozing

It is important that you answer each question as best you can.

Situation   **Chance of Dozing (0–3)**

Sitting and reading _____ _____

Watching TV _____ _____

Sitting, inactive in a public place (e.g., a theater or a meeting) _____ _____

As a passenger in a car for an hour without a break _____ _____

Lying down in the afternoon when circumstances permit _____ _____

Sitting and talking to someone _____ _____

Sitting quietly after lunch without alcohol _____ _____

In a car, while stopped for a few minutes in the traffic _____ _____

THANK YOU FOR YOUR COOPERATION

© M.W. Johns 1990–97, reproduced with permission.
Scale may be accessed here: www.epworthsleepinessscale.com

FIGURE 10–2: Obstructive sleep apnea.

major cause of sleepiness. Drugs or alcohol can disrupt the sleep cycle and produce sleepiness. Other less common conditions include narcolepsy, idiopathic hypersomnolence, and phase alteration syndromes (42).

Following referral to a specialist, diagnostic sleep study tests will be conducted. A full polysomnographic examination with recording of multiple respiratory and neurophysiologic signals during sleep may be conducted, and a positive test must demonstrate recurrent breathing pauses during sleep. A polysomnogram is a multichannel recording of sleep and breathing conducted in a controlled laboratory setting. Electroencephalogram (EEG) arousals, eye movements, chin movements, airflow,

respiratory effort, pulse oximetry, ECG tracings, body position, snoring, and leg movements are monitored and recorded by a qualified technician. The area on a polysomnogram showing no chest movement indicates a lack of ventilation. Arousals are important in determining the fragmentation of sleep. Several key findings are characteristic of OSA including (a) apneic episodes in the presence of respiratory muscle effort lasting 10 seconds or longer, (b) apneic episodes lasting approximately 20 to 40 seconds, (c) apneic episodes most prevalent during REM sleep, (d) apnea or hypopnea or a combination of both, or (e) sleep disruption due to arousals at the termination of an episode of apnea (43).

A full sleep study may not be practical for all patients from a cost perspective. Limited studies that record respiratory and oxygenation patterns overnight without neurophysiologic recording also produce accurate results when conducted by experienced specialists. The use of limited studies as a first line diagnostic test is cost-effective and accurate and allows for treatment to begin quickly. If a limited study does not prove positive in situations that sleepiness is problematic, a full polysomnographic study should be requested to confirm or exclude OSA (42).

Management

The most commonly used treatment is continuous positive airway pressure (CPAP). Administered via a form fitted mask the therapy works by blowing air into the airway and maintaining opening airway pressures of 5 to 20 cm. The use of CPAP has been shown to be effective and improves breathing and sleep quality.

CPAP may be effective in some patients if OSA causes pharyngeal collapse, which then initiates reflex inhibition of respiration. Nasal CPAP is currently the treatment of choice for patients with OSA and upper airway resistance syndrome and all patients should be offered nasal CPAP therapy first. CPAP acts as a pneumatic splint to maintain upper airway patency during sleep by applying continuous positive pressure to the upper airway with a nasal mask, nasal pillows, or oronasal mask. The CPAP device consists of a blower unit that produces positive-pressure airflow applied at the nose. CPAP increases the caliber of the airway in the retropalatal and retroglossal regions and it increases the lateral dimensions of the upper airway and thins the lateral pharyngeal walls, which are thicker in patients with OSA (43). CPAP effectively relieves most symptoms of EDS and improves neuropsychiatric functioning. It also improves heart function and hypertension (43).

Compliance with the use of CPAP may be poor. Initiating the therapy requires patient education and support as the client learns to use the therapy. Multiple masks are available from several different manufacturers and the client should be assisted to find one that fits well. A short daytime trial should be conducted prior to overnight use. This is followed by an overnight monitored trial of CPAP and to establish the pressure required for maintaining the patient's patent airway. Pressure- and airflow-related complications include a sensation of suffocation or claustrophobia, difficulty exhaling, inability to sleep, musculoskeletal chest discomfort, aerophagia, and sinus discomfort. Rare cases of pneumothorax or tympanic membrane rupture have been reported. Mask-related problems include skin abrasions, rash, and conjunctivitis (due to air leaks). The drying nature of the forced air may cause rhinorrhea, nasal congestion, epistaxis, and nasal and/or oral dryness, which can be countered using a heated humidifier. Noise from the blower unit may be troublesome to the patient or their spouse (42, 43). Another option is BiPAP therapy, which permits independent adjustment of the pressures delivered during inspiration and expiration. In a given patient, BiPAP allows the expiratory positive airway pressure level that must be applied to maintain upper airway patency to be lower than the corresponding CPAP level required for maintaining airway patency (42, 43). BiPAP may be better tolerated; however, it is too expensive to be used as first line therapy.

The treatment plan for OSA should include providing client education on the condition and possible factors that aggravate the condition. Inclusion of the partner as well as the client promotes positive lifestyle changes. Weight loss, reduction of alcohol consumption, and withdrawal from sedative medications that reduce airway tone should be incorporated into the management plan. Currently, no pharmacologic interventions are found effective in reducing OSA. Oral appliances, such as the mandibular repositioning splint, have been effective in reducing apneic breathing during sleep, daytime somnolence, and blood pressure. Long-term compliance has been identified as a barrier to the use of oral devices (42, 43). Oral appliances enlarge the upper airway by pulling the tongue forward and thinning the lateral pharyngeal walls by exerting traction. According to the American Sleep Disorders Association guidelines, the major role for oral appliance therapy appears to be the treatment of patients with mild-to-moderate OSA who cannot tolerate CPAP (and BiPAP) therapy (46). These devices are relatively unlikely to benefit patients with severe OSA.

Surgery may be indicated if noninvasive medical therapy fails or is rejected or if the patient desires such therapy. Uvulopalatopharyngoplasty is the most common surgical procedure performed for adults with OSA. Uvulopalatopharyngoplasty involves removal of the tonsils (if present), the uvula, the distal margin of the soft palate, and the redundant pharyngeal tissue, as well as reshaping of the soft tissues in the lateral pharyngeal walls. The surgical success rate is approximately 50% (43). If the patient has OSA that is moderately severe or severe, the patient requires perioperative airway protection with either nasal CPAP or a tracheostomy (43). Tonsillectomy may be effective for children with OSA but rarely affects adults (42). If the condition is linked to morbid obesity, bariatric surgery may correct the problem. Maxillomandibular osteotomy may be indicated for jaw advancement. The midface, palate, and mandible are moved forward in this procedure, increasing the space behind the tongue and increasing tension on the genioglossus muscle. This surgery is more extensive than any of the others described and usually reserved for patients in whom other treatment modalities fail. In extreme cases of obstruction, tracheostomy may be considered; however, comorbid factors must be considered (42, 43).

OSA is associated with an increased risk of upper airway obstruction following an anesthetic or sedation. Patients should be screened for sleep history by the anesthesia provider and precautions taken to prevent an adverse event. Patients with OSA may be more difficult to intubate. It is also noteworthy that a history of difficult intubation may be linked to irregular breathing during sleep.

A major concern of sleep apnea, particularly OSA, is the increased risk of cardiovascular and cerebrovascular events. OSA raises 24-hour mean blood pressure between 4 and 10 mm Hg in patients with recurrent nocturnal hypoxemia. Blood pressure rises with each episode of apnea or hypopnea and also from the associated 24-hour increase in sympathetic tone. Epidemiologic studies show that the rise in blood pressure correlates with a 20% increase in myocardial infarction and 40% increase in stroke. Although observational studies suggest an increase in the risk of myocardial infarction and stroke in untreated OSA, they do not prove an increased vascular risk in normal subjects (42, 43). Additional research in this area is needed to conclusively determine a causal relationship.

OSA is associated with a higher risk of diabetes mellitus. Although obesity is a risk factor for both diabetes and OSA, it does not appear to be the mechanism. Trials suggest that OSA can aggravate diabetes and that increased apneas and hypopneas during sleep are associated with insulin resistance independent of obesity. In addition, uncontrolled trials suggest that OSA can aggravate diabetes and that treatment of OSA in patients who also have diabetes decreases their insulin requirements (44).

Clinical Nurse Specialist Competencies and Spheres of Influence
Coaching/Teaching/Mentoring
Patient education is a major part of the treatment plan for patients with OSA. Because obesity is a predictor, weight reduction reduces the risk of OSA. It is estimated that a 10% reduction in weight leads to a 26% reduction in risk. Weight reduction may lower blood pressure, improve pulmonary function, and improve sleep while decreasing snoring. Sleeping in supine position correlates with increased snoring and OSA (43). For mild disease, a simple device such as sewing a tennis ball to the back of pajamas may discourage the supine position. Patients with marked obesity may benefit from sleeping in an upright position. Additionally, a specially designed pillow is available, which maintains the patient's head and neck position during sleep to optimize upper airway patency.

Patients should be taught to avoid smoking, drinking alcoholic beverages, or taking sedatives as all of these are known to increase OSA. The CNS provides resources and referrals to assist the patient in tobacco cessation. Evaluation and a clear plan that includes pharmacologic interventions, psychosocial support, and education on the benefits of smoking cessation are important.

Clinical Expert/Direct Care and Systems Leadership
Initiating therapy with CPAP is most effective if close contact with the patient is maintained, problems identified, and solutions offered. Many patients with OSA report an immediate improvement in alertness, concentration, and memory, but achieving maximum improvement in neurocognitive symptoms may take as long as 2 months. Follow-up is necessary to ensure compliance and equipment maintenance. Proper mask fitting that prevents excessive leaks is an important consideration. Nasal congestion can be treated with antihistamines and/or topical corticosteroids. Topical saline sprays or heated humidification may alleviate nasal dryness or complaints of the air generated by the unit being too cold.

Because many people are not aware they have OSA, dangerous situations can arise when they are hospitalized for an unrelated illness, injury, or surgical procedure. For example, general anesthesia and opiates for pain management can act synergistically with OSA causing respiratory depression and even lead to respiratory arrest, a source of medical malpractice litigation. CNSs may be instrumental in the development or implementation of risk analysis tools for detection of OSA in undiagnosed individuals. One example from the literature is the STOP-BANG questionnaire (51). The instrument has undergone testing in patients undergoing surgery for cancer during the preoperative evaluation. The acronym stands for **S**noring, **T**iredness during daytime, **O**bserved apnea, high blood **P**ressure, **B**ody mass index, **A**ge, **N**eck circumference, and **G**ender. Researchers have seen promising results with the tool in identifying individuals at higher risk for surgical and anesthesia related complications through detection of occult OSA (51). Implementation of algorithms or practice guidelines that include precautions for patients who test positive for OSA can be life-saving.

PULMONARY HYPERTENSION

Etiology
Pulmonary hypertension is an abnormal elevation in pulmonary artery pressure. This may be the result of left heart failure, pulmonary parenchymal or vascular disease, thromboembolism, or a combination of these factors (52). Normally the pulmonary circulation has low-resistance with normal mean pressures of 10 to 12 mm Hg. Generally, pulmonary hypertension is defined as a mean pulmonary arterial pressure greater than 25 mm Hg at rest or greater than 30 mm Hg during exercise. Typically a progressive and sustained increase in pulmonary vascular resistance eventually leads to RV failure. Pulmonary hypertension is a life-threatening condition if untreated, and therapy is

targeted at the underlying cause and its effects on the cardiovascular system. Pulmonary hypertension was previously classified as primary or secondary pulmonary hypertension (52-54). The WHO proposed one clinical classification of pulmonary hypertension based on similarities in pathophysiology, clinical presentation, and therapeutic options (55).

Primary pulmonary hypertension (PPH) occurs with no apparent cause and is rare. PPH is also termed precapillary pulmonary hypertension or, more recently, idiopathic pulmonary arterial hypertension. The diagnosis is usually made after excluding other known causes of pulmonary hypertension. PPH is responsible for approximately 125 to 150 deaths per year and has an incidence of approximately 1 to 3 cases per 1 million per year. There is no cure for PPH, and left untreated, it leads to right-sided heart failure and death (53). PPH occurs in all races, with a higher occurrence rate in females. Young women and women in their 50s and 60s are more often affected.

Secondary pulmonary hypertension (SPH) may be caused by cardiac or pulmonary disorders, or a combination of both. Cardiac diseases produce pulmonary hypertension via volume or pressure overload. Damage to the pulmonary vessels may also lead to obstruction and vascular resistance. Pulmonary vasoconstriction and perivascular parenchymal changes lead to pulmonary hypertension. Pulmonary hypertension is often seen in patients with severe COPD; an estimated 30,000 persons with COPD die annually of right heart failure secondary to pulmonary hypertension. Cor pulmonale is a term used to indicate RV enlargement secondary to any underlying cardiac or pulmonary disease. Pulmonary hypertension is the most common cause of cor pulmonale and is associated with the development of RV failure (52).

Other contributing factors include interstitial lung disease, cystic fibrosis, sleep apnea syndrome, and pulmonary embolism. A significant number of patients with systemic sclerosis (scleroderma), mixed connective tissue disease, and systemic lupus erythematosus develop SPH. A genetic predisposition is believed to be a factor especially when combined with known risks. Familial pulmonary arterial hypertension is a mutation in the *BMPR2* gene with an autosomal-dominant disease affecting only about 10% to 20% of carriers (56). Although most cases are sporadic, there is a 6% to 12% familial incidence. Fenfluramine and dexfenfluramine have both been identified as potential causative risk factors and relate to the amount and length of exposure. Some diseases may be risk factors for SPH. HIV, portal hypertension and other liver disease, congenital systemic-pulmonary cardiac shunts, and possibly thyroid disorders have all been linked to pulmonary hypertension (52-56). The most common causes of pulmonary hypertension worldwide are sickle cell disease and HIV infection (56).

The U.S. Centers for Disease Control and Prevention Pulmonary Hypertension Surveillance from 1980 to 2002 shows an increase from 5.2 deaths to 5.4 deaths per 100,000 population. Disproportional death rates were identified for women (3.3 deaths to 5.5 deaths per 100,000 population) and blacks (4.6 deaths to 7.3 deaths per 100,000 population) (53).

Pathophysiology

Environmental risks, particularly in susceptible individuals, interact and result in endothelial dysfunction and overproduction of vasoconstrictors, such as thromboxane and endothelin (57, 58). Vasodilators are decreased and vascular growth factors are released that cause changes in the vascular smooth wall called remodeling. Angiotensin II, serotonin, electrolyte transporter mechanisms, and nitric oxide also contribute to the pathogenesis of the disease (58). Pathologic changes result in fibrosis and thickening of the vessel wall. This leads to luminal narrowing and abnormal vasoconstriction. As a result, resistance to pulmonary artery blood flow increases and pulmonary artery pressure rises. The ability of the RV to adapt to increased vascular resistance is influenced by several factors, including age and the rapidity of the development of pulmonary hypertension. Initially the excessive workload on the RV causes RV hypertrophy. As oxygen demand of the hypertrophied muscle increases, RV coronary blood flow decreases, and the RV myocardium becomes ischemic. Coexisting hypoxemia can impair the ability of the ventricle to compensate. The onset of clinical RV failure is usually manifested by peripheral edema. Cor pulmonale follows with eventual death (56, 57, 59).

Clinical Presentation

Pulmonary hypertension is insidious, with the average time from onset to diagnosis approximately 2 years (53). Early symptoms are nonspecific; common symptoms are dyspnea (60%), weakness (19%), and recurrent syncope (13%) (53, 54). Less common symptoms include cough, hemoptysis, or hoarseness (due to compression of the recurrent laryngeal nerve by the distended pulmonary artery [Ortner's syndrome]. Exertional angina is a common symptom occurring in approximately 8.5% of patients secondary to mitral stenosis. This most likely occurs because of the pulmonary artery distention, RV ischemia, or both in combination (53, 54).

Physical examination may reveal a systolic ejection murmur over the left sternal border and an RV heave may be palpated. The pulmonic component of the second heart sound is usually increased, which may demonstrate fixed or paradoxical splitting in the presence of severe RV dysfunction. The physical examination typically reveals increased jugular venous pressure and a reduced carotid pulse. Jugular venous pulsations may be elevated in the presence of volume overload, RV failure, or both. A right-sided fourth heart sound (S_4) with a left parasternal heave may be heard. RV failure leads to systemic venous hypertension and cor pulmonale. A high-pitched systolic murmur of tricuspid regurgitation, hepatomegaly, a pulsatile liver, ascites, and peripheral edema may occur in right heart failure. In this scenario, a RV third heart (S_3) sound is also heard. Lung examination is usually normal. Peripheral cyanosis and/or edema tends to occur in later stages of the disease (52-54).

Severity of the disease is categorized by four classes. Class I are patients who tolerate ordinary physical activity without dyspnea or fatigue. Class II patients are comfortable at rest but experience dyspnea or fatigue, chest pain, or near syncope with ordinary physical activity. Class III patients have marked limitations in physical activity but are comfortable at rest. Class IV patients are unable to perform any physical activity without symptoms and show signs of right-sided heart failure. Dyspnea and/or fatigue may even be present at rest (54).

Diagnosis

Pulmonary hypertension requires an extensive work-up for diagnosis. The evaluation should begin with chest radiography. Typically the images will show enlargement of central pulmonary arteries, attenuation of peripheral vessels, and oligemic lung fields (poorly vascularized lungs). It may also show RV and right atrial dilation. Chest radiography is useful for excluding interstitial and alveolar processes that may cause hypoxia-mediated pulmonary vasoconstriction (53). If the lungs show interstitial markings, consider parenchymal lung disease or veno-occlusive disease. If the lung fields are clear, pulmonary function tests should be completed. This may differentiate the potential diagnosis. If obstructive lung disease is apparent, COPD is most likely the cause. If a restrictive pattern is determined, it is likely to be interstitial lung disease or pulmonary hypertension (52-55).

An ABG should be performed to assess for hypoxemia. Screenings for collagen-vascular disease includes measuring the erythrocyte sedimentation rate, rheumatoid factor levels, and antinuclear antibody levels. Approximately 40% of patients with pulmonary hypertension have a positive ANA. Patients with thyroid disease and HIV infection typically have a higher incidence of pulmonary hypertension; screening should include testing for thyrotropin and HIV status (52, 53). Liver function test results may indicate liver disease associated with portal hypertension. A CBC, biochemistry panel, prothrombin time, and activated partial thromboplastin time should be performed to establish a baseline (54).

Two-dimensional echocardiography is useful to identify signs of chronic RV pressure overload. Positive findings may include increased thickness of the RV with paradoxical bulging of the septum into the LV during systole. Right atrial dilatation and tricuspid regurgitation,

and in late stages, RV dilatation leading to RV hypokinesis may be seen. Doppler echocardiography is also a reliable noninvasive method to estimate pulmonary arterial pressure. Tricuspid regurgitation is identifiable with Doppler studies and generally detected in more than 90% of patients with severe pulmonary hypertension. Right-sided heart catheterization is indicated if Doppler echocardiography cannot obtain a precise measurement of pulmonary hypertension (52-54).

ECG may show signs of RV hypertrophy and include right-axis deviation, an R-to-S wave ratio greater than 1 mm in lead V_1, increased P-wave amplitude, and an incomplete or complete right bundle-branch block pattern. High-resolution chest CT scanning and ventilation-perfusion lung scanning are frequently obtained to help exclude interstitial lung disease and thromboembolic disease (53, 55).

Management

The treatment of pulmonary hypertension is primarily directed at the underlying disease. Effective therapy should be instituted in the early stages, before irreversible changes in pulmonary vasculature occur. Anticoagulation therapy may increase survival rates. Current evidence suggests that in patients with pulmonary hypertension, abnormalities of blood coagulation factors contribute to a prothrombotic state. Coumadin titrated to achieve an international normalized ratio of 1.5 to 2 times the control value is recommended (53). Chronic hypoxemia and acidosis may also increase coagulation. Oxygen supplementation may improve pulmonary function and quality of life. Medicare indications for continuous long-term oxygen therapy are shown in Table 10-15.

Digoxin may be prescribed to improve RV function and diuretics to manage peripheral edema. Digoxin is a cardiac glycoside with direct inotropic effects and indirect effects on the cardiovascular system. Its primary action is

TABLE 10–15 Medicare Indications for Continuous Long-term Oxygen Therapy

Arterial Pao$_2$ of ≤55 mm Hg or an arterial oxygen saturation (Sao$_2$) of ≤88%	Pao$_2$ of 56–59 mm Hg or an Sao$_2$ of 89%, in the presence of evidence of cor pulmonale, right-sided heart failure, or erythrocytosis (hematocrit >55%)

Adapted from McCance K, Huether S. Pathophysiology: The Biologic Basis for Disease in Adults and Children. 6th edition. St Louis, MO: Elsevier Mosby; 2010, Table 33-4 Characteristics of Lung Cancers.

to increase myocardial systolic contractions. Digoxin has been shown to be beneficial for some patients with supraventricular tachycardia–associated LV dysfunction; however, verapamil is generally better for controlling the heart rate (53).

Calcium channel blockers (CCBs) may improve functional status, but they should only be prescribed to patients without overt evidence of right-sided heart failure. A cardiac index of less than 2 L/min/m² or elevated right atrial pressure above 15 mm Hg is evidence that CCBs may worsen RV failure and, thus, are of no benefit (53). CCBs produce vasodilation by inhibiting calcium ions from entering slow channels and voltage-sensitive areas of vascular smooth muscle and the myocardium. Side effects of CCBs include systemic hypotension and lower limb edema (52, 54).

The nonselective endothelin receptor antagonist bosentan has been shown to improve symptoms and exercise tolerance. Therapy is initiated at 62.5 mg twice daily for the first month and then increased to 125 mg twice daily thereafter. Liver function should be monitored monthly due to the high frequency of abnormal hepatic function tests associated with the drug. Bosentan is contraindicated in patients who are on cyclosporine or glyburide concurrently (52).

Sildenafil, a phosphodiesterase-5 inhibitor, improves symptoms and exercise tolerance. Phosphodiesterase-5 is responsible for the hydrolysis of cyclic GMP in pulmonary vascular smooth muscle, the mediator through which nitric oxide lowers pulmonary artery pressure and inhibits pulmonary vascular growth (52). The recommended dose is 20 mg three times daily; the most common side effect is headache. Sildenafil should not be given to patients who are taking nitrate compounds (52).

Clinical trials for intravenous epoprostenol have demonstrated an improvement in symptoms, exercise tolerance, and survival for patients with pulmonary hypertension. Side effects include flushing, jaw pain, and diarrhea, which are generally tolerated by most patients. Treprostinil, an analogue of epoprostenol, has a longer half-life (4 hours), is stable at room temperature, and may be given intravenously or subcutaneously through a small infusion pump. Side effects are similar to those seen with epoprostenol.

Surgical intervention may be indicated for repair of an atrial septal defect, mitral stenosis, or chronic pulmonary thromboembolic disease. Lung transplantation may be indicated in some patients; however, long-term benefits of lung transplantation are only 50% survival at 5 years. Pulmonary endarterectomy has proven to be effective for chronic pulmonary hypertension from thromboembolism. An inferior vena caval filter should be placed to prevent recurrence; the patient must then receive life-long anticoagulants (54).

Clinical Nurse Specialist Competencies and Spheres of Influence
Ethical Decision-Making/Moral Agency/Advocacy and Coaching/Teaching/Mentoring

The prognosis at time of diagnosis for patients with pulmonary hypertension is variable and depends on underlying causes. Patients with severe pulmonary hypertension or right-sided heart failure survive approximately 1 year. Patients with moderate elevations in pulmonary artery pressure (mean pressure less than 55 mm Hg) and preserved right-sided heart function have a median survival of 3 years from diagnosis (53, 54). The patient should undergo frequent evaluation for right heart failure symptoms and adverse effects of medications. The CNS can be an advocate for the patient by providing education and seeking ways to improve the patient's quality of life. Patient education should include instruction on how to administer daily medications, ways to conserve strength, and how to access educational materials and support groups. Palliative care and end-of-life issues should be addressed with sensitivity to the trajectory of the illness and patient/family circumstances; the CNS is often pivotal in initiating this discussion.

LUNG CANCER

Etiology

In 2007, primary carcinoma of the lung affected 114,760 males and 98,620 females in the United States; 86% die within 5 years of diagnosis, making it the leading cause of cancer death in both men and women (60, 61). In the United States, lung cancer death rates are higher than breast cancer, colon cancer, and prostate cancer combined. Lung cancer remains the most common malignancy in the world. An estimated 12% of the global cancer burden is lung cancer and approximately 1.5 million new cases of lung cancer were diagnosed in 2007. Due to advances in combined-modality treatment with surgery, radiotherapy, and chemotherapy, the overall survival rates for lung cancer have increased significantly. Despite improved treatment options, the number of lung cancer deaths is projected to rise. The International Agency for Research on Cancer estimates that the number will continue to rise from 1.18 million deaths in 2007 to 10 million deaths per year by 2030 (60). Primary carcinoma of the lung is a major health problem worldwide.

Most lung cancers are directly linked to inhaled carcinogens of cigarette smoke. The prevalence of smoking in the United States is 28% for males and 25% for females, age 18 years or older; 38% of high school seniors smoke (60, 61). Smokers are 13 times more likely to develop lung cancer than nonsmokers. Long-term passive smoke exposure increases the risk of lung cancer 1.5 times. Although the incidence of lung cancer in males is decreasing, it is stable or increasing in females. This is attributed to an increase in tobacco smoking by women, while there is a decrease in smoking by men compared to 40 years ago. Eighty-five percent of patients with lung cancer are current or former cigarette smokers. About 15% of lung cancers occur in individuals who have never smoked, and most of these are women. Although research has not supported a specific cause, hormones are believed to be a factor. As many as 25% of the lung cancers in persons who do not smoke are believed to be caused by secondhand smoke (62).

A genetic predisposition may contribute to the development of cancer when exposed to carcinogens. Twenty documented lung carcinogens have been identified in cigarette smoke (63). The carcinogens cause the susceptible bronchial cells to develop multiple genetic abnormalities and are responsible for causing 80% to 90% of lung cancers (63, 64). Abnormalities include deletions of chromosomes, activation of oncogenes, and inactivation of tumor-suppressor genes (64). Damage may also occur due to toxic oxygen radicals induced by the smoke. Mutations in the tumor-suppressor gene *p53* have been found in 45% to 55% of non–small cell lung cancers and 75% to 100% of small cell cancers (60, 61). Environmental exposures to air pollution or occupational toxins can also cause genetic mutation, although their role is minor compared to cigarette smoke.

Radiation is also known to be a cause of lung cancer. Radon is a radioactive gas released from the normal decay of uranium in rocks and soil. It is an invisible, odorless, tasteless gas that seeps up through the ground. The gas diffuses into the outdoor air without building enough concentration to cause damage. However, radon can build up sufficient quantity in homes or underground mines to be carcinogenic. In a few areas, depending on local geology, radon dissolves into ground water and can be released into the air when the water is used. Radon decays quickly, giving off tiny radioactive particles that when inhaled can damage the cells that line the lung. Long-term exposure to radon can lead to lung cancer.

Asbestos has been identified as a carcinogen associated with lung cancer, malignant pleural mesothelioma, and pulmonary fibrosis. Asbestos exposure increases the risk of developing lung cancer by as much as five times, particularly the silicate type of asbestos fiber. Asbestos exposure combined with tobacco smoke increases the risk of developing lung cancer 80 to 90 times (60).

Pathophysiology

Tumors arising from the bronchi, bronchioles, and alveoli of the respiratory epithelium are all included in the term *lung cancer* and frequently referred to as bronchogenic. Other pulmonary tumors, sarcomas, lymphomas, blastomas, hematomas, and mesotheliomas, are not included. Lung cancer is divided into two categories: small cell

lung cancer (SCLC) and non–small cell lung cancer (NSCLC). Primary lung neoplasms are predominately from four major cell types and non–small cell cancer comprises 85% to 88% of all lung cancers (60). NSCLC is divided further into adenocarcinoma, squamous cell carcinoma, and large cell carcinoma histologies (61). All of the histologies share similar treatment approaches and prognoses but have distinct histologic and clinical characteristics. Small cell (also called oat cell) carcinoma occurrence rate has declined in the past 25 years; however, adenocarcinoma rates have increased and have the highest incidence. The various cell types have different natural histories, require different therapy, and respond differently to therapy; thus a correct histologic diagnosis by an experienced pathologist is the first step to correct treatment.

Squamous cell carcinoma is usually located in the central bronchi near the hilus and accounts for 30% of bronchogenic cancers (60). The tumors are usually localized and do not metastasize until late in the disease. Surgical resection is the most successful treatment; however, if metastasis is evident, the prognosis is poor. Chemotherapy has limited effectiveness; adjuvant treatment with newer agents may improve survival and quality of life.

Adenocarcinoma is a tumor arising from glands of the lung and constitutes 35% to 40% of all bronchogenic carcinomas. Usually smaller than 4 cm, adenocarcinoma occurs in the peripheral regions of the pulmonary parenchyma. Generally they do not cause symptoms until late in the disease when they may cause a pleuritic chest pain or shortness of breath. Early-stage diagnosis is usually found on a routine chest roentgenogram. Bronchioloalveolar cell carcinoma is a type of adenocarcinoma that usually occurs in the terminal bronchioles and alveoli. Although it is slow growing, metastasis occurs through the pulmonary arterial system and mediastinal lymph nodes. This cell type is not usually linked to smoking (60).

The carcinoma with the strongest link to smoking is the small cell carcinoma. These tumors grow fast, metastasize early, and have the worst prognosis of the lung carcinomas. Survival time for untreated small cell carcinoma is 1 to 3 months; with treatment, however, approximately 10% of individuals are alive at 2 years (65). Small cell carcinoma is associated with ectopic hormone production; this may be production of hormones by tumors of nonendocrine origin or production of an inappropriate hormone by an endocrine gland. Paraneoplastic syndromes are often the first clue to the diagnosis. The most common paraneoplastic syndrome associated with SCLC is the syndrome of inappropriate antidiuretic hormone secretion, which occurs in up to 40% of individuals. Gastrin-releasing peptide, calcitonin, arginine vasopressin, and adrenocorticotropic hormone (ACTH) may also be produced. ACTH production may lead to Cushing syndrome. Signs and symptoms related to this condition include muscular weakness, facial edema, hypokalemia, alkalosis, hyperglycemia, hypertension, and increased pigmentation. Paraneoplastic syndromes are treated primarily with chemotherapy and radiation therapy, resulting in temporary remission (60).

Clinical Presentation

Presentation is most likely due to tumor pressure on surrounding areas or paraneoplastic syndromes. Central tumors are generally squamous cell carcinomas and produce symptoms of a nonproductive cough or hemoptysis, dyspnea, atelectasis, postobstructive pneumonia, wheezing, and hemoptysis. Peripheral tumors are adenocarcinomas and also cause cough and dyspnea; however, the patient may present with symptoms of pleural effusion and severe pain as a result of infiltration of parietal pleura and the chest wall (60). Due to their location, peripheral tumors may first be identified when extrathoracic metastases occurs. These symptoms can include superior vena caval obstruction, hoarseness caused by paralysis of the recurrent laryngeal nerve, and phrenic nerve palsy resulting in paralysis of the diaphragm. Pressure on the esophagus may cause dysphagia, or the tumor could cause a pericardial effusion. Horner syndrome occurs rarely from pressure on the sympathetic plexus, and the patient may present with ptosis, miosis, exophthalmos, and anhidrosis on the affected side. Another paraneoplastic syndrome that is associated with squamous cell carcinomas is hypercalcemia due to parathyroid like hormone production.

Physical examination may reveal enlarged supraclavicular lymph nodes. Facial edema or dusky skin coloration may be a sign of superior vena caval syndrome. Prominent veins on the upper thoracic wall may also be a sign of vena caval syndrome. Respiratory findings vary depending on the location and spread of the tumor. Pleural effusions cause dull and decreased breath sounds. Individual lobes of the lungs may be dull to percussion or have absent breath sounds due to collapse. Cardiac findings are usually due to effusion or tamponade. Liver palpation may reveal tenderness and hepatomegaly; the liver is the most common site of metastasis. The bone is another common site and the patient may complain of bone pain. Percussion of the vertebral column may identify tender spots of possible metastasis. A neurologic exam should be completed to identify deficits caused by brain metastasis or signs of spinal cord compression (60).

Diagnosis

For most lung cancers, diagnosis is suspected based on a history of smoking and a persistent respiratory illness. The initial work-up should begin with a chest radiograph that may reveal an obvious mass, widening of the mediastinum (suggestive of spread to lymph nodes in the thorax), atelectasis (collapse), consolidation (pneumonia), or pleural effusion. If a mass is identified, histology is necessary to confirm the diagnosis. Initially sputum cytology,

bronchoscopy, or guided transthoracic needle biopsy of the mass should be done. Sputum cytology may identify malignant cells from the tumor; it is inexpensive and noninvasive and previously considered the best initial test, especially if squamous cell carcinoma is suspected. However, sputum cytology has a 40% false-negative rate and cannot be used for dependable subtyping. Newer imaging technology allows an accurate needle biopsy and is used more often than sputum cytology.

Correct staging is critical because treatment is directly related to disease stage. The staging of all NSCLCs follows the tumor/node/metastasis (TNM) system used universally for solid tumors. Each of the three criteria is separately listed and paired with a number to indicate the TNM stage. For example, a T1 N2 M0 cancer would be a cancer with one relatively small sized tumor, involvement of some lymph nodes, and no metastases. Table 10-16 defines basic parameters for staging (66, 67).

A CT scan of the chest and upper abdomen including the liver and adrenal glands should be obtained. The liver and adrenals are included since they are common sites for metastasis of non–small cell cancer. If neurologic symptoms are present, a CT scan or magnetic resonance imaging (MRI) of the brain should be considered. MRI is most useful for detection of central nervous system metastasis.

Laboratory tests should include a CBC, electrolytes, and renal function studies. Electrolytes are especially important since paraneoplastic syndromes may alter normal values. Bone is another common site for metastasis, and if the patient complains of bone pain or has an elevated serum calcium and/or alkaline phosphatase level, bone scintigraphy should be obtained.

Positron emission tomography (PET) scans are useful for searching for systemic spread if other diagnostic tests are not conclusive. PET scans appear to be more sensitive and accurate than CT scans for staging mediastinal disease. Recent reports suggest that staging of NSCLC may be influenced by PET scan results in 60% of cases; in approximately 24% of cases, the stage may be moved up indicating surgical resection as a possible curative treatment (60).

Management

Treatment is based on the stage of disease and predicted survival rates. Surgical excision is recommended for stages I and II, but is controversial for stage III. The standard approach is a lobectomy; pneumonectomy is associated with a higher surgical mortality rate (60). A wedge resection may be done if the patient has a low pulmonary reserve; however, the incidence of recurrence is higher with wedge resection. Pulmonary function tests should be conducted prior to surgery to determine the likelihood of tolerating the resection. A lobectomy is possible if an FEV_1 of 1.1 to 2.4 L is achieved. An FEV_1 less than 1 L

TABLE 10–16 Tumor/Node/Metastasis (TNM) System for Staging Lung Cancer

	Tumor	Node	Metastasis	
STAGE 0				
	Carcinoma in situ (early cancer that is present only in the layer of cells in which it began)	No node involvement	No metastasis	
STAGE I				
	T1—<3 cm	N1—Ipsilateral peribronchial, ipsilateral hilar	M1a—Separate tumor nodule(s) in a contralateral lobe; pleural nodules or malignant pleural or pericardial effusion	M1b—Distant metastasis
STAGE II				
	T2—Main bronchus >2 cm from carina, invades visceral pleura, partial atelectasis	N2—Ipsilateral mediastinal, subcarinal		
STAGE III				
	T3—>7 cm; chest wall, diaphragm, pericardium, mediastinal pleura, main bronchus <2 cm from carina, total atelectasis, separate nodule(s) in same lobe	N3—Contralateral mediastinal or hilar, scaleneor supraclavicular		
STAGE IV				
	T4—Mediastinum, heart, great vessels, carina, trachea, esophagus, vertebra; separate tumor nodule(s) in a different ipsilateral lobe			

Adapted from Minna JD, Schiller JH. Neoplasms of the lung. In Fauci AS, Braunwald E, Kasper DL, et al, editors. Harrison's Principles of Internal Medicine. 17th edition. Table 85-2, Tumor, Node, Metastasis International Staging System for Lung Cancer. Retrieved February 4, 2011, from http://www.accessmedicine.com/content.aspx?aID=2899309

indicates that the patient is unlikely to tolerate it and is not considered a candidate for surgery (60).

Radiation therapy may be used if surgery is contraindicated. Adjuvant radiation therapy after resection is controversial. Radiation therapy may reduce local incomplete resection but has not produced a greater survival rate (60). Chemotherapy may be used after surgery and has shown an increased survival benefit; however, a combination of chemoradiation has better overall survival rates compared with either modality used alone (60). Management of lung cancer is best achieved with a multidisciplinary approach. Consultations should be sought from a thoracic surgeon, a radiation oncologist, a medical oncologist, a pulmonologist, and a social worker (60).

Clinical Nurse Specialist Competencies and Spheres of Influence
Clinical Expert/Direct Care, Collaboration, Coaching/Teaching/Mentoring, and Ethical Decision-Making/Moral Agency/Advocacy

For patients with lung cancer, the CNS serves as a link between specialty and general care. When multiple treatment modalities are used, patients may encounter radiotherapists, oncologists, surgeons, intensive care units, and diagnosis centers. CNSs use expert knowledge of the disease and manifestations and the side effects of treatment. Knowing what signs and symptoms of primary disease and paraneoplastic syndromes to anticipate is fundamental; the CNS then systematically interviews and examines the patient to differentiate indications of enlarging or shrinking tumor and effects or undesired side effects of treatment. Collaboration with the oncologist for further care planning follows. Patients and families require teaching and emotional support at every juncture, as treatment of lung cancer is a dynamic process with the potential for many changes in patient condition. In situations when the disease responds poorly to treatment, CNSs are often instrumental in initiating dialogue among the team and between the patient and family on palliative care planning.

CHEST TRAUMA

Etiology

Chest trauma and thoracic injuries result in 20% to 25% of all deaths due to trauma and contribute to another 50% of remaining traumatic deaths. This affects approximately 12 persons per 1 million people per day. Chest trauma is divided into two major categories: blunt trauma and penetrating trauma. Motor vehicle accidents account for the majority of blunt force chest trauma, whereas penetrating injuries such as missile insult from a gunshot wound or a knife injury account for the majority of penetrating chest traumas. Much of the research from penetrating chest injuries has come from combat experience and drug related fighting in urban areas (68-71).

Approximately 70% to 80% of blunt force chest injuries are related to motor vehicle accidents. Acts of violence, pedestrian accidents, falls, and blast injuries have also been associated with blunt chest trauma. The mechanism of action with these injuries typically results in the rapid acceleration or deceleration of the chest cavity organs resulting in direct injury. There are three categories of blunt chest trauma: (a) chest wall fractures and barotraumas, (b) lung injuries, and (c) heart and vasculature injuries (72).

Penetrating chest injuries occur from an outside projectile or object resulting in direct and immediate damage to surrounding tissue. Penetrating chest injuries can be defined as low-, medium-, and high-velocity injuries.

Low-velocity injuries generally include stab wounds and impaled objects and typically only affect the immediate tissue that is damaged. On the other hand, medium- and high-velocity injuries will not only affect the immediate tissue that has been penetrated but also surrounding tissues from the high degree of kinetic energy that is present. The degree of kinetic energy present is proportionally related to the degree of surrounding tissue damage. Typical hand gun injuries are considered as medium velocity injuries, while high-powered military type weapons and shrapnel blasts result in high-velocity injuries (71). Penetrating injuries generally cause more extensive tissue damage than blunt trauma and often have more serious ramifications. In fact, people with penetrating chest trauma who present in cardiac arrest only have an 8% overall survival rate (72). See Table 10-17 for a list of common injuries from penetrating chest trauma.

Clinical Presentation

History is most appropriately addressed while performing management of acute injuries including prioritizing airway, breathing, and circulation. With blunt force injuries, history will be beneficial determining the physics involved in the injuries such as the speed of the automobile on impact, intrusion damage to the vehicle's passenger compartment, or direction of forces from impact. With penetrating trauma, examination of the wounds may be more beneficial in determining the degree of injuries; however, an estimation of the forces of impact (high-powered gunshot wound versus low-velocity stab wound) will be beneficial in determining the degree of tissue damage surrounding the wound.

Although a patient may present with minor signs and symptoms initially, evidence of lung, cardiac, or vasculature injury surfaces quickly. Rapid assessment of vital signs and hemodynamics, airway, breathing, circulation,

TABLE 10–17 Common Injuries From Penetrating Chest Trauma

Hemothorax (may present as bilateral or open)
Hemopneumothorax (May present as bilateral or open)
Pneumothorax (may present as bilateral or open)
Diaphragmatic rupture
Pulmonary contusion
Rib fracture
Subcutaneous emphysema
Sternal fracture
Thoracic wall laceration

Adapted from Inci I, Ozcelik C, Tacyildiz I, et al. Penetrating chest injuries: unusually high incidence of high-velocity gunshot wounds in civilian practice. World J Surg 1998;22(5):438-442.

and neurologic status should be initiated as soon as the individual arrives in the facility, with repeat assessment at frequent intervals. Dyspnea with tachypnea will likely be seen; mental status changes related to hypoxia include confusion, agitation, and/or loss of consciousness. Visual inspection of the entire anterior and posterior chest wall should be performed to identify penetrating wounds, exit wounds, areas of flail chest, or significant bruising. Pneumothorax may be present and will result in asymmetrical chest wall movement. The mechanisms of a pneumothorax are illustrated in Figure 10-3. Flail chest will present with an area of paradoxical movement of the chest wall during inspiration and expiration. It is critical to maintain spinal stabilization during the exam to reduce the risk of spinal cord injury in the event of a spinal fracture. Auscultation may reveal absent sounds in lung fields when a pneumothorax or hemothorax is present.

Diagnosis

Diagnosis depends largely on the history and physical exam. Additionally, basic laboratory and imaging studies are done to identify all the injuries and guide the management plan. Blood is sampled when inserting intravenous catheters for fluid resuscitation. Hemoglobin, hematocrit, red cell and platelet count, and coagulation studies provide an estimate of blood loss and should be repeated at frequent intervals during initial hospitalization to judge the need for supplemental blood or blood products. Blood type and cross-match should be done if administration of blood products is anticipated (72). A basic metabolic profile to assess renal and liver function and electrolytes is indicated. ABGs should be done to determine the adequacy of ventilation, oxygenation, and acid-base balance. Various other tests to consider include serum lactate levels to evaluate tissue perfusion and oxygenation, and serum troponin and myocardial muscle creatine kinase for assessment of myocardial damage from contusion, ischemia, or tamponade.

Standard posterior/anterior and lateral chest radiograph is the first choice of imaging for patients with traumatic chest injuries, which can be done relatively quickly and

easily and often provides enough information to begin emergent treatment. Pneumothorax, hemothorax, chest wall fractures, tamponade, mediastinal shift, and damage to the heart and great vessels are evident on standard images. When stable enough, chest CT scan should be done. In the hemodynamically stable patient, CT scanning has been found to identify injuries in 50% of patients with a normal chest radiograph. Spiral CT scan and aortogram may be used to diagnose aortic injuries. Thoracic ultrasound is another option in the emergency setting with a sensitivity and specificity greater than 90% in detecting pericardial and cardiac injuries (72-76).

Twelve-lead ECG should also be performed on all traumatic chest injuries. ECG findings with blunt trauma may include tachyarrythmias, conduction delays such as heart block or bundle branch block, and R-wave and ST-T wave changes indicative of myocardial and/or pericardial injury (74).

Management

Management of chest trauma is based on the specific type of injury. Key treatment in all trauma patients begins with establishing and maintaining the airway, breathing, circulation, and neurologic function during primary and secondary assessment. Immediate emergency surgical intervention may be required depending on the degree and type of injuries. However, researchers have shown that only 8% of people with blunt traumatic chest injuries require surgical intervention (72). On the other hand, people with penetrating chest trauma often need immediate surgical intervention to explore the chest, repair vessels and other injured structures, and stop bleeding (77).

Rib fractures and chest wall injuries are common in both blunt and penetrating chest trauma and are found in 50% of blunt force injuries. When three or more ribs are fractured in two or more places, it is considered a flail chest and results in an unstable section of the chest wall. There is usually an associated pulmonary contusion, which often results in respiratory distress, sometimes delayed several days after the injury. In addition, severe pain may affect pulmonary function and necessitate endotracheal intubation (71, 73).

For the most part, chest wall injuries alone, although serious, are not typically life threatening. However, fractures of the first and second rib may be seen in high kinetic energy injuries, which occur in conjunction with cranial, thoracic, major blood vessel, and abdominal injuries. These potentially life threatening injuries should be ruled out.

The most common lung injuries are pneumothorax and hemothorax. Either may present individually or concomitantly. A pneumothorax is caused by a loss of negative pressure in the pleural space resulting in collapse of the lung and inability to inflate during inspiration. Treatment is a thoracostomy with chest tube to maintain negative

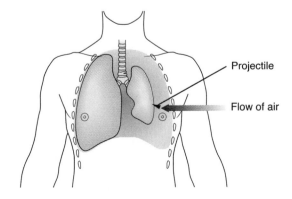

Projectile

Flow of air

FIGURE 10-3: Mechanisms of pneumothorax.

pressure. In certain emergency situations, a tension pneumothorax may occur, resulting in no breath sounds on the a effected side and tracheal deviation to the opposite side of the injury. This requires immediate needle thoracostomy at the midclavicular second intercostal space to evacuate the air. Generally, a massive hemothorax is considered to be more than 1,500 mL of blood and is evacuated with a chest tube. If less than 200 mL of blood has collected, the hemothorax may not show on the chest radiograph. The patient is evaluated clinically for oxygenation and signs and symptoms of respiratory distress and if necessary, a chest tube is indicated for drainage of blood.

As many as 75% to 80% of penetrating chest injuries involve the cervical spine, trachea, and large blood vessels. These injuries are often fatal. Physical findings include respiratory distress, subcutaneous emphysema, hemoptysis, pneumomediastinum, and pneumothorax. Operative repair is essential.

Prognosis of traumatic chest injuries is highly dependent on the degree of insult and the ability of the clinician to properly identify and treat underlying injuries. With blunt force injuries, only 20% of patients require invasive modalities. With penetrating chest trauma, the more stable the patient is on presentation, the more likely they can expect a full recovery.

Clinical Nurse Specialist Competencies and Spheres of Influence
Clinical Expert/Direct Care and Consultation

Patients with traumatic chest injuries often present acutely symptomatic and require rapid decisive life-support interventions such as airway protection, large-bore intravenous catheter insertion, and immediate fluid resuscitation, followed by diagnosis. Although risky for unstable patients, the more rapidly diagnostic tests can be performed, differential diagnoses can be established and appropriate management undertaken. CNSs may orchestrate transport to radiology or surgery for exploratory evaluation or definitive treatment. The CNS who recognizes the significance of the clinical presentation of patients with chest injuries can timely facilitate initial emergency interventions.

Coaching/Teaching/Mentoring

People with significant pneumothorax or hemothorax will require chest tubes. Chest tube management is a relatively complex and high-risk clinical procedure that may not be common for staff on some nursing units. Formal education or competency validation in practice settings may be coordinated or delivered by the CNS and supplemented with informal daily educational support on units where patients are managed. Because not all traumatic injuries are exactly alike and patients may have other system injuries besides the chest, unique presentations and complications can occur. The CNS provides informal education to bedside clinicians using advanced knowledge and grasp of the patient's injuries and potential multisystem affects.

PULMONARY EDEMA

Etiology

Pulmonary edema is the result of extravasation of fluid from the pulmonary vasculature to the interstitial space and alveoli. It is typically the result of one of the following: imbalance of Starling forces, damage to the alveolar capillary barrier, lymphatic obstruction; sometimes the etiology is idiopathic. The result is a V/Q mismatch where proper diffusion of oxygen and carbon dioxide cannot occur. As events continue to cascade, respiratory failure will ensue. Pulmonary edema is most often found as a serious complication of heart failure with overall mortality rates in a high-acuity setting approximately 15% to 20% (95). Pulmonary edema can be subcategorized into (a) cardiogenic pulmonary edema (CPE) and (b) noncardiogenic pulmonary edema (NPE).

Cardiogenic Pulmonary Edema

CPE is the most common type. Starling forces, also known as the Frank Starling law, explain the hydrostatic and oncotic forces of fluid movement across capillary membranes. In CPE, pulmonary edema is caused by increased capillary hydrostatic pressure as a result of elevated pulmonary venous pressure. This results in a disruption within the pulmonary capillary structure from the increased pressure, and fluid in the pulmonary interstitium and alveoli (Table 10-18).

CPE typically occurs as a result of left atrial or LV dysfunction. It may also occur as a result of mitral valve disorders and rarely left atrial tumors. Heart rhythm disorder such as atrial fibrillation and ventricular tachycardia that reduce LV filling is another etiology. Basically, any condition that affects LV ejection fraction may result in pulmonary venous hypertension and pulmonary edema (78).

Noncardiogenic Pulmonary Edema

NPE occurs as a result of changes in the pulmonary capillary membranes from pathology unrelated to cardiac function. NPE accounts for approximately 70 cases per 100,000 population worldwide. Causes include drowning, fluid overload, aspiration, glomerulonephritis, inhalation injuries, allergic reaction, ARDS, and neurogenic pulmonary edema (Table 10-19) (78).

Neurogenic Pulmonary Edema

Neurogenic pulmonary edema, a subset of NPE, is not completely understood, yet has been found to occur in approximately 30% to 70% of patients with subarachnoid and intracerebral hemorrhage. It has also been found in 71% of fatal cases of subarachnoid hemorrhage. In addition, as many as one-third of patients with status epilepticus show evidence of neurogenic pulmonary edema, and more than half of patients with head injuries have complications from neurogenic pulmonary edema (79).

TABLE 10–18 Status of Fluid Accumulation in Cardiogenic Pulmonary Edema (CPE)

Stage I	Elevated left atrial pressure; no change in blood gas exchange
Stage II	Fluid and colloid shift to the lung interstitium; lymphatics attempt to filter liquid; may result in mild hypoxemia
Stage III	Fluid continues to collect in interstitial space and may account for up to 500 mL of fluid shift; fluid crosses the alveolar epithelium in results in alveolar flooding; noticeable abnormalities and gas exchange are present with more severe hypoxemia

TABLE 10–19 Causes of Noncardiogenic Pulmonary Edema

Acute respiratory distress syndrome
Neurogenic pulmonary edema
Pulmonary edema and renal failure
Pulmonary edema and marathon runners
Decompression sickness
Heroin and nalaxone overdose
Cytotoxic chemotherapy
Drowning
Recent lung transplantation
Complications of pregnancy

Etiology for neurogenic pulmonary edema is unclear. However, an increased sympathetic tone may actually result in an increase in left atrial pressure from venous return. This may increase capillary hydrostatic pressure to produce pulmonary edema without affecting pulmonary capillary or left atrial/LV pressures (79).

Clinical Presentation

Cardiac pathology is the most common cause of pulmonary edema. On interview, recent sudden development of shortness of breath, anxiety, and chest pain may be elicited. An immediately preceding cardiac event such as acute myocardial infarction may be present. The patient's history may include diaphoresis, dyspnea on exertion, orthopnea, paroxysmal nocturnal dyspnea, and recent weight gain (80, 81).

Tachypnea and tachycardia is usually evident on physical exam. Hypertension are typically present due to adrenergic effects, but hypotension may be present in severe LV disease. A weak pulse may be present with CPE; however, NCPE usually notes a bounding pulse. Level of hypoxemia is easily assessed with pulse oximetry (82). General observation may reveal shortness of breath such as inability to complete sentences without

rest or with minimal physical exertion. A general degree of anxiousness is noted, with some confusion present in marked hypoxic individuals. Skin color may be pale and diaphoretic. Mottling may also be present and is considered as an independent risk factor in determining in-hospital mortality. Cool extremities may indicate significantly decreased cardiac output. Auscultation of the lungs will likely reveal crackles in the bases. As the disease worsens consolidation and adventitious breath sounds may be found at higher levels. Auscultation of a S_3 heart sound is typically found in CPE and not in NCPE. Murmurs signify valve malfunction and may provide insight to the underlying cause of pulmonary edema. If right-sided heart failure is present, typical findings will include jugular vein distention, hepatomegaly, hepatojugular reflex, and peripheral edema (80, 82).

Diagnosis

The diagnostic plan begins with establishing the presence of pulmonary edema followed by differentiation of CPE and NCPE. A CBC with differential is beneficial in determining if underlying anemia or a septic process is present; high output failure and pulmonary edema are associated with severe anemia, and ARDS is frequently part of sepsis and/or systemic inflammatory response syndrome. Serum electrolytes will identify abnormalities commonly found in patients on diuretic therapy such as hypokalemia and hypomagnesemia. Blood urea nitrogen and creatinine will be helpful in determining baseline renal function, necessary if diuretics are planned for management. ABGs should be performed to evaluate oxygenation and acid-base balance and are useful in determining the need for mechanical ventilation. Respiratory alkalosis may be initially present as a result of hyperventilation (78, 83, 84). Plasma BNP and NT-pro-BNP testing is useful in determining the degree of CPE and underlying heart failure. The levels are also useful in identifying whether the etiology of pulmonary edema is cardiac or pulmonary in nature. BNP is produced by cardiac myocytes and increases as a result of poor cardiac function. Trending BNP levels has been shown to decrease total cost of treatment and hospitalization times (Table 10-20) (85-87).

Chest radiography should be performed and may likely note Kerley B lines and enlarged heart. Other findings may include pleural effusion, basilar edema, and occlusion of proximal bronchi. Some findings in acute CPE may not be present for 12 hours or more after clinical presentation (79-81).

Echocardiography will determine underlying valvular disorders, LV dysfunction, and pericardial conditions. Mechanical causes of pulmonary edema such as acute papillary muscle rupture, ventricular septal defect, cardiac tamponade, and LV rupture are evident on the echocardiogram (80, 81).

Pulmonary artery wedge pressure (PAWP) may also be used to differentiate NCPE from CPE. A pulmonary artery catheter insertion is recommended if the specific etiology of pulmonary edema is unclear. A normal PAWP is 10 to 18 mm Hg. In CPE pressure will typically exceed 25 to 30 mm Hg. Cardiogenic shock may also be present and is defined as a systolic blood pressure less than 80 mm Hg, a cardiac index less than 1.8 L/min/m², and PAWP greater than 18 mm Hg (80, 82, 84, 88).

Management

Treatment of pulmonary edema depends on the type (CPE or NCPE) and the specific etiology. For both types, oxygen should be administered to maintain oxygen saturation greater than 90%; patients in severe distress may require 100% via face mask. Noninvasive ventilation such as CPAP or NPPV will decrease the workload of the heart and rest respiratory muscles. In more severe cases mechanical ventilation with PEEP will have several positive effects: (a) decrease both preload and after load resulting in increased cardiac function; (b) redistribute fluid in the alveoli to the extra-alveolar space, thereby enhancing gas exchange; and (c) increase lung volume to circumvent atelectasis (80, 82).

General care for patients with CPE includes dietary guidelines that promote a low sodium diet. Regular weight measurements should be recorded to monitor fluid retention. Fluid intake and output should be closely monitored (80). Treatment for underlying cardiac conditions is the standard of care for CPE. Table 10-21 lists medications for the treatment of CPE. There are three underlying considerations in treatment: reduction in preload, reduction in afterload, and inotropic support if needed.

Preload Reduction

The first choice for decreasing preload is loop diuretics such as furosemide, bumetanide, or torsemide. These medications typically reduce preload by diuresis in 20 to 60 minutes. Initial dosing for furosemide is 0.5 to 1 mg/kg bolus intravenously. The dose may be doubled if no effect has been achieved in 30 minutes. In chronic heart failure or renal insufficient patients who are currently on diuretic therapy, higher initial dosing may be required (80, 82). Nitrates are beneficial in decreasing preload by acting as venodilators and are considered first line therapy in acute CPE. Nitrates are also useful in patients who present with cardiac-related chest pain because they moderately reduce afterload. Nitrates produce the most predictable and effective reduction in preload, however. They are contraindicated in individuals taking phosphodiesterase type 5 inhibitors such as sildenafil (80, 82). Morphine is a mild venodilator that also provides relief from dyspnea and anxiety. Naloxone should be readily available if adverse side effects occur (89).

Afterload Reduction

Afterload reducers work to decrease the peripheral vascular resistance and increase stroke volume and cardiac output, which in turn relieve fluid from the pulmonary bed. ACE inhibitors have been shown to be effective for heart failure in extensive studies. ACE inhbitors are also beneficial in CPE when hypertension is present. Researchers have shown that short-term and long-term mortality rates decrease for individuals who take ACE inhibitors for heart failure following acute myocardial infarction (82).

TABLE 10–20 Brain Natriuretic Peptide Testing

Normal	0–99 picograms per milliliter (pg/mL) or 0–99 nanograms per liter (ng/L) SI units. No heart failure is present.
Abnormal	100–300 pg/mL or 100–300 ng/L (SI units) suggests heart failure may be present. 300 pg/mL or 300 ng/L (SI units) or higher is considered mild heart failure. 600 pg/mL or 600 ng/L (SI units) or higher is considered moderate heart failure. 900 pg/mL or 900 ng/L (SI units) or higher is considered severe heart failure.

From: Essig MG. Brain Natriuretic Peptide (BNP) Test. Retrieved June 19, 2007, from http://health.yahoo.com/heart-diagnosis/brain-natriuretic-peptide-bnp-test/healthwise—ux1072.html

TABLE 10–21 Medication for Treatment of Cardiogenic Pulmonary Edema

Category	Medication	Dosage and Indication
Preload reducers	Furosemide	• IV bolus 1 mg/kg or 40–100 mg. PO route is not appropriate with CPE due to slow onset.
	Nitroglycerin	• Sublingual 0.4 mg q3–5min • 2% ointment 1–3 inches (absorption may be unreliable) • IV may be initiated a 5–10 mcg/kg/min and titrated appropriately (close blood pressure [BP] monitoring needed)
	Morphine	• 2–4 mg IV bolus may repeat q15min prn
Afterload reducers	Captopril	• Sublingual 12.5–25 mg (BP should be minimum <90 mm Hg)
	Enalapril	• IV bolus 1.25 mg or 1 mg q2h
	Nitroprusside	• IV infusion 0.3-0.5 mcg/kg/min • May titrate q5–10min • Not to exceed 10 mcg/kg/min
Catecholamines	Dobutamine	• IV infusion 2.5 mcg/kg/min • Not to exceed 20 mcg/kg/min
	Dopamine	• IV infusion 5 mcg/kg/min, initially • Not to exceed 20/mcg/kg/min
	Norepinephrine	• IV infusion 8—12 mcg/min initially • 2-4 mcg/min maintenance • Not to exceed 30 mcg/min • Reserved for severe hypotension (BP <70 mm Hg)
Phosphodiesterase enzyme inhibitors: Positive inotropic and vasodilator	Milrinone	• IV loading 50 mcg/kg over 10 min, then continuous infusion 0.375–0.75 mcg/kg/min • Titrate to maintain adequate systolic BP and cardiac output

Angiotensin II receptor blockers have comparable benefits to ACE inhibitors for heart failure. Nitroprusside works on both afterload and preload by directly relaxing smooth muscle. It is also useful for increasing cardiac output and decreasing LV filling pressures and is commonly titrated to achieve a PAWP of 18 mm Hg or less (80, 82, 84).

Inotropic Support
Inotropic support is necessary when attempts to reduce afterload and preload have not been effective or when hypotension is present. Catecholamines such as dobutamine, dopamine, and norepinephrine are frequently used, with dobutamine as the first line choice. Phosphodiesterase inhibitors (PDIs) such as milrinone or inamrinone result in positive inotropic effects with a decrease in afterload and preload. Catecholamines stimulate adrenoreceptors; patients may show a tolerance to the medications and require increasing doses for effectiveness, which carries the risk of undesirable complications such as tachycardia. PDIs do not have this property and can generally be given at a stable dose as initially titrated (82-84).

Invasive Intervention
Intra-aortic balloon pump (IABP) may also be utilized in the treatment of CPE. IABP will improve coronary blood flow during balloon inflation and reduce afterload during balloon deflation. The IABP is used as a temporary procedure for severe cardiogenic shock or cardiomyopathy and sometimes as a bridge to further definitive surgical intervention (80, 82).

Ultrafiltration
Ultrafiltration is a procedure that mimics the natural filtration effect of the kidneys by removing a predetermined amount of fluid from the blood. It has been found to be beneficial in patients who have responded poorly to large doses of diuretics or when diuretics are contraindicated (80, 90).

Clinical Nurse Specialist Competencies and Spheres of Influence
Clinical Expert/Direct Care and Consultation

Due to the potentially life-threatening nature of pulmonary edema, the CNS begins evaluation of the patient with the ABC approach (airway, breathing, circulation) and begins oxygen therapy immediately. Facilitating care by other team members when intubation and ventilator support is necessary must be anticipated. The CNS applies expert knowledge to facilitate the triage of patients presenting with difficulty breathing in the emergency department. In the inpatient units, the CNS assists staff with administration and monitoring hemodynamic response to inotropes and other medications. Vigilance is required when caring for patients with pulmonary edema to detect any changes in condition and avert potential health crises. Overall, the CNS provides and/or assists in the direct care of patients in the ICUs and on the general-care floors, role modeling effective communication and authentic presence.

As a clinical expert, the CNS is consulted by the nursing staff to troubleshoot issues related to care management. Additionally, consultation with the bedside clinician is important to facilitate patient transfers from the ICU to the general care floor to ensure that critical aspects of the care plan such as medications and fluid assessment are addressed.

RESPIRATORY FAILURE

Etiology

Acute respiratory failure is described as inadequate gas exchange by the lungs that is considered to be life threatening. It is characterized by a PaO_2 level less than 60 mm Hg or a $PaCO_2$ greater than 50 mm Hg. Respiratory failure is typically the result of an underlying pathology and may be broken down into two types. Respiratory failure may be acute or chronic in nature, however, chronic failure is more insidious and may not be as apparent on examination. Mortality rates associated with respiratory failure are based on underlying etiology. For example, ARDS carries a mortality rate of approximately 45% and acute exacerbation of COPD carries a mortality rate of approximately 30% (91, 92).

Type I hypoxic respiratory failure results in a PaO_2 of less than 60 mm Hg; however, $PaCO_2$ is normal or low (equal to or less than 49 mm Hg). This is typically seen with acute lung injury, ARDS, pneumonia, pulmonary thromboembolism, acute lobar atelectasis, cardiogenic pulmonary edema, and acute collagen or vascular disease (92).

Type II hypercapnic-hypoxic respiratory failure is the result of airway resistance. This leads to a decrease in oxygen and an increase in CO_2 levels. This is commonly caused by underlying pulmonary disease such as COPD, asthma, respiratory suppression from drugs, Guillain-Barré syndrome, acute myasthenia gravis, spinal cord tumors, and fatigue. Acute onset of type 2 hypercapnic failure usually results in a pH less than 7.3, whereas chronic respiratory failure will typically develop over a longer period of time, allowing renal compensation and only a minimal decrease pH level.

Type III respiratory failure is a result of lung atelectasis. This condition commonly occurs in the perioperative period and has been called perioperative respiratory failure. It is specifically related to atelectasis following general anesthesia. It is typically treated with frequent positional change, chest physiotherapy, and aggressive pain management for abdominal or incisional pain that may limit expiratory volume.

Type IV respiratory failure occurs specifically in shock victims due to hypoperfusion of respiratory musculature. This results in 40% of cardiac output being distributed to respiratory muscles to compensate. In such instances, mechanical ventilation assists the redistribution of cardiac output to support other organ systems (91, 92).

Pathophysiology

The mechanism of respiration may be affected at three physiologic points: diffusion of oxygen across the alveoli, transport of oxygen to the tissue, and diffusion of CO_2 from to the blood to the alveoli. Respiratory failure may occur with any combination of these factors.

Gas exchange occurs at the alveolar capillary level where oxygen and carbon dioxide diffuse to maintain equilibrium of pressure on both sides of the alveolar membrane. Hemoglobin contains four sites for oxygen binding. The quantity of oxygen combined with hemoglobin is dependent upon blood PaO_2. This relationship is known as the oxygen hemoglobin dissociation curve (Figure 10-4).

Carbon dioxide is transported in the blood stream by three routes: (a) simple solution, (b) bicarbonate, and (c) a carbamino compound combined with hemoglobin. With proper gas exchange, blood flow and ventilation result in no alveolar–arterial PO_2 differences. However, these mismatches tend to occur as alveoli are underventilated and overventilated due to physiology location resulting in high V/Q units and low V/Q units, respectively. In other words, the V/Q units are greater in either the alveolar or arterial side of the equation, resulting in the mismatch. V/Q mismatching occurs to some degree in normal lung function; however, increased alveolar to arterial PO_2 greater than 15 to 20 mm Hg indicates a likely pulmonary disease as the cause of hypoxemia.

The three most common causes of acute respiratory failure include hypoventilation, V/Q mismatch, and shunt. Hypoventilation is commonly caused by CNS depression. It is characterized by hypercapnia and hypoxemia and cannot be differentiated from other causes of

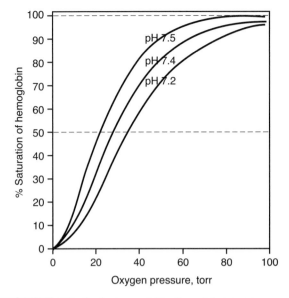

FIGURE 10–4: Oxyhemoglobin dissociation curve.

TABLE 10–22 Common Causes of Respiratory Failure

Type 1 Respiratory Failure	Type 2 Respiratory Failure
Chronic obstructive pulmonary disease	Chronic obstructive pulmonary disease
Pneumonia	Severe asthma
Pulmonary fibrosis	Drug overdose
Asthma	Poisoning
Pneumothorax	Myasthenia gravis
Pulmonary embolism	Polyneuropathy
Pulmonary arterial hypertension	Poliomyelitis
Pneumoconiosis	Primary muscle disorders
Granulomatous lung disease	Porphyria
Cyanotic congenital heart disease	Cervical cordotomy
Bronchiectasis	Head and cervical cord injury
Acute respiratory distress syndrome	Primary alveolar hypoventilation
Fat embolism syndrome	Obesity hypoventilation syndrome
Kyphoscoliosis	Pulmonary edema
Obesity	Acute respiratory distress syndrome
	Myxedema
	Tetanus

Adapted from Kaynar AM, Sharma A. eMedicine. Respiratory Failure. Retrieved May 20, 2009, from http://emedicine.medscape.com/article/167981-overview

hypoxemia by the normal presence of alveolar–arterial PO_2 level. V/Q mismatch is the most common cause of respiratory failure. A low V/Q ratio may occur from a decrease in ventilation or overperfusion during normal ventilation. Administration of 100% oxygen eliminates low V/Q units and will correct hypoxemia. $PaCO_2$ levels are generally not affected with the V/Q mismatch. Shunt is the persistence of hypoxemia with FIO_2 levels at 100% and occurs when deoxygenated blood bypasses the alveoli, resulting in decrease in PaO_2 levels. This may occur as a result of cardiac defects (i.e., ventricular septal defect, atrial septal defect, arteriovenous malformation in the lung) and is also observed in pneumonia, atelectasis, and pulmonary edema. Common causes of respiratory failure are shown in Table 10-22 (91-93).

Clinical Presentation

A thorough history is important to identify the underlying cause of respiratory failure. Recent symptomatology such as chest pain, paroxysmal nocturnal dyspnea, and orthopnea may suggest a cardiogenic pulmonary condition. Noncardiogenic edema may also be present with other comorbid factors such as sepsis, trauma, aspiration, pneumonia, pancreatitis, drug toxicity, and multiple transfusions. The physical examination may reveal underlying causative medical conditions for respiratory failure. Table 10-23 provides a list of common differential diagnoses for respiratory failure.

TABLE 10–23 Differential Diagnosis for Respiratory Failure

Acute respiratory distress syndrome	Pneumonia	Sleep apnea
Asthma	Atelectasis	Cardiogenic shock
Cardiomyopathy	Cor pulmonale	Myocardial infarction/ischemia
Diaphragmatic paralysis	Emphysema	Pneumothorax
Pulmonary edema	Pulmonary embolism	Pulmonary fibrosis
Pulmonary hypertension	Respiratory acidosis	Restrictive lung disease
Shock	Mechanical ventilation	

The most common clinical findings include cyanosis, dyspnea, confusion, and altered level of consciousness. On auscultation, crackles will typically be heard. Cardiac examination may reveal tachycardia and various arrhythmias. Neurologic exam may reveal asterixis (found mostly with severely elevated $PaCO_2$ levels), restlessness, anxiety, confusion, and loss of consciousness.

A patient presenting with suspect respiratory failure should immediately have an ABG analysis. Additional laboratory tests are done to identify underlying causes. A CBC may reveal polycythemia in patients with chronic hypoxemia. A complete metabolic profile panel is done to identify underlying hepatic or renal dysfunction. Electrolyte imbalances may be found that could complicate respiratory failure. A cardiac panel including creatine kinase and troponin I will help to exclude underlying myocardial infarction from causes. Additional laboratory testing should be considered based on patient history and could include drug toxicity levels and thyroid function studies (92, 94).

Imaging studies are also essential in diagnosing the underlying cause of respiratory failure. Portable posterior/anterior and lateral chest radiography should be performed immediately and may provide clinical information on heart size, pleural effusion, distribution of infiltrates, Kerley A and B lines, and peribronchial thickening. If an underlying cardiogenic pathology is suspected, an echocardiogram will be beneficial in determining ventricular dilation, valvular disorders, or cardiac wall motion abnormalities. In addition, normal cardiac findings with pulmonary edema may suggest ARDS.

Other testing may include a 12-lead ECG to evaluate a cardiac pathology. Pulmonary function testing may be performed in patients with chronic respiratory failure; however, many patients will not be able to complete the tests (92, 94).

Management

Initial treatment should consist of oxygen supplementation, which is vital in addressing hypoxemia and decreasing end organ damage. Acute respiratory failure is the most common indication for endotracheal tube intubation and mechanical ventilation. In chronic respiratory failure, a patient may be treated in the ambulatory setting with oxygen supplementation. Outpatient ventilator assistive devices may also be used. (Table 10-24 lists common medications used for treating underlying causes of respiratory failure.)

In acute respiratory failure, the goal is to achieve PaO_2 of greater than 60 mm Hg or SaO_2 greater than 90%. Generally speaking, this is facilitated by ventilator support. Positive pressure ventilation is typically used in an ICU setting. There is very little indication for negative

TABLE 10–24 Common Medications for Treating Underlying Causes of Respiratory Failure

Classification	Medication, Generic (Brand)	Dosage
Diuretics	Furosemide (Lasix)	10–20 mg IV for symptomatic congestive heart failue not currently taking diuretic
		40–80 mg IV in patients already using diuretics
		80–120 mg IV for patients who symptoms are refractory to initial dose after 1 hour
	Metolazone (Zaroxolyn)	10 mg PO before redosing with furosemide
Nitrates	Nitroglycerin (Nitro-bid, Nitrol)	Spray: 1 puff 0.4 mg equivalent; may repeat q3–5min
		Ointment: Apply 1–2 inches of nitro paste to chest wall
		Injection: Started at 20 mcg/min IV and titrate to effect in 5- to 10-mcg increments every 3–5 minutes BP <90 mm Hg
	Nitroprusside sodium (Nitropress)	0.3-0.5 mcg/kg/min mcg/min IV; titrate to effective dose range of 3 -4 mcg/kg/min with systolic BP >90 mm Hg
Analgesics	Morphine sulfate	2–5 mg; repeat q10–15min IV unless respiratory rate is <20
Inotropics	Dopamine	5 mcg/kg/min IV and increase in increments of 5 mcg/kg/min IV to dose of 20 mcg/kg/min

TABLE 10–24 Common Medications for Treating Underlying Causes of Respiratory Failure—cont'd

Classification	Medication, Generic (Brand)	Dosage
	Norepinephrine	8-12 mcg min IV titrated according to hemodynamic response
	Dobutamine	2.5 mcg/kg/min IV, therapeutic range 10–40 mcg/kg/min
Bronchodilators	Terbutaline (Breathaire)	0.25 mg SC; do not exceed 0.5 mg SC q4h
	Albuterol	2.5 mg/ nebulizer solution
	Theophylline	5 mg/kg IN initially 0.2-0.6 mg/kg/hour maintenance
	Ipratropium bromide	0.5 mg/nebulizer treatment
Corticosteroids	Methylprednisolone	10-250 mg IV q6h for first 24–48 hr of therapy

Adapted from Kaynar AM, Sharma A. eMedicine. Respiratory Failure. Retrieved May 20, 2009, from http://emedicine.medscape.com/article/167981-overview

pressure ventilation, and it is poorly tolerated by patients. Ventilation may be controlled or patient initiated. In control mode the ventilator works independently of the patient's effort. However, patient-initiated control works as an assistive action in response to the patient's own inspiratory effort. Positive pressure ventilation may also be regulated based on target pressure versus volume. As the name implies, pressure regulation is the set variable with tidal volume being an independent variable, and with volume regulation tidal volume is set and pressure is the independent variable. PEEP may also be used to maintain a pressure level greater than zero in the alveoli. This in turn works to open atelectatic alveoli and to shift fluid in the lungs to the perivascular interstitial space. In addition, it allows for a reduction in FIO_2 and decrease risk for oxygen toxicity. With improper ventilation, barotrauma may occur and has typically been found to occur when excessive tidal volumes are present. Lower tidal volumes have shown a reduced incidence in barotrauma in mechanically ventilated patients with ARDS.

NPPV has also been used in patients with mild to moderate acute respiratory failure whereby ventilatory support is provided through nasal or full face mask. A patent airway and alert patient is required for this means of ventilation. Studies have shown that NPPV was beneficial in treatment of COPD, asthma, and acute decompensated heart failure with mild pulmonary edema. NPPV has been shown in clinical trials to decrease complications during ICU visits (93-96).

Additional observation and monitoring for acute respiratory failure should include cardiac monitoring, pulse oximetry, blood pressure, and capnometry. Treatment of underlying cause essential in managing acute respiratory failure. Consultation with the pulmonary specialist and

admission to ICU for ventilator support should be performed (94, 95).

Clinical Nurse Specialist Competencies and Spheres of Influence
Clinical Expert/Direct Care, Consultation, and Collaboration

The CNS uses advanced knowledge of underlying disease pathology and other causes of acute respiratory failure, along with accurate interpretation of the physical presentation. Risk factors such as opiate use with patient-controlled analgesia, for example, and chronic pulmonary diseases are considered. Accurate interpretation of chest radiographs, blood gases, and cardiac diagnostics are crucial for correct differential diagnosis and prompt management plan, as patients with acute respiratory failure can deteriorate quickly. Intubation before becoming emergent is better for reducing complications such as bronchospasm or lethal cardiac dysrhythmia. Bedside clinicians may activate the rapid response team for assistance with assessment and management of the patient, who can become extremely anxious during periods of acute hypoxemia. Families may need support when they witness their loved one in distress. The CNS facilitates emergency transfer to the intensive care unit when intubation and mechanical ventilation is required. This is also a time of commotion for families that CNSs mitigate.

Research/Evidence-Based Practice

Reducing ventilator time minimizes complications. Whenever mechanical ventilator support is initiated for patients with acute respiratory failure, goals for weaning and extubation are soon established. Numerous researchers over the past two to three decades have evaluated various methods of mechanical ventilator weaning procedures and tested instruments that predict readiness for weaning. The Burns Weaning Assessment Program (BWAP) is one example that has been tested in a variety of patient populations. The instrument consists of a 26-item checklist of general and respiratory factors used to assess readiness for weaning (97). The spontaneous breathing trial, which requires 30 minutes free of ventilator support, has been tested over multiple patient populations and settings, and shows strong predictability for success with formal, longer weaning trials (98). Results vary with these and other instruments, however, over different patient groups. The CNS must critically appraise the studies in which these instruments have been tested to determine applicability in their practice setting.

Some researchers report success in managing ventilated patients with standardized protocols, resulting in fewer ventilator days and shortened intensive care and/or hospital length of stay. Many hospitals have designated units in which the patients are managed by CNSs using protocols. CNSs provide leadership for continued research to establish best practices for ventilator weaning and predictors of readiness to wean for various patient populations.

Resources for COPD

The Global Initiative for Chronic Obstructive Lung Disease: www.goldcopd.org

American Lung Association: http://lungusa.org/lung-disease/copd

Medline Plus: http://www.nlm.nih.gov/medlineplus/copdchronicobstructivepulmonarydisease.html

Mayo Clinic: http://www.mayoclinic.com/health/copd/DS00916

National Heart, Lung, and Blood Institute: http://www.nhlbi.nih.gov/health/dci/Diseases/Copd/Copd_WhatIs.html

COPD International: http://www.copd-international.com/

E-medicine health: http://www.emedicinehealth.com/chronic_obstructive_pulmonary_disease_copd/article_em.htm

Resources for Sleep Apnea

The American Sleep Apnea Association (ASAA) is dedicated to reducing injury, disability, and death from sleep apnea and to enhancing the well-being of those affected by this common disorder. The ASAA promotes education and awareness. Website: http://www.sleepapnea.org/support/index.html

Resources for Pulmonary Hypertension

Pulmonary Hypertension Association (PHA) is an organization dedicated to research for pulmonary hypertension. Information and links to support groups are available at http://www.phassociation.org/Page.aspx?pid=197

Resources for Lung Cancer

National Cancer Institute Website: http://www.cancer.gov/cancertopics/types/lung

American Cancer Society Website: http://www.cancer.org/docroot/home/index.asp

American Lung Association Website: http://www.lungusa.org/

References

1. Thompson DA. Clinical and economic outcomes of hospital-acquired pneumonia and intra-abdominal surgery patients. Ann Surg 2006;243(4):547-552.

2. Mandell A, Wunderink R, Azueto A, et al: Infectious disease Society of America and American Thoracic Society guidelines or the management of adults with community-acquired pneumonia. Clin Infect Dis 2007;44:S27.

3. Lutfiyya M, Henley E, Chang L. Diagnosis and treatment of community-acquired pneumonia. Am Acad Fam Pract 2006;73(3).

4. Limper AH. Overview of pneumonia. In Goldman L, Ausiello, D, editors. Cecil Textbook of Medicine. 23rd edition. Philadelphia: Saunders; 2007.

5. Schmitt S. Community-Acquired Pneumonia. The Cleveland Clinic Foundation. Retrieved February 7, 2011, from http://www.clevelandclinicmeded.com/medicalpubs/diseasemanagement/infectious-disease/community-acquired-pneumonia/

6. The Merck Manuals Online Library. Hospital-Acquired and Institution-Acquired Pneumonia. Retrieved February 7, 2011, from http://www.merck.com/mmhe/sec04/ch042/ch042c.html

7. American Thoracic Society and the Infectious Diseases Society of America. Guidelines for the management of adults with hospital-acquired, ventilator-associated, and healthcare-associated pneumonia. Am J Respir Crit Care Med 2005;171(4):388-416.

8. Xu J, Kochanek K, Tejada-Vera B. Deaths: preliminary data from 2007. Natl Vital Stat Rep August 19, 2009;58(1). Retrieved February 7, 2011, from http://www.cdc.gov/nchs/data/nvsr/nvsr58/nvsr58_01.pdf

9. The American Thoracic Society. Guidelines for the initial management of adults with community-acquired pneumonia: diagnosis, assessment of severity, and initial antimicrobial therapy. Am J Respir Crit Care Med 2001;163(7):1730-1754.

10. Melsen WG, Rovers MM, Bonten MJ. Ventilator-associated pneumonia and mortality: a systematic review of observational studies. Crit Care Med 2009;37(10):2709-2718.

11. Campbell GD Jr. Blinded invasive diagnostic procedures in ventilator-associated pneumonia. Chest 2000;117(4 suppl 2):207S-211S.

12. American Association of Critical Care Nurses. AACN practice alert ventilator associated pneumonia. Retrieved January 15, 2011, from http://www.aacn.org/WD/Practice/Docs/PracticeAlerts/Ventilator_Associated_Pneumonia_1-2008.pdf

13. American Association of Critical Care Nurses. AACN practice alert for patients at risk for ventilator associated pneumonia. Retrieved January 15, 2011, from http://www.aacn.org/WD/Practice/Docs/PracticeAlerts/oral%20care%2004-2010%20final.pdf

14. Anthonisen N. Chronic obstructive pulmonary disease. In Goldman L, Ausiello D, editors. Cecil Textbook of Medicine. Philadelphia: Saunders; 2004:509-515.

15. World Health Organization (WHO). Chronic obstructive pulmonary disease. Retrieved February 4, 2011, from http://www.who.int/respiratory/copd/en/

16. Reilly JJ Jr, Silverman EK, Shapiro SD. Chronic obstructive pulmonary disease. In Fauci AS, Braunwald E, Kasper DL, et al, editors. Harrison's Principles of Internal Medicine. 17th edition.

Retrieved February 4, 2011, from http://www.accessmedicine.com/content.aspx?aID=2899309

17. Kamangar K, Nikhanj NS. Chronic obstructive pulmonary disease. Retrieved February 4, 2011, http://emedicine.medscape.com/article/297664-overview

18. Global Initiative for Chronic Obstructive Lung Disease (GOLD). Global strategy for the diagnosis, management, and prevention of chronic obstructive pulmonary disease. Bethesda, MD: Global Initiative for Chronic Obstructive Lung Disease (GOLD); 2008:94.

19. Halbert RJ, Natoli JL, Gano A, et al. Global burden of COPD: systematic review and meta-analysis. Eur Respir J 2006;28(3):523-532.

20. United States Centers for Disease Control. Deaths from chronic obstructive pulmonary disease: United States, 2000—2005. MMWR Morb Mortal Wkly Rep 2008;57:1229-1232.

21. US Department of Health and Human Services Public Health Service, National Institutes of Health, National Heart, Lung, and Blood Institute. Morbidity and Mortality Chartbook on Cardiovascular, Lung and Blood Diseases. Bethesda, MD: Author. Retrieved February, 7, 2011, from http://www.nhlbi.nih.gov/resources/docs/cht-book.htm

22. US Department of Labor Occupational Safety and Health Administration. Safety and Health Topics: Cadmium. Retrieved February 4, 2011, from http://www.osha.gov/SLTC/cadmium/

23. Brashers VL. Alterations of pulmonary function. In McCance K, Huether S, editors. Pathophysiology: The Biologic Basis for Disease in Adults and Children. 6th edition St Louis, MO: Elsevier Mosby; 2010:1266-1309.

24. US Preventive Services Task Force. Counseling and interventions to prevent tobacco use and tobacco-caused disease in adults and pregnant women: US Preventive Services Task Force reaffirmation recommendation statement. Ann Intern Med 2009;150(8):551-555.

25. US Food and Drug Administration. Chantix and Zyban to Get Boxed Warning on Serious Mental Health Events. Retrieved February 5, 2011, from http://www.fda.gov/ForConsumers/ConsumerUpdates/ucm170356.htm

26. Bond DC. Clinical nurse specialist–initiated smoking cessation program. Clin Nurse Spec 2005;19(2):68.

27. Ellstrom K, Halsey L, Press D, et al. Soaring to new heights in pulmonary rehabilitation: the CNS as program manager. Clin Nurse Spec 2006;20(2):88-89.

28. Drazen, JM. Asthma. In Goldman L, Bennett C, editors. Cecil Textbook of Medicine. Philadelphia: Saunders; 2008:612-619.

29. Morris MJ. Asthma. eMedicine.com. Retrieved February 7, 2011, from http://emedicine.medscape.com/article/296301-overview

30. Barnes PJ. Asthma. In Fauci AS, Braunwald E, Kasper DL, et al, editors. Harrison's Principles of Internal Medicine. 17th edition. Retrieved February 7, 2011, from http://www.accessmedicine.com/content.aspx?aID=2861512

31. World Health Organization (WHO). Asthma. Retrieved February 7, 2011, from http://www.who.int/topics/asthma/en/

32. American Lung Association. Trends in Asthma Morbidity and Mortality. Retrieved February 4, 2011, from http://www.lungusa.org/finding-cures/our-research/trend-reports/asthma-trend-report.pdf

33. Brim AN, Rudd RA, Funk RH, et al. Asthma prevalence among US children in underrepresented minority populations: American Indian/Alaska Native, Chinese, Filipino, and Asian Indian. Pediatrics 2008;122(1):e217-e222. doi:10.1542/peds.2007-3825

34. Sharma GD, Gupta P. Asthma. Retrieved February 4, 2011, from http://emedicine.medscape.com/article/1000997-overview

35. National Asthma Education and Prevention Program. Expert Panel Report 3: Guidelines for the Diagnosis and Management of Asthma. NIH Publication No. 07-4051. 2007.

36. American Lung Association. Asthma. Retrieved February 7, 2011, from http://www.lungusa.org/lung-disease/asthma/

37. Akinbami LJ, Moorman JE, Liu X. Asthma prevalence, health care use, and mortality: United States, 2005–2009. Natl Health Stat Rep 2011;32(1). Retrieved February 7, 2011, from http://www.cdc.gov/nchs/data/nhsr/nhsr032.pdf

38. Anderson SD, Pearlman DS, Rundell KW, et al. Reproducibility of the airway response to an exercise protocol standardized for intensity, duration, and inspired air conditions, in subjects with symptoms suggestive of asthma. Respir Res. Retrieved February 4, 2011, from http://respiratory-research.com/content/11/1/120

39. National Institutes of Health. Expert PANEL REPORT 3 (EPR-3): Guidelines for the Diagnosis and Management of Asthma. Retrieved February 7, 2011, from http://www.nhlbi.nih.gov/guidelines/asthma/07_sec3_comp4.pdf

40. Global Initiative for Asthma (GINA). Global Strategy for Asthma Management and Prevention. Updated 2010. Retrieved August 8, 2011 from http://www.ginasthma.org/pdf/GINA_Report_2010.pdf.

41. Reddel HK, Taylor DR, Bateman ED, et al. An official American Thoracic Society/European Respiratory Society statement: asthma control and exacerbations: standardizing endpoints for clinical asthma trials and clinical practice. Am J Respir Crit Care Med 2009;180(1):59-99.

42. Douglas NJ. Sleep apnea. In Fauci AS, Braunwald E, Kasper DL, et al, editors. Harrison's Principles of Internal Medicine. 17th edition. Retrieved February 7, 2011, from http://www.accessmedicine.com/content.aspx?aID=2869549

43. Downey R, Gold PM. Obstructive Sleep Apnea. Emedicine.com. 2009. Retrieved February 4, 2011, from http://emedicine.medscape.com/article/295807-overview

44. Downey R, Gold PM, Wickramasinghe H. Obstructive Sleep Apnea. Retrieved February 4, 2011, from http://emedicine.medscape.com/article/295807-overview

45. Johnson EO, Roth T. An epidemiologic study of sleep-disordered breathing symptoms among adolescents. Sleep 2006;29(9):1135-1142.

46. American Academy of Sleep Medicine. International Classification of Sleep Disorders: Diagnostic and Coding Manual. 2nd edition. Westchester, IL: American Academy of Sleep Medicine, 2005.

47. Schwab RJ, Pasirstein M, Pierson R, et al. Identification of upper airway anatomic risk factors for obstructive sleep apnea with volumetric magnetic resonance imaging. Am J Respir Crit Care Med 2003;168(5):522-530.

48. Freedman DS, Khan LK, Serdula MK, et al. Trends and correlates of class 3 obesity in the United States from 1990 through 2000. JAMA 2002;288(14):1758-1761.

49. Becker HF, Jerrentrup A, Ploch T, et al. Effect of nasal continuous positive airway pressure treatment on blood pressure in patients with obstructive sleep apnea. Circulation 2003;107(1):68-73.

50. Shahar E, Whitney CW, Redline S, et al. Sleep-disordered breathing and cardiovascular disease: cross-sectional results

of the Sleep Heart Health Study. Am J Respir Crit Care Med 2001;163(1):19-25.

51. Vasu TS, Doghramji K, Cavallazzi R, et al. Obstructive sleep apnea syndrome and postoperative complications: clinical use of the STOP-BANG questionnaire. Arch Otolaryngol Head Neck Surg 2010;136(10):1020-1024.

52. Rich S. Pulmonary hypertension. In Fauci AS, Braunwald E, Kasper DL, et al, editors. Harrison's Principles of Internal Medicine. 17th edition. Retrieved February 4, 2011, from http://www.accessmedicine.com/content.aspx?aID=2883094

53. Oudiz RJ. Pulmonary Hypertension, Primary, 2010. Retrieved February 4, 2011, from http://emedicine.medscape.com/article/301450-overview

54. Kamangar N, Pirouz S. Pulmonary Hypertension, Secondary, 2010. Retrieved February 4, 2011, from http://emedicine.medscape.com/article/303098-overview 4

55. World Health Organization (WHO). Chronic Respiratory Diseases. Retrieved February 5, 2011, from http://www.who.int/gard/publications/chronic_respiratory_diseases.pdf

56. Battle RW, Davitt MA, Cooper SM, et al. Prevalence of pulmonary hypertension in limited and diffuse scleroderma. Chest 1996;110(6):1515-1519.

57. Hyduk A, Croft JB, Ayala C, et al. Pulmonary hypertension surveillance: United States, 1980-2002. MMWR Surveill Summ 2005;54:1.

58. Gokhale S, Choudhary G. Pulmonary hypertension. In Ferri's Clinical Advisor. Retrieved February 5, 2011, from http://www.merckmedicus.com/pp/us/hcp/thcp_ferri_content.jsp?pg=/ppdocs/us/hcp/content/ferri/B9780323056090000253/ferri-834A.htm

59. Workman LM. Care of patients with noninfectious lower respiratory problems. In Ignatavicius DD, Workman LM, editors. 6th edition. Medical-Surgical Nursing: Patient-Centered Collaborative Care. St Louis: Elsevier Mosby; 2010:508-570.

60. Minna JD, Schiller JH. Neoplasms of the lung. In Fauci AS, Braunwald E, Kasper DL, et al. editors. Harrison's Principles of Internal Medicine. 17th edition. Retrieved February 4, 2011, from http://www.accessmedicine.com/content.aspx?aID=2889473

61. Huq S, Maghfoor I. Lung Cancer, Non-Small Cell. eMedicine. 2010. Retrieved February 4, 2011, from http://emedicine.medscape.com/article/279960-overview

62. American Cancer Society. Cancer Facts and Figures 2008. American Cancer Society. Retrieved February 4, 2011, from http://www.cancer.org/downloads/STT/2008CAFFfinalsecured.pdf

63. Beckles MA, et al. Initial evaluation of the patient with lung cancer: symptoms, signs, laboratory tests, and paraneoplastic syndromes. Chest 2003;97S-104S.

64. Patel J, Bach P, Kris M: Lung cancer in US women: a contemporary epidemic. JAMA 2004;291(14):1763-1768.

65. Zhong L, Goldberg MS, Parent ME, et al. Exposure to environmental tobacco smoke and the risk of lung cancer: a meta-analysis. Lung Cancer 2000;27(1):3-18.

66. American Joint Committee on cancer. Lung. In AJCC Cancer Staging Manual. 5th edition. Philadelphia: Lippincott-Raven; 2007:127-137.

67. Mountain CF. Revisions in the International System for Staging Lung Cancer. Chest 1997;111(6):1710-1717.

68. Mancini MC. Blunt Chest Trauma, 2008. Retrieved February 5, 2011, from http://emedicine.medscape.com

69. Rohit S, Galla JD. Penetrating Chest Trauma, 2008. Retrieved February 5, 2011, from http://emedicine.medscape.com

70. Gavant ML, Menke PG, Fabian T, et al. Blunt traumatic aortic rupture: detection with helical CT of the chest. Radiology 1995;197(1):125-133.

71. Omert L, Yeaney WW, Protetch J. Efficacy of thoracic computerized tomography in blunt chest trauma. Am Surg 2001;67(7):660-664.

72. Parker MS, Matheson TL, Rao AV, et al. Making the transition: the role of helical CT in the evaluation of potentially acute thoracic aortic injuries. AJR Am J Roentgenol 2001;176(5):1267-1272.

73. Centers for Disease Control and Prevention. Accidents/Unintentional Injuries. Retrieved February 7, 2011, from http://www.cdc.gov/nchs/FASTATS/acc-inj.htm

74. LoCicero J 3rd, Mattox KL. Epidemiology of chest trauma. Surg Clin North Am 1989;69(1):15-19.

75. Demetriades D, Kimbrell B, Salim A. trauma deaths in a mature urban trauma system: is "trimodal" distribution a valid concept? J Am Coll Surg 2005;201(3):343-348.

76. Shahani R, Galla J. Penetrating Chest Trauma, 2008. Retrieved October 23, 2008, from www.emedicine.medscape.com

77. Biffl WL, Moore EE, Harken AH. Emergency department thoracotomy. In Mattox KL, Feliciano DV, Moore EE, editors. Trauma. 4th edition New York: McGraw-Hill; 2000:245-258.

78. Gropper MA, Wiener-Kronish JP, Hashimoto S. Acute cardiogenic pulmonary edema. Clin Chest Med 1994;15(3):501-515.

79. Mattu A, Martinez JP, Kelly BS. Modern management of cardiogenic pulmonary edema. Emerg Med Clin North Am 2005;23(4):1105-1125.

80. Morrison LK, Harrison A, Krishnaswamy P, et al. Utility of a rapid B-natriuretic peptide assay in differentiating congestive heart failure from lung disease in patients presenting with dyspnea. J Am Coll Cardiol 2002;39(2):202-209.

81. Ray P, Arthaud M, Birolleau S, et al. Comparison of brain natriuretic peptide and probrain natriuretic peptide in the diagnosis of cardiogenic pulmonary edema in patients aged 65 and older. J Am Geriatr Soc 2005;53(4):643-648.

82. Sacchetti A, Ramoska E, Moakes ME. Effect of ED management on ICU use in acute pulmonary edema. Am J Emerg Med 1999;17(6):571-574.

83. Sovari AA, Kocheril AG, Baas AS. Pulmonary Edema, Cardiogenic. Retrieved April 22, 2008, from www.emedicine.medscape.com

84. Khan AN, Kasthuri RS, MacDonald S. Pulmonary Edema, Noncardiogenic. Retrieved May 7, 2008, from www.emedicine.medscape.com

85. Naik TK, Soo Hoo GW, Sharma S. Pulmonary Edema, Neurogenic. Retrieved September 28, 2009, from www.emedicine.medscape.com

86. Hochman JS, Ingbar DH. Cardiogenic shock and pulmonary edema. In Fauci AS, Braunwald E, Kasper DL, et al, editors. Harrison's Principles of Internal Medicine. 17th edition. Retrieved September 2009 from http://www.accessmedicine.com/content.aspx?aID=2862597

87. Binanay C, Califf RM, Hasselblad V, et al. Evaluation study of congestive heart failure and pulmonary artery catheterization effectiveness: The ESCAPE trial. JAMA 2005;294(5):1625-1633.

88. Ferri FF. Ferri's Clinical Advisor: Instant Diagnosis and Treatment. Pulmonary Edema. Retrieved February 7, 2011, from http://www.merckmedicus.com/pp/us/hcp/thcp_ferri_content.jsp?pg=/ppdocs/us/hcp/content/ferri/B9780323056090000253/ferri-828B.htm

89. Essig MG. Brain Natriuretic Peptide (BNP) Test. Retrieved June 19, 2007, from http://health.yahoo.com/heart-diagnosis/brain-natriuretic-peptide-bnp-test/healthwise—ux1072.html

90. Costanzo MR, Guglin ME, Saltzberg MT, et al. Ultrafiltration versus intravenous diuretics for patients hospitalized for acute decompensated heart failure. J Am Coll Cardiol 2007;49(6):675-683.

91. Anthonisen N. Chronic obstructive pulmonary disease. In Goldman L, Bennett C, editors. Cecil Textbook of Medicine. Philadelphia: Saunders; 2008:619-627.

92. Esteban A, et al: Noninvasive positive-pressure ventilation for respiratory failure after extubation. N Engl J Med 2004;350:2452.

93. Harrison's Practice: Answers on Demand. Principles of Critical Care Medicine. Retrieved February 7, 2011, from http://www.unboundmedicine.com/hpmerck/ub/view/Harrison's_Principles_of_Internal_Medicine_17th_Edition/Principles_of_Critical_Care_Medicine/395261/2

94. Ata MK, Sat S. Respiratory Failure. Retrieved May 20, 2009, from http://emedicine.medscape.com

95. Girault C, Briel A, Benichou J, et al. Interface strategy during noninvasive positive pressure ventilation for hypercapnic acute respiratory failure. Crit Care Med 2009;37(1):124-131.

96. Keenan SP, Kernerman PD, Cook DJ, et al. Effect of noninvasive positive pressure ventilation on mortality in patients admitted with acute respiratory failure: a meta-analysis. Crit Care Med 1997;25(10):1685-1692.

97. Burns SM, Fahey SA, Barton DM, et al. Weaning from mechanical ventilation: a method for assessment and planning. AACN Clin Iss 1991;2:372-387.

98. Hanneman SK. Weaning from short-term mechanical ventilation. Crit Care Nurse 2004;24:70-73.

Endocrine Problems

Celia Levesque, RN, MSN, CNS-BC, CDE, BC-ADM

INTRODUCTION

The endocrine system consists of five glands situated throughout the body, to include the pituitary, thyroid, parathyroid, pancreas, and adrenal glands. There are a host of diseases and conditions that arise from endocrine gland dysfunction and these are generally discreet, with differing clinical presentation and management approaches depending on the endocrine gland of concern. Most, however, cause multisystem involvement, owing to the complicated positive or negative feedback systems that suppress or stimulate hormone secretion and the effect on the target end-organs. This chapter focuses on the more common pathologies and includes diabetes mellitus types 1 and 2, adrenal insufficiency, hyper- and hypoparathyroidism, hyper- and hypothyroidism, syndrome of inappropriate antidiuretic hormone, and diabetes insipidus. Numerous problems stem from diabetes mellitus alone, including diabetic ketoacisosis, hyperglycemic hyperosmolar nonketotic syndrome, and hypoglycemia, which will also be covered in the chapter.

Life-threatening complications can occur from all of these disorders, and as a result, clinical nurse specialists (CNSs) are often called upon to assist with clinical management to prevent these problems and to intervene during emergent situations. Coaching, teaching, and mentoring patients and nurses are important parts of prevention. Systemwide implementation of research-based practice guidelines is another important role played by CNSs when caring for this patient population.

TYPE 1 AND TYPE 2 DIABETES MELLITUS

Etiology

Diabetes is a heterogeneous group of metabolic disorders caused by a defect in insulin secretion, insulin action, or both. Although many types of diabetes exist, all are associated with abnormal carbohydrate, protein, and fat metabolism and with hyperglycemia. Hyperglycemia

increases the risk of long-term diabetes complications such as cardiovascular disease (CVD), diabetic retinopathy, diabetic nephropathy, and neuropathy. Most diabetes cases fall into one of two categories: type 1 diabetes mellitus (T1DM) or type 2 diabetes mellitus (T2DM) (1, 2). T1DM is subcategorized into types 1A and 1B (2).

Normal fasting glucose levels are maintained between 70 and 100 mg/dL via a negative-feedback system. Insulin, produced by pancreatic beta cells, is the primary hormone that suppresses hepatic glucose production, lipolysis, and proteolysis. Basal plasma insulin maintains hepatic glucose release at a rate of 1.9 to 2.1 mg/kg/min, a rate that provides adequate glucose for the brain, which uses approximately 50% of basal glucose. Insulin facilitates the transport of glucose into adipocytes and myocytes and stimulates glycogen synthesis. In the postprandial state, approximately 85% of ingested glucose enters the systemic circulation, increasing the arterial glucose concentration and stimulating insulin release. Insulin travels from the pancreas to the liver, via the portal vein, where it undergoes the first-pass effect. During this process, half of the insulin is extracted by the liver, which suppresses hepatic glucose release. The unextracted insulin enters the systemic circulation, stimulating glucose uptake (primarily by muscle) and decreasing lipolysis and proteolysis. If blood glucose levels fall below basal concentrations, insulin production decreases, which triggers glucagon production to increase hepatic glucose release (3).

Other hormones help regulate blood glucose. Somatostatin, for example, controls insulin and glucagon release. Epinephrine and norepinephrine regulate glucose metabolism from storage depots, promoting glycogenolysis and lipolysis and the release of free fatty acids. Cortisol, a catabolic steroid hormone released in response to hypoglycemia or heavy exercise, causes gluconeogenesis, inhibits protein synthesis, and promotes the release of free fatty acids. Growth hormone stimulates cells to grow and divide, stimulates protein synthesis, and increases the rate of fat usage by cells. It also enhances synthesis of glucose in the liver, decreasing insulin's ability to stimulate the uptake of glucose in peripheral tissues. Thyroxin regulates the metabolism of lipids, proteins, and carbohydrates in cells, enhances protein synthesis and lipid metabolism, and stimulates cells to use carbohydrate as an energy source. It helps convert glycogen to glucose and enhances absorption of glucose from the intestines. (See Table 11-1.)

In the United States, 23.6 million people over age 20 (10.7% of the age group) have diabetes: 17.9 million are diagnosed and 5.7 million are undiagnosed. Another 57 million Americans have prediabetes. In 2007, Americans newly diagnosed with diabetes included 1.6 million over age 20 and 186,300 less than age 20. One of every six overweight American adolescents have prediabetes (4).

TABLE 11–1 Hormones Involved in Maintaining Normal Glucose Homeostasis (5)

Hormone	Produced by:	Function	Effect on blood glucose
Insulin	Beta cell of the islets of Langerhans	Anabolic hormone that lowers glucose Stimulates glycogenesis Increases protein synthesis Facilitates diffusion of glucose into cells Antagonistic to gluconeogenesis	Decreases
Glucagon	Alpha cells of the islets of Langerhans	Stimulates the liver to release glucose by glycogenolysis Involved in glucogenolysis	Increases
Somatostatin	Delta cells of the islets of Langerhans	Controls glucose metabolism by inhibiting secretion of insulin and glucagon	Neutral
Epinephrine/ norepinephrine	Adrenal medulla	Regulates glucose metabolism from storage depots Promotes glycogenolysis Promotes lipolysis and release of free fatty acids	Increases
Cortisol	Cells of the middle layer of adrenal cortex	Catabolic steroid hormone that is released in response to hypoglycemia or heavy exercise Causes gluconeogenesis Inhibits protein synthesis Promotes release of free fatty acids	Increases
Growth hormone (somatotropin)	Anterior pituitary	Stimulates cells to grow and divide Stimulates protein synthesis Increases the rate of fat usage by cells Decreases the rate of usage of carbohydrate by cells	Increases
Thyroxine	Follicular cells of the thyroid	Regulates the metabolism of lipids, proteins, and carbohydrates in cells Enhances protein synthesis and lipid metabolism and stimulates cells to use carbohydrate as an energy source	Decreases

T1DM is one of the most common chronic diseases in children and adolescence; 1 of every 400 to 600 U.S. children and adolescents has T1DM (4). Approximately 90% of T1DM cases are immune-mediated (type 1A), and 10% are idiopathic (type 1B) (5). More than 13,000 new cases are diagnosed in the United States annually. The highest incidence of T1DM occurs in Scandinavia and northern Europe, where the incidence in those younger than 14 years is 37 per 100,000 (6). The peak incidence for the development of T1DM occurs at age 14 years, although the disease may occur at any age (2). Two million U.S. adolescents aged 11 to 19 years have prediabetes (4). In those with T2DM aged 20 years or older, 14.9 million (9.8%) are non-Hispanic whites and 3.7 million (14.7%) are non-Hispanic African Americans (4). The American Indian Service conducted a national survey from 2004 to 2006 to determine the number of people with diagnosed diabetes according to race (7, 8). (See Table 11-2.)

Multiple factors come into play in determining the cause of T1DM, including the presence of several genes known to increase the risk of T1DM and the absence of protective genes. Because some people with high-risk genes do not develop T1DM, it is theorized that a "trigger" causes the autoimmune attack of the pancreatic beta cells. Although 80% of people with T1DM do not have a family history of the disease, having such a history increases the risk of development (Table 11-3).

Having another autoimmune disease such as thyroid disease or celiac disease also increases the risk. Studies are under way to determine whether exposure to cow's milk during the first year of life increases the likelihood of

TABLE 11–3 Familial Risk of Developing Type 1 Diabetes Mellitus (2)

Relationship to proband	Risk (%)
Identical twin	25–50
Dizygotic twins	6
Father	6
Sibling	5
Offspring	5
Mother	3
General population	0.2–0.4

developing T1DM. Furthermore, viruses such as coxsackie B, enterovirus, adenovirus, rubella, cytomegalovirus, and Epstein-Barr have been linked to the development of T1DM (7). Factors that increase the likelihood of developing T2DM include increasing age, obesity, physical inactivity, members of certain racial/ethnic populations, a history of hypertension, high-density lipoprotein (HDL) cholesterol level of less than 35 mg/dL or triglycerides level of greater than 250 mg/dL, a family history of T2DM, and previous gestational diabetes (5).

The cost of medical care for people with diabetes is 2.3 times higher than the cost for those who do not have the disease. The total direct cost of diabetes in the United States in 2007 was estimated to be $116 billion: $27 attributed to direct medical expenses, $58 billion for treatment of chronic diabetes-related complications, and $31 billion for excess general medical costs (Figure 11-1).

Of the cost for direct diabetes care, 50% was due to hospitalization, 11% for diabetes medication and supplies,

TABLE 11–2 Indian Health Service 2004–2006 Survey: Diabetes Statistics Age 20 Years and Older (4, 7)

Race	Percentage With Diagnosed Diabetes
Non-Hispanic white	6.6
Asian American	7.5
Hispanic	10.4
Non-Hispanic African American	11.8
American Indian and Alaska Native	14.2
Cuban	8.2
Mexican American	11.9
Puerto Rican	11.6

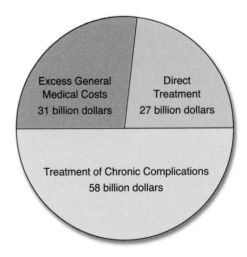

FIGURE 11–1: Cost of diabetes mellitus in the United States.

11% for prescriptions to treat chronic diabetes-related complications, and 9% for physician office visits. In addition, the cost of lost productivity at work was about $31.1 billion, and the cost of lost productivity from premature death was about $26.9 billion (Figure 11-2).

Many indirect costs were not included in these estimates such as those for over-the-counter medications, pain, suffering, reduced quality of life for the patient and significant others, care provided by nonpaid caregivers, medical costs of undiagnosed diabetes, diabetes research, administrative costs, and clinical training programs (9).

Pathophysiology

Type 1A diabetes is a genetically influenced and immunologically mediated disease with a variable pre-type 1 stage. The human leukocyte antigen (HLA) region is a cluster of genes on chromosome 6 that encode proteins used by the immune system to differentiate self from nonself. The HLA region is part of the major histocompatibility complex (MHC), a large gene family that plays an important role in the immune system and autoimmunity. Proteins that are encoded by the MHC are expressed on cell surfaces and display chains of amino acids called antigens that are analyzed by T cells. MHC class I chains assemble from inside cells, whereas MHC class II chains assemble from outside the cells.

T cells normally bind to and attack foreign threats such as viruses, bacteria, and tumor cells. In autoimmune diseases such as T1DM, T cells bind to chains from the body's healthy cells. HLA alleles in T1DM may increase or decrease the risk of diabetes or have no effect (10). The presence of certain HLA alleles can account for more than half of the genetic risk of developing T1DM. The genes encoding MHC class II proteins are most strongly linked with diabetes and include *HLA-DR*, *HLA-DQ*, and *HLA-DP*. Only half of the general population inherits a copy (allele) of the *DR* gene (*DR3* or *DR4*), and less than

3% have two alleles. Approximately 95% of individuals with T1DM have at least one *DR3* or *DR4* allele; those possessing both *DR3* and *DR4* alleles are particularly susceptible to developing T1DM. Inheriting the *DR2* allele, however, is protective. The alleles of the *DQ* gene either increase or decrease the risk of T1DM. The protective alleles of *DR* and *DQ* tend to be inherited together. (See Table 11-4.)

One or more markers of beta cell destruction can be detected in 85% to 90% of individuals with T1DM at the onset of hyperglycemia and include islet cell autoantibodies, autoantibodies to insulin, autoantibodies against the 65-kDa isoform of glutamic acid decarboxylase (GAD65), and autoantibodies to tyrosine phosphatases IA-2 and IA-2beta (Table 11-5).

Autoimmune destruction of beta cells may be triggered by an environmental factor such as mumps, rubella, coxsackie B4, toxic chemicals, exposure to cow's milk in infancy, and cytotoxins (3). Progressive impairment of insulin release occurs until approximately 85% of the beta cells are destroyed. Once 85% to 90% of the beta cells are destroyed, hyperglycemia develops, causing signs and symptoms of overt diabetes. Once insulin therapy is initiated, the patient may have a "honeymoon" period, during which beta cell function temporarily improves insulin secretion. Eventually, all beta cells are destroyed, causing absolute insulin deficiency (Figure 11-3).

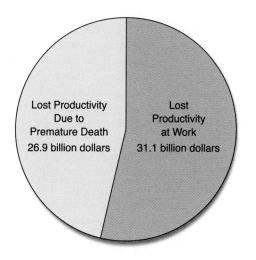

FIGURE 11-2: Lost productivity secondary to diabetes mellitus.

Lost Productivity Due to Premature Death 26.9 billion dollars

Lost Productivity at Work 31.1 billion dollars

TABLE 11-4 Risk of Type 1A Diabetes Based on DR and DQ Haplotypes

DRB1	DQA1	DQB1
HIGH RISK		
0401, 0403, or 0405	0301	0302 (DQ8)
0301	0501	0201 (DQ2)
MODERATE RISK		
0801	0401	0402
0404	0301	0302
0101	0101	0501
0901	0301	0303
STRONG PROTECTION		
1501	0102	0602 (dq6)
1401	0101	0503
0701	0201	0303

HLA-DRB1, -DQA1, and -DQB1 loci are the major genetic determinants of type 1 diabetes. Specific combinations of alleles determine risk.

TABLE 11–5 Comparison of Islet Autoantibodies and Genetics in Type 1A, Type 1B, and Type 2 Diabetes Mellitus

Type	Islet Autoantibodies	Genetics	Comment
1A	Positive >90%	30–50% have DR3 and DR4 90% have DR3 or DR4 <3% have DQBI*0602	90% non-Hispanic white children 50% black children 50% Latino-American children
1B	Negative	Unknown	Rare in whites
2	Negative	Not fully understood	If Ab+, consider latent autoimmune diabetes in adults (LADA) and human leukocyte antigen (HLA) similar to T1DM

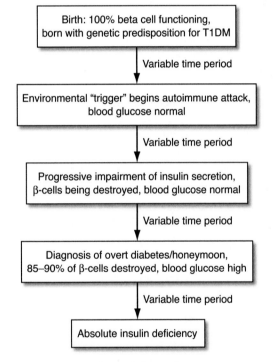

FIGURE 11–3: Beta cell destruction.

T2DM occurs when the beta cells cannot secrete enough insulin to maintain euglycemia because of a combination of factors that include relative insulin deficiency and peripheral and hepatic insulin resistance that leads to hyperglycemia. It is unclear whether insulin resistance leads to beta cell dysfunction or whether beta cell dysfunction leads to insulin resistance because both occur long before hyperglycemia. Early in the disease process, hyperinsulinemia is present with hyperglycemia, primarily due to hepatic insulin resistance. At diagnosis, insulin levels may be low, normal, or high. Autoimmune destruction of beta cells does not occur with this type of diabetes; however, insulin secretion is defective. Decreased insulin secretion reduces insulin signaling in its target tissues; in response, levels of glucose and fatty acids increase, further reducing insulin secretion and enhancing insulin resistance.

Most people with T2DM are obese, and obesity is strongly associated with insulin resistance. Excess fat, however, is stored not only in adipocytes, but also in myocytes, and intramyocellular lipids have been associated with skeletal muscle insulin resistance. Adipose tissue is not merely a site for the storage of excess energy in the form of triglycerides; it secretes a variety of endocrine and panacrine substances that effect metabolism. Leptin, for example, a 16-kDa protein synthesized mainly in adipose tissue, suppresses feeding behavior. People with mutations associated with leptin are morbidly obese and insulin-resistant. Adiponectin, a protein hormone secreted into the bloodstream and produced exclusively by adipose tissue, modulates many metabolic processes, including glucose regulation and fatty acid metabolism. Low levels of adiponectin are associated with obesity and increased risk of myocardial infarction.

Resistin is also produced and released by adipose tissue, and serum levels increase with obesity. Elevated resistin levels are linked to insulin resistance and contribute to the inflammatory response by causing the release of proinflammatory cytokines such as interleukin (IL)-1, IL-6, IL-11, and tumor necrosis factor-α (TNF-α). IL-6 is secreted by T cells, macrophages, and adipocytes and acts as a proinflammatory and anti-inflammatory cytokine. High levels of IL-6 are correlated with increased adiposity, insulin resistance, hepatic glucose production, lipolysis, and fatty acid oxidation (5). TNF-α is released by multiple tissues, including adipocytes, and performs various functions on many organ systems. For example, TNF-α induces insulin resistance by promoting serine phosphorylation in insulin receptor substrate-1, causing impairment of insulin signaling. Monocyte chemotactic protein-1, also present in adipose tissue and at levels proportional to the amount of this tissue, increases insulin resistance by inhibiting insulin action.

A positive family history of T2DM increases the risk of developing T2DM 2- to 4-fold. Genetically, T2DM consists of a monogenic and a polygenic form; most people with this disease have the polygenic form.

Clinical Presentation

The presence and/or severity of the signs and symptoms of T1DM and T2DM are directly related to the severity and duration of hyperglycemia. Many individuals with T2DM have no symptoms, especially those who are obese, whereas signs and symptoms are often severe in people with T1DM, particularly when newly diagnosed (11) (Table 11-6). Common signs and symptoms include glycosuria, polyuria, nocturnal enuresis, polydipsia, polyphagia, weakness, fatigue, weight loss, blurred vision, vulvovaginitis, pruritis, peripheral neuropathy, impotence, and diabetic ketoacidosis (DKA). Glycosuria occurs when the blood glucose level increases above the renal threshold (usually 160 to 180 mg/dL) and the proximal tubules are unable to reabsorb all of the glucose. Polyuria

TABLE 11–6 Clinical Connections: Type 1 and Type 2 Diabetes

Clinical Manifestations	Pathophysiology	Assessment Finding	Laboratory Diagnostic Tests	Treatment
Hyperglycemia	Relative or absolute lack of insulin	Blood glucose level >116 mg/dL fasting or >200 mg/dL postprandial	Blood glucose	Diet, exercise, medications
Polyuria	Osmotic diuresis occurring when the blood glucose level exceeds the renal threshold	Frequently urinates large volumes of urine	Output measurement	Control blood glucose to below the renal threshold
Polydipsia	The hypothalamus regulates thirst in the ventromedial nucleus by sensing serum osmolality and relaying it to the cortex used by the serum. Serum osmolality increases with hyperglycemia and dehydration from osmotic diuresis.	Person with diabetes drinks an excessive amount of fluid secondary to increased thirst	Intake measurement	Control blood glucose to below the renal threshold
Polyphagia	Can be caused by weight loss from hyperglycemia or hypoglycemia	Person with diabetes reports excessive hunger and consumes an increased amount of food	Subjective medical history	Control blood glucose to below the renal threshold
Weight loss	The lack of insulin causes cell starvation with subsequent breakdown of adipose tissue into free fatty acids and ketones.	Positive urine ketone, decreased body weight	Weight	Control blood glucose to below the renal threshold

Continued

TABLE 11–6 Clinical Connections: Type 1 and Type 2 Diabetes—cont'd

Clinical Manifestations	Pathophysiology	Assessment Finding	Laboratory Diagnostic Tests	Treatment
Glycosuria	Blood glucose level has exceeded the renal threshold	Urine glucose positive	Urinanalysis	Control blood glucose to below the renal threshold
Weakness, fatigue	Hyperglycemia	Person with diabetes reports weakness/fatigue	Subjective medical history	Control blood glucose to below the renal threshold
Blurred vision	Lens in the eye is sensitive to fluctuations in blood glucose level	Decreased visual acuity	Snellen eye chart	Control blood glucose to prevent wide fluctuations in blood glucose
Increased infections and delayed wound healing	Hyperglycemia impairs immune cell response to injury	Increased risk of infection and delayed healing	Medical history, physical, specific tests for various infections	Control blood glucose
Diabetic ketoacidosis	Insulin deficiency causes breakdown of fat into ketones	Signs and symptoms of diabetic ketoacidosis (Table 11-48)	See Table 11-48	Insulin therapy, electrolyte replacement

is secondary to osmotic diuresis caused by glucose excretion into the urine. Nocturnal enuresis is common in young children newly diagnosed with T1DM. Polydipsia, weakness, fatigue, and blurred vision are secondary to the hyperosmolar state. Polyphagia with weight loss is common with T1DM, whereas polyphagia with weight gain is common in T2DM. Women with T2DM often have vulvovaginitis; men may have impotence. Neurotoxicity from sustained hyperglycemia may cause neuropathies. If insulin deficiency is severe, DKA may occur, causing severe dehydration, anorexia, nausea, vomiting, Kussmaul respiration, acidosis, altered consciousness, severe circulatory collapse, and death.

Diagnosis

Until recently, diabetes was diagnosed on the basis of blood glucose levels alone (Table 11-7).

A fasting blood glucose level of greater than 125 mg/dL or a postprandial blood glucose level of greater than 199 mg/dL is still diagnostic of diabetes; however, use of the hemoglobin A1c (HbA1c) test can also be diagnostic. In the past, the HbA1c test was not used to diagnose diabetes because it had not been standardized. The International Expert Committee, made up of experts appointed by the American Diabetes Association, the European Association for the Study of Diabetes, and the International Diabetes Federation, met in 2008 to consider both current and future methods for diagnosing diabetes. The experts agreed that an HbA1c test result of 6.5% or greater, determined by a method certified by the National Glycohemoglobin Standardization Program and traceable to the Diabetes Control and Complications Trial (DCCT) reference assay, is diagnostic of diabetes in nonpregnant people. An HbA1c result of greater than 6.5% is also correlated with increased risk of retinopathy. Point-of-care HbA1c tests are not recommended for diagnosis of diabetes because they are not certified by the National Glycohemoglobin Standardization Program. The patient does not need to fast for the HbA1c test. If the result is 6.5% or greater, the test should be repeated to rule out laboratory error. The HbA1c can be inaccurate in people with hemolytic anemia, blood loss, and hemoglobinopathies (Table 11-8), so in these cases, the blood glucose level will need to be used for diagnosis (3, 6).

The HbA1c test is based on measurement of chronic hyperglycemia. In the normal 120-day life span of the red blood cell, glucose molecules join hemoglobin, forming glycated hemoglobin. Once a hemoglobin molecule is

TABLE 11–7 Diagnostic Criteria for Diabetes in the Nonpregnant Person

In the absence of unequivocal hyperglycemia, these criteria should be confirmed by repeat testing on a different day.

Fasting plasma glucose, ≥125 mg/dL (7.0 mmol/L). "Fasting" is defined as no caloric intake for at least 8 hrs.

Or

Symptoms of hyperglycemia and a casual plasma glucose >199 mg/dL (11.1 mmol/L). "Casual" is defined as any time of day without regard to time since last meal.

Or

2-hr plasma glucose, ≥200 mg/dL (11.1 mmol/L) during an oral glucose tolerance test. The test should be performed as described by the World Health Organization by using a glucose load containing the equivalent of 75 g of anhydrous glucose dissolved in water.

Or

Hemoglobin A1c (HbA1c), ≥6.5% on 2 occasions

TABLE 11–8 Factors Interfering With Chromatographic Measurement of Glycohemoglobin

Substances that cause falsely high values
Prehemoglobin A1c (reversible aldimine intermediate)
Carbamoylated hemoglobin (uremia)
Hemoglobin F
Conditions that cause falsely low values
Hemoglobinopathies (hemoglobins C, D, and S)
Reduced life span of erythrocytes
Hemorrhage or therapeutic phlebotomies
Hemolytic disorders

familiar with when they perform home glucose monitoring (6). Point-of-care testing has shown to produce improved outcomes in diabetes self-management (11-15).

Serum fructosamine, formed by nonenzymatic glycosylation of serum proteins (predominately albumin), is used to measure the average glucose level over a 2- to 3-week period. It is useful in looking at glycemic control at conception, during pregnancy, and when evaluating glycemia after a treatment change is desired sooner than the HbA1c would reflect (1). Table 11-9 provides a risk assessment for gestational diabetes and Table 11-10 provides an explanation for interpretation of blood glucose values in in diagnosing gestational diabetes.

Besides management of pregnant women, assessment of fructosamine levels may be uselful in the presence of abnormal hemoglobins or hemolytic states. Caution is advised in the interpretation of these values, as fruc-

glycated, it remains that way. A buildup of glycated hemoglobin within the red blood cell reflects the average level of glucose to which the cell has been exposed during its life cycle. Measuring HbA1c assesses the effectiveness of therapy by monitoring long-term serum glucose regulation. The HbA1c level is proportional to the average blood glucose concentration over the previous 1 to 3 months. The test assumes that the red blood cell life span is normal, that no blood loss or transfusions have occurred recently, and that the mix of hemoglobin subtypes is normal.

The American Diabetes Association recommends testing HbA1c at diagnosis and every 3 months until the patient's glycemic targets have been reached and twice yearly in those who have achieved glycemic targets and are stable. Results should be reported to patients using the same terms (e.g., mg/dL or mmol/L) that patients are

TABLE 11–9 Risk Assessment for Gestational Diabetes

Those meeting the following criteria do not need glucose testing at the time of assessment.
Age <25 years
Normal body weight
No first-degree relatives with diabetes
No history of abnormal glucose metabolism
No history of poor obstetric outcome
Not members of an ethnic/racial group with a high prevalence of diabetes (e.g., Hispanic American, Native American, Asian American, African American, Pacific Islander)

TABLE 11–10 Diagnosis of Gestational Diabetes With a 75-Gram or 100-Gram Glucose Load

Two or more of the venous plasma concentrations must meet or exceed the limits for a diagnosis to be made. The patient should be fasting for 8–14 hours after a 3-day unrestricted diet of at least 150 grams of carbohydrate per day and unrestricted activity. The patient should sit during the test and refrain from smoking.

Glucose Load	mg/dL	Mmol/L
100-g		
Fasting	95	5.3
1 hr	180	10
2 hr	155	8.6
3 hr	140	7.8
75-g		
Fasting	180	5.3
1 hr	155	10
2 hr	140	8.6

tosamine levels are usually falsely low if a person is malnourished, severely burned, or has low albumin, hyperthyroidism, hemolysis, or erratic fluctuations in blood glucose level. Fructosamine levels are often falsely high when levels of serum albumin or IgA are elevated or in patients with cirrhosis or hepatitis (15, 16). Estimated Average Glucose (EAG), developed in the A1c-Derived Average Glucose (ADAG) study, is the ratio between HbA1c and the average glucose level (17). The correlation of EAG, using two methods of measurement, mg/dl and mmol/L, and fructosamine is found in Table 11-11.

Historically, ketone testing of urine and blood was a mainstay of the diagnostic plan and evaluation of treatment effectiveness. However, there is limited usefulness of ketone testing in the management of diabetes and it is not used in the diagnostic work-up. Commercial products that test for urine ketones such as Ketostix use nitroprusside, which reacts only with acetoacetate, not with beta-hydroxybutyrate. These two ketones normally exist in equilibrium, but beta-hydroxybutyrate levels are 3 to 5 times greater in DKA. This test for ketones is useful only in diagnosing early DKA; it is not useful in monitoring response to DKA treatment because the excess beta-hydroxybutyrate is converted back to acetoacetate as the patient improves biochemically. Ketones may appear in the urine for other reasons besides DKA such as starvation, high-fat diets, alcoholic ketoacidosis, fever, and other conditions that increase metabolism. Serum ketone can be used to detect levels of beta-hydroxybutyrate, as well as acetone and acetoacetate levels. The Precision Xtra Blood Glucose & Ketone Monitoring System (Abbott Diabetes Care, Inc., Alameda, CA) gives patients the ability to test for beta-hydroxybutyrate at home.

Management
Treatment Goals

The ultimate goal of diabetes treatment is to prevent or delay acute and chronic complications. This means hyperglycemia must be managed, as well as the comorbid conditions associated with diabetes. Choosing target blood glucose and HbA1c goals is the first step in managing hyperglycemia, using either standard values or with a customized approach. Custom glycemic targets are important for people with a limited life expectancy, history of severe hypoglycemia, advanced macrovascular or microvascular complications, or significant comorbid conditions. Custom glycemic targets are also important for patients who have long-standing and difficult-to-control diabetes, even after they receive diabetes self-management education, follow an appropriate diabetes medication regimen, and use glucose self-monitoring.

TABLE 11–11 Comparison of HbA1c, Estimated Average Glucose, and Fructosamine

HbA1c (%)	Estimated Average Glucose (mg/dL)	Estimated Average Glucose (mmol/L)	Fructosamine (µmol)
5	97	5.4	199
6	116	7.0	258
7	154	8.6	317
8	183	10.2	375
9	211	11.8	461
10	240	13.4	493
11	269	14.9	552
12	298	16.5	611

In patients who do not need custom target blood glucose goals, the premeal blood glucose level should be 70 to 140 mg/dL, the 2-hour postprandial level should be less than 160 mg/dL, and the bedtime level should be 100 to 140 mg/dL. The American Diabetes Association recommends an HbA1c level of less than 7%, and the International Diabetes Federation recommends a level of less than 6.5% for most patients; neither of these HbA1c levels is in the nondiabetic range. These recommended HbA1c levels were based on several trials, including the Diabetes Control and Complications Trial (DCCT) (18), the Stockholm Study (19), the United Kingdom Prospective Diabetes Study (UKPDS) (20), and the Kumamoto study (21). None of these studies were able to maintain HbA1c levels in the nondiabetic range, even in the intensive management arm, yet they were able to demonstrate improved outcomes for those in the intensive-management arm (22). The goal of the Action to Control Cardiovascular Risk in Diabetes (ACCORD) study was to achieve an HbA1c level of less than 6.0% in the intensive-management arm versus less than 7.9% in the control arm. The intensive-management arm had excess CVD mortality (23). The Action in Diabetes and Vascular Disease: Preterax and Diamicron MR Controlled Evaluation (ADVANCE) trial (24) and the Veterans Affairs Diabetes Trial (25) used different interventions but showed no increase in CVD death rates in those who achieved HbA1c levels of 6.5%.

Patient History and Recommended Laboratory Evaluations/Examinations

In addition to the usual medical history taken at the first patient visit (e.g., past medical, surgical, family, and social histories), the history for an individual with diabetes should include age, date and characteristics of the onset of diabetes, diet history, nutritional status, physical activity habits, diabetes education history, previous treatment regimens and response to therapy, current treatment of diabetes, current blood glucose monitoring habits and previous results and the patient's response to glucose results, any episodes of DKA, mild and severe hypoglycemia, diabetes-related microvascular complications (including retinopathy, nephropathy, and sensory and autonomic neuropathy) and macrovascular complications (including CVD, cerebrovascular disease, and peripheral vascular disease), psychosocial issues such as depression, and routine health maintenance such as eye examinations, dental visits, and foot care.

The physical examination should include height, weight, body mass index (BMI), waist-to-hip ratio, blood pressure, assessment of arterial pulses for bruits or other signs of atherosclerosis, and thyroid palpation. The skin should be examined for acanthosis nigricans and insulin injection site. A comprehensive foot examination should also be performed, including palpation of dorsalis pedis and posterior tibial pulses and testing of the patellar and Achilles reflexes, proprioception, vibration, and monofilament sensation.

Laboratory evaluation includes HbA1c, fasting lipid profile, liver function tests, urine albumin excretion with spot urine albumin-to-creatinine ratio, serum creatinine, calculated glomerular filtration rate (GFR), and thyroid-stimulating hormone (TSH) in those with T1DM or in women older than 50 years. Other tests that may be considered include C-peptide, antibodies such as islet cell antibody 511 and glutamic acid decarboxylase, electrocardiogram (ECG), chest radiograph, complete blood count, and urinalysis.

The patient should be referred for an annual dilated eye examination (at diagnosis in patients with T2DM and after 5 years in patients with T1DM), to a registered dietitian for medical nutrition therapy (MNT), for diabetes self-management education, for a dental examination, to a mental health professional if needed, and to an obstetrician who specializes in diabetes (for women planning pregnancy).

MNT is an essential component of treating diabetes that can reduce HbA1c levels by approximately 1% in those with newly diagnosed T1DM and by 2% in those with newly diagnosed T2DM; MNT can also reduce low-density lipoprotein (LDL) cholesterol levels by 11% to 16% and triglycerides by 8%; furthermore, in those with hypertension, MNT can reduce systolic blood pressure by 5 mm Hg and diastolic pressure by 2 mm Hg (26). Nutritional requirements of those with diabetes are identical to those without diabetes. Currently, there is no "American Diabetes Association diet" that applies to every person with diabetes. The meal plan is based on performing an assessment, choosing therapy goals, and applying techniques that meet the patient's needs.

Preferably, MNT is provided by a registered dietitian familiar with the components of diabetes MNT. Continued support is required in order for most people to experience positive long-term clinical improvements. It is not necessary to prescribe a particular caloric intake or nutrient distribution. Several visits are usually necessary to help the person with diabetes learn how to eat a variety of healthy foods in various situations. See Table 11-12 for nutritional recommendations.

At diagnosis, many people are frightened and commonly want to be told what to eat. Initially, published materials such as preprinted food lists, meal planning books, cookbooks, and reputable diabetes Web sites and videos may be helpful until the patient can see a registered dietitian for an individualized meal plan. Initial MNT should consist of teaching basic nutritional guidelines: making healthy food choices based on the food guide pyramid and basic carbohydrate counting. Patients should be advised to eat similar amounts of carbohydrate throughout the day and from day to day; they should also be advised to eat portion sizes to prevent weight gain or in overweight individuals, to reduce weight. Keeping a

TABLE 11–12 American Diabetes Association General Recommendations for Medical Nutrition Therapy for People With Diabetes

Fat	Saturated fat: <7% of total calories
	Trans fats should be avoided
Carbohydrates	Monitoring carbohydrate intake is a key strategy in glycemic control
	Use of glycemic index or glycemic load may be usuful for some individuals
Fiber	Recommendation is 14 grams per 1,000 calories
Alcohol sugar	Considered to be safe when consumed within the amounts recommended by the FDA
Alcohol	Limit to <1 drink per day for women and <2 drinks per day for men
Supplements	Supplementation with antioxidants, such as vitamins E, C, and carotene, and chromium is not recommended because of the lack of evidence of efficacy and safety.
Non-nutritive sweetners	FDA has approved these non-nutritive sweeteners

- Acesulfame K^+
- Aspartame
- Neotame
- Saccharin
- Sucralose

food journal helps patients learn how much food they are consuming, and comparing the food journal with a blood glucose log helps patients learn how various foods affect their blood glucose level.

At subsequent visits, MNT training can build on previous visits and may include topics such as carbohydrate, fat, or calorie counting, the use of exchange lists, and lifestyle changes. Advanced MNT training can include topics such as carbohydrate counting with insulin-to-carbohydrate ratios, structured lifestyle-change programs, or medically supervised very-low-calorie diets. The key principle of MNT for those with T1DM is synchronizing insulin with food and activity and using glucose self-monitoring results to adjust therapy.

Most people with T1DM are not overweight or obese at diagnosis; however, people with T1DM can become overweight and obese over time, so making healthy food choices in the correct portion sizes to maintain desired body weight is a goal. Monitoring glucose, HbA1c, lipids, microalbumin, and blood pressure is important. If any of these levels are abnormal, the meal plan can be adjusted along with other treatment to help achieve the desired goal (27).

Most people with T2DM are obese at diagnosis, so attaining and maintaining desired body weight (not necessarily ideal body weight) is a goal. Even modest weight loss has been shown to reduce insulin resistance and improve glycemic control. Low-carbohydrate calorie-restricted or low-fat calorie-restricted diets may be effective in some individuals short-term (up to 1 year). If the patient is following a low-carbohydrate diet, lipids,

protein intake, and renal function must be monitored closely. No study has shown an optimal mix of macronutrients that work for every person with diabetes. Total calories, regardless of the macronutrient content, must be appropriate for weight management. Long-term weight loss is challenging, and most do not maintain weight loss. Assessing readiness to commit to a life-long treatment plan for weight reduction and maintenance is vital for success.

Pharmacologic agents for obesity can be useful but cannot replace lifestyle changes; these agents are recommended only when the BMI is greater than 27 kg/m^2 in the presence of a cormorbid condition or is greater than 30 kg/m^2 when no cormorbid condition is present. Bariatric surgery can be considered in adults with T2DM and a BMI greater than 35 kg/m^2. It has been shown to normalize blood glucose levels in 55% to 95% of patients with T2DM, depending on the surgical procedure. Procedures that only constrict the stomach had a lower rate of glucose normalization than did procedures that bypass portions of the small intestine (27-29).

Physical Activity

The American Diabetes Association recommends at least 150 minutes per week of moderate-intensity aerobic physical activity, and in the absence of contraindications, those with T2DM should perform resistance exercise 3 times per week. Regular exercise improves blood glucose control, lowers HbA1c levels, helps with weight loss, reduces CVD risk, and improves the feeling of well-being. Aerobic and resistance exercise have the same beneficial effect on insulin resistance (30). Before recommending activity, assess for risk factors for CVD. If the patient does not have any of the risk factors found in Table 11-13 and is younger than 35 years, moderate or vigorous activity may be recommended; if the patient does not have any of the risk factors found in Table 11-13 and is older than 35 years, moderate activity may be recommended; however, if the patient wants to engage in vigorous activity, he or she should first undergo an exercise stress test. If the patient has any of the risk factors mentioned previously, low-intensity/low-impact activity may be recommended; however, if the patient has any of these risk factors and wants to begin a moderate or vigorous exercise program, he or she should undergo an exercise stress test (31).

Contraindications to exercise include hyperglycemia in the presence of ketones. Glucagon is released during exercise and causes glycogenolysis, gluconeogenesis, lipolysis, protein degradation, amino acid catabolism, and ketogenesis, increasing both glucose and ketone levels. For those using insulin therapy and/or a secretagogue and have adequate insulin levels, exercise will lower glucose and can cause hypoglycemia. These patients should test their blood glucose level before exercising and should ingest carbohydrate if necessary to prevent hypoglycemia. In those with proliferative diabetic retinopathy or severe nonproliferative diabetic retinopathy, vigorous aerobic or resistance exercise may be contraindicated because it may trigger vitreous hemorrhage or retinal detachment. If the patient has severe peripheral neuropathy, the risk of injury, skin breakdown, Charcot joint, and infection is increased. In these cases, activities such as swimming, bicycling, or upper body exercises may be better.

Autonomic neuropathy increases the risk of reduced cardiac responsiveness, postural hypotension, impaired thermoregulation, impaired night vision, and delayed gastric emptying; it is also highly correlated with CVD. Those who are starting an exercise program or intensifying their existing program should first undergo a cardiac evaluation. Exercise increases urinary protein excretion, but no studies have shown that exercise increases the rate of progression of diabetic kidney disease.

Patients should be advised to maintain safety during exercise, specifically, to wear appropriate attire, especially well-fitted shoes with socks, and to examine their feet after exercise for any reddened or irritated areas or breaks in the skin. They should also be instructed to check their blood glucose level before and during exercise to determine whether hypoglycemia develops and to carry carbohydrate, maintain adequate hydration, and wear some form of medical identification (31, 32). They should be instructed to ingest carbohydrates if hypoglycemia develops.

Diabetes Self-Management Education

Diabetes self-management education improves clinical outcome and quality of life and is therefore critical for all people with diabetes. For this reason, the American Diabetes Association developed national standards (updated in January 2009) for establishing quality diabetes education programs as well as evidence-based guidelines for teaching diabetes self-management (33). In addition, the American Association of Diabetes Educators (AADE) developed a model for diabetes education called AADE7, which includes seven self-care behaviors (34, 35). This

---

TABLE 11–13 Recommendation for Exercise Tolerance Test Before Prescribing Moderate or Vigorous Activity

If any of the following are present, recommend an exercise tolerance test before beginning moderate or vigorous activity:

- Anginal equivalent pain or discomfort of the chest, neck, jaw, arms
- Shortness of breath at rest or with mild exertion
- Dizziness or syncope
- Orthopnea or paroxysmal nocturnal dyspnea
- Ankle edema
- Palpitations or tachycardia
- Intermittent claudication
- Unusual fatigue or shortness of breath with usual activities
- Any macrovascular disease
- Any microvascular disease
- Peripheral vascular disease
- Hypertension
- Smoking
- Hyperlipidemia
- Family history of cardiovascular disease

model, based on systematic literature reviews, includes tools and references for educators and describes the following health care behaviors: healthy eating, being active, monitoring, taking medication, problem solving, reducing risk, and healthy coping.

Diabetes self-management education, an empowerment-based model, helps patients take an active role in their own health care by helping them make informed decisions, encouraging healthy self-care behaviors, teaching problem-solving skills, and encouraging active collaboration with the health care team. Measurable behavior change is the desired outcome of diabetes education, so behavior goal-setting by the patient followed by evaluation is a vital part of the AADE7 model.

Education strategies should be based on a thorough patient assessment that includes learning style, learning ability, literacy, cultural background, age, environmental

stressors, family support, financial constraints, physical ability, work environment, coping skills, and degree of depression. Diabetes education should be performed by diabetes educators who not only are knowledgeable about the disease, but also possess skills in communication, counseling, patient education, and self-management training.

Medications for Glycemic Control

Although lifestyle interventions are an effective means of controlling blood glucose, most patients will require medications for glycemic control. These medications (27) must be individualized to each patient, and since T2DM is progressive, the regimen will need to be changed as needed to attain or maintain blood glucose and HbA1c goals. See Table 11-14 for expected decreases in HbA1c levels and the associated advantages and disadvantages of each class of diabetes medication.

TABLE 11–14 Classes of Diabetes Medications: Expected Effect on HbA1c, Advantages and Disadvantages

Intervention	Expected Decrease in HbA1c (%)	Advantages	Disadvantages
Lifestyle changes to decrease weight and increase activity	1.0–2.0	Increases insulin sensitivity	Most patients do not adhere to lifestyle changes
Metformin	1.0–2.0	Weight neutral	Multiple adverse effects and contraindications
Insulin	1.5–3.5	No dose limit; rapidly effective, improved lipid profile	1–4 injections per day; glucose monitoring, weight gain, hypoglycemia, analogs are expensive
Sulfonylurea	1.0–2.0	Rapidly effective	Weight gain, hypoglycemia
Thiazolidinediones	0.5–1.4	Improved lipid profile (pioglitazone), potential decrease in myocardial infarction (pioglitazone)	Fluid retention, congestive heart failure, weight gain, bone fractures, expensive, potential increase in myocardial infarction (rosiglitazone)
GLP-1 agonist	0.5–1.0	Weight loss	2 injections per day; frequent GI adverse effects, long-term safety not established, expensive
Glucosidase inhibitor	0.5–0.8	Weight neutral	Frequent GI adverse effects; 3 × per day dosing; expensive
Glinide	0.5–1.5	Rapidly effective	Weight gain; hypoglycemia; 3 × per day dosing; expensive
Pramlintide	0.5–1.0	Weight loss	3 injections daily; frequent GI adverse effects; long-term safety not established; expensive
DPP-4 inhibitor	0.5–0.8	Weight neutral	Long-term safety not established, expensive

GI, Gastrointestinal.

Metformin, introduced into the U.S. market in 1995, is the most widely prescribed oral agent for T2DM. It decreases hepatic glucose output and lowers fasting glucose by activating AMP-activated protein kinase, which inhibits the production of glucose by liver cells. As monotherapy, metformin lowers HbA1c levels by approximately 1.5% and does not cause hypoglycemia or weight gain. The UKPDS showed a beneficial effect of metformin on CVD outcome. Common adverse effects include diarrhea, nausea, vomiting, flatulence, asthenia, indigestion, abdominal discomfort, anorexia, and metallic taste. A serious but uncommon reaction is megaloblastic anemia because the drug interferes with vitamin B_{12} absorption and lactic acidosis. Metformin is contraindicated for hypersensitivity to the drug, renal dysfunction, metabolic acidosis, DKA, lactic acidosis, hypoxemia, dehydration, sepsis, surgery, and in patients undergoing radiographic studies involving iodinated contrast material. Metformin should be used cautiously in those with heart failure, in those with a history of alcohol abuse, in elderly patients, and in those using secretagogues or insulin. In the United States, single-therapy metformin is available in several forms (Table 11-15); the drug is also available in several combinations with other agents (Table 11-16).

Sulfonylureas, available since the 1950s, cause insulin release by binding to sulfonylurea receptors on functioning pancreatic beta cells. The binding closes the linked ATP-sensitive K^+ channels, decreasing K^+ influx and the subsequent depolarization of the beta cell membrane. The voltage-dependent calcium (CA) channels open, and the influx of CA causes translocation and exocytosis of secretory granules of insulin to the cell surface. This group of medications is divided into first- and second-generation drugs. As monotherapy, sulfonylureas lower HbA1c levels by approximately 1.5%. Common adverse effects include hypoglycemia and weight gain. Hypoglycemia from sulfonylureas is rarely life-threatening, but when it is, it is usually in elderly patients; these patients are

TABLE 11–15 Metformin Forms: Starting and Maximum Dose

Name	Dose Available (mg)	Starting Dose (mg)	Maximum Dose (mg)
Metformin (Glucophage)	500, 850, 1,000	500 bid or 850 qd	2,550
Metformin (Extended-Release Glucophage XR)	500, 750	500 bid or 750 qd	2,550
Metformin liquid (Riomet)	100 mg/mL	5 mL bid or 8.5 mL qd	2,550

TABLE 11–16 Combination Forms of Metformin: Initial and Maximum Doses

Name	Dose Available (mg)	Starting Dose (mg)	Maximum Dose (mg)
Actos with metformin (ACTOplus met)	15/500; 15/850	15/500 qd or bid; 15/850 qd or bid	45/2,550
Avandia with metformin (Avandamet)	1/500; 2/500; 4/500; 2/1,000; 4/1,000	2/500 qd or bid	8/2,000
Glipizide with metformin (Metaglip)	2.5/250; 2.5/500; 5/500	2.5/250 qd If BG 280–320 mg/dL start 2.5/500 qd	20/2,000
Glyburide with metformin (Glucovance)	1.25/250; 2.5/500; 5/500	1.25/250 qd or bid	20/2,500
Sitagliptin phosphate with metformin (Janumet)	50/500; 50/1,000	50/500 bid	100/2,000

most prone to severe, prolonged, hypoglycemia from sulfonylureas, especially when the drug is combined with chlorpropamide or glyburide. When sulfonylureas are used as monotherapy, the glucose-lowering response to this drug is more rapid than the response to thiazolidinediones is; however, over time, maintaining glycemic targets with use of sulfonylureas is not as effective as with use of thiazolidinedione or metformin. The maximum benefit of sulfonylureas is realized at half-maximum doses, so higher doses should be avoided if possible (Table 11-17).

Meglitinides stimulate insulin secretion; however, they bind to a different site within the sulfonylurea receptor and have a shorter circulating half-life than sulfonylureas.

They are administered with meals. Repaglinides decrease HbA1c levels by approximately 1.5% and carry a higher risk of hypoglycemia than nateglinide, which is less potent; weight gain is similar with the two drugs (Table 11-18).

Glucosidase inhibitors (Table 11-19) inhibit alpha-glucosidase enzymes in the brush border of the small intestines and pancreatic alpha-amylase, reducing the rate of digestion of complex carbohydrates. The drugs inhibit the breakdown of complex carbohydrates into smaller glucose molecules, therefore helping to slow the rise in postprandial glucose. Reducing HbA1C levels by 0.5% to 0.8%, glucosidase inhibitors are less effective than metformin or the sulfonylureas. Also, since glucose is increased in the colon with use of glucosidase

TABLE 11–17 Sulfonylurea Forms: Starting and Maximum

Generic	Brand	Dosage strengths (mg)	Starting dose (mg)	Doses per day	Max dose (mg)	Duration of effect	Active metabolite
Glipizide	Glucotrol	5, 10	5	1–2	40	10–24 hr	No
Glipizide	Glucotrol XL	2.5, 5, 10	5	1	20	24 hr	No
Glyburide	Diabeta, Micronase	1.25, 2.5, 5	2.5–5	1–2	20	16–24 hr	Yes
Glyburide micronized	Glynase	1.5, 3, 4.5, 6	1.5–3	1–2	11	11–24 hr	Yes
Glimepiride	Amaryl	1,2,4	1–2	1	8	24 hr	Yes

TABLE 11–18 Meglitinide Forms: Starting and Maximum

Name	Dose available (mg)	Usual start dose	Comments
Natelinide (Starlix)	60, 110	110 mg tid;	Max dose: 360 mg qd; can start at 60 mg tid if A1c near target
Repaglinide (Prandin)	0.5, 1, 2	0.5 mg ac if A1c <8	Max dose: 16 mg qd; caution hepatic/renal impairment

TABLE 11–19 Glucosidase Inhibitors Forms: Starting and Maximum Doses

Name	Dose available (mg)	Usual start dose	Comments
Acarbose (Precose)	25, 50, 100	25 mg tid	Max dose: Adult: 150 mg/day <60 kg, 300 mg/day >60 kg
Miglitol (Glyset)	25, 50, 100	25 mg tid	Max dose: 300 mg

inhibitors, gas production increases, causing gastrointestinal symptoms. Approximately 25% to 45% of patients discontinue use as a result of this adverse effect.

Thiazolidinediones, introduced into the U.S. market in 1990, bind to peroxisome proliferator-activated receptors gamma (PPARγ), a group of receptor molecules inside the cell nucleus. The ligands for the PPARγ receptors are free fatty acids and eicosanoids, and when activated, the receptors migrate to the DNA, activating transcription of a number of specific genes. When PPARγ is activated, insulin resistance decreases, adiponectin levels increase, adipocyte differentiation is modified, levels of certain interleukins such as IL-6 decrease, vascular endothelial growth factor (VEGF)–induced angiogenesis is inhibited, and leptin levels decrease. The result is increased insulin sensitivity in the muscle, fat, and liver, leading to a 0.5% to 1.4% reduction in HbA1c levels that lasts longer than with sulfonylureas. The subcutaneous adipose tissue increases and the visceral adipose tissue decreases. Adverse effects include weight gain, fluid retention, peripheral edema, a 2-fold increase in congestive heart failure, and increased bone fracture in women.

Pioglitazone, one type of thiazolidinedione, has a beneficial effect on atherogenic lipid profiles compared with rosiglitazone, another thiazolidinedione that has a neutral effect (Table 11-20). The Prospective Pioglitazone Clinical Trial in macrovascular events (PROactive), however, showed no significant effects of pioglitazone compared with placebo for primary diabetic vascular disease outcomes after 3 years of follow-up but suggested a possible beneficial effect on CVD risk. Rosiglitazone, in contrast, was found to carry a 30% to 40% relative increased risk for myocardial infarction, according to a meta-analysis. Rosiglitazone is also available combined with glimepiride (a sulfonylurea) (Table 11-21).

Dipeptidyl peptidase 4 (DPP-4) inhibitors block DDP-4, which increases incretin levels (glucagon-like peptide-1 [GLP-1] and gastric inhibitory polypeptide also known as glucose-dependent insulinotropic peptice [GIP]). These incretin hormones inhibit glucagon release, increase insulin secretion, and decrease gastric emptying. The first DPP-4 inhibitor was introduced in the United States in 2007. The HbA1c-lowering effect is 0.5% to 0.8%. The adverse effects were similar to those of the placebo, except for rare nausea and common cold-like symptoms (Table 11-22).

The GLP-1 agonist (exenatide), approved by the FDA in 2005, lowers HbA1c levels by 0.5% to 1.0%. Produced by the L cells of the small intestine, GLP-1 is a naturally occurring peptide that potentiates glucose-stimulated insulin secretion by binding with the GLP-1 receptor on the beta cell of the pancreas, causing glucose-mediated insulin secretion. Injected twice daily before the two largest meals, exenatide helps to lower postprandial glucose by decreasing gastric emptying, inhibiting inappropriate hyperglucagonemia and potentiating glucose-stimulated insulin secretion. It has beta cell–proliferative, antiapoptotic, and differentiation effects (5). Of patients who use exenatide, 30% to 45% experience nausea, vomiting, or diarrhea, which tends to decrease over time. Exenatide is associated with a 2- to 3-kg weight loss over 6 months. A small number of patients using exenatide have developed pancreatitis, but it is unclear whether exenatide was the cause. Therapy should be initiated in

TABLE 11–20 Thiazolidinedione Forms: Starting and Maximum Doses

Name	Dose available (mg)	Usual start dose	Comments
Pioglitazone (Actos)	15, 30, 45	15 mg or 30 mg qd	Max dose: 45 mg qd; contraindicated in class III or IV HF
Rosiglitazone (Avandia)	2, 4, 8	4 mg qd or 2 mg bid	Max dose: 8 mg qd

TABLE 11–21 Combination Form of Rosiglitazone and Glimepiride: Initial and Maximum Doses

Name	Dose available (mg)	Usual start dose	Comments
Rosiglitazone with glimepiride (Avandaryl)	4/1; 4/2; 4/4	4 mg/1 mg qd	Max dose: 8 mg/4 mg

TABLE 11–22 DPP-4 Forms: Starting and Maximum Doses

Name	Dose available (mg)	Usual start dose	Comments
Sitagliptin phosphate (Januvia)	25, 50, 100	100 mg qd	Max dose 100 mg; Cr Cl 30–50, 50 mg qd; Cr Cl <30, 25 mg qd
Saxagliptin (Onglyza)	2.5, 5	5 mg qd	Reduce dose for moderate renal disease with Cr Cl of ≤50

patients with T2DM by administering 5 mcg before a large meal twice daily for 1 month, after which the dose should be titrated as tolerated to 10 mcg before a large meal twice daily (Table 11-23). Exenatide is approved for use with sulfonylureas, metformin, and/or thiazolidinediones; however, hypoglycemia may occur when exenatide is used in combination with a sulfonylurea.

Amylin agonist (pramlintide), approved by the FDA in 2005, is a synthetic amylin analog. The beta cells of the pancreas produce amylin in a glucose-dependent fashion and lower postprandial blood glucose levels by inhibiting glucagon production and slowing gastric emptying. Pramlintide acts as an amylinomimetic agent, preventing postprandial increase of glucagon and modulating gastric emptying leading to satiety, reduction in caloric intake, and potential weight loss. The HbA1c level decreases by 0.5% to 0.7%. Adverse effects include hypoglycemia nausea, which tends to subside over time. Weight loss of 1 to 1.5 kg is associated with pramlintide over 6 months. It is approved for use with insulin in patients with T1DM or T2DM.

The recommended starting dose of pramlintide for those with T2DM is 60 mcg injected with meals. The dose of insulin before the meals, including regular, rapid-acting analog, and premixed insulin, should be reduced 50% when initiating pramlintide (Table 11-24). When the patient has no clinically significant nausea for 3 to 7 days, the dose of pramlintide should then be increased to 120 mcg injected before meals. If there is significant nausea with 120 mcg, reduce the dose to 60 mcg. Once the target dose of pramlintide is achieved, adjust the insulin doses and review the blood glucose levels weekly to achieve target glucose control.

For patients with T1DM, a beginning dose of 15 mcg is injected with meals and titrated by 15-mcg increments until a maintenance dose of 60 mcg is reached. Patients should be instructed to reduce their preprandial rapid- or short-acting insulin and fixed-mix insulin by 50%. Blood glucose levels should be monitored premeal, postprandially, and at bedtime. The dose of pramlintide may be increased if there is no clinically significant nausea for 3 days. If clinically significant nausea occurs with 45 or

TABLE 11–23 Forms of GLP-1 Agonist: Starting and Maximum Dose

Name	Dose available	Usual start dose	Comments
Exenatide (Byetta)	5-mcg pen 10-mcg pen	5 mcg before a large meal twice daily for the first mo, after which the dose is increased to 10 mcg before a large meal twice daily if tolerated. Use within 60 min before meals at least 6 hr apart.	Hypoglycemia with sulfonylureas, nausea, vomiting, dizziness, feeling jittery, headache.
Liraglutide (Victoza)	6 mg/mL pen containing 3 mL	0.6 mg subcutaneous daily for 1 week, then increase dose to 1.2 mg subcutaneous daily. The dose may be increased to a maximum 1.8 mg if blood glucose control is suboptimal	Inject once daily

GLP-1, Glucagon-like peptide-1.

TABLE 11–24 Amylin Agonist Forms, Starting and Maximum Dose

Name	Dose Available (mcg)	Usual Start Dose	Comments
Pramlintide	1.5-mL disposable multi-dose SymlinPen 60 pen-injector containing 1,000 mcg/mL; 2.7 mL disposable multidose SymlinPen 110 pen-injector containing 1,000 mcg/mL; 5-mL vial containing 600 mcg/mL	Type 2 diabetes mellitus: 60 mcg, titrate up in 30-mcg increments to 110 mcg; type 1 diabetes mellitus: 15 mcg, titrate up in 15-mcg increments to 60 mcg	Potential for severe hypoglycemia when used with insulin. When using an insulin syringe to draw up Pramlintide from a vial, see the conversion chart.

60 mcg, reduce the pramlintide dose by 15 mcg. If at least 30 mcg cannot be tolerated, consider discontinuing pramlintide. If a target dose of pramlintide can be achieved, the insulin doses should be adjusted until glucose targets are achieved. If the vial form is being used, the conversion chart in Table 11-25 can be used to instruct patients on the units of pramlintide to draw into the U-100 insulin syringe for the desired mcg dose.

Insulin, the original diabetes medication, was introduced into the U.S. market in 1922. Since 1982, most of the newly approved insulin preparations have been produced by inserting portions of recombinant DNA into laboratory-cultivated bacteria or yeast, creating complete human insulin. The structure of the even newer analog insulins differs slightly from human insulin by one or two amino acids. The changes in amino acid sequence cause the insulin to act differently in its onset, peak, and duration. The published data on the onset, peak, and duration of the various insulins is merely an approximation; variability in insulin action occurs between different individuals and within the same person from day to day.

TABLE 11–25 Conversion of Pramlintide Dose to Insulin Unit Equivalents

Dosage of pramlintide prescribed (mcg)	Increment using a U-100 insulin syringe (units)
15	2.5
30	5
45	7.5
60	10
110	20

More than 20 types of insulin products are available on the market (Table 11-26). When choosing one or more insulins to prescribe, the insulin action should be matched to the patient needs. The intermediate- and long-acting insulins are designed to replace basal insulin requirements, whereas the rapid- and short-acting insulins are designed to replace prandial (bolus) requirements. There is no maximum dose of insulin. It can be titrated up until the HbA1c goal is achieved. Insulin therapy can cause hypoglycemia, especially in those who have achieved target HbA1c levels. Weight gain often occurs as glycosuria improves. Insulin therapy can also improve triglyceride and HDL cholesterol levels, especially in those with poor control (34).

Insulin Needs of Patients With T2DM

Most patients with T2DM will require combination therapy. When additional antihyperglycemic medications are needed, choosing medications with various mechanisms of action will produce the greatest synergy. For example, combining metformin with a sulfonyurea is particularly effective while limiting weight gain. A consensus algorithm for the management of T2DM was developed by the American Diabetes Association and the European Association for the Study of Diabetes in 2009. The algorithm was divided into Tier 1, with well-validated therapies, and Tier 2, with less well-validated therapies (Table 11-27).

Step 1 of Tier 1 recommends lifestyle interventions and metformin at diagnosis. If metformin is not tolerated, then lifestyle interventions are attempted as monotherapy. If the HbA1c target is not achieved after 2 to 3 months, then step 2 is initiated.

Step 2 of Tier 1 is either adding a second medication if metformin was used in step 1 or administering metformin as a first medication if it was not used in step 1. The second medication can be either a sulfonylurea or insulin, depending on the HbA1c level. If the HbA1c level is above 8.5% and symptoms of hyperglycemia are

TABLE 11–26 Insulins on the U.S. Market, Time Action, and Storage Recommendations

Name	Onset	Maximum Effect	Duration	Available Forms	Storage Recommendation
Humalog (lispro)	15 min	30–90 min	3–5 hr	Lilly: vial, disposable pen, penfill cartridge	28 d once in use
Novolog (aspart)	10–20 min	60–110 min	3–5 hr	NovoNordisk: vial, disposable pen (Flexpen), penfill cartridge	28 d once in use
Apidra (glulisine)	10–20 min	1–2 hr	3–4 hr	Sanofi-Aventis: vial, Penfill cartridge (Opticlix)	28 d once in use
Humulin regular	0.5–1 hr	2–3 hr	4–11 hr	Lilly: vial	28 d once in use
Novolin regular	0.5–1 hr	2–3 hr	Up to 8 hr	Novo/Nordisk vial, penfill cartridge, InnoLet	28 d once in use
Neutral protamine Hagadorn (NPH)	1.5–4 hr	4–11 hr	Up to 24 hr	Lilly: vial, disposable pen; NovoNordisk: vial, penfill cartridge, InnoLet	Vial 28 d once in use; pen 14 d once in use
Lantus (glargine)	1–2 hr	Flat	24 hr	Sanofi-Aventis: vial, penfill cartridge (Opticlix). Do not mix Lantus with any other insulin	28 d once in use
Levemir (detemir)	0.8–2 hr	3.2–9.3 hr (dose dependent)	Up to 24 hr	NovoNordisk: vial, disposable pen (Flexpen)	Vial and pen: 42 d once in use

TABLE 11–27 Algorithm for Management of Type 2 Diabetes Mellitus

Tier 1: Well-validated

Step 1	*Step 2*	*Step 3*
At diagnosis: Lifestyle interventions + metformin (if tolerated)	2–3 months after step 1 if HbA1c > target: Add a sulfonylurea if HbA1c is <8.5%, or initiate insulin if HbA1c is >8.5% to the step 1 regimen	2–3 months after step 2 if HbA1c is > target: If insulin was not initiated in step 2, initiate insulin. If insulin was initiated in step 2, intensify the insulin regimen

Tier 2: Less well-validated

Step 1	*Step 2*
Lifestyle + metformin + pioglitazone Or Lifestyle + metform + GLP-1 agonist	Lifestyle + metformin + pioglitazone + sulfonylurea Or Lifestyle + metformin + basal insulin

GLP-1, Glucagon-like peptide-1.

present, basal insulin with a morning or bedtime long-acting (detemir or glargine) insulin or a bedtime intermediate-acting (neutral protamine Hagadorn [NPH]) insulin is recommended. The recommended starting dose is either 10 units or 0.2 unit/kg. The dose is titrated on the basis of the fasting blood glucose level and should be increased by 2 units every 3 days until the fasting blood glucose level is 70 to 130 mg/dL. If the fasting blood glucose level is above 180 mg/dL, the dose can be increased by 4 units. If hypoglycemia occurs, the dose should be reduced by 10% or 4 units, whichever is greater. The HbA1c level should be rechecked in 2 to 3 months.

Step 3 of Tier 1 includes further adjustments with metformin and a sulfonylurea if the HbA1c level is above target; adding a third oral agent can be considered if the HbA1c level is close to 7%. The disadvantages to adding a third agent include cost and little additional benefit to the HbA1c level. If insulin therapy has not been started, it should be initiated as outlined above. If insulin therapy has been instituted, intensified therapy may be necessary. Once the fasting blood glucose level is in target range, the blood glucose level should be checked again before lunch and dinner and at bedtime. If the blood glucose was elevated pre-lunch, 4 units of a rapid-acting insulin should be added at breakfast. The dose is titrated by 2 units every 3 days until the pre-lunch blood glucose level is in the target range. If the pre-dinner level is above the target blood glucose, 4 units of NPH insulin at breakfast or 4 units of a rapid-acting insulin at lunch may be added. The dose is titrated by 2 units every 3 days until the pre-dinner blood glucose level is in the target range. If the pre-bedtime blood glucose level is above target, 4 units of a rapid-acting insulin may be added at dinner and titrated by 2 units every 3 days until the pre-bedtime blood glucose is in the target range. If the HbA1c level remains elevated at 7% or above, the pre-meal blood glucose levels should be rechecked and if above target, another injection may need to be added. If the HbA1c level continues to be above target, the 2-hour postprandial blood glucose level should be checked and adjusted with preprandial rapid-acting insulin. Once insulin is initiated, the sulfonylurea should be discontinued (22).

Step 1 of Tier 2 may be considered in clinical settings in which hypoglycemia is very undesirable. Lifestyle with metformin and pioglitazone or lifestyle with metformin and a GLP-1 agonist can be used. If promotion of weight loss is a major consideration and HbA1c is less than 8%, a GLP-1 agonist may be preferred. If the HbA1c remains above target with step 1 of Tier 2, then step 2 of Tier 2 recommends adding a sulfonylurea with lifestyle, metformin and pioglitizone, or discontinuing the GLP-1 agonist and adding basal insulin to lifestyle

and metformin. For patients with severely uncontrolled blood glucose levels, consider that the patient may not have T2DM but may have unrecognized T1DM, latent autoimmune diabetes in adults (LADA), or severely insulin-deficient T2DM.

Insulin Needs of Patients With T1DM

Since patients with T1DM produce little or no insulin, insulin therapy is initiated at diagnosis. Many different insulin regimens are used. At diagnosis, many patients choose either a 2-injection/day regimen or a basal/bolus 4- or 5-injection/day regimen. MNT is vital to balance carbohydrates with the insulin doses. Regular insulin may be substituted for rapid-acting insulin if cost is a factor. As mentioned earlier, shortly after diagnosis and initiation of insulin therapy, the patient may have a "honeymoon" period, during which the insulin requirements are reduced. The honeymoon is temporary, however, and the duration varies among patients.

A split-mixed regimen using a short- or rapid-acting insulin with NPH insulin twice daily (at breakfast and dinner) requires a consistent schedule, regular mealtimes, and less than 10 hours between breakfast and dinner. Premixed insulin is not advised in T1DM. If ketones are not detected or are at a moderate level, treatment should begin with a total daily dose of 0.5 unit of insulin per kilogram of body weight. If the ketone levels are high, 0.7 unit of insulin per kilogram should be used. Of the total daily dose, give two-thirds pre-breakfast, and give one-third pre-dinner. The pre-breakfast dose should consist of one-third short- or rapid-acting insulin and two-thirds NPH insulin; the pre-dinner dose should be half short- or rapid-acting insulin and half NPH insulin. Adjust the insulin doses on the basis of blood glucose patterns. See Table 11-28 for dose adjustment recommendations. Table 11-29 lists insulin dosing adjustments for split-mixed insulin regimens according to blood glucose levels.

A multiple daily insulin dose regimen, consisting of basal insulin injected once daily in the morning or evening or given twice daily in the morning and evening along with pre-meal injections of short- or rapid-acting insulin, may help those who have erratic or inconsistent schedules, variable carbohydrate intake, greater than 10 hours between breakfast and dinner, infrequent snacks or the desire to eliminate snacks, shift work, frequent travel, or post-meal hypoglycemia.

The goal of a basal/bolus insulin regimen is to mimic normal physiologic insulin secretion. If urine ketones are negative to moderate, treatment should begin with a total daily dose of 0.5 unit of insulin per kilogram of body weight. If the urine ketone levels are high, 0.7 unit of insulin per kilogram should be used. After determining the total daily insulin requirements, distribute 50% as basal insulin and 50% as bolus insulin. The basal insulin

TABLE 11–28 Starting a Split-Mixed Insulin Regimen for Type 1 Diabetes Mellitus

Calculate the total daily dose based on:
0.5 units/kg for negative to moderate ketones
0.7 units/kg for large ketones

	AM	Noon	PM	Bedtime
Distribution of total daily dose	2/3	0	1/3	0
Short-/rapid-acting insulin–to–neutral protamine Hagadorn (NPH) ratio	1:2	0	1:1	0

TABLE 11–29 Adjustment of Insulin Dose for a Split-Mixed Regimen for Type 1 Diabetes Mellitus

Type	Blood Glucose	Insulin Adjustment
a.m.	<70 mg/dL	Decrease PM NPH insulin 1–2 units
a.m.	<140 mg/dL	Increase PM NPH insulin 1–2 units
Mid-day	<70 mg/dL	Decrease AM short/rapid insulin 1–2 units
Mid-day	<140 mg/dL	Increase AM short/rapid insulin 1–2 units
p.m.	<70 mg/dL	Decrease AM NPH 1–2 units
p.m.	<140 mg/dL	Increase AM NPH insulin 1–2 units
Bedtime	<100 mg/dL	Decrease PM short/rapid insulin 1–2 units
Bedtime	<140 mg/dL	Increase PM short/rapid insulin 1–2 units
Move the PM NPH insulin to bedtime if nocturnal hypoglycemia occurs.		

NPH, Neutral protamine Hagadorn.

is used to control the fasting blood glucose levels, and the bolus insulin controls post-meal blood glucose. A correction factor or sensitivity factor should be calculated to correct pre-meal hyperglycemia (see "Insulin delivery methods" section).

If the patient is switching from a split-mixed regimen, reduce the current total insulin dose by 20% and distribute 50% as basal insulin and 50% as bolus insulin. Depending on blood glucose patterns, some patients may benefit by receiving their long-acting insulin at a certain time of day or by splitting it into two doses. Adjust the insulin doses based on blood glucose patterns. See Table 11-30 for dose adjustment recommendations.

Insulin Delivery Methods

An insulin pump is a mechanical medical device that delivers insulin subcutaneously via a disposable infusion set that has a metal or plastic catheter that is placed under the skin. It is an alternative to multiple daily insulin injections. An advantage of insulin pump therapy is the use of only short- or rapid-acting insulin, both of which have less variability of insulin action than do intermediate- and long-acting insulins. Since the pump is able to deliver very tiny doses (as small as 0.025 unit) at a time, the doses can be adjusted in smaller increments. This allows more flexibility in eating and activity than do alternative insulin regimens.

Most patients find that the insulin pump is more convenient and discreet than injections. In addition, many pumps have advanced features such as the ability to calculate the pre-meal bolus on the basis of the pre-meal blood glucose level, the carbohydrate grams that will be eaten, and insulin-on-board. See Table 11-31 for a comparison of insulin pumps on the U.S. market. Some disadvantages of insulin pump therapy include cost and possible DKA if the pump was not designed according to the protocol for prevention of DKA.

If insulin pump therapy is desired, the patient needs to work with medical personnel who are experienced in initiating this therapy and in making adjustments to the pump as needed; the medical team must also be available to provide educational support to the patient. Requirements for insulin pump candidates include a willingness to check blood glucose 4 or more times per day, as well as the ability to quantify food by either a fixed meal plan or carbohydrate counting, to learn pump operation and

TABLE 11–30 Adjustment of Insulin Dose for a Basal/Bolus Regimen for Type 1 Diabetes Mellitus

Type	Blood Glucose	Insulin Adjustment
a.m.	<70 mg/dL	Decrease bedtime long-acting insulin 1–2 units
a.m.	<140 mg/dL	Increase bedtime long-acting insulin 1–2 units
Mid-day	<70 mg/dL	Decrease AM short/rapid-acting insulin 1–2 units
Mid-day	<140 mg/dL	Increase AM short/rapid-acting insulin 1–2 units
p.m.	<70 mg/dL	Decrease mid-day short/rapid-acting insulin 1–2 units
p.m.	<140 mg/dL	Increase mid-day short/rapid-acting insulin 1–2 units
Bedtime	<100 mg/dL	Decrease PM short/rapid-acting insulin 1–2 units
Bedtime	<140 mg/dL	Increase PM short/rapid-acting insulin 1–2 units
Consider splitting long-acting insulin if 24-hr coverage is not provided.		

TABLE 11–31 Comparison of Insulin Pumps on the U.S. Market

Insulin Pump Manufacturer	Insulet	Johnson & Johnson	Medtronic	Roche	Sooil
Brand Name	Omnipod	Animas	Revel	Accuchek Spirit	DiabecareIIS
Dimensions/wt	41 × 61 × 18 PDA: 66 × 10 × 26 OmniPod 1.2 oz PDA 4 oz	51 × 77 × 18 3.9 oz	5x: 51 × 79 × 20 3.5 oz 7x: 51 × 91 × 20 3.8 oz	80 × 47 × 24 4.8 oz	46 × 77 × 19 1.9 oz
Reservoir Volume Units	200	200	176 or 300	315	300
Reservoir to Infusion Set Connection	Built in	Luer lock	Proprietary	Luer lock	Proprietary
Basal Rates Units/hr	0.05–30	0.025	0.05–35	0.1–25.0	0.1–16.0
Total Number of Basal Rates Per Day Per Column	48	11	48	24	24
Number of Alternate Basal Columns	7	4	3	5	1

Continued

TABLE 11–31 Comparison of Insulin Pumps on the U.S. Market—cont'd

Insulin Pump Manufacturer	Insulet	Johnson & Johnson	Medtronic	Roche	Sooil
Temporary Basal Rates	% or U/hr (1–11 hr, in 30-min increments)	–90% to +200% in increments of 10% for 0.5–24 hr (30-min increments)	0.025–35.0 U/hr as single basal rate for 0.5–24 hr or as % of current basal	In 10% increments from 0% to 200%, and 15 min–24 hr	10% increments from 0% to 200% and up to 11 hr
Bolus Increments (units)	0.05, 0.1, 0.5, 1.0	0.05 visual or audio, 0.1, 1.0, 5.0 audio	0.1 visual, 0.5 or 1.0 visual, audio, or remote	0.1, 0.2, 0.5, 1.0, 2.0	0.1, .05, 1.0
Carb and Correction Factor	Yes	Yes, carb and bg values can be entered into the pump or meter-remote	Yes, manual carb, BG direct from BD or One Touch meter or manual entry	Yes, manual carb, BG from Accu-Chek BG monitor	Yes, manual carb
Bolus Type	Meal, correction, meal & correction; normal, extended, combination	Units or carbs: standard, extended, combination	Units or carbs: standard, extended, combination	Quick, scroll, extended, multiwave	Normal, extended, combination
1 Unit Bolus Duration (seconds)	40	1 or 3	40	40	11
Battery	AAA × 2 (PDA)	AA lithium or alkaline × 1	AAA for pump, A23 for remote	AA × 1 alkaline or rechargeable	½ AA 3.6v lithium
Battery Life	4 wk	4–6 wk with lithium, 2–4 with alkaline	3 wk	4 wk	8–10 wk
Memory	90 days of data (up to 5400 records)	Nonvolatile: 500 boluses, 270 basals, 110 daily totals, 60 alarms, 60 primes, 900 BG levels	4,000 events, volatile (basal & history loss can occur): 24 boluses, 7 day totals	Nonvolatile: 90 days (4,500 events); history recall of last 30 boluses, alerts, daily insulin totals, and temporary basal rate increases	Last 500 boluses, primes and daily totals. Last 100 alarms (all time- and date-stamped)

TABLE 11–31 Comparison of Insulin Pumps on the U.S. Market—cont'd

Insulin Pump Manufacturer	Insulet	Johnson & Johnson	Medtronic	Roche	Sooil
Software Download	None	ezManager Max, downloads in 3 min with dongle and software that are available at Animas	Medtronic CareLink® Therapy Management System and ParadigmPA L™ 3.0 Software at Medtronic	Pocket Compass with Bolus Calculator, insulin pump configuration software, IR Communication Port	None
Water	Watertight	11 ft for 24 hr	Splash-resistant	IPX 8, 60 min at 2.5 meters	Watertight
Warranty	4 years	4 years	4 years	4 years	4 years

troubleshooting, and to make safe decisions when the blood glucose levels are out of the target range or if the pump alarms.

The insulin pump starting doses are based on a generally recommended mathematical calculation and safe starting point. Adjustments to the rates are based on blood glucose patterns once pump therapy has been initiated. When the patient is transitioning to the insulin pump, any long-acting insulin that the patient received before insulin pump initiation will affect blood glucose levels for several days; hence, initial pump calculations are based on a reduced total daily dose (10% to 25%), with most patients requiring a dosage increase after several days to 2 weeks.

To determine the initial total daily insulin pump dose, the amounts of all types of insulin that the patient is currently using daily are totaled first. If the patient uses a variable amount from day to day, the current total daily insulin dose is based on the daily average of the total insulin used during the week just prior to initiation of the insulin pump. Once the total daily insulin dose is determined, it is reduced 10% to 25% to obtain the initial total daily insulin pump dose.

To calculate the initial total basal rate, the total daily insulin pump dose is divided in half. Active patients may need less basal and more bolus insulin, whereas inactive patients may need more basal and less bolus insulin. The other half of the total daily dose is for meal boluses. There are several ways to determine the meal bolus. One is to divide the total bolus dose by three and have the patient take a fixed meal bolus; however, the patient is required to eat a fixed amount of carbohydrate at each meal to match the bolus. Most patients want the flexibility

to vary the amount of carbohydrates they eat from day to day, which can be achieved with use of the "500 Rule," a method for determining the initial insulin-to-carbohydrate ratio. For this method to work, the basal rate must be approximately 50% of the total daily dose, and the patient must be able to correctly count grams of carbohydrate. The total daily insulin dose is divided into 500 to get the initial insulin-to-carbohydrate ratio. For example, if the total daily insulin dose before pump therapy is 50 units, 50 is divided into 500, which equals 10. The initial insulin to carbohydrate ratio would be 1 unit per 10 grams of carbohydrate. If the person consumed 45 grams of carbohydrate, the insulin pump bolus would be 4.5 units. (See Figure 11-4.)

A sensitivity factor, also called a correction factor, is used to correct hyperglycemia. The sensitivity factor is the amount (in mg/dL) that the blood glucose level decreases per 1 unit of short- or rapid-acting insulin and it is determined more accurately in patients with T1DM whose basal and meal bolus rates are set correctly. The sensitivity factor is not as accurate in those with T2DM because of their insulin resistance and variable amount of endogenous insulin production. If regular insulin is used, the "1500 Rule" is commonly used: the total daily insulin dose is divided into 1500 to determine the sensitivity factor. For example, if the total daily dose is 50 units, then 50 is divided into 1500 which would equal 30. If the target blood glucose was 100 mg/dL and the current blood glucose was 160 mg/dL, then 2 units would be needed to decrease the blood glucose from 160 mg/dL to 100 mg/dL. If rapid-acting insulin is used, the "1800 Rule" is commonly used: the total daily insulin dose is divided into 1800 to determine the sensitivity factor. For

Initial Insulin Pump Basal and Meal Dosage Calculations

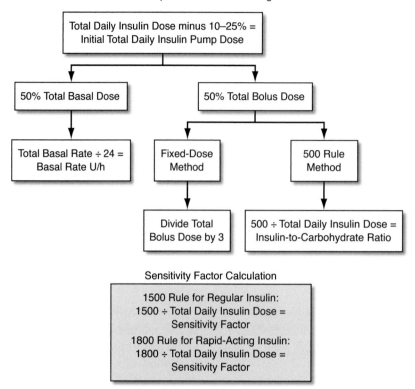

FIGURE 11–4: Initial Insulin Pump Basal and Meal Dosage Calculations.

example, if the total daily dose was 90 units per day, then 90 is divided into 1800, which would equal 20. If the target blood glucose is 100 mg/dL and the current blood glucose is 180 mg/dL, then 4 units would be needed to decrease the blood glucose from 180 mg/dL to 100 mg/dL. The target blood glucose is customized for each patient. See Figure 11-4 for a summary of the initial insulin pump dosage calculations.

Insulin dosing adjustments after insulin pump initiation are based on glucose patterns. The patient may wear a continuous glucose monitor to assist with adjustment. Since the purpose of basal insulin is to maintain normoglycemia during the fasting state, the blood glucose level during periods of fasting is evaluated. The patient should be able to avoid a bedtime snack or skip a meal and not experience an increase or decrease in blood glucose by more than 30 mg/dL from baseline.

The overnight basal rate should be evaluated first. Have the patient check his or her blood glucose levels before bedtime, in the middle of the sleep period, and again on awakening for 3 consecutive days. If the overnight blood glucose level increases greater than 30 mg/dL from baseline, have the patient increase the basal rate 10% to 20% 1 to 2 hours before the increase in blood glucose occurs and return to the original basal rate 1 to 2 hours before the blood glucose decreases. After the rate is adjusted, have the patient continue to perform the overnight basal test until the blood glucose level does not increase or decrease greater than 30 mg/dL from the bedtime blood glucose.

The morning basal rate is then adjusted. Begin the test when the blood glucose level is in the target range. Have the patient skip breakfast and check blood glucose levels at 2, 4, and 6 hours after the start of the test. If at any time the blood glucose level decreases to less than 70 mg/dL, end the test and reduce the morning basal rate 10% to 20%. If the blood glucose level increases to greater than 250 mg/dL, end the test and increase the morning basal rate by 10% to 20%. If the blood glucose level increases or decreases greater than 30 mg/dL during the test, have the patient adjust the basal rate 10% to 20% and perform the test again.

The afternoon basal rate is then adjusted. Begin the test when the blood glucose level is in the target range. Have the patient skip lunch and check blood glucose levels at 2, 4, and 6 hours after the start of the test. If at any time the blood glucose level decreases to less than 70 mg/dL, end the test and reduce the afternoon basal rate 10% to 20%. If the blood glucose level increases to greater than 250 mg/dL, end the test and increase the afternoon basal rate by 10% to 20%. If the blood glucose level increases or decreases greater than 30 mg/dL during the test, have the patient adjust the basal rate 10% to 20% and perform the test again.

The evening basal rate is then adjusted. Begin the test when the blood glucose level is in the target range. Have the patient skip dinner and check blood glucose levels at 2, 4, and 6 hours after the start of the test. If at any time the blood glucose level decreases to less than 70 mg/dL, end the test and reduce the evening basal rate 10% to 20%. If the blood glucose level increases to greater than 250 mg/dL, end the test and increase the evening basal rate by 10% to 20%. If the blood glucose level increases or decreases greater than 30 mg/dL during the test, have the patient adjust the basal rate 10% to 20% and perform the test again.

Once the basal rates are adjusted, the insulin-to-carbohydrate ratio is then adjusted. Most patients require one insulin-to-carbohydrate ratio for the entire day; some require a different ratio at different meals. Begin the test when the blood glucose level is in the pre-meal target range. Instruct the patient to eat a known amount of carbohydrate and bolus appropriately. Have the patient recheck blood glucose levels at 1, 2, 3, and 4 hours after eating. The blood glucose level should increase 30 to 50 mg/dL. If it increases greater than 50 mg/dL, have the patient increase the carbohydrate ratio (the number will be smaller) by 10% to 20%. For example, if the patient is using a starting ratio of 1 unit per 10 grams of carbohydrate and the blood glucose level increases greater than 50 mg/dL after eating, change the ratio to 1 unit per 9 grams of carbohydrate or 1 unit per 8 grams of carbohydrate. If the increase occurs in the third or fourth hour instead of in the second hour, have the patient try an advanced bolus feature, in which part of the bolus is delivered immediately and the rest is delivered over a specified amount of time. Each insulin pump company calls this feature by a different name; see Table 11-31 for examples.

Once the insulin-to-carbohydrate ratio is adjusted, test the sensitivity factor. Have the patient begin the test only if the blood glucose level is 50 mg/dL or more above target, no bolus has been given in the past 4 hours, no food has been consumed in the past 4 hours, and the patient can continue for the next 4 hours without food or a bolus. Have the patient repeat the test until the 4-hour blood glucose level is within 30 mg/dL of the target. Table 11-32 summarizes the key points of patient instructions for pump dose testing.

Insulin pens are the most widely used insulin-delivery method in the world, except in the United States, where the syringe and vial are most commonly used. Many

TABLE 11–32 Patient Instructions for Performing Insulin Pump Dose Testing

Do not perform insulin pump dose testing if:

- The blood glucose is outside of the target range.
- Illness is present.
- Strenuous exercise has been performed in the past 24 hours unless this amount of exercise is performed every day.

Stop the insulin pump adjustment exercise if:

- The blood glucose decreases to <70 mg/dL or increases to >300 mg/dL.

When performing basal testing:

- Eat a known amount of carbohydrate and bolus as prescribed.
- Do not eat mixed meals such as casseroles or high-fat foods such as pizza.
- When performing the overnight basal test, the bedtime blood glucose must be 100 mg/dL to 250 mg/dL, and the blood glucose during the night must be >90 mg/dL to 250 mg/dL.

When performing meal bolus testing

- Begin with the pre-meal blood glucose in the target range.
- Eat a known amount of carbohydrate and bolus as prescribed.
- Repeat the test until the blood glucose level does not increase >50 mg/dL 2 hours after the test begins.

When performing the sensitivity factor testing

- Perform the test when the blood glucose is at least 50 mg/dL above target.
- Perform the test only if no bolus has been taken in the past 4 hours, no food has been consumed in the past 4 hours, and the patient can continue for the next 4 hours without food or a bolus.
- Repeat the test until the 4-hour glucose value is within 30 mg/dL of the target blood glucose.

different insulin pens are on the U.S. market (Table 11-33) and offer many advantages. Some pens are prefilled and the entire pen is disposed of when the insulin is used or if it has been opened for the recommended time, whereas others are not disposed of and the patient changes a cartridge of insulin. Most pen needles can be used with any pen. The pen needles are screwed onto the pen, used once, and discarded. Needle lengths range from 5 to 11.7 mm, and gauges range from 29 to 31. Since the needle contains space, the pen needs to be "primed" before every injection by dialing and injecting 2 units into the air to fill the dead space in the needle and prevent inaccurate dosing. Pen needles need to be discarded after each use. If using a pen with an inserted cartridge follow the product instructions carefully in order to load the insulin cartridge correctly. Pens are generally easy to use. If using NPH or a premixed insulin, the pen needs to be shaken gently to ensure that the insulin is well mixed before injection. Compared with syringes, pens offer repeatable dose accuracy, especially in patients with reduced visual acuity.

TABLE 11–33 Insulin Pens on the U.S. Market

Lilly	Humalog Original Prefilled Pen	Disposable, 3 mL, prefilled
	Humalog Mix 75/25 Original Prefilled Pen	Disposable, 3 mL, prefilled
	Humalog Mix 50/50 Original Prefilled Pen	Disposable, 3 mL, prefilled
	Humalog KwikPen	Disposable, 3 mL, prefilled
	Humalog Mix 75/25 KwikPen	Disposable, 3 mL, prefilled
	Humalog Mix 50/50 KwikPen	Disposable, 3 mL, prefilled
	Pen for prefilled cartridges	3-mL cartridges inserted into a nondisposable pen
	Humalog cartridge	
	Neutral protamine Hagadorn (NPH) cartridge	
	HumaPen MEMOIR	3 mL cartridges inserted into a nondisposable pen allow a patient to record and review the 16 most recent doses, including priming doses
	HumaPen LUXURA HD	3-mL cartridges inserted into a nondisposable pen can deliver ½-unit increments
Novo Nordisk	Levemir FlexPen	Disposable, 3 mL, prefilled
	Novolin N InnoLet	Disposable, 3 mL, prefilled
	Novolin R Innolet	Disposable, 3 mL, prefilled
	Novolin 70/30 Innolet	Disposable, 3 mL, prefilled
	Novolog FlexPen	Disposable, 3 mL, prefilled
	Novolog Mix 70/30 FlexPen	Disposable, 3 mL, prefilled
	NovoPen 3	3-mL cartridges inserted into a nondisposable pen
	Novolin R PenFill	
	Novolin N PenFill	
	Novolin 70/30 Penfill	
	NovoPen 4	3-mL cartridges inserted into a nondisposable pen
	Novolin R PenFill	
	Novolin N PenFill	
	Novolin 70/30 PemFill	
	NovoPen Junior	3-mL cartridges inserted into a nondisposable pen can deliver ½-unit increments
	Novolin R PenFill	
	Novolin N PenFill	
	Novolin 70/30 Penfill	
Sanofi Aventis	Lantus Solostar	Dispose of remaining insulin after 28 days of use
	Opticlik	Uses insulin cartridges
	Lantus for OptiClik	Dispose of remaining insulin after 28 days of use
	Apidra for OptiClik	

Management of Hyperglycemia in the Hospitalized Patient

Approximately 38% of all hospitalized patients have hyperglycemia, one third of whom have no history of diabetes. Inpatient management of patients with hyperglycemia is important since hyperglycemia is a marker for poor clinical outcome and mortality (3). The glucose goal for hospitalized patients with hyperglycemia or diabetes is to maintain near-normal blood glucose levels while avoiding hypoglycemia. Kitabchi, Freire, and Umpierrez (36) suggested a goal of fasting and pre-meal blood glucose values of 100 to 130 mg/dL and random glucose levels of less than 180 mg/dL. The biggest barrier to achieving these target glucose values is hypoglycemia. Some patients will require alternate glucose goals at a higher level to prevent hypoglycemia.

Most patients with diabetes will require insulin therapy while hospitalized. Metformin must be discontinued if the patient is having surgery or tests involving injected dye, can receive nothing by mouth (is NPO) for a prolonged period, or has an elevated creatinine level. Sulfonylurea therapy may place the patient at increased risk for hypoglycemia, especially if the patient is not eating. Oral agents require a prolonged adjustment period, whereas insulin therapy is effective and flexible and can be changed quickly to meet rapidly changing requirements.

The normal pancreas produces approximately half of the daily amount as basal insulin and the other half as bolus insulin. During the fasting state, the body receives glucose from stored sources such as liver glycogen. The purpose of basal insulin is to maintain normal fasting glucose levels by metabolizing stored fuels converted to glucose during the fasting state. Bolus insulin is produced in response to the digestion of nutrients and maintains normal postprandial glucose levels. Patients with T2DM continue to produce endogenous insulin. In some cases, prolonged fasting in these individuals may reduce the overall insulin requirements to the point at which no basal insulin is required. However, patients with T1DM who produce no endogenous insulin will always require basal insulin to prevent DKA. In cases of prolonged fasting, T1DM patients may require a reduced amount of basal insulin (37). Sliding-scale insulin regimens are associated with erratic and poor control and should not be used as a monotherapy (38, 39).

An effective insulin regimen includes three components: basal insulin, bolus insulin, and correction insulin. The first step in designing a subcutaneous insulin regimen is to determine the total daily insulin requirement.

For people with T2DM, if prehospital insulin doses are known, begin with that total daily dose. If that information is not available, calculate the total daily dose based on body weight in kilograms. Begin with 0.3 unit of insulin per kilogram of body weight, with 50% of that dose in the form of basal insulin and the other 50% for

bolus insulin (37). The dose will likely need to be increased because most people with T2DM require more than 0.3 unit per kilogram of body weight.

For people with T1DM, the total daily dose is usually known. The basal requirements are usually 40% to 50% of the total daily dose. If the insulin regimen before admission is more than 50% of the basal rate, dose readjustment may be needed. It is not uncommon for people with T1DM to use basal insulin to cover ingested carbohydrates. In this situation, if the patient becomes NPO, the basal insulin level will cause hypoglycemia. A good question to ask the patient before determining a hospital insulin regimen is "can you skip a meal without having hypoglycemia?" If the answer is "no," then a readjustment is needed. Most patients with T1DM will need approximately 0.5 unit of insulin per kilogram of weight.

Conditions that may reduce total daily insulin requirements include renal impairment, prolonged fasting, malnutrition, weight loss, liver impairment, and sepsis. In contrast, steroid therapy and many other medications will increase insulin requirements. Steroids increase basal and bolus requirements, with an increase in postprandial glucose levels even higher than fasting glucose levels. Short-acting steroids, however, may require no extra insulin or a small dose of 70/30 insulin. The intermediate- and long-acting steroids often require an increase in both the basal and bolus insulin doses. The total bolus requirements are usually 60% to 75% of the total daily dose (37). See Table 11-34 for the dose equivalent and biologic half-life of steroids.

TABLE 11–34 Dose Equivalent and Biologic Half-Life of Steroids

Glucocorticoid	Approximate Equivalent Dose (mg)	Biologic Half-Life
SHORT-ACTING		
Cortisone	25	8–11
Hydrocortisone	20	8–11
INTERMEDIATE		
Methylprednisolone	4	18–36
Prednisolone	5	18–36
Prednisone	5	18–36
Triamcinolone	4	18–36
LONG-ACTING		
Betamethasone	0.6–0.75	36–54
Dexamethasone	0.75	36–54

Once the total daily dose and the percentage of basal and bolus doses are determined, the next step is choosing the type of insulin. If the patient is a predictable eater, then a premixed insulin may be used before breakfast and dinner.

If the patient is eating little or will be having tests or procedures requiring NPO status, a regimen of basal insulin dosed in a scheduled manor without regard to meals dosed once daily or divided into 2 doses with short- or rapid-acting insulin given every 4 to 6 hours to correct hyperglycemia is a safer alternative. To calculate a correction dose, if the patient is not taking steroids, divide the total daily insulin dose into 1800 to determine the sensitivity or correction factor. For example, if a person requires 60 units of insulin per day, using the 1800 Rule (1800 ÷ 60), the sensitivity factor will be 30. If the target blood glucose is to remain less than 180 mg/dL, then for every 30 mg/dL that the blood glucose is above 180 mg/dL, 1 unit of short- or rapid-acting insulin should be given (37).

Intravenous (IV) insulin infusion may be required in certain patients, such as those in the intensive care unit (ICU) with DKA, a hyperglycemic hyperosmolar non-ketotic state, dehydration, or critical illness, or are undergoing surgery (especially those with T1DM), receiving high-dose glucocorticoid treatment, or are posttransplantation (37). A number of insulin infusion protocols have been published; however, a single standard insulin infusion protocol is currently not available. (See Table 11-35 for an example of an insulin infusion protocol.)

When the patient is ready to return to subcutaneous insulin, several methods can be used to determine the

TABLE 11–35 Example of Insulin Drip Protocol for Adults Patients in the ICU Setting

Algorithm 1		Algorithm 2		Algorithm 3		Algorithm 4	
Glucose	Units/hr	Glucose	Units/hr	Glucose	Units/hr	Glucose	Units/hr
<60 = Hypoglycemia. Follow hypoglycemia treatment protocol							
<70	Off	<70	Off	<70	1	<70	Off
70–109	0.2	70–109	0.5	70–109	2	70–109	1.5
110–119	0.5	110–119	1	110–119	3	110–119	3
110–149	1	110–149	1.5	110–149	4	110–149	5
150–179	1.5	150–179	2	150–179	5	150–179	7
180–209	2	180–209	3	180–209	6	180–209	9
210–239	2	210–239	4	210–239	8	210–239	11
240–269	3	240–269	5	240–269	10	240–269	16
270–299	3	270–299	6	270–299	11	270–299	20
300–329	4	300–329	7	300–329	14	300–329	24
330–359	4	330–359	8	330–359	16	330–359	28
>360	6	>360	11	>360	1	>360	32

This algorithm is not intended to be used for individuals with type 1 diabetes, diabetic ketoacidosis, or hyperglycemic hyperosmolar states.

Target range for glycemic control: 80–140 mg/dL (generally 110 mg/dL)

Standard drip of 100 units/100 mL of 0.9% NaCl.

Start IV insulin therapy when glucose is above target range.

Insulin infusions should be discontinued when:

Patient has no history of diabetes and is receiving <1 unit/hr.

Patient receives first dose of subcutaneous basal + bridging dose of fast analog or Regular. Bolus dose and initial infusion rate: divide initial glucose level by 100, then round to nearest 0.5 units for bolus AND initial infusion rate.

Examples: Initial glucose = 326 mg/dL: 326 ÷ 100 = 3.26, round to 3.5: IV bolus 3.5 units + start infusion @ 3.5 units/hr.

Initial glucose = 174 mg/dL: 174 ÷ 100 = 1.74, round to 1.5: IV bolus 1.5 units + start infusion @ 1.5 units/hr.

Intravenous fluids

Most patients will need 5–10 g glucose per hour

D5W or D5W½NS at 100–200 mL/hr or equivalent in TPN or enteral feeding.

TABLE 11–35 Example of Insulin Drip Protocol for Adults Patients in the ICU Setting—cont'd

Adjusting the infusion:
  Algorithm 1: Start here for most patients.
  Algorithm 2: Start here for patients not controlled with Algorithm 1; if they have undergone coronary artery bypass graft surgery or solid organ or islet cell transplantation; have received glucocorticoids; or have diabetes and receive >80 units/day of insulin before hospitalization.
  Algorithm 3: For patients not controlled with Algorithm 2. No patient should start here without authorization from the endocrine service.
  Algorithm 4: For patients not controlled with Algorithm 3. No patient should start here.

proper regimen. One is to evaluate the insulin requirements before the IV insulin infusion and restart the previous doses (39). Another method is to calculate the total daily insulin requirements based on body weight and determine the regimen as outlined insulin needs in the previous paragraphs (39). Both of these methods assume that the patient's current status is similar to that before the insulin drip. If substantial changes occurred while the patient was undergoing insulin infusion, such as steroid treatment, altered nutritional status or renal function, or weight fluctuation, there is another way to determine total daily insulin dose: determine the amount of insulin (in units) received by IV drip during the 24 hours before the drip was discontinued and multiply by 0.8 to arrive at the new total daily dose for the subcutaneous regimen. Whatever approach is used, the subcutaneous insulin regimen must be initiated before discontinuing the insulin drip to prevent rebound hyperglycemia.

In those requiring total parenteral nutrition (TPN), several methods can be used to control blood glucose levels. Regular insulin can be added to the solution, 1 unit per 10 to 15 grams of carbohydrate, and/or subcutaneous injections of Regular insulin can be ordered to correct hyperglycemia. The dose in the TPN solution can be adjusted, depending on the blood glucose values and the amount of subcutaneous Regular insulin needed to correct hyperglycemia. If too much insulin is added to the TPN and hypoglycemia occurs, either another drip with dextrose must be initiated or the TPN must be discarded. Another method is to have no Regular insulin in the TPN solution and begin a separate insulin drip to determine the concentration of insulin required, and then add that amount to the TPN. The amount of Regular insulin in the TPN should cover only the amount of carbohydrate in the solution without providing all of the patient's insulin requirements. Likewise, the basal insulin should not cover the amount of carbohydrate in the TPN solution. With the separate insulin infusion method, if the

TPN is suddenly stopped or the rate of TPN administration is changed and the amount of Regular insulin in the bag is correct, the blood glucose levels will not be adversely affected (39).

The principle in managing blood glucose levels in patients receiving enteral feedings is similar to that in patients receiving food orally. The insulin should cover only the carbohydrate in the formula, not basal needs. The first step is to calculate the amount of carbohydrate contained in the prescribed formula. If the enteral feeding is continuous, then the carbohydrate will be distributed throughout the day, and long-acting insulin is an appropriate choice. However, enteral feedings are often suddenly discontinued or changed for many reasons, so giving the long-acting insulin in divided doses is a safer choice. Begin with a total dose of 0.3 units per kilogram of body weight or 1 unit per 6 to 8 grams of carbohydrate. Divide the total dose of insulin by 4, and give every 6 hours; or divide the total dose by 3 and give every 8 hours.

A combination of Regular and NPH insulins constitutes 70/30 insulin and is commonly used during enteral feeding because of the rapid onset of the Regular insulin component and the shorter duration of the NPH component. Hold the dose if the tube feeding is stopped. Change the dose if the tube feeding rate is changed. The patient may need only 2 or 3 injections every 6 to 8 hours while receiving enteral feeding. The patient's need for basal insulin will persist if it is needed before initiation of the enteral feeding. Some patients receive enteral feeding and still consume food by mouth. In that case, the patient will require prandial short- or rapid-acting insulin for the amount consumed orally. Correction doses of short- or rapid-acting insulin may be required to treat hyperglycemia (39). Carbohydrate content for various enteral formulas is listed in Table 11–36.

If the patient is NPO, basal insulin is required in T1DM patients. After the patient fasts for approximately 16 hours, the basal insulin requirements may decrease, so

TABLE 11-36 Carbohydrate Content of Common Enteral Formulas

Osmolite 1.2	158 grams CHO/L
Fibersource HN	160 grams CHO/L
Isosource 1.5	170 grams CHO/L
Diabetisource AC	100 grams CHO/L
Novosource Renal	200 grams CHO/L
Vivonex RTF	175 grams CHO/L
Peptamen AF	107 grams CHO/L
Peptamen 1.5	188 grams CHO/L
Resource Breeze	230 grams CHO/L or 53 for 240 mL per can
Glytrol	100 grams CHO/L or 24 for 240 mL per Can

the patient should be monitored closely. If the patient usually takes basal insulin once daily, the basal insulin may need to be divided into 2 doses. If the basal insulin requirements decrease, the next dose can be reduced or omitted. Because the person with T2DM produces endogenous insulin, some T2DM patients may need a reduction in basal insulin after prolonged fasting to the point that no basal insulin is required.

Surgery and anesthesia cause a neuroendocrine stress response. Counterregulatory hormones including epinephrine, glucagon, cortisol, growth hormone, and inflammatory cytokines are released, causing insulin resistance, decreased peripheral glucose utilization, impaired insulin secretion, increased lipolysis, and protein catabolism. This stress response can cause hyperglycemia and ketosis. When assessing the individual for surgery, several things should be considered, such as the extent and duration of surgery, type of anesthesia, and other surrounding factors such as steroid use, hydration of the patient, complications such as infection, and the use of IV dextrose or TPN. There is no consensus on a blood glucose target range for patients after surgery. Since patients with T1DM are insulin-deficient, they will require continuous insulin and frequent glucose monitoring. Avoidance of hypoglycemia and DKA is a top priority. If the basal insulin dose is correct before surgery, then theoretically 100% of the usual basal insulin can be delivered. If the patient must fast for more than 16 hours, a basal reduction may be needed since the liver glucose output decreases after 16 hours of fasting. After surgery, a person with T2DM will require 50% to 100% of the basal insulin dose that was needed before surgery (39). Oral diabetes agents are discontinued before surgery.

An insulin drip can be used during surgery and is most effective if started the night before to establish euglycemia before surgery. In some patients, especially cardiothoracic surgery patients, the best outcomes are achieved if the insulin drip is continued for days after the procedure (40).

Clinical Nurse Specialist Competencies and Spheres of Influence

CNSs work within the three spheres of influence (patients/families, nurses/other professionals, and system/organization) using the core competencies of direct clinical care, expert coaching/teaching/mentoring, collaboration, consultation, research/evidence-based practice, systems leadership, and ethical decision-making/moral agency/advocacy to provide health care for patients with diabetes (41, 42). CNS practice has been shown to be effective in improving outcomes in patient satisfaction, readmissions, cost, health status, and complications in patients with diabetes (43).

Numerous examples of the various functions and competencies of the CNS are found in the literature. An example of the coaching/teaching/mentoring competency is described by Campbell-Fleming, Catania, and Courtney (44), who were faced with the dilemma of helping staff nurses keep pace with current practice. Because of competition for time, patient care demands on nurses, and limited resources for education, staff education can be challenging. In response to these challenges, the authors developed a learning program based on self-direction of the learner and on adult learning principles by creating a traveling journal board. An article was selected and posted on the board. The board was taken to seven ambulatory sites where the nurses could read the article when it was best for them rather than trying to attend a scheduled journal club meeting.

Kelly (45) addressed the requirement for knowledge and application of genomics in nursing education. She described the CNS as a change agent in this process, working from the bottom up at the basic clinical level and from the top down through professional organizations and health care policy.

Application of the consultation and collaboration competencies is evident in the Care Coordination Model, developed by two CNSs. To facilitate and enhance positive patient outcomes, the model was developed as an individual practice, based on the organizational system within which the CNSs worked. The model involved synchronizing a comprehensive, multidisciplinary plan that included identifying problems in the processes of patient care leading to prolonged stay, recommending resolution to the problems, implementing a plan for resolution, and evaluating the intervention (46).

CNSs combine the attributes of clinical and metrics expert in the role of knowledge management. This involves identification of the task at hand, and use of autonomy and innovative methods to continually learn, teach, and produce quality outcomes. Knowledge management involves identification, sharing, and developing knowledge to make decisions, to improve performance, to provide quality services, and to increase productivity and workplace satisfaction. Data collection and analysis of current statistics and trends provide a basis for quality-improvement projects, research studies, and the development of patient care algorithms (47).

Hospital discharge, during which several core competencies are typically applied, provides an opportune time for CNS intervention. The CNS functions as an expert coach, applying evidence-based teaching-learning strategies when educating patients, families, and other health care workers. The teaching-learning approaches are based on an assessment of the learners' readiness to learn, ability to learn, and learning style. The CNS may serve as a consultant when other specialties need the CNS's expertise to meet the patient's needs for discharge. Frequently, the CNS collaborates with numerous other health care team members to properly prepare patients for discharge, given the complex patient care needs (43). Finally, CNSs provide evidence-based interventions for the management of patient diseases and the prevention of complications (43).

These general examples of CNS practice can be applied specifically to the role of the CNS in caring for patients with diabetes. Depending on the employment setting, the role of the endocrine CNS can vary considerably; therefore, this chapter includes only a partial list of the CNS's functions.

The diabetes CNS provides direct clinical care to patients with diabetes by conducting a comprehensive medical history and physical assessment based on evidence-based techniques and tools to diagnose and treat diabetes. Professional organizations such as the American Diabetes Association and the American College of Clinical Endocrinologists publish specific guidelines for patient care.

When consulting, the CNS should review the patient's case, offer alternative approaches to patient care, and help implement planned changes in lifestyle, medications, and other aspects of diabetes management. The CNS should obtain the necessary resources to achieve the goal of the consult and communicate the consult findings to the appropriate colleagues. Because diabetes management is dependent on patients knowing how to care for themselves, the CNS implements a patient/family teaching plan based on established evidenced-based national standards. Diabetes self-management education is critical for all people with diabetes; it is effective for improving clinical outcomes and quality of life. The American Diabetes Association established evidence-based national standards for diabetes self-management training, which were updated in January 2009. The purpose of the standards includes defining quality diabetes programs and assisting diabetes educators by providing evidence-based education guidelines (33). The American Association of Diabetes Educators developed a model for diabetes education called AADE7 (35) that was based on systematic literature reviews; they also developed tools and references for educators. Education strategies should be based on a thorough assessment including learning style, learning ability, literacy, cultural background, age, environmental stressors, family support, financial constraints, physical ability, work environment, coping, and depression.

Coaching/teaching/mentoring of nursing staff is also important since most nurses are not familiar with the current standards of diabetes care, and many errors can occur with diabetes medications. The CNS identifies the learning need and implements a creative teaching method based on the learner's needs and learning style. Diabetes has been extensively researched, and many associations such as the American Diabetes Association, American College of Clinical Endocrinologists, and American Association of Diabetes Educators publish the most recent findings, recommendations, and consensus statements.

The role of the diabetes CNS in clinical and professional leadership involves responsibility for innovation and change in the patient care system such as implementing a hospitalwide hypoglycemia protocol or spearheading a committee for developing algorithms for the care of patients with diabetes within the hospital. The collaboration role may involve organizing and participating in multidisciplinary team meetings involving pharmacists, patient educators, social workers, physicians, and many others.

The CNS may participate in diabetes research, having important roles in leading evidence-based practice changes and serving as primary investigator for studies that improve patient care, quality of life, and prevention of complications.

The CNS may contribute to ethical decisions involving diabetes patients, such as those affecting the allocation of resources. Patients with diabetes, for example, may require access to care, equipment, and supplies but have limited financial means. Another situation may involve organ transplants for patients with end-stage renal disease or CVD, particularly elderly patients and those with multisystem organ dysfunction; these difficult decisions are often encumbered by ethical conflict.

COMPLICATIONS OF DIABETES MELLITUS

Etiology

Diabetes mellitus is the leading cause of blindness in those aged 20 to 74 years and the leading cause of chronic kidney disease and amputations. Pathologic changes

CASE STUDY 11–1

CHIEF COMPLAINT: Increased thirst, urination, hunger, fatigue, and weight loss of 40 pounds.

HISTORY OF PRESENT ILLNESS: An 18-year-old white male presents with blurred vision and a 40-pound weight loss, as well as extreme polydipsia, polyphagia, and polyuria that began 1 month previously.

FAMILY HISTORY: No family history of diabetes

CURRENT MEDICATIONS: None

REVIEW OF SYSTEMS AND PHYSICAL EXAM:
VITAL SIGNS
Blood pressure: 100/58 mm Hg
Pulse: 104/min
Respirations: 22/min
Temperature: 37.2°C
Height: 188 cm
Weight: 63.6 kg
BMI: 19 kg/m^2.
LABORATORY
Random blood glucose: 417 mg/dL (normal: 70–110 mg/dL)
HbA1c: 11.6% (normal: 4–6%)
C-peptide: <0.5 ng/dL (normal: 0.9–4.3 ng/dL)
Antibodies ICA 511, IA, IAA, GAD65: drawn, results pending
Urine glucose: 3+
Urine ketones: moderate
Urine specific gravity: 1.05 (normal: 1.002–1.028)
BUN: 26 mg/dL (normal: 8–20 mg/dL)
Creatinine: 1.1 mg/dL (normal: 0.7–1.3 mg/dL).
GENERAL: Thin, appears fatigued
HEENT: Decreased visual acuity, mucous membranes dry
CARDIOVASCULAR: Tachycardia, pulse thready
RESPIRATORY: Increased rate
INTEGUMENTARY: Skin dry
GASTROINTESTINAL: Mild abdominal discomfort
GENITOURINARY: Polyuria, nocturia

QUESTIONS (See DavisPlus for answers)

1. What diagnosis do you suspect?

2. After discussing various options for insulin regimens, the patient chooses a multiple daily insulin regimen. What would be the beginning total daily insulin dose, the percent of basal insulin versus bolus insulin, the units of bolus insulin per meal, the sensivity factor for correcting pre-meal blood glucose above target, and the target blood glucose before meals and bedtime?

3. One week after beginning insulin therapy, the patient returns and presents his blood glucose diary. The average pre-breakfast blood glucose level is 200 mg/dL. Which insulin would you change and why?

4. The patient will be undergoing a procedure requiring him to be NPO after midnight, and he will not be able to eat until the afternoon of the next day. What adjustments need to be made in the prescribed insulin regimen?

CASE STUDY 11-2

CHIEF COMPLAINT: A 43-year-old Hispanic female presents for a general checkup and has no specific complaints. She is currently not taking any medications. After the laboratory results were reviewed and the patient questioned, the patient revealed that she has fatigue, nocturia, polydipsia, polyphagia, and weight gain.

FAMILY HISTORY: Mother and maternal grandfather: diabetes, hyperlipidemia, hypertension, coronary artery disease; 2 sisters and 1 brother have diabetes.

SOCIAL HISTORY: The patient is a married homemaker, mother of 2 daughters aged 23 and 20 years. She has no history of smoking or illegal drug use and does not drink alcohol.

CURRENT MEDICATIONS: None

REVIEW OF SYSTEMS AND PHYSICAL EXAM:
VITAL SIGNS
Blood pressure: 146/88 mm Hg
Pulse: 88/min
Respirations: 18/min
Temperature: 37°C
Height: 162.6 cm
Weight: 94 kg
BMI: 35 kg/m^2.
LABORATORY
Fasting blood glucose: 173 mg/dL (normal: 70–110 mg/dL)
HbA1c: 7.6% (normal: 4–6%)
Urine glucose: 1+
Urine ketones: negative
Urine protein: negative
Urine microalbumin: 28 mg/day (normal: <31 mg/day)
BUN: 16 mg/dL (normal: 8–20 mg/dL)
Creatinine: 0.7 mg/dL (normal: 0.7–1.3 mg/dL)
ALT: 100 IU/L (normal: 8–50 IU/L)
AST: 92 IU/L (normal: 8–46 IU/L)
Total cholesterol: 289 mg/dL (normal: <200 mg/dL)
Triglycerides: 228 mg/dL (normal: <150 mg/dL)
LDL: 162 mg/dL (normal: <100 mg/dL)
HDL: 38 mg/dL (normal female >60 mg/dL).
GENERAL: Obese
CARDIOVASCULAR: Mild fatigue with exertion, pedal pulses 1+
RESPIRATORY: Mild dyspnea on exertion
INTEGUMENTARY: Skin dry, especially on lower extremities; acanthosis nigricans present on the neck
NEUROLOGICAL: Diminished sensation on both feet with 10 gram monofilament
GASTROINTESTINAL: Obese
GENITOURINARY: Increased urination, nocturia

QUESTIONS (See DavisPlus for answers)
1. What type of diabetes does the patient most likely have and why?

2. Should the patient be started on diabetes medications in addition to therapeutic lifestyle changes as the initial treatment plan for diabetes? If so, which one(s)?

3. In addition to lifestyle therapeutic changes, should the patient be treated with medications for hyperlipidemia at this visit? If yes, which one(s)?

4. In addition to making lifestyle therapeutic changes, should the patient be treated with medications for hypertension at this visit? If yes, which one(s)?

occur over time that involve the vascular system, nervous system, skin, bones, joints, and lens. Diabetes mellitus also increases the risk of certain types of infections. See Table 11-37 for a list of common chronic complications of diabetes mellitus.

According to the American Diabetes Association, 65% of those with diabetes die of heart disease and stroke. The heart disease death rate in these patients is 2 to 4 times higher than in those without diabetes. The risk of stroke is 2 to 4 times higher, and dying from stroke is 2.8 times higher. Most patients (73%) with diabetes have hypertension (blood pressure of greater than 130/80 mm Hg) or use prescription antihypertension medications. Diabetic retinopathy is the cause of 11,000 to 23,000 new cases of blindness each year. In 2005, nearly 47,000 people with diabetes developed chronic kidney disease requiring dialysis or a transplant. Approximately 60% to 70% of people with diabetes have neuropathy. In 2004, approximately 71,000 nontraumatic lower-limb amputations were performed (60% of all cases) in people with diabetes. Periodontal disease incidence is twice the incidence in healthy patients, and 30% of all people with diabetes have severe periodontal disease, with loss of greater than 5 mm attachment of the gums to the teeth. Among patients with diabetes aged 60 years or older, the number of those unable to walk one-quarter mile, climb stairs, or do housework and of those requiring a mobility aid is 2 to 3 times

higher than in those without the disease. Other complications with a higher incidence in people with diabetes include sexual dysfunction in men and women, DKA, hyperosmolar coma, and certain infections (48). (See Table 11-37.)

The U.S. economic burden due to diabetes complications in 2007 was $58 billion (excluding the cost of lost productivity). Other costs associated with diabetes mellitus include $2.6 billion for increased absenteeism, $20 billion for reduced productivity while at work, $0.8 billion for lost productivity for those no longer employed, $7.9 billion for unemployment from disease-related disability, and $26.9 billion for lost productivity from early mortality (9).

Pathophysiology

Microvascular complications involve the small blood vessels, capillaries, and precapillary arterioles. These complications commonly cause diabetic retinopathy, diabetic nephropathy, cardiomegaly, and heart failure (48). The duration and magnitude of hyperglycemia is the most important factor in the development of microvascular complications, which are caused by thickening of the capillary basement membrane. Intacellular hyperglycemia develops in endothelial cells. Unlike other cells, endothelial cells cannot down-regulate glucose transport when exposed to extracellular hyperglycemia. Vascular smooth muscle cells, on the other hand, are not damaged by hyperglycemia.

TABLE 11–37 Common Chronic Complications of Diabetes Mellitus

Eyes	Retinopathy (nonproliferative and proliferative)
	Cataracts (subcapsular and nuclear)
Kidneys	Intercapillary glomerulosclerosis (diffuse and nodular)
	Infection (pyelonephritis, perinephric abscess, renal papillary necrosis)
	Renal tubular necrosis
Nerves	Peripheral neuropathy (distal, symmetric sensor loss)
	Motor neuropathy (foot drop, wrist drop, mononeuropathy multiplex)
	Autonomic neuropathy (postural hypotension, resting tachycardia, loss of sweating, gastroparesis, diabetic diarrhea, urinary bladder atony, impotence)
Skin	Diabetic dermopathy
	Necrobiosis lipoidica diabeticorum
	Candidiasis
	Foot and leg ulcers (neurotropic, ischemic)
Cardiovascular	Heart disease (myocardial infarction, cardiomyopathy)
	Gangrene of the feet (ischemic ulcers, osteomyelitis)
Bones/joints	Diabetic cheiroarthropathy
	Dupuytren's contracture
	Charcot joint
Infection	Necrotizing fasciitis
	Necrotizing myositis
	Mucor meningitis
	Emphysematous cholecystitis
	Malignant otitis externa

Early in the course of diabetes, before structural changes are evident, hyperglycemia causes abnormalities in blood flow and vascular permeability in the retina, glomerulus, and peripheral nerve vasa nervorum. The increase in blood flow and intracapillary pressure is believed to be caused by hyperglycemia-induced nitric oxide production on the efferent side of the capillary beds and possibly by increased sensitivity to angiotensin II. As a consequence of increased intracapillary pressure and endothelial cell dysfunction, retinal capillaries exhibit increased leakage, and glomerular capillaries have an elevated albumin excretion rate.

Similar changes occur in the vasa vasorum of the peripheral nerve. Early in the course of diabetes, increased permeability is reversible; however, it can become permanent. Progressive narrowing and occlusion of the vascular lumina results in inadequate perfusion and function of the affected tissue. Microvascular hypertension and increased vascular permeability contribute to irreversible damage via periodic acid–Schiff–positive, carbohydrate-containing plasmaproteins deposited in the capillary wall, stimulating perivascular cells and mesangial cells. The extravasation of growth factors stimulates overproduction of the extracellular matrix, possibly causing apoptosis. In the retina, microvascular disease induces programmed cell death of Müller cells, ganglion cells, pericytes, and endothelial cells. In the glomerulus, capillary occlusion and podocyte loss occurs. In the vasa nervorum, endothelial cell and pericyte degeneration occur. Progression of microvascular complications can occur even in the presence of normal glucose homeostasis. Genes may also play a role in the development of microvascular complications. Although no genes have been identified, approximately 40% of people with diabetes may be at increased risk for microvascular complications via their genetic makeup (3, 5).

Macrovascular disease involves the large blood vessels and increases the incidence of myocardial infarction, stroke, and accelerated atherosclerosis. The pathophysiology of macrovascular disease in the person with diabetes is the same as in those without diabetes; however, the process is accelerated in those with diabetes (3, 5). Even when factoring in hypertension and dyslipidemia, diabetes confers a 75% to 90% increased risk of macrovascular complications (49). The United Kingdom Prospective Diabetes Study revealed that hyperglycemia is not the central determinant in diabetic macrovascular disease as it is in microvascular disease (20).

Insulin resistance is present in those with T2DM and prediabetes; both groups have a similar increased risk of macrovascular disease. Insulin resistance is associated with a lipid profile that has a high level of very-low-density lipoprotein (VLDL), low HDL, and high LDL. Increased free fatty acid release by insulin-resistant adipocytes causes hepatocyte stimulation of VLDL secretion. Excess VLDL, in the presence of cholesteryl ester transfer protein, transfers significant amounts of triglyceride to both HDL and LDL while depleting HDL and LDL of cholesterol ester. The resultant triglyceride-enriched HDL carries less cholesteryl ester for reverse cholesterol transport to the liver, and loss of Apo1A-1 from these particles reduces the total concentration of HDL available for reverse cholesterol transport. The triglyceride-enriched, cholesteryl ester–depleted LDL is smaller and denser than normal LDL, allowing it to penetrate the vessel wall and be oxidized more easily. Atherosclerotic plaque develops, which contains lipids, inflammatory cells, smooth muscle cells, connective tissue, and calcium deposits.

All stages of atherosclerosis are the result of an inflammatory response to injury, primarily endothelial injury. Turbulent blood flow leads to endothelial dysfunction, causing nitric oxide inhibition and production of adhesion molecules that recruit and bind inflammatory cells (monocytes and T cells). These inflammatory cells migrate to the subendothelial space and initiate a vascular inflammatory response. Monocytes in the subendothelial space transform into macrophages. LDL and VLDL also bind to the endothelial cells and are oxidized in the subendothelium. Uptake of oxidized lipids and macrophage transformation into lipid-laden foam cells result in the typical early atherosclerotic lesions called fatty streaks. Macrophages have elaborate proinflammatory cytokines that recruit smooth muscle cell migration from the media and that further attract and stimulate the growth of macrophages. Various factors promote smooth muscle cell replication and increase production of dense extracellular matrix. The result is a subendothelial fibrous plaque with a fibrous cap, made of intimal smooth muscle cells surrounded by connective tissue and intracellular and extracellular lipids. A process similar to bone formation causes calcification within the plaque. Atherosclerotic plaques may be stable or unstable. Stable plaques regress, remain static, or grow slowly over several decades until they may cause occlusion (3, 5).

Clinical Presentation

The clinical presentation of early nonproliferative diabetic retinopathy includes microaneurysms, cotton wool spots, hard exudates, intraretinal microvascular abnormalities, and venous caliber abnormalities. Visual acuity will be unaffected unless macular edema is present. Proliferative retinopathy develops when new abnormal blood vessels grow and fibrous tissue develops within the retina and into the vitreous chamber causing retinal hypoxia, which stimulates more new abnormal blood vessel growth.

Diabetic nephropathy is initially manifested by microalbuminuria followed by macroalbuminuria. As kidney function declines, creatinine and blood urea nitrogen levels increase and glomerular filtration rate decreases. The patient will not exhibit symptoms of diabetic nephropathy until stage 5 (Table 11-38). Microalbuminuria correlates with increase blood pressure, increasing the risk of CVD morbidity (50).

TABLE 11–38 Stages of Chronic Kidney Disease

Stage	GFR(mL/min/1.73 m^2)
Stage 1: Kidney damage with normal or elevated GFR	>90
Stage 2: Kidney damage with mild reduction in GFR	60–89
Stage 3: Moderate decreased GFR	30–59
Stage 4: Severely decreased GFR	15–29
Stage 5: Kidney failure	<15 or dialysis

GFR, Glomerular filtration rate.

Diabetic neuropathy affects the pain fibers, motor neurons, and autonomic nerves and therefore can affect every organ since every organ is innervated. Sensorimotor peripheral neuropathy is the most common form of diabetic neuropathy. Sensory involvement causes a bilateral and symmetrical decrease in perception of pressure, vibration, and temperature. The patient may report numbness, tingling, dull ache, or burning of the hands and feet. Longer nerves are affected before shorter nerves, so symptoms appear in the toes bilaterally first and then extend upward. Loss of sensation increases the risk of foot ulcers and bone fractures, which can lead to Charcot joint. If motor nerves are involved, reflexes may be diminished or absent, dorsiflection of the toes leading to hammer toes may occur, and muscle loss in the hands may occur.

Autonomic neuropathy can affect the heart and the gastrointestinal and genitourinary systems. Patients with autonomic neuropathy may have orthostatic hypotension and loss of sinus respiratory variation (a normal change in heart rate with normal breathing). If both of these conditions exist, the patient has autonomic neuropathy to the heart. Gastrointestinal manifestations may cause gastroparesis, nausea, bloating, and diarrhea. Genitourinary manifestations may include urinary frequency, urgency, incontinence, and retention. Urine retention can cause infections, bladder diverticula, stones, and reflux nephropathy.

Cranial neuropathy manifestations include oculomotor palsy, leading to abrupt frontal or periorbital pain and then diplopia. All of the oculomotor muscles innervated by the third cranial nerve may be affected except those that control pupil size. The abducens nerve, innervating the lateral rectus muscle of the eye moving the eye laterally, is also commonly affected. Mononeuropathies of the thoracic or lumbar spinal nerves can occur and lead to painful syndromes that mimic myocardial infarction, cholecystitis, or appendicitis. Entrapment neuropathies such as carpal tunnel syndrome are common.

The clinical presentation of coronary artery disease can be silent. If symptoms are present, it is usually angina pectoris; discomfort in the chest, jaw, arm, or other sites associated with myocardial ischemia; acute myocardial infarction; dyspnea; fatigue; lower extremity edema; arrhythmias; sudden death; peripheral arterial embolism; and/or third heart sound. Cerebrovascular disease can produce transient ischemic attack and stroke. Peripheral arterial disease can produce pain in the calf muscles when walking, poor wound healing, or decreased pulses in the feet.

Diagnosis

Diagnostic testing for retinopathy includes visual acuity, dilated retinal exam, optical coherence tomography, digital retinal screening, slit lamp biomicroscopy retinal screen, and fluorescein angiography.

Diagnostic testing for diabetic nephropathy includes analysis of urine microalbumin (via a random or 24-hour urine collection), spot urine-to-creatinine ratio, blood urea nitrogen (BUN), urine creatinine, and blood creatinine (50).

Diagnostic testing for neuropathy includes a through foot examination, which involves use of a 10-gram monofilament for feeling and a tuning fork to test vibratory sense as part of sensory nerve conduction studies, possible radiographs if bone fracture is suspected, electromyography, and nerve biopsy. If autonomic neuropathy is suspected, ultrasound for bladder emptying and gastric emptying studies may be considered.

Diagnostic testing for coronary artery disease includes an ECG, which is often normal. The presence of Q waves almost always indicates myocardial infarction. The ECG may also show changes suggestive of pericarditis, left ventricular hypertrophy, right heart strain, and atrial fibrillation. The chest radiograph is also often normal, but having a normal baseline chest radiograph may be valuable later for comparison. If cardiac failure is present, the cardiothoracic ratio will be increased or pulmonary venous congestion present. The aortic contour may show aortic dissection or thoracic aortic aneurysm. The chest radiograph can also show pleural shadowing, masses in the lung fields or mediastinum, fluid at the level of the hiatus hernia behind the heart, and radiographic features of pulmonary hypertension. Blood testing includes complete blood cell count, thyroid function, urea, electrolytes, full lipid profile, and glucose. Optional cardiac and noncardiac tests to rule out coronary artery disease include upper gastrointestinal endoscopy; barium studies or abdominal ultrasound; lateral radiograph of the thoracic or cervical spine; computed tomography (CT) or magnetic resonance imaging (MRI) of the chest to examine the aorta, lung fields, and mediastinum; and an echocardiogram if a murmur is present or for another specific reason. After a myocardial infarction, an echocardiogram may be used to document left ventricular function, regional wall motion abnormalities, mitral regurgitation, ischemic septal defect, or left ventral thrombus. An exercise test can show abnormal ST-segment depression and heart rate and blood pressure response to exercise. Radioisotope myocardial perfusion scanning provides imaging of myocardial perfusion. A coronary calcification score, obtained via fast electron beam CT scanning, allows noninvasive calculation of coronary calcification. Stress echocardiography reveals changes in regional wall motion over left ventricular function during exercise and/or pharmacologic stress.

Diagnostic testing for cerebrovascular disease includes MRI, CT, ultrasound of the carotid arteries, ECG to identify arrhythmias, Holter monitor to identify intermittent arrhythmias, and angiogram of the cerebral vasculature.

Diagnostic testing for peripheral vascular disease includes ankle brachial pressure index, Doppler ultrasound angiography, and multislice CT scan.

Management

The relationship of blood glucose control to the development of long-term diabetes complications has been studied extensively. Several landmark trials have shown that microvascular complications are highly correlated with elevated HbA1c levels and that near-normal HbA1c levels reduce the incidence and severity of disease (18-21). Therefore, management of serum glucose level is an important component of managing microvascular complications.

Management of diabetic retinopathy begins with referral for an initial dilated ophthalmic examination. The initial examination, performed by a qualified optometrist or ophthalmologist, is recommended at diagnosis for adults with T2DM and 5 years after a diagnosis of T1DM for those aged 10 years or older. Subsequent examinations are performed annually unless the optometrist or ophthalmologist recommends less frequent checkups. More frequent examinations may be required if the patient has retinopathy, other progressive ocular complications, or is undergoing treatment for ocular conditions. Women with preexisting diabetes who are pregnant should be examined as soon as the pregnancy is discovered; those planning pregnancy should be examined before becoming pregnant. Subsequent examinations and treatment may be needed throughout the pregnancy and postpartum.

Laser photocoagulation is indicated for patients with high-risk severe nonproliferative diabetic retinopathy, proliferative diabetic retinopathy, or vision-threatening macular edema. Intraocular steroid injection is a new treatment for macular edema that may be used in combination with laser treatments; multiple treatments may be needed. Cryotherapy may be used if the vitreous is clouded by blood, thus removing the need for laser treatment. Cryotherapy helps to shrink the new abnormal blood vessels and bond the retina to the back of the eye. Vitrectomy is used to remove blood-filled vitreous. Intensive diabetes management has been shown to help prevent and/or delay the onset and progression of retinopathy. Reducing blood pressure reduces the progression of retinopathy.

Management of diabetic nephropathy depends on the stage of kidney disease (Table 11-38). The management of microalbuminuria (31 to 299 mg/day) includes the treatment of hypertension and dyslipidemia and strict blood glucose control. In patients with T1DM, angiotensin-converting enzyme (ACE) inhibitors have been shown to delay the progression of nephropathy, and in patients with T2DM, both ACE inhibitors and angiotensin receptor blockers (ARBs) have been shown to delay the progression to macroalbuminuria. Since proteinuria is a risk factor for coronary heart disease, the patient should undergo a baseline ECG, echocardiogram, dobutamine stress test, urine culture, fluorescein angiography, and Doppler limb flow. The patient should also be assessed for comorbid conditions, including angina, congestive heart failure, cardiomyopathy, respiratory disease, ocular complications, autonomic neuropathies, cerebrovascular disease, musculoskeletal disorders such as renal bone disease, infections, and hematologic problems other than anemia. After implementing treatment, monitoring should be continued for urinary protein, creatinine clearance, retinopathy, cataracts, cardiac integrity, bone density, peripheral perfusion, neurologic stability, and psychosocial adjustment.

Adults with macroalbuminuria (greater than 299 mg/day) are likely to progress to chronic kidney disease. A referral to a nephrologist should be considered for those who are at high risk for progression to chronic kidney disease or who have advanced kidney disease (stage 4) or if there is uncertainty about etiology. In patients with T2DM, ARBs have been shown to delay the progression of nephropathy. Hypertension and dyslipidemia may worsen, so multiple medications will probably be needed. Diuretics may be needed to control edema. Blood glucose control may deteriorate. As renal function declines, the half-life of insulin is prolonged and renal response to hypoglycemia is impaired, so prevention of hypoglycemia is important. Oral antihyperglycemic agents should be chosen carefully. Prolonged hypoglycemia may occur in those treated with sulfonylureas. Metformin is contraindicated if the creatinine level is greater than 1.5 in men or greater than 1.4 in women. The use of nonsteroidal anti-inflammatory drugs and cyclooxygenase-2 inhibitors should be avoided. Anemia may require intervention. A reduction of dietary protein intake to 0.8 to 1.0 g/kg/day may improve renal function. Continued monitoring is needed for urine albumin excretion, serum creatinine, and estimated glomerular filtration rate (GFR) and K+ levels. If the estimated GFR is less than 60 mL/min/1.73 m², screening is needed for anemia, malnutrition, and metabolic bone disease. If the patient is likely to progress to chronic kidney disease, vaccination against hepatitis B is needed. Patients requiring renal replacement therapies have many options, including home or facility hemodialysis, peritoneal dialysis, renal transplantation, or combined pancreas-kidney transplantation (50). See Table 11-39 for diabetic nephropathy screening and treatment recommendations.

The goal of managing diabetic neuropathy is to ameliorate symptoms and prevent progression. Screening for distal symmetric polyneuropathy should be done at diagnosis and annually thereafter by using a 10-gram monofilament for testing pressure sensation, a 118-Hz tuning fork to test vibration, and a reflex hammer to test ankle reflexes. Screening for signs and symptoms of cardiovascular autonomic neuropathy should be performed at diagnosis of T2DM and 5 years after diagnosis of

TABLE 11–39 Diabetic Nephropathy Screening and Treatment Recommendations

Risk reduction

- Optimize blood glucose control
- Optimize blood pressure control

Screening

- Annual screening of urine albumin excretion in patients with T1DM with a duration of >5 years and all patients with T2DM at diagnosis
- Use a random spot urine collection for albumin-to-creatinine ratio
- Normal: <30 µg/mg creatinine
- Microalbuminuria: 30–299 µg/mg creatinine
- Macroalbuminuria: >300 µg/mg creatinine
- Measure serum creatinine annually
- Use creatinine to estimate GFR and stage the level of chronic kidney disease if present

Nonpregnant patients with micro or macroalbuminuria

- ACEI or ARB (if one class is not tolerated, the other should be substituted)

T1DM with HTN and albuminuria

- ACEI has shown to delay the progression of CKD
- Intensive diabetes management
- Tight blood pressure control

T2DM, hypertension, and microalbuminuia

- ACEI or ARB (if one class is not tolerated, the other should be substituted)
- Intensive diabetes management
- Tight blood pressure control

T2DM, hypertension and macroalbuminuria

- ARBs have been shown to delay the progression of CKD
- Intensive diabetes management
- Tight blood pressure control

Individuals intolerant to ACEI or ARB

- Consider these medications to control blood pressure:
- Beta-blocker
- Diuretics
- CA channel blockers

TABLE 11-39 Diabetic Nephropathy Screening and Treatment Recommendations—cont'd

Dietary protein restriction

- Early CKD: 0.8–1.0 g/kg/day
- Advanced CKD: 0.8 g/kg/day

Continued evaluation of CKD

- Urine albumin excretion to assess response to therapy and progression of disease
- If ACEI or ARB is used, monitor serum creatinine and K^+

Refer to physician experienced in CKD

- Uncertain about the etiology of CKD
- Active urine sediment
- Absence of retinopathy
- Rapid decline in GFR
- Difficult management issues
- Advanced kidney disease

ACEI, Angiotensin-converting enzyme; *ARB,* angiotensin receptor blocker; *HTN,* hypertension; *CKD,* chronic kidney disease.

T1DM. Common signs and symptoms include resting tachycardia, exercise intolerance, orthostatic hypotension, constipation, diarrhea, gastroparesis, erectile dysfunction, sudomotor dysfunction, impaired neurovascular function, and hypoglycemia autonomic failure. Improving blood glucose control may slow progression but not reverse neuronal loss; however, treatment of symptoms of neuropathy is recommended. Medications such as tricyclic antidepressants, anticonvulsants, 5-hydroxytryptamine and norepinephrine uptake inhibitors, and substance P inhibitors can be used to treat symptoms of diabetic polyneuropathy. Gastroparesis symptoms may improve with dietary changes or with medications such as metoclopramide or erythromycin. Erectile dysfunction treatment may include phosphodiesterase type 5 inhibitors, intracorporeal or intraurethral prostaglandins, vacuum devices, or penile prostheses (27).

Macrovascular complications are the result of multiple metabolic abnormalities such as hypertension and dyslipidemia, and merely normalizing glucose is not enough for prevention and management. Many of the macrovascular complications are present at diagnosis of T2DM. Control of blood glucose level, blood pressure, and lipid level is vitally important. The goals for HbA1c, blood pressure, and lipids are different in patients with diabetes versus those with CVD alone and are outlined in Table 11-40.

Hypertension increases CVD morbidity and mortality. If hypertension is diagnosed, lifestyle modifications

TABLE 11-40 American Diabetes Association Goals for Diabetes Management

Blood glucose: nonpregnant	Preprandial capillary plasma glucose: 70–130 mg/dL (3.9–7.2 mmol) Peak postprandial capillary plasma glucose: <180 mg/dL (<10.0 mmol/L)
Blood glucose: GDM	Preprandial: <95 mg/dL (5.3 mmol/L)
	• 1-hr postmeal: <140 mg/dL (7.8 mmol/L)
	or
	• 2-hr postmeal: <110 mg/dL (6.7 mmol/L)
Blood glucose: pregnant with preexisting T1DM or T2DM	The following is optimal glycemic control if they can be achieved without excessive hypoglycemia:
	• Premeal, bedtime, and overnight glucose: 60–99 mg/dL • Peak postprandial glucose: 100–119 mg/dL

Continued

TABLE 11–40 American Diabetes Association Goals for Diabetes Management—cont'd

HbA1c: nonpregnant	<7%
HbA1c: GDM	<6%
HbA1c: pregnant with preexisting T1DM or T2DM	<6% if achievable without excessive hypoglycemia
Blood pressure: not pregnant	130/80 mm Hg
Blood pressure: pregnant with chronic hypertension	Systolic: 110–119 mm Hg Diastolic: 65–79 mm Hg
Lipids in low-risk adults	LDL cholesterol: <100 mg/dL HDL cholesterol: >50 mg/dL Triglycerides: <150 mg/dL
Lipids in high-risk adults	LDL cholesterol: <100 mg/dL HDL cholesterol: >50 mg/dL Triglycerides: <150 mg/dL
LDL in those with diabetes and overt cardiovascular disease	<70 mg/dL (1.8 mmol/L)
Drug treated patients not reaching targets on maximal tolerated statin therapy	A reduction in LDL cholesterol of >30–40% from baseline is an alternative goal

GDM, Goals for diabetes management; *HDL,* high-density lipoprotein; *LDL,* low-density lipoprotein; *T1DM,* type 1 diabetes mellitus; *T2DM,* type 2 diabetes mellitus.

should be reviewed; the patient should also be referred to a dietitian and/or to tobacco cessation counseling/treatment if needed. Weight reduction, healthy eating with sodium restriction, consumption of omega-3 fatty acids, physical activity, and limiting alcohol consumption to less than 2 drinks per day for men and less than 1 drink per day for women will help lower blood pressure. The patient should begin taking antihypertensive medications if systolic blood pressure is greater than 140 mm Hg or diastolic blood pressure is greater than 90 mm Hg. See Table 11-41 for recommendations for treating hypertension in adults with

diabetes. Most adults with diabetes and hypertension will require combination therapy, which uses smaller doses of multiple medications and allows complementary mechanisms of action while reducing the incidence of adverse effects (51, 52).

Diabetes is a coronary heart disease risk equivalent; therefore, lipid goals in adults with diabetes are the same as in adults with coronary artery disease. Dyslipidemia in diabetes, a modifiable risk factor for CVD, generally consists of a moderate elevation of triglycerides, low HDL, and high LDL. In adults with T2DM, dyslipidemia is often present before the diagnosis of diabetes. Most do

TABLE 11–41 Suggested Hypertension Treatment in Adults With Diabetes

If systolic blood pressure is 130–139 mm Hg and diastolic pressure is 80–89 mm Hg

- Lifestyle therapy for maximum of 3 months.
- If target not achieved in 3 months, add pharmacologic agents.

If systolic blood pressure is >140 mm Hg and diastolic pressure is >90 mm Hg
Begin with lifestyle therapy plus pharmacologic agents.

- Titrate every 4–8 weeks to at least ½ maximum dose.
- On average, at least 3 agents will be needed.
  - ✓ Hypertension alone: ACEI, ARB, beta-blocker, or diuretic.
  - ✓ Presence of microalbuminuria or macroalbuminuria: ACEI or ARB is strongly recommended.
  - ✓ Consider verapamil or diltiazem in patients with proteinuria unable to tolerate ACEI or ARBs.

TABLE 11–41 Suggested Hypertension Treatment in Adults With Diabetes—cont'd

- Adults older than 55 years with hypertension, or those without hypertension but with a cardiovascular risk fastor:
  ✓ After recent myocardial infarction: beta-blocker.
  ✓ African American: start ACEI in combination with diuretic or CA channel blocker.
  ✓ If systolic blood pressure is >145 and/or diastolic blood pressure is >90 mm Hg, begin with combination therapy
- Reassess blood pressure in 4–8 weeks

If Blood Pressure Targets Are Not Met:

- Verify adherence to regimen.
- Add diuretic <u>or</u> CA channel blocker <u>or</u> beta-blocker.
  ✓ If choosing a diuretic: use thiazide if creatinine is <1.8 mg/dL, a loop diuretic if creatinine is >1.8 mg/dL.
  ✓ If choosing a beta-blocker: choose without intrinsic sympathomimetic activity.
  ✓ If choosing a CA channel blocker: diltiazem or verapamil. Do not use dihydropyridine if using ACEI or ARB.
- Reassess blood pressure in 4–8 weeks.

If Blood Pressure Targets Are Still Not Met:

Add an additional agent from another class not used in the above classes, or

- Consider referral to a specialist, or
- Add an α blocker, hydralazine, or clonidine

If Pregnant With Chronic Hypertension:

- Do not use ACEI or ARB.
- Agents that may be used during pregnancy: methyldopa, labetalol, diltiazem, clonidine, or prazosin.
- Use of diuretics has been associated with restricted maternal plasma volume and may reduce uteroplacental perfusion.

ACEI, Aangiotensin-converting enzyme inhibitor; *ARB,* angiotensin receptor blocker.

not achieve target goals for lipids with monotherapy and will require combination therapy. Smaller doses of combination therapy are preferable to high-dose monotherapy. Common therapeutic combinations include a statin with one of the following: niacin, fibrate, bile acid sequestrant, omega-3 fatty acid, or ezetimibe; another common combination is ezetimibe with a fibrate (53-56). Table 11-42 outlines recommendations for dyslipidemia management in adults with diabetes; Table 11-43 compares lipid modifying medications; and Table 11-44 compares dose equivalency of the statin medications.

Coronary heart disease is the leading cause of morbidity and mortality in adults with diabetes; therefore, prevention, early diagnosis, and treatment are vital. The Framingham Risk Score includes the following risk factors: sex, total cholesterol, HDL, systolic blood pressure, cigarette smoking, and age. The American Diabetes Association recommends screening of adults with typical or atypical chest pain, abnormal ECG suggestive of ischemia or infarction, peripheral or carotid arterial occlusive disease, age older than 35 years with a sedentary lifestyle who want to start an exercise program, and two or more risk factors in addition to diabetes (dyslipidemia, hypertension, tobacco use, family history of premature coronary arterial disease, or proteinuria). Assessment of traditional risk factors alone does not detect those with silent ischemia; however, the American Diabetes Association does not recommend routine screening of asymptomatic patients with T2DM and normal ECGs (49). See Table 11-45 for American Diabetes Association recommendations for coronary heart disease treatment.

Clinical Nurse Specialist Competencies and Spheres of Influence
Clinical Expert/Direct Care

The CNS provides direct clinical care of the patient with diabetes complications by conducting a comprehensive history and physical assessment based on evidence-based

TABLE 11–42 Lipid Treatment for Adults With Diabetes

- Lifestyle modifications for all with abnormal lipid levels:
  - Reduce saturated fat, trans fat, and cholesterol intake.
  - Lose weight if indicated.
  - Increase physical activity.

All patients with overt CVD or those without CVD who are older than 40 years and have >1 CVD risk factor:

- Begin statin therapy (*contraindicated in pregnancy).

Patients younger than 40 years without overt CVD and LDL >100 mg/dL (2.6 mmol/L), or multiple CVD risk factors:

- Begin statin therapy (*contraindicated in pregnancy).

LDL in those with diabetes and overt CVD not achieving LDL <70 mg/dL:

- Consider high-dose statin (*contraindicated in pregnancy).

LDL in those who do not achieve goal on maximum tolerated doses of statins (*contraindicated in pregnancy):

- Consider adding niacin (can elevate blood glucose).
- Consider adding fenofibrate.
- Consider adding ezetimibe.
- Consider adding bile acid sequestrants.

Patients with hypertriglyceridemia:

- Consider fibric acid derivative.
- Consider niacin (can elevate blood glucose).
- Consider fish oil.

Patients With Low HDL and LDL of 100–119 mg/dL:
- Consider gemfibrozil.
- Consider niacin (can elevate blood glucose).

If goals are not achieved after adjustment, consider referring to a lipid specialist.
Combination therapy using a statin, niacin, and a fibrate increases the risk of abnormal transaminase levels, myositis, and rhabdomyolysis.

CVD, Cardiovascular disease; LDL, low density lipoprotein.

TABLE 11–43 Comparison of Lipid-Modifying Medications

Medication Class	LDL-C	HDL-C	Triglycerides
Statins	↓ 18–55%	↑ 5–15%	↓ 7–30%
Bile acid resins	↓ 15–30%	↑ 3–5%	↑ 0–15%
Absorption inhibitors	↓ 18–20%	↑ 3%	↓ 8%
Nicotinic acid	↓ 5–25%	↑ 15–35%	↓ 20–50%
Stanol ethers	↓ 5–14%	No change	No change
Fibrates	↓ 5–20%	↑ 10–20%	↓ 25–50%
Omega-2 fatty acid	↓ 2–5%	No change	↓ 30–40%

HDL-C, High-density-lipoprotein cholesterol; LDL-C, low-density-lipoprotein cholesterol.

TABLE 11–44 HMG Co-A Reductase Inhibitors (Statins) LDL-C Equivalency in LDL % Reduction

Fluvastatin (mg)	Pravastatin (mg)	Lovastatin (mg)	Simvastatin (mg)	Atorvastatin (mg)	Rosuvastatin (mg)	Ezetibe/ Simvastatin (mg)	Approximate ↓ % LDL Reduction
20	10	10					15–20
40	20	20	5–10				21–29
80 XL	40–80	40	20	10			30–38
		80	40	20	5–10	10/10	39–47
			80	40	20	10/20	48–54
				80	40	10/40	55–59
						10/80	>59

LDL-C, Low density lipoprotein cholesterol; *HMG Co-A,* 3-hydroxy-3-methyl-glutaryl-CoA reductase.

TABLE 11–45 American Diabetes Association Recommendations for Coronary Heart Disease (CHD) Treatment for Individuals With Diabetes

Primary prevention in those at increased risk of CVD (assess for risk factors annually):

- Smoking cessation
- Blood pressure control
- Lipid control
- Antiplatelet agents for adults older than 40 years with additional risk factors such as the following (26):
  - Family history of CVD
  - Hypertension
  - Smoking
  - Dyslipidemia
  - Albuminuria
  - Cardiac autonomic neuropathy
- Treat with aspirin at 75–162 mg/day.
- Those with documented aspirin allergy should consider clopidogrel at 75 mg/day.

After acute coronary syndrome:

- Consider: Aspirin at 75–162 mg/day and clopidogrel at 75 mg/day for up to 1 year.

CHD screening in asymptomatic patients:

- Evaluate risk factors and stratify patients by 10-year risk.
- Treat risk factors.

Known CVD:

- ACE inhibitor
- Aspirin
- Statin therapy

Prior myocardial infarction:

- Add beta-blocker if not contraindicated

Patients >40 years old with another risk factor listed above:

- Add aspirin and statin

Patients with congestive heart failure:

- Thiazolidinediones are contraindicated

Stable congestive heart failure and renal function is normal:

- Metformin may be used

Candidates for cardiac testing:

- Typical or atypical cardiac symptoms
- Abnormal testing electrocardiogram

ACE, angiotensin-converting enzyme; *CVD,* Cardiovascular disease.

techniques and on tools to diagnose and treat diabetes complications. Professional organizations such as the American Diabetes Association and the American College of Clinical Endocrinologists publish specific guidelines to assist in these assessments and guide management. The CNS should refer patients to a specialist for management of certain complications (as listed in Table 11-46). For example, the CNS would not be able to provide a dilated eye examination and would need to refer the patient to an ophthalmologist or optometrist. The diabetes CNS's role in clinical and professional leadership regarding diabetes complications may include

TABLE 11–46 Clinical Connections: Complications of Diabetes

Clinical Manifestations	Pathophysiology	Assessment Finding	Laboratory Diagnostic tests	Treatment
Retinopathy	Increased intracapillary pressure and endothelial cell dysfunction causes retinal capillary leakage	Microaneurysms, soft exudates, hard exudates, macular edema, neovascularization	Dilated eye exam by a specialist	Laser photocoagulation, intraoccular medications, cryotherapy, vitrectomy, tight blood glucose control
Nephropathy	Increased intracapillary pressure and endothelial cell dysfunction causes albumin excretion by the glomerular capillaries	No early symptoms, albuminuria, late nephropathy (weakness, poor appetite, nausea, vomiting, reduced diabetes medication doses, sleep difficulty)	Microalbumin, 24-hour urine, urine-to-creatinine ratio, creatinine	Blood glucose control, ACEI or ARB, blood pressure control, lipid control, low protein diet, low Na diet, avoidance of nephrotoxic substances
Neuropathy	Increased intracapillary pressure and endothelial cell dysfunction in the vasa vasoum in the peripheral nerve	Tingling, numbness, burning, pain; decreased sensation to vibration, pressure, and temperature; diminished reflexes, muscle atrophy, orthostatic hypotension, inability to empty bladder, gastroparesis, diabetic diarrhea, loss of sinus respiration variation, gustagory sweating, lack of sweating, Charcot joint, carpal tunnel, erectile dysfunction	History, foot exam, reflexes, Monofilament, tuning fork, EMG, nerve biopsy, bladder ultrasound	Blood glucose control: tricyclics, anticonvulsants, 5-hydroxytryptamine, norepinephrine uptake inhibitors, and substance p inhibitors. Modified diet for gastroparesis. Surgery for carpal tunnel. Erectile dysfunction: phosphodiesterase type 5 inhibitors, intracorporeal or intraurethral prostaglandins, vacuum devices, or penile prostheses

Continued

TABLE 11–46 Clinical Connections: Complications of Diabetes—cont'd

Clinical Manifestations	Pathophysiology	Assessment Finding	Laboratory Diagnostic tests	Treatment
Hypertension	In T1DM: Usually presents with nephropathy; in T2DM: volume expansion, increased salt sensitivity, loss of nocturnal dipping of blood pressure	Elevated blood pressure (>130/80 mm Hg)	Blood pressure (>130/80 mm Hg)	Lifestyle therapy. One or moreof the following anti-hypertension medications: ACEI, ARB, beta blocker, diuretic, CA channel blocker. If not met by combination therapy with the above agents, add: α blocker, hydralazine, or clonidine. Pregnancy: methyldopa, labetalol, diltiazem, clonidine, or prazosin
Hyperlipidemia	Insulin resistance causes adverse lipid profile	Elevated triglycerides, total cholesterol, LDL or VLDL; decreased HDL	Lipid panel	Lifestyle therapy. Medications: statin, niacin, fibric acid derivative, ezetimibe, bile acid sequestrants, and fish oil
Coronary heart disease	Adverse lipid profile, hypertension, genetics, age, and modifiable risk factors increase risk of atherosclerosis	Angina, acute myocardial infarction, heart failure	Electrocardiogram, echocardiogram, chest radiograph, CBC, thyroid function, urea, electrolytes, lipid panel, glucose, exercise cardiac stress test, radionucleide stress test, stress echocardiography, physiologic stress test	Smoking cessation. Blood pressure control: ACEI or ARB Lipid control: Statin, antiplatelet agents, beta-blocker

ACEI, Angiotensin-converting enzyme inhibitor; *ARB,* angiotensin receptor blocker; *LDL,* low density lipoprotein; *VLDL,* very low density lipoprotein.

helping to develop a foot care program to prevent ulcers while the patient is hospitalized. In the outpatient area, there may be a need for the CNS to develop assessment tools to remind the clinician to record diabetes health maintenance activities such as eye examination and microalbumin screening results. Chart audits for the screening of diabetes complications should be conducted, and the results can be the basis for quality-improvement initiatives.

Collaboration

The collaboration role of the CNS may involve working with cardiologists for patients with CVD, pharmacists for medications to treat complications, or the wound care team to help manage patients with ulcers. Keeping the patient and family informed about the schedule for screening for complications of diabetes is important to prevent or discover the complication as early as possible. If the patient does develop complications, education about treatment is needed. For example, if microalbuminuria is discovered, the patient needs to know the new blood pressure, blood glucose, and lipid goals; medications such

as an ACE inhibitor or an ARB should be started; and if needed, a statin to lower the LDL to less than 70 mg/dL should be initiated since microalbuminuria is a cardiac risk factor. Since those with microalbuminuria commonly have other microvascular complications, screening for retinopathy and neuropathy is also vital. The CNS involved in research of diabetes complications can keep a database of complications on the patient population being served. Trends can be tracked and reported, and the research data can be used for publications, poster presentations, and oral presentations to implement new programs, change policy, or develop algorithms.

DIABETIC KETOACIDOSIS

Etiology

DKA is a life-threatening condition caused by severe insulin deficiency leading to hyperglycemia, electrolyte imbalances, dehydration, and metabolic acidosis. The development of DKA is more common in those with

---

CASE STUDY 11–3 | Diabetes Complications

CHIEF COMPLAINT: The patient has just moved to town and needs to establish medical care.

HISTORY OF PRESENT ILLNESS: A 70-year-old African American male has a history of T2DM diagnosed 25 years ago, hypertension diagnosed 30 years ago, hyperlipidemia diagnosed 25 years ago, myocardial infarction diagnosed 15 years ago, chronic kidney disease diagnosed 5 years ago, and peripheral neuropathy diagnosed 20 years ago.

FAMILY HISTORY: Mother: heart disease, breast cancer; father: diabetes, heart disease, hypertension; grandparents: history unknown; brother: T2 DM and heart disease; sister: breast cancer.

CURRENT MEDICATIONS: metformin at 1,000 mg PO bid, glyburide at 5 mg PO daily, pioglitazone at 30 mg PO daily, losartan at 100 mg PO daily, hydrochlorothiazide at 25 mg PO daily, and atorvastatin at 20 mg PO daily

REVIEW OF SYSTEMS AND PHYSICAL EXAM
VITAL SIGNS
Blood pressure: 142/84 mm Hg
Pulse: 88/min
Respirations: 16/min
Temperature: 37°C
Height: 177.8 cm
Weight: 94.8 kg
BMI: 30 kg/m².
LABORATORY
Fasting blood glucose: 132 mg/dL (normal: 70–110 mg/dL)
HbA1c: 7.5% (normal: 4–6%)
Urine glucose: 1+
Urine ketones: negative
Urine protein: positive
Urine microalbumin: 754 mg/day (normal: <31 mg/day)
BUN: 26 mg/dL (normal: 8–20 mg/dL)

CASE STUDY 11-3 | Diabetes Complications—cont'd

GFR: 78 mL/min (normal: >90 mL/min)
Creatinine: 1.6 mg/dL (normal: 0.7–1.3 mg/dL)
ALT: 11 IU/L (normal: 8–50 IU/L)
AST: 14 IU/L (normal: 8–46 IU/L)
Total cholesterol: 226 mg/dL (normal: <200 mg/dL)
Triglycerides: 188 mg/dL (normal <150 mg/dL)
LDL: 110 mg/dL (normal <100 mg/dL)
HDL: 32 mg/dL (normal male >40 mg/dL).
GENERAL: Obese
HEENT: History of bilateral lens replacement, nearsighted
CARDIOVASCULAR: Fatigues easily with exertion, occasional chest discomfort with exertion, history of myocardial infarction
RESPIRATORY: Exertional dyspnea when climbing stairs
NEUROLOGIC: Reflexes: patellar and Achilles 1+, decreased sensation to a 10-gram monofilament to both feet, and unable to distinguish touch from vibration when touched with a tuning fork
INTEGUMENTARY: Skin dry lower extremities and feet
GASTROINTESTINAL: Obese
GENITOURINARY: Frequency, history of enlarged prostate

QUESTIONS (See DavisPlus for answers)
1. Should the dose of any diabetes medications be reduced or should any diabetes medications be discontinue and why?

2. Should any diabetes medications be increased or added and why?

3. Should the antihypertensive medications be adjusted? If yes, which ones and why?

4. Are the lipids acceptable? If not, what should be changed?

T1DM younger than 19 years, but it can occur in any type of diabetes and at any age. Males and females are equally affected. In 1994, DKA was listed as the primary hospital admission diagnosis for 89,000 patients and was the underlying cause of death in 1701 patients, with an age-adjusted mortality rate of 20.2 per 100,000 (57). The most common cause is illness (40%), followed by omission of insulin (25%) and newly diagnosed diabetes (15%). The approximate cost of DKA per hospitalization is $13,152, which represents 1 of every 4 health care dollars spent on T1DM (58).

Pathophysiology

The basic cause of DKA is profound insulin deficiency. Although small amounts of insulin may be circulating, the presence of large amounts of stress hormones (glucagon, catecholamines such as epinephrine and norepinephrine, cortisol, and growth hormone) renders the insulin less effective. Carbohydrate, protein, and fat metabolism are all markedly affected. Insulin deficiency in the postprandial state impairs glucose uptake in the peripheral tissues (mainly muscle) and liver, leading to hyperglycemia. During fasting, insulin deficiency results in excess hepatic glucose production that can also lead to hyperglycemia. Insulin deficiency causes impaired protein synthesis and excessive protein degradation. The resulting increase in gluconeogenic amino acids leads to increased hepatic glucose production (by means of gluconeogenesis) and finally hyperglycemia. The failure to build new protein and the increased breakdown of already formed protein are the reasons for the loss of lean body mass in uncontrolled diabetes.

Severe insulin deficiency and increased counterregulatory hormones cause excessive hydrolysis of triglycerides, the stored form of fat, releasing increased amounts of free fatty acids and glycerol. This metabolic pathway is called lipolysis. Glycerol is an important gluconeogenic precursor to increasing hepatic glucose production and further hyperglycemia. Excessive amounts of ketone bodies (beta-hydroxybutyric acid and acetoacetic acid) are formed in the liver from the free fatty acids with resulting ketonemia and metabolic acidosis. Low levels of insulin permit ketogenesis, not only by providing more free fatty acids but also by enhancing certain critical hepatic enzymes that change free fatty acids into ketone bodies.

Hyperglycemia leads to osmotic diuresis, which causes hypotonic fluid losses and dehydration as well as electrolyte depletion. Ketone bodies are weak acids that can be used by most tissues, but only to a limited extent. When this capacity is exceeded, the ketone bodies must be neutralized (buffered). As ketones continue to accumulate, the buffering capacity of the body is exhausted and acidosis supervenes. Ketonuria leads to more electrolyte depletion because cations must be eliminated along with the anionic ketone bodies to maintain electrical neutrality. Twelve to 24 hours of insulin deficiency in patients with T1DM (depending on the hyperglycemic state) causes profound fluid and electrolyte losses.

Clinical Presentation

The symptoms of hyperglycemia may mimic other diseases or conditions. Although the symptoms of poorly controlled diabetes may be present for several days, the metabolic alterations typical of DKA usually occur within a short timeframe. Occasionally, DKA may develop more acutely with no prior signs or symptoms. Manifestations of hyperglycemia are polyuria, polydipsia, blurred vision, polyphagia (if insulin deficiency is present long enough, i.e., days to weeks), and weight loss. Nonspecific symptoms include weakness, lethargy, malaise, and headache. Gastrointestinal symptoms are nausea, vomiting, and abdominal pain. The cause of these symptoms is unclear, but they are probably related to the ketosis and/or acidotic state. Respiratory symptoms may include hyperpnea and deep respirations termed Kussmaul respirations and reflect a pulmonary response to acidosis. Acetone breath may be present. Acetoacetate, one of the ketone bodies, is converted to acetone, which is excreted by the lungs. It has a fruity odor that can sometimes be detected on the breath of the patient. This hyperventilation produces respiratory alkalosis in a partial, but not completely successful, attempt to correct the metabolic acidosis by blowing off carbon dioxide.

There are no specific signs of DKA; rather, a constellation of evidence should suggest the possibility of DKA. Hypothermia is often found; therefore, the presence of fever suggests associated infection. Dehydration (intravascular volume depletion) is a common sign. Dehydration can be assessed by observing for decreased neck vein filling from below when the patient is lying absolutely flat. Orthostatic hypotension (a decrease in systolic blood pressure of 20 mm Hg after 1 minute of standing) may occur as a result of decreased intravascular volume from dehydration. Poor skin turgor is seen earlier in children. Acute abdomen is a common condition marked by tenderness to palpation, diminished bowel sounds, and some muscle guarding, especially in children. A few patients may have more severe signs such as absent bowel sounds, rebound tenderness, and board-like abdomen that suggest a surgical emergency. However, in virtually every case, these signs are due to profound DKA and disappear after treatment.

Mentation changes may be present. Patients may be alert, obtunded, stuporous, or in frank coma. Mentation seems to correlate best with serum osmolality and less well with glucose concentrations, and least with pH changes. Hyporeflexia, or decreased reflexes, if not present initially, may occur if during treatment, the potassium level falls below normal. Hypotonia, uncoordinated ocular movements, and fixed, dilated pupils are all late signs that suggest a poor prognosis.

Diagnosis

Immediately at the bedside, order a blood glucose and beta-hydroxybutyrate by meter if available. Implement continuous ECG monitoring. Determine levels of serum glucose, BUN, creatinine, calcium, magnesium, phosphate, ketones, lactate, and creatine phosphokinase; also, conduct liver function tests, urinalysis, upright chest radiography, complete blood cell count, and arterial blood gases. Other tests may be ordered, depending on clinical findings. If the patient has new-onset T1DM, order islet cell antibodies, insulin auto antibodies, anti-GAD antibodies, C-peptide, and insulin. See Table 11–47 for usual initial laboratory findings for DKA.

TABLE 11–47 Initial Laboratory Findings for Diabetic Ketoacidosis (DKA)

Blood glucose	Usually >300 mg/dL
pH	<7.3
PCO_2	<35 mm Hg reflects the hyperventilatory response to the metabolic acidosis
Bicarbonate	0–15 mEq/L vc
Total serum ketones	Positive at 1:2 dilution
Initial K^+	May be high, normal, or low (total body depletion)
WBC	May be high; >10% band formation usually signifies severe infection
Phosphate	May be normal or low
Na	May be low, normal, or high (total body depletion)
Chloride	May be high

TABLE 11–47 Initial Laboratory Findings for Diabetic Ketoacidosis (DKA)—cont'd

Serum amylase (predominant form is of salivary gland origin)	May be high, but lipase is not
BUN and creatinine	May be high
Arterial oxygen levels	May be low
Aspartate aminotransferase, alanine aminotransferase	Can be elevated
Urine ketone testing	Positive. Nitroprusside reacts only with acetoacetate, not with beta-hydroxybutyrate. These two ketones exist in equilibrium, with the amount of beta-hydroxybutyrate 3 to 5 times greater than that of acetoacetate in DKA. This test for ketones can only be used to diagnose DKA; it is not useful in monitoring response to therapy because the excess beta-hydroxybutyrate is converted back to acetoacetate as the patient improves biochemically.
Na	Concentration at a particular time will reflect the relative amounts of water and Na lost and replaced up to that point. If the deficit of water is greater than that of Na, the Na level will be high; if the deficit of Na is greater than that of water, the Na level will be low; if the deficits are approximately equal, the Na level will be normal.
K^+	Can be low, normal, or high despite a profound loss of K^+. The K^+ level does not reflect the relative amounts of water lost but depends on the balance between the amount of K^+ lost in the urine and other factors that raise the K^+ level, such as the lack of insulin, which allows K^+ to remain in the circulation rather than enter cells. If K^+ transferring from the cells into the circulation exceeds excretion, the serum K^+ level may be high. Total body depletion of K^+ always occurs regardless of the initial serum level.
Phosphate	Usually high or high-normal initially, and decreases, sometimes markedly, to very low levels over the next day or two.
BUN and creatinine	Creatinine and BUN concentrations are usually mildly increased because of the dehydration and prerenal azotemia. After rehydration, elevated creatinine and BUN levels indicate the presence of renal insufficiency before DKA.
Hemoglobin, hematocrit, and total protein	Often mildly elevated, reflecting the decreased plasma volume (dehydration).
White blood cell count (WBC)	Usually increased, occasionally to very high levels. This increase does not necessarily reflect an ongoing infection, since DKA itself often causes an increase in white cell count. However, if a differential count is performed, a >10% band formation (immature WBC) almost always denotes a severe infection, whereas <10% band formation usually does not.
Amylase	Values are usually increased. This increase does not reflect pancreatitis because in DKA, salivary glands, not the pancreas, release most of the amylase. Liver function tests often produce mildly elevated values. This elevation does not necessarily reflect acute or chronic liver damage because the values usually return to normal in several weeks.

Management

The goal of DKA treatment is to correct fluid and electrolyte disturbances, provide adequate insulin to restore and maintain normal blood glucose metabolism and correct acidosis, prevent complications resulting from the treatment of DKA, and provide patient and family education and follow-up. Begin by inserting an IV catheter and drawing blood for laboratory analyses. If physical evidence of dehydration is present (hypotension, decreased skin turgor, or dry mucous membranes), in most adults, give 1 liter of normal saline over 1 hour and then decrease the rate to 200 to 500 mL/hr until hypotension resolves and adequate circulation is maintained. If hypotension is causing evidence of hypoperfusion and does not respond to normal saline, lactated Ringer's solution should be considered, along with invasive hemodynamic monitoring. If no hypotension is present and there is no concern about kidney function, give 1 liter of one-half normal saline over the first hour. Once laboratory test results return, further therapy may be indicated. Calculate the corrected sodium level according to the following formula: sodium concentration = measured sodium + 0.016 × (glucose − 100). The sodium is usually low because of the osmotic effects of glucose.

Severe hypertriglyceridemia can cause a false decrease in the serum sodium concentration by approximately 1.0 mEq/L at a serum lipid concentration of 460 mg/dL. Calculated water deficit in liters = 0.6 × weight in kg × [(Na/140) − 1]. After the initial 1 liter of fluid, replace urinary fluid losses with one-half normal saline and one-half of the calculated water deficit over the next 11 to 24 hours by using 5% dextrose. Once the blood glucose levels decrease to 250 to 300 mg/dL, switch all IV fluids to 5% dextrose to maintain that blood glucose range for approximately 24 hours.

Replacement of insulin should be given via IV infusion at 0.1 unit/kg/hr. A 10-unit IV bolus initially will help to saturate insulin receptors to decrease the time in achieving a steady state. If the blood glucose does not decrease at least 10% or 50 mg/dL in the first hour, give another IV bolus of insulin and increase the rate by 50% to 100%. Once the blood glucose level falls to 250 mg/dL, decrease the insulin infusion rate and administer dextrose to help clear ketones. Once the patient begins to eat, switch IV insulin to subcutaneous insulin. Administer the rapid-acting insulin 30 minutes before the meal and before discontinuing the IV insulin. Potassium shifts from intracellular to extracellular during acidosis and is lost to osmotic diuresis. Initial laboratory results may show normal or high potassium levels; the level will decrease as the DKA is treated.

Monitor the ECG for signs of hyperkalemia; if hyperkalemia is absent and the serum potassium level is less than 5.5 mEq/L, administer potassium. If the patient is oliguric, do not administer potassium unless the serum potassium level is less than 4 mEq/L or the ECG shows signs of hypokalemia. Potassium is usually replaced at 10 to 20 mEq/L/hr, half as potassium chloride and half as K⁺ phosphate. Monitor potassium levels every 2 hours initially, and monitor the ECG. The serum bicarbonate level is always low in DKA; however, a deficit does not exist because the ketoacid and lactate anions are metabolized to bicarbonate during therapy. Bicarbonate is not routinely used. It is sometimes used if the pH is less than 6.9 or if the pH is less than 7.1 and the patient is hemodynamically unstable and the ECG shows hyperkalemia. When given, the dose of 1 mEq/kg of bicarbonate is administered intravenously over 10 to 15 minutes. Monitor for hypokalemia after administration of bicarbonate. Repeated doses of bicarbonate are based on blood gases every 30 to 120 minutes. Identifying the underlying cause of the DKA (such as infection, myocardial infarction, or stroke) and treating the cause appropriately is a priority once the patient is stabilized. See Table 11-48 for a synopsis of the clinical presentation, underlying pathophysiology, assessment and diagnostic findings, and treatment plan.

Clinical Nurse Specialist Competencies and Spheres of Influence
Clinical Expert/Direct Care; Consultation; System Leadership; Coaching Teaching/Mentoring

DKA is a life-threatening emergency that requires the intervention of a physician; it should not be independently treated by an advanced practice nurse. However, the CNS should be knowledgeable about the treatment of

---

TABLE 11–48 Clinical Connections: Diabetic Ketoacidosis (DKA)

Clinical Manifestations	Pathophysiology	Assessment Finding	Laboratory Diagnostic tests	Treatment
Hyperglycemia; See Table 11-6 for related clinical manifestations of type 1 and type 2 diabetes	Relative or absolute lack of insulin	Blood glucose levels usually >300 mg/dL	Blood glucose	IV insulin

Continued

TABLE 11–48 Clinical Connections: Diabetic Ketoacidosis (DKA)—cont'd

Clinical Manifestations	Pathophysiology	Assessment Finding	Laboratory Diagnostic tests	Treatment
Dehydration	Massive fluid loss secondary to polyuria and vomiting	Increased heart rate, increased respiration, decreased sweating, decreased urination, increased body temperature, extreme fatigue, muscle cramps, headaches, nausea	Serum osmolality, BUN, creatinine, urine specific gravity	IV fluids
Hyperkalemia	Hyperglycemia causes K^+ to leave the cell and enter the serum	Reduced p waves, peaked t waves, wide QRS complex,	K^+	IV insulin
Hypokalemia	Once DKA treatment is implemented, insulin facilitates K^+ into the cells, causing hypokalemia	Muscle weakness, myalgia, muscle cramps, constipation, flaccid paralysis, hyporeflexia, tetany, rhabdomyolysis, and respiratory depression	K^+	IV K^+
Glycosuria	When blood glucose exceeds the renal threshold, the kidneys excrete glucose into the urine	Polyuria	Urine glucose	Insulin therapy to reduce the glucose below the renal threshold
Acidosis	As ketones accumulate and buffers are exhausted, serum pH deceases	Weakness, lethargy, malaise, headache, nausea, vomiting, abdominal pain, Kussmaul respiration	Serum pH, P_{CO_2}, bicarbonate, serum ketones, anion gap	Correction of the DKA; bicarbonate should not be used unless the patient experiences cardiac arrest
Tachycardia	Dehydration, volume depleation	Heart rate >100	Pulse	IV fluids

TABLE 11–48 Clinical Connections: Diabetic Ketoacidosis (DKA)—cont'd

Clinical Manifestations	Pathophysiology	Assessment Finding	Laboratory Diagnostic tests	Treatment
Kussmaul respiration	Hyperventilation produces respiratory alkalosis in a partial attempt to correct the metabolic acidosis by blowing off carbon dioxide	Deep and rapid respiration	Respirations	Correct acidosis
Mentation change	Mentation changes in DKA best correlated with elevated serum osmolality	Decreased mentation	None	Correct serum osmolality
Nausea/vomiting	Acidosis, dehydration, and extreme hyperglycemia causes nausea and vomiting	Nausea and vomiting	None	Correct acidosis, hyperglycemia, and dehydration
Hyporeflexia	Decreased serum K^+	Decreased reflexes	Reflexes	Correct K^+

DKA. The CNS may identify precipitating factors for DKA, helping the patient to avoid DKA in the future. When consulting, the CNS should review the patient's case, offer alternative approaches to patient care, and help implement planned change. The CNS should obtain the necessary resources to achieve the goal of the consult and communicate the consult findings to the appropriate colleagues.

The diabetes CNS role in clinical and professional leadership involves responsibility for innovation and change in the patient care system such as implementing a hospitalwide DKA treatment protocol or serving on a committee for developing algorithms for the care of patients with DKA. A collaboration role may involve multidisciplinary team meetings composed of pharmacists, patient educators, social workers, physicians, and other providers. Since most DKA cases are preventable, educating patients would include helping them identify the precipitating events that contribute to the development of DKA. Patients should be taught how to prevent DKA, recognize it early, and know what steps to take if they are developing DKA. The staff nurses caring for the patient in the hospital will need to be instructed on the DKA treatment protocol. Data on the number of admissions to the hospital for DKA, the precipitating events causing DKA, the method of treatment, and outcomes can be tracked to help identify potential areas for improvement.

For example, the numerous admissions due to patients omitting insulin on sick days could prompt a program that focuses on teaching patients to use insulin properly on sick days. If DKA occurred because the patient could not afford the insulin, the CNS can assist by completing forms for the patient to obtain insulin from the manufacturer or by directing the patient to the proper services to receive coverage for insulin and other diabetes supplies.

HYPERGLYCEMIC HYPEROSMOLAR NONKETOTIC SYNDROME

Etiology

Hyperglycemic hyperosmolar nonketotic syndrome (HHNS) is a metabolic derangement that occurs mainly in elderly persons with T2DM and is characterized by hyperglycemia, severe dehydration, hyperosmolarity, and neurologic deficits. In the United States, the incidence of HHNS is less than 1 per 1,000 person-years and carries a mortality rate of 10% to 20% (10 times greater than DKA) because many of those with HHNS are older and have comorbid conditions (53). Those who live in nursing homes who have dementia are at highest risk. The mean age at onset is 70, with women having a slightly higher prevalence than men. Incidence of disease in

African Americans, Hispanics, and Native Americans is disproportionately high. Commonly, this condition occurs in people who are unable to care for themselves and have gradually deteriorating mental function; these people typically do not consume enough fluids yet continue to urinate due to hyperglycemia until they are profoundly dehydrated. Significant ketones are absent. If left untreated, people with HHNS will develop confusion, coma, and death. Pneumonia and urinary tract infections are the most common predisposing factors. Other conditions that increase the likelihood of developing HHNS include cerebrovascular accident, myocardial infarction, burns, recent surgery, or certain drugs such as phenytoin, diazoxide, glucocorticoids, and thiazide diuretics (3).

Pathophysiology

In patients with insulin deficiency or insulin resistance, an infection or other acute event can cause an increase in insulin requirements. Reduced glucose utilization by muscle, fat, and the liver leads to hyperglycemia and hyperglucagonemia. Glucagon release causes hepatic glucose release. Decreased oral intake of fluids combined with increased urine output from osmotic diuresis secondary to hyperglycemia leads to profound dehydration. Renal insufficiency develops, limiting renal glucose excretion and contributing to the increase in serum glucose levels and osmolality. Once the serum osmolality exceeds 320 to 330 mOsm/kg, water is drawn out of cerebral neurons, causing mental obtundation and coma.

Clinical Presentation

The clinical presentation of HHNS is typically in the elderly adult with T2DM, as described above. The signs and symptoms commonly occur gradually over days or weeks and may include weakness, lethargy, polyuria, polydipsia, reduced fluid intake, profound dehydration, dry mucous membranes, warm and dry skin with poor skin turgor and absence of sweating, orthostatic hypotension, increased pulse, supine tachycardia, frank shock, confusion, hallucinations, coma, absence of ketoacidosis, and Kussmaul respiration (unless superimposed DKA).

Diagnosis

The main diagnostic tests for HHNS are listed in Table 11-49. However, additional tests to discover the underlying cause will be required.

Management

Fluid replacement in HHNS is fundamental. If circulatory collapse is present, use isotonic saline. In all other patients, use hypotonic saline since the serum osmolality is increased. As much as 4 to 6 liters may be needed in the first 8 to 10 hours. Careful monitoring of intake and output, pulse, and blood pressure is important. Placement of a central venous pressure or pulmonary artery catheter may be needed. Small insulin doses are usually needed to reduce blood glucose. Once the blood glucose level reaches 250 mg/dL, 5%

TABLE 11-49 Diagnostic Tests for Hyperglycemic Hyperosmolar Nonketotic Syndrome and Results Indicating Disease

Test	
Blood glucose	Usually 800–2400 mg/dL
Urine ketones	Usually absent, or small
Osmolality	Usually 330–340 mosm/kg
Serum Na	Usually >140 mEq/L

dextrose should be added. Serum potassium may be normal initially, but as insulin lowers blood glucose, serum potassium levels will decrease, and replacement is usually necessary. If the patient has adequate urine output and the initial potassium level is not elevated, then potassium chloride is usually added to the initial IV bag. If the phosphate levels decrease to less than 1 mg/dL during insulin therapy, phosphate may be replaced if urine output is adequate. Identify and treat the underlying precipitating factor. A summary of clinical presentation, underlying pathophysiology, diagnostic tests, and treatment is included in Table 11-50.

Clinical Nurse Specialist Competencies and Spheres of Influence
Clinical Expert/Direct Care; Consultation; System Leadership; Coaching Teaching/Mentoring

With expert endocrine knowledge, the diabetes CNS, along with the critical care CNS, may provide direct clinical care of the patient with HHNS, since this condition is life-threatening. The diabetes CNS may identify precipitating factors for HHNS and may help treat this condition, according to guidelines. The collaborative role may also involve working with the ICU team, nutrition specialists, patient educators, and others. Since the person with HHNS is generally unable to care for himself or herself, teaching is directed toward the patient's caregivers and may require additional resources to prevent HHNS and DKA from recurring.

Ethical Decision-making/Moral Agency/Advocacy

Ethical decision making with HHNS may involve evaluating the ability of the patient's caregivers to care for the patient. Professional organizations such as the American Diabetes Association and the American College of Clinical Endocrinologists publish specific guidelines for the care of patients with HHNS.

TABLE 11–50 Clinical Connections: Hyperglycemic Hyperosmolar Nonketotic Syndrome

Clinical Manifestations	Pathophysiology	Assessment Finding	Laboratory Diagnostic tests	Treatment
Dehydration	Decreased oral intalke combined with increased urine output	Increased heart rate, increased respiration, decreased sweating, decreased urination, increased body temperature, extreme fatigue, muscle cramps, headaches, nausea	Serum osmolality, BUN, creatinine, urine specific gravity	IV fluids
Hyperglycemia	Relative or absolute lack of insulin	Blood glucose levels usually >600 mg/dL	Blood glucose	IV hydration, low-dose IV insulin
High serum osmolality	Dehydration and hyperglycemia cause high serum osmolality	Elevated serum osmolality	Serum osmolality	Correct dehydration and hyperglycemia
Hypernatremia	Decreased oral fluid intake	Elevated serum Na	Serum Na	Fluid replacement

Consultation

When consulting, the CNS should review the patient's case, offer alternative approaches to patient care, and help implement planned changes. The CNS should obtain the necessary resources to achieve the goal of the consult and communicate the consult findings to the appropriate colleagues. The diabetes CNS's role in clinical and professional leadership can include such activities as working in an interdisciplinary workgroup to develop treatment protocols.

HYPOGLYCEMIA

Etiology

Hypoglycemia is a true medical emergency that requires prompt treatment to prevent brain and other organ damage. It is a frequent cause of emergency department admissions and is the most common cause of coma in insulin-treated patients. Mild hypoglycemia occurs when the blood glucose level decreases to less than 70 mg/dL; at this point, the person is able to treat himself or herself. Severe hypoglycemia renders the person unable to treat him or herself, and 75% of all cases occur during sleep. Relative hypoglycemia occurs when a person has symptoms of hypoglycemia, but the blood glucose level is greater than 70 mg/dL. Asymptomatic hypoglycemia occurs when the blood glucose level is less than 70 mg/dL with no symptoms (59).

Adults with diabetes who are at highest risk for hypoglycemia include those who have T1DM, low C-peptide level, duration of diabetes longer than 5 years, advanced age, autonomic neuropathies, liver disease, renal disease, congestive heart failure, cardiomyopathy, hypothyroidism, adrenal insufficiency, hypopituitarism, impaired counterregulation, illness that causes decreased food intake, and/or stress; those who take oral agents that cause increased insulin secretion, oral agents combined with insulin, and/or pramlintide combined with insulin; those who practice prolonged fasting, excessive intake of alcohol, and/or high-level physical activity; and/or those who experience unplanned events that interfere with the usual dietary pattern (60).

Errors made by the person administering the diabetes medication can cause hypoglycemia. Insulin brands can accidently be switched or the amount in the syringe can be drawn incorrectly. Correction doses of short- or rapid-acting insulin may be given too frequently, causing the insulin peak and duration to overlap. In rare instances, extra insulin may be purposefully administered, resulting in hypoglycemia. Conditions that are rare but can increase the risk of hypoglycemia include isolated growth hormone deficiency, isolated glucagon deficiency, non-endocrine tumors such as large mesenchymal tumors, inborn errors of carbohydrate metabolism such as glycogen storage disease and gluconeogenic enzyme deficiencies, and autoimmune hypoglycemia.

Pathophysiology

The body maintains a narrow range of blood glucose, and once the blood glucose level decreases to less than 70 mg/dL, counterregulatory hormones come into play. In the adult without diabetes, once the blood glucose level is less than 80 mg/dL, insulin release shuts off, mediated by sympathetic innervations of beta cells and the alpha adrenergic effects of circulating catecholamines. This causes decreased muscle and adipose glucose uptake, increased glycogenolysis, and increased gluconeogenesis. Once the blood glucose level decreases to less than 70 mg/dL, the autonomic nervous system is activated. When insulin levels decrease, glucagon secretion increases, causing glycogenolysis, increased gluconeogenesis, and lipolysis. Once the blood glucose level decreases to less than 60 mg/dL, growth hormone, adrenocorticotropic hormone (ACTH), and cortisol are released, causing lipolysis and muscle breakdown. Those who either inject insulin or take a secretagogue are unable to decrease the insulin levels in response to hypoglycemia. Therefore, glucagon is not released appropriately. Table 11-51 shows the body's response to blood glucose levels of less than 70 mg/dL in people without diabetes or with diabetes but not taking insulin or a secretagogue compared with the body's response to these levels in those who are taking insulin or a secretagogue (59, 60).

Clinical Presentation

Clinical presentation varies among individuals. Table 11-52 outlines the typical clinical presentation correlated with blood glucose levels; however, symptoms can vary at different blood glucose levels. Symptoms of adrenergic hypoglycemia include hunger, trembling, pallor, sweating, shaking, palpitations, and anxiety. Symptoms of neuroglycopenic hypoglycemia include dizziness, poor concentration, drowsiness, weakness, confusion, lightheadedness, slurred speech, blurred vision, double vision, unsteadiness, and poor coordination; behavioral symptoms of neuroglycopenic hypoglycemia include tearfulness, confusion, fatigue, irritability, and aggression (2).

Diagnosis

A blood glucose level of less than 70 mg/dL is diagnostic of hypoglycemia. If a C-peptide level and an insulin level are drawn at the time of hypoglycemia and the C-peptide

TABLE 11–52 Usual Clinical Presentation of Hypoglycemia*

Blood Glucose Level (mg/dL)	Clinical Presentation
70	Counterregulatory hormone release
60	Adrenergic symptoms
50	Neuroglycopenic symptoms
40	Lethargy
30	Coma
20	Seizure
10	Permanent damage (blindness, paralysis)

*NOTE: Clinical presentation may vary in individuals.

TABLE 11–51 Comparison of Body's Response to Blood Glucose at <70 mg/dL in Adults

Adults without diabetes or those with diabetes not taking insulin or a secretagogue	Adults with diabetes who are taking insulin or secretagogue
1. Low insulin level	1. Elevated insulin level
2. Glucagon secreted by pancreas	2. Glucagon not secreted by pancreas
3. Epinephrine release	3. Epinephrine release
4. Norepinepherine release	4. Norepinepherine release
5. Cortisol release	5. Cortisol release
6. Growth hormone release	6. Growth hormone release
7. Neurotransmitter release	7. Neurotransmitter release

is normal or elevated, the hypoglycemia was likely caused by exogenous insulin or a secretagogue (2).

Management

If the blood glucose level is less than 70 mg/dL and the adult with diabetes can swallow, give 15 grams of carbohydrate orally, wait 15 minutes, recheck the blood glucose, and if the blood glucose level remains less than 70 mg/dL, give another 15 grams of carbohydrate orally. Keep repeating all of these steps until the blood glucose level is greater than 70 mg/dL. Examples of 15 grams of carbohydrate include 4 glucose tablets, ½ cup of regular soda or juice, 5 crackers, or 4 pieces of candy. Choose low-fat items since high-fat items may slow absorption of carbohydrate.

If the adult with diabetes cannot swallow carbohydrate, give 1 mg of glucagon intramuscularly (IM) or subcutaneously in the deltoid or anterior thigh. Place the person on their side because vomiting after glucagon administration is common. Once glucagon is administered, blood glucose levels rise quickly but can decrease again after 30 minutes, so give carbohydrate orally and check the blood glucose every 15 minutes until it is stable. Because of the risk of nausea and vomiting after glucagon is administered, use carbohydrate forms that are easily digested, and avoid high-fat foods or drinks. Good choices include drinks sweetened with table sugar such as regular soda, sweetened electrolyte drinks, or natural sugar drinks such as juices. Usually in several hours, the person feels well and is able to resume their usual diet.

If the person has IV access, ½ ampule of 50% dextrose can be administered in place of the IM or SC administration of glucagon. The blood glucose level needs to be rechecked 15 minutes after administration of dextrose. If the blood glucose level remains less than 70 mg/dL, then repeat the 50% dextrose administration until the level is greater than 70 mg/dL. Identifying the cause of the hypoglycemia will determine the plan for reducing the risk of future hypoglycemia. Patient education based on the cause and subsequent plan will be required (5). A summary of the clinical picture and management approach for hypoglycemia is listed in Table 11-53.

Clinical Nurse Specialist Competencies and Spheres of Influence
Clinical Expert/Direct Care

The diabetes CNS provides direct clinical care of the patient with hypoglycemia by recognizing and treating with oral carbohydrate, IV dextrose, or glucagon. The CNS identifies precipitating factors for hypoglycemia, helping the patient avoid hypoglycemia in the future. When consulting, the CNS should review the patient's case, offer alternative approaches to patient care, and help implement planned change. The CNS should obtain the necessary resources to achieve the goal of the consult and communicate the findings to the appropriate colleagues.

Systems Leadership, Collaboration

The clinical leadership role may include developing a hospitalwide hypoglycemia protocol. The collaboration role may involve working with the nursing leaders of the hospital for implementation of the hypoglycemia protocol, pharmacists to have glucagon and 50% dextrose available at all times, nutrition support staff to help the patient obtain adequate nutrition, and patient educators to teach the patient/family.

Coaching/Teaching/Mentoring

Patient/family education is required for all patients with diabetes who take medications that could potentially cause hypoglycemia. The patient needs to be instructed to carry a form of oral carbohydrate at all times, and if hypoglycemia occurs, must know the amount of carbohydrate to consume. If the patient is at risk for severe hypoglycemia, a glucagon kit should be prescribed and a significant other trained to know when and how to use it. The nursing staff needs to be instructed on the hospital-wide hypoglycemia protocol. Research-related activities might involve collecting data on the incidence of hypoglycemia, conducting a literature review of other hospital-wide hypoglycemia protocols, and evaluating the current hypoglycemia hospitalwide hypoglycemia protocol for efficacy. Patients may need assistance with obtaining a glucagon kit because many insurance providers require a phone call by the CNS or physician for authorization.

TABLE 11–53 Clinical Connections: Hypoglycemia

Clinical Manifestations	Pathophysiology	Assessment Finding	Laboratory Diagnostic tests	Treatment
Hypoglycemia	Glucose level of <70 mg/dL due to increased insulin level relative to glucose	Serum glucose level of <70 mg/dL	Serum glucose	Carbohydrate by mouth, IV dextrose, or glucagon SC, IM, or IV

IM, Intramuscular; *IV,* intravenous.

ADRENAL INSUFFICIENCY

Etiology

Adrenal insufficiency occurs when inadequate amounts of steroid hormones are produced. Two major types include primary and secondary adrenal insufficiency; it can also be congenital or acquired or the result of iatrogenesis. Primary adrenal insufficiency is very uncommon and occurs when the gland itself is dysfunctional. Secondary adrenal insufficiency occurs when the hypothalamus secretes inadequate amounts of corticotrophin-releasing hormone and/or the pituitary gland secretes inadequate amounts of adrenocorticotropic hormone. Iatrogenic adrenal insufficiency results from abrupt cessation of exogenous sources of corticosteroids used to treat a wide variety of medical conditions.

Adrenal insufficiency occurs in approximately 50 of every 1 million people and is most common in middle-aged women. Approximately 6 million people in the United States are believed to have undiagnosed adrenal insufficiency, which is only clinically significant during times of physiologic stress, when the adrenal hormones are depleted. Adrenoleukodystrophy, a congenital form of adrenal insufficiency, is limited to males because it is X-chromosome linked. Secondary adrenal insufficiency affects males and females equally. The most common cause of primary adrenal insufficiency is autoimmune destruction of the adrenal cortex. The most common cause of secondary adrenal insufficiency is long-term glucocorticoid administration. Other causes of adrenal insufficiency include tuberculosis, treatment with megestrol acetate, amyloidosis, cancer, critical illness–related corticosteroid insufficiency, kidney injury, head injury, genetics, radiotherapy, surgical and trauma induced resection, meningitis, congenital hypopituitarism, congenital hypoadrenalism, adrenal hemorrhage, exposure to etomidate, and familial glucocorticoid deficiency. In patients with thalassemia who have received multiple transfusions, iron deposition in the pituitary and/or adrenal glands may lead to adrenal insufficiency. Adrenal insufficiency is a potentially fatal disease if unrecognized and untreated; death is usually caused by hypotension or cardiac arrhythmia secondary to hyperkalemia.

Pathophysiology

The adrenal glands sit on top of the kidneys; their primary function is to regulate the stress response via the synthesis of corticosteroids, mineralcorticoids, and catecholamines. The medulla is the central core and is surrounded by the cortex. It is derived from nerve cells and produces catecholamines. The chromaffin cells of the medulla produce epinephrine and norepinephrine. The outer cortex, regulated by neuroendocrine hormones secreted by the pituitary gland, hypothalamus, and renin-angiotensin system, produces corticosteroid hormones

from cholesterol, androgens, and aldosterone. Some of the cells belong to the hypothalamic-pituitary-adrenal axis and are the source of cortisol and corticosterone synthesis. The zona glomerulosa is the main site of mineralcorticoid production; the zona fasciculata produces glucocorticoids; and the zona reticularis produces androgens. The rennin-angiotensin system primarily regulates the secretion of aldosterone, a mineral corticoid. Hyperkalemia can also stimulate aldosterone secretion. Cortisol secretion is regulated by ACTH, which is regulated by corticotropin-releasing hormone (CRH) from the hypothalamus. Serum cortisol inhibits the secretion of both CRH and ACTH to prevent excessive secretion of cortisol. Adrenal androgen secretion is partially regulated by ACTH.

Primary adrenal insufficiency is due to impairment of the adrenal glands. The most common subtype is idiopathic, which causes adrenal atrophy and hypofunction. It is an organ-specific autoimmune disease. Autoantibodies specific to cells of the adrenal cortex are present in 50% to 70% of cases. A genetic defect in immune surveillance mechanisms causes a deficiency of immune-suppressor cells, which causes proliferation of immunocytes directed against specific antigens within the adrenocortical cells. Many individuals with idiopathic adrenal insufficiency have other autoimmune disorders such as Hashimoto thyroiditis, pernicious anemia, and idiopathic hypoparathyroidism. The adrenal gland is smaller than normal, and microscopically, the cortex shows atrophy with diffuse cortical lymphocytic infiltrates while the medulla is normal.

Secondary adrenal insufficiency is caused by inadequate adrenal stimulation, adrenal atrophy, and decreased corticosteroidogenesis. In the case of iatrogenic adrenal insufficiency, caused by long-term administration of glucocorticoids, only a 2-week exposure to glucocorticoids can suppress the CRH-ACTH-adrenal axis. Acute adrenal crisis can occur if corticosteroids are abruptly stopped. The hyperpigmentation seen in some cases of adrenal insufficiency is due to increased secretion of ACTH, beta-lipotropin, and melanocyte-stimulating hormone, which causes pigment changes in epithelial cells. Vitiligo is due to autoimmune destruction of melanocytes. Hypotension results from hypoaldosteronism causing increased renal sodium loss and decreased blood volume. Gastrointestinal disturbances, weakness, and fatigability that generally progress throughout the day stem from electrolyte imbalances, altered hormonal levels, and impaired glucose metabolism.

Hypoglycemia is caused by the absence of cortisol, which decreases gluconeogenesis, liver glycogen storage, and metabolism of proteins and increases insulin sensitivity. Na loss from the kidneys and the inability to excrete a water load causes hyponaturemia, which results from mineralocorticoid defect and glucocorticoid deficiency.

Chronic mineralocorticoid deficiency with the inability to excrete potassium and acid causes hyperkalemia and acidosis. Increased calcium absorption due to the lack of glucocorticoid effect on the gut causes hypercalcemia. When mineralocorticoid deficiency is present, renin levels are elevated. Addison crisis occurs with the combined effects of hypocortisolism, hypoaldosteronism, extracellular volume depletion, a precipitating stressor, and decreased vasomotor tone due to cortisol deficiency.

Clinical Presentation

The symptoms of adrenal insufficiency are primarily caused by hypocortisolism and hypoaldosteronism. The disease is frequently undiagnosed for long periods because of the slow progression of symptoms. Common signs and symptoms include fatigue, loss of appetite, nausea, vomiting, hypoglycemia, diarrhea, abdominal pain, weight loss, muscle weakness, dizziness when standing, dehydration, cold intolerance, salt craving, altered mental status, adrenal calcifications on radiography or CT scan of the adrenal glands, anxiety, depression, and increased skin pigmentation especially in the areola, genitalia, scars, moles, palmar creases, and axillae. Women lose pubic and underarm hair and stop having normal menstrual periods. Unfortunately, significant symptoms are usually not noticed until about 90% of the adrenal cortex has been destroyed (61).

Adrenal crisis may present with severe abdominal pain, diarrhea, vomiting, profound muscle weakness and fatigue, extremely low blood pressure, weight loss, kidney failure, and changes in mood and personality. Shock and death may occur without prompt intervention.

Diagnosis

Laboratory tests are used to differentiate whether there is inadequate cortisol secretion by the adrenals and whether the causes are due to the lack of ACTH. The peak value of cortisol occurs between 4 a.m. and 8 a.m. and nadir values are in the evening. Basal morning serum cortisol levels of less than 3 mcg/dL are suggestive of adrenal insufficiency. Random serum cortisol levels at other times of the day are not helpful unless they are in the high-normal range, which indicates that the hypothalamic-pituitary-adrenal axis is intact.

The most commonly used test to assess adrenal function is the cosyntropin stimulation test. Serum cortisol levels greater than 18 mcg/dL to 20 mcg/dL obtained 30 or 60 minutes after IV or intramuscular injection of 250 mcg of synthetic cosyntropin rules out primary adrenal insufficiency. An insufficient cortisol response is diagnostic of adrenal insufficiency. Cosyntropin test results may be normal if the test is administered after recent onset of secondary adrenal insufficiency. It may take weeks for the adrenal glands to atrophy after acute disruption of ACTH secretion. The low-dose cosyntropin stimulation test has been suggested as more sensitive and specific. It is performed in the same manner as the cosyntropin stimulation test, but with the low-dose test, only 1 mcg of synthetic cosyntropin is administered. An ACTH level is drawn at the same time as the cortisol. A low cortisol level and high ACTH level (greater than 200 pg/mL) are suggestive of primary adrenal insufficiency (Table 11-54).

Steroid replacement interferes with the serum cortisol results. Therefore, the patient should be switched to dexamethasone the day before the test. The insulin tolerance test is not used routinely because it requires close monitoring of the patient for dangerous hypoglycemia, which can develop during the test. It is contraindicated in patients with a history of seizure, susceptibility to seizure, or CVD.

The metyrapone stimulation test is also not commonly used. It is most useful in confirming secondary adrenal insufficiency. It should not be performed in patients who have known severe cortisol deficiency because it can cause adrenal crisis. The standard and low-dose cosyntropin stimulation test correlates well with the insulin tolerance test and usually reveals adrenal insufficiency.

Serum adrenal antibodies may be positive in autoimmune adrenal insufficiency. Very-long-chain fatty acids are elevated in adrenoleukodystrophy. Low gonadotropin and sex steroid levels suggesting hypogonadotropic hypogonadism may be seen with congenital adrenal hypoplasia. After a laboratory diagnosis has revealed the type of adrenal insufficiency, radiologic tests may be done if needed. If autoimmune adrenal insufficiency is diagnosed, radiologic tests are not needed. If the diagnosis is chemical primary adrenal insufficiency, CT of the adrenal

TABLE 11-54 Laboratory Results of Primary Versus Secondary Adrenal Insufficiency

Hormone	Primary Adrenal Insufficiency	Secondary Adrenal Insufficiency
ACTH	High	Low
Angiotensin	High	Normal
Cortisol	Low	Low
Aldosterone	Low	Normal

gland is helpful in identifying inflammation suggestive of infection, hemorrhage, or malignancy. MRI of the brain to image lesions in the pituitary or hypothalamus is done if secondary adrenal insufficiency is diagnosed.

Laboratory results may suggest the following conditions in patients with adrenal insufficiency, but are not diagnostic for adrenal insufficiency: hyponatremia, hyperkalemia, acidosis, hypercalcemia, hypoglycemia, and elevated rennin levels.

Management

Glucocorticoid replacement at physiologic levels is given along with mineralocorticoid replacement in those with primary adrenal insufficiency. Chronic treatment for those with primary or secondary adrenal insufficiency requires glucocorticoid replacement with 15 to 30 mg of hydrocortisone by mouth per day, or prednisone at 5 to 7.5 mg by mouth daily, or dexamethasone at 0.75 to 1.25 mg by mouth daily (Table 11-55).

The dose of hydrocortisone is usually given once in the morning; however, if the dose is divided, the larger dose is given in the morning and the smaller one in the afternoon. The dose is adjusted to reduce the symptoms of fatigue, weight loss, and hyponatremia, and in cases of primary adrenal insufficiency, hyperpigmentation. Excess glucocorticoid replacement can result in weight gain, osteoporosis, and a compromised immune system. Steroids should be given with a meal or with milk to prevent gastric upset or ulcers. During illness, the need for steroids will increase. The patient needs to be strictly advised against discontinuing therapy and to wear a Medic Alert bracelet. Follow-up care includes frequent monitoring of blood glucose and urinary acetone levels.

Mineralocorticoid replacement with fludrocortisone at 0.05 to 0.2 mg daily is also given. Management of adrenal crisis includes IV fluids, IV steroids, and rest. See Table 11-56 for steroid treatment for adrenal crisis management. Table 11-57 provides a summary of the clinical presentation and treatment for adrenal insufficiency.

Clinical Nurse Specialist Competencies and Spheres of Influence
Clinical Expert/Direct Care

The CNS provides direct clinical care of the patient with adrenal insufficiency by recognizing signs and symptoms,

---

TABLE 11–55 Steroid Maintenance Treatment for Adrenal Insufficiency

- Hydrocortisone at 15–30 mg PO daily, or
- Prednisone at 5.0–7.5 mg PO daily, or
- Dexamethasone at 0.75–1.25 mg PO daily

TABLE 11–56 Steroid Treatment Options for Adrenal Crisis Management

- Hydrocortisone (Cortef), 20–35 mg
- Prednisone (Deltasone), 7.5 mg
- Prednisolone (Delta-Cortef), 7.5 mg
- Methylprednisolone (Medrol), 6 mg
- Dexamethasone (Decadron), 0.25–1 mg

Mineralcorticoid deficiency (low aldosterone)

- Fludrocortisone (Florinef)

---

ordering the correct diagnostic tests, and treating appropriately. If adrenal crisis occurs, early recognition and prompt treatment are vital to patient survival. When consulting, the CNS reviews the patient's case, offers alternative approaches to patient care, and helps implement planned change. The CNS should obtain the necessary resources to achieve the goal of the consult and communicate the consult findings to the appropriate colleagues.

Systems Leadership

The clinical leadership role may include serving on a committee to develop hospitalwide treatment guidelines and plans for nursing education. Another example of the leadership role includes participating in professional organizations such as the National Adrenal Disease Foundation, American Autoimmune Related Diseases Association, and the National Endocrine and Metabolic Diseases Information Service.

Collaboration, Coaching/Teaching/Mentoring

The collaboration role may involve working with endocrinologists, the primary care team, pharmacists, and patient educators to teach the patient/family. Patient/family education is required for all patients with adrenal insufficiency. Education includes teaching the patient to carry identification stating his or her condition in case of an emergency. The identification card should alert emergency personnel about the need to inject 100 mg of cortisol if its bearer is found severely injured or unable to answer questions. The identification card should also include the physician's name and telephone number and the name and telephone number of the nearest relative to be notified. The patient should be instructed to carry injectable cortisol, a needle, and a syringe in case of emergency. The patient may need assistance in obtaining injectable cortisol and in gaining access to medical care for follow-up. The nursing staff needs to be instructed on the hospitalwide adrenal crisis guidelines. Examples of research-related activities include collecting data about the incidence of adrenal insufficiency and crisis, conducting a literature

TABLE 11–57 Clinical Connections: Adrenal Insufficiency

Clinical Manifestations	Pathophysiology	Assessment Finding	Laboratory Diagnostic tests	Treatment
Constitutional: Fatigue, muscle weakness that is progressive throughout the day	Unknown	Subjective complaints	None	Treatment of adrenal insufficiency with hydrocortisone, prednisone, or dexamethasone
Gastrointestinal: loss of appetite, nausea, vomiting, salt craving	Unknown	Subjective complaints	None	Treatment of adrenal insufficiency with hydrocortisone, prednisone, or dexamethasone
Hypoglycemia	Absence of cortisol decreases gluconeogenesis, liver glycogen storage, decreased metabolism of proteins, and increased insulin sensitivity	Blood glucose level of <70 mg/dL	Blood glucose	Treatment of adrenal insufficiency with hydrocortisone, prednisone, or dexamethasone
Hyponatremia	Na loss from the kidneys and the inability to excrete water causes hyponaturemia	Serum Na <135 mEq/L	Serum Na	Treatment of adrenal insufficiency with hydrocortisone, prednisone, or dexamethasone
Hyperkalemia and acidosis	Chronic mineralocorticoid deficiency with the inability to excrete K^+ and acid causes hyperkalemia and acidosis	K^+ above normal limits for laboratory reference range	Serum K^+	Treatment of adrenal insufficiency with hydrocortisone, prednisone, or dexamethasone
Hypotension	Hypoaldosteronism causes increased renal Na loss and decreased blood volume	Lightheadedness, dizziness, fainting, blood pressure lower than the patient's usual blood pressure	Blood pressure	Treatment of adrenal insufficiency with hydrocortisone, prednisone, or dexamethasone
Increased skin pigmentation and vitiligo	Increased secretion of ACTH, beta-lipotropin and melanocyte-stimulating hormone causes pigment changes in epithelial cells. Vitiligo is due to	Increased skin pigmentation, expecially in the areola, genitalia, scars, moles, palmar creases, and axillae, vitiligo	None	Treatment of adrenal insufficiency with hydrocortisone, prednisone, or dexamethasone

Continued

TABLE 11–57 Clinical Connections: Adrenal Insufficiency—cont'd

Clinical Manifestations	Pathophysiology	Assessment Finding	Laboratory Diagnostic tests	Treatment
	autoimmune destruction of melanocytes.			
Adrenal crisis: severe abdominal pain, diarrhea, vomiting, profound muscle weakness, fatigue, extremely low blood pressure, weight loss, kidney failure, changes in mood and personality, shock, and death	The combined effects of hypocortisolism, hypoaldosteronism, extracellular volume depletion, a precipitating stressor, and decreased vasomotor tone due to cortisol deficiency.		Serum CA, glucose, electrolytes, BUN, creatinine, cortisol, thyroid function tests, CBC, chest radiographs, CT scan, adrenocorticotropic hormone stimulation test (after patient is stable), ECG, 24-hour urinary cortisol (after patient is stable)	IV fluids, IV steroids, and rest. Use supportive measures as necessary. Correct electrolyte abnormalities. Perform judicious volume resuscitation.

CT, Computed tomography; *ECG,* electrocardiogram.

review of other hospitalwide adrenal crisis guidelines, and evaluating current outcomes.

HYPERPARATHYROIDISM

Etiology

The parathyroid glands are small glands located on the posteroid surface of the thyroid. Rarely, the parathyroid can be within the thyroid or in the chest. The number of glands is usually 4; however, it can vary from 2 to 6. Three cell types exist in the parathyroid gland: parathyroid chief cells, which manufacture parathyroid hormone (PTH); oxyphil cells, which have an unknown function; and adipocytes, which contain fat. The function of the parthyroid glands is to maintain the body's calcium level within a narrow range. Calcium is regulated by a negative-feedback system. PTH is released in response to low blood calcium and increases blood calcium levels by stimulating

---

CASE STUDY 11-4 | Adrenal Insufficiency

CHIEF COMPLAINT: The patient is tired all the time, does not feel well, and is losing weight.

HISTORY OF PRESENT ILLNESS: The patient is a 42-year-old white female who reports fatigue, loss of appetite, nausea, diarrhea, abdominal pain, weight loss, muscle weakness, dizziness when standing, and cold intolerance. The symptoms have been vague for years; however, in the past few months, the symptoms seem to be worsening.

CURRENT MEDICATIONS: None

REVIEW OF SYSTEMS AND PHYSICAL EXAM:
VITAL SIGNS
Blood pressure: 92/54 mm Hg
Pulse: 88/min

CASE STUDY 11-4 | Adrenal Insufficiency—cont'd

Respirations: 16/min

Temperature: 37°C

Height: 177.8 cm

Weight: 94.8 kg

BMI: 30 kg/m².

LABORATORY

Fasting blood glucose: 68 mg/dL (normal: 70–110 mg/dL)

BUN: 26 mg/dL (normal 8–20 mg/dL)

GFR: 78 mL/min (normal: >90 mL/min)

Creatinine: 1.6 mg/dL (normal: 0.7–1.3 mg/dL)

ALT: 11 IU/L (normal: 8–50 IU/L)

AST: 14 U/L (normal: 8–46 U/L)

Total cholesterol: 226 mg/dL (normal: <200 mg/dL)

Triglycerides: 188 mg/dL (normal: <150 mg/dL)

LDL: 110 mg/dL (normal: <100 mg/dL)

HDL: 32 mg/dL (normal male: >40 mg/dL).

GENERAL: Anxious, reports weight loss

INTEGUMENTARY: Increased skin pigmentation of the areola, genitalia, scars, moles, palmar creases, and axillae

ENDOCRINE: Cold intolerance

NEUROLOGIC: Occasional dizziness when standing

GASTROINTESTINAL: Diarrhea, abdominal pain

GENITOURINARY: Decreased pubic hair; irregular, light menstrual cycles

MUSCULOSKELETAL: Decreased muscle strength, weakness

QUESTIONS (See DavisPlus for answers)

1. What is the most significant complication of adrenal insufficiency?

2. What labs should be ordered to determine whether there is inadequate cortisol secretion by the adrenals and whether the causes are due to the lack of ACTH?

3. If secondary adrenal insufficiency is diagnosed, what test should be ordered?

4. If the patient has adrenal crisis, which corticosteroids and dosages can be used?

osteoclasts to break down bone and release calcium, activating vitamin D and prompting calcium uptake by the kidneys (3, 62). See Table 11-58 or the actions of hormones involved in calcium regulation.

Hyperparathyroidism can be primary, secondary, or tertiary. In most cases of hyperparathyroidism, the cause is unknown; only 5% of cases are linked to a genetic problem. Approximately 100,000 cases of hyperparathyroidism are diagnosed each year in the United States, which is 0.04% of the population. Twice as many women develop hyperparathyroidism as men. Two of 1,000 people older than age 60 years will develop hyperparathyroidism. The most common age at diagnosis is 30 to 50 years. Risk factors for hyperparathyroidism include low-dose external beam irradiation to the neck, chronic use of furosemide, lithium use, and a family history of multiple endocrine neoplasia (MEN) (62).

Pathophysiology

Primary hyperparathyroidism is the most common form of hyperparathyroidism. Adenoma is the most common cause of primary hyperparathyroidism. Other causes include hyperplasia of all parathyroid glands, adenomas in more than one gland, parathyroid carcinoma, familial hyperparathyroidism, and multiple endocrine neoplasia types 1 and 2A. The parathyroid gland overproduces PTH, and calcium levels are high. Secondary hyperparathyroidism occurs when the parathyroid gland produces an increased compensatory amount of PTH secondary to a hypocalcemia-producing abnormality, such as chronic renal failure, renal absorption disorders, vitamin D deficiency, osteogenesis imperfect, Paget's disease, multiple myeloma, carcinoma with bony metastasis, pituitary basophilism, and osteomalacia. The abnormality causes resistance to the metabolic action of PTH. Tertiary hyperparathyroidism occurs when secondary

TABLE 11–58 Actions of Hormones Involved in CA Regulation

	PTH	Vitamin D	Calcitonin
Released in response to:	Low blood CA	PTH	High blood CA
Kidneys	CA reabsorbed	CA reabsorbed	High blood CA
	Vitamin D activated		
Intestines	Negligible	CA absorbed	Negligible
Bones	CA released	CA trapped	CA trapped

CT, computed tomography; PTH, Parathyroid hormone.

hyperparathyroidism is no longer responsive to treatment or medication (61-63).

Clinical Presentation

Some patients may have no symptoms or vague symptoms. The progression of primary hyperparathyroidism is slow. Symptoms usually occur at a serum calcium level of greater than 11 mg/dL and include bone and joint pain, renal stones with hematuria, decreased bone mineral density, and nephrolithiasis (62, 63).

Diagnosis

Recommendations for diagnosis of primary hyperparathyroidism from the American Association of Clinical Endocrinologists and the American Association of Endocrine Surgeons include serum calcium, immunoassay of the intact PTH, 24-hour urinary collection for calcium and creatinine excretion, and bone density screening (63). The localization study of choice is the sestamibi scan, which has a sensitivity of 80% to 90% and specificity approaching 100%. With this test, it is possible to perform three-dimensional single-photon emission computed tomography (SPECT) imaging of deep cervical and mediastinal parathyroid tissue. False-positive results can occur in the presence of thyroid nodules, which is significant since 25% of patients have associated thyroid disease. This problem can be minimized by the use of iodine or pertechnetate subtraction techniques. False-negative results are more of a problem and can occur with small adenomas and hyperplasia. The accuracy of sestamibi scans may be reduced to 35% in the setting of multigland hyperplasia. In addition, radionuclide scans have the advantage of being inexpensive (comparable to ultrasound) (3, 62).

Management

Patients with mild hyperparathyroidism without symptoms who do not undergo surgery should be followed up with calcium, creatinine, and PTH analyses as well as urinalysis every 6 to 11 months and with bone density screening every 11 months. Oral intake for calcium should be 1 gram or less. The use of bisphosphonate inhibits bone resorption and the release of ionized calcium from the skeleton and protects bones against demineralization and pathologic fracture. In postmenopausal women, estrogen increases bone density but does not affect serum calcium.

If hypercalcemia causes mental status changes such as confusion or delusions, saline-furosemide diuresis, bisphosphonates, and calcitonin therapy can be implemented, which consists of 4 to 10 L of normal saline given every 24 hours along with 40 to 80 mg of furosemide given every 4 to 6 hours. Bisphosphonates that may be given include zoledronic acid 8 mg over 15 minutes IV for 3 days or pamidronate 90 mg as a 24 hour infusion or 90 mg over 90 to 120 minutes. Calcitonin 4 to 8 international units/kg of may be given intramuscularly or subcutaneously every 6 to 8 hours. Hemodialysis may also be required. Chronic renal failure is associated with low levels of vitamin D, hyperphosphatemia, and hyperparathyroidism and is treated with calcium salts (which bind phosphorous) and with vitamin D supplementation.

Surgery offers the only curative treatment for hyperparathyroidism. No evidence supports the long-term use of medical management. The treatment of choice for tertiary hyperparathyroidism is the surgical removal of three and half of one parathyroid gland. Surgery is used in those with symptoms of hyperparathyroidism, a serum calcium level of 1 to 1.6 mg/dL above normal, a history of life-threatening hypercalcemia, a creatinine clearance of less than 70% of normal, kidney stones on radiography, a markedly elevated urine calcium level, a bone density of greater than 2 standard deviations below expected, and a coexistent illness that complicates management; surgery is also used in patients younger than 50 years and in those who request it. Parathyroidectomy has a morbidity of 1% and cures hypercalcemia in 95% of cases. In the setting of renal failure, the cure rate decreases to 50% to 85%. Indications for surgery include renal osteodystrophy or pathologic fractures, intractable bone pain or pruritius, and calciphylaxis unresponsive to hemodialysis or medications (3, 5, 62, 63). See Table 11-59 for a summary of the presentation and management of hyperthyroidism.

TABLE 11–59 Clinical Connections: Hyperparathyroidism

Clinical Manifestations	Pathophysiology	Assessment Finding	Laboratory Diagnostic tests	Treatment
Hypercalcemia, nausea, vomiting, excessive thirst, frequent urination, constipation, abdominal pain, muscle weakness, muscle and joint aches, irritability, depression, confusion, lethargy and fatigue	The parathyroid glands overproduce PTH, causing hypercalcemia. The severity of symptoms correlates with the severity of hypercalcemia	Elevated CA, elevated PTH	Serum CA, serum PTH	If mild and patient not undergoing surgery, limit CA intake and biphosphonates. If hypercalcemia causes mental status changes: saline-furosemide diuresis, bisphosphonate, calcitonin, and possibly hemodialysis; surgery is the only cure.
Bone: bone and joint pain, decreased bone mineral density	Activity of PTH on bones causing calcium to be absorbed out	Subjective complaints; dexascan shows bone loss	Dexascan	Correct hypercalcemia and hyperparathyroidism
Renal: stones with hematuria	Filtering of large amounts of calcium will cause calcium to collect within the renal tubules, leading to kidney stones	Colicky flank pain, hematuria, fever, chills	Helical CT scan, urinalysis	Correct hypercalcemia and hyperparathyroidism

PTH, Parathyroid hormone; *CT,* computed tomography.

Clinical Nurse Specialist Competencies and Spheres of Influence
Clinical Expert/Direct Care

The CNS provides direct clinical care for the patient with hyperparathyroidism by recognizing signs and symptoms, ordering the correct diagnostic tests, and treating according to evidence-based recommendations. For example, the CNS should know that although serum calcium levels respond to fluids and furosemide, therapy to reduce calcium has no effect on the underlying pathophysiologic cause of hypercalcemia. When consulting, the CNS should review the patient's case, offer alternative approaches to patient care, and help implement planned change. The CNS should obtain the necessary resources to achieve the goal of the consult and communicate the consult findings to the appropriate colleagues.

Systems Leadership

The clinical leadership role may include serving on a committee to develop hospital-wide treatment guidelines and plans for nursing education. Another example of the leadership role includes participating in professional organizations such as the American Association of Clinical Endocrinologists, American Association of Endocrine Surgeons, The American Society for Bone and Mineral Research, The Endocrine Society, The Paget Foundation for Paget's Disease of Bone and Related Disorders, and The National Endocrine and Metabolic Diseases Information Service.

Collaboration, Coaching/Teaching/Mentoring, Research/Evidence Based Practice

The collaboration role may involve working with emergency department personnel, endocrinologists, and surgeons. Patient/family education for patients with hyperparathyroidism includes the treatment options, prescribed medications, and the importance of periodic laboratory and radiologic testing. The nursing staff needs to be instructed on the care of patients with hypercalcemia and on the postsurgic care of patients after hyperparathyroidectomy. Examples of research-related activities include collecting data about the incidence of hyperparathyroidism, conducting a literature review for evidence-based medical guidelines, and evaluating current outcomes.

HYPOPARATHYROIDISM

Etiology

Hypoparathyroidism is a rare condition secondary to inadequate PTH production. Hypoparathyroidism can be secondary to surgical removal of the parathyroid glands or type 1 polyglandular autoimmune syndrome and can present as idiopathic hypoparathyroidism, familial hypoparathyroidism, or pseudohypoparathyroidism (65). The most common cause is the removal of or injury to the parathyroid glands during parathyroid or thyroid surgery. Hypoparathyroidism after surgery may be transient or permanent. Approximately 250,000 cases occur after surgery each year. Women and those in the fifth decade of life have a greater incidence (65).

The most common nonsurgical cause of hypoparathyroidism is autoimmune invasion and destruction, which occurs in autoimmune polyendocrine syndromes. Other causes include hemochromatosis, chromosome 22q11 microdeletion syndrome (DiGeorge syndrome, Shprintzen syndrome, velocardiofacial syndrome), magnesium deficiency, familial hypoparathyroidism, irradiation to the neck, infiltration of the gland by heavy metals, metastatic tumors or Riedel thyroiditis, type 1 polyglandular autoimmune syndrome, metastatic cancer, HIV infection, idiopathic secretion of biologically inactive PTH, and resistance to PTH (pseudohypoparathyroidism) (5). High maternal calcium can cause suppression of developing parathyroid glands in the fetus.

Pathophysiology

Decreased PTH causes hypocalcemia and hyperphosphatemia. Those with congenital hypoparathyroidism are born without parathyroid tissue due to atypical genes that encode anomalous forms of either PTH or its receptor; this is caused by aberrant conduction of cell signals from the PTH receptor to the nucleus or by abnormal gland development before birth. Babies born of mothers who have hypercalcemia can have temporary suppression of the parathyroid gland function at birth.

Acquired hypoparathyroidism due to immune system antibody development and destruction of the parathyroid gland can be a part of a syndrome that affects many glands. An antibody binding to the calcium sensor of the parathyroid gland may cause the gland to sense a high blood level of ionized calcium and therefore quit making PTH. Hypomagnesemia can lead to hypocalcemia because magnesium is important to the normal production of PTH by parathyroid cells. Pseudohypoparathyroidism is caused by the loss of function of one allele of the gene encoding the stimulatory G protein α or GNAS1, which causes a 50% reduction in levels of the α-subunit of the heterotrimeric G_s subunit, which couples the PTH receptor to adenyl cyclase. Several variants of pseudohypoparathyroidism exist. Type 1A is the most understood and consists of a markedly blunted response of urinary cyclic adenosine monophosphate (cAMP) to administration of PTH, resulting in a generalized disorder of hormonal unresponsiveness (3, 5).

Clinical Presentation

The clinical presentation of hypoparathyroidism is associated with calcium levels. Mild symptoms may include tingling in the hands, fingers, toes, and circumoral paresthesias. Moderate symptoms include carpopedal spasms; pain in the face, legs, feet, and abdomen; dry hair; brittle nails; dry, scaly skin; cataracts; weakened tooth enamel in children; and painful menstruation. As symptoms become more severe, irritability, confusion, delirium, tetany, spasms of the larynx, and seizures may occur. On physical examination, a positive Chvostek sign (sensitivity rate of 27% and false-positive rate of 25%) or Trousseau sign (sensitivity rate of 66% and false-positive rate of 4%) may be present. Impetigo herpetiformis, a form of acute pustular psoriasis associated with hypocalcemia during pregnancy, may be present (3, 5, 65).

Diagnosis

Blood tests include PTH, serum calcium, ionized calcium, albumin, 25-hydroxy vitamin D, magnesium, and phosphorus. Urine tests include cAMP after an IV dose of PTH, which may help differentiate hypoparathyroidism from other causes. An ECG can be used to identify heart arrhythmias secondary to hypocalcemia. In patients with hypoparathyroidism, levels of serum total calcium and ionized calcium will be decreased, serum phosphorus will be greater than 5.4 mg/dL, and PTH will be decreased. Since the calcium ion is highly bound to protein, a total calcium level cannot be interpreted without a total protein or albumin level. Hypoalbuminemia causes a decrease in total calcium; however, the ionized fraction may be normal. In conditions such as multiple myeloma and paraproteinemias (elevated protein states), the total calcium may be elevated and the ionized fraction normal.

Primary hypoparathyroidism is diagnosed by low levels of serum PTH and serum calcium. In pseudohypoparathyroidism, the serum PTH level is high. In secondary hypoparathyroidism, the level of serum PTH is low and of serum calcium is high. Measuring 25-hydroxy vitamin D is important since deficiency can cause hypocalcemia. Measuring magnesium is important since hypomagnesemia is a cause for PTH deficiency. The phosphorous levels increases if the PTH level is low (3, 5, 65).

Management

Acute, severe hypocalcemia is life-threatening and demands prompt treatment with IV calcium gluconate via a central venous catheter. The patient is monitored closely for heart arrhythmias, seizures, and larynx spasms. Once the patient is stable, IV treatment is switched to oral treatment. For non–life-threatening hypocalcemia in primary hypoparathyroidism, a diet rich in calcium and vitamin D_3 is the mainstay of treatment. calcium supplementation of 1.5 to 3 grams by mouth per day is commonly prescribed. Vitamin D supplementation is typically given as 50,000 to 100,000 international units of ergocalciferol by mouth daily. If the cause of the hypoparathyroidism is hypomagnesemia, magnesium supplementation is prescribed. Levels of calcium and 25-hydroxy vitamin D, as well as renal function, should be monitored (3, 5, 65). The clinical presentation and management of hypoparathyroidism is summarized in Table 11-60.

Clinical Nurse Specialist Competencies and Spheres of Influence
Clinical Expert/Direct Care

The CNS provides direct clinical care for the patient with hypoparathyroidism by recognizing signs and symptoms, ordering the correct diagnostic tests, and treating according to evidence-based recommendations. For life-threatening hypocalcemia, the CNS should know that prompt treatment with IV calcium gluconate via a central venous catheter is required. When consulting, the CNS should review the patient's case, offer alternative approaches to patient care, and help implement planned change. The CNS should obtain the necessary resources to achieve the goal of the consult and communicate the consult findings to the appropriate colleagues.

Systems Leadership

The clinical leadership role may include serving on a committee to develop hospital-wide treatment guidelines and plans for nursing education. Another example of the leadership role includes participating in professional organizations such as the American Association of Clinical Endocrinologists, The American Society for Bone and Mineral Research, The Endocrine Society, and The National Endocrine and Metabolic Diseases Information Service.

TABLE 11–60 Clinical Connections: Hypoparathyroidism

Clinical Manifestations	Pathophysiology	Assessment Finding	Laboratory Diagnostic tests	Treatment
Hypocalcemia and hyperphosphatemia	Decreased PTH causes hypocalcemia and hyperphosphatemia	Tingling in the hands, fingers, toes, and circumoral paresthesias; carpopedal spasms; pain in the face, legs, and feet; abdominal pain; dry hair; brittle nails; dry, scaly skin; cataracts; weakened tooth enamel in children; painful menstruations; irritability, confusion, delirum, tetany, spasms of the larynx, and seizures	PTH, serum CA, ionized CA, albumin, 25-hydroxy vitamin D, Mg, phorphorus. Urine cAMP after an IV dose of PTH to differentiate hypoparathyroidism from other causes. Other tests: ECG	CA and vitamin D_3 supplementation, and if needed, Mg supplementation. Acute, severe hypocalcemia: IV CA gluconate via a central venous catheter

Collaboration, Coaching/Teaching/Mentoring

The collaboration role may involve working with emergency department personnel and the endocrinology service. Patient/family education for patients with hypoparathyroidism includes teaching patient/family members that the patient needs to consume a diet rich in calcium and how to take prescribed calcium and vitamin D. Patients should be informed that they have a lifelong risk of symptomatic tetany and that without access to calcium, death may occur. They should be encouraged to wear a chain or bracelet that identifies them as having hypoparathyroidism. They should also be informed that diuretic use may alter calcium homeostasis. Patients may need assistance in obtaining medical follow-up. Examples of research-related activities include collecting data about the incidence of problems associated with hypoparathyroidism, conducting a literature review for evidence-based practice guidelines, and evaluating current outcomes.

THYROID DISEASE

The thyroid gland is located inferior to the thyroid cartilage at approximately the level of the cricoid cartilage and produces two thyroid hormones (thyroxine [T_4] and triiodothyronine [T_3]) via a negative-feedback system) and calcitonin. The hypothalamus secretes thyrotropin-releasing hormone (TRH), stimulating the anterior pituitary gland to secrete thyroid-stimulating hormone (TSH). The TSH enables the thyroid gland to produce and release T_4, which is converted in the peripheral tissues into T_3. Circulating T_4 and T_3 negatively inhibit TRH and TSH secretion. The thyroid hormones regulate metabolism and affect the growth and rate of function of many body systems. Iodine and tyrosine are used to form T_3 and T_4. The most common forms of thyroid disease are hypothyroidism and hyperthyroidism (5, 61, 66).

Hypothyroidism
Etiology

Hypothyroidism results from a deficiency of thyroid hormone and is a common endocrine disorder. Primary hypothyroidism occurs when the thyroid gland produces insufficient amounts of thyroid hormone. The most common causes include Hashimoto thyroiditis and radioiodine therapy for hyperthyroidism. Secondary hypothyroidism is due to inadequate TSH secretion from the pituitary gland. The most common cause is damage to the pituitary gland such as tumor, radiation, or surgery. Tertiary hypothyroidism, also called hypothalamic-pituitary axis hypothyroidism, results when the hypothalamus fails to produce sufficient TRH. Cretinism refers to congenital hypothyroidism. Subclinical hypothyroidism, common in elderly persons, is defined as a normal serum free T_4 with a slightly high serum TSH. According to the National Health and Nutrition Examination Survey III (NHANES III), elevated TSH levels occur in approximately 4.6% of the U.S. population and are more common in women who had a small body size at birth and a low BMI during childhood. The prevalence is higher in whites than in Hispanics or African Americans. Women are 2 to 8 times more likely to develop hypothyroidism than are men, and the likelihood of developing hypothyroidism increases with age (3, 5, 63, 66, 67).

Pathophysiology

Hashimoto thyroiditis is an autoimmune response manifested by lymphocytic infiltration and progressive destruction of the gland. In approximately 95% of cases, patients have positive antibodies to thyroid tissue. Antithyroid peroxidase antibodies are more common than antithyroglobulin antibodies.

Postpartum thyroiditis may occur 2 to 10 months after delivery and is usually transient. Women with lymphocytic thyroiditis, however, have a higher likelihood of developing hypothyroidism permanently. It occurs in approximately 10% of postpartum women and up to 25% of those with T1DM. High levels of antithyroid peroxidase antibodies are common in postpartum thyroiditis.

Inflammatory conditions or viral syndromes may cause a transient hyperthyroidism followed by transient hypothyroidism. The patient usually has a fever, malaise, and a painful gland. Medications such as amiodarone, interferon alpha, thalidomide, lithium, and stavudine may induce primary thyroidism. Hypothyroidism also occurs after the use of radioactive iodine for treatment of Graves disease, after thyroidectomy, and after external neck irradiation. Iodine deficiency is the most common cause of primary hypothyroidism worldwide. Excess iodine inhibits iodide organification and thyroid hormone synthesis. Rarely, inborn errors of thyroid hormone synthesis can cause primary hypothyroidism. Secondary and tertiary hypothyroidism can be caused by pituitary adenoma, tumors impinging on the hypothalamus, brain irradiation, dopamine, and lithium (1, 5, 63, 67).

Clinical Presentation

All metabolically active cells require thyroid hormone. Common symptoms of hypothyroidism include cold intolerance, puffiness, decreased perspiration, coarse skin, nerve entrapment syndromes, paresthesia, blurred vision, decreased hearing, fullness of the throat, neck pain, sore throat, low-grade fever, galactorrhea, constipation, menstrual disturbances, impaired fertility, fatigue, muscle pain, joint pain, weakness in the extremities, decreased appetite, hair loss, depression, emotional lability, mental impairment, impaired memory, inability to concentrate, sleepiness, and obstructive sleep apnea secondary to macroglossia.

Common signs of hypothyroidism include hypothermia, weight gain, slow speech, slow movements, dry skin, jaundice, pallor, dull facial expression, coarse facial features, periorbital puffiness, macroglossia, goiter, hoarseness, decreased systolic blood pressure, increased diastolic blood pressure, bradycardia, pericardial effusion, abdominal distention, nonpitting edema, pitting edema of the lower extremities, and painless thyroid enlargement. Also seen are hyporeflexia with delayed relaxation, ataxia, or both; coarse, brittle, stawlike hair; and loss of scalp, axillary, or pubic hair.

Metabolic abnormalities include anemia, dilutional hyponatremia, hyperlipidemia, and reversible increase in creatinine level. Hypothyroidism in pregnancy is associated with preeclampsia, anemia, postpartum hemorrhage, cardiac ventricular dysfunction, spontaneous abortion, low birth weight, impaired cognitive development, and fetal mortality. Myxedema coma signs and symptoms include altered mental status, hypothermia, bradycardia, hypercarbia, hyponatremia, cardiomegaly, pericardial effusion, cardiogenic shock, and ascites (3, 5, 63, 67).

Diagnosis

Blood tests include TSH, total T_4, and free T_4. The TSH normal range is 0.40 to 4.2 m/IU/L; serum levels peak in the evening and are lowest in the afternoon. T_4 is highly protein-bound, and levels of binding proteins can vary according to hormonal status, inheritance, and various disease states. Free T_4 is a measure of unbound hormone but is unreliable if severe illness is present. Thyroid autoantibodies (antimicrosomal and antithyroglobulin) may be useful in determining the etiology of hypothyroidism or in predicting future hypothyroidism.

Elevated TSH and decreased free T_4 levels occur in primary hypothyroidism. Those with elevated TSH but normal free T_4 have subclinical hypothyroidism. In people with hypothalamic or pituitary dysfunction, the TSH level does not rise in proportion to the low free T_4 levels (3, 5, 63, 67-69).

Management

Supplemental thyroid hormone replacement is the treatment for hypothyroidism, with the goal of restoring the TSH and free T_4 to the normal range. Thyroid hormone replacement can precipitate adrenal crises in patients with untreated adrenal insufficiency. If suspected, the presence of adrenal insufficiency should be ruled out or treated before treatment of hypothyroidism. The adult dose of levothyroxine ranges from 1 to 2 mcg/kg/day. The average starting dose is 50 to 100 mcg/day. The initial dose depends on multiple factors including age, weight, and cardiac status. The American Association of Clinical Endocrinology advocates the use of a high-quality brand of levothyroxine and the use of the same brand name for each refill. Dose adjustments in increments of 25 to 50 mcg are made every 6 to 8 weeks based on subsequent free T_4 and TSH levels. The initial dose of levothyroxine for those older than 50 years is 25 to 50 mcg/day. Dose adjustments are made at 6- to 8-week intervals. The initial starting dose for elderly persons with

cardiac disease is 11.5 to 25 mcg/d, with gradual dose increase at 4- to 6-week intervals (3, 5, 63, 66, 67).

Achieving a normal TSH level may take months because of the hypothalamic-pituitary axis readaptation. Follow-up, after initial stabilization, can be annual and should include a review of signs and symptoms of overtreatment (tachycardia, palpitation, nervousness, tiredness, headache, increased excitability, sleeplessness, tremors, and angina). Management of hypothyroidism in pregnancy includes increasing the levothyroxine dose by 30% at the beginning of the pregnancy and then adjusting the dose based on the TSH level. In those with hypothyroidism before pregnancy, the TSH level should be tested every 3 to 4 weeks during the first half of the pregnancy and every 6 weeks thereafter. After each dose adjustment, retest the TSH level, and test the free T_4 level 3 to 4 weeks later (3, 5, 63, 66, 67).

Myxedema coma is an acute medical emergency that should be treated in the ICU since most patients require intubation and mechanical ventilation. Those who are older and have long-standing, untreated hypothyroidism with a concurrent illness are at greatest risk of myxedema coma, and this condition is more common during cold weather. Signs and symptoms include hypothermia, bradycardia, severe hypotension, seizures, and coma.

Definitive diagnosis of myxedema coma is difficult; however, because survival is dependent on rapid treatment, initial treatment should be started before the test results are available and based on clinical evidence. T_4 at 50 to 100 mcg should be given every 6 to 8 hours as an IV bolus, and then the dose should be changed to 75 to 100 mcg IV daily. Hydrocortisone at 100 mg IV should be given initially, followed by 50 mg every 12 hours or 25 mg every 6 hours until coexistent adrenal insufficiency can be ruled out. Once the patient is able to eat, the medication form should be changed to oral. The caregiver needs to monitor cardiac function, correct hypothermia, monitor blood gases closely, support ventilatory function, hydrate with normal or hypertonic saline, and treat any coexisting conditions (3, 5, 63, 67).

The American Thyroid Association recommends screening at age 35 years and every 5 years thereafter, with closer attention be given to patients at high risk (e.g., pregnant women, women older than 60 years, patients with T1DM or other autoimmune disease, and patients with a history of neck irradiation (64). The American Association of Clinical Endocrinologists recommends that TSH be measured in all women of childbearing age before pregnancy or during the first trimester. The U.S. Preventive Task Force concludes that the evidence is insufficient to recommend for or against routine screening for thyroid disease in adults. Because screening prevents a delay in recognizing and treating cretinism, governmental bodies frequently mandate screening of neonates (66). A detailed listing of assessment findings, pathophysiology, and treatment of hypothyroidism is found in Table 11-61.

TABLE 11–61 Clinical Connections: Hypothyroidism

Clinical Manifestations	Deficiency in thyroid hormone
Pathophysiology	Thyroid unable to produce sufficient thyroid hormone due to autoimmune attack of the thyroid, inflammatory conditions, viral syndromes, certain medications, thyroidectomy, neck irradiation, iodine deficiency, inborn errors in thyroid hormone synthesis, pituitary adenoma, tumors impinging on the hypothalamus, or brain irradiation
Assessment Finding	Cold intolerance, puffiness, decreased perspiration, coarse skin, nerve entrapment syndromes, paresthesia, blurred vision, decreased hearing, fullness of the throat, neck pain, sore throat, low-grade fever galactorrhea, constipation, menstrual disturbances, impaired fertility, fatigue, muscle pain, joint pain, weakness in the extremities, decreased appetite, hair loss, depression, emotional lability, mental impairment, impaired memory, inability to concentrate, sleepiness, and obstructive sleep apnea secondary to macroglossia, hypothermia, weight gain, slow speech, slow movements, dry skin, jaundice, pallor; coarse, brittle, stawlike hair; loss of scalp, axillary, or pubic hair; dull facial expression, coarse facial features, periorbital puffiness, macroglossia, goiter, hoarseness, decreased systolic blood pressure, increased diastolic blood pressure, bradycardia, pericardial effusion, abdominal distention, nonpitting edema, pitting edema of the lower extremities; hyporeflexia with delayed relaxation, ataxia, or both; painless thyroid enlargement, anemia, dilutional hyponatremia, hyperlipidemia, and reversible increase in creatinine
Laboratory Diagnostic tests	TSH, total T_4, and free T_4
Treatment	Supplemental thyroid hormone replacement

TSH, Thyroid-stimulating hormone.

Clinical Nurse Specialist Competencies and Spheres of Influence
Clinical Expert/Direct Care

The CNS provides direct clinical care for patients with hypothyroidism by recognizing signs and symptoms, ordering the correct diagnostic tests, and treating according to evidence-based recommendations. If myxedema coma occurs, the CNS should recognize it as a medical emergency requiring intensive care and usually intubation. When consulting, the CNS should review the patient's case, offer alternative approaches to patient care, and help implement planned change. The CNS should obtain the necessary resources to achieve the goal of the consult and communicate the findings to the appropriate colleagues.

Systems Leadership

The clinical leadership role may include serving on a committee to develop hospitalwide treatment guidelines and plans for nursing education. Another example of the leadership role includes participating in professional organizations such as the American Association of Clinical Endocrinologists, The Endocrine Society, and The National Endocrine and Metabolic Diseases Information Service, American Thyroid Association, and the Hormone Foundation.

Collaboration, Coaching/Teaching/Mentoring

The collaboration role may involve working with emergency department personnel, ICU staff, and the endocrinology service. Patient/family education for patients with hypothyroidism includes teaching the patient to take thyroid hormone replacement medication on an empty stomach each morning 30 minutes before eating breakfast. The patient also needs to know the signs and symptoms of hypothyroidism and hyperthyroidism in case the dose needs to be adjusted. Periodic thyroid function studies will be needed for adjustment of the doses. Examples of research-related activities include collecting data about the incidence of complications and undiagnosed hypothyroidism, conducting a literature review for evidence-based practice guidelines, and evaluating current outcomes.

Hyperthyroidism
Etiology

Hyperthyroidism occurs when free T_4 and/or T_3 is overproduced. Approximately 60% to 80% of those with hyperthyroidism have Graves disease. Other causes include multinodular goiter; toxic thyroid adenoma; a single functional, autonomous, hyperfunctioning nodule; iodine and drugs containing iodine; subacute thyroiditis; painless thyroiditis; surreptitious ingestion of thyroid hormone; ectopic thyroid tissue; and TSH-secreting pituitary adenoma. The incidence of Graves disease in women is approximately 0.5 per 1,000 each year, which is 10 times higher than in men. Overall, hyperthyroidism occurs in 1 in 1,000 women and 1 in 3,000 men. It is found in whites and Asians more often than in African Americans. The peak age is 40 years. Risk factors include a positive family history, female, other autoimmune disorders, and iodide repletion after iodide deprivation (3, 5, 63, 67).

Pathophysiology

Graves disease is an autoimmune disorder caused by antibody attack of the TSH receptors causing stimulation and hyperfunction of the thyroid gland and hyperplasia and hypertrophy of the thyroid follicles. Three types of autoantibodies are known to attack the TSH receptor: thyroid-stimulating immunoglobulins, which are long-acting thyroid stimulants that activate cells more slowly than TSH does; thyroid growth immunoglobulins, which bind directly to the TSH receptor, causing growth of thyroid follicles; and thyrotrophin-binding inhibitory immunoglobulins, which inhibit the normal union of TSH with its receptor, acting like TSH. Antibodies may develop against thyroglobulin, T_3, and T_4. Diffuse goiter develops as lymphocytes invade.

Ocular manifestations are believed to be caused by the thyroid gland and the extraocular muscles, which share a common antigen recognized by the antibodies. This results in edema and inflammation of the extraocular muscles and an increase in the orbital connective tissue and fat. Edema occurs due to the hydrophilic action of glycosaminoglycans secreted by fibroblasts, and inflammation occurs secondary to infiltration by lymphocytes and macrophages.

Nontoxic multinodular goiter can develop into toxic multinodular goiter if one or more of the nodules achieve functional autonomy. Solitary functioning nodules occur due to somatic mutations in the TSH receptor gene, causing progressive growth, and sometimes originate from a long-standing simple goiter that transitions from a nontoxic multinodular thyroid gland into an autonomous functional state (3, 5, 63).

Clinical Presentation

Clinical presentation depends on severity of the disease, age of the patient, and the underlying cause. General signs and symptoms include goiter, bruit over the thyroid, hyperactivity, sleep disturbance, heat intolerance, increased sweating, fatigue, exertional intolerance, hair loss, and palmar erythema. Nervous system manifestations include nervousness, irritability, mental disturbance, fine tremor, hyperreflexia, muscle weakness and wasting, and sudden paralysis. Manifestations of the eyes include Graves ophthalmopathy, eye dryness, blurred vision, photophobia, diplopia, and exophthalmos. Gastrointestinal signs include increased stool frequency and diarrhea, weight loss or gain, and alteration in appetite. Reproductive system changes include oligomenorrhea, amenorrhea, infertility, and loss of libido. Cardiovascular changes include palpitations, sinus tachycardia, atrial fibrillation, congestive heart failure, dependent lower-extremity edema, pretibial myxedema, exacerbation of coronary artery disease, and dyspnea (3, 5, 63, 67).

Diagnosis

TSH screening is the best tool for detecting hyperthyroidism. A result of greater than 0.1 mIU/L excludes clinical hyperthyroidism. Determining the free T_4 level helps assess the extent of hyperthyroidism. An elevated free T_4 level with a decreased TSH is diagnostic of hyperthyroidism. In a person with symptoms of hyperthyroidism, if the free T_4 level is normal and the TSH is suppressed to 0.1 mIU/L, the person may have triiodothyronine toxicosis; in this situation, the T_3 level should be measured as well. A thyroid scan may be helpful to distinguish Graves disease from nodules and thyroiditis. Autoantibody analysis may also be helpful. Antibodies are positive in 80% of those with Graves disease (3, 5, 63, 67).

Management

Treatment options include radioactive iodine ablation, antithyroid medications, and subtotal thyroidectomy. Surgery has not been used often in recent years unless the patient has thyroid cancer, the patient is pregnant and intolerant of antithyroid drugs, or the patient refuses radioactive iodine treatment and is a good candidate for surgery. Methimazole at 10 to 40 mg/day once daily and propylthiouracil at 200 to 600 mg/day in 3 or 4 divided doses inhibit thyroid peroxidase and block production of thyroid hormone. Elderly persons and those with cardiac disease may need medication treatment before radioactive iodine treatment. Radioactive iodine treatment is the treatment of choice for most people with hyperthyroidism. It is contraindicated in pregnancy and in those breastfeeding. Ablative therapy quickly resolves hyperthyroidism and usually causes hypothyroidism. Some endocrinologists may attempt a smaller dose to attempt to reestablish euthyroid.

Thyroid storm is an acute life-threatening condition that occurs when hyperthyroidism is severe and causes marked hypermetabolism. Rapid recognition and treatment is vital for survival of the patient. Causes include infections, stroke, DKA, thyroid surgery, discontinuation of antithyroid medications, radioactive iodine treatment, pregnancy, excessive thyroid hormone replacement, and acute myocardial infarction and other cardiac emergencies. Signs and symptoms include weakness, nausea, vomiting, diarrhea, hyperthermia, tachycardia, arrhythmias, chest pain, heart failure, shortness of breath, anxiety, irritability, disorientation, and coma. Management includes determining TSH and FT4 levels for diagnosis and administering propylthiouracil or methimazole orally or via nasogastric tube every 6 hours. Propylthiouracil and methimazole prevent the conversion of T_4 to T_3. At 1 to 2 hours after initiating treatment, the patient should be given 1 to 2 drops of a saturated solution of K$^+$ iodide or 0.5 mg of iopanoic acid, and this dosing schedule should be repeated every 11 hours. Lithium may be used in patients with iodine allergy. Atrial fibrillation is common during thyroid storm, so cardiac monitoring is required. Beta-blockers will reduce palpitations, tremors, and anxiety. Verapamil may be used if the patient has severe heart failure or asthma. If adrenal insufficiency is present, IV glucocorticoids are indicated. If infection is present,

antibiotics should be used. Aggressive hydration, cooling, and analgesics should be used to treat symptoms, but not aspirin (3, 5, 67). See Table 11-62 for a summary of the assessment findings and treatment of hyperthyroidism.

Clinical Nurse Specialist Competencies and Spheres of Influence
Clinical Expert/Direct Care
The CNS provides direct clinical care for patients with hyperthyroidism by recognizing signs and symptoms, ordering the correct diagnostic tests, and treating according to evidence-based recommendations. If thyroid storm occurs, the CNS should recognize it as a medical emergency. When consulting, the CNS should review the patient's case, offer alternative approaches to patient care, and help implement planned change. The CNS should obtain the necessary resources to achieve the goal of the consult and communicate findings to the appropriate colleagues.

Systems Leadership
The clinical leadership role may include serving on a committee to develop hospitalwide treatment guidelines and plans for nursing education. Another example of the leadership role includes participating in professional organizations such as the American Association of Clinical Endocrinologists, The Endocrine Society, and

TABLE 11–62 Clinical Connections: Hyperthyroidism

Clinical Manifestations	Overproduction of thyroid hormone
Pathophysiology	Autoimmune antibody attack of the TSH receptor, causing stimulation and hyperfunction of the thyroid gland
Assessment Finding	Goiter, bruit over thyroid, hyperactivity, nervousness, irritability, mental disturbance, sleep disturbance, heat intolerance, increased sweating, fatigue, exertional intolerance and dyspnea, weakness, weight loss or gain, alteration in appetite, palpitations, Graves ophthalmopathy, eye dryness, blurred vision, photophobia, diplopia, exophthalmos, increased stool frequency, diarrhea, oligomenorrhea, amenorrhea, infertility, loss of libido, sinus tachycardia, atrial fibrillation, fine tremor, hyperreflexia; warm, moist skin; hair loss, muscle weakness and wasting, sudden paralysis, congestive heart failure, dependent lower-extremity edema, pretibial myxedema, exererbation of coronary arter disease, palmar erytherma, onycholysis, and periodic paralysis
Laboratory Diagnostic tests	TSH, free T_4, T_3
Treatment	Radioactive iodine ablation, antithyroid medications, and/or subtotal thyroidectomy

TSH, Thyroid-stimulating hormone.

The National Endocrine and Metabolic Diseases Information Service, American Thyroid Association, and the Hormone Foundation.

Collaboration, Coaching/Teaching/Mentoring, Research/Evidence-based Practice

The collaboration role may involve working with emergency department personnel, ICU staff, and the endocrinology service. Patient/family education for patients with hyperthyroidism includes instruction in the use of various treatment options and in how to take prescribed medications. If the treatment for hyperthyroidism causes hypothyroidism, then the patient will require treatment. Examples of research activities include collecting data about the incidence of hyperthyroidism-related complications, conducting a literature review for evidence-based medical guidelines, and evaluating current outcomes.

SYNDROME OF ANTIDIURETIC HORMONE

Etiology

The body normally maintains sodium balance by regulating a balance of water intake, renal excretion of sodium antidiuretic hormone (ADH)-mediated feedback mechanisms of the renin-angiotensin-aldosterone system, and variation of renal handling of filtered sodium. Hyponatremia can result if any of these components of sodium balance is abnormal. Increased ADH, also called arginine vasopressin, occurs appropriately when vascular baroreceptors sense a decrease in the effective circulatory volume associated with cirrhosis, nephritic syndrome, congestive heart failure, and plasma volume depletion. The hypovolemia overrides osmotic signals, causing excess vasopressin release and resulting in hyponatremia (5).

Syndrome of inappropriate antidiuretic hormone (SIADH) secretion is characterized by hyponatremia, elevated urine osmolality level (greater then 200 mOsm/kg), excessive urine sodium excretion (greater than 30 mEq/L), and decreased serum osmolality. This condition occurs in the absence of diuretic therapy and edema, in the presence of normal cardiac, renal, adrenal, hepatic, and thyroid function, and in the presence of euvolemia. The cause is excessive water, not a sodium deficiency (70).

Hyponatremia is the most common electrolyte abnormality in hospitalized patients. It occurs in an estimated 1% to 4% of patients, and approximately two-thirds of cases are hospital-acquired. The mortality rate in patients with hyponatremia is 7- to 60-fold higher than in those who do not have this abnormality because hyponatremia is a measure of underlying illness (3). The highest mortality rates are in those with acute-onset hyponatremia. Symptomatic hyponatremia occurs more commonly in females, but there is no racial preference. Very old and very young patients develop symptoms of hyponatremia sooner than do those in other age groups. The most common cause of euvolemic hyponatremia is SIADH (71). The causes of SIADH are found in Table 11-63. The most common cause is idiopathic.

TABLE 11–63 Causes of Syndrome of Inappropriate Antidiuretic Hormone

Central Nervous System

- Tumor
- Head trauma
- Infection
- Cerebrovascular accident
- Subarachnoid hemorrhage
- Guillain-Barré syndrome
- Delirium tremens
- Multiple sclerosis
- Acute intermittent porphyria
- Hydrocephalus
- Infection: meningitis, encephalitis, abscess

Pulmonary

- Tumor
- Pneumonia
- Chronic obstructive pulmonary disease
- Lung abscess

Continued

TABLE 11–63 Causes of Syndrome of Inappropriate Antidiuretic Hormone—cont'd

- Tuberculosis
- Cystic fibrosis
- Positive-pressure ventilation

Medication

- Bromocriptine mesylate
- Carbamazepine
- Chlorpropamide
- Clofibrate
- Cyclophosphamide
- Desmopressin
- Diuretics
- Exogenous vasopressin
- Nonsteroidal anti-inflammatory drugs
- Opiates
- Oxytocin
- Phenothiazines
- Selective serotonin reuptake inhibitors
- Thioridazine
- Tricyclic antidepressants
- Vinblastine
- Vincristine

Neoplasms

- Duodenal carcinoma
- Lymphoma
- Mesothelioma
- Olfactory neuroblastoma
- Pancreatic carcinoma
- Prostate carcinoma
- Small cell carcinoma of the lung
- Thymoma

Miscellaneous

- HIV
- Nausea
- Neuropsychiatric disorders
- Increased thirst
- ADH release at a lower osmolality
- Increased renal sensitivity to ADH
- Pain
- Postoperatively
- Ecstasy
- Nicotine

HIV, Human immunodeficiency virus; *ADH,* antidiuretic hormone.

Pathophysiology

Secreted by the posterior pituitary gland, ADH affects the kidneys, mediated by vasopressin V2 receptors on the basolateral surface of the principal cells of the collecting duct, cyclic AMP, protein kinase A, and a molecular dynein motor. Insertion of water channels in the principal cells of the collecting duct is the key action of ADH. The water channels allow free water to be reabsorbed from the collecting duct within the hypertonic renal medulla and include aquaporin-2, located at the apical membrane, and aquaporin-3, located at the basolateral membrane. SIADH enhances reabsorption of water, produces concentrated urine, causes the inability to excrete water, and causes hyponatremia (3, 5, 70).

Clinical Presentation

Signs and symptoms of hyponatremia are related to central nervous system dysfunction caused by cerebral edema and increased intracranial pressure from osmotic fluid shifts. The symptoms are greater if the decrease in serum sodium is rapid and severe. Symptoms usually occur once the serum sodium drops to less than 115 mEq/L and include anorexia, nausea, malaise, headache, irritability, confusion, muscle cramps, weakness, obtundation, seizures, and coma. If the serum sodium level drops to less than 105 mEq/L, death may occur (3, 71).

Obtaining a patient history is important in determining the cause of hyponatremia. Details such as food and fluid intake, gastrointestinal losses, amount of urinary output, and medications can help determine whether the condition is acute or chronic. Before making a diagnosis of SIADH, numerous conditions capable of causing hyponatremia (congestive heart failure, hepatic dysfunction, adrenal insufficiency, renal failure, and thyroid disease) are excluded (3,71).

Since SIADH occurs in a euvolemic state, edema in the presence of hyponatremia should lead the clinician to consider congestive heart failure, cirrhosis, and nephritic syndrome. Blood pressure will be normal without orthostatic instability, mucous membranes will be moist, and skin turgor will be normal. Other physical findings include myoclonus, asterixis, depressed reflexes, generalized seizures, and coma (3, 70).

Diagnosis

Blood tests include serum electrolytes, BUN, creatinine, TSH, cortisol, and glucose. The sodium level will be less than 135 mEq/L, and K^+ and bicarbonate levels will be normal. Hypokalemia and metabolic alkalosis suggest diuretic therapy or vomiting. Hyperkalemia and metabolic acidosis coexisting with hyponatremia suggest adrenal insufficiency. Blood urea nitrogen and serum uric acid levels are usually low because of plasma dilution and increased excretion of nitrogenous products. Elevated glucose levels decrease the serum sodium levels by 1.6 mEq/L for every 100 mg/dL above normal. Glucose draws water into the intravascular space by osmosis, and once the glucose is corrected, the sodium levels return to normal. The serum osmolality will be less than 280 mOsm/kg, the urine osmolality will be greater than 100 mOsm/L, and the urine sodium level will be greater than 20 mmol/L (3, 5).

SIADH is diagnosed via exclusion of other causes of hyponatremia. Plasma ADH levels are inappropriately elevated relative to plasma osmolality. When assessing renal, adrenal, and thyroid function, the creatinine, cortisol, and TSH must be normal in SIADH. If severe hyperlipidemia with hyperproteinemia (greater than 10 g/dL) exists, as seen in multiple myeloma, pseudohyponatremia occurs. Chest radiographs may reveal pulmonary disease or lung carcinoma that may cause SIADH. CT scan of the head may show cerebral edema or a CNS disorder that is causing SIADH and may rule out other causes of acute neurologic status changes (3)(5) (70).

If the serum sodium level is greater than 115 mEq/L, a water load test may be performed by giving 20 mL/kg of water to be ingested in 10 to 20 minutes. If the patient is unable to excrete 80% in 4 hours and/or fails to dilute urinary osmolality to less than 100 mOsm/kg, the test is abnormal. Improvement of serum sodium after water deprivation or no significant improvement of serum sodium with volume expansion is suggestive of SIADH (71).

Management

In general, the serum sodium should not be corrected to greater than 120 mEq/L and should not exceed 11 mmol/L in the first 24 hours to minimize the risk of osmotic central pontine myelinolysis (CPM), which can occur one to several days after aggressive treatment of hyponatremia. Signs and symptoms of CPM include spastic quadriparesis, pseudobulbar palsy, confusion, and coma. Since patients with hepatic failure, K^+ depletion, large burns, and malnutrition have an increased risk for CPM, the correction of hyponatremia in these patients should be restricted to 10 mmol/L/24 hr (71).

Acute hyponatremia can be corrected by using 3% NaCl at a rate of 1 to 2 mEq/hr if severely symptomatic (i.e., seizures) or if the serum Na concentration is less than 120 mEq/L; however, the total rate of correction should not exceed 15 mEq/L/24 hr. An initial infusion rate of 3% saline can be estimated by the following formula: (patient's body weight [kg]) × (the rate of increase in serum sodium [mmol/L/hr]). Acute treatment should be discontinued when the patient's symptoms resolve, when a sodium level of 120 mEq/L is achieved, or when a total correction of 18 mmol/L is achieved (71). Furosemide given at 1 mg/kg will increase excretion of free water and can be used in conjunction with isotonic or hypertonic saline. Once normal renal function is ascertained, try to normalize K^+ levels before or concurrent with the correction of hyponatremia. Monitor serum and urine electrolyte levels every 2 to 4 hours during the active phase of treatment. Therapy should be stopped when the serum sodium concentration is 110 to 130 mEq/L, when symptoms resolve, or when the serum sodium concentration increases by 15 mEq/L in 24 hours or less.

Fluid restriction to 500 to 1,000 mL/day is the main treatment for patients with chronic hyponatremia with sodium levels greater than 115 mEq/L. Pharmacologic agents may be used in patients with chronic hyponatremia and a serum sodium level of less than 115 mEq/L who are unable to comply with the water restriction or in whom the condition is refractory to water restriction treatment. Demeclocycline is usually used in consultation with a nephrologist or primary care physician and is not used acutely in the emergency department since its action is delayed by more than 1 week. This drug impairs the action of cyclic AMP and induces diabetes insipidus. Urea is an osmotic diuretic that elevates the osmolarity of the glomerular filtrate and hinders the tubular reabsorption of water. Loop diuretics are used in patients with hypervolemic hyponatremia. They increase the excretion of water by interfering with the chloride-binding cotransport system, causing inhibition of sodium and chloride reabsorption in the ascending loop of Henle and distal renal tubule. Vasopressin receptor antagonists such as conivaptan, an IV dual V1a/V2 antagonist, increase free water diuresis without natriuresis or kaliuresis in patients with SIADH (3, 63, 70). The treatment of SIADH is detailed in Table 11-64.

Clinical Nurse Specialist Competencies and Spheres of Influence
Clinical Expert/Direct Care
The CNS provides direct clinical care for the patient with SIADH by recognizing signs and symptoms, ordering the correct diagnostic tests, and treating according to evidence-based recommendations. Severe acute hyponatremia is a medical emergency requiring careful intervention to prevent CPM. When consulting, the CNS should review the patient's case, offer alternative approaches to patient care, and help implement planned change. The CNS should obtain the necessary resources to achieve the goal of the consult and communicate the consult findings to the appropriate colleagues.

Systems Leadership
The clinical leadership role may include serving on a committee to develop hospitalwide treatment guidelines and plans for nursing education. Another example of the leadership role includes participating in professional organizations such as the American Association of Clinical Endocrinologists, The Endocrine Society, and The National Endocrine and Metabolic Diseases Information Service.

Collaboration, Coaching/Teaching/Mentoring, Research/Evidence-Based Practice
The collaboration role may involve working with the endocrinology service, emergency department personnel, ICU staff, and nutrition. Patient/family education for patients with SIADH includes teaching the causes of the

TABLE 11-64 Clinical Connections: Syndrome of Increased Antidiuretic Hormone

Clinical Manifestations	Hyponatremia
Pathophysiology	Signs and symptoms of hyponatremia are related to central nervous system dysfunction caused by cerebral edema and increased intracranial pressure from osmotic fluid shifts.
Assessment Finding	Anorexia, nausea, malaise, headache, irritability, confusion, muscle cramps, weakness, obtundation, seizures, coma, and death
Laboratory Diagnostic tests	Electrolytes, BUN, creatinine, TSH, cortisol, and glucose
Treatment	The serum Na should not be corrected above 110 mEq/L and should not exceed 11 mEq/L in the first 24 hours;]3% NaCl only for acute hyponatremia; furosemide. For chronic hyponatremia: fluid restriction of 500–1,000 mL/day, or medications: demeclocycline, urea, loop diuretics, and conivaptan

TSH, Thyroid-stimulating hormone; *BUN,* blood urea nitrogen.

condition, the importance of following the prescribed fluid restriction, and the necessity of taking medications, if prescribed. Examples of research activities include conducting a literature review for the implementation of evidence-based practice guidelines and evaluating current outcomes.

Ethical Decision-Making/Moral Agency/Advocacy

Ethical decision making with regard to treatment of SIADH in conjunction with end-stage lung cancer may be necessary. This involves helping the patient and family realize that treatment of SIADH may be part of a palliative plan of care that will help resolve symptomatology and contribute to quality of life but will not alter the course of the cancer.

DIABETES INSIPIDUS

Etiology

Diabetes insipidus (DI) is characterized by excessive thirst and dilute polyuria. It is a relatively uncommon condition that occurs when the kidneys are unable to conserve water. The defect in regulation of water balance is secondary to either decreased pituitary secretion of ADH (central DI, also called neurogenic DI) or to a failure to respond to ADH (nephrogenic DI).

Central DI is the most common form and is usually caused by damage to the hypothalamus or pituitary gland. Familial cases of vasopressin deficiency have been reported and are usually autosomal dominant; more than 20 mutations have been identified. Common causes of damage include head injury, infection, surgery, and tumor. Dispogenic DI is due to a defect or damage to the thirst mechanism located in the hypothalamus causing increased thirst. Additionally, iatrogenic DI may be induced by certain medications (3, 5, 63, 72).

Nephrogenic DI usually occurs during infancy in males secondary to an X-linked defect in the V2 receptor that binds ADH or to an autosomal dominant or recessive defect in the aquaporin-2 gene that encodes an ADH-responsive water channel. Nephrogenic DI may also be caused by chronic renal failure, chronic renal medullary disease, pyelonephritis, obstructive uropathy, polycystic kidney disease, and renal transplantation. Other conditions that may lead to nephrogenic DI include electrolyte disturbances such as chronic hypokalemia and chronic hypercalcemia; pregnancy, multiple myeloma, sickle cell disease, and protein starvation. The use of certain drugs, including lithium, amphotericin B, colchicine, demeclocycline, gentamicin, loop diuretics, and methoxyflurane are atrogenic causes of nephrogenic DI.

Pathophysiology

The hypothalamus regulates urine production via the production of ADH in the supraoptic and paraventricular nuclei. Transported in neurosecretory granules down the axon of the hypothalamic neurosecretory granules to the posterior lobe of the pituitary gland, ADH is stored and released as needed. The hypothalamus regulates thirst sensation in the ventromedial nucleus by sensing serum osmolality and relaying the information to the cortex. The kidney helps to regulate fluid homeostasis. Antidiuretic hormone increases water permeability in the collecting ducts and distal convoluted tubule and acts on proteins call aquaporins. Aquaporins open and allow water into the collecting duct cells, increasing permeability and allowing water reabsorption into the bloodstream; this results in concentrated urine. Normally, ADH release is suppressed at plasma osmolalities less than 285 mOsm/kg. At greater than 285 mOsm/kg, ADH secretion increases linearly with plasma osmolality. At a plasma osmolality of approximately 295 mOsm/kg, the urine is maximally concentrated, even if the serum ADA levels continue to rise. Thirst also increases linearly with increasing plasma osmolality, protecting the body against hypertonicity. If there is an absolute or relative deficiency in the circulating levels or bioactivity of ADH, diabetes insipidus occurs (3, 5, 72).

Clinical Presentation

The main signs and symptoms of DI include polyuria resulting in greater than 3 L/day and polydipsia. The patient may show signs of dehydration or crave cold water or ice. If hypernatremia is present, symptoms may include weakness, altered mental status, hyperreflexia, muscle twitching, seizure, and coma (3, 5, 63, 72).

Diagnosis

Blood tests include blood glucose to rule out diabetes mellitus as the cause of the polyuria and polydipsia, bicarbonate, calcium, and electrolytes. The sodium level will be normal or elevated. The serum osmolality will usually be greater than 295 mOsm/kg. Hypokalemia in the presence of hypercalcemia suggests nephrogenic DI. Urine tests should include urinalysis. The specific gravity of urine will be less than 1.010, and the urine osmolality will be less than 200 mOsm/kg. A fluid deprivation test will reveal whether the DI is caused by excessive fluid intake, a defect in ADH production, or a defect in the kidneys' response to ADH. Those with DI will continue to urinate large amounts of dilute urine, although they are fluid-deprived. The ADH level is sometimes measured during the fluid deprivation test (3, 5, 63, 72).

Management

Desmopressin (DDAVP) is used to treat central and gestational DI; however, it is not used for dipsogenic or nephrogenic DI. Carbamazepine can also be used. Gestational DI tends to resolve spontaneously within 4 to 6 weeks after delivery. Occasionally, those treated with DDAVP should withdraw from treatment to confirm the reoccurrence of polyuria and polydipsia.

Nephrogenic DI is treated with a sodium-restricted diet and hydrochlorothiazide or indomethacin. To help prevent hypokalemia, amiloride is sometimes used in combination with hydrochlorothiazide. If the nephrogenic DI is caused by a drug, the offending agent is discontinued. Adequate hydration is important for those with DI (3, 5, 63,72). A summary of assessment and diagnostic findings and treatment plan is described in Table 11-65.

Clinical Nurse Specialist Competencies and Spheres of Influence
Clinical Expert/Direct Care
The CNS provides direct clinical care for the patient with DI by recognizing signs and symptoms, ordering the correct diagnostic tests, and treating according to evidence-based recommendations. When consulting, the CNS should review the patient's case, offer alternative approaches to patient care, and help implement planned change. The CNS should obtain the necessary resources to achieve the goal of the consult and communicate the consult findings to the appropriate colleagues.

Systems Leadership
The clinical leadership role may include serving on a committee to develop hospitalwide treatment guidelines and plans for nursing education. Another example of the leadership role includes participating in professional organizations such as the American Association of Clinical Endocrinologists, The Diabetes Insipidus Foundation, Inc, The Diabetes Insipidus and Related Disorders Network, National Organization for Rare Disorders (NORD), Nephrogenic Diabetes Insipidus Foundation, The Endocrine Society, and The National Endocrine and Metabolic Diseases Information Service.

Collaboration, Coaching/Teaching/Mentoring
The collaboration role may involve working with the endocrinology service, emergency department personnel, ICU staff, and nutritionists. Patient/family education for patients with SIADH includes teaching the causes of this condition, the importance of following the prescribed fluid restriction, and the necessity of taking medications (if prescribed).

TABLE 11–65 Clinical Connections

Clinical Manifestations	Absolute or relative deficiency in the circulating levels or bioactivity of ADH
Pathophysiology	The defect in the regulation of water balance is secondary to either decreased pituitary secretion of ADH (central DI) or the failure to respond to ADH (nephrogenic DI).
Assessment Finding	Polyuria >3 L/day, polydipsia, and extreme thirst, dehydration, crave cold water or ice, weakness, altered mental status, hyperreflexia, muscle twitching, seizure, and coma
Laboratory Diagnostic tests	Bicarbonate, CA, electrolytes, serum osmolality, urine specific gravity, fluid deprivation test with ADH
Treatment	Central or gestational DI: Desmopressin or carbamazepine and adequate hydration. Nephrogenic DI: Na-restricted diet and hydrochlorothiazide or indomethacin. To help prevent hypokalemia, amiloride is sometimes used in combination with hydrochlorothiazide. If the nephrogenic DI is caused by a drug, the offending agent is discontinued.

ADH, = Antidiuretic hormone; *DI,* = diabetes insipidus.

References

1. Bode B. Medical Management of Type 1 Diabetes Mellitus. 4th Edition. Alexandria, VA: American Diabetes Association; 2004.

2. American Diabetes Association. Diagnosis and classification of diabetes mellitus. Diabetes Care 2010;33:S62-S69.

3. Gardner D, Dolores S. Greenspan's Basic & Clinical Endocrinology. 8th Edition. New York: McGraw Hill; 2007.

4. American Diabetes Association. Total Prevalence of Diabetes and Pre-diabetes. Retrieved March 13, 2009, from http://www.diabetes.org/diabetes-statistics/prevalence.jsp

5. Kronenberg H, Meimed, S, Polonsky, K, et al. Williams Textbook of Endocrinology. 11th Edition. Philadelphia: Saunders Elsevier; 2008.

6. Nathan D. International expert committee report on the role of the A1 c assay in the diagnosis of diabetes. Diabetes Care 2009;32:1327-1334.

7. United States Department of Health and Human Services Centers for Disease Control and Prevention. Epidemiology of Type 1 and Type 2 Diabetes Mellitus among North American Children and Adolescents. Retrieved March 13, 2009, from http://www.cdc.gov/DIABETES/projects/cda2.htm

8. National Diabetes Information Clearinghouse. National Diabetes Statistics 2007. Retrieved March 15, 2009, from http://diabetes.niddk.nih.gov/DM/PUBS/statistics/#allages

9. American Diabetes Association. Direct and indirect cost of diabetes in the United States. Diabetes Care 2008;31:596-615.

10. Dean L, McEntyre J. The Genetic Landscape of Diabetes. Retrieved March 16, 2009, from http://www.ncbi.nlm.nih.gov/books/bv.fcgi?rid=diabetes.section.104

11. Eisenbarth G. Prediction of Type IA Diabetes: The Natural History of the Prediabetic Period. Retrieved March 16, 2009, from http://www.barbaradaviscenter.org/

12. Bry L, Chen P, Sacks D. Effects of hemoglobin variants and chemically modified derivatives on assays for glycohemoglobin. Clin Chem 2001;47:153-163.

13. Rohlfling C, Wiedmeyer H, Little R, et al. Defining the relationship between plasma glucose and HbA1c: an analysis of glucose profiles and HbA1c in the Diabetes Control and Complications Trial. Diabetes Care 2002;25:275-278.

14. Goldstein D, Little R, Lorenz R, et al. Tests of glycemia in diabetes. Diabetes Care 2004;27:1761-1773.

15. Smaldone A. Glycemic control and hemoglobinopathy: when A1c may not be reliable. Diabetes Spectrum 2008;21(1):46-49.

16. Wilkipedia. Fructosamine. Retrieved March 23, 2009, from http://en.wikipedia.org/wiki/Fructosamine

17. Nathan D, Kuenen J, Borg R, et al. Translating the A1c-assay into estimated average glucose values. Diabetes Care 2008;31: 1473-1478.

18. Diabetes Control and Complications Trial Research Group. The effect of intensive diabetes treatment on the development and progression of long-term complications in insulin-dependent diabetes mellitus: The Diabetes Control and Complications Trial. N Engl J Med 1993;329:978-986.

19. Reichard P, Nilsson B, Rosenqvist U. The effect of long-term intensified insulin treatment on the development of microvascular complications of diabetes mellitus. N Engl J Med 1993;329:304-309.

20. UK Prospective Diabetes Study (UKPDS) Group. Intensive blood glucose control with sulphonylureas or insulin compared with conventional treatment and risk of complication in patients with type 2 diabetes mellitus. Lancet 1998;352:854-865.

21. Ohkubo Y, Kishikawa H, Araki E, et al. Intensive insulin therapy prevents the progression of diabetes microvascular complications in Japanese patients with NIDDM: a randomized prospective 6-year study. Diabetes Res Clini Pract 1995;28:103-117.

22. Nathan D, Buse J, et al. Medical management of hyperglycemia in type 2 diabetes mellitus: a consensus algorithm for the initiation and adjustment of therapy:—a consensus statement of the American Diabetes Association and the European Association for the Study of Diabetes. Diabetes Care 2009;32:193-203.

23. The Action to Control Cardiovascular Risk in Diabetes Study Group. Effects of intensive glucose lowering in type 2 diabetes mellitus. N Engl J Med 2008;358:2545-2559.

24. The Advance Collaborative Group. Intensive blood glucose control and vascular outcomes in patients with type 2 diabetes mellitus. N Engl J Med 2008;358:2560-2572.

25. Abraira C, Duckworth W, Moritz T. Glycaemic separation and risk factor control in the Veterans Affairs Diabetes Trial: an interim report. Diabetes Obes Metab 2008;11:150-156.

26. Leboitz H. Therapy for Diabetes Mellitus and Related Disorders. 4th Edition. Alexandria, VA: American Diabetes Association; 2004.

27. American Diabetes Association. Standards of medical care in diabetes–2009. Diabetes Care 2009;32:S13-S61.

28. Buchwald E, Fahrbach K, Banel D, et al. Weight and type 2 diabetes mellitus after bariatric surgery: systematic review and meta-analysis. Am J Med 2009;112:248-256.

29. Lyznicki J, Young D, Riggs J, et al. Obesity: assessment and management in primary care. Am Fam Phys 2001;63:2191-2196.

30. Sigal R, Kenny G, Wasserman D, et al. Physical activity/exercise and type 2 diabetes mellitus. Diabetes Care 2004;27:2518-2539.

31. Texas Diabetes Council: Publication Number: E45-11166: Exercise Algorithm: Type 2 Diabetes Mellitus Prevention & Therapy. Retrieved January 22, 2009, from http://www.dshs.state.tx.us/diabetes/PDF/algorithms/EXERCISE.PDF

32. Wasserman E, Zinman B. Exercise in individuals with IDDM. Diabetes Care 1994;17:924-937.

33. Funnell M, Brown T, Childs B, et al. National standards for diabetes self-management education. Diabetes Care 2009;32: S87-S94.

34. U.S. Food and Drug Administration (2002). Insulin Preparations. Retrieved April 5, 2009, from http://www.fda.gov/fdac/features/2002/chrt_insulin.html

35. American Association of Diabetes Educators. AADE7 Self-care Behaviors. Retrieved April 9, 2009, from http://www.diabeteseducator.org/ProfessionalResources/AADE7/

36. Kitabchi A, Freire A, Umpierrez G. Evidence for strict inpatient blood glucose control: time to revise glycemia goals in hospitalized patients. Metab Clin Exp 2008;57:116-110.

37. Campbess K, Braithwaite. Hospital management of hyperglycemia. Clin Diabetes 2004;22:81-84.

38. Wexler D, Cagliero E. Inpatient diabetes management in non-ICU settings. Curr Diabetes Rev 2007;3:239-243.

39. John R, Fogelfeld L. Inpatient management of diabetes and hyperglycemia. Disease-a-Month. ;50(8):438-479. doi:10.1016. Retrieved August 11, 2011 from http://www.citeulike.org/user/iskanbasal/article/910828.

40. Texas Diabetes Council. IV insulin infusion protocol for critically-ill adult patients in the ICU setting. Publication number 45-11063. Revised October 25, 2007. Retrieved 8-15, 2009, from http://www.dshs.state.tx.us/diabetes/PDF/algorithms/iv%20insulin%20infusion.pdf

41. Baldwin K, Lyon B, Clark A, et al. Developing clinical nurse specialist practice competencies. Clin Nurse Specialist 2007;21:297-302.

42. Zuzelo P. Clinical Nurse Specialist Practice–Spheres Of Influence–Educaton. Retrieved May 22, 2009, from http://findarticles.com/p/articles/mi_m0FSL/is_2_77/ai_98134861/?tag=content;col1

43. Cooke L, Gemmill R, Grandt M. Advanced practice nurses core competencies: a frameowk for developing and testing an advanced practice nurse discharge intervention. Clin Nurse Specialist 2008;22:221-225.

44. Campbell-Fleming J, Catania K, Courtney L. Promoting evidence-based practice through a traveling journal club. Clin Nurse Specialist 2009;23:16-20.

45. Kelly P. The clinical nurse specialist and essential genomic competencies: Charting the course. Clin Nurse Specialist 2009;23:145-150.

46. Tringali C, Murphy T, Osevala M. Clinical nurse specialist practice in a care coordination model. Clin Nurse Specialist 2008;22:231-239.

47. Barton A. Knowledgement and the clinical nurse specialist. Clin Nurse Specialist 2009;23:113-114.

48. American Diabetes Association. Complications of diabetes in the United States. Retrieved April 9, 2009, from http://www.diabetes.org/diabetes-statistics/complications.jsp

49. Roelker E. Screening for coronary artery disease in patients with diabetes. Diabetes Spectrum 2008;21:161-171.

50. National Kidney Foundation Kidney Disease Outcomes Quality Initiative. Clinical Practice Guidelines for Chronic Kidney Disease: Evaluation, Classification, and Stratification. Retrieved March 30, 2009, from http://www.kidney.org/Professionals/Kdoqi/guidelines_ckd/p4_class_g1.htm

51. American Diabetes Association. Treatment of hypertension in adults with diabetes. Diabetes Care 2002;25:S71-S73.

52. Texas Diabetes Council. Publication number 45-11167. Hypertension Algorithm for Diabetes Mellitus in Adults. Retrieved April 11, 2009, from http://www.dshs.state.tx.us/diabetes/PDF/algorithms/HYPER.PDF

53. Texas Diabetes Council. Publication number 45-10777. Lipid Algorithm for Type 1 and Type 2 Diabetes Mellitus in Adults. Retrieved April 11, 2009, from http://www.dshs.state.tx.us/diabetes/PDF/algorithms/lipid.PDF

54. Solano M, Goldberg R. Lipid management in type 2 diabetes mellitus. Clin Diabetes 2006;24:27-32.

55. National Heart, Lung, and Blood Institute Expert Panel. Third report of the Expert Panel on Detection, Evaluation, and Treatment of High Blood Cholesterol in Adults (ATP III Final Report). Retrieved April 11, 2009, from http://www.nhlbi.nih.gov/guidelines/cholesterol/atp3_rpt.htm

56. Khera A, McLean B. The moving LDL target: getting your patients to goal. Best Practices in Primary Care Conference, Houston, TX, June 13-14, 2008.

57. Maldonado M, Chong E, Oehl M, et al. Economic impact of diabetic ketoacidosis in a multiethnic indigent population. Diabetes Care 2003;26:1165-1169.

58. Kotsanos J, McDonald R, Baron A, et al. DKA Costs Relative to Medical Costs of Patients with Type 1 Diabetes Mellitus. AHSR FHSR Annual Meeting Abstract Book, 1996, Indianapolis: Eli Lilly & Co. Retrieved April 13, 2009, from http://gateway.nlm.nih.gov/MeetingAbstracts/ma?f=102222250.html

59. Cryer P, Davis S, Shamoon H. Hypoglycemia in diabetes. Diabetes Care 2003;26:1902-1911.

60. Cryer P. Diverse causes of hypoglycemia-associated autonomic failure in diabetes. N Engl J. Med 2004;350:2272-2279.

61. Meszaros G. Crash Course: Endocrine and Reproductive Systems. Phildelphia: Mosby; 2006.

62. National Endocrine and Metabolism Disease Institute. NIH Publication No. 6-3425. Hyperparathyroidism. Retrieved April 30, 2009, from http://www.endocrine.niddk.nih.gov/pubs/hyper/hyper.htm

63. Henderson K, Baranski T, Bickel P. The Washington Manual Subspecialty Consult Series: Endocrinology Subspecialty Consult. Philadelphia: Lippincott Williams & Wilkins; 2005.

64. American Thyroid Association. Treatment Guidelines for Patients with Hyperthyroidism. Retrieved May 16, 2009, from http://hyper.thyroidguidelines.net/hyperthyroidism

65. BMJ Group. Hypoparathyroidism. Retrieved May 8, 2009, from https://online.epocrates.com/u/2923132/Hypoparathyroidism/Basics/Epidemiology

66. American Thyroid Association. Treatment Guidelines for Patients with Hypothyroidism. Retrieved May 16, 2009, from http://hyper.thyroidguidelines.net/hypothyroidism

67. AACE Task Force. American Association of Clinical Endocrinologists Medical Guidelines for Clinical Practice for the Evaluation and Treatment of Hyperthyroidism and Hypothyroidism. Retrieved May 16, 2009, from http://www.aace.com/pub/pdf/guidelines/hypo_hyper.pdf

68. Ceresini G, Lauretani F, Maggio M, et al. Thyroid function abnormalities and cognifive impairment in elderly people: results of the Invecchiare in Chianti Study. J Am Geriatr Soc 2009;57:89-93.

69. American Thyroid Association. American Thyroid Association Guidelines for Detection of Thyroid Disease: Screening for Thyroid Dysfunction. Retrieved May 16, 2009, from http://dysfunction.thyroidguidelines.net/screening

70. Holm E, Bie P, Ottesen M, et al. Diagnosis of syndrome of inappropriate secretion of antidiuretic hormone. South Med J 2009;102:380-384.

71. Verbalis J, Goldsmith S, Greenberg A, et al. Hyponatremia treatment guidelines 2007: expert panel recommendations. Am J Med 2007;110:S1-21.

72. Makaryus A, McFarlane S. Diabetes insipidus: Diagnosis and treatment of a complex disease. Cleve Clin J Med 2006;73:65-71.

CHAPTER 12

Gastrointestinal Problems

Stephen D. Krau, PhD, RN, CNE

INTRODUCTION

Some of the most seemingly benign gastrointestinal (GI) problems can rapidly turn into the most devastating issues for a patient and constitute some of the most challenging conditions for the bedside nurse and the clinical nurse specialist (CNS). In the early stages, many clinical manifestations of GI disorders are nonspecific and can be caused by a variety of pathologic processes (1). This adds to the challenge for the CNS.

To address the needs of the patient, the CNS will need to rely on advanced practice skills and knowledge of factors leading to GI problems. The CNS fosters optimal patient care through coordination of disciplines and activities that are patient focused, evidence-based, and designed to shape optimal outcomes for the patient. In order to achieve favorable outcomes, the CNS will need to utilize competencies among several domains. Clearly, the importance of direct care competency is essential in assessing the patient, differentiating a diagnosis, planning appropriate management, and evaluating the efficacy of the management plan. With the insidious nature of many GI problems, assessment skills are crucial to an overall effective outcome. Competencies related to collaboration, leadership, and consultation clearly play a vital role; however, knowing when and how to evoke these competencies appropriately are largely contingent upon the data obtained through direct care.

IRRITABLE BOWEL SYNDROME

Irritable bowel syndrome (IBS) is a chronic condition that has gained considerable attention in the health care milieu in the past two decades due to its increasing prevalence, potentially debilitating effects, and varied symptom presentation (1). IBS belongs to a broader classification of GI diseases referred to as functional bowel disorders (FBDs) as classified by the Rome Foundation, an international organization dedicated to research and education in the field of GI disorders (1, 2). Additionally, the World Health Organization (WHO) has given IBS its own classification as indicated in the *International Classification of Diseases: 10th Edition (ICD-10)*, which validates the significance of the syndrome.

The American College of Gastroenterology (ACG) defines IBS as abdominal discomfort associated with altered bowel habits (3). The disorder is characterized by alterations in serotonin signaling and alterations in the enteric nervous system, which lead to abnormalities in the motility of GI smooth muscle and visceral hypersensitivity. Patients with IBS will present with a myriad of symptoms that might include diarrhea, constipation, straining, sense of incomplete evacuation, bloating, or even fecal urgency. There have been attempts to classify IBS by bowel patterns such as diarrhea predominant or constipation predominant, but, these subgroupings have not been clinically validated.

Etiology

Potential risk factors for IBS include genetics, psychological or psychiatric causes, GI infections, and medications, including antibiotics or estrogens (4, 5). Although the symptoms are bothersome, only about 30% of patients with IBS seek medical attention, with most of them being managed in a primary care setting (6). The syndrome transcends cultural and geographic boundaries but is most prevalent in Western populations and occurs primarily in women. The prevalence in Western general populations ranges from 10% to 26% (7). Age-related onset of IBS occurs in patients younger than 45 years but then the prevalence increases again in the elderly (1). The most common psychiatric disorders associated with IBS are depression and anxiety (1). Many patients diagnosed with IBS meet the criteria for at least one primary psychiatric disorder (8).

There are other factors that are being considered as contributing to the incidence of IBS, including diverticular disease, ingestion of coffee or other stimulants, smoking, and certain medications, including nonsteroidal anti-inflammatory drugs (NSAIDs). Additionally, dietary factors are being considered such as dietary fat intake, sulfur intake, and milk allergies (9).

Pathophysiology

The precise pathophysiology of IBS is still unclear; however, there are some physiologic factors that are known to contribute to the development of this chronic disease process that involve the neurotransmitter serotonin. The limbic system, along with the paralimbic structures, connects the gut bidirectionally with the central nervous system through the autonomic nervous system. This allows the transmission of emotional states from the central nervous system to the gut and the perception of GI changes, such as bloating, pain, and cramping to the central nervous system (1). The release of the neurotransmitters serotonin and acetylcholine as part of the enteric nervous system is independent of the connections from the central nervous system (10). The main neurotransmitter that regulates GI motility is serotonin (5-HT), which is released from cells in the GI mucosa to stimulate acetylcholine release, which stimulates GI motility (1). There are variant serotonin receptors involved in the enteric nervous system transmission, primarily 5-HT$_3$ and 5-HT$_4$, each with specific signaling patterns. Serotonin signaling is interrupted by a specific serotonin transporter (SERT) located on the enterocytes within the intestinal mucosa. There is evidence to support that a decrease in SERT consistently leads to dysfunction in humans through increased serotonin levels (11). As a result, serotonin receptors constantly stimulate the receptors, leading to dysregulated dilations and contractions of the GI tract (1). This aberrant signaling is responsible for the symptoms and clinical presentation of persons with IBS.

Diagnosis and Clinical Presentation

The clinical symptoms of IBS provide the diagnostic criteria for IBS and distinguish IBS from other GI disorders. In general, IBS is identified as a functional disorder of the GI tract associated with abdominal pain and altered bowel activity in the absence of pathologic organic changes. IBS does not cause inflammatory effects that could be identified with laboratory testing of the blood or feces or visualization of damage to the GI tract through imaging.

The diagnosis of IBS is based on symptom presentation and thorough evaluation to eliminate other disease conditions. Symptoms that predominate in IBS include unspecific abdominal pain or discomfort, frequent or infrequent or alternating patterns of bowel movements, alleviation of pain and discomfort with defecation, and onset of symptoms with changes in stool frequency and appearance. These are the symptoms that are used to make a differential diagnosis of IBS in conjunction with the Rome II and Rome III criteria. The most common

symptom associated with IBS is pain in the left lower quadrant (LLQ) of the abdomen (12).

The two dominate subtypes of IBS include diarrhea (IBS-D) and constipation (IBS-C). There is a mixed subtype (IBS-M) that occurs less frequently (1). Regardless of the type, there is a slow onset of IBS over weeks and months and a strong correlation with stress disorders, especially depression and anxiety. IBS that is associated with an infection is classified as postinfectious IBS (PI-IBS). As opposed to other forms of IBS, patients with PI-IBS can present with altered GI immune function in the form of increased lymphocytes and inducible nitric oxide synthase in the feces (1).

Management

IBS management is contingent on the symptoms that are presented and accompanying conditions such as lifestyle, diet, and stress disorders. Management and treatment goals are centered on normalizing GI motility, regardless of the classification of IBS. Before pharmacologic treatment is considered, lifestyle issues and diet indices should be evaluated as potential triggers for IBS. An overview of considerations is presented in Table 12-1.

The pharmacologic management of IBS is complex and based on the presenting symptoms of the patient. Each medication can be used as a single entity, may be used in conjunction with other medications, and may be used in conjunction with nonpharmacologic interventions. These medications follow predominant symptom presentation and are related to symptom management, as opposed to causative treatment. Table 12-2 provides an overview of commonly used medications in the management of IBS.

Clinical Nurse Specialist Competencies and Spheres of Influence
Clinical Expert/Direct Care

Assessing and evaluating outcomes related to patients with IBS have strong implications for direct patient care. Because of the nebulous nature of IBS, and the fact that IBS warrants a functional diagnosis, it is extremely important to attain a thorough yet focused history and physical exam. The clinician must be attuned to even the subtlest cues as the patients share information related to their diet, lifestyle, and use of medications. Many of the symptoms of IBS are associated with pathologic processes that have variable and potentially devastating complications such as Crohn's sisease, ulcerative colitis, or malignancy.

Coaching/Teaching/Mentoring

The clinician must be astute to the impact of IBS on the patient, family, and the overall context in which the patient and family live. The clinician must know what treatment options are available, and which will work best for this patient. The clinician must be able to evaluate the response to options that are initiated to know

TABLE 12–1 Nonpharmacologic Treatment and Management of Irritable Bowel Syndrome (IBS)

Dietary Suggestions	Avoid specific foods that might be triggers to symptomatic IBS. Typically, these foods include alcohol, eggs, nuts, foods with caffeine, wheat products, and beverages with sorbital or fructose. If lactose intolerance is an issue, milk products should be avoided, but calcium supplements might be warranted. Large meals might be cramping. Patients with IBS or suspect IBS should eat smaller, more frequent meals. Meals should be eaten slowly to avoid swallowing air, which also causes abdominal pain. Adequate hydration is essential for persons with IBS-D to prevent dehydration. Hydration is also important for patients with IBS-C as this might lead to softer stools and alleviate symptoms. Drinking carbonated beverages increases pain and distention. Probiotics have shown to modestly improve bloating. No specific probiotic strain appears to be superior to another. Altering fiber contents in the diet is controversial and, if done, should be done gradually. Insoluble fiber is effective in increasing stool size and bulk. Soluble fibers form a gelatin-like substance in the bowel and increase water content. The type of fiber consumed should be guided by the symptoms the patient presents.
Psychotherapy	Psychotherapeutic interventions are usually reserved for persons with severe forms of IBS that accompany a psychological disorder or when a known comorbidity of anxiety or depression exists. Recent studies show that hypnotherapy and stress management have a high rate of success.
Acupuncture	Studies indicate that the effect of acupuncture on IBS is variable and at this time inconclusive.

TABLE 12–2 Pharmacologic Treatment of IBS Based on Symptoms

Symptom Target for the Medication	Medication and Dose	Considerations
ANTISPASMODICS (ANTICHOLINERGIC AGENTS)		
	Dicyclomine 10–20 mg PO tid Hyoscyamine 0.125 mg PO or SL prn or qid (sustained release) 0.037 mg or 0.75 mg PO bid	These medications are commonly used despite lack of evidence of good efficacy
ANTIDIARRHEAL AGENTS		
	Loperamide 2 mg PO tid–qid (this medication is an upload) Diphenoxylate with atropine 2.5 mg PO qid (this medication is an opioid agonist)	Hydration is always a consideration when the patient presents with diarrhea
FIBER SUPPLEMENTS		
	Bran, psyllium, methycellulose, or polycarbophil	May cause increased bleeding It is also essential that no gastrointestinal strictures are present Take with full glass of water.

Continued

TABLE 12–2 Pharmacologic Treatment of IBS Based on Symptoms—cont'd

Symptom Target for the Medication	Medication and Dose	Considerations
OSMOTIC LAXATIVES		
	Milk of Magnesia Polyethylene glycol	Milk of Magnesia is rarely prescribed as there are other osmotic laxatives with less risk Polyethylene glycol has fewer side effects than most osmotic laxatives
TRICYCLIC ANTIDEPRESSANTS		
	Nortriptyline, desipramine, imipramine, or trazodone Begin at 10 mg at bedtime. Increase gradually 25–50 mg at bedtime as tolerated	Not recommended for predominant constipation IBS
SELECTIVE SEROTONIN REUPTAKE INHIBITORS		
	Sertraline 50–150 mg PO daily Fluoxetine 20–40 mg PO daily	Not recommended for patients who present with predominant diarrhea
DRUGS USED WHEN PATIENT DOES NOT RESPOND TO CONVENTIONAL THERAPIES		
	Tegaserod 6 mg PO bid Alosetron 0.5-3 mg PO bid	For constipation as predominant symptom (IBS-C) For diarrhea as predominant symptom (IBS-D) Use judiciously as this drug interacts with many over-the-counter drugs and herbal supplements
NOT YET APPROVED, UNDER STUDY		
	Muscarinic receptor antagonists (darifenacin, zamifenacin)	Some have been FDA approved for overactive bladder, but not yet for IBS treatment.

when more rigorous intervention is warranted or when to test further for other underlying causes.

Consultation

Consultation competencies are also important to achieve optimal outcomes for patients with IBS. In situations where dietary modifications are justified, consultation to a dietician would provide expertise necessary for the patient. In cases of severe IBS associated with psychological issues, as IBS strongly correlates with depression and anxiety, an advanced psychiatric mental health CNS or nurse practitioner, a psychologist, or a psychiatrist

might provide the appropriate intervention for this patient.

APPENDICITIS

Etiology

Appendicitis is an acute inflammation of the vermiform appendix and is one of the most common causes of abdominal pain in patients who come to emergency departments. Appendicitis is the leading cause of litigation related to abdominal pain in emergency centers and one of the overall leading causes of litigation (13). More than 250,000 cases of appendicitis are diagnosed in the United States each year, and an appendectomy is the most common emergent surgery performed worldwide (13). The incidence of appendicitis varies from 12% to 28%, and although it is more prevalent in persons in their second or third decade of life, it can occur at any age. The prevalence is slightly higher in men (8.6%) than in women (6.7%) (13). The mortality associated with appendicitis is low (1%) if the appendix is not ruptured, but in cases of rupture the mortality is closer to 3%. Because diagnosing appendicitis is more difficult in the elderly, the chance of mortality increases among the elderly to 15% (14).

Pathophysiology

The typical process in the development of acute appendicitis is usually the result of an obstruction in the lumen of the appendix. With the advent of an obstruction, inflammation of the appendix occurs, which leads to infection as bacteria invade appendix wall. The cause of the obstruction varies with age. In children, lymphoid hyperplasia, which can be exacerbated by infection and dehydration, is thought to be the primary cause (13). In adults, fecaliths, gallstones, or foreign materials as well as twisting and spasm can be a common cause. Once the appendix becomes inflamed, through the inflammation process, fluids build up and microorganisms proliferate. As this process continues, the appendix begins to swell. Purulent exudates form and the circulation in the appendix diminishes as the appendix becomes ischemic and necrosis begins. With this process, the capillary permeability of the appendix increases, allowing bacteria and toxins to escape the cell wall and leak into the surrounding area. The leaking bacteria contribute to the formation of abscesses or peritonitis in the immediate area. As the wall of the appendix weakens, it is susceptible to perforation or rupture, allowing contents of the appendix to enter the peritoneal cavity and leading to the life-threatening condition of peritonitis. Although the risk of perforation occurs during the first 24 hours of developing appendicitis, the risk rises rapidly after 48 hours. Elderly persons are more prone to perforations, due to the aging of tissues and the fact that presenting symptoms of appendicitis are less pronounced in the elderly than they are in younger patients. The subtly of symptoms can lead to delayed intervention and increase the mortality rate of peritonitis due to appendicitis (15).

Clinical Presentation

No singular sign or symptom is reliable to confirm or deny the diagnosis of appendicitis. The nebulous presentation of appendicitis contributes to the incidence of misdiagnosis and subsequent legal issues. In many cases, the patient presents with symptoms of right lower quadrant (RLQ) pain and tenderness. As the anatomical location of the appendix varies to some degree from person to person, the precise location of pain and tenderness is difficult to conclusively identify. The pain is often accompanied by nausea, vomiting, and anorexia. When the appendix ruptures, the pain subsides temporarily, then as peritonitis develops, pain increases steadily. With the onset of peritonitis, the patient presents with a rigid abdomen, tachycardia, and hypotension. Additionally, low-grade fever and leukocytosis with a shift to the left provide compelling evidence for the need of prompt surgical intervention.

Diagnosis

The variant symptom profile in patients with appendicitis makes it difficult to diagnose. There are no symptoms or laboratory tests available to conclusively deny or confirm appendicitis. The clinician must be acutely aware of the cumulative features of the patient's history and physical exam to determine the relative probability that the patient is experiencing appendicitis. The physical signs of rigidity, RLQ tenderness, the psoas sign, and rebound tenderness of the abdomen contribute to a high likelihood that appendicitis is present (13).

Along with blood profiles demonstrating leukocytosis, computed tomography (CT) is recommended as a tool to diagnosis appendicitis in adults (16). CT is suggested for patients in whom the risks associated with the procedure and radiation exposure are low. In cases where CT is too risky, ultrasound is recommended.

There are scoring scales that have been developed to increase the accuracy of appendicitis diagnosis. These scales attach weighted value to specific signs, symptoms, and laboratory results. The most widely used tool is the Alvarado Score, known also as the MANTRELS (Migration of pain, Anorexia, Nausea/vomiting, Tenderness in the RLQ, Rebound tenderness, Elevated temperature, Leukocytosis, Shift to the left) (17). Another scale available is the Ohmann scoring system, which uses a variety of signs and symptoms to predict appendicitis in adults and children over the age of 6 years (18). The scoring systems help the clinician decide on the future management to include observation alone, imaging, or whether immediate surgical intervention is indicated (13, 19).

In the past 10 years, imaging has had increasing utility in the diagnosis of suspected appendicitis. CT has a greater accuracy than ultrasound, as plain abdominal radiographs are rarely used now for the diagnosis of appendicitis (13). Findings from a CT scan indicative of appendicitis include an appendix greater than 6 mm, thickening of the appendix wall, RLQ inflammatory changes such as fat stranding, and the presence of appendicoliths (20).

Management

Monitoring the patient with acute appendicitis is a mainstay of management. In the event of a ruptured appendix, the surgical timing becomes paramount. Nonsurgical management of the patient with appendicitis is presented in Table 12-3.

TABLE 12–3 Nonsurgical Management of Appendicitis

Management Intervention	Rationale
Prepare the patient for potential emergency surgery.	Throughout nonsurgical management of the patient, the clinician must keep in mind that indications for emergency surgery can occur at any point. The patient should be physically and emotionally prepared for emergent surgery.
Patient should be kept NPO.	This decreases the probability of aspiration should emergent surgery be necessary.
Patient should receive intravenous fluids.	Prevents dehydration due to nausea, vomiting, anorexia, and NPO status
Keep patient in semi-Fowler's position.	This keeps abdominal drainage in the lower right abdomen.
Antibiotics should be administered.	Antibiotics used for wound prophylaxis are initiated preoperatively and often not continued when the patient has an uncomplicated postsurgical course.
	If the appendix perforates preoperatively, broad-spectrum antibiotics should be initiated and continued post surgery.
Avoid the use of laxatives or enemas.	Laxatives and enemas can cause perforation of an inflamed appendix.
Never apply heat to the area.	Heat causes the circulation to the area to increase, which can result in increased inflammation and perforation.

Surgical Management

Appendectomy is typically achieved by one of two methods. Most uncomplicated appendectomies are performed via laparoscopy. A laparoscopy is also sometimes used to rule out appendicitis and is a procedure where several small incisions are made near the umbilicus through which an endoscope is placed. A laparotomy is an open approach with a much larger abdominal incision, which is the typical method of choice for appendicitis that is atypical or complicated or for appendicitis associated with peritonitis. The care of the patient postsurgically is similar to that of any patient who has undergone surgery under general anesthesia.

Clinical Nurse Specialist Competencies and Spheres of Influence
Clinical Expert/Direct Care and Consultation

A thorough history and initial assessment of the patient with appendicitis will provide evidence for further diagnosis and etiology. Key findings on assessment along with laboratory data will assist in ensuring the patient is quickly and safely treated before the situation worsens. As litigation related to appendicitis is a prominent risk, prompt and safe action from the CNS and the nursing staff for consultation with a surgeon are essential. Additionally, clinicians must keep in mind that the patient's condition can deteriorate at any time and should keep the patient and family prepared for surgery. As the coordinator of care, it is important to assemble the surgical team when necessary.

CHOLECYSTITIS

Cholecystitis in its varied forms is one of the most prevalent causes of surgical intervention in industrialized countries. The most common cause of cholecystitis is the formation of gallstones, or cholelithiasis. Inflammation as the result of stones is referred to as cholecystitis. When the stones migrate to the common bile duct, the condition results in choledocholithiasis. Autopsy results indicate that approximately 11% to 35% of American adults have gallstones, while 1% to 2% of people with cholelithiasis experience symptoms and complications (20). About 2% to 15% of acute cholecystitis cases occur as the result of something other than stone formation.

Etiology

Gallstones arise from the precipitation of cholesterol and calcium salts in supersaturated bile. Additionally, it is theorized that a crystallization process contributes to the formation of the stones. The stones are classified based on their content as cholesterol stones or pigmented stones. The pigmented stones are typically brown or black. The brown gallstones that are more commonly found in Asian populations are associated with disorders of biliary motility and bacterial infection. Black gallstones, typically consisting of calcium and unconjugated bilirubin, are small and tarry and commonly associated with cirrhosis and hemolytic disorders including sickle cell anemia and spherocytosis (20).

The prevalence of gallstones varies widely around the world and among different ethnic groups. In the United States, the incidence of gallstone formation is higher among Caucasians, Native Americans, and Hispanics than among African Americans. The average age for a person developing gallstones ranges from about 40 years to 80 years, and as the individual ages, there is greater risk for the development of gallstones. A familial or genetic tendency has a role in the development of cholelithiasis, but this may be due to family nutrition or lifestyle habits as opposed to actual chromosomal similarity. Women are three times more likely than men to develop gallstones, and women who are multiparous, are taking estrogen therapy, or use oral contraceptives are at increased risk of developing gallstones (21-23). Oral contraceptives, estrogens, and cofibrate are all known to increase biliary cholesterol saturation.

Although the incidence of cholecystitis is higher in women than in men, the severity of acute cholecystitis is higher in men (24). Additionally, the incidence of gallstone formation is more prevalent among obese persons, persons who lose weight rapidly, persons with hypercholesterolemia, or persons taking antilipid medications. Cholelithiasis is often seen in other disease states that affect metabolic function, such as diabetes, regional enteritis, and various blood dyscrasias. There is early evidence that indicates that exercise might ameliorate the incidence of gallstones. Additionally, the consumption of coffee is thought to decrease gallstone formation. Coffee consumption triggers the release of cholecystokinin, which promotes gallbladder emptying, a mechanism that is thought to prevent the incidence of gallstone formation. To date, it is unclear whether it is the caffeine in coffee that exerts this effect or some other ingredient in the coffee.

Other causes of obstructive cholecystitis, not necessarily associated with the formation of gallstones, include primary tumors of the gallbladder or common bile duct, gallbladder polyps, parasites, metastatic tumors to the gallbladder or to the periportal lymph nodes, or foreign objects such as bullets (21, 25, 26). In these cases, the obstruction is not directly related to the formation of gallstones, but the effect of the obstruction in the bile duct is similar in presentation and pathophysiology to that of gallstones.

Pathophysiology

Regardless of the presenting factors, prolonged obstruction of the gallbladder outlet leads to cholecystitis. The formation of gallstones is usually the result of a disruption among the balance of bile salts, lecithin, and cholesterol. With this disruption, cholesterol has a tendency to precipitate. The process is further complicated by the production of mucin glycoprotein, which traps cholesterol particles (23). Supersaturation of the bile with cholesterol also inhibits gallbladder motility and contributes to stasis. As the gallbladder concentrates the bile, supersaturation of stone components along with stasis further worsens the process (27).

Obstruction of the gallbladder neck leads to increased intraluminal pressure, which results in venous congestion, compromised perfusion, and impaired lymphatic drainage. The mucosa becomes ischemic and releases mediators of inflammation particularly prostaglandins I_2 and E_2 (21). Localized trauma causes the release of phospholipase, which converts lecithin, and usually protects the mucosa against bile salts, to lysolecithin. Unlike lecithin, lysolecithin is a detergent and exerts a toxic effect to the mucosa of the gallbladder. This results in wall thickening, edema, further vascular congestion, and intramural hemorrhage.

Clinical Presentation

Typically, an acute attack is the result of a large fatty meal. The patient will identify a relatively sudden, severe, and continual pain in the epigastric area that might dissipate some over 12 to 18 hours. In about 75% of patients with acute cholecystitis, vomiting occurs, which affords variable relief in about 50% of these patients (28). Additionally, patients often present with a low- to moderate-grade fever and accompanying tachycardia. Up to 15% to 25% of patients have a palpable distended gallbladder (21, 28). The classic Murphy sign, the abrupt inhibition of inspiration concurrent with palpation directly over the gallbladder fossa, is common. In the presence of abdominal wall guarding or rigidity, the clinician must consider the possibility of gangrenous cholecystitis or perforation (21). Flatulence, eructation, and dyspepsia are commonly seen in patients experiencing cholecystitis.

Jaundice occurs in about 25% of these cases and most commonly among persons with chronic cholecystitis. When the jaundice is persistent or severe, there is a strong possibility there is an underlying choledocholithiasis, or it may be the result of a compressed common bile duct or hepatic duct by a cystic duct that is inflamed due to the presence of a stone (28).

Diagnosis

Laboratory values are generally nonspecific for diagnosing cholecystitis. In the differential diagnosis, one must rule out disease processes with similar symptoms of cholecystitis such as pancreatitis or peptic ulcer disease. In many cases, a mild to pronounced leukocytosis is evident with a left shift. Bilirubin, alkaline phosphatase, aspartate amino-transferase (AST), and lactate dehydrogenase (LDH) may be elevated. If there is pancreatic involvement, the serum amylase and lipase levels are elevated. A total bilirubin level greater than 3 mg/dL should raise concerns for choledocholithiasis. (21).

Plain films of the abdomen are of minimal value in diagnosing cholecystitis and show radiopaque gallstones in about 15% of the cases (28). Ultrasound of the right upper abdomen is sensitive and specific for the diagnosis of acute calculus cholecystitis, with the identification of stones, or sludge, and wall thickening (>4 mm), or the presence of pericholecystic fluid (21). The size of the common bile duct is also an important consideration in the diagnosis of cholecystitis. Although the size of the bile duct increases with age, a bile duct with a diameter greater than 8 mm could be the result of a common bile duct obstruction. CT scan of the abdomen may reveal many of the features of cholecystitis, but it is much less sensitive, more expensive, and more time consuming than ultrasound (21).

Currently, the HIDA scan (^{99m}Tc-HIDA cholescintig-raphy) is considered the most accurate test for cholecysti-tis, with a sensitivity of 97% and specificity of 87% (29). This scan allows for visualization of the gallbladder in about 30 minutes, and the absence of the radiotracer uptake for 4 hours is indicative of cystic duct occlusion. With ultrasound being about 67% sensitive and 82% spe-cific, most clinicians will reserve the use of the HIDA scan for situations where there is diagnostic ambiguity (29).

Management

Treatment of acute calculus cholecystitis usually consists of intravenous fluid resuscitation, refraining from oral intake, analgesia, and antibiotic therapy. The role of antibi-otics in uncomplicated acute cholescystitis has not been completely determined when surgical intervention can be done in a timely fashion (29). When it is difficult to deter-mine if secondary bacterial infection is evolving or whether the cholecystitis has progressed to gangrene or perforation, the use of broad-spectrum antibiotic coverage is warranted. Commonly used regimens include ampicillin-sulbactam, piperacillin-tazobactam, ampicillin with gentamicin, a third- or fourth-generation cephalosporin, or a third-generation fluroquinolone, such as moxifloxacin (21). Cefoperazone, a third-generation cephalosporin is often prescribed and given at 1 to 2 g every 12 hours intravenous-ly (28). Controversy ensues over the best analgesics for use in these patients. Meperidine may be preferable to mor-phine for analgesia as it causes less activity of the sphincter of Oddi in the duodenum where pancreatic and bile ducts enter (28). However, it is known that meperidine breaks down into a toxic metabolite (normeperidine) that has con-vulsive properties. All opioids have the potential to cause some degree of sphincter spasm (30).

Anticholinergic drugs are sometimes given to relax smooth muscles and decrease ductal tone and subsequent spasm. Anticholinergic medications such as dicyclomine (Bentyl, Biclomine, Dibent, Di-Spaz, Lomine) should be avoided for use in the elderly. These medications com-monly result in constipation, dry mouth, confusion, blurred vision, and urinary retention. Ketorolac (Toradol, Acular) is an NSAID that alleviates discomfort and should be used in older adults. Antiemetics might be necessary to control nausea and vomiting.

Nonsurgical Treatment

One method used to remove gallstones involves dissolving gallstones through the infusion of a solvent such as mono-octanoin, or methyl tertiary butyl ether (MTBE). There are a variety of methods by which the solvent is introduced into the gallbladder. Other nonsurgical methods of remov-ing gallstones include stone removal by instrumentation and lithotripsy. There are two main methods of removal by instrumentation: inserting a catheter and instrument with a basket-like device into a T-tube or fistula formed at the time of T-tube insertion. The basket apparatus is used pri-marily for stones that were not removed during the time of a cholecystectomy or have become lodged in the common bile duct, and it retrieves and removes the stones lodged in the common bile duct.

Lithotripsy can be performed via either intracorpore-al or extracorporeal methods with the use of shock waves. The intracorporeal lithotripsy involves using a probe that delivers electrical sparks in rapid pulses, which create an expansion of the liquid environment surrounding the gallstones. This results in pressure waves that cause the stones to fragment (31). Extracorporeal lithotripsy is a procedure in which shock waves are transmitted through the patient's body to the proposed site of the stones. The waves are transmitted either through fluid-filled bags placed on the patient's body or by immersing the patient into water. The procedure often requires numerous visits and several sessions and has been largely replaced by the laparoscopic cholecystectomy.

Surgical Treatment

Laparoscopic cholecystectomy is currently the definitive management for acute calculous cholecystitis and per-formed far more often than the traditional open approach. This procedure is considered a minimally invasive surgery, and the advantages of this procedure are numerous. Complications of laparoscopic cholecystectomy are uncom-mon; the death rate is very low, bile duct injuries are rare, pain is less severe, the patient is unlikely to experience paralytic ileus, and patient recovery is quicker (32). Approximately 500,000 patients in the United States require surgery each year for gallbladder removal and 80% to 90% are candidates for laparoscopic cholecystectomy (33).

The procedure is commonly done on an ambulatory care basis in a same-day surgery setting with the patient under general anesthesia. During the procedure, the surgeon makes a small midline puncture at the umbilicus. In some cases, additional small incisions are needed. The incisions provide openings for about 3 to 4 liters of carbon dioxide to be insufflated into the abdominal cavity to allow visualization and introduction of instruments into the area. More recently, the use of abdominal wall–lifting devices have become more popular and result in improved pulmonary and cardiac function. Once prepared, a trocar catheter is introduced into the abdomen, followed by a laparoscope. The laparoscope is attached to a video camera, which allows the abdominal organs to be viewed on monitor. Once located, the gallbladder is dissected from the liver bed and the cystic artery, and the duct is closed. At this point, bile is aspirated and any large stones are crushed, followed by extraction of the gallbladder through the umbilical opening.

There are multiple advantages to the laparoscopy approach: the procedure takes about 90 minutes but is more expensive than the traditional cholecystectomy. However, the shorter hospital stay for patients undergoing laparoscopic cholecystectomy offsets the higher costs. The postoperative sequelae are often more benign and is commonly manifested by mild shoulder pain, which are the result of nerve irritation from distention of the carbon dioxide gas that was introduced. The discomfort is alleviated in most patients with mild analgesics.

Traditional Cholecystectomy

In selected patients with comorbid factors or a more tenuous prognosis due to inflammation, the traditional or open cholecystectomy is performed. In this procedure, the gallbladder is removed through an abdominal incision once the cystic duct and artery are ligated. In some patients, a drain is placed proximal to the gallbladder bed and brought through to the body surface if there is a bile leak. Use of a T-tube inserted into the common bile duct during this procedure was once common but is now used primarily for situations where a complication ensues.

In about 5% to 10% who begin their cholecystectomy via a laparoscopic procedure, the decision is made to convert to an open cholecystectomy (34, 35). Conversion may occur as the result of indefinable anatomy or of poorly progressing laparoscopic surgery or if complications are encountered. Postoperative care of the patient who has undergone an open cholecystectomy is similar to the care of any patient who has undergone abdominal surgery.

Clinical Nurse Specialist Competencies and Spheres of Influence
Coaching/Teaching/Mentoring and Systems Leadership

The need for expert assessment skills in determining subtle patient changes in evolving cholecystitis is clearly evident. The CNS is pivotal in educating staff nurses about the pathophysiology of cholelithiasis and the nonsurgical management of patients with cholecystitis. It is through this teaching that changes in the patient might be identified, at which time surgical intervention is warranted. CNSs are in key positions to lead evidence-based protocols and to assure positive outcomes for patients with cholecystitis.

DIVERTICULAR DISEASE

Diverticula are pouchlike herniations of the mucosa through the muscular wall most commonly found in the colon. The term "diverticulosis" denotes the presence of many pouchlike herniations, or diverticula, and the term "diverticulitis" indicates an inflammation in one or more of the diverticula. Colonic diverticulosis is mainly an asymptomatic disease of Western countries.

Etiology

In 95% of cases, diverticula are located in the sigmoid and left colon (36). Right-sided colonic diverticula are rare in Western countries, but with increasing age there is a propensity for diverticula to not only increase in quantity but also develop more proximally in the colon. Asian countries demonstrate populations with predominance for right-sided colon diverticula, indicating a genetic predilection for diverticula as well. Most diverticula are acquired and associated with increasing age. Less than 2% of patients 30 years of age or younger have diverticulosis, whereas more than 40% of persons over the age of 60 have diverticula. The incidence increases further with age, as 60% of patients who reach 80 years have acquired diverticula (36). Early findings suggested diverticular disease might be more common in men than in women, but more recent findings indicate that the reverse is true (37). Diverticulosis is more prevalent in societies where low-fiber/high-fat diets are consumed; however, the exact cause of diverticulosis is not known. Diverticulitis occurs in about 10% to 20% of the population with diverticulosis and occurs when food and bacteria become trapped in the diverticula and become inflamed or infected (38). This can result in impaired drainage, perforation, or abscess formation. Not only has the etiology of diverticulitis become more complex than previously understood, but the treatment guidelines have also evolved. Less invasive procedures have taken the forefront in the management of the disease, where once surgical dogma guided treatment options (39).

Pathophysiology

The precise pathophysiologic processes that lead to the development of diverticula is disputed. However, a variety of anatomical factors that may work in conjunction with increased intraluminal pressures and motility changes within the colon are thought to contribute to the development of diverticula. The anatomy of the structure of the colon in humans predisposes to the formation of diverticula as the colon is surrounded by only one layer of muscle coat, which is a circular layer. This is unlike the small intestine and rectum, which are surrounded by two sheaths of smooth muscle in the muscularis propria, an inner circular and outer longitudinal layer. The blood vessels from the mesentery that supply the mucosa and submucosa of the colon run from the mesentery to either side of the bowel wall and penetrate the circular muscle. Where this occurs, the colon wall is weakest, and mucosal herniations can occur through these vascular portals (40). Diverticula typically 5 to 10 mm in diameter form in two to four parallel rows and vary in number from 1 or 2 to up to 100 in more severe cases (40).

Another anatomical difference found in patients with diverticula relates to the thickness of the colon and the fact that collagen cross-linking increases as humans age. Whereas it was once thought that the wall of the colon became thickened due to hypertrophy, studies have shown that there is no evidence that hypertrophy or hyperplasia occurs in the colon (36, 40). The thickening of the muscle is now attributed to an increased deposit of elastin, which results in highly contractile muscle and increased luminal colon pressures. Aging has been associated with collagen cross-linking, making the colon more rigid with a loss of compliance needed to accommodate increased luminal pressures. This is exacerbated by straining, increased constipation, and low colonic volume (fiber-deficient contents).

Most patients with diverticulosis will remain asymptomatic throughout their lifetime until diverticulitis develops. Diverticulitis is the most common cause of the symptoms that affect about 10% to 25% of persons with diverticula and bring them into the health care system for treatment. Diverticulitis occurs when the neck of the diverticulum becomes obstructed due to the presence of trapped fecal matter. This results in accumulated mucus secretion, bacterial overgrowth, and diminished blood supply, which culminate in local infection. Bleeding and hemorrhage are common complications of diverticular disease when ulceration is mild. As the condition worsens, there can be erosion of the vasa recta close to the diverticula that can lead to hemorrhage. Diverticulitis may lead to abscesses, serositis, adhesions, strictures, and obstructions. Inflamed diverticula can also perforate the lining of the colon and cause peritonitis. In some cases, the localized inflammation can spread systemically, resulting in bacteremia or sepsis (40).

Diverticulitis can usually be differentiated as complicated or uncomplicated. Complicated diverticular disease is commonly identified when an abscess, fistula, or obstruction exists or when localized perforations occur, which is usually an indication for surgical intervention. Uncomplicated diverticulitis presents with evidence of wall thickening or pericolonic inflammatory changes such as fat stranding (41).

Clinical Presentation

The patient with diverticulosis is typically asymptomatic, and in many cases, unless there is pain or bleeding, the condition goes undiagnosed. In mild cases, the patient may report intermittent periods of diarrhea, bloating or abdominal distention, nausea, or anorexia. Occasionally, there may be some slight tenderness identified when the abdomen is palpated; frequently chronic constipation precedes the development of diverticulosis.

The patient with diverticulitis often presents with abdominal pain, particularly localized to the LLQ, that is intermittent and over time becomes more constant. In some cases, the pain may be just above the pubic bone and occur on just one side. When there is generalized abdominal pain, the clinician should suspect the possibility of peritonitis. Nausea, and vomiting can occur, as does a fever that may range from low grade to 101°F (38.3°C) (32). On physical exam, a tender mass in the LLQ is the most common finding. Patients with severe diverticulitis may present with hypotension and other signs of peritonitis on physical exam (42).

Diagnosis

The diagnosis of diverticulitis begins with a thorough history and physical exam. The clinician should have the patient try to characterize any pain that he or she is experiencing, or has experienced, in order to determine any possible complications of the disease. Differential diagnosis for lower abdominal pain that should be considered include appendicitis, urinary tract infection, IBS, nephrolithiasis, gynecologic problems, infectious or ischemic colitis, inflammatory bowel disease, and the presence of malignancies (36).

Laboratory evaluation should include a complete blood cell count with a differential analysis and a urinalysis. The blood work usually reveals a leukocytosis with a left shift. Even in the presence of insidious bleeding, decreased hematocrit and hemoglobin are common; stool should be tested for possible bleeding. Urinalysis may reveal a few red blood cells if the ureter is near a perforated diverticulum.

Radiologic Studies

Radiologic imaging for diverticulitis is necessary for the diagnosis of diverticulitis as well as determining the severity of the diverticulitis and the presence of complications. Various radiologic options for the evaluation of the colon include barium or water-soluble enemas, CT scan, endoscopic procedures, ultrasound, and magnetic resonance colonography (MRC). An overview of the studies along with the advantages and disadvantages is found in Table 12-4.

TABLE 12-4 Overview of Radiologic Studies in the Diagnosis of Diverticulitis

Type of Test	Considerations	Advantages	Disadvantages
COLONIC CONTRAST STUDIES			
	Water-soluble enema contrast study should be a low-pressure single-contrast study. If the contrast material is visualized outside of the colon, or into a fistula, there is strong indication of diverticulitis. Barium is contraindicated if there is a suspicion of localized peritonitis, or pericolic abscess. Barium that extravasates in the abdomen via an opening in the colon is extremely toxic.	Water-soluble enema and barium enema can confirm the diagnosis of diverticulitis.	As diverticulitis is mostly an extraluminal process, the usefulness of these studies is limited. These studies do not reveal the severity of inflammation or presence of an abscess.
COMPUTED TOMOGRAPHY (CT) SCAN			
	Considered the imaging modality of choice for the diagnosis of diverticulitis. It is also the most specific imaging modality for the diagnosis of acute diverticulitis. Also used adjunctively to treatment when combined with CT-guided drainage.	As a diagnostic test for diverticulitis, CT has a sensitivity ranging from 85-97%. CT scan images transmural and extraluminal disease. Allows for patient comfort. Provides gradient data to classify the disease for appropriate management.	
ULTRASOUND			
	Requires that other etiologies for colonic mural thickening and pericolic inflammation be ruled out. What is visualized could be attributed to such disease processes as Crohn's disease, colon cancer, ischemic colitis, or other inflammatory conditions.	Is low cost and noninvasive.	Completely "operator" dependent and images may be hard to evaluate. In complicated diverticulitis, it is difficult to visualize the diverticulum.
ENDOSCOPIC PROCEDURES			
	Useful for patients who have been treated for diverticulitis. Should be used primarily when	Useful for visualization. Pediatric scopes available for adults who present with	Risk for colon perforation in patients with acute diverticulitis.

Continued

TABLE 12–4 Overview of Radiologic Studies in the Diagnosis of Diverticulitis—cont'd

Type of Test	Considerations	Advantages	Disadvantages
ENDOSCOPIC PROCEDURES			
	inflammatory bowel disease, ischemic colitis, or carcinoma is suspected.	inflammation that does not allow the adult scope to pass.	Difficulty passing the scope through the colon for visualization.
MR COLONOGRAPHY (MRC)			
	New imaging technique for persons with diverticulitis. Allows visualization of the complete colon. Involves basic colonoscopy preparation, then a tube is passed and the colon is filled with 2–2.5 liters of water. Before and after an injection of gadolinium-based contrast agents, three-dimensional images are obtained via magnetic resonance imaging.	Has a high sensitivity for diverticulitis. Patients are not exposed to ionization radiation. Ability to evaluate entire colon.	Length of time to perform is longer than a CT. Patients with lower abdominal pain may not be able to remain still. Motion artifacts can distort images.

Management

Nonsurgical Management

Patients with mild symptoms and noncomplicated diverticulitis are typically managed on an outpatient basis. A combination of drug therapy, hydration, and rest to decrease inflammation and promote tissue perfusion are the goals of nonsurgical management. Broad-spectrum antibiotics that target aerobic and anaerobic gram-negative rods are typically prescribed. These would include amoxicillin-clavulanate potassium (875 mg/125 mg orally twice a day), or metronidazole (7.5 mg/kg orally three times a day), plus either ciprofloxacin (500 mg orally twice a day) or trimethoprim-sulfamethoxazole (160/800 mg orally twice a day) for 7 to 10 days (38). For initial episodes of diverticulitis, about 50% to 80% of patients respond well to antibiotics, averting surgical intervention. About 15% to 30% of patients who are admitted for their first episodes of diverticulitis require surgery during that particular hospitalization (42).

Pain is a strong benchmark for admission to the hospital for uncomplicated diverticulitis. The patient should then have nothing by mouth. Antibiotics and fluids to prevent dehydration should be initiated intravenously. For patients with moderate to severe diverticulitis, an opioid analgesic should be used. As laxatives and enemas increase intestinal motility, they should be avoided. Additionally, the clinician should monitor for the common side effect of antibiotic therapy, diarrhea. During acute phases of the illness, the patient should be reminded to refrain from lifting, straining, or coughing as this increases intra-abdominal pressure which might result in perforation of the diverticulum (32).

An intra-abdominal abscess may form when a diverticulum perforates, as indentified by a CT scan (Table 12-4). Typically, if the abscess is small and localized, it is treated effectively with antibiotics. In cases where the abscess is large, or there is not an effective response to antibiotics, a CT scan–guided percutaneous drainage tube might be indicated (42), which is considered a palliative procedure only and allows stabilization of the patient. It is used to control sepsis immediately without the need for general anesthesia and can allow the patient to be prepared properly for a one-stage procedure as opposed to two-stage procedure involving an interval colostomy. Once this procedure is done, a resection should be performed in about 4 weeks (42).

Surgical Treatment

Diverticulitis accounts for nearly one-third of all colectomies and colostomies. The frequency of emergency operative intervention has decreased over time while the frequency of percutaneous drainage procedures has increased (43). There are various discussions about the type of surgical resection that should follow when a patient does not respond to nonsurgical management. There are two types of surgeries that are typically considered to either treat acute complications or ameliorate the incidence of further inflammation: the one-stage resection and the multiple-stage procedure. With the one-stage resection, the inflamed area is removed and a primary end-to-end anastomosis is completed. The multiple-stage procedure involves the construction of a colostomy at the proximal end of intestine once the affected area is removed, and a distal stoma is created with no anastomosis. This "double-barreled" temporary colostomy is anastomosed in a subsequent procedure.

Clinical Nurse Specialist Competencies and Spheres of Influence
Clinical Expert/Direct Care and Collaboration

As with many GI problems, the expert assessment skills of the CNS are paramount to the overall patient outcome. As the pattern of diverticulitis is nebulous until it is extreme or, in some cases, life-threatening, early intervention is directly correlated to positive patient outcomes. CNSs should be able to identify persons who are at high risk for the development of diverticula that can lead to diverticulitis. Collaboration with dietitians is an important aspect of the long-term management of diverticulosis, as diets high in fiber can ameliorate the incidence of diverticulitis.

ACUTE ABDOMEN: BOWEL OBSTRUCTION, ISCHEMIC BOWEL, AND PERITONITIS

When discussing issues related to an "acute abdomen" the clinician must look at all possible causes for a myriad of symptoms. Although pain is the predominant symptom with which the patient presents, it is important to discern other symptoms as this helps to determine the underlying cause. Pain can be a symptom of diverticulitis, appendicitis, and cholecystitis, as well as bowel obstruction, ischemic bowel and peritonitis. All of these processes must be considered as a potential cause of acute abdominal pain, or acute abdomen.

Bowel Obstruction

Obstructions can occur anywhere along the GI tract, but are primarily found at the pyloric area of the stomach, or in the small intestine, due to adhesions in the ileum. Over 70% of small bowel obstructions (SBOs) are the result of adhesions that have occurred as the result of prior surgery (44). Hernias account for about 25% of

SBOs, and neoplasms account for approximately 10% (45). Large bowel obstructions (LBOs) are typically the result of malignancies, with colon cancer being the most common cause (60%), and other causes being diverticular strictures and colonic volvulvus (44, 46). Bowel obstruction occurs when the normal flow of intestinal contents is interrupted by a mechanical blockage anywhere along the intestines (44). When this occurs, the digestion and absorption of the GI contents are impaired and blocked. Then, GI fluids become hypertonic, and fluid accumulates in the intestinal lumen as the result of osmotic loss from the body. This results in nutritional and fluid and electrolyte alterations and distention of the intestine. The intestine proximal to the blockage is further distended by the accumulation of swallowed air, gas as the result of bacterial fermentation, and luminal secretions (44). These lead to a cascade of events that cause further complications and worsen the condition. The pressure on the intestine due to the distention decreases perfusion to the intestine, which can result in ischemia, followed by necrosis of the intestinal tissue, which increases the possibility of a perforation and sepsis.

The pain caused by an SBO is typically a colicky type pain that is intermittent and cramps. Frequently, the pain is accompanied by nausea, vomiting, distention, and obstipation. Because of the bacterial overgrowth in the intestine, emesis associated with bowel obstructions is usually very feculent (44). Physical findings typically include high-pitched and intermittent bowel sounds above the obstruction and sometimes "rushes" of luminal fluid. Rigidity, rebound tenderness, guarding, or severe pain when the patient moves is suggestive of peritonitis. Additionally, it is common for patients with bowel obstructions to have decreased skin turgor, concentrated urine, and hemoconcentration, all of which are the result of the fluid shift and intravascular volume depletion (44, 45).

Diagnosis

Laboratory findings in patients with SBO are nonspecific but typically include leukocytosis with a left shift, electrolyte abnormalities, and elevated blood urea nitrogen due to fluid shifts. Plain upright and supine radiographic studies are beneficial in diagnosing a bowel obstruction as typical findings include air-fluid levels, small bowel distention, and paucity of air toward or in the rectal vault (44). The presence of free air under the diaphragm is suggestive of intestinal perforation (45). Although most cases can be diagnosed with plain films, there are instances in which these films are insufficient and CT scans might be most beneficial in diagnosing SBO and revealing the underlying cause (44).

Management

The specific cause of the obstruction should be identified immediately so that appropriate treatment can be instituted and complications from the obstruction prevented. Activity may be limited due to the pain or complications (45). The goals of treatment are aimed at decompressing the abdominal area via nasogastric tube and supporting hydration and electrolytes with intravenous fluids. Pharmacologic interventions might include antibiotics to prevent or treat infection, analgesics for pain relief, antiemetics, and GI stimulants such as metoclopramide or dexpanthenol preoperatively to minimize paralytic ileus (44).

Surgical intervention is indicated when the complete bowel obstruction does not resolve; however, there are cases in which the inflammatory processes subside, and the obstruction resolves without surgery. Paralytic ileus associated with bowel obstruction usually dissipates in 2 to 3 days without treatment (44). In cases where the cause of the obstruction is unknown or when bowel resection is the only logical course of treatment, surgical intervention is warranted.

Ischemic Bowel

Mesenteric ischemia comprises different clinical syndromes that are essentially characterized by inadequate perfusion to the bowel (47). The small bowel ischemia that results from mesenteric arterial hypoperfusion, thrombosis, or impaired venous drainage constitutes an emergency and is one of the most serious abdominal conditions in the elderly (48). Regardless of the events determining a mesenteric ischemia, the final result is a broad spectrum of bowel damage, ranging from minimal and reversible alterations to complete hemorrhagic necrosis of the intestinal wall (49). There are several small intestinal disease processes that complicate the issue further and may mimic ischemia both clinically and radiographically. These alternative diagnoses must be considered in differential diagnoses and can be categorized as infectious, inflammatory, or infiltrative processes as presented in Table 12-5.

Pathophysiology

During mesenteric ischemia, there are two mechanisms that mediate the alteration of the bowel. These mechanisms include the actual ischemia, as a result of lack of perfusion to the bowel, as well as reperfusion to the bowel. Reperfusion injury is associated with increased microvascular permeability, increased epithelial permeability with

TABLE 12–5 Disease Processes Considered for Differential Diagnosis for Small Bowel Ischemia

Process or Agent	Type of Process	Explanation
Mycobacterium avium-intracellulare	Infectious	Affects multiple organs and has been referred to as "pseudo-Whipple" because it presents with similar histology, radiologic, and clinical findings.
Cytomegalovirus	Infectious	This virus is a member of the herpes virus group and is transmitted via sexual contact. This virus can remain dormant in the host, but when activated mucosal ulcerations within the small bowel are typical and can result in hemorrhagic enteritis.
Cryptosporidosis (*Cryptosporidium*)	Infectious	*Cryptosporidium* is a gastrointestinal parasite. In patients with AIDS, the parasite is responsible for diffuse watery diarrhea.
Giardiasis (*Giardia lamblia*)		*Giardia lamblia* is a multiflagellate protozoan that is known to cause severe diarrhea and malabsorption. The protozoan inhabits primarily the duodenum and jejunum.
Whipple Disease	Infectious	This disease is caused by a gram-positive bacilli and is a chronic multisystem condition. Clinical presentation includes malabsorption syndrome and chronic diarrhea. Histologic findings reveal infiltration of the small bowel mucosa and submucosa with foamy microphages that contain periodic acid–Schiff–positive glycoprotein granules.
Crohn Disease	Inflammatory	Crohn disease is a transmural inflammatory bowel disease that can involve the small bowel at the terminal ileum.

TABLE 12–5 Disease Processes Considered for Differential Diagnosis for Small Bowel Ischemia—cont'd

Process or Agent	Type of Process	Explanation
Celiac Disease	Inflammatory	Celiac disease is the result of the host's sensitivity to gluten products. This leads to villous atrophy of the small bowel, as patients usually present with diarrhea and weight loss and sometimes abdominal pain.
Small Bowel Diverticulitis	Inflammatory	Although diverticular disease is primarily associated with the large intestine, it does occur in the small bowel as well. Small bowel diverticula are either acquired or congenital, with acquired small bowel diverticula primarily found in the jejunum.
Radiation Enteritis	Inflammatory	Radiation enteritis is the result of radiation to the abdomen. This typically results in ischemic and subsequent fibrotic injury, secondary to obliterative arteritis.
Graft-Versus-Host Disease	Inflammatory	This is a life-threatening complication of allogeneic bone marrow transplantation. This is thought to be the result of the host forming an immune response to the graft. The small bowel can be affected as the patient usually presents with abdominal cramps and diarrhea.
Small Bowel Malignancy	Neoplasm and infiltrative	Tumor involvement of the small bowel is most likely the result of metastasis from another site, as primary small bowel malignancies are rare.
Amyloidosis	Neoplasm and infiltrative	Amyloid is deposited around the small vessels of the small intestine. This results in decreased motility and normal intestinal secretion.
Other Considerations (include scleroderma, lymphangiectasia, intramural hemorrhage, and angioedema)		

leaking of fluid into the bowel, and decreased intestinal flow. There are cases in which reperfusion injury is actually worse than continual ischemia (49).

Acute Mesenteric Ischemia

Acute mesenteric ischemia is a potentially life-threatening condition with a mortality rate from 30% to 65% (47). The vast majority of people affected with acute mesenteric ischemia are over 60, and the most common presenting symptom is abdominal pain (47). Other symptoms include nausea, vomiting, diarrhea, and tachycardia. Melena stool or occult blood is prevalent in up to 75% of patients with acute mesenteric ischemia. Fever is indicative of bowel necrosis.

In patients with acute mesenteric ischemia, it is imperative to identify if the cause is occlusive, such as the result of embolism or thrombosis, or nonocclusive. The vast majority of patients with acute mesenteric ischemic a present with an occlusive form of ischemia. The presence of an embolism accounts for 50% of these cases, with arterial thrombosis the cause of about 25 % (47). Acute mesenteric ischemia due to arterial occlusion warrants immediate surgical intervention, whereas nonocclusive ischemia can be treated nonoperatively unless there is evidence of a gangrenous bowel (47).

Diagnosis

Leukocytosis, elevated lactate and amylase levels, and high anion gap metabolic acidosis are the most common, but nonspecific, findings in persons with acute mesenteric ischemia (47). There are studies under way that show promise for the use of low serum D-dimer levels in diagnosing acute mesenteric ischemia (5). Recent recommendations suggest that the biphasic CT is the diagnostic test of choice, which allows the clinician to define the arterial anatomy and to evaluate secondary signs of mesenteric ischemia (50).

Nonocclusive causes of acute mesenteric ischemia are discerned when the mesenteric vessels are patent. Conditions that pose risk factors for nonocclusive causes include low cardiac output associated with, for example, heart failure, cardiac arrhythmias, shock, hemodialysis, medications (particularly digoxin, cyclosporine, and vasopressors), and postoperative cardiac bypass surgery (47). Mesenteric vasoconstriction occurs with low perfusion and is further activated by intrinsic angiotensin and vasopressin. If vasoconstriction occurs for longer than 30 minutes, ischemia is irreversible (47).

Management

Fluid resuscitation with an isotonic crystalloid solution, advancing to blood products if necessary, should begin immediately for patients with acute mesenteric ischemia (50). Electrolyte imbalances should be corrected, and the patient should be invasively monitored for urine output, continuous central pressure, and arterial pressures, to ensure that all parameters are optimized prior to intravenous contrast diagnostics or surgery (50). Broad-spectrum antibiotics are indicated to guard against translocated flora and potential sepsis, and heparin should be given to maintain a partial thromboplastin time greater than twice normal (50).

In the event of sepsis or organ dysfunction, the management is much like in any other septic situation, with the exception of vasopressors. Vasopressors often used for sepsis and shock conditions in the presence of ischemic bowel can worsen the ischemia and intensify visceral vasospasm (50). If vasoconstrictors are necessary, better options include dobutamine, low-dose dopamine, and, in some cases, epinephrine. In all cases of acute mesenteric ischemia, pure adrenergic agonists should be avoided (50).

Surgical Treatment

Surgical exploration is recommended for all patients who have evidence of any threatened bowel, regardless of etiology. Surgical procedures used for acute mesenteric ischemia might include an embolectomy, where the offending clot is removed, or vascular bypass to enhance revascularization of the affected area. There is a relatively new hybrid procedure that combines revascularization involving the superior mesenteric artery and potential resection of the bowel. These procedures require extensive patient consideration and skill and experience in both vascular and bowel surgery by the surgeon.

Peritonitis

Peritonitis is either a local inflammation or a generalized inflammation of the peritoneum, and it can be classified as primary, secondary, or tertiary. Primary peritonitis is an infection that develops in the absence of a break in the intestinal tract, which is usually the result of hematogenous or lymphatic seeding or bacterial translocation (51). Secondary peritonitis is a peritoneal infection that develops in conjunction with an inflammatory process of the GI tract or its extensions and is usually associated with a perforation (51). Tertiary peritonitis is a persistent or recurring peritoneal infection that develops after initial treatment of secondary peritonitis.

Pathophysiology

The peritoneum is a semipermeable membrane that allows the flow of fluids and electrolytes between the bloodstream and peritoneal cavity. When peritonitis occurs, fluid can shift rapidly into the abdominal cavity at a rate of 300 to 500 mL/hr in response to acute inflammation (23).

Peristalsis slows or decreases in response to the shunting of blood to the inflamed area to dampen the potential impact of bacteria in that area. As a result, the bowel fills with gas and fluid. The alterations in circulatory changes can be devastating and include capillary leak, hypovolemia, and electrolyte imbalance, particularly when shock develops. The loss of circulatory volume is proportional to the severity of peritoneal involvement, and the fluid becomes more purulent as the condition progresses, with additional bacterial proliferation. The bacteria can enter the blood and cause septicemia (23).

Escherichia coli is the most common organism that is isolated from patients with intra-abdominal infections. Other bacteria associated with peritonitis include gram-negative organisms *Klebsiella pneumoniae* and *Enterococcus,* and gram-positive bacteria *Streptococcus pneumoniae* (52).

Clinical Presentation

The clinical manifestations of peritonitis include local or diffuse pain with rebound tenderness, guarding, and rigidity. Distention and paralytic ileus may ensue as the inflammation progresses but are not always present. Fever and abdominal pain occur in about two-thirds of the patients with peritonitis (52). Other systemic signs may include leukocytosis, nausea, vomiting, and signs of early shock such as tachycardia, tachypnea, oliguria, restlessness, pallor, weakness, and diaphoresis (23). Symptoms are evident in about 80% to 90% of peritoneal cases, and about 10% are asymptomatic (52).

Diagnosis

The diagnosis of peritonitis is made primarily on the basis of symptom pattern, abdominal history, and laboratory findings, including blood and ascites samples when ascites is present. Radiographic studies may show abnormalities in air patterns in the abdomen. White blood cell counts are often elevated to 20,000/mm^3 or higher (23).

Treatment

Source control is the general term used for interventional procedures used to control or eliminate the focus of an intra-abdominal infection (51). This would include any procedure that involves debridement, drainage of fluid or abscesses, or removal of an organ or a portion of an organ that is responsible for the peritonitis. Antimicrobial therapy is generally considered an adjunct to source control procedures, and in cases when the source control is deferred, antimicrobial therapy is more definitive. For example, patients with neutrocytic ascites should be started on antimicrobials regardless of the symptoms. The guiding principle for these patients is to use agents effective against the aerobic/facultative, anaerobic gram-negative bacilli, aerobic gram-positive cocci, and obligate anaerobic organisms commonly encountered in abdominal infections (51). Typically, a third-generation cephalosporin such as cefotaxime 2 g intravenously every 8 to 12 hours is used. If enterococcal infection is suspected, ampicillin is added (52).

Patients with tertiary peritonitis are prone to infections that are highly resistant to antimicrobials. Such patients commonly need multiple drug regimens and should be started on broad-spectrum antimicrobial therapy that can be altered based on subsequent culture results (52). The treatment of patients with complicated intra-abdominal infections using a combination of source control and appropriate antimicrobial therapy has produced satisfactory results, with success rates estimated at 78% to 86% with an overall mortality of 2% to 3% (51).

Clinical Nurse Specialist Competencies and Spheres of Influence

Clinical Expert/Direct Care

CNSs must rely heavily on assessment skills when the patient presents. The posture of the patient sometimes gives subtle cues to the type and location of pain and which positions are most comfortable. Fundamental principles of assessment are key to early identification of an acute abdominal problem; the clinician should observe before touching, then auscultate before palpating. Palpation may alter a physiologic process and lead to adventitious sounds that could mask the signs of something much more severe. Knowing when to collaborate with a surgeon is important when dealing with persons presenting with an acute abdomen. The situation can worsen in a short time without prompt and conclusive intervention.

For cases with high probability of infection, cultures should be drawn before initiating empirical antimicrobials

so that the results are not corrupted. It is imperative that proper medications are prescribed for the proper organisms; broad-spectrum antimicrobials should be initiated early on and then changed with definitive culture results.

It is important to keep in mind that many older patients can present with muted symptoms initially, as it takes longer for their immune system to respond to infection and inflammation. For this group, the clinician must pay additional attention to what is occurring with the patient and be astute to verbal cues. The potential to misdiagnose, mistreat, or offer no treatment at all is tremendous when symptoms are vague.

Coaching/Teaching/Mentoring

Teaching staff nurses the signs and symptoms of worsening abdominal conditions is essential for positive outcomes for these patients. The idea that the patient is a candidate for surgery at any moment guides much of the care for these patients as it relates to feeding and preparation; often nothing by mouth is indicated until surgery is ruled out. Family members must be kept informed and reassured that the patient is being monitored and prepared for anticipated surgery or other treatment as the condition changes. Because pain is associated with all forms of acute abdomen, this is often particularly difficult for family members to witness. The pathophysiologic process, diagnostic and treatment plan, and possible outcomes should be explained to the family, and proper medications for pain given to the patient. As pain is a strong indication of changes that might be occurring, the balance of providing comfort and the ability for the patient to express pain and other symptoms vital for a definitive diagnosis is sometimes difficult to obtain. Medication regimens for other symptoms such as nausea and vomiting should be carefully considered.

PEPTIC ULCER DISEASE

Peptic ulcer disease (PUD) is a problem of the GI tract characterized by mucosal damage due to pepsin and gastric acid secretion (53). It occurs primarily in the stomach and proximal duodenum, and less frequently in the lower esophagus, the distal duodenum, and jejunum (53). Ulcers are five times more common in the duodenum than the stomach, and in the stomach benign ulcers are most common in the antrum (60%), at the junction of the antrum and the body on the lesser curvature (25%) (54). Currently it is thought that up to 10% of ulcers are idiopathic (54).

Etiology

The epidemiology of PUD is difficult to determine as only the more symptomatic forms of PUD are presented and reported (55). However, in the United States, approximately 500,000 persons develop PUD annually, and in 70% of these patients, PUD occurs between the ages of 25 and 64 years (53). The most common causes of PUD are *Helicobacter pylori (H. pylori)* and the use of NSAIDs (53, 56-58). The incidence of PUD is declining, and this is thought to be the result of an increased use of proton pump inhibitors (PPIs) and decreasing rates of *H. pylori* infection. A variety of other infections and comorbidities are associated with the risk of PUD, such as cytomegalovirus, tuberculosis, Crohn disease, hepatic cirrhosis, renal failure, and sarcoidosis (53). There are other medicinal agents that also contribute to the incidence of PUD such as steroids, bisphosphates, potassium chloride, and some chemotherapeutic agents such as intravenous fluorouracil (53). Smoking is thought to increase the risk of ulcer recurrence and slows the healing process (53).

Pathophysiology

Studies show a strong correlation between *H. pylori* infection and duodenal and gastric ulcers. Permanent cure of peptic ulcers associated with the eradication of the *H. pylori* infection was the evidence that demonstrated this to be a main cause of PUD. More than 50% of the world's population has *H. pylori* infection in the gastric mucosa, yet only 5% to 10% ever actually develop ulcers (56). *H. pylori* bacteria, which adhere to the GI mucosa, contain an outer inflammatory protein and a cytotoxin-associated gene island that increases its virulence and its ulcerogenic potential (53). Patients with *H. pylori* infection have increased resting and meal stimulated gastrin levels and a decrease in the protective mucous production along with a decrease in duodenal mucosal bicarbonate secretion. These conditions favor ulcer formation (53). The actual interactions between the host and *H. pylori* are very complex and become more volatile with certain risk factors. It has been shown that eradicating *H. pylori* cures both gastric and duodenal ulcers and prevents relapses (56).

The prevalence of gastric ulcers in persons who take NSAIDs on a long-term basis is about 10% to 20%, and the prevalence for the development of duodenal ulcers in long-term NSAID users is about 2% to 5% (54). NSAIDs damage the stomach mainly by suppressing prostaglandin synthesis. Prostaglandins have protective cyclooxygenase 2–mediated effects such as enhancing gastric mucosal protection by stimulating mucus and bicarbonate secretion. Additionally, prostaglandins aid in epithelial cell proliferation and increase mucosal blood flow to the stomach and duodenum. Persons taking NSAIDs have a four-fold increase in risk of ulcer complications such as bleeding compared with persons who do not take NSAIDs (56). The use of NSAIDs accounts for about half of perforated ulcers, which occur most commonly in older patients (53). PPIs and misoprostol (Cytotec) reduce the ulcerogenic potential of NSAIDs and ulcer recurrence (53). There is also a synergistic effect between NSAIDs and *H. pylori* in the production of ulcers. By eradicating the bacteria, ulcers heal easier in cases where NSAIDs must be used to treat conditions such as arthritis (55).

Clinical Presentation

Epigastric pain or dyspepsia is a major symptom of PUD and is evident in 80% to 90% of PUD cases. Nocturnal pain wakens about two-thirds of patients with duodenal ulcers and one-third of patients with gastric ulcers (54). There is periodicity associated with pain symptoms where patients may report symptomatic pain for several weeks with intervals of months to years in which they are pain free. It is important to identify how the pain correlates with eating, sleeping, stress, and medication timing and regimens as this can sometimes help identify the type of ulcer.

Less common symptoms include vomiting (which could arise from an obstruction), loss of weight (which usually occurs from fear of eating when eating causes pain), intolerance of fatty foods, and family history (53). Deep palpation might reveal mild, localized tenderness (54).

Diagnosis

If the clinical presentation is suggestive of PUD, the patient should be evaluated for anemia, hematemesis, melena, or heme-positive stool suggestive of bleeding. These symptoms are cause for alarm and require further evaluation and intervention. Typically, severe pain that radiates to the back is indicative of perforation (53). In cases where these symptoms are seen, the patient should be referred for prompt endoscopy. The preferred test, esophagogastroduodenoscopy (EGD), is a more sensitive and specific test for PUD than an upper GI barium study and it allows for biopsy of gastric lesions when deemed necessary (54, 59).

Patients younger than 55 years with no severe symptoms should be tested for *H. pylori* and advised to discontinue smoking and NSAID, alcohol, and illicit drug use. The presence of *H. pylori* can be determined with serum enzyme-linked immunosorbent assay (ELISA), stool antigen test, urea breath test, or endoscopic biopsy (53). The ELISA is the least accurate test and is limited to diagnosing only the initial infection, whereas the stool antigen test and breath test are highly accurate and can be used to determine the eradication of *H. pylori* (53). The fecal antigen immunoassay test and the C-urea breath test have a sensitivity and specificity of about 90%. For these tests, a positive result indicates an active infection, and although they cost more to perform than the serologic tests, they may be cost-effective in reducing unnecessary treatment in persons without the infection (54).

Management

The treatment of patients with *H. pylori*–associated PUD is aimed at eradicating the infection. Eradication is usually achieved with a combination of antimicrobials and acid-inhibiting medications. Antibacterial therapy alone does not facilitate healing, but healing is accelerated by adding acid suppressants (56). Pharmacologic therapy for patients with ulcers and no *H. pylori* infection is aimed at healing the ulcer. A table of recommended drug regimens for patients with PUD and active *H. pylori* infection is presented as Table 12-6.

For persons with PUD in the absence of *H. pylori* infection, the use of PPIs and histamine$_2$ (H$_2$) receptor agonists is effective. This is also the regimen that persons taking NSAIDs should consider to reduce the risks of both gastric and duodenal ulcers. PPIs are better than standard-dose H$_2$ receptor agonists for the prevention of duodenal ulcers (56). Misoprostol is better than standard-dose H$_2$ receptor agonists in preventing gastric, but not duodenal, ulcers (56).

Surgical intervention is indicated in cases of complicated PUD, which include perforations, penetration, gastric outlet obstruction, and bleeding that cannot be controlled by endoscopy (54).

Surgery is also indicated when patients cannot tolerate medications or do not comply with medication regimens, and for patients who are at high risk for developing complications such as persons on long-term steroids or dependent on NSAIDs. Persons with PUD who have multiple medication regimens should be considered for surgical intervention (53). Surgical procedures for duodenal ulcers include truncal vagotomy and drainage, selective vagotomy, and drainage, which preserves the hepatic and celiac branches of the vagus, highly selective vagotomy, or partial gastrectomy. Surgery for gastric ulcers typically involves a gastrectomy (53).

Clinical Nurse Specialist Competencies and Spheres of Influence
Research/Evidence-Based Practice

The more recent discovery of *H. pylori* as a cause of PUD changed a whole paradigm of thinking about PUD. Whereas historically the cause of PUD was thought to be stress, a bacterial etiology with strong research evidence challenged traditional thinking. This was a model (and a Nobel Prize–winning exemplar) for prompting all health care providers to think about nontraditional approaches to well-defined issues. There are still many interventions and protocols based on tradition and theory that have not been supported in evidence. Health care professionals should explore and challenge traditional practices through research. Persons caring for patients are ideally positioned to identify those practices that are questionable and lack evidence. The CNS is in a key role to identify such practices

TABLE 12-6 Pharmacologic Regimen for Persons with PUD and Active *H. pylori* Infection

Acute treatment for 7–14 days with one of the following:

Triple Therapy Regimen
Proton pump inhibitor before meals.
  Omeprazole 20 mg PO bid *OR*
  Lansoprazole 30 mg PO bid *OR*
  Raberprazole 20 mg PO bid *OR*
  Pantoprazole 40 mg PO bid *OR*
  Esomeprazole 40 mg once daily

PLUS
Antimicrobials
  Clarithromycin 500 mg PO bid *AND*
  Amoxicillin 1 Gram PO bid *OR*
  Metronidazole 500 mg PO bid
  (For persons with penicillin allergies)

Quadruple Therapy Regimen
Proton pump inhibitor before meals.
  Omeprazole 20 mg PO bid *OR*
  Lansoprazole 30 mg PO bid *OR*
  Raberprazole 20 mg PO bid *OR*
  Pantoprazole 40 mg PO bid *OR*
  Esomeprazole 40 mg once daily

PLUS
Bismuth subsalicylate (2 tablets) PO qid

PLUS
Tetracycline 500 mg PO qid

PLUS
Metronidazole 250 mg PO qid (for 14 days)
  Quadruple therapy is recommended in patients for whom an initial attempt at eradication with triple therapy failed.
Continue treatment for 4–8 weeks with:
  Omeprazole 20 mg PO bid *OR*
  Lansoprazole 30 mg PO bid *OR*
  Raberprazole 20 mg PO bid *OR*
  Pantoprazole 40 mg PO bid *OR*
  Esomeprazole 40 mg once daily

and to formulate questions to expand the science of the nursing profession.

GASTROINTESTINAL BLEED

Because the GI system is lengthy and contains numerous structures, bleeding is usually described by its location as an upper GI bleed (UGIB) or a lower GI bleed (LGIB). The point of demarcation for this anatomical separation is the ligament of Treitz, often referred to as the "suspensory muscle of the duodenum," which is a band of smooth muscle that extends from the junction of the duodenum and jejunum to the diaphragm at the left crus and functions as a suspensory ligament. Structures proximal to the ligament are considered upper GI (UGI), and structures distal to the ligament considered lower GI (LGI).

Etiology

UGI bleeding is a common, potentially life-threatening condition that is the primary cause of approximately 300,000 hospital admissions and about 30,000 deaths in the United States each year (60). PUD accounts for about half of UGIBs (61), with variceal hemorrhage causing about 10% to 25%. Other relatively common conditions associated with UGIB include cancerous and other lesions of the UGI tract, Mallory-Weiss tears, Dieulafoy lesions, and angiodysplasia (61). Mallory-Weiss tears account for 5% to 10% of UGIBs (62).

The exact incidence of LGIB is not known, but the annual incidence of hospitalization is estimated to be 20 to 27 episodes per 100,000 persons per year (63). The incidence of LGIB rises with age, which may in part be explained by the increase in the incidence of diverticulosis and colonic angiodysplasia as people age. The mean age of persons with LGIB ranges from 63 to 77 years, with a reported mortality rate of 2% to 4% (64). The most common causes of LGIB include diverticulosis (50%), vascular ectasias (5% to 10%) hemorrhoids, ischemic colitis, and angiodysplasia (64, 65). Table 12-7 provides a list of the most common causes of both UGIBs and LGIBs.

Clinical Presentation

Prompt and accurate assessment is crucial for patients who have UGIB, as the information will provide guidance to the appropriate management of the bleed. When assessing UGIB, it is important to determine any prior history of GI bleeding, any accompanying symptoms, the character of the bleeding, and medications the patient is taking that might have an impact on the bleed, along with the social habits and medical comorbidities (61). Signs of chronic liver disease indicate the bleeding is most likely due to portal hypertension, although a different lesion is commonly identified in 25% to 50% of the patients with cirrhosis (62). A history of heavy alcohol ingestion along with vomiting, retching, or coughing is indicative of bleeding due to Mallory-Weiss lesions (61, 62).

Pain is a symptom in many cases of UGIB. Epigastric pain is commonly associated with PUD; abdominal pain that is initially relieved by eating but reoccurs in 1 to 2 hours postprandially is often indicative of an ulcer specific to the duodenum (61). Mesenteric ischemia with UGIB often presents with severe abdominal pain, whereas most other forms of GI bleeding are typically relatively painless (61). The character of the stool and emesis is also

TABLE 12–7 Typical Causes of Upper and Lower Gastrointestinal Bleeding

Causes of Upper Gastrointestinal Bleeding
Peptic ulcer disease
Esophageal and gastric varices
Stress-related erosive syndrome
Mallory-Weiss tear
Esophagitis
Duodenitis
Angiodysplasia
Neoplasm
Anastomic Ulcers
Aortoenteric fistula
Cameron lesion
Dieulafoy lesion
Hemobilia
Hemosuccus pancreaticus
Kaposi sarcoma
Post-procedural causes:
    Nasogastric tube
    Endoscopic biopsy
    Polypectomy
    Endoscopic sphincterotomy

Causes of Lower Gastrointestinal Bleeding
Diverticulosis
Angiodysplasia
Neoplasm
Inflammatory bowel disease
Vascular ectasias
Trauma
Infectious colitis
Radiation colitis or proctitis
Ischemia
Aortoenteric fistula
Hemorrhoids
Stercoral ulcers
Portal colopathy
Colonic varices
Endometriosis
Dieulafoy lesion

an indication of GI bleeding. If emesis is bright red, UGIB is suspected, as hematemesis occurs in about 50% of cases (61). Moderate amounts of "coffee grounds" or altered blood emesis are indicative of more limited bleeding than bright red bleeding (61). Keep in mind that some of this blood is digested and will contribute to the similar features of stools of patients with LGIB. Melana, or black and tarry stools, should be differentiated from patients who are taking iron supplements or bismuth. Patients with gross UGIB have melana in about 75% of cases (61). Melana can be indicative of both UGIBs and LGIBs; however, bright red blood per rectum (hematochezia) is usually limited to a lower GI source, which is typically associated with hemorrhoids. In some cases, hematochezia can be the result of massive UGIB, which is often accompanied by signs of hypovolemia and hypoperfusion due to rapid blood loss (61).

The physical exam is aimed at identifying findings relevant to GI bleeding, regardless of the source. The severity of blood loss is generally estimated by the hemodynamic status of the patient along with other crucial signs. Orthostatic hypotension, an increase in the pulse greater than 20 beats/min, and a decrease in systolic blood pressure of more than 20 mm Hg from recumbency to standing are indicative of a loss of blood volume of 15% or more. Hypotension is associated with a blood loss volume of around 40% (66). The abdomen should be assessed for bowel sounds, abdominal tenderness, and the presence of ascites. Hepatomegaly, splenomegaly, palmar erythema, caput medusa, spider angiomata, and peripheral edema are all indications that there may be chronic liver disease or portal hypertension (61).

Diagnosis

All patients require complete history and physical exam and laboratory testing. Laboratory tests should include a complete blood cell count with a differential, INR, prothrombin time (PT), serum creatinine, and liver enzymes. The patient should also be typed and cross-matched for 2 to 4 units of red packed blood cells, especially in cases of UGIB (62, 63, 65).

Differentiating between UGIB and LGIB is important as 2% to 15% of patients who have presumed LGIB actually have UGIB (63). This can be determined via insertion of a nasogastric tube, which should be reserved for patients who have brisk bleeding in whom an upper endoscopy is not anticipated. Nasogastric lavage containing gross blood, blood-tinged fluid, or strongly positively guaiac dark fluid is a strong indicator of UGIB. EGD is the definitive standard for excluding an UGIB (63).

Management

For patients who present with LGIB, aspirin and other NSAIDs should be discontinued (65). For persons with an active UGIB, a medication regimen of intravenous PPIs such as esomeprazole, lansoprazole, or pantoprazole 80-mg bolus, followed by 8 mg/hr for 72 hours, is indicated (62). For bleeding related to portal hypertension, octreotide is recommended with a 100-mcg bolus, followed by 50 to 100 mcg/hr. High doses of oral PPIs are also effective for persons who are able to swallow and are allowed oral intake (65).

For patients who are hemodynamically compromised, resuscitation should be immediate. Patients with active bleeding should receive a 500-mL bolus of saline or another crystalloid to maintain blood pressure during the first 30 minutes. This takes place while the patient's blood is being crossed and matched (61). There is no absolute hematocrit level that indicates a transfusion is necessary; multiple factors such as age, presence of comorbidities, cardiovascular status, tempo of the bleeding, and evidence of hypoperfusion should be considered when determining the need for a transfusion (61). The rate of the transfusion is determined by the severity of hypovolemia.

Bleeding can be exacerbated by the presence of coagulopathy and should be treated with fresh frozen plasma (FFP) as needed. To replace lost coagulation factors, a useful guideline is to transfuse 1 unit of FFP for every 4 units of packed red blood cells transfused (63).

Other guidelines related to coagulopathies include the following: (1) an international normalized ratio (INR) of less than 1.5 does not require therapy, (2) mild thrombocytopenia (50,000 to 90,000 platelets/μL usually does not require platelet transfusion, and (3) for platelet counts less than 50,000 μL in the presence of active bleeding, platelet transfusion should be considered (61).

Invasive and Surgical Procedures

There are a variety of invasive and surgical procedures that are used to stop bleeding. One procedure that can be used for UGIB that may eliminate the need for surgery is transendoscopic coagulation with laser, heat probe, or a sclerosing agent. For UGIB related to esophageal varices, there are a number of procedures that are used to control bleeding, including banding and insertion of a portocaval, mesocaval, or splenorenal shunt. The choice of intervention is based upon the clinical presentation and visualization of the bleed and its source.

Interventions for LGIB can range from sclerosing the bleeding vessels to a bowel resection. The decision is made based on the patient's overall health status, the site, and the degree of bleeding evident in the LGI tract.

Clinical Nurse Specialist Competencies and Spheres of Influence
Clinical Expert/Direct Care

Patients with GI bleeding are among the most challenging patients that a CNS will encounter. Expert assessment skills and knowledge of the condition at the early stages of clinical presentation can have a tremendous impact on the overall outcome for these patients.

Collaboration and Coaching/Teaching/Mentoring

Knowing when to initiate resuscitation or when to intervene to prevent the need for resuscitation requires communication, collaboration, and cooperation from the family as well as the patient. Rapid response teams are often led by CNSs, who are instrumental in educating front-line clinicians about patient conditions that warrant summoning the team to prevent catastrophic events. Many hospitals encourage families to call the rapid response team, which is potentially lifesaving for patients with sudden GIB.

LIVER CIRRHOSIS

Etiology

Cirrhosis is a chronic disease of the liver that is characterized by deformation of the normal hepatic structure by bands of connective tissue and by nodules of regenerating liver cells unrelated to the normal vasculature of the liver. Essentially, there is liver scarring that is usually the result of hepatic inflammation and necrosis that develops slowly and with a destructive course that usually ends in hepatic failure or end-stage liver disease. The most common causes of cirrhosis in the United States are alcoholic liver disease and hepatitis C (67). Worldwide, hepatitis B and hepatitis D are the leading causes. Without liver transplantation, cirrhosis is usually fatal, and it is the tenth leading cause of death in the United States (68, 69).

Pathophysiology

As cirrhosis develops, the tissue in the liver becomes nodular, and these nodules can block the bile flow and blood flow. These nodules form a histologic classification that includes micronodular, macronodular, and mixed forms of cirrhosis. The micronodular cirrhosis usually contains regenerating nodules that are less than or equal to 1 mm and is typical of alcoholic liver disease, or Laenec's cirrhosis. Macronodular cirrhosis is characterized by the presence of larger nodules up to several centimeters in diameter and may contain central veins. This form of cirrhosis corresponds to posthepatic or postnecrotic cirrhosis but may not follow episodes of massive necrosis (69). Apart from the histologic classification, cirrhosis can also be classified based on the causative disease. Laenic's cirrhosis, or alcoholic cirrhosis, is attributed to chronic alcoholism.

Postnecrotic cirrhosis is usually the result of hepatitis, hepatotoxic drugs, and hepatotoxic chemicals. Biliary cirrhosis, also called cholestatic cirrhosis, is caused by chronic biliary obstruction, usually from gallbladder disease. Cardiac cirrhosis, although caused by heart failure, is a rare complication (67).

The complications associated with cirrhosis are proportionate to the extent of liver damage. In cases where the liver is scarred but can perform its essential functions without obvious symptoms, the condition is said to be "compensated cirrhosis." In cases where there is impairment of liver function and obvious signs of liver failure, the cirrhosis is referred to as "decompensated cirrhosis" (67). There are a myriad of complications that are associated with cirrhosis due to the loss of hepatic function. Table 12-8 provides an overview of common complications and their pathophysiological underpinnings.

Clinical Presentation

As all of these symptoms in Table 12-8 can be attributed to cirrhosis, they are also part of the presentation for chronic hepatic failure. These symptoms will be discussed further in the next section within the context of hepatic failure that occurs in chronic conditions.

HEPATIC FAILURE

The management of liver failure is complex and intense and often involves the combined efforts of many specialists in order to achieve optimal outcomes for the patient. Hepatic failure encompasses a broad range of disease, from acute liver failure in patients with no history of disease, to those patients with end-stage decompensated cirrhosis (70). The spectrum of liver failure from acute to chronic can present with poor prognosis, involve many organ systems, and warrant comprehensive primary and intensive care services.

TABLE 12–8 Complications Associated With Liver Cirrhosis

Complication	Physiologic Cause and Considerations
Portal hypertension	Manifestation of portal hypertension is defined as a sustained elevation of pressure in the portal vein above the normal level of 6 to 12 cm water. Blood meets pressure resistance and flows back into organs with lower pressure. In the spleen, the result is splenomegaly. Veins in the stomach, esophagus, abdomen, and rectum become dilated. This can result in ascites, esophageal varices, prominent abdominal veins, and hemorrhoids.
Ascites	Ascites is the accumulation of serous fluid within the peritoneal cavity, which is usually the result of the back pressure in the portal system. Distended abdomen with shifting dullness to percussion and positive fluid wave are indicative of ascites. With the shift of fluid and albumin into the peritoneal cavity, the serum colloidal osmotic pressure in the vasculature is decreased. Severe ascites can cause renal constriction activating the renin-angiotensin dynamic, which leads to more ascites as sodium and water are retained.

TABLE 12–8 Complications Associated With Liver Cirrhosis—cont'd

Complication	Physiologic Cause and Considerations
Esophageal varices	The blood backs up from the liver, putting pressure on thin-walled vessels in the esophagus, resulting in varices. Varices affect more than half of persons with cirrhosis and it is estimated that 30% of these patients will experience an episode of variceal hemorrhage within 2 years of diagnosis. The size of the varix is important in determining the patient's risk of bleeding, as hemorrhage from varices accounts for 20% to 30% of the deaths in persons with cirrhosis.
Portal hypertensive gastropathy (PHG) (PHG)	PHG is the most common gastric mucosal injury in patients with liver cirrhosis; it can cause both acute and chronic upper gastrointestinal bleeding even in the absence of esophageal or gastric varices. The pathogenesis of PHG is unclear and it is not known whether PHG correlates more with portal hypertension or with liver dysfunction.
Coagulopathies	Bile production is decreased, which inhibits the absorption of vitamin K, which is necessary for the synthesis of clotting factors II, VII, IX, and X. Without these factors, patients have high bleeding times and are more prone to bruising and bleeding.
Jaundice	Yellow-green staining of tissues by bilirubin results from compromised bilirubin metabolism, which is a heralding sign of liver impairment. Yellow sclera or yellow tint to skin or mucous membranes is indicative of jaundice.
Portal-systemic encephalopathy (PSE)	PSE is the result of rising levels of toxic substances normally metabolized and excreted by the liver. There are four stages of PSE based on patient status, ranging from prodromal to coma.
Hepatorenal syndrome	The pathophysiology of this disorder is not well understood; however, it manifests in decreased urine output and an increased serum creatinine level, which usually occur acutely. The prognosis for the patient is poor because therapies to improve renal function usually are ineffective.
Spontaneous bacterial peritonitis	This can be a complication attributed to the increasing development of ascites and the translocation of intestinal flora through the capillaries, or it can be the result of paracentesis that is performed as a therapeutic measure for ascites.

As acute liver failure and chronic liver failure are clinically different entities, they will be discussed separately.

Acute Liver Failure
Etiology

Acute liver failure (ALF) is defined as the abrupt loss of liver function, characterized by hepatic encephalopathy and coagulopathy, within 26 weeks of the onset of symptoms in a patient without previous liver disease (71, 72). ALF is further subdivided into hyperacute liver failure, when the interval from jaundice to encephalopathy is less than or equal to 7 days; into acute liver failure, when the interval from jaundice to encephalopathy is 8 to 28 days; and into subacute liver failure, when the same interval is greater than 28 days. The subcategories are important as they relate to possible etiologies and outcomes. For example, patients with hyperacute liver failure are more likely to survive without a liver transplant, and the cause is more likely to have been the result of acetaminophen overdose or acute hepatitis A. Persons presenting with symptoms indicative of hyperacute liver failure are more likely to develop cerebral edema (73, 74). Acute liver failure subclassification is usually the result of hepatitis B, or drug ingestion, and has a moderate survival rate. Cerebral edema is less common in this category than in patients presenting with hyperacute liver failure. Patients with subacute liver failure have a poorer rate of survival, are more likely to have liver injury due to idiosyncratic drug reactions or indeterminate etiologies, and more frequently show signs of chronic liver failure such as ascites, peripheral edema, or renal failure (73). Another classification related to liver failure encompasses the notion of fulminant hepatic failure (FHF), which is an acute form of liver failure typically identified by the development of encephalopathy within 8 weeks from the appearance of any signs of hepatic failure in patients without a history of hepatic disease (72).

In the United States, the actual incidence of acute hepatic failure or fulminant hepatic failure is about 2000 cases per year (73, 75). In the last several years, the outcome of these patients has improved largely due to evidence-based treatments and clearer understanding of the pathophysiology. The goal in the management of ALF is aimed at determining the etiology of the failure and should be focused on the prevention of systemic infection, multiorgan failure, hepatic encephalopathy, and brain edema. At this time, the ideal standard of treatment for fulminant hepatic failure is orthotopic liver graft (OLT), which has been shown to have a 5-year survival rate of about 90%.

Pathophysiology

The specific pathogenesis of liver injury depends on the etiology. There are similarities in the changes that occur in the liver regardless of the cause, in which an injury to the hepatocytes causes cell damage or death by necrosis or apoptosis or both (71). The presence or absence of adenosine triphosphate (ATP) seems to make a difference in the pathogenesis of ALF, as ATP triggers the mitochondrial permeability transition injury of the liver cell and is associated with apoptosis if ATP stores are preserved and by necrosis if ATP stores are depleted. Reye's syndrome and acute Wilson's disease represent disease processes in which the mitochondrial injury is associated with apoptosis (71).

Necrotic injury of the hepatocytes leads to loss of cell membrane integrity and eventual rupture, which results in cell death with the release of cytosolic proteins including LDH, alanine aminotransferase (ALT), AST, and ferritin (71). With the release of these compounds into the systemic circulation, serum levels of these enzymes and ferritin are helpful in diagnosing not only hepatic injury but also the degree of injury. The release of these substances further leads to oxidative injury and inhibits the ability of the liver to conjugate and detoxify some toxic substances. Along with this, other detoxification mechanisms are compromised, including the transport mechanism for bilirubin, which leads to cholestasis and conjugated hyperbilirubinema (71). An additional important aspect of both chronic and acute liver failure is the inhibition or loss of Kuppfer cell function that results in increased serum endotoxins and other substrates that extend the damage to the liver and increase the risk for infection. Hence, not only are liver and systemwide protective mechanisms compromised, but also there is further assault by the released toxins.

The site of injury within the liver is an important consideration in determining the ability of the liver to regenerate. Arterial blood and portal blood, which contain oxygen and requisite nutrients, are supplied in the portal tract. This is where the progenitor cells, ductal hepatocytes, or oval cells are present. Injury to the portal zone hinders the regenerative response. Injury to the central zone of liver, where the portal zone is unaffected, permits more frequent and spontaneous recovery and is susceptible to ischemic injuries. Other toxic injuries vary in their sites of action due to the differences in metabolism of central hepatocytes and portal hepatocytes (71).

Toxins

Acetaminophen overdose is the most common cause of toxic liver injury in the United States and the United Kingdom (70, 71). Acetaminophen is metabolized in hepatocytes by cytochrome enzymes. When overdose of acetaminophen is confirmed, *N*-acetylcysteine (NAC) should be initiated immediately. NAC decreases the injury to the liver by augmenting glutathione synthesis, which results in less formation of acetaminophen's hepatotoxic intermediate. There is evidence that administration of NAC may be beneficial even after 16 hours from the ingestion of acetaminophen (70). It is also thought that NAC might have a beneficial effect on the microcirculation in the liver and improve outcomes. NAC has traditionally been administered via the oral route; however, there is parenteral NAC now available that is preferable in these cases because intravenous routes improve the bioavailability of the drug and are not subject to absorption, especially in patients who have received activated charcoal or adsorbents (71).

Amanita poisoning, from the heat-stable toxin produced by the mushroom *Amanita phalloides,* may lead to acute liver injury. Usually there is initial vomiting and diarrhea followed by liver damage and then development of secondary injury to other organs. Mortality of amanita poisoning approaches 10% to 30%. Early treatment with silibinin or with penicillin G in high doses may lessen the degree of hepatic injury (71).

There are other drugs and herbal supplements that may cause acute liver injury. There is the possibility of some persons having idiosyncratic effects to certain drugs or have a predisposition to develop liver injury due to a unique metabolic process for that individual when exposed to the drug. Examples of some of these drugs include isoniazid, ketoconazole, disulfuram, amiodarone, and valproate, among others. Other toxic injuries can result in severe immune-mediated liver injury; halothane is one example (71).

Viral Infections

Viral infections with hepatotropic viruses such as hepatitis A, B, and E are often associated with liver injury with good chances of recovery. However, a small percentage of persons infected with these viruses will develop ALF. Although there are no specific therapies for hepatitis A or E, there are antiviral agents that inhibit the replication of hepatitis B (71). The degree of efficacy of these antivirals in reducing the risks for the development of ALF remains in debate. For patients who have hepatitis B virus (HBV) infection with liver failure, antiviral drugs should be considered as part of the plan of care, as they might reduce the risk for infection in a potential graft if the patient receives a transplant. Acute HBV may be more severe if there is a concurrent infection with hepatitis D virus (HDV). Outbreaks of HBV and HDV have been associated primarily with injectable drug use (71). The use of injectable drugs is another important aspect of transplant screening. The nature and use of certain drugs may prevent a patient from being a viable transplant candidate. Other viruses associated with ALF include herpes simplex, varicella zoster virus, and cytomegalovirus (76). Rarely, ALF is caused by Epstein-Barr virus (EBV) infection (71).

Metabolic Etiologies

Pathophysiologic processes may result in liver failure; copper toxicosis as seen in Wilson's disease is an example. ALF caused by Wilson's disease is typically accompanied by a nonimmune hemolytic anemia and may be recognized by a lower than normal alkaline phosphatase–to–bilirubin ratio (<4) and ALT-to-AST ratio of less than 2, elevated serum copper greater than 200 μg/dL, and 24-urine copper level often greater than 200 μg (71, 77).

Acute fatty liver of pregnancy (AFLP) is a disorder in which there is a metabolic disruption that results in maternal-fetal distress (78). Typically occurring in the third trimester, this disorder presents with marked elevation in liver function tests and may progress rapidly to jaundice and liver failure. Fifty percent of these patients have preeclampsia (71). Fatty liver may be suspected with imaging studies. However, because the type and percent of fat content cannot be substantiated through imaging, liver biopsy is required for diagnosis, with fatty concentration found in the centrilobular hepatocytes. Typically, delivery of the fetus is necessary for maternal and fetal survival (71).

Vascular Etiologies

Acute obstruction of hepatic venous outflow, or Budd-Chiari syndrome, is a vascular disorder, often recognized by hepatomegaly, that may result in ALF (71). The hepatomegaly is frequently accompanied by new and rapid onset of ascites and imaging studies that demonstrate hepatic venous thrombosis. Immediate decompression of the obstruction with a transhepatic, intrahepatic, or portosystemic shunt or surgical portosystemic shunt procedure may be indicated to prevent further hepatic injury (71). In cases of underlying cirrhosis or continuing decompensation, immediate transplantation might be the only viable option. Budd-Chiari syndrome is often associated with hypercoagulable states or disorders.

Ischemic hepatitis or shock liver is associated with liver injury that occurs mainly in the central zone of the liver. Usually there is significant hypotension that is antecedent to the development of the injury; treatment of the underlying condition is essential for hepatic recovery (71).

Autoimmune

Autoimmune hepatitis, which may result in ALF, may be either acute or, in cases where an earlier disease or injury went undetected, might be chronic. Up to 30% of patients who present with acute presentation of autoimmune hepatitis do not have typical serum markers for autoimmune hepatitis, thus confounding the diagnosis. Some patients respond to high-dose steroids following the exclusion of viral hepatitis, which may be diagnostic (71).

Clinical Presentation and Diagnosis

The most critical aspect to patient survival with ALF is the early recognition of the disease process and early identification of the etiology. This allows the clinician to base management on targeted interventions to ameliorate the course of the disease and improve patient outcomes.

The first phase of an evaluation should be a thorough history and physical exam. In cases where the patient has altered mental status, the history should be obtained from other reliable sources such as knowledgeable family members and past medical records. Physical exam should include the patient's mental status, liver and spleen size, and presence or absence of ascites. Any evidence of encephalopathy should be graded using standard scoring systems such as the Glasgow Coma Scale or West Haven Criteria. It is essential to establish a baseline as many presenting signs including mental status may show only subtle changes. In patients who have a rapidly accelerating disease process, neurologic evaluation should be done frequently as changes may occur in hours, if not minutes (71).

Initial laboratory testing and imaging should be performed on patients who have ALF. The tests will help identify the degree of impairment of the liver and the impact on other organs such as the kidney. Table 12-9 lists the tests commonly performed for diagnosis and evaluation of ALF.

Social work and psychiatric evaluations are important in patients with suspected history of substance abuse or when there are indications of an underlying psychiatric disorder. This is an essential aspect of the evaluation when considering the patient's viability for transplantation. This information is also helpful when considering sedation parameters if patients require sedatives during hospitalization.

Management

The overall management of liver failure mandates an interdisciplinary approach involving advanced practice nurses, physicians, surgeons, dietitians, psychologists,

TABLE 12-9 Initial Laboratory Tests for Patients With Acute Liver Failure

Blood Testing

Complete blood cell count with platelets and differential
Electrolytes and renal function panel
International normalized ratio
Factors V and VII
Ammonia levels
Bilirubin, total
Alanine aminotransferase
Alkaline phosphatase
Antimitochondrial antibody
Ceruloplasmin
Gamma glutamyltranspeptidase
Hepatitis serologies
Leucine aminopeptidase
Ornithine carbamyoltransferase
Viral markers
Blood cultures
Pregnancy testing (in females)
Uric acid
Serum copper

Diagnostic Studies and Imaging

Liver scan
Liver biopsy
Liver ultrasonography
Chest radiograph
Electrocardiogram
Echocardiogram with estimation of pulmonary artery pressures

Toxicology Screen

Acetaminophen
Opiates
Barbiturates
Cocaine
Alcohol

Other Specimens

Urine analysis
Urine cultures
Urine copper

intensivists, and other specialists. The multisystem impact of ALF can be profound. Frequent assessment of mental status, assessment of hepatic synthetics, glucose, and coagulation studies is necessary (70). Unless an invasive procedure is planned, or there is evidence of overt bleeding, coagulopathies in ALF do not usually require correction. FFP can mask the deterioration of liver function, is only partially effective in correcting coagulopathies, and is typically short lived. Also, FFP is associated with risk of cytomegalovirus infection and may exacerbate volume overload and pulmonary edema in the presence of compromised renal function (70).

Infection

Infections are a common cause of death in patients with ALF and commonly precipitate multiorgan system failure, the most common cause of death (73, 79). Patients experiencing ALF are particularly vulnerable to severe infection due to immunologic alterations that occur during the disease process. Because of the patient's immunocompromised state, the response to infection is atypical in that fever or leukocytosis occurs in only about 30% of these patients. Pneumonia (50%), urosepsis (22%), intravenous catheter–induced bacteremia (12%), and spontaneous bacteremia (16%) account for the majority of infections in patients with ALF (70, 73, 80, 81). There is much ongoing debate about the use of prophylactic antibiotics in patients with ALF (70, 73). Although there is evidence that parenteral antibiotics are associated with a lower incidence of infection, there are limited data to support the value of prophylactic antibiotics for all patients with ALF (70, 73). When culture results are not yet available, patients with ALF who present with progressive high-grade encephalopathy, renal failure, or any component of the systemic inflammatory response syndrome (SIRS) should be given broad-spectrum antibiotics (73). In any ALF patients receiving antibiotics, the number of intravenous lines should be minimized and the care of the intravenous lines should be done with only strict aseptic technique. In severely ill patients, surveillance of blood, urine, and sputum cultures are recommended along with frequent chest radiographs (73).

Cerebral Edema and Intracranial Hypertension

Cerebral edema can result in death for patients with ALF. Although the mechanism of edema is multifaceted and poorly understood, the uptake of ammonia by astrocytes resulting in an accumulation of osmotically active glutamine is involved, followed by a passive influx of water (82).

In patients with cirrhosis and hyperammonemia, where intracranial hypertension (ICH) rarely occurs, it is thought that a slower rate of glutamine accumulation is offset by the export of organic osmolytes from the astrocytes to maintain osmotic balance. Interventions to minimize the risks and complications associated with ICH should be applied to all patients with ALF with hepatic encephalopathy. The head of the bed should be elevated to 30 degrees. Elevations higher than this is contraindicated as cerebral blood flow may be compromised when when the head of the bed is higher than 30 degrees. To promote venous return from the cranium, the neck should be kept in straight alignment to keep the internal jugular veins in the correct anatomical position. Painful stimuli, including suctioning, should be avoided, and a state of mild respiratory alkalosis is recommended (to a PCO_2 of 30 to 35 mm Hg) (73). There is ongoing debate related to the placement of ICP monitors, and practices vary from institution to institution. However, the U.S. Acute Liver Failure Study Group recently endorsed the placement of ICP monitors in patients with ALF who are at high risk for ICH, including nontransplant candidates who fall into groups that have shown high spontaneous survival rates (hepatitis A or acetaminophen overdose patients) (83).

ICH parameters form the basis for the administration of mannitol, an osmotic diuretic that draws water from astrocytes into the intravascular space. Most patients with ALF who maintain high levels of ICH, despite described interventions, progress to brain herniation and death (73). There are other approaches that are considered "salvage maneuvers" that are used to lower ICH, such as the induction of a barbiturate coma, the use of paralytic agents and deep sedation, and intravenous indomethacin (25-mg boluses). Intractable ICH can also result in brain herniation during transplantation as increased ICH frequently occurs with the dissection of the native liver and following reperfusion of the transplanted liver (73). Therapeutic hypothermia is a method that has commonly been used to improve cerebral edema in other conditions where ICH contributes to brain injury. In some experimental models with ALF patients, the induction of hypothermia has been shown to be neuroprotective, with numerous benefits on a variety of physiologic targets (84). Before there is widespread adoption of the practice, there is a need for more research to validate the efficacy of hypothermia for ICH in patients with ICH.

Bleeding Diathesis

Even though abnormal PT and abnormal INR results are common in patients with ALF and are part of the definition of ALF syndrome, spontaneous, significant bleeding rarely occurs. This is where a large distinction can be seen between patients with ALF and those with chronic conditions resulting in liver failure. Patients with ALF have essentially normal portal pressures, and bleeding generally occurs from the superficial mucosa as opposed to varices (73). The administration of histamine$_2$ receptor antagonists, which suppress gastric acid secretion, has been shown to decrease the risk of mucosal bleeding, resulting in a decrease in the transfusion requirements of persons with ALF.

There are limited data related to the coagulopathy in patients with ALF and complications associated with bleeding during invasive procedures. Additionally, evidence-based guidelines related to INR goals do not exist, although many experts agree that the INR should be corrected to equal or less than 1.5 (73). It is important to consider that PT/INR results poorly reflect the bleeding risk in ALF patients because liver-derived anticoagulants decrease proportionately to the procoagulant factors produced in the liver. Although there are no data to support the correction of coagulopathy before invasive procedures in patients with ALF, the practice is nearly universal (73).

Liver Assist Devices and Transplantation for ALF

There are currently two general types of liver assist devices that are available for persons with ALF. These devices are either biologic devices, which use living hepatocytes to replace liver function, or artificial devices, such as the molecular absorbent recirculating device (MARS), which removes injurious substances from circulation (70). However, a recent meta-analysis found that MARS offers no significant survival benefit over standard medical therapy (85). There have been numerous clinical trials involving porcine hepatocytes and some involving human hepatocytes. The overall results thus far indicate that they are quite costly and have not resulted in improved liver synthetic function or survival for persons with ALF.

Patients with ALF receive the utmost priority for liver transplantation when they have no prior history of liver disease and fulfill the criteria for ALF with poor prognosis. In patients who are potential candidates, the importance of avoiding complications that could preclude transplantation becomes a priority. With consideration of transplantation it is imperative that the patient's social network, mental stability, compliance with medical management, and personal wishes be considered. Psychiatric stability and evidence of a strong social support are important considerations in determining a potential transplant patient's status. It is important to identify and document any active drug or alcohol abuse, suicidal attempts, or current suicidal ideations, as all of these are contraindications for a liver transplant (70).

Chronic Liver Failure
Etiology

Patients with chronic liver conditions have a poor survival rate when they are admitted to intensive care units, even when they survive the initial intensive care unit stay. Acute hepatic decompensation in patients with chronic liver disease, acute-on-chronic liver failure (AoCLF), is usually the result of sepsis or hemorrhage (70). In addition, the dysregulation of the liver and inability to perform life-sustaining functions are further insulted by an increased physiologic demand, which leads to life-threatening conditions such as infection, renal failure, ascites, and bleeding (70). An initial and vital step in the management of persons with AoCLF is the identification of the precipitating events and factors that led to the acute episode of decompensation.

Pathophysiology

Portal Hypertensive Bleeding

Bleeding as the result of portal hypertension is a serious complication for persons with chronic liver disease. Bleeding in patients with AoCLF often originates from gastroesophageal varices or portal hypertensive gastropathy or, less frequently, from portal colopathy, duodenal, or rectal varices (70). Acute variceal hemorrhage occurs in 30% to 35% of patients with cirrhosis and carries a high mortality rate.

Hepatic Encephalopathy

GI bleeding for patients with AoCLF is a common precipitant to hepatic encephalopathy (HE). Other conditions or factors that contribute to HE include medications, infections, dehydration, electrolyte disturbances, constipation, and worsening liver function (70). Spontaneous bacterial peritonitis is the most common infection in persons with AoCLF, and sometimes HE is the only manifestation of spontaneous bacterial peritonitis (70).

Infection

As in patients with ALF, systemic bacterial infections complicate about 35% to 66% of the cases of patients with AoCLF. This often leads to sepsis, septic shock, and multisystem organ dysfunction.

Spontaneous Bacterial Peritonitis

Spontaneous bacterial peritonitis (SBP) is a frequent and severe complication of chronic liver disease, especially for persons who have cirrhosis and ascites. Mortality and morbidity in SBP are highly correlated with accompanying renal failure, and worsening HE, which often culminates in hemodynamic collapse in critically ill patients (70). Renal complications related to SBP result from a decrease in circulating blood volume, surges in inflammatory mediators, and the activation of the renin-angiotensin mechanism. Presence of bacteria in the ascitic fluid is thought to be the result of transmigration of intestinal flora due to a variety of mechanisms. Risk factors for the development of SBP include a previous history of SBP, advanced liver disease, gastric bleeding, and a total protein count of less than or equal to 1 g/dL (70).

Ascites

Ascites is the result of altered hemodynamics commonly found in individuals with cirrhosis and portal hypertension. It is associated with a 50% 2-year survival (70). Ascites presents with a myriad of potential complications, including increased pressure on the thoracic space, making breathing more difficult. Massive ascites can worsen renal failure by placing pressure on the renal arteries and diminishing perfusion to the kidneys.

Renal Failure

Renal failure in cirrhotic patients with massive ascites is characterized by hepatorenal syndrome (HRS) and occurs in about 20% of cirrhotic patients (87). There are two types of HRS differentiated by the extent of renal failure and the rapidity in which the process develops. HRS I occurs when there is a rapid and severe deterioration of renal function. In these cases survival is measured in days to weeks (70). HRS II is a slower and more stable renal dysfunction. Classifications of HRS are determined by a variety of laboratory data and diagnostic testing, including creatinine levels, urine protein, red blood cells, and osmolarity, along with imaging studies negative for primary renal disease, with no evidence of sustained improvement in renal function after hydration. Renal vasoconstriction is the result of a compensatory mechanism brought on by splanchnic arteriolar vasodilation and central vasodilation. Renal vasoconstriction results in a decreased glomerular filtration rate accompanied by an increase in sodium and water retention (70).

Management

Successful outcomes for patients experiencing portal hypertensive bleeding depend on prompt identification of the bleeding source, control of bleeding, prompt resuscitation, hemodynamic support, and management of complications.

The administration of lactulose is typically first-line therapy for HE for the reduction of ammonia levels. It is effective when given orally and titrated to a dose that prompts three or four bowel movements daily. When a patient still manifests signs of HE, even when lactulose is effective in achieving adequate bowel movements, nonabsorbable antibiotics such as neomycin or rifaxamin have been shown to be beneficial (70).

Another treatment aimed at ameliorating HE includes the use of supplemental zinc. Zinc is a cofactor for the urea cycle and can increase the clearance of ammonia, although zinc levels are frequently decreased in patients with HE and cirrhosis. Supplemental zinc sulfate 600 mg/day normalizes zinc levels, decreases ammonia, and improves HE (70).

Management of systemic infection and SBP associated with chronic liver failure is the same as any other etiology of sepsis and follows the principles of early, goal-directed therapy described in Chapter 15. Additionally, there have been clinical trials showing that antibiotic prophylaxis targeted at enteric organisms is effective in the prevention of post-bleeding infections in persons with cirrhosis.

Uncomplicated ascites is frequently managed through a combination of interventions. Sodium restriction

(<88 mmol/day) and potassium-sparing diuretics such as aldactone alone or in combination with a loop diuretic such as furosemide are recommended (70). When diuretic therapy is used, doses are increased until therapeutic efficacy is reached or limited by worsening renal function or hyponatremia. In these cases, large-volume paracentesis with albumin or shunts might be used. Although the latter interventions are helpful in improving ascites, they do not improve survival (70, 86). Albumin with large-volume paracentesis helps maintain intravascular volume and minimizes postparacentesis circulatory dysfunction. Large-volume paracentesis with albumin infusions should be reserved for patients with massive ascites who are experiencing respiratory difficulties or impaired renal perfusion. When infusions of albumin, other colloids, and large volumes of crystalloids are used without concomitant large-volume paracentesis, the ascitic condition worsens (70).

Management of renal failure is consistent with management approaches for other etiologies of renal failure. Renal replacement therapy in the acute setting may be accomplished by one of several methods of continuous, slow dialysis, or filtration, whereas intermittent dialysis is typically used in long-term management. A description of each is detailed in Chapter 13.

Clinical Nurse Specialist Competencies and Spheres of Influence
Clinical Expert/Direct Care
Management of patients with acute or chronic hepatic failure is a challenge. Multisystem involvement, complex etiology, and potential mental health and substance abuse issues must be recognized early. Often the CNS is pivotal in evaluation of the patient through the trajectory of the disease process, recognizing subtle changes over time.

Collaboration
Ultimate treatment for many persons with chronic liver disease is transplantation. Collaboration among a large network of providers ranging from transplant surgical services to the United Network of Organ Sharing (UNOS) requires skill in principles of case management. The CNS is pivotal in this process, with knowledge of the patient's history and current health status, recognizing changes in the patient that may place him or her higher on the list for transplantation or, conversely, make the patient ineligible for transplantation. The CNS coordinates care, interagency transfer, and communication among health care professionals and organizations to ensure prompt and accurate treatment of persons with acute and chronic liver failure.

Coaching/Teaching/Mentoring
Symptom recognition and prompt intervention while awaiting transplantation or spontaneous recovery are critical for satisfactory outcomes in patients with acute or chronic liver disease. The CNS must educate frontline nurses in fundamental interventions such as head of bed levels, strict fluid intake and output measurements, and safety measures necessary for patients with altered mental status.

Liver Transplantation
Orthotopic liver transplantation (OLT) was initially developed as a treatment for persons dying of end-stage hepatic failure and is now used routinely for patients with acute liver failure. Liver transplantation is currently considered an option for any patient who has progressive, irreversible acute or chronic hepatic disease in which therapeutic interventions show no efficacy. There are a variety of diseases associated with hepatic failure for which transplantation is considered; however, the most common indications for liver transplantation in adults are alcohol-induced liver disease and chronic viral hepatitis (88). The 1-year survival rate for patients undergoing liver transplantation is from 66% to 77% (89), with a 5-year survival rate of 70% or greater.

Candidate selection for liver transplantation is complex on many levels. Considerations include the patient's immediate health status, surgical risk, and predicted survival of the effects of long-term immunosuppression. (90). Some of the relative contraindications for liver transplantation include older than 70 years, certain malignancies outside of the liver, HIV-positive status, peripheral vasculature disease, severe infection, brain death, and psychosocial behaviors indicating noncompliance to medical regimens (90, 91). The criteria for patient placement on a transplantation list include evidence that the patient has a life expectancy of less than 7 days without a transplant, is 18 years of age or older (but less than 70), had an onset of HE within 8 weeks of the first symptoms of liver disease, is currently in an intensive care unit, has limited preexisting liver disease, and has at least one of the following: (1) ventilator dependence, (2) renal replacement therapy, or (3) INR greater than 2.0 (91).

There are several types of liver transplants that can be performed, which depends on the availability of the donor organ. These types include transplantation from a deceased donor, living donor split grafts, variable ABO status, and auxiliary liver transplants. As there continues to be a shortage of organs available for transplant, the risk of mortality while waiting for an organ should be the main consideration when weighed against the risk of complications or failure using an alternative graft (91). Different types of liver transplantation, with an explanation about each, are presented in Table 12-10.

Clinical Nurse Specialist Competencies and Spheres of Influence
Systems Leadership
Regardless of the type of liver transplantation, the CNS is in a key position to provide continuity and constancy of care for patients undergoing transplantation.

TABLE 12–10 An Overview of Types of Liver Transplantation

Type of Liver Transplant	Explanation and Considerations
Deceased liver donor transplantation or "orthotopic liver transplant"	In cases where an individual does not have an option of a living donor, the patient may receive a liver from an individual who through some misfortune is brain dead, and the liver can be harvested while it is still viable. This is typically referred to as an "orthotopic liver transplant," where the individual who is the recipient has his or her liver removed and the donor's liver is placed into the cavity created by the extraction of the recipient's liver. This is the most common procedure for liver transplantation but is not always a viable option for many patients with liver disease, as the demand for viable organs far exceeds the supply.
Living donor liver transplantation (LDLT)	Adult-to-adult LDLT has been performed primarily with patients who present with cirrhosis and has a survival rate of 73% to 90%. Right lobe transplantation has a higher success rate; however, there are more complications with right lobe transplantation than with left lobe transplantation, including biliary leaks, seromas, and wound infections. Donor complications range from 8% for persons donating left lobes to 32% for right lobe donation. A donor mortality of 0.2% has been associated with right lobe donation. This is rapidly becoming more commonly used in children with hepatic failure as livers that are comparable in size are in short supply.
ABO-incompatibility grafts	ABO-identical grafts are preferred. ABO-incompatible grafts occur when the graft is O and the recipient is a blood type other than O. There are multiple complications associated with this type of transplantation that primarily affect the graft itself such as rejection, vascular thrombosis, or biliary injury. The degree of posttransplant outcomes when comparing ABO-compatible to ABO-incompatible remains controversial.
Auxillary transplantation	This occurs when a partial left or partial right lobe is transplanted from a donor and provides temporary support for the recipient's liver, which remains in place. Once the liver of the recipient recovers, the transplanted lobe is either removed or allowed to naturally atrophy. In most cases, immunosuppressant therapy can be halted once the native liver recovers.

This can be executed in the role of transplant coordinator, transplant case manager at the hospital level, or transplant nurse for donor services. The roles vary, and all warrant the clinical expertise and judgment of an advanced practice nurse. The CNS is central to the selection, evaluation, and ongoing assessment of patients at all phases of transplantation and must be cognizant of the legal and ethical ramifications of transplantation. The CNS must remain attuned to the standards set forth by the UNOS and evaluate the patient in terms of those standards for the patient's eligibility as an organ recipient.

Coaching/Teaching/Mentoring

Because most patients who receive liver transplants take life-long immunosuppressants, there is a great deal of patient and family teaching that follows. Evaluation of immunosuppressant therapy side effects and complications and monitoring for signs of potential rejection are critical aspects of patient/family education.

Enteral Nutrition

There remains much discussion about the appropriate substrate and timing of enteral nutrition in patients who are acutely and critically ill. Other issues surrounding enteral nutrition include questions about the delivery of nutrition, gastric versus small-bowel tube placement, and concerns about what markers accurately indicate intolerance to enteral nutrition (92). It is well understood that illness, especially critical illness, results in an increased metabolic state in patients, resulting in a condition often referred to as "stress hypermetabolism." This can lead to malnutrition, which has been associated with increased mortality and morbidity. The generally accepted goals of nutritional delivery in critically ill patients are to provide nutritional support consistent with the patient's condition, prevent nutrient deficiencies, avoid complications related to delivering nutrition, and improve patient outcomes (93).

Nutritional support involves a variety of methods by which nutrients are administered to patients to encourage optimal nutritional status. In patients who are unable to swallow for any variety of reasons, there are two main forms of delivery. Enteral nutrition refers to the introduction of nutrients directly into the alimentary tract via a nasogastric tube, an orogastric tube, or a tube that is placed in the alimentary tract through a surgical procedure such as a gastrostomy tube or jejunostomy tube. Parenteral nutrition involves introducing nutrients into the patient's vasculature preferably through a central line or sometimes through a peripheral line. Whenever possible, the enteral route is preferred as "bowel rest" that occurs with parenteral nutrition interferes with the immunologic and barrier function of the GI tract. Enteral nutrition enhances mucosal integrity, maintains intestinal blood flow, and contributes to the maintenance of the immune system (94). Additionally, the intestinal stimulation by enteral nutrients further maintains bowel integrity; decreases translocation of bacterial flora in the intestine, which further results in less infectious sequelae; and decreases length of hospital stay (95). For patients in whom enteral nutrition is possible, there is no disease state that is known to benefit from parenteral nutrition over enteral nutrition (96).

Indications for and Implementation of Enteral Nutrition

All patients who are not expected to take a full oral diet within 72 hours should receive enteral nutrition (97). Prior to initiating enteral nutrition, assessment should include evaluation of weight loss, previous nutrient intake before the disease and severity of disease, comorbid conditions, and function of the GI tract. Keep in mind that traditional nutritional assessment tools such as albumin, prealbumin, and anthropometry are not validated in the critical care setting (98).

Tube feeding should be initiated slowly (20 ml/hr) with permissive underfeeding for the first 3 to 5 days of 15 to 20 kcal/kg/day and then advanced to a goal of 20 to 25 kcal/kg/day as the patient's condition improves. Patients with severe undernutrition should receive enteral nutrition up to 25 to 30 kcal/kg/day. If these target values are not met, supplemental parenteral nutrition should be given (97). Should the patient require significant hemodynamic support, including high-dose inotropes, alone or in combination with large-volume or blood product resuscitation, enteral nutrition should be withheld until the patient is stable. For patients in critical care areas, neither the presence or absence of bowel sounds, nor the passage of flatulence or stool is a prerequisite to the initiation of enteral nutrition (98). Assessment data provide a baseline but should not dictate the initiation of enteral nutrition.

Either gastric or small bowel feeding is appropriate in acute and critical care areas, as the route should be guided by patient risk for aspiration. In some cases, withholding enteral nutrition for repeated high gastric residual volumes alone may constitute sufficient rationale for switching from a gastric tube to a small bowel feeding tube (98). Otherwise, there is no significant difference in the efficacy of jejunal versus gastric feeding (97). If at all possible, additional parenteral nutrition in patients who tolerate enteral nutrition should be avoided and are fed approximate to the target values. If the patient cannot be fed sufficiently via the enteral route, use supplemental parenteral nutrition at a level that meets, but does not exceed, the nutritional needs of the patient.

There are no current data indicating improvement in outcomes for patients who receive early enteral nutrition. However, the current recommendation is that critically ill patients who are hemodynamically stable and have a functioning GI tract should be fed in less than 24 hours, using the appropriate amount and type of formula (97, 98).

Type of Formula

As no advantage of peptide-based formula is evident, whole protein formula is the appropriate choice for most patients (97). Immune-modulating formulas, those enriched with argine, nucleotides, and omega-3 fatty acids, are superior to standard formulas for patients who have undergone elective GI surgery, in patients with mild sepsis, in patients with trauma, and in patients with head and neck cancer. Patients with acute respiratory distress syndrome and severe acute lung injury should be placed on enteral formula containing anti-inflammatory lipids (omega-3 fish oils, borage oil) and antioxidants. For the patient to receive maximum benefit of the immune-modulating formulas, at least 50% to 65% of the goal energy requirements should be delivered (98). Immune-modulating formulas are not recommended in patients with severe sepsis or in critically ill patients who do not tolerate more than 700 mL enteral formula per day, as immune-modulating formulas may be detrimental (97). In burn-injured patients, formulas containing higher than standard doses of copper, selenium, and zinc should be considered. Trauma and burn patients should receive formula with added glutamine (97). In cases where diarrhea ensues, soluble fiber or small peptide formulas are indicated, but further evaluation for the etiology of the diarrhea is warranted. Insoluble fiber formulas should be avoided in all critically ill patients, and both soluble and insoluble fiber should be avoided in patients who are at risk for bowel ischemia or severe dysfunction in GI mobility (98).

Monitoring the Tolerance and Adequacy of Enteral Nutrition

For hospitalized patients, evidence of bowel motility is not required to initiate enteral nutrition, although assessment baseline parameters should be identified. Patients receiving enteral nutrition should be monitored for tolerance of the formula, which can be determined from patient complaints of pain or distention, passage of flatus and stool, as well as abdominal radiographs (98). As inappropriate cessation of enteral nutrition should be avoided, it is imperative that the clinician understand and recognize indications that warrant continuance and cessation of enteral nutrition. Avoid withholding enteral nutrition for gastric residual volumes less than 500 mL in the absence of other signs, although this in and of itself is not an indication to withhold formula. Enteral feeding protocols have been shown to increase the overall percentage of goal calories and should be implemented (98). Additionally, protocols abet consistency among nurses in the delivery of enteral nutrition.

Patients placed on enteral nutrition should be assessed for aspiration risk and steps to reduce this risk should be implemented. Measures that have shown to reduce the risk of aspiration include the following: (1) In all patients in critical care units who are intubated, the head of the bed should be elevated 30 to 45 degrees. (2) Continuous infusion of enteral nutrition should be implemented for patients who are at high risk for aspiration or who are intolerant to gastric feeding. (3) Prokinetic agents used to promote motility such as metoclopramide and erythromycin (97, 98) or narcotic agonists such as naloxone or alvimopan should be initiated if clinically feasible. (4) Diversion of the level of feeding by post pyloric tube placement, such as a Dobhoff tube, should be considered (98). If using erythromycin to promote motility, the clinician must outweigh this benefit to the possible risk of bacterial resistance. The use of chlorhexidine mouthwash twice a day reduces the risk of ventilator-associated pneumonia. Blue food coloring and glucose oxidase strips, which once were popular surrogate markers for aspiration, should not be used (98).

Clinical Nurse Specialist Competencies and Spheres of Influence
Clinical Expert/Direct Care and Coaching/ Teaching/Mentoring

Several enteral nutrition practices are directly influenced by CNSs. Advocating for enteral nutrition as opposed to parenteral nutrition when indicated, identifying the times to increase volumes, preventing aspiration through implementation of evidence-based protocols, and preventing feeding tube occlusions fall within the purview of the advanced practice nurse. As such, it is imperative for the CNS to teach nurses at the bedside procedures and standards of care for patients receiving enteral nutrition. As protocols have shown consistency and improvement in patient outcomes, the CNS is ideally postured to develop evidence-based protocols for efficient enteral nutrition delivery, optimizing outcomes, and eliminating complications. The CNS must have information about which types of formulas are indicated in which circumstances, and should share this information with nurses and other clinicians.

Research/Evidence-Based Practice

The Joint Commission (TJC) has mandated that evidence-based practice initiatives be launched as part of hospital performance improvement; administration of enteral nutrition provides an important opportunity for use of evidence to improve care. There are numerous research studies under way, and there are replications of older studies to determine the most beneficial formulas, most efficient methods of delivery, and measures to minimize risks associated with enteral nutrition. The CNS must stay abreast of the literature to ensure that protocols created for use in the clinical environment are effective and safe and demonstrate positive patient outcomes. A comprehensive model of nutrition delivery can be created through collaboration with dietitians and other health care professionals.

ABDOMINAL TRAUMA

Blunt Abdominal Trauma
Etiology

There are typically two classifications of abdominal trauma. One type is blunt abdominal trauma (BAT), which is historically encountered more frequently in the emergency department than the other type of trauma referred to as "penetrating" abdominal trauma. BAT is most typically the result of motor vehicle collision and, when combined with pedestrian-related accidents, accounts for 75% of BAT (100). Falls and direct abdominal blows account for the other 25% (100, 101). Blunt trauma occurs when there is a force to the abdomen that does not leave an open wound. Examples of blunt trauma are compression and shearing trauma. Compression trauma is the result of a direct blow, such as being thrust against a steering wheel or pressure from a seat, and shearing trauma occurs when anatomical parts of the body move in opposite directions or when one part remains stationary while another portion of the body moves forward (acceleration/deceleration injury). Penetrating trauma occurs when there is an open wound to the abdomen, such as in cases of a gunshot wound or a stab wound or when an object is impaled into the abdomen, leaving a wound.

Management

There are interventions common to both BAT and penetrating abdominal trauma, regardless of the etiology. As with any other type of trauma, the patency of airway, the presence and quality of breathing, and any problems related to circulation should be identified and treatment initiated in a timely manner (102). Should there be any indication of protruding viscera, they should be covered with a sterile dressing moistened with normal saline. There are other interventions for either type of abdominal trauma, including intravenous infusion of normal saline, or lactated Ringer's solution, and insertion of an indwelling catheter, unless there is evidence of an injury to the urinary tract. Pain should be controlled as much as possible without sedation so that the patient is awake and alert enough to describe subjective changes and provide information that alerts the clinician to subjective changes in status (102). Analgesics such as morphine and meperidine are good medication choices for controlling pain without sedation. Other recommendations once blood is drawn for appropriate laboratory data include the insertion of a gastric tube when there is no evidence of contraindications, such as accompanying head trauma, and administration of tetanus prophylaxis (102).

Due to the nature of the injury, BAT is more difficult to detect than penetrating trauma, and correct diagnosis is contingent upon expert assessment skills. The spleen is the most injured organ and may be the only injured organ in over 60% of patients with intra-abdominal injury, followed by liver and then hollow viscous injuries. Physical exam is the cornerstone of primary assessment of BAT. In patients who are stable and conscious, a complete assessment is possible including inspection, auscultation, percussion, and palpation. For patients who are not stable or who are unconscious, the clinician may need to rely on inspection data.

Inspection includes the detection of any distention, contusions, abrasions, lacerations, as well as penetrating wounds, or abdominal asymmetry. In motor vehicle-related cases, trauma caused by a seatbelt is usually revealed by a contusion or abrasion across the lower abdomen, known as the "seat belt sign" (102). Ecchymosis around the umbilical area (Cullen's sign) or flanks (Grey-Turner sign) are often indicative of retroperitoneal hemorrhage but may be delayed presentations.

If not hampered by resuscitation efforts, bowel sounds should be auscultated, with attention to detecting an abdominal bruit. Auscultation in all four quadrants is preferred before percussion and palpation as these procedures can alter the frequency of bowel sounds. The absence of bowel sounds may indicate intraperitoneal damage, as blood and bacteria and chemical irritants can cause diminished or absent bowel sounds. Bowel sounds in the thorax are indicative of a ruptured diaphragm with small bowel herniation into the thoracic space. Bruits that are auscultated in the abdomen could be the result of arterial damage or signal the presence of an aneurysm (102).

After auscultation, if the patient is stable and alert, the patient should be asked to identify areas of pain. Examine those areas last, and if the pain is severe, do not palpate or percuss as this may worsen the pain and injury; diagnostic studies are warranted in order to accurately evaluate the abdomen (102). In patients who are hemodynamically stable and awake, abdominal pain, tenderness, and peritoneal signs are the most reliable findings for intra-abdominal injury as they are found in 90% of patients experiencing abdominal injury (100).

Dull sounds over solid organs and fluid-filled structures and tympany over air-filled areas are normal abdominal findings. Loss of dullness over solid organs indicates the presence of air, which may indicate bowel perforation. Dullness over regions that are normally tympanic may indicate an accumulation of fluid or blood. When pain accompanies light percussion, the clinician should suspect peritoneal inflammation. The presence of Ballance's sign, which is fixed dullness in the left flank, shifting dullness in the right flank while the patient is lying on his or her left side, indicates blood around the spleen or spleen injury (102).

Gentle palpation should begin in an area that has not been identified as painful. One quadrant at a time should be palpated for involuntary guarding, tenderness, rigidity, spasm, and localized pain (102). Absence of findings may be the result of an uninjured abdomen or could be masked by the presence of alcohol or other traumatic injuries such as spinal cord trauma, retroperitoneal hematoma, or decreasing level of consciousness. Discomfort during palpation may indicate peritonitis. Though inspection, auscultation, percussion, and palpation are fundamental to initial assessment, they may have limited use in patients with abdominal trauma. The absence of physical findings early especially does not exclude injury and the need for further evaluation and diagnostic testing (103, 104).

Diagnosis

Most hematologic and blood studies serve only as adjuvants in the management of patients with abdominal trauma; however, they do serve as baseline data and may provide parameters for worsening or stable conditions. As in the cases of any suspected hemorrhage, blood typing should be sent in case a transfusion is warranted. Pancreatic enzymes, liver function tests, and white blood cell counts have traditionally been used as markers of intra-abdominal injury; however, current studies show these have limited usefulness in the acute decision-making for patients with abdominal trauma (100, 105). Urinalysis showing the presence of erythrocytes indicates renal injury. Toxicology studies have little value in the management of abdominal trauma, but are useful in ruling out causes of altered mental status.

When a patient with BAT is hemodynamically unstable, identification of the need for emergent surgical intervention is a priority. CT is considered the standard of care in diagnosing abdominal injury and is the preferred method in hemodynamically unstable patients (106, 107). The issue of contrast versus no contrast and the method of contrast pose controversy in the use of CT. Focused abdominal sonography for trauma (FAST) offers an alternative to CT that is portable, fast, and noninvasive and does not require exposure to radiation. It is considered by some to be an effective screening tool in the hypotensive patient and when coupled with other data, can effectively rule out intra-abdominal injury that warrants surgery. Some authorities have identified that for stable patients, a negative FAST, coupled with a physical exam that is negative for abdominal findings, followed by an observation period of 12 to 24 hours, essentially excludes intra-abdominal injury. There are some trauma experts who recommend serial abdominal ultrasound studies to increase the sensitivity of the FAST exam (100).

In a recent study (2009) concerned with ionizing radiation exposure, expense, and overall feasibility with the use of CT for all persons with potential BAT, it was concluded that persons with no high-risk variables for abdominal injury are unlikely to benefit from abdominal CT scanning for confirming a diagnosis. Instead, the researchers identified hypotension, Glasgow Coma Scale score less than 14, costal margin tenderness, abdominal tenderness, femur fracture, hematuria level greater than or equal to 25 red blood cells/high-power field (RBCs/hpf), hematocrit less than 30%, and rib fracture or pneumothorax on radiograph as predictors of high risk for abdominal injury related to BAT (107).

Penetrating Trauma
Etiology

The incidence of penetrating trauma is increasing due to the increase of violence in our society. Stab wounds are three times more prevalent than gunshot wounds but, due their lower velocity and less invasive patterns, carry a lower mortality (100). Because of their force and movement trajectories, gunshot wounds account for up to 90% of the mortality associated with penetrating abdominal trauma. The solid organs of the abdomen can bleed profusely when injured, whereas the hollow organs are less likely to bleed significantly but are more likely to cause peritonitis when damaged.

Clinical Presentation

It is imperative that persons sustaining penetrating trauma be thoroughly undressed and be examined for injury. In the case of gunshot wounds, patients will often present with an obvious entry wound in the anterior abdomen and may have an exit, or secondary, wound in the axilla, perineum, scalp, back, or skinfold that could go unnoticed, which might be lethal. Various types of guns and bullets produce variant patterns when in contact with the target, and in some cases, what look like minor exit and entry wounds can accompany tremendous internal damage due to the trajectory pattern of the bullet that passed through the patient.

Management

With object impalement, immediate surgical intervention is indicated. The need for surgical intervention is less apparent in cases of stabbings or gunshot wounds. In the presence of hemodynamic instability or the presence of peritoneal signs on physical exam, immediate laparotomy is indicated (100, 108). In the presence of evisceration, surgical intervention is warranted, especially when the evisceration is the result of a gunshot wound, as there is more diffuse trauma and higher risk of contamination associated with these injuries.

Diagnosis

Penetrating injuries as the result of stab wounds produce peritoneal violation in about 70% of the cases, but only about 25% of these patients will require surgery. For patients without complications such as peritonitis, evisceration, and hemodynamic instability, options such as wound exploration, CT, laparoscopy, or ultrasound along with physical exam can eliminate the need for surgical intervention (100). Some centers will use a FAST study or diagnostic laparoscopy to determine the need for surgery. Diagnostic laparoscopy is less expensive and associated with a shorter length of hospital stay than an exploratory laparotomy. Diagnostic peritoneal lavage determines the presence of peritoneal violation and injury. This is a rapid but invasive test that reveals information regarding potential injury to the solid viscous, bowel, or diaphragm (100). Whereas there is some controversy, the consensus is that the presence of greater than 10,000 RBCs/hpf is indicative of visceral injury.

When penetrating abdominal trauma is the result of a gunshot wound, it is important to identify the number of bullet perforations and use radiographic studies to determine the path and pattern of the bullet is indicated. A three-dimensional estimation trajectory path can be created through the use of radiopaque markers and anteroposterior radiographic films (100). For every entry wound, there should be a corresponding exit wound, or the bullet or missile is still inside the patient's body. CT is also used to determine the trajectory of the bullet and organ damage and helps determine the need for surgical intervention. The use of laparoscopy to determine peritoneal violation and to inspect the diaphragm is increasing (100).

Clinical Nurse Specialist Competencies and Spheres of Influence
Clinical Expert/Direct Care and Systems Leadership

The evaluation and management of abdominal trauma require the expertise of an advanced practice nurse. The development of protocols for the treatment of both blunt and penetrating abdominal trauma allow the health care team to provide standardized care that can be implemented quickly, save process time, and increase the likelihood of desired outcomes. In many cases of abdominal trauma, an alert patient can quickly decompensate. Rapid evaluation of the patient with an abdominal injury must be executed, using advanced assessment skills because there may be no outward signs of trauma at all. Knowing when to intervene during decompensation

with resuscitative efforts is a critical aspect of patient care that is often led by the CNS.

ABDOMINAL COMPARTMENT SYNDROME

Although commonly thought of as a problem confined to injured extremities, compartment syndrome is also important to consider when pressure increases within the abdomen. There is an increased awareness of abdominal compartment syndrome (ACS) over the past decade. Whereas the condition was previously recognized as only an issue related to blunt trauma patients, it is now appreciated that abdominal pressure elevations can occur in a variety of patients. It is essential that clinicians know the signs and symptoms of ACS and understand the importance of prompt and evidence-based interventions. The underlying issue related to ACS is the potential for the intra-abdominal pressure (IAP) to reach a point where blood flow to end organs is compromised, resulting in organ dysfunction or failure. To understand the dynamics of ACS, some basic concepts and terms are described in Table 12-11.

TABLE 12–11 Concepts and Terms Related to Abdominal Compartment Syndrome

Term or Concept	Explanation
Intra-abdominal Pressure (IAP)	This is the pressure located within the abdominal cavity. It is normally <5 mm Hg but can range under normal conditions from 0.2 mm Hg to 16.2 mm Hg. Increases with body mass index, but usually, sustained pressures greater than 15 mm Hg have been associated with impaired cardiac, respiratory, gastrointestinal, and central nervous system function.
Abdominal Perfusion Pressure (APP)	APP is the mean arterial pressure (MAP) minus the IAP. This is an index not only for the severity of the IAP but also the patient's perfusion status. Failure to maintain an APP of at least 60 mm Hg in patient with intra-abdominal hypertension (IAH) is correlated to an increased mortality.
Increased Abdominal Hypertension (IAH)	This is defined by the World Society of Abdominal Compartment Syndrome as the sustained increase in IAP of greater than or equal to 12 mm Hg, based on three standardized measurements completed 4-6 hours apart, with or without an APP of 60 mm Hg.
Abdominal Compartment Syndrome (ACS)	Sustained increase in IAP of greater than or equal to 20 mm Hg, with or without an APP <6 0 mm Hg and single or multiple organ system failure not previously present.
Primary ACS	A condition associated with an injury or disease in the abdominopelvic region that usually requires early surgical or radiologic intervention, or a condition that follows abdominal surgery. Characterized by the presence of acute or subacute IAH specific to intra-abdominal causes.

Continued

TABLE 12–11 Concepts and Terms Related to Abdominal Compartment Syndrome—cont'd

Term or Concept	Explanation
Secondary ACS	Caused by conditions not originating in the abdomen but result in signs and symptoms associated with primary ACS. Some conditions that prompt secondary ACS include sepsis, major burns, or other conditions that require massive fluid resuscitation.
Recurrent ACS	Develops following prophylactic or therapeutic treatment (medical or surgical) or primary or secondary ACS.

Etiology

Any abnormality that elevates the pressure within the abdominal cavity can result in IAH. Some of these conditions include abdominal surgery, massive fluid resuscitation (more than 5 liters in 24 hours), intra-abdominal infection, pneumoperitoneum, (including the result of a laparoscopy), hemoperitoneum, and intestinal ileus that can be paralytic, mechanical, or pseudo-obstructive in nature (109-112). There are a variety of common clinical conditions that warrant prospective monitoring due to the high risk of IAH. Some of these conditions include postoperative abdominal surgery, blunt or penetrating abdominal trauma, pelvic fractures with retroperitoneal bleeding, patients with multiorgan dysfunction, or sepsis-related organ failure who are mechanically ventilated (113). There is an increased risk of developing ACS in any patient with increased abdominal contents including patients with ascites or liver dysfunction.

Pathophysiology

The pathophysiology of ACS is similar to the genesis of compartment syndrome in other body regions. The abdominal compartment is bounded. The lower aspect of the compartment is the pelvic floor; the abdomen is circumferentially bounded by the abdominal wall and superiorly by the diaphragm. Although the diaphragm is not a rigid structure, pressure within the abdomen typically raises the diaphragm and puts pressure within the thoracic space.

Organ damage sustained from IAH is usually clinically significant before organ dysfunction is evident. As with extremity compartmental syndromes, however, there is a threshold at which the microvascular derangement becomes self-propagating. When the elevations in IAP increase, resulting in venous outflow resistance, there results a venous congestion and further increase in intra-compartmental pressures (113). When the IAP is greater than 20 mm Hg, there is a drastic reduction in perfusion, which leads to tissue ischemia and the activation of inflammatory mediators. This leads to an increase in intra-abdominal pressure as an influx of fluid into the intra-abdominal compartment occurs as the result of intravascular fluid loss caused by capillary fluid leak into the abdomen. Additionally, the lymphatic system to the area is impaired, leading to an increase in intestinal edema (113, 114). There are multiple pathophysiologic changes that are associated with IAH and ACS. See Table 12-12 for an overview of these changes.

TABLE 12–12 Pathophysiologic Changes Associated With Intra-abdominal Hypertension and Abdominal Compartment Syndrome

System	Physiologic Changes
Cardiovascular	Hemodynamic compromise can occur when IAP exceeds 20 mm Hg, as this elevation can alter preload, afterload, and intrathoracic pressures. Preload is reduces as the result of caval compression that reduces cardiac output. High IAP compresses the abdominal vascular beds, which results in an increase in afterload. An elevated diaphragm due to increased abdominal pressures will result in compression of the pericardium and a decrease in left ventricular end-diastolic volume. Increases in intrathoracic pressures associated with ACS can cause indirect measures of cardiac performance, such as

TABLE 12-12 Pathophysiological Changes Associated With Intra-abdominal Hypertension and Abdominal Compartment Syndrome—cont'd

System	Physiological Changes
	central venous pressure and pulmonary artery occlusion pressure, to become falsely elevated.
Pulmonary	Increased IAP and ACS cause diaphragmatic elevations and decreases in thoracic space and wall compliance and can lead to respiratory failure.
Renal	IAP pressures from 15 to 20 mm Hg have been shown to lower renal flow and glomerular filtration, resulting in oliguria. Anuria can occur with pressures about 30 mm Hg. This is the result of renal vascular resistance as well as decreased perfusion due to cardiovascular alterations. Plasma levels of aldosterone, renin, and antidiuretic hormone are elevated in ACS, with resultant sodium and water retention, and increased urine osmolarity.
Gastrointestinal	Elevations in IAP has a detrimental effect on splanchnic perfusion with decreased blood flow and tissue hypoxia. Elevations in IAP can reduce flow to all abdominal viscera, leading to bowel ischemia and mucosal acidosis. The progression of this ischemia can lead to mesenteric thrombosis.
Neurological	IAH is a risk factor for the development of secondary brain injury in persons with traumatic brain injury. Increases in IAP have been shown to increase intracranial pressure as the result of increased central venous pressure and functional obstruction to cerebral outflow.

Clinical Presentation

Understanding the pathophysiology of ACS provides the basis for understanding of presenting symptoms seen in these cases. The classic signs of ACS include decreased arterial oxygenation, elevations in partial pressure of carbon dioxide, high peak inspiratory pressures, oliguria or anuria, and a massively distended or tense abdomen (115). As many critical care patients experience some of these symptoms for other reasons, it is very difficult to identify the presence of ACS without diagnostic testing specific for ACS.

Diagnosis

The diagnosis of IAH and ACS is difficult because the clinical findings are poor indicators of IAP. There are a myriad of diagnostic tests that have been used to measure IAP including gastric pressure from a nasogastric tube, inferior vena cava pressure, rectal pressure, direct IAP via puncture, and use of the ultrasound to evaluate the quality and respiratory variation of the inferior vena cava (113). Elevations in IAP and even the presence of ACS might be discerned based on computed tomography findings; however, the current mainstay for the diagnosis of ACS is the measurement of IAP with an an indwelling transurethral catheter to measure intravesicular pressure (113, 115).

The standard technique to measure IAP via the bladder involves instilling 25 to 50 mL of sterile water into the bladder via a transurethral catheter. With the patient in a supine position, at end inspiration, 50 mL has been shown to be the most valid and accurate assessment (116). The catheter tubing is clamped, and the needle is inserted into the specimen collection port proximal to the clamp and attached to a pressure transducer. The zeroing point for the transducer is controversial, with some authorities suggesting that the transducer should be zeroed at the mid-axillary line (109, 113), and others suggesting it be zeroed at the symphysis pubis (115, 117). Patients identified at risk for ACS should have a baseline measurement IAP completed and documented and the anatomical structure used for zeroing the transducer included in the documentation for consistency.

Management

The best management of ACS is prevention. Patients with ACS or impending ACS can be managed medically and/or surgically. The management depends on the severity of IAH with regard to the grading system for IAH. An explanation of the grading system can be found in Table 12-13. For patients at level 1 and 2 (IAH less

TABLE 12–13 Grades of Intra-abdominal Hypertension

Grade	IAP Reading	Management
I	I AH 12–15 mm Hg	Normovolemic resuscitation and continued monitoring
II	IAH 16–20 mm Hg	Hypervolemic resuscitation, continued monitoring, ensure adequate oxygenation and ventilation, and consideration of surgical decompression
III	IAH 21–25 mm Hg	Hypervolemic resuscitation and surgical decompression at bedside or in the operating room
IV	IAH >25 mm Hg	Hypervolemic resuscitation and decompression in the operating room

than 20 mm Hg), medical management might be all that is warranted. However, when a patient reaches level 2, the possibility of impending surgery must be considered. Until surgical intervention is warranted, there are some nonsurgical treatment options useful in lowering IAH. These options include gastric decompression via nasogastric suction, rectal decompression through the use of enemas, or rectal drainage catheters or tubes, sedation, neuromuscular blocking, positioning, or paracentesis. Other medications such as prokinetic agents for the stomach such as cisapride, metoclopramide, domperidone, or erythromycin might be used, whereas prokinetic agents for the colon such as prostigmine might be effective. Additionally, diuretics used either alone or in combination with 25% human albumin might be useful, as well as venovenous hemofiltration or ultrafiltration (113).

As ACS evolves, the self-propagation mechanism is created whereby increases in abdominal pressure promote further exacerbation of abdominal pressure. As the underlying problem is an increase of volume in the abdominal cavity with limited space, the immediate solution to ACS is to enlarge the space. The current standard to alleviate IAP is decompressive laparotomy with temporary abdominal wall closure to enlarge the peritoneal space, thus reducing the level of intra-abdominal pressure. However, there is a grading system with recommendations for management based on that grading system as identified in Table 12-13.

A significant complication associated with sudden decompression of the abdomen is reperfusion syndrome that could result in severe hypotension and possibly cardiac arrest. To ameliorate the incidence of reperfusion syndrome, there must be adequate volume resuscitation before opening the abdomen. Although hypervolemic resuscitation would seem to exacerbate the issue, this is done at and beyond stage II when a decompressive laparotomy is being considered or indicated. Despite the potential complications, decompressive laparotomy has been shown to be very successful in restoring normal physiological function (115).

Clinical Nurse Specialist Competencies and Spheres of Influence
Clinical Expert/Direct Care and Consultation

Early detection of ACS is imperative to prevent adverse sequelae. CNS competencies in diligent assessment, evaluation, and anticipation of this and other complications are imperative. The competencies of clinical expert and consultation in the patient and nurse spheres of influence are priorities at this time. Diligent assessment of the patient as well as education for the bedside nurse about the signs of IAH has a definitive impact on progression of ACS an overall patient outcome. The CNS applies expert knowledge in quickly assessing surrounding events and recognition of the complication and consultation with the medical practitioner for definitive intervention.

References

1. Grundman O, Yoon SL. Irritable bowel syndrome: epidemiology, diagnosis, and treatment: an update for healthcare practitioners. J Gastroenterol Hepatol 2009;25:691-699.

2. Drossman DA. Introduction. The Rome Foundation and the Rome III. Neurogastroenterol Motil 2007;19:783-786.

3. Schoenfeld P. Efficacy of current drug therapies in irritable bowel syndrome: what works and what does not work. Gastroenterol Clin North Am 2005;34:319-335.

4. Saito YA, Petersen GM, Locke GR, et al. The genetics of irritable bowel syndrome. Clin Gastroenterol Hepatol 2005;3(11):1057-1065.

5. Grover M, Herfarth H, Drossman DA. The functional-organic dichotomy: postinfectious irritable bowel syndrome and inflammatory bowel disease–irritable bowel syndrome. Clin Gastroenterol Hepatol 2009;7:48-53.

6. Jellema P, Van der Wint DAWM, Schellevis FG, et al. Systemic review: accuracy of symptom-based criteria for diagnosis of irritable bowel syndrome in primary care. Aliment Pharmacol Therap 2009;30:695-706.

7. Hillila MT, Farkkila MA. Prevalence of irritable bowel syndrome according to different diagnostic criteria in a non-selected adult population. Aliment Pharmacol Therap 2004;20:339-345.

8. Croghan A, Heitkemper MM. Recognizing and managing patients with irritable bowel syndrome. J Am Acad Nurse Pract 2005;17(2):51-59.

9. Korzenik JR. Past and current theories of the etiology of IBD: toothpaste, worms, and refrigerators. J Clin Gastroenterol 2005;39(4 suppl 2):S59-S65.

10. Gershon MD. Nerves, reflexes, and the enteric nervous system: pathogenesis of irritable bowel syndrome. J Clin Gastroenterol 2005;39(5 suppl 3):S184-193.

11. Coates MD, Mahoney CR, Linden DR, et al. Molecular defects in mucosal serotonin content and decreased serotonin reuptake transporter in ulcerative colitis and irritable bowel syndrome. Gastroenterology 2004;136:1657-1664.

12. Brophy L, Ignatavicius DD. Care of patients with noninflammatory intestinal disorders. In Ignatavicius DD, Workman ML, editors. Medical Surgical Nursing: Patient Centered Collaborative Care, 6th ed. St Louis: Saunders; 2010:1289-1314.

13. Vissers RJ, Lennarz WB. Pitfalls in appendicitis. Emerg Med Clin North Am 2010;28:103-118.

14. Yeh B. Does this adult have appendicitis? Ann Emerg Med 2008;52:301-303.

15. Ruschman K. (2010). Care of patients with inflammatory intestinal disorders. In Ignatavicius DD, Workman ML, editors. Medical Surgical Nursing: Patient Centered Collaborative Care, 6th ed. St Louis: Saunders; 2010:1315-1343.

16. Doria AS, Moineddin R, Kellenberger CJ, et al. US or CT for diagnosis of appendicitis in children and adults? A meta-analysis. Radiology 2006;241:83-94.

17. Alvarado A. A practical score for the early diagnosis of acute appendicitis. Ann Emerg Med 1986;15:557-564.

18. Ohmann C, Franke C, Yang Q, et al. Clinical benefit of a diagnostic score for appendicitis: results of a prospective interventional study. Arch Surg 1999;134:993-996.

19. McKay R, Shepard J. The use of the clinical scoring system by Alvarado in the decision to perform computed tomography for acute appendicitis in the ED. Am J Emerg Med 2007;25:489-493.

20. Rao PM, Rhea JT, Novelline RA, et al. Effect of continuous computed tomography of the appendix on treatment of patients and use of hospital resources. N Engl J Med 1998;338:141-146.

21. Elwood DR. Cholecystitis. Surg Clin North Am 2008;88:1241-1252.

22. Good EW, Sands JK. Gallbladder and exocrine pancreatic problems. In Monahan FD, Neighbors M, Sands JK, et al, editors. Phipp's Medical-Surgical Nursing: Health and Illness Perspectives, 8th ed. St Louis: Mosby; 2008:1285-1302.

23. Sands JK. (2003). Gallbladder and exocrine pancreatic problems. In Phipps WJ, Monahan FD, Sands JK, et al, editors. Phipp's Medical-Surgical Nursing: Health and Illness Perspectives, 7th ed. St Louis: Mosby; 2003:1115-1135.

24. Lee HK, Han H, Min SK. The association between body mass index and the severity of cholecystitis. Am J Surg 2009;197:455-458.

25. Kuzu MA, Ozturk Y, Ozbek H, et al. Acalculous cholecystitis: ascariasis as an unusual cause. J Gastroenterol 1996;31(5):747-749.

26. Langley RG, Bailey EM, Sober AJ. Acute cholecystitis from metastatic melanoma to the gallbladder in a patient with low risk melanoma. Br J Dermatol 1997;136(2):279-282.

27. Trotto NE. Contemporary management of gallstone disease. Patient Care 1999;33(20):90-106.

28. Friedman LS. Cholecystitis, acute. In Papadakis MA, McPhee SJ, editors. Current Consult Medicine. New York: McGraw-Hill, Lange; 2007:220-221.

29. Johannsen EC, Madoff LC. Infections of the liver and biliary system. In Mandell GL, Bennett JE, Dolin R, editors. Principles of Practice of Infectious Diseases, 6th edition. Philadelphia: Elsevier; 2005:951-958.

30. Holcomb SS. Stopping the destruction of acute pancreatitis. Nursing 2007;37(6):43-48.

31. Smeltzer SC, Bare BG, Hinkle JL, et al. Assessment and management of patients with biliary disorders. In Suddarth's Textbook of Medical-Surgical Nursing, 11th ed. Philadelphia: Lippincott Williams & Wilkins; 2008:1334-1374.

32. Ignatavicius DD, & Pettus S. (2010). Care of patients with problems of the biliary system and pancreas. In Ignatavicius DD, Workman ML, editors. Medical Surgical Nursing: Patient Centered Collaborative Care, 6th ed. St Louis: Saunders; 2010:1366-1385.

33. Kelly KA, Sarr MG, Hinder RA, editors. Mayo Clinic Gastrointestinal Surgery. Philadelphia: Saunders; 2004.

34. Csikesz NG, Tseng JF, Shah SA. Trends in surgical management for acute cholecytitis. Surgery 2008;144(2):283-289.

35. Livingston EH, Rege RV. A nationwide study of conversion from laparoscopic to open cholecystectomy. Am J Surg 2004;188:205-211.

36. Touzios JG, Dozois EJ. Diverticulosis and acute diverticulitis. Gastroenterol Clin North Am 2009;38:513-525.

37. Heise CP. Epidemiology and pathogenesis of diverticular disease. J Gastrointest Surg 2008;12:1309-1311.

38. McQuaid KR. Diverticulitis. In Papadakis MA, McPhee SJ, editors. Current Consult Medicine. New York: McGraw-Hill, Lange; 2007:322-323.

39. Chapman J, Davies M, Wolff B, et al. Complicated diverticulitis: is it time to rethink the rules? Ann Surg 2005;242:576.

40. Ye H, Losada M, West AB. Diverticulosis coli: update on a "western" disease. Adv Anat Pathol 2005;12(2):74-80.

41. Nelson RS, Ewing BM, Wengert TJ, et al. Clinical outcomes of complicated diverticulitis managed nonoperatively. Am J Surg 2008;196:969-974.

42. Dominguez EP, Sweeney JF, Choi YU. Diagnosis and the management of diverticulitis and appendicitis. Gastroenterol Clin North Am 2006;35:367-391.

43. Salem L. Anaya DA, Flum DR. Temporal changes in the management of diverticulitis. J Surg Res 2005;124:318-323.

44. Flasar MH, Goldberg E. Acute abdominal pain. Med Clin North Am 2006;90:481-503.

45. Swearingen PL. Manual of Medical Surgical Nursing Care: Nursing Interventions and Collaborative Management, 6th ed. St Louis: Mosby; 2007.

46. Kahi CJ, Rex DR. Bowel obstruction and pseudo-obstruction. Gastroenterol Clin North Am 2003;32(4):1229-47.

47. Paterno F, Longo WE. The etiology and pathogenesis of vascular disorders of the intestine. Radiol Clin North Am 2008;46:877-885.

48. Umphrey H, Canon CL, Lockhart ME. Differential diagnosis of small bowel ischemia. Radiol Clin North Am 2008;46:943-952.

49. Bartone G, Severino BU, Armelino MF, et al. Clinical symptoms of intestinal vascular disorders. Radiol Clin North Am 2008;46:887-889.

50. Wyers MC. Acute mesenteric ischemia: diagnostic approach and surgical treatment. Semin Vasc Surg 2010;23(1):9-20.

51. Mazuski JE. Intra-abdominal infections. Surg Clin North Am 2009;89:421-437.

52. McQuaid KR. Peritonitis, spontaneous bacterial. In Papadakis MA, McPhee SJ, editors. Current Consult Medicine. New York: McGraw-Hill, Lange; 2007:720-721.

53. Ramakrishnan K, Salinas RC. Peptic ulcer disease. Am Fam Phys 2007;76(7):1005-1012.

54. McQuaid KR. Peptic ulcer disease. In Papadakis MA, McPhee SJ, editors. Current Consult Medicine. New York: McGraw-Hill, Lange; 2007:716-717.

55. Leong RW. Difference in peptic ulcer between the east and west. Gastroenterol Clin North Am 2009;38:363-379.

56. Gustafson J, Welling D. "No acid, no ulcer": 100 years later: a review of the history of peptic ulcer disease. J Am Coll Surg 2010;210(1):110-116.

57. Malfertheiner P, Chan FK, McCall KE. Peptic ulcer disease. Lancet 2009;374:1149-1461.

58. Barkum A, Leontiadis G. Systemic review of the symptom burden, quality of life, impairment and costs associated with peptic ulcer disease. Am J Med 2010;123 (4):358-366.

59. Talley NJ, Vakil NB, Moayyedi P. American Gastroenterological Association technical review on the evaluation of dyspepsia. Gastroenterology 2005;129:156-180.

60. Fallah MA, Prakash C, Edmundowicz S. Acute gastrointestinal bleeding. Med Clin North Am 2000;84(5):1183-1208.

61. Cappell MS, Friedel D. Initial management of acute upper gastrointestinal bleeding: from initial evaluation up to gastrointestinal endoscopy. Med Clin North Am 2008;92: 491-509.

62. McQuaid K. Gastrointestinal bleeding, acute upper. In Papadakis MA, McPhee SJ, editors. Current Consult Medicine. New York: McGraw-Hill, Lange; 2007:400-401.

63. Tariq SH, Mekhjian G. Gastrointestinal bleeding in older adults. Clin Geriatr Med 2007;23:769-784.

64. Bounds BC, Kelsey PB. Lower gastrointestinal bleeding. Gastrointest Endosc Clin North Am 2007;17:273-288.

65. McQuaid K. Gastrointestinal bleeding, acute lower. In Papadakis MA, McPhee SJ, editors. Current Consult Medicine. New York: McGraw-Hill, Lange; 2007:398-399.

66. Kupfer Y, Cappell MS, Tessler S. Acute gastrointestinal bleeding in the intensive care unit: the intensivist's perspective. Gastroenterol Clin North Am 2000;29(2):275-307.

67. Ignatavicius DD. (2010) Care of patients with liver problems. In Ignatavicius DD, Workman ML, editors. Medical Surgical Nursing: Patient Centered Collaborative Care, 6th ed. St Louis: Saunders; 2010:1334-1365.

68. Kelso LA. Cirrhosis: caring for patients with end stage liver failure. Nurse Pract 2008;33(7):24-30.

69. Friedman LS. Cirrhosis. In Papadakis MA, McPhee SJ, editors. Current Consult Medicine. New York: McGraw-Hill, Lange; 2007:230-231.

70. Rinella ME, Sanyal A. Intensive management of hepatic failure. Semin Respir Crit Care Med 2006;27(3):241.

71. Schilsky ML, Shyoko H, Arnott L, et al. ICU management of acute liver failure. Clin Chest Med 2008;30:71-87.

72. Trey C, Davidson C. The management of fulminant hepatic failure. Progr Liver Dis 1970:282-298.

73. Stravitz RT. Critical management decisions in patients with acute liver failure. Chest 2008;134(5):1092-1102.

74. O'Grady JG, Schalm SW, Williams R. Acute liver failure: redefining the syndromes. Lancet 1993;342:273-275.

75. Gagliardi G, Laccania G, Boscolo A, et al. Intensive care unit management of fulminant hepatic failure. Transpl Proc 2006; 38:1389-1393.

76. Ostapowicz G, Fontana RJ, Schiodt FV, et al. Results of a prospective study of acute liver failure at 17 tertiary care centers in the United States. Ann Intern Med 2002;137: 947-54

77. Roberts E, Schilsky ML. A practice guideline on Wilson disease. Hepatology 2008;47:2089-2111.

78. Castro MA, Fasset MJ, Reynolds TB, et al. Reversible peripartum liver failure: a new perspective on the diagnosis, treatment, and cause of acute fatty liver of pregnancy based on 28 consecutive cases. Am J Obstet Gynecol 1999;181:389-395.

79. Rolando N, Wade J, Davalos M, et al. The systemic inflammation response syndrome in acute liver failure. Hepatology 2000;32: 734-739.

80. Rolando N, Philpott-Howard J, Williams R. Bacterial and fungal infection in acute liver failure. Semin Liver Dis 1996;16:389-402.

81. Rolando N, Gimson A, Wade J, et al. Prospective controlled trial of selective parenteral and enteral antimicrobial regimen in fulminant liver failure. Hepatology 1993;17:196-201.

82. Blei AT. The pathophysiology of brain edema in acute liver failure. Neurochem Int 2002;47:71-77.

83. Stravitz RT, Kramer AH, Davern T, et al. Intensive care of patients with acute liver failure: recommendations of the U.S. Acute Liver Failure Study Group. Crit Care Med 2007;35: 2498-2508

84. Vaquero J, Blei AT. Mild hyperthermia for acute liver failure: a review of mechanisms of action. J Clin Gastroenterol 2005;39 (suppl);S147-S157.

85. Khuroo MS, Farahat KL. Molecular adsorbent recirculating system for acute and acute-on-chronic liver failure: a meta-analysis. Liver Transpl 2004;10:1099-1106.

86. Choudhury J, Sanyal AJ. Treatment of ascites. Curr Treat Options Gastroenterol 2003;6:481-491.

87. Gines P, Cardenas A, Arroyo V, et al. Management of cirrhosis and ascites. N Engl J Med 2004;350:1646-1654.

88. Bloom RD, Goldberg LR, Want AY, Faust, TW, Kotloff, RM. An overview of solid organ transplantation. Clin Chest Med 2005;26(4):529-543.

89. Thuluvath PJ, Guidinger MK, Fung JJ, et al. Liver transplantation in the United States 1999-2008. Am J Transpl 2010;10(part 2): 1003-1019.

90. Urden LD, Stacy KM, Lough ME Gastrointestinal disorders and therapeutic management. In Priorities in Critical Care Nursing, 5th ed. St Louis: Mosby; 2008.

91. Liou IW, Larson AM. Role of liver transplantation in acute liver failure. Semin Liver Dis 2008;28 (2):201-209.

92. Bourgalt AM, Ipe L, Weaver J, et al. Development of evidence-based guidelines and critical care nurses' knowledge of enteral feeding. Crit Care Nurse 2007;27(4):17-29.

93. Stapleton RD, Jones N, Heyland DK. Feeding critically ill patients: what is the optimal amount of energy? Crit Care Med 2007;35 (9):S535-S540.

94. Ros C, McNeill L, Bennett P. Review: Nurses can improve patient nutrition in intensive care. J Clin Nursing 2008;18:2406-2415.

95. Gunnar E, Schadler D, Christoph E, et al. Current practice in nutritional support and its association with mortality in septic patients: results from a national, prospective multicenter study. Crit Care Med 2008;36(6):1762-1767.

96. Zaloga GP. Parenteral nutrition in adult in patients with functioning gastrointestinal tracts: assessment of outcomes. Lancet 2006;367:1101-1111.

97. Kreyman KG, Berger MM, Deutz NEP, et al. ESPEN guidelines on enteral nutrition: intensive care. Clin Nutr 2006;25:210-223.

98. Martindale RG, McClave SA, Vanek VW, et al. Guidelines for the provision and assessment of nutrition support therapy in the adult critically ill patient: Society of Critical Care Medicine and American Society for Parenteral and Enteral Nutrition: executive summary. Crit Care Med 2009;37(5):1757-1761.

99. Marik PE. Death by TPN . . . the final chapter? Crit Care Med 2008;36(6):1964-1965.

100. Isenhour JL, Marx J. Advances in abdominal trauma. Emerg Med Clin 2007;25:713-733.

101. Demetriades DE, Murray JA, Brown C, et al. High-level falls: type and severity of injuries and survival outcome according to age. J Trauma 2005;58:342-345.

102. Blank-Reid C. Abdominal trauma: dealing with the damage. Emerg Dept Insider 2007:4-11.

103. Poletti PA, Mirvis SE, Shanmuganathan K, et al. Blunt abdominal trauma patients: can organ injury be excluded without performing computed tomography? J Trauma 2004;57:1072-1081.

104. Salim A, Sangthong B, Martin M, et al. Whole body imaging in blunt multisystem trauma patients without obvious signs of injury: results of a prospective study. Arch Surg 2006;141:468-473.

105. Asimos AW, Gibbs MA, Marx JA, et al. Value of point-of-care blood testing in emergent trauma management. J Trauma 2000;48:1101-1108.

106. Wise BV, Mudd SS, Wilson ME. Management of blunt abdominal trauma in children. J Trauma Nursing 2002;9(1):6-14.

107. Holmes JF, Wisner DH, McGahan JP, et al. Clinical prediction rules for identifying adults at very low risk for intra-abdominal injuries after blunt trauma. Ann Emerg Med 2009;54(4):575-584.

108. Ahmed N, Whelan J, Brownlee J, et al. The contribution of laparoscopy in evaluation of penetrating abdominal wounds. J Am Coll Surg 2005;201:213-216.

109. Cheatham ML, Malbrain ML, Kirkpatrick A, et al. Results from the International Conference of Experts on Intra-Abdominal Hypertension and Abdominal Compartment Syndrome: II. Recommendations. Intens Care Med 2007;33:951-962.

110. Malbrain ML, Cheatham ML, Kirkpatrick A, et al. Results from the International Conference of Experts on Intra-Abdominal Hypertension and Abdominal Compartment Syndrome: I. Definitions. Intens Care Med 2006;32:1722-1732.

111. Balough Z, De Waele JJ, Kirkpatrick A, et al. Intra-abdominal pressure measurement and abdominal compartment syndrome: the opinion of the World Society of the Abdominal Compartment Syndrome. Crit Care Med 2007;35:677-678.

112. Kimball EJ, Kim W. Cheatham ML, et al. Clinical awareness of intra-abdominal hypertension and abdominal compartment syndrome in 2007. Acta Clin Belg Suppl 2007;1:66-73.

113. An G, West MA. Abdominal compartment syndrome: a concise clinical review. Crit Care Med 2008;36(4):1304-1310.

114. Lattuda M, Hedenstierna G. Abdominal lymph flow in an endotoxin sepsis model; influence of spontaneous breathing and mechanical ventilation. Crit Care Med 2006;34:2792-2798.

115. Teicher EJ, Pasquale MD, Cipolle MD. Abdominal compartment syndrome. Oper Techn Gen Surg 2008:39-59.

116. Fusco MA, Martin RS, Chang MC. Estimation of intra-abdominal pressure by bladder pressure measurement: validity and methodology. J Trauma 2001;50:297-302.

117. Walker J, Criddle LM. Pathology and management of abdominal compartment syndrome, Am J Crit Care 2003;12(4):367-371.

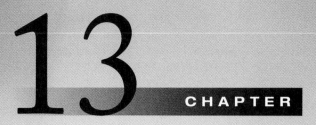

CHAPTER

Renal Problems

Margaret M. Ecklund, MS, RN, CCRN, ACNP-BC, Marvin Grieff, MD, and Paul Bernstein, MD

INTRODUCTION

The renal system, from the kidneys to the bladder to the urinary meatus, functions to filter and excrete waste products and contribute to fluid and electrolyte balance. This chapter will explore renal function and common problems encountered in acute care.

FLUID AND ELECTROLYTE DISORDERS

Cellular processes are regulated by fluid and electrolytes. Renal regulation contributes to the balance of electrolytes and imbalances can create system chaos. Imbalances often appear in combination, but to understand and treat effectively, each electrolyte is described in this section. Evaluation of fluid and electrolyte imbalances includes history, physical examination, serum laboratory values and urinary electrolyte concentrations, and serum osmolality (1). See Table 13-1 for the calculation of fractionated excretion of urine values.

Fluids as Medicine

Fluids are medicine. They are as essential and as important part of patient care as antibiotics, oxygen, pain killers, or vasopressors. Used injudiciously, they are a source for iatrogenic morbid events, which can be prevented with careful forethought and monitoring.

Step one is recognizing the patient's deficit or surfeit, followed by tailoring selected fluids to run at an appropriate rate for an appropriate time to achieve a preselected goal. The goal is determined by estimated losses at the time, in addition to estimated ongoing losses. Often, the best choice is no intravenous (IV) therapy at all if the patient is recovering with oral intake. That may be referred to as: "Don't just do something; stand there." Intravenous fluids are not a compulsory part of hospital admission. On a daily basis, patients are given saline in the morning and diuretics in the evening, which, with rare clinical exception, is the *sine qua non* for misunderstanding salt and water needs.

The Relationship of Sodium and Water

The next key concept is the complete separation of salt and water prescription. The former is essentially a synonym for volume and results in pulmonary or peripheral edema when in excess and in orthostasis or hypotension when lacking. Underperfused organs as a result of hypotension should be considered a "salt-lacking" emergency. Water, on the other hand, which adds little or nothing to blood pressure, except in extreme circumstances, simply balances osmotic pressure affecting the serum sodium concentration.

The serum sodium concentration, expressed as a fraction in mEq per liter, can be increased or decreased by both the sodium itself, (the numerator) or the liters of

TABLE 13–1 Urine Evaluation

Urine concentration of an electrolyte indicates renal function of excreting or retaining the electrolyte.
The 24-urine collection for quantifying the daily electrolyte excretion—gold standard
Fractional excretion (FE) is calculated from a spot urine sample and provides information quickly

$$FE\ electrolyte\ \% = \frac{Urine\ electrolyte/Serum\ electrolyte}{Urine\ Cr/Serum\ Cr} \times 100$$

water in which the sodium is dissolved (the denominator). An abnormal serum sodium concentration is often an issue of water adjustment (the denominator). This normal balance, between 135 and 145 mEq/L, is all the health care provider needs to know to choose the water prescription. If the sodium concentration is greater than 145 mEq/L, the patient needs water. The goal is to increase the denominator to drive the number down. This is separate from salt needs. Volume status is not considered when addressing a water excess or deficit. The blood pressure is irrelevant. If the serum sodium is greater than 145 mEq/L, osmotic balance is reestablished and water administered, returning the serum sodium to within the normal range. The rate of fall of the serum sodium will be dependent on water delivery and any ongoing losses and will be addressed in a later chapter. Although it may seem counterintuitive to run an IV solution of D5W in a grossly edematous patient, if the sodium level is elevated or rising quickly, this is clinically indicated (1).

If the serum sodium is less than 135 mEq/L, there is a water excess. This is the denominator indicating the liters of water is too great for the sodium. Water should be restricted. This is independent of blood pressure or edema, both of which are salt issues. Therefore, it is easy to deduce that the computer decides the water balance via the serum sodium concentration obtained from the chemistry laboratory apart from the patient assessment of need or excess. However, the health care provider can decide salt balance by history, physical exam, symptoms, and select laboratory values.

One may easily grasp the complete lack of interdependence of salt and water states by imagining any nine possible clinical scenarios for salt and water: a patient may present with salt overload, which is hypervolemia, combined with too much, just right, or too little water; with appropriate salt stores, as euvolemia, with too much, just right, or too little water; or with low salt stores present as hypovolemia with too much, just right, or too little water. Some of the possible clinical presentations are presented in Table 13-2, providing nine possible suggestions. In practice, patients often present with more common scenarios. For example, it is common to see frail elderly patients who have fallen at home with a salt deficit and who are hypotensive and have a water deficit with a serum sodium greater than 145 mEq/L. If this is the case, it may be helpful to separate the water and salt prescription and run two simultaneous lines: one for the salt needs, usually saline, and one for the water needs, typically D5W (1).

Another key concept is recognizing that salt and water taken by mouth is equivalent to salt and water given via vein. A liter of 0.9% saline is 0.9 g/dL of sodium, or 9 g/L dissolved in 1000 mL of water (Table 13-3). To calculate, multiply numerator and denominator by 10. Nine grams of sodium and 1 L of water, given by mouth, accomplishes the same result, at a different rate. Note that this is close to a typical hospital diet of 3.5 to 4 grams of sodium. Absorption of sodium in the gastrointestinal tract is immediate and complete. It is a common understanding that in critical care, if a patient is on feeding per nasogastric tube, this fluid is considered intake. However, if we were to blenderize a normal meal into a "soft meal," no one would consider this as fluid so long as the patient consumes it with a spoon. Whether it is a "full" lunch taken orally or a liquid meal administered tube per nasogastric tube, the components should be broken down into their salt and water constituents to decipher the contribution to the patient's salt and water stores. The consistency of the food is immaterial.

The same is true with water. Water is realized by the body equally regardless of the route of intake. With extremely rare exception, everything we drink is water to the body. Ginger ale, coffee, tea, or pomegranate juice—they are all water. Even sports drinks designed with "extra

TABLE 13–2 Clinical Presentations of Fluid Imbalance

Independence of Salt and Water Balance	High Salt Stores (Hypervolemic)	Appropriate Salt Stores (Euvolemic)	Low Salt Stores
Water Excess: (serum sodium <135 mEq/L	Cirrhotic with ascites or typical	Syndrome of inappropriate antidiuretic hormone (pure water gain)	Nausea and vomiting with lots of ginger ale and water as replacement fluids
Water "balance" (serum sodium between 135 and 145 mEq/L)	CHF (with pulmonary edema on exam) High salt meal/intake with water to match per thirst.	Normal person on a daily basis	Acute upper GI bleed before resuscitation
Water deficit: serum sodium >145 mEq/L	High-salt meal but no fluids at the table!	Diabetes insipidus with limited water intake (pure water loss)	Sweating in the desert with no water intake

TABLE 13-3 What's in the Bag?

Type of Fluid	Na, mEq/L	Cl, mEq/L	Ca, mEq/L	K, mEq/L	Lactate, mEq/L	pH Range	Osmoles, mOsm/L	Dextrose, g/L
Normal saline	154	154	0	0	0	4.5–7.0	308	
Lactated Ringer's	130	109	2.7	4	28	6.0–7.5	273	
D5W	0	0	0	0	0	3.2–6.5	252	50

electrolytes" and sugar are essentially water to the body. Very large salt losses cannot be repleted by sports drinks. Any drink with serious salt or potassium content is unpalatable and, therefore, unmarketable. An example is a mouthful of seawater consumed while swimming. Even sweat, typically about one-quarter normal saline, which contains more water than salt, tastes disturbingly salty.

The exception is fruit juices with remarkably high glucose content. Especially in the absence of an appropriate insulin response, the sugar content, raising the blood sugar level, may promote water movement out of the cells and act as an osmotic diuretic, dragging electrolytes into the urine. This may even contribute to salt losses and therefore hypovolemia. Normal insulin response or administration in diabetics protects against this possibility and renders fruit juices similar to other drinks.

The converse is true as well, in that saline infusion should be guided by best guess clinical endpoint, and not the serum sodium concentration. A hypotensive patient with serum sodium of 160 mEq/L still needs saline, as well as water. The amount and rate of saline replacement depends on assessed losses on arrival and perceived ongoing losses at the time of therapy.

Body Compartments

Saline as the preferable fluid to elevate blood pressure is a result from its property to remain in the extracellular space. Consider that our body fluids are compartmentalized. Blood pressure is a function only of the fluid that is found in the intravascular space, outside of any cells. Intracellular fluid does not contribute to blood pressure. In replenishing this space, fluids are chosen to maximize this advantage. In the average 70-kg adult, 60% or 42 L (kg) is fluid. Of this, about two-thirds or 28 L is intracellular, consisting of mostly muscle and organ cells, and one third or about 14 L is extracellular. Of the extracellular fluid, approximately one fourth is intravascular totaling about 3.5 to 4 L. The remainder of the extracellular fluid is extravascular, or interstitial, and does not contribute to blood pressure. Therefore, the blood pressure compartment contains only about one-twelfth of the total body fluids. Water, unlike saline, is not confined to any compartment. It is distributed to both intracellular and extracellular compartments and both intravascular and extravascular spaces (1). Therefore, any amount of water delivered only contributes to blood pressure by one-twelfth its volume or 8%. At the end of a liter-bag of D5W, 8%, or 83 mL, has been added to the extracellular, intravascular space. If the patient has approximately 4 L in this space, then it has been expanded by 83 mL/4000 mL, or about 2%. This is why it is a poor choice for hypotensive patients. Table 13-4 details how the compartments of the body are changed after a 1-L bag of IV fluids is completely infused.

TABLE 13-4 Changes in Compartment Volume After Fluid Infusion

1000 mL Intravenous (IV) Fluid (Type)	ICF	ECF	IF	IV	Change IV/L
D5W	667 mL	333 mL	250 mL	83 mL	8.3%
0.45%	333 mL	667 mL	500 mL	167 mL	16.7%
0.9%	0 mL	1000 mL	750 mL	250 mL	25%
3%	−1.57 L	2.57 L	1.93 L	640 mL	64%
PRBCs	0 mL	1000 mL	0 mL	1000 mL	100%

ICF, Intracellular fluid; *ECF,* extracellular fluid; *IF,* interstitial fluid; *PRBCs,* packed red blood cells.

Note that the 3% saline, which has three-fold more sodium than normal saline, will "steal" water from the intravascular space. Packed red blood cells (PRBCs) remain an ultimate volume expander but obviously must be reserved for appropriate clinical settings. The dextrose in D5W disappears rapidly in the presence of insulin, leaving 0 osmol/L, which is water (1).

Consider the patient's needs in deciding which fluids to choose. Lactated Ringer's, for example, has the advantage of containing potassium and calcium as well as some buffering capacity with lactate, resulting in a more physiologic pH range. However, if the patient is hyperkalemic, additional potassium may be contraindicated. Consider your patients' salt and water needs and sources of intake and reevaluate with weights, physical exam, and laboratory values.

Sodium

Now that fluid balance is reviewed, we will turn attention to sodium. Sodium is the major extracellular cation with a positive charge. With reduced sodium intake, extracellular volume decreases to stimulate the renin-angiotension-aldosterone system, reducing atrial natriuetic peptide (ANP) and reducing sodium elimination. With hypovolemia, the glomerular filtration rate (GFR) is decreased and the loop of Henle reabsorbs sodium. Sodium reabsorption in the distal tubule and ascending loop of Henle is primarily regulated by flow and less by hormonal mediation. Because of these factors, changes in these segments do not often play a large role, unless loop diuretics such as furosemide are used, reducing the loop reabsorption and increasing fluid delivery to the distal tubule. Blocking distal reabsorption with thiazide diuretics can create increased sodium transport in the collecting tubules, responding to change in flow (1, 2).

Hyponatremia

Hyponatremia (serum sodium less than 135 mEq/L) reflects an excess in water, relative to sodium. It is due to an inability to excrete ingested or infused water. It is the most common electrolyte abnormality in hospitalized patients. Causes of hyponatremia include volume depletion, thiazide diuretic use, and syndrome of inappropriate antidiuretic hormone secretion (SIADH) due to medication effects such as selective serotonin reuptake inhibitors (SSRIs), hypothyroidism, and adrenal insufficiency (1).

Symptoms of acute hyponatremia reflect the neurologic dysfunction as a result of cerebral edema. Osmotic swelling of brain cells occur from the fall in plasma osmolality, as water moves into the cells. The severity of symptoms is relative to the degree of overhydration, including nausea and malaise as early symptoms, followed by headache, lethargy, and obtundation. Seizures, coma, and respiratory arrest can be associated with serum sodium levels below 120 mEq/L. With chronic hyponatremia, cerebral adaptation allows an individual to appear asymptomatic despite serum sodium levels below 120 mEq/L. Nonspecific symptoms are fatigue, nausea, dizziness, unsteady gait, forgetfulness, confusion, and muscle cramps. In the elderly, falls are associated with chronic hyponatremia (1, 3).

The symptoms from the cerebral edema can be corrected with the correction of sodium. There are potentially deleterious effects if the sodium is corrected too rapidly. The reuptake of brain solutes during the correction is a slow process, and correction of less than 0.5 mEq/hr or 12 mEq in a 24-hour period is recommended. Osmotic demyelination syndrome may occur with rapid replacement of sodium. Treatment of chronic hyponatremia may include salt tablets, fluid restriction, and/or oral vasopressin receptor antagonist to improve neurologic symptoms (4, 5).

Hypernatremia

Hypernatremia (serum sodium greater than 145 mEq/L) is a water deficit, relative to the level of serum sodium. It is caused by failure to replace losses of water volume. Hypernatremia leads to cellular dehydration as there is an osmotic movement of water from the cells into the extracellular fluid. There can be an acute water movement out of the brain, potentially causing rupture of cerebral veins. Increased urine output with hypernatremia suggests diabetes insipidus. Diabetes mellitus can also contribute to hypernatremia (1).

The early symptoms of hypernatremia include lethargy, weakness, and irritability progressing to twitching, seizures, and coma. Thirst, followed by water intake, is the first defense for rising sodium levels. Symptoms may begin with serum sodium levels above 155 mEq/L. Urine osmolality can help determine renal versus nonrenal water loss (2, 6). Chronic hypernatremia does not usually produce neurologic symptoms. Water deficit is calculated, and fluids replaced. Free water deficit is calculated:

$$\text{Free water deficit} = 0.6 \times \text{weight in kg} \times [(\text{current serum Na}/140) - 1]$$

As with hyponatremia, correction of sodium should be done slowly to avoid cerebral edema. Correction should not exceed 12 mEq/L per day (2).

Potassium

Potassium is the major intracellular cation. The normal serum value of potassium is 3.5 to 5.5 mEq/L. Potassium affects the action potential of muscles. The resting membrane potential is related to the ratio of intracellular to the extracellular potassium concentration (1).

Hypokalemia

Hypokalemia symptoms present when the serum potassium fall below 3 mEq/L. A reduction in the extracellular potassium will hyperpolarize the cell membrane, making it more negative, increasing the sodium permeability, and making the membrane more excitable. Hypokalemia can delay the ventricular repolarization, increasing the relative refractory period and increasing arrhythmia potential. Hypomagnesemia may be a cause of hypokalemia and can contribute to arrhythmias. Severe muscular weakness that can be progressive toward rhabdomyolysis appears as the potassium drops to the range of 2.5 mEq/L. Respiratory, gastrointestinal or skeletal muscles can be affected. Hypokalemia can also produce cardiac arrhythmias. Classic changes on the electrocardiogram (ECG) include ST-segment depression, decreased T-wave amplitude, and an increased U-wave amplitude at the end of the T wave. Arrhythmias such as premature atrial and ventricular beats, sinus bradycardia, paroxysmal atrial or junctional tachycardia, atrioventricular block, and ventricular tachycardia or fibrillation can all manifest as a result of hypokalemia. Causes of hypokalemia include renal or nonrenal losses. Diuretics can exacerbate potassium loss in the urine. Measuring potassium in the urine can differentiate renal versus gastrointestinal loss. Severe potassium depletion can also lead to rhabdomyolysis with extreme muscle exertion (2, 7).

Resolution of symptoms accompanies potassium replacement. The degree of potassium loss affects the severity. Treatment of hypokalemia includes replacement while monitoring ECG changes. Oral replacement is indicated for those individuals on diuretics. Caution is used when replacing potassium when potassium-sparing diuretics, such as spironolactone, as hyperkalemia can develop rapidly. Serum potassium can transiently rise up to 1.5 mEq/L after an oral dose of 40 to 60 mEq. Potassium can be given multiple times in the course of a 24-hour period. Potassium replacement is monitored by serum potassium values. Intravenous potassium chloride is preferred when gastrointestinal symptoms limit oral replacement or in individuals with severe hypokalemia and profound loss. Concentrations of 20 to 40 mEq/L added to fluids can be infused through peripheral veins. Potassium chloride can incite local burning with infusion. Larger concentrations or intermittent replacement may be best tolerated via larger central venous access. The maximum recommended rate of IV potassium administration is 10 to 20 mEq/hr diluted in a nondextrose solution. Safety measures to prevent hyperkalemia include administration by pump and pharmacy-controlled solution mixtures. For individuals with chronic loss, dietary modifications to increase potassium intake in foods may assist with preventing hypokalemia (1, 2).

Hyperkalemia

Hyperkalemia is when the serum potassium exceeds 5 mEq/L and is often secondary to retention due to renal insufficiency. Medications that contribute to hyperkalemia include angiotensin-converting enzyme (ACE) inhibitors, angiotensin II receptor blockers (ARBs), nonsteroidal anti-inflammatory drugs (NSAIDs), and potassium-sparing diuretics. Hyperkalemia related to potassium moving out of the cells is caused by uncontrolled hyperglycemia. Hyperosmolity, insulin deficiency and metabolic acidosis contribute to the shift of potassium. Hyperkalemia is often without symptoms until the serum potassium exceeds 7 mEq/L, but should be monitored when levels are above 6 mEq/L. Muscle weakness and fatigue occur. ECG changes include tall, peaked T waves and shortened QT interval that progress to prolonged PR and QRS duration. Polyuria and polydipsia occur with hyperglycemia (2).

Therapy to correct hyperkalemia aims to stimulate potassium loss includes fluid administration. Resin binders, such as polystyrene, can bind the potassium and promote gastrointestinal excretion. Medication adjustment, such as eliminating potassium replacements and fluids, correct the hyperkalemia. To urgently facilitate entry of potassium intracellularly, Dextrose 50% and insulin may be administered. A renal consult may assist with management of severe hyperkalemia (2).

Calcium

Calcium is a major cation and is bound to principally albumin in the serum. Calcium plays a role in muscle contraction and nerve conduction. Normal serum levels range 8.5 to 10.2 mg/dL. Since the serum levels are affected by variance in albumin levels and nutritional status of the critically ill, an ionized calcium level may normal. The serum level of calcium falls approximately 0.8 mg/dL for every 1-g/dL drop in serum albumin. Hypoalbuminemia with critical illness or malnutrition can create normal serum calcium when the serum ionized calcium is high. A calculation used to correct for albumin is (1):

$$\text{Corrected Ca} = (0.8 \times 4 \text{ [normal albumin]} - \text{patient's albumin}) + \text{serum Ca}$$

Hypocalcemia

Hypocalcemia can either be acute or chronic and symptoms will vary according to severity. It can be mistaken for a neurological disorder. Symptoms include paresthesias, spasms, tetany, and seizures. Signs include Chvostek's (tapping of facial nerve anterior to the ear that elicits facial muscle contraction) or Trousseau's sign (carpal spasm as a result of brachial artery occlusion), bradycardia, prolonged QT interval, and decreased cardiac contractility. Hypoparathyroidism is a common cause of hypocalcemia and occurs with abnormal parathyroid gland development, surgical removal, or impaired PTH function (1).

Correction of acute symptomatic hypocalemia includes replacement of IV calcium, with ECG monitoring. As calcium values normalize, oral replacement can follow. Supplement range is 1,500 mg to 2,000 mg per day in divided doses of elemental calcium given in the form of calcium carbonate or calcium citrate. Calcium gluconate can be replaced intravenously at a rate of 1 to 2 g over 10 to 20 minutes. This is equivalent to 90 to 180 mg elemental calcium. The serum calcium is raised for up to 3 hours, so follow-up dosing is planned, as the cause of hypocalemia is identified. Concurrent correction of magnesium levels will aid the success of therapy. If serum magnesium is low, correct that first in an intermittent, then continuous infusion, to raise the serum magnesium level greater than 0.8 mEq/L. Vitamin D supplements are necessary for hypocalemia due to hypoparathyroidism. The amount of supplementation varies among individuals. Calcitriol is an active metabolite that is given to patients with hypoparathyroidism, lacking PTH. PTH stimulates renal calcium reabsorption. Monitoring of serum and urinary calcium is necessary. Other vitamin D analogues include alfacalcidol, dihydrotachysterol, and calcidiol (8).

Hypercalcemia

Hypercalcemia is excess serum calcium above 10.5 mg/dL. It occurs when there is more entry of calcium into circulation than elimination by the kidney or deposited into the bone, since calcium is absorbed in the small intestine by active and passive transport. Hypercalcemia is diagnosed by measuring elevated ionized or free calcium. Approximately 40% to 45% of calcium is bound to protein (albumin). Increased protein binding can cause an increase in the total calcium, as measured on basic chemical profile. With the binding, the ionized calcium concentration is not altered, which is referred to as pseudohypercalcemia. Hyperparathyroidism and malignancy are the most common causes. Malignancies can precipitate hypercalcemia, both solid tumors and leukemias and myeloma. The pathology is bone resorption. With metastases, there is direct induction of local osteolysis by tumor cells. Other causes of hypercalcemia include thyrotoxicosis, immobility, Paget disease of the bone, estrogen therapy for cancer, and hypervitaminosis A (9).

An elevated intact PTH is an indicator of primary hyperparathyroidism, possibly secondary to malignancy. If the PTH is less than 20 pg/mL, vitamin D metabolites (25-hydroxyvitamin D, calcidiol; 1,25-dihydroxyvitamin D, 1,25-D calcitrol) are measured for vitamin D intoxication (9).

The treatment of hypercalcemia is correction of the underlying cause with the goal of lowering serum calcium by inhibiting bone resorption, increasing urinary calcium excretion, and decreasing intestinal calcium absorption. Hypercalcemia of malignancy accounts for 90% of cases, with rapid appearance of symptoms. A review of medication, history, laboratory values, and diet contributes to the differential diagnosis and treatment (9).

The degree of hypercalcemia drives the intensity of treatment. Mild hypercalcemia, with a measured calcium less than 12 mg/dL, can be treated by avoiding drugs that exacerbate the calcium levels, including thiazide diuretics, lithium carbonate, avoiding volume depletion, prolonged immobility, and a high calcium diet. Increasing water intake eases the elevation.

Moderate hypercalcemia, with levels of calcium between 12 and 14 mg/dL, presents with symptoms based on the speed of the level change. Calcitonin, administered intramuscularly or subcutaneously, increases renal calcium excretion and interferes with osteoclast maturation. Combination therapy may be more effective using normal saline hydration and bisphosphonates. Bisphosphonates such as pamidronate are analogues of pyrophosphate, adsorb to the surface of the bone to inhibit calcium release, and interfere with bone resorption. This class of drug carries side effects of flulike symptoms, ocular inflammation, hypocalcemia, and impaired renal function. Glucocorticoids such as prednisone may be added to reduce calcium levels in 2 to 5 days in hypercalcemia related to dietary intake or granulomatous disease or lymphoma. Gallium nitrate infusions may also assist with calcium reduction but carry a risk of renal toxicity. Other treatments include calcimimetics to treat the hyperparathyroidism such as cincalcet. Hemodialysis or peritoneal dialyses are options for individuals with chronic renal failure (CRF) with hypercalcemia (2, 8).

Phosphate

Phosphate is the major intracellular anion, with a normal serum value of 2.2 to 4.5 mg/dL. It is important to proper cellular function. The kidney is the most important regulator of the serum phosphate level. PTH decreases the absorption of phosphate in the proximal tubule while 1,25-dihydroxyvitamin D increases tubular phosphate reabsorption. Volume expansion and corticosteroid administration decrease tubular reabsorption. In the gastrointestinal system, active vitamin D and PTH stimulate absorption. Both can stimulate phosphate release from the bone. Phosphorus metabolism is related to calcium metabolism (1)

Hypophosphatemia

Hypophosphatemia can arise with decreased net absorption, acute intracellular movement, and increased urinary excretion. When serum phosphate is decreased, the kidneys increase the reabsorption in the proximal tubule, using the sodium-phosphate cotransporter (10).

The diagnosis can be obtained through history. Measurement of urinary phosphate can be via a 24-hour sample or calculated by a random sample, by fractional excretion of filtered phosphate. Daily excretion of phosphate is less than 100 mg. The differential diagnosis of low phosphorus excretion includes increased cellular entry if the patient received glucose or insulin. This can also appear with the increased insulin of refeeding syndrome and acute respiratory alkalosis. Chronic diarrhea causes loss of phosphate from intestinal secretions. Chronic antacid intake promotes phosphate binding to magnesium or calcium, forming nonabsorbing insoluble salts.

Treatment of the underlying cause may include vitamin D supplementation and phosphate supplementation. Oral supplementation is preferred over IV due the risks of sudden hypocalcemia, renal failure, and arrhythmias (2, 11).

Hyperphosphatemia

Hyperphosphatemia is due to renal insufficiency and chronic kidney disease. Renal failure can cause hyperphosphatemia, as 5% to 20% of filtered phosphate is via the kidneys. As the GFR decreases, less phosphate is filtered and excreted. Since phosphate is the major intracellular anion, conditions with marked tissue breakdown will increase extracellular volume of phosphate. Increase in phosphate can trigger hypocalcemia as it precipitates in tissue. Conditions that trigger may include rhabdomyolysis, tumor lysis syndrome, hemolysis, diabetic ketoacidosis, and lactic acidosis (12).

Hyperphosphatemia may also be triggered by large ingestion of phosphate-containing laxatives such as Fleet's phosphosoda, causing volume-depleting diarrhea and renal insufficiency. With acute phosphate nephropathy, acute renal failure (ARF) follows laxative ingestion for procedures such as colonoscopy. Hyperphosphatemia is treated with restricting phosphorus in the diet and administration of phosphate binders (2, 12).

Magnesium

Magnesium plays a function for cellular metabolism and nerve conduction. Normal serum value is 1.5 to 2.4 mg/dL. Approximately one-third is bound to protein and two-thirds exists as a free cation. Altered magnesium levels provoke hypokalemia and hypocalcemia (1,2).

Hypomagnesemia

Hypomagnesemia is often due to renal or gastrointestinal losses. Renal losses are often secondary to diuretic use. Hypomagnesemia is suspected with chronic diarrhea, hypocalcemia, refractory hypokalemia and ventricular arrhythmias, especially in the setting of an ischemic event. Hypomagnesemia occurs in 12% of hospitalized patients, affecting up to 60% of critical care patients. In addition to history, a serum magnesium and urinary magnesium can differentiate between gastrointestinal and renal loss (13).

Signs of hypomagnesemia include generalized weakness, anorexia, hypokalemia, hypocalcemia, positive Chvostek and Trousseau signs, delirium and tetany. Magnesium depletion can change the electrocardiogram, widening the QRS and creating peaked T waves. As the loss becomes more severe, the PR interval lengthens and QRS widens. Ventricular arrhythmias manifest during myocardial injury or cardiopulmonary bypass (14).

Treatment of hypomagnesemia varies as to clinical symptom severity, and the key is treating the underlying disease. Slow IV magnesium replacement is indicated for severe loss with gastrointestinal intolerance. Oral replacement is indicated for asymptomatic patients, in a sustained release formation. If the cause of loss is diuretic therapy, adding a potassium-sparing diuretic such as amiloride may be beneficial (13).

Hypermagnesemia

Hypermagnesemia occurs in two settings: individuals with end-stage renal disease and with excessive intake. With renal failure, there is no protection from excess magnesium as there are no alternative mechanisms to regulate. In healthy adults, magnesium is readily excreted in the urine. High magnesium is triggered with exogenous ingestion with laxatives or antacids; therefore these agents are contraindicated in renal disease. Women with severe preeclampsia can receive magnesium, and if in excess, can trigger hypermagnesemia. Laxative abuse can create hypermagnesemia with increased intake. Other causes of hypermagnesemia include primary hyperparathyroidism, familial hypocalciuria, hypercalcemia, diabetic ketoacidosis, hypercatabolic states and theophylline or lithium toxicities (1).

Treatment of hypermagnesemia includes correction of the underlying cause. Magnesium is limited in diet and drugs for individuals with end stage renal disease. Reducing intake suffices for those with normal renal function. In an emergent situation, IV calcium can be administered to antagonize magnesium's effects. Dialysis can be considered for the renal failure patient (1,2).

Chloride

Chloride is the negative ion that partners with sodium. Normal serum chloride is 98 to 108 mEq/L. Evaluation of chloride does not occur as a separate electrolyte, but in the calculation of anion gap (2).

ACID-BASE DISTURBANCES

Cooperation of several systems ensures consistency of the blood pH despite many types of insults that pressure the pH up or down. The acid-base disturbance is emblematic of an underlying insult. Fixing the disturbance without identifying the cause accomplishes little.

The disturbances may be acute or chronic, acidotic or alkylotic in nature, metabolic or respiratory. Acidosis is more commonly seen in acute care. The most common acid-base disturbance is as a result of buffer loss in the form of bicarbonate in diarrhea.

Acidosis

Each day we have to balance the acid we accumulate because of what we eat that is sulfur-rich (converted from sulfur-containing amino acids). The buffer, bicarbonate, is consumed in this process but "re-made" by the kidney, provided there is adequate kidney function. The secondary buffers may be proteins that can accept the acid load (H+) and intracellular shift in desperate situations. It is a myth that H+ ions are switched for K+ ions, except in rare circumstances such as infusion of nonorganic acid. Because the lungs excrete carbon dioxide, derived from carbonic acid, we have an additional organ system to raise or lower pH by its effects on retaining or "blowing off" carbon dioxide, giving rise to the Henderson-Hasselbach equation, which describes this relationship: (H+) = 24 (pCO_2/HCO_3). Therefore, knowing either the bicarbonate or the pCO_2 value is insufficient information to determine an acid-base equation. There is an expected response by the body to return to as close to normal a pH as possible, consistent with a recognized constant relationship between the pCO_2 and the bicarbonate. If there is a sudden acid load, initially the bicarbonate will drop, increasing the above fraction and therefore the concentration of H+. As pH drops with increasing H+ concentration, the pH falls. The response intuitively, over time, is that the pCO_2 will go down, restoring the ratio, decreasing the H+ concentration and therefore normalizing the pH. Note that the body does not drop the pCO_2 down sufficiently to return pH back to normal. After an acid load, if there is an uncomplicated and appropriate drop in the pCO_2, then the pCO_2 = 1.5 (HCO_3) + 8 +/- 2. If this is not the case, then there may be an additional disturbance, or the person may be incapable of enough pulmonary reserve to eliminate pCO_2. In that case, the pH will not return to as normal a value as it should. Clinically, as the bicarbonate drops when the patient is acidemic, the pulmonary response to rid the body of CO_2 may be life saving, as the above equation suggests compounding a decrease in HCO_3 with an increase, or failure to decrease in pCO_2 will affect the H+ concentration dramatically. Note that we are much better adapted to breathe off pCO_2 to help normalize an acid load, then to retain pCO_2 to balance an alkalotic insult. Since the individual still needs oxygen delivery, respiratory rate cannot be limited in an attempt to retain pCO_2 (15).

With this as a background, every time a set of routine electrolytes is ordered, a simple check of the anion gap should be calculated. This is simply the difference between all the cations and all the anions in the body. We use sodium as the major cation and subtract from it the addition of chloride and bicarbonate (Na—(chloride + bicarbonate). Since individuals must be electroneutral, this difference of about 8-12 mEq/L must represent anions that we are not measuring, typically from proteins, predominantly albumin. Therefore, as the serum albumin drops, so should the "anion gap." If the anion gap is greater than 12 mEq/L, some acid is suspected and investigated (15).

All approaches to acid-base problems should be driven by clinical scenario. If the patient is diabetic and has measurable ketones in blood or urine, then this acid insult should be reflected in a decreased bicarbonate and an increased respiratory rate, resulting in a decreased pCO_2. As the ketosis represents an acid insult, the pH of the blood should be reduced proportionately, while the compensation of the diminished pCO_2 attempts correction toward normal. Established nomograms may be used to better understand these relationships.

All acid loads that result in an elevated anion gap are intuitively called, an anion gap acidosis. Life threatening ingestions, such as methanol, salicylates, or ethylene glycol cause anion gap acidosis. Other acid disturbance, most notably diarrhea, which wastes bicarbonate in the GI tract, yields an acid pH in the blood, but without the anion gap. It should be understood however, that the loss of bicarbonate from the system is equivalent to gaining acid. Typically in these scenarios, the chloride will rise as the bicarbonate drops, as the kidney will raise its absorption of chloride to compensate for the lost bicarbonate (15).

In terms of management, replacement of the bicarbonate to correct the pH has never shown to be of any value when kidney function is normal or near normal. When treating lactic acidosis, diabetic or alcoholic ketoacidosis, reversing the underlying illness will quickly reverse the situation, obviating the need for the addition of bicarbonate. Conversely, if there is little or no renal function return anticipated, there is equally little chance of rapid reversal of bicarbonate deficit and addition of bicarbonate, in either an anion gap or non–anion gap acidosis. Finally recall that acidosis may not be clinically detrimental at all. A 100 meter sprinter at race's end has a lactate buildup and a low pH. During a grand mal seizure, acid builds up very quickly compounded by poor respiratory function disabling the lungs from accelerating rate sufficient to "breathe off" pCO_2, creating respiratory acidosis and limiting compensatory response. Arterial blood gases performed during a seizure show remarkably low pH, in the range of 6.9, but the patient suffers no ill effects as a result of the pH and no increase in serum potassium.

Alkalosis

Almost universally as a result of two clinical possibilities, we handle pH shift upward with limited response from the lungs. As is the case with acidosis, but in reverse, the rare addition of alkali or the loss of acid will result in an alkalosis. The lungs, by breathing off an "acid equivalent" (CO_2) may generate an alkaline pH as respiratory alkalosis or excreting acid through the GI tract or kidneys results in a metabolic alkalosis.

GI losses, in nausea and vomiting or nasogastric suctioning, remove HCl, leaving elevated levels of bicarbonate in the serum. Aldosterone rises acutely with gastric content loss, and this relative hypovolemia with high bicarbonate content overwhelms the renal tubule's ability to reabsorb this filtered load, and promotes acid secretion simultaneously. Both the aldosterone and the presence of the alkalai promote H+ secretion, as well as potassium loss. Once the relative hypovolemia is treated, the return to balance of the normal chloride and bicarbonate concentration allows the kidney to quickly dump the "excess" bicarbonate and the pH returns to normal. Therefore, alkalosis is typically described in terms of generation of the alkalosis by nasogastric suction or diuretics and maintenance of the alkalosis secondary to maintenance of the volume depletion. Diuretics that make the patient waste sodium and chloride via the specific transporters blocked by diuretics such as furosemide and hydrochlorthiazide, force relative high concentrations of bicarbonate in the serum in addition to H+ loss in the form of exchange with sodium in the kidney at the distal tubule. The low serum potassium independently promotes alkalosis because this upregulates ammonia production, the main vehicle to excrete acid. Regardless of either of these two mechanisms, the treatment is the same: the administration of sodium and chloride. The patient at risk is vigorously diuresed with rising bicarbonate levels, low potassium levels and sudden weight loss attributable to "fluid weight" loss, not caloric weight loss. Less commonly are disorders of the kidney tubule, ingestion of high numbers of calcium carbonate pills, or even acute relief of the pCO_2-retaining patient when intubated, whose high bicarbonate levels represent a compensatory maneuver to respiratory acidosis. In the short time after intubation, with the serum bicarbonate still elevated and the pCO_2 acutely down, there is a post-hypercapneic alkalosis (15).

Central to analysis of all acid base issues, is the use of an arterial blood gas. This is the litmus test to the actual pH and testimony to how the lungs and the kidney are attempting to return the pH toward "normal" for that patient. Remember that there may be acute and chronic, respiratory and metabolic, acidosis and alkalosis simultaneously.

Case Report

An end stage COPD is oxygen-dependent who gets septic, hypotensive and intubated after days of diarrhea. Based on the clinical scenario, it is possible that there is a combination of:

- Elevated pCO_2, i.e., chronic respiratory acidosis as a baseline
- Elevated serum HCO_3, i.e., chronic metabolic alkalosis in compensation (the arterial blood gas would show an acidotic pH if we stopped here)
- Elevated lactate level from sepsis, i.e., an acute anion-gap metabolic acidosis
- Posthypercapneic metabolic alkalosis, i.e., the pCO_2 is driven down acutely from baseline to a much lower level

(relative respiratory alkalosis) leaving the elevated serum bicarbonate with nothing to "compensate for"

- Chronic non–anion gap acidosis from loss of bicarbonate in the diarrhea. How these sort out ultimately, and their relative contributions can only be discerned from the arterial blood gas; everything else is theoretical.

CALCIPHYLAXIS

Calciphylaxis is associated with renal disease and hyperphosphatemia. A more definitive term is calcific uremic arteriolopathy. It arises with abnormal mineral metabolism that manifests with tissue calcification in the vascular and soft tissues. The prevalence is increasing since 1962, as more individuals are being treated for hyperparathyroidism with calcium-based phosphate binders and vitamin D analogues (16).

Histologic findings are small vessel mural calcification with or without endovascular fibrosis, extravascular calcification and vascular thrombosis, which leads to tissue ischemia. Obesity can create excess stress on the dermal tissue arterioles and precipitate vessel calcification. It can also occur with individuals with chemotherapy treated breast cancer, alcoholic liver cirrhosis, cholangiocarcinoma, Crohn disease, rheumatoid arthritis, primary hyperparathyroidsm, malignancies, and systemic lupus erythematosus (17, 18).

Clues to diagnosis include patients with end-stage renal diseases, who are receiving vitamin D supplementation, have hyperphosphatemia, and hyperparathyroidism. The precipitating event is local skin trauma or injections. Ischemic necrotic areas develop in the dermis, adipose tissue, and rarely muscle. The lesions on the trunk, buttocks, or on a proximal extremity can be quite painful. Ischemic myopathy may develop (16).

There are no specific laboratory findings that confirm the diagnosis. Laboratory values to provide a clue with diagnostics include elevated PTH, elevated phosphate, and elevated calcium. Radiographs or high-resolution CT scans can differentiate calcium from surrounding tissue. Skin biopsies have limited usefulness in diagnosis, but may be a necessity to rule out other diagnoses (18).

There are no controlled prospective studies that compare treatment strategies for calciphylaxis. A plan may include wound care and pain control, including limiting local tissue trauma. Correcting the electrolyte abnormalities, using non–calcium phosphate binders such as sevelamer or lanthanum carbonate. Monitor and normalize the PTH as able. Cincalet may be more effective than vitamin D analogues. A parathyroidectomy may be considered for refractory elevations in PTH, with life-threatening symptoms of tissue necrosis and infection. Sodium thiosulfate may be administered intravenously. Therapy response is monitored by physical examination and symptom control (18).

Clinical Nurse Specialist Competencies and Spheres of Influence

Having a background in understanding of the complexities of fluid, electrolyte, and acid-base balance, the CNS in acute care can be proactive with a thorough history. Each imbalance has an underlying cause, and the history can offer clues.

Coaching the multidisciplinary team for accurate measurements of intake, output, and weight provide through data. Reassessing laboratory values helps determine correction of imbalance. For sodium replacement, monitoring serum sodium values helps to monitor the pace of correction.

Teaching patients and families about rationale for dietary and fluid restrictions, and medication action promotes potential understanding and compliance to treatment plans. The CNS leads the multidisciplinary team to assure all interventions are coordinated to promote excellent patient care.

Case Report

Flora is a 56-year-old woman with a history of CHF, CAD with multiple coronary stents, chronic renal insufficiency, obesity, anxiety, depression, lower extremity cellulitis, type 2 diabetes, celiac disease, obstructive sleep apnea, anemia, hypertension, atrial fibrillation.

Over the course of the past 6 months, her hospital admissions for chest pain and CHF management have increased. She lives alone, and despite home care services, she was unable to successfully follow a treatment plan, including medications and mental health follow-up.

This hospital admission for CHF and chest pain resulted in a 48-hour intubation and renal consult for worsened renal function. Her serum creatinine was 4.7 mg/dL, BUN 53 mg/dL and binatriuric peptide (BNP) 2,030 pg/mL. A furosemide infusion at 5 mg/hour helped stimulate diuresis, and her oxygenation was stable with her baseline CPAP unit with 12 cm H_2O support and 3 liters of oxygen. Nephrologists discussed the risks/benefits and alternatives to hemodialysis. This conversation mirrored many prior conversations of the likelihood of eventual dialysis. She agreed to a fistula, and she had a surgical procedure of a plastic loop fistula. Since her numbers were "stable" and she was managing a diuresis, a temporary catheter was not placed, and she was followed for medical management until fistula maturity.

In the 6 weeks post fistula, several electrolyte imbalances were monitored and corrected by medication management. Diet alterations included fluid intake restriction with phosphorus limitations, while providing protein supplements.

Hyperparathyroidism, suspected with an intact PTH of 659pg/mL, combined with a low vitamin D 25-hydroxy of 25 ng/mL, may have contributed to painful patches in her inner thigh adipose tissues. Calciphylaxis was of concern, and treatment was intensified to reduce her phosphorus of 5.1 mg/dL and supplemental calcium. Flora's calcium was 7 mg/dL, and

albumin 2.2 mg/dL, calculating corrected calcium of 8.4 mg/dL. Her medication plan included calcitrol 0.25 mcg daily, lanthanum carbonate 500 mg with meals, cinacalcet 30 mg daily, and calcium carbonate 500 mg with each meal. Over the next three weeks, Flora's pain improved. She continued with intermittent furosemide and metolazone. Her fistula healed and matured for use. Repeat intact PTH was 358 mg/dL, phosphorus 3.9 mg/dL, corrected calcium 8.8 mg/dL. At this point, the cinacalcet and calcitrol were stopped and doxercalciferol 4 mcg subcutaneously was started. Her hemodialysis treatments started successfully, and ongoing monitoring of her electrolytes continued.

Summary of Medications:

Calcitrol	manages hypocalcemia in CRF to promote the absorption of calcium and phosphorus; a form of vitamin D
Lanthanum	carbonate reduces serum phosphorus by acting as a phosphorus binder
Cinacalcet	a calcimimetic causing parathyroid to produce less PTH to reduce calcium levels
Calcium carbonate	calcium replacement
Doxercalciferol	synthetic vitamin D that lowers PTH by promoting the absorption and use of calcium and phosphorus

ACUTE RENAL FAILURE

The kidney serves as a filter. When the filter fails, ARF develops. Multifactorial issues contribute to the filter's function, and differentials are key to treatment. ARF is broadly defined as a decrease in GRF over a period of time of hours to weeks. It can be an abrupt or rapid decline in renal function. Waste products such as urea and creatinine accumulate when the filtering malfunctions, with possible cessation of urine production (19).

Clinical Presentation

While there is no universal definition, the consensus definition and classification for ARF is using RIFLE. The RIFLE classification in Table 13-5 includes the range of disease: Risk, Injury, Failure, Loss, and End-stage kidney disease. RIFLE considers GFR and urine output combined with clinical outcomes.

The incidence of ARF increases with age. It is 3.5% for over the age of 70. Despite advances in critical care and renal replacement therapy (RRT), mortality for ARF has not changed in 40 years and remains at 75% (19).

In the elderly, the aging kidney sets up risk for development of acute tubular necrosis Changes in morphology and function include cortical atrophy, changes in the glomeruli and proximal tubules. Functional changes include decreased renal blood flow and GFR. Other associated risks are diabetes, hypertension, and hyperlipidemia. Iatrogenic complications include exposure to nephrotoxins (20). (See Table 13-6.)

TABLE 13-5 RIFLE Classification for ARF Management

Class	GFR Criteria (patient's creatinine in equation)	Urine Output
Risk	Serum creatinine × 1.5	<0.5 mL/kg/hr × 6 hr
Injury	Serum creatinine × 2	<0.5 mL/kg/hr × 12 hr
Failure	Serum creatinine × 3	<0.5 mL/kg/hr × 24 hr
	Or 4 mg/dL with an acute rise	Or anuria × 12 hr
Loss	Persistent ARF >4 wk	
End-stage kidney disease	End-stage kidney disease >3 mo	

TABLE 13-6 Nephrotoxins

- Acyclovir
- Allopurinol
- Amphetatmines
- Antibiotics
- Aminoglycosides, tetracycline, amphotericin B, cefalosporins, sulfonamides, ciprofloxacin, penicillins, trimethoprim, bacitracin, and polymixin

- Analgesics
- Salicylates, acetaminophen, NSAIDs
- Anesthetics
- Cimetidine
- Contrast dyes
- Cyclosporine
- Dextran, mannitol
- Furosemide

- Heavy metals
- Interleukin-2
- Organic solvents
- Ethylene glycol, gasoline, kerosene, turpentine, tetrachorethylene
- Poisons
- Mushrooms, herbicides, insecticides, snake venom
- Probenecid
- Phenytoin
- Rifampin
- Thiazide diuretic

Acute kidney injury affects 2000—3000 individuals per million per year. RRT involves 200—300 individuals per million yearly. Four to five % of the critical care patients will be treated with RRT, and up to 2/3 will develop ARF using RIFLE classification. Considering surviving patients with RRT, 5 to 20% will remain dialysis dependent upon discharge from the hospital. (20).

Pharmacologic therapy for repair of ARF has been unsuccessful, but the kidney has the ability to regenerate after acute injury if a critical number of cells is preserved. Research is promising in the use of mesenchymal and hematopoetic stem cells that differentiate into tubular epithelial cells (21).

Markers of Kidney Function

Creatinine is the most widely used marker of ARF, but is not always reflective of the GFR. Creatinine is influenced by muscle mass, catabolism, and drugs. Urea is a marker of renal function, but is affected by effective circulating volume, increased dietary protein, critical illness and gastrointestinal bleeding (19, 22).

An ideal marker for GFR would be endogenous, non-toxic without protein binding, freely filtered at the glomerulus, and excreted unchanged (not filtered or reabsorbed) in the urine. Cystatin C is a nonglycosolated protein used as a marker for GFR. It is unaffected by age, body mass, infection or inflammation. In the clinical setting, the marker is best suited when it can be obtained from specimens easy to recover (urine and serum), and is rapid and inexpensive, but not fully tested or available in general practice (19, 22).

Cause of ARF/Approach to Diagnosis

ARF can be categorized as prerenal, indicating altered perfusion to the kidney. Intrarenal indicates damage within the kidney. Postrenal indicates alteration in flow from the kidney. Each will be discussed further.

Prerenal

The etiology of 21 to 30% of all ARF in hospitalized elders is a prerenal source. The elderly are at high risk with decreased autoregulation. Causes of decreased prefusion to the kidney include conditions that decrease circulating blood volume, including gastrointestinal loss, decreased fluid intake, diuretic administration, decreased cardiac output, and vasodilation. The use of NSAIDS can cause renal vasoconstriction. ACE-inhibitor use with underlying renal artery stenosis can contribute to hypoperfusion. Prerenal urine characteristics are observation of bland urine sediment, FE_{na} (fractional excretion of sodium) less than 1%, FE_{urea} (fractional excretion of urea) less than 35%, and urine osmolality greater than 500 mOsm/kg (19, 21).

Intrarenal

The intrarenal cause of ARF is acute tubular necrosis from ischemic or toxic injury. Sources of the injury are sepsis as the leading cause and nephrotoxic drugs. Glomerulonephritis is usually due to an immune process which causes inflammation in the glomerulus and can rapidly progress to renal failure requiring emergent dialysis. Causes of glomerulonephritis include vasculitis, systemic lupus erythematosus, Wegener's granulomatosus, and Goodpasture's disease. Wegener's granulomatosus and Goodpasture's disease are associated with both kidney and lung disease and can present with hemoptysis. Vascular causes of ARF are hypertension and atheroembolic disease, occurring after having an angiogram. Acute interstitial nephritis can follow an exposure to a medication with consequent inflammation within the kidney. This can be accompanied by release of eosinophils, rash, and pyuria.

The urine characteristics of intrarenal ARF are active urine sediment with tubular or granular casts, FE_{na} greater than 2 %, FE_{urea} greater than 35% and urine osmolality 250 to 300 mosm/kg. An elevated sediment rate and leukocytosis in the complete blood count are diagnostic clues (19, 21).

Postrenal

Postrenal ATN is diagnosed with clinical history and physical findings. Renal diagnostic imaging can reveal stones in the upper urinary system or malignancy. Lower obstruction has likely causes of benign prostatic hypertrophy, malignancy, or stricture. Once the postobstructive cause is removed, diuresis follows. Urology consultation is appropriate for postrenal ARF.

The hallmark of prerenal ARF is the improvement with volume repletion, while the hallmark of postrenal ARF is improvement after relief of the obstruction (19, 21).

Management

ARF is treated based on the cause. ATN is treated by avoiding nephrotoxins, optimizing fluid and electrolyte status, and providing nutritional support. The use of dopamine is not universally supported. Studies support the use of acetylcysteine for prevention of ARF for contrast studies (21). The need to dialyze is determined by the nephrologist's consult. Renal replacement therapy will be addressed later in the chapter.

Influence

A thorough history and initial assessment of the patient with ARF will provide clues for accurate diagnosis and etiology. Key initial laboratory tests of urinalysis and FE_{na} with serum chemistries in a timely fashion, and staff members coached in collection will assist accuracy.

In the multidisciplinary plan of care the APN can consider age-related changes in the GFR and renal blood flow when prescribing drugs to the elderly and individuals with diabetes, chronic renal insufficiency, and heart failure. Caution is advised with drugs with a narrow therapeutic index or nephrotoxic. Teaching awareness of nephrotoxic drugs can raise awareness for complications. Careful attention to fluid balance and admission medication lists can prevent dehydration and ARF progression. Drugs to focus awareness on to adjust dosing include ACE inhibitors, ARB, NSAIDS, contrast dyes, and aminoglycosides.

HYPERTENSION

Renal function can affect or be affected by cardiovascular changes. Renal blood flow affects GFR, which has an impacts on renal function. Most hypertension is unexplained. Secondary causes of hypertension include chronic kidney disease, renal vascular disease, primary hyperaldosteronism, pheochromocytoma, and Cushing disease. Renal vascular hypertension is secondary to renal artery stenosis or renal infarction. The decrease in renal blood flow activates the renin-angiotensin-aldosterone system to increase blood pressure. Renal hypertension with parenchymal disease occurs with glomerulonephritis, polycystic disease, and pyelonephritis. The kidney's ability to excrete salt and water is limited (20).

Systolic hypertension results in nephrosclerosis. When hypertension is uncontrolled for over five years, there are degenerative changes in arterioles and intralobular arteries. There is a correlation between the duration and degree of increased blood pressure and the severity of vascular disease. Renal disease can slowed with diet and blood pressure control (20).

DIALYSIS: THE NEED FOR RENAL REPLACEMENT THERAPY (RRT)

Pathophysiology

Dialysis is the term used for renal replacement therapy. The main functions of the kidneys can be broadly defined as control of volume status, regulation of electrolytes; and elimination of toxic wastes. The need for dialysis is determined by the inability of the kidneys to function adequately to keep these under control. Lack of control of volume status with kidney failure is usually associated with volume overload, which results in any of the following: edema, hypertension and congestive heart failure. Inability to regulate blood chemistry by the kidney may result in the following: hyperkalemia, acidosis, hypocalcemia, and hyperphosphatemia. Uremic syndrome presents when toxic wastes rise, manifested by nausea, vomiting, or confusion, known as uremic encephalopathy. Uremic pericarditis is the accumulation of toxins around the heart, causing inflammation. This may result in chest pain, a pericardial friction rub, and/or a pericardial effusion. The specific toxins which cause these symptoms are not known, though the levels of these toxins in the blood often correlate with the blood urea nitrogen (BUN) concentration. It must be noted that urea is not the "uremic" toxin and that patients can develop the uremic syndrome with relatively low levels of BUN.

Indications for Dialysis

Dialysis is indicated when the glomerular filtration rate (GFR) is less than 15 mL/min. Absolute indications for urgent dialysis, which reflect alterations in renal function, are commonly severe volume overload leading to pulmonary edema unresponsive to diuretics, hyperkalemia, uremic pericarditis, and uremic encephalopathy. It is common to begin dialysis before patients have these absolute indications (24).

In chronic kidney disease, early referral to a nephrologist ensures care of medical issues such as hypertension, anemia of chronic kidney disease, and secondary hyperparathyroidism. A nephrologist addresses the issues of initiating RRT, selecting a dialysis modality, and referral for renal transplantation when indicated (25).

Dialysis Modalities

Dialysis modality depends on the clinical indication and the forms of dialysis support provided by the hospital. Acute dialysis is usually performed with either intermittent hemodialysis or slow continuous therapies. Peritoneal dialysis can be performed for acute dialysis but is used less frequently for this indication, as access is not ready to use on an emergent basis Chronic dialysis is usually performed with intermittent hemodialysis or peritoneal dialysis.

The dialysis modality decision is based on medical history, functional ability, lifestyle and financial and social situation. Intermittent hemodialysis is usually done in a designated treatment center, and care is provided by medical personnel. Programs are emerging to support home hemodialysis, allowing more individual independence, Peritoneal dialysis is considered a home treatment, allowing more independence, gentler fluid removal, and less dietary restrictions.

Intermittent Hemodialysis

Intermittent hemodialysis is the most commonly performed type of dialysis in both ARF and end-stage renal disease. It is usually done three times weekly for 3 to 4½ hours per treatment. In this form of dialysis, blood is circulated in an extracorporeal circuit of about 200 mL. This circuit is made up of tubing threaded through air and pressure detectors to a dialysis membrane. The dialysis membrane is made up of hollow fibers with blood running through the hollow fibers as dialysate, a balanced electrolyte solution, circulates on the other side of the membrane moving in a countercurrent direction. Metabolic toxins and electrolytes, such as potassium, diffuse through pores in the membrane from the blood side to the dialysate and are thus removed. Pores limit the size of molecules that can be removed through the filter. Toxin removal, electrolyte balance, and reachieving an estimated dry weight are goals of dialysis (26). Excess volume is removed as the dialysis machine generates negative pressure. Potassium concentrations vary in the dialysate solution according to the serum electrolyte values prior to treatment. Plasma removal rate depend on goals, blood pressure, and patient tolerance. Slow continuous therapy treatments are called continuous renal replacement therapies (CRRT). In critical care, hemodialysis may be performed continuously. The technique is similar to intermittent hemodialysis with blood pumped through a dialysis membrane and dialysate circulates on the other side of the membrane, but the treatments are done with a low blood flow, often 200 mL/min with a low steady rate of fluid removal. The slow continuous nature of these treatments is advantageous in the patient who is hemodynamically unstable and may not tolerate rapid fluid removal and those who have large fluid volume overload. Access for dialysis for slow continuous therapies is a hemodialysis catheter. Treatment is initiated with a nontunneled catheter (26).

Access for Dialysis

Access for hemodialysis into the blood stream must allow delivery of blood to the dialysis circuit at rates of 250 to 450 mL/min. For individuals with end-stage renal disease, this is usually accomplished with an arteriovenous fistula or synthetic graft or a tunneled hemodialysis catheter into a central vessal. For patients needing urgent dialysis, a percutaneously placed nontunneled catheter may be secured by sutures to the patient's skin. Nontunneled catheters are temporary and should be replaced by a tunneled hemodialysis catheter when possible and appropriate. The bacteremia rate of nontunneled catheters is approximately 5% after 3 weeks of placement in the internal jugular vein and 11% after 1 week in the femoral vein (27).

Peritoneal Dialysis

This form of dialysis is usually done at home and is used in the hospital setting when a patient who uses this modality is hospitalized. Peritoneal dialysis involves placement of dialysis solution into the peritoneal cavity.

Peritoneal dialysis solutions are provided in defined sizes and with glucose concentrations of 1.5%, 2.5%, and 4.25%, and varied glucose concentrations allow for removal of fluid volume with each exchange. The peritoneal membrane serves as the dialysis membrane. Usually 2 to 2.5 L of peritoneal dialysis solution is placed in the peritoneal cavity and left in for 2 hours or more. The fluid is removed at defined periods and more fluid is instilled. Each exchange is done in a clean environment with the patient or caregiver using sterile technique. Contamination of the fluid can lead to peritonitis (26).

Access for Peritoneal Dialysis

Access for peritoneal dialysis is a surgically placed catheter, which leads into the peritoneal cavity. It has one or two Dacron cuffs, which over time become adherent to the abdominal wall tissue and tether the catheter to the patient. The catheter is placed by a provider with insertion competency. To allow an adequate seal to form around the catheter and between the abdominal tissues and the Dacron cuff, the catheter is not used for at least 2 weeks after catheter placement. Temporary hemodialysis may be needed if renal replacement is needed earlier.

Common Complications of Dialysis
Hemodialysis

Hypotension after dialysis is common and usually due to excess or rapid fluid removal. Other causes of hypotension include sepsis and cardiac disease including ischemia or pericardial disease. Medications administered prior to dialysis can effect hypotension, and alterations in timing may limit the degree of hypotension and dialysis tolerance (24).

Hemodialysis access clotting is diagnosed by lack of pulsation on palpation and lack of a bruit by auscultation. A clotted access constitutes an emergency, and the access must have a thrombolysis procedure, which can be done in a radiology department, or the clot is surgically removed. If the access cannot be repaired, a temporary hemodialysis catheter may need to be placed (26).

Patients on hemodialysis are at an increased risk of infection. Possible causes of the sepsis syndrome in dialysis patients include an infected dialysis access, as well as the usual differential diagnosis in the general population with other similar comorbidities such as cellulitis, diabetic foot infections, or pneumonia (27, 28).

Peritoneal Dialysis

Peritoneal dialysis–related peritonitis occurs less often than once every 24 months and can usually be treated successfully with antibiotics. Patients present with cloudy fluid and/or abdominal pain with possible fever. A sample of the peritoneal fluid with more than 100 white blood cells (WBCs)/mm^3 with polymorphonuclear leukocytes indicates peritonitis. Empirical antibiotics are given intraperitoneally. Antibiotic choices include vancomycin and an aminoglycoside to cover both gram-positive and gram-negative organisms. Peritonitis is usually presumed to be due to contamination by the patient or caregiver, but often the exact source of infection cannot be identified. A surgical cause of the peritonitis may be suspected when culture of the peritoneal dialysis fluid reveals more than one organism. Patients with peritoneal dialysis–related peritonitis need to be observed carefully by the peritoneal dialysis staff. Lack of improvement in the patent may indicate that the peritoneal dialysis catheter is infected and that it must be removed. If the peritoneal catheter is removed, a temporary hemodialysis catheter is placed until the infection is treated and a peritoneal catheter can be reinserted and matures (26, 28). As with hemodialysis, excess fluid removal can result in hypotension. Other possible causes of hypotension include sepsis and cardiac disease (26).

Peritoneal dialysis may precipitate hyperglycemia due to the high glucose concentrations in the peritoneal dialysis solutions. Over time, with each exchange, some glucose is absorbed from the peritoneal cavity into the systemic circulation. Glucose control may be achieved with medication adjustments (26).

Inpatient Management of the RRT Patient

Care of the inpatient dialysis patient can be complex and is best achieved by collaboration between the primary and dialysis teams. Patients on both hemodialysis and peritoneal dialysis need to follow a strict diet. The most important restrictions per day are for 3 g sodium, less than 2.5 g potassium, and 1 g phosphorus. Control of the serum potassium and phosphorus is essential. Protein is not restricted, and many people require protein supplementation to maintain their protein stores. Although a fluid restriction is often imposed, thirst stimulates excess fluid intake is due to high salt intake. Dietary issues include no orange juice due to high potassium content to treat hypoglycemia and no salt substitutes as they are high in potassium. A broadly stated "renal diet" for inpatients will include many of the above restrictions. Phosphorus binder is added to medications and given at meal times. Patients on slow continuous therapies need to have their nutritional status monitored very carefully. Due to the long duration of dialysis, patients may experience hypokalemia and hypophosphatemia (26).

Hemodialysis access is the patient's lifeline and must be protected. No IV lines should be inserted or blood pressures measured on that arm. Care should be taken to not apply pressure on that arm or have the patient lie on that arm. It is beneficial in the hospital setting to have that arm marked with a loose wrist bracelet with those instructions and to have a sign indicating that as well over the patient's bed and on the medical record.

The hemodialysis catheter should be kept clean and dry. Catheter dressings are changed regularly by the hemodialysis staff. Redness, tenderness, and discharge over the catheter exit site indicate the possibility of infection and necessitate treatment by the dialysis team. Central line protocols may provide structure to the care of tunneled catheters.

Most dialysis teams discourage use of tunneled dialysis catheters for non-dialysis purposes. Accessing the catheter by nondialysis staff increases the risk of infection of these catheters, with potential clotting of the catheter. Protocols may permit use of the hemodialysis catheter with permission of the staff nephrologist only if no other venous access can be obtained. These catheters may have large doses of concentrated heparin instilled in them, and this heparin must be withdrawn before use.

The peritoneal dialysis catheter should be kept clean and dry. At home, it is the patient's or caregiver's responsibility to take care of the exit site daily. When hospitalized, exit site care is usually undertaken by nurses familiar with peritoneal dialysis catheter care. Exit sites are covered with nonocclusive gauze attached by tape. Redness, tenderness, and discharge over the catheter exit site indicate the possibility of infection and necessitate treatment by the dialysis team.

A stable outpatient hemodialysis patient usually has serum chemistry and hematology evaluation on a monthly basis. These assessments include assessment of dialysis adequacy, anemia management, bone metabolism, and electrolytes. Additional laboratory values are based on clinical need.

Chronic treatments of anemia and bone disease are often attended to by the nephrologist and renal team. Hemodialysis patients will frequently receive erythropoietic agents, such as erythropoietin and darbopoietin, to stimulate production of red blood cells and treat anemia. The efficacy of this treatment is questioned for the critically ill individual. Intravenous vitamin D analogues such as calcitriol, hectoral, and doxercalciferol and IV iron compounds are administered with treatments (26).

Other medications can be given on dialysis depending on patient need and alternative access. It is common to administer IV antibiotics such as cefazolin, aminoglycosides (e.g., gentamicin and tobramycin), and vancomycin with treatments.

Due to the prolonged nature of CRRT, medication doses may need to be increased as medications may be removed with prolonged dialysis treatment. It is best to consult with the nephrologist, renal team, and pharmacist as the dosing will vary depending on the medication. Timing may vary according to the dialyzability of the medication and the impact on blood pressure during treatment.

The issue of bacteremia is critical for patients with invasive lines. While tunneled catheters minimize risk, altered immune systems and repeated access into central circulation create high risk.

Clinical Nurse Specialist Competencies and Spheres of Influence

The APN is positioned to coordinate the efforts of the multidisciplinary team. For the inpatient, scheduling care in concert with CRRT is important to achieve goals. Since critically ill patients are fatigued after CRRT, it may be advantageous to organize therapies and activities around the treatment schedule. Medication dose adjustments and doses to hold are important to CRRT tolerance. Teaching patient and family about catheter care, diet, and scheduling will help with plan of care. The APN can champion adherence to protocols for line care. Teaching and quality monitoring can help with excellence in patient care. Protocols and standard order sets for the inpatient with RRT can improve care and promote safety.

METABOLIC EMERGENCIES

Diabetic Ketoacidosis

Diabetic ketoacidosis (DKA) is an acute life-threatening emergency that usually occurs in patients with type 1 diabetes but can manifest with type 2 diabetics. It is due to insulin deficiency and/or insulin resistance. It presents with the triad of hyperglycemia, ketosis, and acidemia. DKA develops quickly, within as little as 24 hours. Patients can present with vomiting and abdominal pain, with a history of polyuria and polydypsia (29).

The most common precipitating event in DKA is infection, although other potential causes include noncompliance with insulin regimens, myocardial infarction, and cardiovascular accident. Precipitating factors for DKA should be investigated and treated appropriately (29).

Initial Treatment

Isotonic saline is given to replete the fluid deficit, which is estimated to be between 2 and 3 L. When the blood glucose falls below 270 mg/dL the IV solution is changed to 5% dextrose, often in saline. The aim is to prevent the blood glucose from falling below 180 mg/dL. Care must be undertaken in administering this fluid in the elderly as well as in patients with underlying cardiac or renal disease. Intravenous insulin is given to achieve a steady decrease in the serum glucose.

Potassium depletion is usually present and is due to the hyperglycemia and resulting urinary potassium losses. The serum potassium may not be low as hyperglycemia and insulin deficiency will cause potassium to shift out of cells. It is important to include potassium in IV fluids after the first liter of fluid. The fluid deficit is usually replaced within 24 hours. The insulin infusion should be continued until the patient can eat and drink normally (29).

Hyperosmolar Nonketotic State

Hyperosmolar nonketotic state (HONK) is a life-threatening emergency that occurs in patients with type

2 diabetes. It is due to insulin deficiency and/or insulin resistance. It presents with severe hyperglycemia; the serum glucose is often greater than 900 mg/dL. In contrast to DKA, HONK develops over days to weeks. Patients can present with polyuria and polydypsia and often present with confusion (29).

The most common precipitating event in HONK is infection, although other potential causes include noncompliance with insulin regimens, myocardial infarction, and cardiovascular accident. Precipitating factors for DKA should be investigated and treated appropriately.

Treatment of HONK

The primary defect in HONK is often volume depletion, as opposed to DKA, in which the primary defect is a lack of insulin or the development of insulin resistance. Thus, the fluid deficit is higher in HONK than in DKA and is estimated to be about 5 L. Care must be undertaken in administering isotonic saline in the elderly as well as in patients with underlying cardiac or renal disease (29).

As HONK is usually due to volume depletion, the glucose level will often fall with administration of fluids. Insulin need not be given as a bolus and can be infused with an insulin drip. Serum potassium should be followed carefully as it may drop with insulin administration.

Potassium depletion is usually present and is due to the hyperglycemia and resulting urinary potassium losses. The serum potassium may not be low as hyperglycemia and insulin deficiency will cause potassium to shift out of cells. It is important to include potassium in IV fluids once the potassium falls below 5.2 mmol/L.

Poisonings

Treatment of poisonings is usually done in consultation with a medical toxicologist. Treatments may include acute hemodialysis in cases in which the substance is free in the blood and not heavily protein bound, which can diffuse across a dialysis membrane. The efficacy of dialysis to remove a poison is often suggested by a relatively low volume of distribution. Peritoneal dialysis is not usually a treatment for intoxications. Hemodialysis is often indicated when there is a severe toxicity and when hemodialysis treatment can increase total body elimination of the toxin by 30% or more. It is often advisable to contact nephrology regarding these patients to discuss indications for dialysis. Intoxications for which hemodialysis can be used include lithium, salicylates and toxic alcohols such as methanol and ethylene glycol (30).

Case Report

A 54-year-old male patient, who has been on lithium for his psychiatric illness for 20 years, presents to the emergency department with confusion and myoclonic jerking. He had been started on hydrochlorothiazide for his hypertension about 6 months ago and developed diarrhea about 1 week ago. He was found, confused, on the floor by his wife. In the emergency department, his creatinine was found to be 2.0 mg/dL, and his lithium level was 3.0 mEq/L.

Nephrology is consulted and a urinalysis is done, which reveals no blood or protein, and on microscopic examination, there are no cells, crystals, or casts. A creatinine kinase is checked to exclude rhabdomyolysis, which is normal. Hemodialysis is initiated immediately via a femoral hemodialysis catheter, and the patient's mental status and muscular shaking improve markedly.

Because of worry over a rebound in lithium level, a lithium level is drawn the next day, and it is found to be low enough not to necessitate another hemodialysis session. The APN asks the nephrologist about the need for keeping the femoral hemodialysis catheter, and it is decided to have it removed. The patient receives IV saline, on the presumption of prerenal ARF, and his kidney function returns to normal by the next day.

Clinical Nurse Specialist Competencies and Spheres of Influence

The APN should be aware of several issues here: (a) lithium is renally excreted, and diuretics may result in increased retention of lithium by the kidney; (b) the importance of determining whether an intoxication can be treated with hemodialysis; and (c) the importance of working with the nephrology team to determine the ongoing need for hemodialysis access.

THE STABLE PATIENT WITH CKD HOSPITALIZED FOR ANOTHER REASON

Cardiac Catheterization

Intravascular contrast administration for cardiac catheterization is a common cause of hospital-acquired ARF. The risk of ARF from IV contrast, contrast medium–induced nephropathy (CIN), may be as low as less than 1% to 2% in patients with normal renal function but as high as 45% in some studies of patients with underlying chronic kidney disease and diabetes mellitus. Contrast nephropathy results in an immediate rise in the serum creatinine, which is detected within 24 to 48 hours after contrast administration and often peaks at 3 to 5 days, and then begins to fall. Most, but not all patients, are nonoliguric and most recover renal function over the next days. In some patients, CIN results in the need for temporary hemodialysis and it may result in an increase in mortality (31).

Prevention

Prevention of CIN is based on avoiding contrast when possible and limiting the volume of contrast administration. For example, cardiologists often limit the volume of contrast administered during cardiac catheterization by analyzing ventricular and valvular function with an echocardiogram rather than a ventriculogram. NSAIDs and diuretics, if possible, should be withheld shortly before and after contrast administration. Metformin should be held before contrast administration and only restarted after it is clear that CIN has not occurred (31).

Strategies to Prevent Contrast Nephropathy

Isotonic sodium bicarbonate (154 mmol/L) given at 3 mL/kg for 1 hour preprocedure and then continued at 1 mL/kg for 6 hours after contrast administration has been shown in some studies to be better than isotonic IV saline. At dosages between 600 to 1,200 mg twice daily starting before contrast administration and continuing for 4 doses has been shown to prevent CIN in some studies (31).

Patients with chronic kidney disease, who are not on dialysis, are at an increased risk of ARF with changes in blood pressure and fluid status. Surgical procedures in patients with chronic kidney disease should be planned carefully with careful attention to the patient's volume status. Specific recommendations for fluid and electrolyte management are patient specific and should be made with the patient's nephrologist. Other issues that need careful attention include (a) use non-nephrotoxic antibiotics, (b) dose all medications for the patient's kidney function and avoid completely some medications that accumulate with kidney disease, (c) avoid NSAIDs, and (d) monitor renal function and serum electrolytes frequently.

Case Report

A 56-year-old white diabetic man with chronic kidney disease and a GFR of 20 mL/min is admitted because of right toe cellulitis. Home medications including lisinopril, furosemide, and insulin are continued. He is initially treated with vancomycin and gentamicin. He is put on low-molecular-weight heparin prevention of venous thrombosis. Vascular surgery is consulted and finds by noninvasive vascular studies that the circulation to that toe may be compromised. They request an angiogram of that leg. The first night after admission his glucose is found to be 40 and he is given orange juice. The next morning, his creatinine is found to be elevated with a potassium level of 6 mEq/L, and his nephrologist is consulted.

The patient's nephrologist requests that the gentamicin, lisinopril, furosemide, and low-molecular-weight heparin be stopped. The low-molecular-weight heparin is stopped because of the increased risk of bleeding with this medication in patients with this level of chronic kidney disease. Instructions to prevent contrast nephropathy are given.

INFECTIONS IN THE URINARY TRACT

Infections can affect any portion of the genitourinary system. This section will focus on the diagnosis and management of urinary tract infections (UTIs). UTIs can be divided into upper tract infections, involving the kidneys. Lower UTI involves the bladder, urethra, or prostate. Primary pathogens are enteric bacteria. Nosocomial UTIs, or catheter-associated urinary tract infections (CAUTIs), will be discussed later in the chapter.

The urinary tract, from the kidneys to the urethral meatus, is sterile and resistant to bacterial colonization despite frequent exposure to bacteria. Protective mechanisms include the acidity of urine, the process of bladder emptying, sphincters, and mucosal barriers; 95% of UTIs are ascending etiology (32).

Lower Urinary Tract Infection

In both men and women, UTIs are diagnosed with pyuria (urine with pus), dysuria, urgency, and frequency. In the elderly, UTIs can be asymptomatic or present with confusion and sepsis (32).

Rapid diagnosis is achieved with a fresh, unspun microscopic sample of clean voided urine. A Gram stain can be helpful with initial antimicrobial choices. Bacteriuria (greater than 1 organism per oil immersion field) or pyuria (greater than 8 leukocytes per high power field) or cultures yielding more than 10^5 bacteria/mL correlate with infection. However, colony counts of 10^2 to 10^4 may indicate infection in women with acute dysuria (33).

Escherichia coli causes more than 75% of community-acquired UTIs; *Staphylococcus saprophyticus* causes 10%. In hospitalized patients, *E. coli* accounts for 50%, with 40% due to several other species of nosocomial gram-negative organisms, and the remaining 10% are of gram-positive origin. A complicated UTI is present with underlying factors predisposing to infection. An uncomplicated UTI has no compromised urine flow or underlying abnormality. Risk factors for UTI are situations that expose the meatus to bacteria such as intercourse, use of spermicidal condoms, and fecal incontinence (32).

When candiduria is present, it is crucial to distinguish infection from colonization, which does not require treatment. Symptomatic candiduria with pyuria and those at high risk for developing candidemia should receive fluconazole 100 to 200 mg daily orally for 5 days. Amphotericin bladder irrigations clear funguria but are not supported by evidence to treat infection (2). Concern for asymptomatic candiduria is the concern of ascending development of kidney infection. Symptoms of kidney infection include flank or abdominal pain, costovertebral angle, and abdominal tenderness. Chronic candidal infections follow a subacute to chronic course. Individuals with predisposing urinary tract abnormalities are at highest risk. Prevention includes glucose control for diabetics and changing or removing the indwelling Foley catheter (33).

Asymptomatic bacteriuria is defined differently for men and women. There are no presenting symptoms of urgency, frequency, fever, tenderness, or dysuria. It is the isolation of a specific amount of bacteria in a collected urine sample that minimizes contamination. For women, two consecutive voided samples with the same amount (100,000 CFU/mL) and type of bacteria, or a single catheterized sample with one bacteria species quantified 100 CFU/mL. For men, samples may include a single collection of urine that minimizes contamination with a bacterial colony count of 100,000 CFU/mL or a single catheterized specimen of 100 CFU/mL bacterial count. Patients without treatment are followed if symptoms change (34).

Acute Cystitis

Acute cystitis is an infection of the bladder usually due to *E. coli*. It is usually ascending infection from the urethra. Cystitis is rare in men and is usually pathologic with infected stones, prostatitis, or chronic urinary retention. Presenting symptoms include irritative voiding (frequency, urgency and dysuria), afebrile, positive urine culture, possible positive blood cultures, and suprapubic discomfort. Gross hematuria may be a possible symptom after sexual intercourse. The physical exam is unremarkable except for suprapubic tenderness. The urinalysis has pyuria and bacteriuria and varying degree of hematuria. A positive urine culture determines pathogen. No diagnostic studies are indicated unless the symptoms are recurring. Hematuria usually resolves once cystitis is treated (33).

Differential diagnoses in women are vulvovaginitis and pelvic inflammatory disease. In men the differentials are urethritis and prostatitis. Noninfectious causes include pelvic irradiation, chemotherapy, bladder cancer, interstitial cystitis, voiding dysfunction, and psychosomatic disorders. Prevention for cystitis is the prescribing of prophylactic antibiotics for recurrence after treatment of UTI (women with more than three episodes per year). An anatomical abnormality is ruled out as a cause. Scope of coverage is to eliminate pathogenic bacteria from the fecal and introital reservoir and not create bacterial resistance. Dosing is a single dose at bedtime or prior to intercourse. Drugs include trimethoprim-sulfamethoxazole 40 mg/200 mg, nitrofurantoin, and cephalexin (35).

The treatment for uncomplicated infections in women is short-term single-drug therapy for 1 to 3 days. Fluoroquinolones and nitrofurantoin are now the drugs of choice. Men are more likely to have complicated UTIs; thus duration may vary. Adjunct therapies include sitz baths and phenazopyridine (33).

Acute Pyelonephritis

Acute pyelonephritis is an infectious, inflammatory disease involving renal parenchyma and pelvis. Gram-negative bacteria are the most common pathogens. They ascend from lower urinary tract, with exception of *S. aureus*, which has a hematologic origin. Twenty percent of community-acquired bacteremias are from pyelonephritis. The kidney can enlarge due to inflammation, and the infection is focal and patchy (32, 33).

Signs of acute pyelonephritis include fever, flank pain, shaking chills, and voiding dysuria. Other symptoms include nausea and vomiting, diarrhea, fever, and tachycardia. Laboratory values include a CBC showing leukocytosis with a left shift. The urinalysis has evidence of pyuria, bacteriuria, and hematuria; WBC casts are likely. Colony counts of bacteria exceed 10^5. A renal ultrasound may be necessary for complicated cases to rule out hydronephrosis (36).

Differential diagnosis can be challenging because presenting signs and symptoms mimic those found in numerous other disorders. With acute intra-abdominal disease, the patient will have a normal urinalysis; with gastrointestinal disorders, the patient will have abnormal liver function tests that will not be present with pyelonephritis. A chest radiograph may confirm pneumonia. With men, other differential diagnoses include acute epididymitis, acute prostatitis, and acute cystitis. Physical examination helps with differential.

Treatment may require hospitalization for severe cases. Intravenous antibiotics are selected according to pathogen. Outpatient treatment includes oral antibiotics. Fever may persist for up to 72 hours. Catheter drainage may be necessary for urinary retention and nephrostomy drainage for obstruction. Antibiotics are continued intravenously for 24 hours after fever and oral antibiotics for a 14-day course. A good prognosis is anticipated with proper treatment; however, a complication of untreated cystitis is sepsis (36).

Evaluation for Infection

Urinalysis is one of the most important tools available and has been cited as a poor man's renal biopsy. A clean catch urine sample minimizes contamination risk. The procedure of washing the urethral opening with a mild disinfectant and dried, followed by catching the specimen mid stream. Spreading the labia or retracting the foreskin minimizes contact with the urinary stream. Best collections are having the individual begin to void, stop the stream, and then collect the specimen. Bladder catheterization can help with samples that cannot be obtained in a moderately clean format. It is optimal to examine the urine within 1 hour to avoid destruction of formed elements (32, 33). Refer to Table 13-7 for urinalysis overview.

A urinalysis is crucial in the diagnosis of acute kidney injury. The first step in urinalysis is the chemical dipstick. Findings of hematuria and proteinuria may suggest a particular form of renal disease. On microscopy the following findings may be suggestive of specific clinical scenarios: (a) granular casts suggest acute tubular necrosis, which may be due to hypotension, sepsis, or adverse effects of medications including contrast; (b)

TABLE 13–7 Considerations of Evaluating a Urinalysis

DIPSTICK AND MICROSCOPIC EXAM

Dipstick includes urinary pH, protein, hemoglobin, glucose, ketones, nitrites and leukocyte esterase, and specific gravity

pH—values >7 may indicate infection

Protein—may be false positive with a high white blood cell load; physical exertion and fever can cause proteinuria; seen with nephrotic syndrome and glomerulonephritis

Glucose—most positives indicate diabetes mellitus

Hemoglobin—screen for hematuria is not specific for erythrocytes; can indicate glomerulonephritis

Ketones—are positive in a catabolic or starvation state

Bacteria—tested by having positive nitrites in the urine

Leukocyte esterase—indicates the presence of white blood cells; if negative, there is low likelihood of infection

Microscopy searches for all for elements, including crystals cells, casts, and infecting organisms

Leukocytes—significant if >5 per high power field

Erythrocytes—microscopic hematuria is significant—strenuous exercise, inflammation of surrounding organs, vaginal bleeding

Casts are formed in the distal tubules and collecting ducts, not seen in normal urinary sediment, and usually indicate renal disease

Casts

Hyaline = concentrated urine, febrile disease, after strenuous exercise, diuretics

RBC = glomerulonephritis

WBC = pyelonephritis, interstitial nephritis

Renal tubular cell casts = acute tubular necrosis, interstitial nephritis

Coarse, granular casts = nonspecific

Broad, waxy casts = CRF—stasis in tubules

Casts and epithelial cells = acute tubular necrosis

WBC with neutrophils and eosinophils and protein = interstitial nephritis and pyelonephritis

---

pyuria suggests infection or allergic interstitial nephritis; (c) hematuria and proteinuria suggest a glomerulonephritis; and (d) a completely normal urinalysis in the face of ARF suggests low kidney perfusion pressure, adverse effects of medications, or urinary tract obstruction. The finding of hematuria on chemical dipstick but no red blood cells on microscopy suggests the diagnosis of rhabdomyolysis.

The appearance and color of urine can be affected by medications. Red urine does not always indicate hematuria. Hematuria is ruled out by urinalysis. Cloudy urine is not always pyuria and may be reflective of amorphous phosphates or crystallization of salts. Without pyuria, the specimen clears with addition of acid (32).

Microscopic examination is useful but not definitive. Pyuria is greater than 8 WBCs/microliter of uncentrifuged urine. This is equivalent to 2 to 5 WBCs/high power field in a centrifuged sample. Samples containing bacteria without pyuria are likely contaminated. WBC casts indicate inflammatory reaction. Microscopic hematuria is more common than gross hematuria (32). A high number of epithelial cells suggest contamination. Low colony counts of bacteria could be due to

prior antibiotic exposure, dilute urine, or obstruction to flow (32).

Urine Electrolytes in Acute Kidney Injury

Urine sodium and creatinine are often measured in patients with acute kidney injury (AKI). A low urine sodium is often present when the patient has low renal perfusion and is hypovolemic. It may also be low when hypovolemia is not present, such as in AKI after contrast exposure and in AKI due to rhabdomyolysis. A fractional excretion of sodium is often calculated to distinguish acute tubular necrosis from prerenal ARF, which would be expected to get better with repletion of intravascular volume. See Table 13-1 for the calculation. A level of less than 1% is consistent with prerenal ARF. Both the urine sodium and fractional excretion of sodium rise after diuretic exposure, making it an insensitive test for prerenal ARF in the presence of diuretics (1).

Hematuria

Microscopic hematuria is often detected on urinalyses. This can be due to glomerular or extraglomerular causes. Glomerular causes include glomerulonephritis and are often accompanied by changes in renal function and proteinuria. Urine microscopy would reveal red blood cell casts and/or dysmorphic red blood cells and/or proteinuria. The finding of glomerular hematuria indicates the need for nephrology evaluation. Extraglomerular causes of hematuria include renal as well as urothelial malignancies, nephrolithiasis, and infection. Extraglomerular hematuria is suggested by the passage of clots if there is gross hematuria. Extraglomerular hematuria needs to be evaluated with computed tomography, urography, urine cytology, and referral to a urologist, often for cystoscopy (37).

Catheter-Associated Urinary Tract Infections

The urinary system accounts for approximately 40% of all hospital-acquired infections. Infections of the urinary tract are the most common types of health care–acquired infection in medical-surgical units and critical care units, and approximately 80% are associated with the use of an indwelling urinary catheter. The Centers for Medicare & Medicaid Services (CMS) identified CAUTIs as one of eight conditions that, when hospital acquired, will no longer qualify for additional reimbursement in the acute care facility. The Centers for Disease Control and Prevention (CDC) reports that there are 561,667 CAUTIs per year. For fiscal year 2006, there were 11,780 reported cases of Medicare patients who had a CAUTI as a secondary diagnosis. The cases had average charges of $40,347 for the entire hospital stay. According to a study by Stamm (1991) published in the *American Journal of Medicine*, CAUTI is the most common nosocomial infection, accounting for more than 1 million cases in hospitals and nursing homes nationwide. Nosocomial UTI necessitates one extra hospital day per patient or nearly 1 million extra hospital days per year. It is estimated that each episode of symptomatic UTI adds $676 to a hospital bill. In total, according to the study, the estimated annual cost of nosocomial UTI in the United States ranges between $424 and $451 million (38, 39).

Having an indwelling catheter increases the risk of CAUTI. Other risk factors include patients with other active infections, prolonged hospital stay, diabetes, malnutrition, ureteral stent, females, abnormal serum creatinine, and improper technique in catheter care and handling. CAUTI is a common source of gram-negative bacteremia in hospitalized patients (39).

The primary measure to prevent CAUTI is catheter removal as quickly as possible. Prevention measures include aseptic technique for insertion and maintaining a closed drainage system. In patients with chronic indwelling catheter, bacteriuria is inevitable and long-term antimicrobial suppression simply selects for multidrug-resistant bacteria. Such patients should be treated with systemic antimicrobials only when symptomatic infection with pyuria is evident (33). Treating UTIs with antibiotics increase resistance and the risk of developing *C. difficile* infection. If feasible, using intermittent straight catheterizations for patients with urinary retention will provide less risk than long-term indwelling Foley catheters (39-41).

Clinical Nurse Specialist Competencies and Spheres of Influence

With the attention on elimination of CAUTIs, APNs are positioned to lead evidence-based practice initiatives to ensure optimal outcomes. The following interventions can reduce the incidence of CAUTI: staff education about catheter management and monitoring of the incidence of CAUTIs. APNs can lead an institution-wide program to ensure catheters are used only when needed and removal in a timely fashion. APNs can lead teaching the importance to all direct caregivers of the importance of daily cleansing at the meatus with soap and water or a perineal cleanser. An intact, closed urinary drainage system can reduce CAUTI. There is limited evidence for routine catheter changes for patients having long-term catheters. The following were not supported for reducing the incidence of CAUTI: sterile technique for insertion, use of antiseptic solutions or ointments with routine meatal care, and the use of dual-chamber collection devices (41).

APNs can also lead initiatives with provider colleagues for protocols to either prompt early removal of catheters or automatic removal for specified conditions. Policy development can guide use and indication for catheters.

The APN can lead the consideration of catheter alternatives with the team, including condom catheters for men without bladder obstruction. Intermittent catheterization may also reduce the infection risks. Without catheters, urinary incontinence can lead to skin maceration and breakdown. Prevention, with multidisciplinary skin care protocols, is proactive for excellent patient care. In caring for the elderly population, clinical suspicion for UTI is strong for an individual presenting with acute-onset delirium, without other cause.

For recurrent infections unrelated to CAUTI, the APN can work with the individual on prevention strategies based on history. Teaching about medication and hygiene practices may influence behavior and reduce risk.

RENAL TRANSPLANTATION

Renal transplantation is a rapidly evolving field that necessitates support and choreography from a designated transplant center. Transplant centers rely on a range of medications known collectively as immunosuppressives, which handcuff the body's immune system to hinder attack on the foreign tissue. There are a range of medical issues that must concern the health care provider whenever a transplant recipient is admitted. These would include, but are not limited to, issues in how the transplant or graft and the respective medications affect the patient and how patient's illness affects the graft. Every patient is followed by a nephrologist who is familiar with the patient's transplant history and medications. Contact this person as soon as possible for guidance, as well as someone within your system who may care for transplant patients. Critical information must be gathered that extends beyond just medications; this may include baseline GFR, previous infections associated with the graft or that developed subsequently, and obviously clinical history as well.

The issues that remain a concern include:

1. *Medication adjustment:* The immunosuppressant medications are followed very carefully and often involve testing levels to ensure therapeutic range, which may vary according to time since transplant was performed. Many medications may be added or discontinued when a patient is admitted and require retitration potentially of these medications. Be sure to involve a pharmacy that has experience with these medications. If the cause of admission results in a change of kidney function, as with any patient with ARF, adjustments must be made.

2. *Acute rejection:* Although often feared given the investment in the graft, unless there is a history of the patient specifically either choosing to or incapable of taking their medications before admission, this worry can be avoided with a minimal amount of attention. Bridging with prednisone, though not ideal, can be done in an emergency especially in light of the fact that many patients will receive stress-dose steroids for their acute illness. The best help again is through contacting a transplant nephrologist.

3. *Infection:* Immunosuppressive medications work in very specific ways, and the transplant patient is at risk for specific "opportunistic" infections depending on time since transplant and specific immunosuppressives used. The post transplant time period is broken up into first month, 1 to 6 months, and after 6 months of therapy. Immediate post transplant infections either come with the graft or are related to the surgery itself. Often these are not the result of immunosuppression at all. Between 1 and 6 months, certain viral infections and opportunistic infection occur such as *Pneumocystis pneumonia.* Beyond 6 months, fewer viral infections crop up, and those that do are often community acquired respiratory viruses. (42).

4. *Metabolic consequences of transplantation:* These include hypertension, gout, bone disease, hyperkalemia, hypocalcemia, hyperphosphatemia, renal tubular acidosis, gingival hyperplasia, and coronary artery disease. Some, but not all, malignancies occur at a higher rate, compared to the nontransplant population. Many of these are related to cumulative immunosuppression and may in fact result from the immunosuppression directly, such as post transplant lymphoproliferative disorders (PTLD).

5. *Recurrence of the disease that caused renal failure:* Certain types of glomerulonephritis, thrombotic microangiopathies, light chain diseases, and their systemic effects. Diabetes and hypertension may be exacerbated by transplant-related medications, although many of the immunosuppressents treat rheumatologic diseases, recurrence of lupus, or vasculitis should be considered if applicable.

6. *Sequelae of the chronic kidney disease if the GFR is diminished.*

7. *Transplant pyelonephritis:* This is a true emergency with a single kidney in a patient on immunosuppressant medication. On examination of the graft, typically in the right or left lower quadrant of the abdomen, if there is tenderness or if the graft feels "boggy," obtain urine and blood cultures and begin broad-spectrum antibiotic treatment immediately, including coverage for gram-negative rods (43).

The obvious dilemma ensues when the provider is unclear as to whether infection plays a part of the hospital admission. The health care provider may be stuck in the unenviable position considering whether to back off on immunosuppressive agents to aid treatment of a serious infection or to maintain or even increase these same medications for a systemic flare of a rheumatologic disease. The need to be aggressive with procuring cultures, including, if necessary, bronchial lavage may actually help tailor treatment more expediently. Injudicious use of antibiotics without cultures or defining diagnosis may be a set up for prolonged and unhelpful treatment.

RHABDOMYOLYSIS

Etiology

Rhabdomyolysis is muscular injury that can lead to pigment nephropathy, or myoglobinuric ARF (1). ARF may develop in 13% to 50% of cases of rhabdomyolysis (44). The common thread in the cause of rhabdomyolysis is the interruption of normal muscular cell metabolism as a result of ischemia. With muscle injury causing lysis, myoglobin and other intracellular proteins and electrolytes are released into circulation. Myoglobin is filtered by the glomeruli, leading to increased urinary myoglobin, which can cause ARF. Rhabdomyolysis is cited in early German literature as Meyer Betz disease presenting as a triad of muscular pain, weakness, and brown urine (45).

The etiology of rhabdomyolysis is broad, with striated or skeletal muscle injury the common denominator. It can be associated with diseases, injuries, medications, and trauma or with crush injuries. Rhabdomyolysis can occur with vascular compromise of an extremity, occurring during a prolonged surgical procedure or sustained fall. Surgical positions creating risk due to venous flow obstruction include lithotomy and lateral decubitus positions. Exertional muscle use can precipitate rhabdomyolysis, exacerbated in extreme temperatures with possible limited training prior to the exercise. McArdle syndrome is a hereditary disease in which the individual is unable to breakdown glycogen, and people with this syndrome are at risk for rhabdomyolysis (46). Table 13-8 cites causes of rhabdomyolysis.

The economic considerations of treatment are in the acute stage of early recognition and treatment to avoid progression to ARF, which is a complicated treatment course. Identifying rhabdomyolysis with early recognition and prompt treatment helps to predict the course of recovery (44).

Pathophysiology

There is a limited understanding of the full mechanism for rhabdomyolysis, but it is a major cause of ARF. It is estimated to cause 7% to 10% of all cases of ARF in the United States (45). Rhabdomyolysis is the release of injured skeletal muscle components into circulation. Prolonged muscle ischemia results in anaerobic metabolism, decreasing adenosine triphosphate (ATP) production, and release of anaerobic by-products and inflammatory mediators into the microvascular circulation (44, 45).

When muscle cells disintegrate, striated muscles release contents into circulation and extracellular fluid. Myoglobin, which resembles hemoglobin, is loosely bound to plasma globulins and only small amounts reach the urine. With the large amount of myoglobin release with the muscle injury, it exceeds the binding capacity of the plasma proteins. The glomeruli are filtering myoglobulin, which causes obstruction of tubules and renal dysfunction. Myoglobin exerts a direct cytotoxic effect in the proximal tubules. Acute tubular necrosis results from the oxidative stress in the cells of the tubules. ATP reduction facilitates the toxic effect of myoglobin, causing morphological and functional cellular changes. Myoglobinuria occurs only in the context of rhabdomyolysis, but not all cases of rhabdomyolysis are associated with myoglobinuria (44).

Clinical Presentation

The individual presenting with a muscle tenderness and fatigue following a recent injury, fall, or exercise can be suspected for rhabdomyolysis. Initial laboratory values of creatine phosphokinase (CPK) elevation, with tea-colored urine raises clinical suspicion. Up to 50% of patients will present without symptoms or with vague descriptions (44).

Rhabdomyolysis can be considered as a differential diagnosis in the presentation of ARF. A thorough history is a key to swift diagnosis. The majority of people presenting with exertional rhabdomyolysis have recently participated in an exertional exercise they had not trained for, or hydrated adequately if temperatures are high. The person exhibits obvious muscle damage, often in an extremity. A swollen extremity may suggest compartment syndrome and the suspicion for muscle injury and rhabdomyolysis. Fifty percent of patients present with injury of the thighs, calves, and lower back. The extremity presents with possible paralysis with extensive necrosis or hyperkalemia (47).

Diagnosis

Serum CPK measures the release of the protein CPK into the bloodstream from damaged skeletal muscles. The rise of CPK begins 2 to 12 hours after the injury, peaks in 1 to 3 days, and declines in 5 days. Elevations of

TABLE 13–8 Causes of Rhabdomyolysis

- Muscle Injury
  - Trauma
  - Burns
  - Electrocution
  - Immobilization
  - Metabolic disorders
  - DKA
  - Electrolyte disorders
- Ischemia
  - Compression
  - Vascular injury
  - Exercise or exertion
  - Repetitive muscle injury
  - Sickle cell disease
- Medications/drugs
  - Alcohol
  - Cocaine
  - Amphetamines
  - Statins
  - Neuroleptics
  - Amphotericin B
- Toxins
  - Isopropyl alcohol
  - Tetanus toxin
  - Quail
- Increased muscular activity
  - Sports
  - Seizures
  - Status asthmaticus
  - Infections
  - Inflammatory myopathies
- Metabolic myopathies
  - Hypothermia and hyperthermia

concern vary, but rhabdomyolysis can cause elevations up to 5 times normal value (50,000 U/L). A CPK that is greater than 20,000 units/L triggers early and aggressive treatment is instituted to avoid renal failure. The MM isoenzyme reflects muscular tissue involvement (44).

The urinalysis reveals an acid pH, with microscopic evidence of no red blood cells or less than 5 per high power field and urinary dipstick that is positive for blood. Because of the difference in myoglobin and hemoglobin, the dark pigment of the urine suggests the brown sediment contains casts and myoglobin that are filtered easily through the glomeruli. Hemoglobin saturates haptaglobin, and that complex is not filtered easily in the kidney (49).

The FE_{na} is the fractional excretion of sodium, calculated from urine and serum sodium. In rhabdomyolysis, the FE_{na} is greater than 1%, as the urine sodium concentration is elevated (greater than 20 mEq/L) (44).

Management

The goals of therapy are fluid resuscitation maintaining hemodynamic stability and urine output. Large volumes of crystalloid fluid are administered to correct the hypovolemia and hyperkalemia. Studies do not support a specific choice of solution (1). Early, aggressive volume replacement is important, especially in situations of crush injuries. Establishing a large-bore peripheral IV line or central access ensures adequate IV access. Volumes of normal saline of 400 mL/hr may be appropriate, based on clinical condition (44).

Studies also do not validate or dispute the use of sodium bicarbonate or mannitol. Sodium bicarbonate is given to alkalize the urine, decrease cast activity, and reduce myoglobin toxicity. The goal is to raise the urinary pH above 6.5. No potassium is added to solutions, and no lactate solutions are recommended for volume replacement (48, 49).

Mannitol (Osmitrol) is an osmotic diuretic acting to increase renal blood flow and assist in myoglobin clearance. It attracts fluid from the interstitial compartment, counteracting the hypovolemia and reducing muscle swelling. The drug also serves to act as a free radical scavenger to restore function to renal tissue. Mannitol is given as volume is restored and urine production begins. Loop diuretics such as furosemide increase tubular flow and decrease myoglobin precipitation. Loop diuretics act to acidify urine and promote calcium loss and therefore are added cautiously in the rhabdomyolysis treatment plan. Early hyperkalemia may be treated with insulin and dextrose to drive potassium into the cell. Ongoing correction of hyperkalemia may include binders or CRRT. Monitoring for arrhythmias is concurrent with potassium alterations. CRRT is considered if resistant hyperkalemia continues or patient displays cardiac arrhythmias or oliguria (44). Early hypocalcemia is not treated, as the calcium corrects as rhabdomyolysis is treated and resolves (49). While treatment goals are aggressive, identifying and correcting the underlying cause are imperative. For trauma injuries, considering a fasciotomy or limb amputation may be life saving (50). (See Table 13-9.)

TABLE 13-9 Considerations in Triage and Treatment of Rhabdomyolysis

Outcomes

- Urine output at 200 mL/hr
- Urine pH between 6 and 7
- Hemodynamic stability

Interventions

- Serum CPK—begin treatment if >10,000 U/L.
- IV fluids—crystalloid infusion
- Urine output monitoring
- Urine pH monitoring
- Monitor for fluid volume overload, with possible hemodynamic monitoring for at-risk patients
- Monitor serum potassium and calcium and correct
- Diuresis
- Consideration of
  - Mannitol administration
  - Sodium bicarbonate if urine pH is <6
  - If hyperkalemia, oliguria, and arrhythmias, consult nephrology for
    - Possible continuous renal replacement therapies

The progression to ARF is signaled by acidosis, oliguria, and hyperkalemia despite aggressive fluid resuscitation and possible bicarbonate administration. Timing of CRRT is based on nephrology input.

Safety Issues

Rhabdomyolysis progressing to ARF is potentially reversible. Early keys to diagnosing rhabdomyolysis with urinalysis and serum CPK, can lead to rhabdomyolysis protocols of fluid volume resuscitation and treatment. Careful reassessment for fluid volume overload and return of urine output avoids congestive heart failure. Diuretics without urine output can cause further hemodynamic compromise. Establishing early adequate IV access ensures fluid and medication use. Aseptic technique for access decreases bacteremia risk. Mannitol administration with use of micron filter per institution protocol filters the drug for administration. While monitoring urine output is imperative, UTI is reduced without catheter placement or early removal (46).

Clinical Nurse Specialist Competencies and Spheres of Influence

The APN can influence the care of patients with rhabdomyolysis by ensuring evidence-based protocols for recognition and treatment of patients. APN in the direct care role can ensure adequate access and monitoring of patients with rhabdomyolysis. The most important element in the plan of care is to closely follow electrolyte imbalance, and monitor hemodynamic response of fluid resuscitation (44).

APNs are positioned to partner with community first responders to ensure rapid recognition and fluid administration to trauma victims. Establishing access and initiating fluid resuscitation prior to extrication have shown to improve outcomes.

Case Report

Jim, a 53-year-old runner, logs in 20 miles per week with cross-training for core muscle groups. He participated this morning in a relay race, where his 6-mile "leg" of the race was entirely downhill at a grade of 45 degrees. He completed his portion in 55 minutes at moderate pace for his training. Temperature and humidity were high, and he did consume water at two intervals during the race and at the finish. At the relay point where he finished the run, he consumed 240 mL of water but did not urinate. His body temperature was warm, and he was profusely diaphoretic. An hour after his run, he complained of muscle pain and fatigue. Emergency responders triaged him to be transported to the emergency department at the local hospital. The triage nurse, gaining his history, and assessing his sore, edematous legs, obtained labwork, including a CPK and serum chemistries and urinalysis. His urine sample was tea colored. She initiated the hospital's rhabdomyolysis protocol; she inserted a large-bore peripheral IV line and infused 0.25% normal saline at 250 mL/hr. His oral temperature was 39°C. His heart rate was 88 and regular, and blood pressure was 98/58 mm Hg. His serum CPK was 18,000 U/L. His urine dipstick revealed a pH of 5.9 and no red blood cells. Serum sodium was 148 mEq/L and potassium was 4.8 mEq/L.

With evaluation by the nurse practitioner and physician, exertional rhabdomyolysis was confirmed. Sodium bicarbonate was added to the IV infusion, and mannitol 20% bolus given with a micron filter. Jim was transferred to the medical telemetry unit, and hourly intake and output and vital sign monitoring were continued. With no cardiac history for Jim, his risk of congestive heart failure was minimized with the fluid volume resuscitation. Four hours after treatment initiation, his urine output was 1,000 mL, of a lighter brown urine. A chest radiograph confirmed clear lung fields. His temperature and vital signs were in normal parameters.

Within the following 4 hours, fluids with sodium bicarbonate and mannitol continued, and urine output averaged 200 mL/hr. His serum sodium was 143 mEq/L and potassium was 4.5 mEq/L. CPK was 20,000 U/L. His urine pH was 6.5. IV fluids were continued for the next 24 hours with every-4-hour monitoring of urine output, urine pH, and serum laboratory values and vital signs.

Jim continued with stable vital signs, and urine output that was greater than 200 mL/hr of clear yellow urine. His renal function was within normal range and his IV fluids were titrated to off. His muscular swelling gradually improved as he continued with significant fatigue. He was discharged home, with gradual resumption of activity and continued oral hydration.

References

1. Cho KC, Fukagawa M. Kurokawa K. Fluid and electrolyte disorders. In McPhee SJ, Papadakis MA, editors. Current Medical Diagnosis and Treatment. 48th ed. New York: McGraw-Hill; 2009:766-793.

2. Rose BD, Post TW. Clinical Physiology of Acid-Base and Electrolyte Disorders. 5th ed. New York: McGraw-Hill; 2001:551-558, 583-588, 628-633, 749-761.

3. Yeates KE, Singer M, Morton AR. Salt and water: a simple approach to hyponatremia. CMAJ 2004;170:365.

4. Sterns RH, Cappuccio JD, Silver SM, et al. Neurologic sequelae after treatment of severe hyponatremia: a multicenter perspective. J Am Soc Neprol 1994;4:1522.

5. Sterns RH, Silver SM. Brain volume regulation in response to hypo-osmolality and its correction. Am J Med 2006;119:S12.

6. Adrogue HJ, Madias NE. Hypernatremia. N Engl J Med 2000;342:1493.

7. Lindner G, Funk GC, Schwarz C, et al. Hypernatremia in the critically ill is an independent resk factor for mortality. Am J Kidney Dis 2007;50:952.

8. Cooper MS, Gittoes NJ. Diagnosis and management of hypocalcaemia. BMJ 2008;336:1298.

9. Meric F, Yap P, Bia MJ. Etiology of hypercalcemia in hemodialysis patients on calcium carbonate therapy. Am J Kidney Dis 1990;16:459.

10. Goltzma D, Cole DEC. Hypoparathyroidism. In Primer on the Metabolic Bone Diseases and Disorders of Mineral Metabolism. 6th ed. Washington, D. C.: American Society of Bone and Mineral Research; 2006:36:216.

11. Holick MF. Vitamin D deficiency. N Engl J Med 2007;357:266.

12. Beloosesky Y, Grinblat J, Weiss A, et al. Electrolyte disorders following oral sodium phosphate administration for bowel cleansing in elderly patients. Arch Intern Med 2003;163:803.

13. Tong GM, Rude RK. Magnesium deficiency in critical illness. J Intens Care Med 2005;20:3.

14. Agus ZS. Hypomagnesemia. J Am Soc Nephrol 1999;10:1616.

15. Toto KH. Complex acid base disorders and associated electrolyte imbalances. In Carlson KK, editor. Advanced Critical Care Nursing. St Louis, MO: Elsevier; 2009:865-885.

16. Angelis M, Wong LL Myers SA, et al. Calciphylaxis in patients on hemdialysis: a prevalence study. Surgery 1997;122:1083.

17. Nigwekar SU, Wolf M, Sterns RH, et al. Calciphylaxis from nonuremic causes: a systematic review. Clin J Am Soc Nephrol 2008;3:1139.

18. Pollock B, Cunliffe WJ, Merchant WJ. Calciphylaxis in the absence of renal failure. Clin Exp Dermatol 2000;25:389.

19. Cheung CM, Ponnusamy A, Anderton JG. Management of acute renal failure in the elderly patient. Drugs Aging 2008;25 (6):455-476.

20. Hoste EAJ, Schurgers M. Epidemiology of acute kidney injury: how big is the problem? Crit Care Med 2008;36(4):S146-S151.

21. Needham E. Management of acute renal failure. Am Fam Phys 2005;72:1739-1746.

22. Bagshaw SM, Gebney N. Conventional markers of kidney function. Crit Care Med 2008;36(4):S152-S158.

23. Molzahn AE. Management of clients with renal disorders. In Black JM. Hawks JH. Medical-Surgical Nursing: Clinical Management for Positive Outcomes. 8th ed. Philadelphia, PA: Elsevier 2009:780-805.

24. Hakim RM, Lazarus MJ. Initiation of dialysis. J Am Soc Nephrol 1995;6:1319-1328.

25. Pereira B. Optimization of pre-ESRD care: the key to improved dialysis outcomes. Kidney Int 2000;57:351-365.

26. Tonelli M, Manns B, Wiebe N, et al. Continuous renal replacement therapy in adult patients with acute renal failure: systematic review and economic evaluation. Can Agency Drugs Technol Health 2007:1-30. Retrieved from http://www.cadth.ca/index.php/en/publication/732

27. Oliver MJ, Callery SM, Thorpe KE, et al. Risk of bacteremia from temporary hemodialysis catheters by site of insertion and duration of use: a prospective study. Kidney Int 2000;58(6):2543-2545.

28. Lew SQ, Ing TS. Vascular access: Past, present, and future. Int J Artif Organs 2008;31:382-385.

29. Kearney T, Dang C. Diabetic and endocrine emergencies. Postgrad Med J 2007;83:79-86.

30. Kraut JA, Kurtz I. Toxic alcohol ingestions: Clinical features, diagnosis, and management. Clin J Am Soc Nephrol 2008;3:208-225.

31. Barrett BJ, Parfrey PS. Preventing nephropathy induced by contrast medium. N Engl J Med 2006;154:379-386.

32. Beers MH, Porter RS, Jones TV, et al. Merck Manual of Diagnosis and Therapy. 18th ed. Retrieved from http://online.statref.com/Document.aspx?fxid=21&docid=803

33. Lawrence SJ, Mundy LM. Treatment of infectious disease. In Green GB, Harris IS. Lin GA, et al, editors. The Wash Man of Medical Therapeutics. 31st ed. Philadelphia: Lippincott Williams and Wilkins; 2004:292-325.

34. Saint S, Meddings JA, Calfee D, et al. Catheter-associated urinary tract infection and the medicare rule changes. Ann Intern Med. 2009;150:877-884.

35. Kreder K, Williams RD. Urologic laboratory examination. In Tanagho EA, McAninch JW, editors. Smith's General Urology. 17th ed. Retrieved from http://online.statref.com/document.aspx?fxid=12&cocid=29

36. Pinson AG, Philbrik JT, Lindbeck GH, et al. Fever in the clinical diagnosis of acute pyelonephritis. Am J Emerg Med 1997;15:148.

37. Cohen RA, Brown RS. Microscopic hematuria. N Engl J Med 2003;348:2330-2338.

38. Stamm WE. Catheter associated urinary tract infection: epidemiology, pathogenesis and prevention. Am J Med 1991;91:65S.

39. Centers for Disease Control and Prevention (CDC). Urinary incontinence among hospitalized persons aged 65 years and older—United States, 1984-1987. MMWR Morb Mortal Wkly Rep 1991;40(26):433-436.

40. Hess CT Rook LJ. Understanding recent regulatory guidelines for hospital-acquired catheter-related urinary tract infections and pressure ulcers. Ostomy Wound Manage 2007;53(12):34-42.

41. Wilson M, Wilde M, Webb ML et al. Nursing interventions to reduce the risk of catheter –associated urinary tract infection; part 2: Staff education, monitoring and care techniques. J Wound Ostomy Continence Nurs 2009;36(2):137-154.

42. Rubin RH. The changing pattern of infections following transplantation. ASN Renal Week. November 2005.

43. Radovich P. Liver, kidney and pancreas transplantation. In Carlson KK, edition. Advanced Critical Care Nursing. St Louis, MO: Elsevier; 2009:832-837.

44. Bosch X, Poch E, Grau JM. Rhabdomyolysis and acute kidney injury. N Engl J Med 2009;361:62-72.

45. Bagley WH, Yang H, Shah KH. Rhabdomyolysis. Int Emerg Med 2007;2:210-218.

46. Chatzizisis Y, Misirli G, Hatzitolios G, et al. The syndrome of rhabdomyolysis: complications and treatment. Eur J Intern Med 2008;19:568-574.

47. Russell TA. Acute renal failure related to rhabdomyolysis: pathophysiology, diagnosis and collaborative management. Nephrol Nurs J 2005;32:409-418.

48. Malinoski DJ, Slater MS, Mullins RJ. Crush injury and rhabdomyolysis. Crit Care Clin 2004;20:171-192.

49. Singh D, Chander V, Chopra K. Rhabdomyolysis. Methods Find Exp Clin Pharmacol 2005;27:39-48.

50. Schulman CS. Trauma. In Carlson KK, editor. Advanced Critical Care Nursing. St Louis, MO: Elsevier; 2009:1134-1188.

CHAPTER 14

Hematology and Oncology Problems

Brenda K. Shelton, MS, RN, CCRN, AOCN, CNS

INTRODUCTION

Disorders of the hematopoietic system involve abnormal structure or function of the hematopoietic or blood-forming cells. Each specific defect has unique risk factors and pathophysiology that will predict clinical symptoms, diagnosis, and management. There are similarities in assessment and nursing care that are translatable across disorders. Hematological disorders affect the red blood cells (RBCs), white blood cells (WBCs), platelets, or coagulation and present with manifestations of altered protection with inadequate tissue oxygenation, infection, bleeding, or clotting. Suppression of all hematopoietic cells is termed myelosuppression, but many patients with hematological disorders will have suppression of one or two of these cellular components. This chapter addresses the deficiencies separately within the hematological disorders section, but the cumulative effects of all cells suppressed is described within the hematological-oncological disorders. Complex multisystem symptoms also occur due to blood cell dysfunction or inadequate cellular activities. Clinicians must recognize the common and unique risks and manifestations in order to plan optimal individualized nursing care. A comprehensive knowledge of protective strategies, blood component transfusions, hemostatics, and antimicrobials is essential.

Oncological disorders that may require acute and critical care nursing management include a vast array of malignant conditions that affect all body organ systems and structures. Since most cancers of the organs, called solid tumors, have similar features to the other medical-surgical disorders in that body system, they are addressed elsewhere. Patients with hematological cancers have malignant transformation of the blood-forming cells and immunological system and are termed hematological malignancies. The hematological malignancies include: leukemia, lymphoma, and multiple myeloma. Symptoms and management of hematological malignancies require specialized knowledge and skills beyond those required for care of patients with hematological disorders.

Oncological emergencies are defined as emergent conditions highly associated with the presence of malignancy. Some relate to the mass effect of tumors compressing or eroding into body tissues and termed structural oncological emergencies (e.g., carotid artery erosion, superior vena cava syndrome [SVCS]). Metabolic emergencies are complications that arise from physiological changes in metabolism and common organ dysfunction. Oncological emergencies occur with different types of malignancies and are considered core knowledge in the management of each specific malignant condition. Common oncological emergencies and their unique features are described in a dedicated oncological emergency subheading.

Hematological-oncological conditions have some shared risk factors, but many have clearly different risks. Patients at risk for hematological-oncological complications most commonly have specific genetic abnormalities or exposure to carcinogenic agents. Individuals with autoimmune disorders or immunosuppression are at high risk for these complications due to abnormal immune responses. Each disorder is associated with specific risks that are defined in the discussion of that disorder. A general hematological-oncological assessment for risk includes the personal/family history findings and key clinical findings as outlined elsewhere (1, 2).

Hematological-oncological complications may be the primary or secondary disorder that brings an individual to acute care settings. Many individuals with hematological-oncological complications are admitted to specialized clinical areas with dedicated specialty trained nurses. This practice is ideal when the primary reason for admission is exacerbation or acute management of that hematological-oncological disorder; however, it may not be practical in emergency care, smaller community hospitals, or when the patient's initial clinical presentation is or mimics another medical-surgical disorder. The acute care advanced practice nurse (APRN) provides a bridge between specialty and general medical-surgical care for these patients.

When hematological-oncological patients are admitted to an acute care setting, special considerations in their care include the need for special blood components, heightened bleeding and infection prevention precautions, and complex multisystem symptoms assessment. A summary of the unique needs of these patients and how it affects patient care is included. Most nursing orientation programs do not provide education regarding the specialized care of patients with hematological-oncological complications, yet a high number of patients are affected by some aspect of these abnormalities. The clinical nurse specialist (CNS) provides an important link between this specialty practice and routine medical-surgical acute care. Oncology specialty organizations provide resources for the CNSs to obtain the most up-to-date clinical management of these patients.

There are some common clinical features among patients with hematological-oncological disorders; both often present with abnormal numbers or function of the hematological cells. The most common manifestations of reduced RBCs are hypoxemia and inadequate tissue perfusion. WBCs are essential for resistance to microbial invasion and their absence leads to infection. Low or dysfunctional platelets are needed to provide the initial platelet plug response in clotting and, when inadequate, leads to bleeding risk.

Many hematological-oncological disorders are assessed using similar diagnostic tests. The most common screening tool for many disorders is the complete blood count (CBC). It provides a global overview of the production and function of the RBCs, WBCs, and platelets. This test will identify numbers of cells, helping identify anemia, leukopenia, and thrombocytopenia. There are also morphological alterations (e.g., Dohl bodies in inflammation and certain cancers, Heinz bodies in hepatic failure, schistocytes in hemolysis) that signal a variety of hematological and medical-surgical disorders that affect the blood cells. The RBC indices (mean corpuscular volume [MCV], mean corpuscular hemoglobin [MCH], mean corpuscular hemoglobin concentration [MCHC]) and WBC differential provide clues to precise abnormalities in specific disease states.

If it is suspected that a hematologic-oncological disorder is related to inadequate or abnormal production and maturation of cells, a bone marrow aspirate and biopsy may be performed. Bone marrow procedures are usually performed in the posterior iliac crest but may also be sampled from the anterior iliac crest or sternum. Localized anesthesia is usually adequate analgesia for this procedure. An incision of the skin is made, followed by insertion of a large coring needle into the bone. When through the outside bone, the liquid red bone marrow is aspirated and then a coring needle draws bone fragments called spicules for examination. This test is also essential for diagnosis of hematological malignancies.

HEMATOLOGICAL DISORDERS: ANEMIA, SICKLE CELL ANEMIA, THROMBOCYTOPENIA, HEMOPHILIA, DISSEMINATED INTRAVASCULAR COAGULATION, AND BONE MARROW SUPPRESSION

Hematological disorders involve the blood-forming cells and their activities. The disorders in this group include altered numbers and function of RBCs, WBCs, platelets, and the coagulation factors. The consequence of inadequate number and function of cells results in altered protection. Specific deficits include poor oxygen delivery to tissues, inability to combat microbial invasion, and inadequate or inappropriate clotting and bleeding. Each disorder has a variety of etiologies with some common and other unique manifestations.

Clinical Nurse Specialist Competencies and Spheres of Influence
Clinical Expert/Direct Care and Consultation
The acute care CNS is in an ideal role to be informed and available for clinical consultation for nurses caring for patients having these unusual medical disorders. The genetic hematological disorders occur in less than 1% of the population; however, the consequence of single-component deficiencies occur with much greater frequency as secondary clinical complications. The problems of anemia, leukopenia, and thrombocytopenia are often related to medical-surgical diseases and treatments. The CNS will help nursing staff explore the potential risk factors and specialized clinical testing that may be required to diagnose the etiology. In general medical-surgical units, nurses may also require assistance in planning specialized infection prevention or bleeding precautions for these patients. Standard patient education is an essential component of care for these chronically ill patients, and complex discharge planning and medication education may be needed.

Coaching/Teaching/Mentoring
In hematological disorders, management often involves transfusion of blood components. Frequent transfusions necessitate administration of specialized products, unique

administration procedures (e.g., blood warming), and observation for higher incidence of transfusion reactions. The CNS is often responsible for clinical education and will be a key individual for development of educational products or competency validation relating to these special patient needs. Some of these chronic disorders are also associated with challenging emotional responses that may require support and assistance for patient and family adherence to the plan of care. The CNS is an expert in management of vulnerable populations and family dynamics and can assist staff in coping with these barriers to best care.

Systems Leadership, Collaboration, and Research/Evidence-Based Practice

The CNS in acute care is an expert in multidisciplinary collaboration that is required for basic management of many patients with hematological disorders. The chronicity and complexity of symptoms often require physical therapy, occupational therapy, nutrition support, and pharmacy coordination. The costs of care and need for multiple specialty consultations place these patients at risk for medication errors and breaks in continuity of care.

The CNS involved in care of patients with hematological disorders will likely be involved in the validation and standardization of administration of hematopoietic growth factors. There are precise clinical indications for which these agents will be reimbursed by insurers, and the implications of breaks in medication administration can be life-threatening. Standard orders or checklists can be used to provide the necessary quality control.

ANEMIA

Etiology

Anemia is defined as an inadequate number or function of RBCs. As a general symptom, it is one of the most common findings in primary care and can be a complication of many medical or surgical conditions such as gastrointestinal disease, hepatic disease, renal failure, and gynecological disorders (1, 3). Many medications also affect the production and function of RBCs, precipitating anemia. Due to the association of this disorder to poor nutrition, it is prevalent among the elderly, small children, economically disadvantaged persons, and addicted individuals (4). While some nutritional support strategies may be uncomplicated, barriers to their implementation offer challenges for health care providers. Additionally, the supplemental RBC interventions such as RBC transfusions and erythrocyte stimulating factors (ESAs) are costly and introduce the risk of potentially life-threatening complications.

Pathophysiology

Anemia occurs due to inadequate circulating functional RBCs. The rationales for absent or dysfunctional RBCs are grouped into several categories based on the pathophysiological mechanism. They include bone marrow production failure, abnormal structure with failure to mature and differentiate, inappropriate sequestration or destruction, and blood loss. It is essential to understand the etiology of anemia to predict unique signs and symptoms, assess appropriate diagnostic tests, and plan targeted therapy. Risk factors for specific types of anemia provide clues to guide further assessment. A summary of types of anemia and their unique clinical features is included in Table 14-1 (1, 2, 4). Table 14-2 provides an overview of etiology for anemias.

Clinical Presentation

Anemia with low circulating RBCs presents with signs and symptoms of inadequate RBC function, symptoms reflecting compensatory mechanisms, and late symptoms of organ failure. Symptoms of early abnormalities can be differentiated from late symptoms by the presence of compensation. RBCs are responsible for carrying oxygen to tissues and removing cellular carbon dioxide. With small decreases in RBC capacity, blood is shunted to the vital organs of heart, lung, and brain, but in more severe or prolonged deficits, all organs demonstrate dysfunction. This is seen as oliguria, decreased bowel sounds, altered cognition, dyspnea, or cardiac ischemia. The loss of oxygen- and carbon dioxide–carrying capacity results in hypoxemia and acidosis. The body responds to lower blood oxygen and high blood carbon dioxide by attempting to improve tissue perfusion through tachypnea, dyspnea, tachycardia, full bounding pulses, heart murmurs, cool extremities, and vascular constriction (hypertension). When compensation fails and inadequate RBCs are not corrected, organ systems fail due to poor perfusion. Anemia can lead to respiratory distress, heart failure, hypotension, renal failure, hepatic failure, skin and soft tissue ischemia, or coma (1).

Diagnosis

Diagnosis of anemia is initiated by consideration of risk factors and targeted physical examination. The risks and symptomatology will then guide selection of diagnostic tests. The acuity of symptoms and risk of continued loss of functional RBCs will also contribute to diagnostic decision-making.

When blood loss is suspected, endoscopic procedures are used to attempt to locate bleeding vessels. It is essential that blood be cleared as much as possible to permit optimal visualization during the procedure. The patient will be placed on a nothing-by-mouth (NPO) diet (upper endoscope) and have enemas (lower endoscope). Bleeding sites may diagnosed and treated through cauterization, injected with normal saline, or cryodestroyed at the same time. When scopic procedures do not readily show the location of bleeding,

(Text continued on page 599)

TABLE 14-1 Overview of Anemia

Type of Anemia	Pathophysiology	Risk factors	Common Clinical Findings	Diagnostic Test Results
Bone marrow suppression of red blood cell (RBC) production	Damage to the bone marrow leads to decreased production of RBCs. Radiation therapy exposure of axial skeleton (long bones, sternum, iliac crest slows stem cell commitment and RBC production.	Regimens containing alemtuzumab, cladribine, doxorubicin, gemcitabine, imatinib, interferon, interleukin-2, irinotecan, platinols, topoisomerase inhibitors, taxanes, and trastuzumab are more likely to cause severe anemia than other agents. The most significant contributors to anemia are the platinol agents. Other medications causing anemia: Allopurinol, antiretroviral agents, trimethoprim-sulfamethoxazole, anticonvulsants, and antidysrhythmic agents Radiation exposure—therapeutic radiation involving bones that develop cells, generalized occupational radiation exposure, toxic exposures such as radiation leaks from nuclear power plants	Infection, bleeding and fatigue. Degree/severity and length of time marrow has been suppressed will predict symptoms.	Bone marrow aspiration/biopsy shows low level of erythroblasts and other RBC precursors Serum leukopenia, thrombocytopenia and anemia The onset of RBC cell depletion may not occur immediately after chemotherapy is administered, since the normal life expectancy of RBCs is 120 days. Anemia from chemotherapy is best assessed by the hemoglobin level, and usually peaks in incidence 4 weeks after myelosuppressive therapy. Erythropoietin levels are usually low in all patients with cancer and do not necessarily rise in relation to erythropoietin therapy, and hence are not monitored during treatment.
Nutritional anemia—iron deficiency	Iron stores are inadequate for? RBC development, hemoglobin deficiency from incomplete development of the heme molecule	Occurs in 10%–30% of all adults in the United States. Primarily due to dietary deficiency. Common in infants, adolescents, elderly, pregnant and lactating women, socioeconomically disadvantaged. Can be caused by malabsorption disorders such as diarrhea, Crohn' disease.	Fatigue, headache, smooth red tongue (painful), cracks in corners of the mouth, pica Late—symptoms of cardiopulmonary compromise	Decreased hemoglobin Decreased MCV, decreased MCH/MCHC Decreased ferritin Decreased or normal serum iron Increased total iron binding capacity (TIBC) Decreased transferrin saturation
Nutritional anemia—folate deficiency	Malabsorption of folic acid due to lack of intake or absorption.	Primarily due to dietary deficiency. Common in infants, adolescents, elderly, pregnant an lactating women, socioeconomically disadvantaged. Can be caused by malabsorption disorders such as diarrhea, Crohn' disease.	Fatigue, paresthesias, headache, difficulty concentrating/cognitive impairment	Decreased serum folate level (<4 mg/dL) Decreased hemoglobin Increased MCV

Nutritional anemia—B$_{12}$ deficiency	Pernicious anemia is decreased gastric production of HCl and intrinsic factor	Familial incidence is related to autoimmune gastric mucosal atrophy with decreased intrinsic factor production. Occurs with other autoimmune diseases such as systemic lupus erythematosus, Graves disease. Common after gastric surgery, especially in base of stomach or near pylorus. More common in Northern Europeans. Rare in children	Affects production of all blood components, and although begins with decreased RBCs, leukopenia and thrombocytopenia also occur over time. These patients display paresthesias and peripheral neuropathies in addition to other symptoms of anemia. Demyelination of the spinal cord can result in profound weakness.	Vitamin B$_{12}$ deficiency is evidenced by: increased MCV, and a positive Schilling' test.
Anemia of chronic illness (ACD), cancer-associated anemia (CAE)	Inflammatory cytokines and other mediators can cause red blood cell (RBC) hemolysis. Cancer associated anemia is also thought to be related to chronically depleted erythropoietin levels.	Inflammatory gastrointestinal disease, liver failure, acute or chronic infections or malignancies. Severe sepsis is a common cause. Renal failure (acute and chronic) causes reduced erythropoietin production.	Common signs and symptoms of nonspecific anemia—fatigue, malaise, tachycardia, full bounding pulses, palpitations, heart murmurs, dyspnea, tachypnea, hypoxemia, cool extremities, decreased bowel sounds, constipation, oliguria, cognitive dysfunction, somnolence	Increased erythrocyte sedimentation rate (ESR) Increased bilirubin (total and direct) Erythropoietin levels are low, but unclear whether serum erythropoietin levels reflect the severity of anemia. The absence of an elevated reticulocyte count signals the chronicity of the disorder and lack of bone marrow reserve.
Immune hemolytic anemia	Immune destruction of RBCs outside of normal hepatosplenic hemolysis	Autoimmune diseases are most common causes—systemic lupus erythematosis, Graves disease, etc.	Enlarged and tender liver and/or spleen, jaundice, pruritis	Decreased transferrin Decreased haptoglobin Increased urine urobilinogen levels Increased schistocytes

Continued

TABLE 14-1 Overview of Anemia—cont'd

Type of Anemia	Pathophysiology	Risk factors	Common Clinical Findings	Diagnostic Test Results
	Intravascular hemolysis causes cell lysis, serum circulating cell fragments, excess release and serum levels of heme. Cell components must be bound and recycled or removed by the spleen and liver—cell neutralization causes excess circulating bilirubin and increased binding to haptoglobin and transferrin.	Organ transplant patients have autoantibodies created by the host in response to the transplanted organ and result in immune destruction of RBCs. Certain medications (e.g., phosphenytoin, rasburicase) cause autoimmune antibody production in sensitive individuals. Foreign implanted devices (e.g., heart valves, stents) can trigger autoimmune destruction of RBCs. Infusion of major mismatched blood products can cause hemolysis. Other known causes of extrasplenic hemolysis include severe hypertension, extremes in temperature (hypothermia/hyperthermia)		RBC survival studies- Indium tagged RBCs administered and scanned for abnormal hepatic or splenic uptake
Blood loss anemia	Failure of normal hemostasis, or traumatic injury to blood vessels leads to blood loss through impairment of vascular integrity.	Ulcerative gastrointestinal disease (e.g., gastritis, peptic ulcer, ulcerative colitis), neoplasm	Common signs and symptoms of anemia plus signs and symptoms of decreased circulating blood volume—dizziness, tachycardia, orthostasis, hypotension. Evidence of bleeding from orifices, into body spaces.	Rapid decrease in hematocrit and hemoglobin seen within hours of the blood loss. Increased serum reticulocyte count occurs as a compensatory mechanism for replacing the circulating mass of RBCs.
Sickle cell anemia	Instability of the "S" fragment or strand of the hemoglobin molecule causing cell collapse and sickling of the cell when it becomes	Autosomal recessive inheritance pattern of abnormal hemoglobin structure that predisposes the individual to adverse effects of sickled cells.	Usual signs and symptoms of anemia and hemolysis. Early in life, joint swelling, abdominal pain, hypoxemia are most common.	Definitive diagnosis of sickle cell disease (genetic abnormality of hemoglobin) diagnosed by hemoglobin electrophoresis. Disease stability and response to treatment may be monitored by fetal hemoglobin

hypoxic. The sickled cell is less able to move freely in small vessels, and is less able to carry and transfer oxygen on its hemoglobin molecule.

The most common symptoms of sickling involve pain. Pain in bones and joints, abdomen, chest are most common sites. "Chest syndrome" due to pulmonary constriction and hypoxemia leads to late pulmonary hypertension and chronic hypoxemia. The frequency of chest syndrome crisis events predicts poor outcomes. Sickled cells lead to intravascular hemolysis with all signs and symptoms similar to other hemolytic anemias. Late effects of chronic hyperviscosity include splenic infarction, pulmonary hypertension, hypertension, heart failure, thrombotic diseases (myocardial infarction, pulmonary embolism, deep vein thrombosis, stroke). Chronic infections related to poor circulation are common.

levels, LDH, C-reactive protein. In children, bilirubin may be elevated, and reticulocytes may be elevated, but the capacity to create these abnormalities diminishes over time. Acute sickling episodes may be accompanied by signs of poor perfusion with elevated lactic acid levels. Long-term monitoring of organ function may inform for organ atrophy or dysfunction.

TABLE 14–2 Etiologies of Anemia

Etiology	Description	Unique Clinical Findings
Extrasplenic hemolysis	Extrinsic red blood cell (RBC) defects (e.g., hypertension, severe hyperthermia), defective RBC membrane function (e.g., sickle cell disease), or antibody-induced RBC destruction causes RBCs to prematurely die.	Increased total and direct bilirubin indicates extrasplenic hemolysis that occurs in primary hemolytic disorders such as sickle cell anemia. Autoimmune hemolysis or splenic sequestration may also occur with hematological malignancies and autoimmune disease and is detectable by the presence of autoantibodies.
Medications other than anticancer agents		Most medication-induced anemia interferes with RBC production in the bone marrow. Other special clinical features may be reflective of the unique pathophysiological mechanism.
Nutritional defects	Common protein-calorie malnutrition from poor intake is most likely to result in iron deficiency anemia. Functional iron deficiency anemia occurs in anemia of chronic illness or inflammation. A specific deficit of fruits and vegetables is likely to also result in folic acid deficiency. When gastric malabsorption is present, vitamin B_{12} is poorly absorbed and results in vitamin B_{12} deficiency (pernicious anemia).	Iron deficiency produces reduced mean corpuscular hemoglobin, mean corpuscular volume (MCV), and reduced hemoglobin. In absolute iron deficiency, serum iron levels, ferritin levels, and total iron binding capacity are low. Total serum iron levels and ferritin are often falsely normal in patients with cancer, so the transferring saturation level <20% may be used as an alternative measure. In addition to common clinical findings is the presence of "pica," a craving for nonfood substances. Folic acid deficiency is identified by a folate level <4 mg/dL and an increased MCV. Folic acid deficiency also presents with paresthesias and peripheral neuropathy. Vitamin B_{12} deficiency is evidenced by increased MCV and a positive Schilling' test. These patients display paresthesias and peripheral neuropathies in addition to other symptoms of anemia.
Radiotherapy	Radiotherapy involving the long bones containing red bone marrow suppresses production of RBCs. Highest incidence of anemia has been reported in patients receiving radiotherapy for colorectal, lung, and cervical cancers.	The effects of radiation on RBC production may be slow to onset and lasts for up to 3 months after cessation of therapy.
Renal disease	Renal insufficiency leads to decreased erythropoietin production. Decreased erythropoietin levels lead to decreased RBC production.	Erythropoietin levels are decreased, but iron levels are normal.

angiograms with injection of dye into the circulation may demonstrate the location of blood loss. Another invasive test used to diagnose RBC production abnormalities is bone marrow aspiration and biopsy. Low numbers of RBCs and red cell precursors indicate lack of normal early production.

Many noninvasive or minimally invasive blood tests are helpful in differentiating types of anemia. A summary of the specialty RBC blood tests used to diagnose types of anemia is included in Table 14-3 (1, 2). Miscellaneous laboratory values useful in diagnosing anemias are found in Table 14-4.

TABLE 14–3 Diagnostic Tests in Anemia

Test	Description and Purpose	Normal Values
Hb	Measurement of gas-carrying capacity of red blood cells (RBCs)	Women: 12–16 g/dL (120–160 g/L) Men: 13.5–18 g/dL (135–180 g/L)
Hct	Measure of packed cell volume of RBC expressed as a percentage of the total blood volume	Women: 38%–47% (0.38–0.47) Men: 40%–54% (0.40–0.54)
Total RBC count	Count of number of circulating RBCs	Women: 4–5 × 10^6/μL (4–5 × 10^{12}/L) Men: 4.5–6 × 10^6/μL (4.5–6 × 10^{12}/L)
Red cell indices $MCV = \dfrac{Hct \times 10}{RBC \times 10^6}$	Determination of relative size of RBC; low MCV reflection of microcytosis, high MCV reflection of macrocytosis	82–98 fL
$MCH = \dfrac{Hb \times 10}{RBC \times 10^6}$	Measurement of average weight of Hb/RBC; low MCH indication of microcytosis or hypochromia, high MCHC indication of macrocytosis	27–33 pg
$MCHC = \dfrac{Hb}{Hct} \times 100$	Evaluation of RBC saturation with Hb; low MCHC indication of hypochromia, high MCHC evident in spherocytosis	32%–36% (0.32–0.36)
RBC morphology	Examination of the shape, size, and hemoglobin saturation of the RBCs	No variation in RBC morphology
WBC count	Measurement of total number of leukocytes. When the WBC count is very low, machine counting may be inaccurate, and laboratory personnel may hand-count the WBCs on the slide.	4000–11,000/μL (4–11 × 10^9/L)
WBC differential	Determination of whether each kind of WBC is present in proper proportion, determination of absolute value by multiplying percentage of cell type by total WBC count and dividing by 100. When calculating the absolute neutrophil count, both mature neutrophils (segmented neutrophils) and bands are included in the calculation. In addition to the common WBCs, immature neutrophils, called bands may be noted as a percentage of the total WBC count.	Neutrophils: 50%–70% (0.50–0.70) Neutrophil bands: <20% of total WBC count Eosinophils: 2%–4% (0.02–0.04) Basophils: 0%–2% (0–0.02) Lymphocytes: 20%–40% (0.20–0.40) Monocytes: 4%–8% (0.04–0.08)
Platelet count	Measurement of number of platelets available to maintain platelet clotting functions (not measurement of quality of platelet function)	150,000–400,000/μL (150–400 × 10^9/L)

Hb, Hemoglobin; *Hct,* hematocrit; *MCH,* mean corpuscular hemoglobin; *MCHC,* mean corpuscular hemoglobin concentration; *MCV,* mean corpuscular volume; *RBC,* red blood cell; *WBC,* white blood cell.

TABLE 14–4 Miscellaneous Laboratory Blood Studies

Study	Description and Purpose	Normal Values
Absolute lymphocyte count CD3 cells CD4 cells	Monitoring for HIV disease progression, response to therapy	$CD3^+$: 2-3 yr: 55%–92% 4-8 yr: 53%–93% 12-23 yr: 48%–84% >23 yr: 51%–91% $CD4^+CD3^+$: 2-3 yr: 53%–80% 4-8 yr: 30%–79% 12-23 yr: 36%–70% >23 yr: 32%–68%
HIV antibody	Screening for antibodies to the HIV virus	Nonreactive, negative
HIV culture and p24 antigen testing	Assessment for HIV "core antigen" DNA	Negative
HIV viral load	Detection of HIV viral DNA, number of copies. Test unable to test more than 200 copies	Negative
ESR	Measurement of sedimentation or settling of RBCs in 1 hr; inflammatory processes cause an alteration in plasma proteins, resulting in aggregation of RBCs and making them heavier; the faster the sedimentation rate, the higher the ESR	Women: 1–20 mm in 1 hr Men: 1–15 mm in 1 hr
Reticulocyte count	Measurement of immature RBCs; reflection of bone marrow activity in producing RBCs	0.5%–1.5% of RBC count (0.005–0.015 of RBC count)
Bilirubin	Measurement of degree of RBC hemolysis or liver's inability to excrete normal quantities of bilirubin; increase in indirect bilirubin with hemolytic problems	Total: 0.2–1.3 mg/dL (3.4–22 µmol/L) Direct: 0.1–0.3 mg/dL (1.7–5.1 µmol/L) Indirect: 0.1–1 mg/dL (1.7–17 µmol/L)
LDH	An enzyme released with RBC breakdown that may indicate hemolysis.	25-75 mg/dL
Iron Serum iron	Reflection of amount of iron combined with proteins in serum; accurate indication of status of iron storage and use	50–150 µg/dL (9–26.9 µmol/L)
Total iron-binding capacity	Measurement of percentage of saturation of transferrin, a protein that binds iron; evaluation of amount of extra iron that can be carried	250–410 µg/dL (45–73 µmol/L)
Ferritin level	As a precursor to iron in the body, the level reflects the body's ability to create new iron stores	20–200 mcg/dL
Folate level	Degree of folic acid/folate available for RBC production	5.4–24 ng/mL
Cobalamin (B_{12}) level	Absolute level of vitamin B_{12} available for production of new RBCs	

TABLE 14–4 Miscellaneous Laboratory Blood Studies—cont'd

Study	Description and Purpose	Normal Values
Vitamin B$_{12}$ level, serum	Assess absorption of vitamin B$_{12}$	200–900 pg/mL
Transferrin level	Essential element used to bind to and recirculate iron from hemolyzed cells	200–400 mg/dL
Haptoglobin level	Essential element used to bind to and recirculate the heme molecule from hemolyzed cells	60–270 mg/dL
Hemoglobin electrophoresis	Proteins involved in development of the hemoglobin molecule have a definitive pattern of separation on electrophoresis. This pattern is altered with abnormal hemoglobin synthesis such as with sickle cell anemia or thalassemia.	Normal hemoglobins A and S
Hemoglobin A1C level	Detection of abnormal hemoglobin S or C seen with sickle cell trait	4.5%–6.1%
Hemoglobin A2	Screen for thalassemia when there is unexplained microcytosis, and hemoglobin S A1C is inconclusive for subtype of abnormal hemoglobin	2.2%–3.4%
Hemoglobin heat test	Assess for unstable hemoglobin characteristic of hemolytic anemia	Negative
Coombs test	Differentiation among types of hemolytic anemias; detection of immune antibodies; detection of Rh factor	Negative
Direct	Detection of antibodies that are attached to RBCs	Negative
Indirect	Detection of antibodies in serum	Negative

ESR, Erythrocyte sedimentation rate; *LDH,* lactic dehydrogenase.

Management

Anemia may be acute or chronic, and the most important assessments required for patients are those reflecting the degree of organ perfusion deficit. Patients with mild anemia may demonstrate non–life-threatening symptoms such as fatigue, headache, or somnolence. More serious signs and symptoms of perfusion deficit signal the need for increased assessment complexity and frequency and rapid escalation of diagnostic interventions to prevent organ failure. In patients with anemia, assessment of skin and excrement for ecchymoses, petichiae, hematomas, or frank bleeding when the etiology of anemia is suspected to be blood loss.

The first interventions in anemia are assessment for tolerance of low RBC count. Patients with few symptoms and a correctable cause should be monitored while treating the etiology of the anemia. Most patients with anemia of unclear etiology should have blood drawn for type and crossmatch of donor blood products if needed.

Placing blood products on hold for potential transfusion may also be implemented for patients who may need urgent treatment. Intravenous (IV) access should be maintained until concerns of acuity have been resolved. If blood loss anemia is suspected, IV fluids are started with an isotonic solution until fluid replacement needs have been confirmed and RBCs are available for infusion.

Patients with anemia may not always require treatment if the etiology is quickly discovered and corrected. However, many causes of anemia are related to the absence of specific nutrients needed for RBC development (2, 4-6). When anemia is symptomatic and determined to need treatment, clinicians may administer ESAs.

ESAs, also known as erythrocyte growth factors, are hormones that stimulate the production of erythrocyte colony stimulating factor that regulates the bone marrow production of RBCs. These agents are administered by subcutaneous or intramuscular injection every 2 to 3 weeks but are only indicated when the hemoglobin (Hgb) falls below 10 mg/dL or when the patient exhibits severe non-compensatory symptoms at a more modestly reduced Hgb level (7). They have only been licensed for use in a select group of patients—cancer patients with chemotherapy-related anemia, individuals with renal failure, and patients with HIV disease and anemia related to antiretroviral therapy (8). These agents are tightly controlled due to their cost, and risks associated with unintentional polycythemia such as thromboses, hypertension, pulmonary embolism, and stroke (9).

When anemia is symptomatic, RBC transfusions may be administered to replace the normal functions of RBCs. The infusion of concentrated RBCs is preferred over whole blood when only RBCs are needed. They are associated with less frequent transfusion reactions and infection risk. In addition to careful monitoring for transfusion reactions through physical examination and vital signs monitoring; fluid overload, iron overload, hypocalcemia, and hypothermia may occur. The other concern with transfusions is that the influx of RBCs provides feedback to normal erythrocyte stimulating mechanisms that they can turn off, and when the transfused RBCs die, the anemia may be actually worse due to lack of persistent triggering (10).

In some cases, anemia can be preventable or reduced in severity with proactive risk assessment and education of supportive care measures. Assessment of nutrition, bleeding, and medications is particularly important for recognition of possible etiologies of anemia. In addition, clinical disorders such as sickle cell disease, renal failure, malabsorption syndrome, and hepatic disease may reveal chronic conditions that contribute to anemia (1, 3). Patients are advised to maintain a diet high in protein, B and C vitamins, iron, and zinc for maximal RBC development.

The frequency and diversity of patients with anemia are likely to increase in the upcoming years. Patients surviving with chronic disease, autoimmune disorders, HIV disease, and organ transplant have increased. The economy and nutritional state of the U.S. population also suggest that nutritional anemias may be more prevalent in the future. Anemia management in the future is likely to be based on a number of sophisticated laboratory diagnostic tests that more precisely define the RBC deficit and which interventions will be most effective. The staff nurse and CNS will need to acquire more advanced skills in laboratory test interpretation.

There has been a recent trend in reduction of the use of ESAs to treat anemia. This has correlated to several studies identifying an increased risk for complications and death among patients who received high-dose ESAs to a goal Hgb of 14 to 15 g/dL. These studies were translated to a broader population of patients, and the indication to start ESAs has been reduced to lower than 10 g/dL (11). Recently, the Food and Drug Administration (FDA) implemented consent forms and mandatory education for patients prescribed ESAs with oversight from a central agency. This practice will be demanding of nursing and pharmacy time.

Clinical Nurse Specialist Competencies and Spheres of Influence
Clinical Expert/Direct Care and Consultation
The acute care CNS is a key expert clinician to identify patients who are at risk for anemia and encourage assessment and evaluation of patients. Some of these patients do not clearly have hematological disease, and so may not be immediately recognized. Medical-surgical patients with concomitant anemia may be overlooked because of the significance of their primary medical disorder. Admission assessment and discharge planning forms designed by CNSs can incorporate cues to guide daily clinical practice.

The CNS will be involved in multidisciplinary planning for diagnostic tests, therapeutic interventions, and follow-up. It is important for the CNS to discuss discharge plans for patients who have nutritional anemias and may require assistance to ensure they correct their dietary deficits. A unique role of the CNS in discharge planning also involves assessment of appropriate indications and insurance coverage for ESAs (8). These agents are considered "medications" rather than therapeutic treatments and cost thousands of dollars per month. Often, they will not be covered by insurers unless the defined clinical indications are present. Some insurance companies provide support of the cost when administered in the clinic but not in the home setting.

Coaching/Teaching/Mentoring
Nurses are taught signs and symptoms of disease but may not have the expertise to differentiate early and late or noncompensatory symptoms of anemia. The CNS will assist staff to recognize signs and symptoms and their associated acuity in patients with anemia. For nursing staff who do not frequently administer blood transfusions in daily practice, care of these patients may require clinical updates or competency assessment of best practices in transfusion medicine. The CNS should also be able to act as a resource to staff regarding transfusion alternatives at times when patients object to receiving blood transfusions. Nursing staff are likely to require the assistance of the CNS to interpret new and unusual diagnostic tests that may be performed in patients with anemia.

Systems Leadership, Collaboration, and Research/Evidence-Based Practice
Patients with high risk for clinically significant anemia are identifiable patient groups who could benefit from standard plans of care or standard teaching plans. The implementation of best practice in ESA use is an ideal area of responsibility and collaboration of the CNS with

medical staff and pharmacists. Standard orders for ESAs with optimal dosing plans, embedded indications for ESAs, and check systems to ensure reimbursement is validated prior to patient discharge can optimize outcomes and reduce costs.

Quality improvement projects surrounding safe transfusion practices are conducted by many institutions, and are important for ensuring prudent resource utilization of blood components. The CNS working with patients having anemia may further evaluate this practice to include validated indications, consistent blood consents, and administration procedures.

The CNS is a key team member to coordinate risk assessment and recognition of patients who should have dietary referrals or hematology consultations when anemia may be amenable to early detection and management.

SICKLE CELL ANEMIA

Etiology

Sickle cell anemia is an autosomal recessive genetic disorder of Hgb S that results in RBC sickling in the presence of hypoxia. This genetic aberration is most prevalent in individuals of African or Mediterranean descent and is reported to occur in up to 8% of the African American population (12, 13). As an autosomal recessive disorder, the disease is present only when both parents contribute an abnormal gene. This means that the gene must be carried as "sickle cell trait" or present as disease in both parents. Even the presence of the carrier gene causes sickle cell trait that is associated with a number of major health conditions such as arteriosclerosis, hypertension, hyperlipidemia, diabetes mellitus type 2, renal medullary carcinoma, and thrombotic tendency (13). There are distinct geographic regions within the United States where this disease is more prevalent, and evaluation of families in the public health system enables family planning and enhanced care for affected infants and children. Public policy developed within the past two decades has been instrumental in providing screening, access to care, and enhanced outcomes, particularly in children (13). At one time, this disease was fatal for more than 50% of affected individuals before the fourth decade of their life (13). Individuals with sickle cell anemia having regular health care intervention and support can expect to live longer and healthier lives, and today more than 50% of patients are alive beyond 50 years of age (13). Annual mortality rates for sickle cell disease average 5.6% to 18.4%, and are most highly associated with renal failure, concomitant asthma, and escalating incidents of chest syndrome (13). The most common causes of death are pneumococcal disease and stroke (13). This chronic disease is associated with significant demands of health care maintenance and frequent exacerbations and illnesses requiring hospitalization. Healthy living has been shown to improve the overall health of these individuals and reduces their health care costs.

Pathophysiology

Hemoglobin is divided into two strands: Hgb A and Hgb S. The Hgb portion of the molecule carries oxygen to the tissues. In this disorder, when tissue hypoxia is present, the Hgb S molecule collapses and the RBC becomes sickled in shape. This abnormally shaped RBC is less flexible and able to travel freely through the capillaries. The sickled cells occlude small capillaries, causing thrombosis (12, 14). Tissues that become occluded with sickled cells become ischemic and produce pain. The pain is translated into the complication called sickle cell crisis (15). Painful crises also result in organ damage. The severity of hypoxemia, extent of vascular occlusion, length of time for tissue ischemia, and frequency of sickling episodes predict the disability and life expectancy for patients with this disease. Recognition and avoidance of health problems that precipitate crises can be instrumental in optimizing health and prolonging life.

Many of the late effects of sickle cell disease are related to frequent sickling, organ ischemia, and progressive tissue destruction. Patients with long-term sickle cell disease develop arthritic joints, heart failure, strokes, renal dysfunction, chronic infections, splenic infarction and destruction, pulmonary hypertension, and hepatic failure (12, 13, 16, 17).

Clinical Presentation

Sickle cell crisis can produce pain in many parts of the body, but the smallest vessels are the most prone, and pain has been commonly reported in the chest, abdomen, and joints. Pain often occurs prior to laboratory confirmation of sickling, and there may be few other outward symptoms. The severity this pain may reach is often frightening to the patient and may result in anticipatory anxiety. This presents conflicts for health care providers who are providing care. Studies have shown that the amount of analgesics used is lower when health care providers trust and treat the pain perceptions of the patient at an early age (15).

After frequent sickling episodes, some organs become thrombosed and dysfunctional. Older individuals with sickle cell disease may develop chronic renal insufficiency, osteoarthritis with severe joint impairment, pulmonary hypertension with dyspnea and hypoxemia, cerebral thromboses with mental status or motor changes, or dysfunctional spleen.

Each sickling episode and individual response produces a different amount of cells that become sickled, a variable number of cells that respond, and some cells that reverse to normal with correction of tissue hypoxia. Those sickled cells that are permanently misshapen must be removed from circulation. Normal removal of senescent RBCs is via the liver and spleen. Fragmented RBCs are hemolyzed outside the normal liver and spleen removal process and produce unique symptoms. Hemolysis causes excess direct bilirubin and lactic dehydrogenase (LDH). This leads to jaundice, hyperbilirubinemia, hepatomegaly, splenomegaly, and abdominal pain. Since the iron is recirculated and hemolysis leads to anemia, replacement blood transfusions can cause iron overload and worsen hepatic dysfunction (12).

Infections are a common problem for patients with sickle cell disease. For some, vaso-occlusion leads to altered circulation and impaired skin integrity and wound healing. Perhaps more importantly, the vascular damage to the spleen progressively destroys essential phagocytes that recognize encapsulated bacteria. Before enhanced therapies for sickle cell disease, most patients died of infection such as pneumonia and meningitis. Infection prevention measures and vaccination have greatly reduced both morbidity and mortality (18).

Chest syndrome is a common cluster of pain symptoms in which the patient has exacerbation of pulmonary hypertension with chest pain. Hypoxemia is common and must be differentiated from cardiac ischemia. Patients are frequently admitted and placed on continuous monitoring. Chest syndrome usually signifies progressive pulmonary fibrosis and pulmonary hypertension, and increasing frequency of chest syndrome episodes is considered a poor prognostic sign (17).

The most dangerous complication and a significant cause of death is both hemorrhagic and thrombotic stroke. Approximately one-fourth of all patients with sickle cell disease have a stroke before the age of 45 years (19). If patients present with mental status changes, unequal motor responses, or severe hypertension, computed tomography (CT) scans and magnetic resonance imaging (MRI) are performed to diagnose potential neurological complications.

Diagnosis

The definitive diagnostic test to confirm sickle cell anemia is Hgb electrophoresis. This demonstrates the presence of abnormal genes and can show the presence of disease or trait. Other diagnostic tests are used to monitor the disease severity, the presence of sickling episodes, or long-term complications. Patients with sickle cell trait should have early preventive health screening and monitoring for cardiovascular complications. It is common for patients with sickle cell disease to have periodic testing of complete blood count, reticulocyte count, erythrocyte sedimentation rate, iron binding saturation, C-reactive protein, lactate, fetal Hgb levels, chemistry panel with full hepatic profile, and enzymes (12, 20). Since organ dysfunction is also a common complication of progressive organ dysfunction during frequent crises, many patients also receive routine electrocardiograms (ECGs), CT scans of head and abdomen, MRI of joints, and echocardiogram.

Management

When patients are initially diagnosed with sickle cell disease, they are usually young. Joint swelling and abdominal pain are common, but subside as the cause of pain; instead progressive necrosis of the joints or splenic infarction causes severe pain in the older person with sickle cell disease. When a patient presents in sickle cell crisis, the most important assessment is to identify the severity of the crisis and response to interventions via pain ratings and descriptions. Nurses are responsible for identification of the various locations of pain and their specific characteristics. Some pain will be resolved with only IV fluids and oxygen therapy, but others may require more directive interventions. It is possible that no diagnostic evaluation will ever reveal a specific organ abnormality that triggers pain, and the sign of resolving crisis is only the absence of pain.

Because there is great concern that a patient in sickle cell crisis will experience a life-threatening thrombotic event such as myocardial infarction or stroke, thorough physical assessment is performed to establish baseline and performed frequently until the crisis begins to resolve. Complete neurological examination includes awareness, cognition, memory, motor skills, and pupillary responses.

Whenever a patient presents with sickle cell crisis, the immediate priority is to correct the thromboses causing the pain. Oxygen therapy to achieve an oxygen saturation of 92% to 94% is usually implemented, but since the true pathophysiology is poor perfusion, IV fluids are more likely to achieve this goal than oxygen. Isotonic fluids such as Ringer's lactate or 0.9% normal saline are infused at 125 to 200 mL/hr. Blood is drawn to assess markers of RBC loss, hemolysis, and inflammation, and a lactate level reflects adequacy of tissue perfusion. Ongoing monitoring of organ function with laboratory and radiological tests is incorporated as appropriate.

The next priority at presentation is to identify the potential etiology of crisis and implement treatments to reverse the disorder. The infection, excessive cold exposure, or other trigger will continue to cause cellular hypoxemia and sickling if not immediately addressed. All stabilizing interventions may be ineffective without resolution of the etiology of crisis.

Patients who present with chest syndrome are placed on continuous cardiac and oxygen saturation monitoring. Frequent vital signs supplement this information. If refractory hypoxemia and chest pain are present, more invasive interventions are implemented. Chest syndrome, however, is a unique clinical complication of sickle cell disease that may require more extensive clinical management than fluids and pain control. The central vasodilator epoprostenol sodium (Flolan) via IV infusion also inhibits platelet aggregation, providing direct clinical benefit for these patients, as has inhaled nitric oxide (16).

While sickle cell disease is not treated specifically with medications, analgesic medications are a core component of managing sickle cell crises. Due to the nature of the pain experienced by patients, this visceral and ischemic pain is only moderately responsive to any interventions. True pain relief is achieved by halting the sickling process. Potent opioid analgesics have shown the greatest promise in alleviating painful exacerbations. Initially, pain is anticipated to be severe, constant, and prolonged, necessitating continuous or frequent dosing of long-acting agents. As the crisis resolves, pain may become more intermittent or variable and manageable with intermittent injections of shorter-acting agents.

Chronic sickle cell disease causes a number of concomitant health problems that may warrant medical and pharmacological treatment. Patients receive medications for heart failure (e.g., diuretics, digoxin), hypertension (e.g., angiotensin-converting enzyme inhibitors, calcium channel blockers), iron-chelating agents, or glycoprotein inhibitors. Patients are provided influenza and pneumococcal vaccines to prevent life-threatening infections (18).

The majority of treatments for sickle cell anemia are supportive and reactive to symptoms. The individual inherits the disease and its specific severity, and this cannot be prevented. Some newer therapies for progressive and refractory disease have shown promise. Hematopoietic stem cell transplantation (HSCT) has been performed with some early success at replacing the deformed hemoglobin with donor hemoglobin (12). Complications of transplantion such as immunosuppression and rejection continue to challenge the long-term survival of these patients. Too few patients have undergone this therapy to ascertain optimal disease-free survival relapse rate.

On occasion, the cardiac workload of pulmonary hypertension also causes some degree of heart failure. In these patients with complicated chest syndrome, noninvasive positive pressure ventilator support with continuous positive airway pressure (CPAP) has been effective at reducing the workload on the heart until other interventions are effective.

Sickle cell disease is a major public health problem in some communities. While the disease cannot be prevented, family planning can help individuals anticipate and proactively address the challenges if their child has sickle cell disease. A large number of individuals are not aware that they have sickle cell trait and do not realize how this disease is imparted to their children. Having proactive genetic testing may also address health disorders that are also common for individuals with sickle cell trait. Important as well is to establish a comprehensive health care plan for children before they are born so that early diagnosis and healthy lifestyles can be established. For children with sickle cell disease, there are continuous challenges in maintaining a healthy lifestyle to minimize sickling crises. It may necessitate altered living conditions, commitment to keep the house warm, support for healthy eating, or family counseling to manage symptoms.

As the scientific understanding of the individual variations in sickle cell disease and crisis precipitation improves, so will symptom control. In the past two decades, improvement in pain management has resulted in less physical dependency on pain medications. In the future decades, it is hoped that genetic transformation, gene transplantion, and similar therapies may minimize the clinical effects or remove the defective gene in affected individuals (21). Supportive corrective therapies such as joint replacement surgery or dialysis therapies are likely to extend and enhance quality of life for these patients.

Clinical Nurse Specialist Competencies and Spheres of Influence
Clinical Expert/Direct Care and Consultation

Sickle cell disease is not a common disorder and will present a multitude of challenges for medical-surgical, emergency, and critical care nurses who may infrequently encounter these patients. The CNS who is knowledgeable about this disease and its trajectory will guide staff in implementing priority interventions and designing a plan of care. Staff nurses may be unaware of some of the subtle problems encountered by these patients. Unique clinical problems such as chest syndrome, high risk for stroke, or prior splenic infarction and subsequent high risk for infections with encapsulated organisms are potential consultative concerns.

Since there are usually only a few of these patients in most communities, the CNS with expertise in their care may become a consultant to medical-surgical units and provide case management of these patients. The CNS is available to assist in planning care and addressing discharge concerns. Pain management is often complex and complicated by the patient's anxiety and emotional responses in the context of chronic illness. Chronic health problems and frequent hospitalizations may necessitate behavioral contracts to address adherence with treatments.

Coaching/Teaching/Mentoring

The CNS is a key support to staff who must care for patients with complex life-threatening disorders. The patient with sickle cell disease presents with multiple symptoms, often paired with anxiety or distrust of the health care system. The CNS can help normalize their feelings of frustration and help them establish concrete plans of care. It has been shown that consistency of caregivers with this patient population is a positive predictor for enhanced health, reduced hospitalizations and adherence to the plan of care. Specialized care such as epoprostenol sodium infusions may require inservice education, standard orders or nursing protocols coordinated by the CNS to ensure proper administration, titration, and monitoring among nurses who have infrequent exposure to this therapy.

Systems Leadership, Collaboration, and Research/Evidence-Based Practice

Patients with sickle cell disease usually comprise a small number of patients but represent a large number of hospital visits to the emergency department and hospitalizations for complications. The CNS may be instrumental in minimizing these costly interactions by providing consistency through consultation and establishment of standards such as pain management algorithms. Due to the multisystem nature of the disease, coordination of care for these patients is costly and time-consuming and will involve many professionals and outside hospital clinics. The CNS can ease this process for patients, families, and nursing staff through coordination.

There are some newer therapies emerging in management of refractory sickle cell disease. Dissemination of new information regarding best pain management, prostacyclin infusions, or HSCT will help nursing staff stay abreast of these changes.

LEUKOPENIA

Etiology

The WBCs are responsible for inflammatory responses and combating infections. The normal total WBC count is 5000 to 10,000/mm^3. The total WBC count is composed of granulocytes (neutrophils, eosinophils, basophils), monocytes, and lymphocytes. Each WBC has a specific function that is lost when that cell is depleted. The most common WBC cytopenia is neutropenia (22). The neutrophil is the most prominent and important cell for recognizing and destroying bacteria. Lymphopenia has been associated with viral illnesses including human immunodeficiency virus (HIV) and with immunosuppressant agents such as corticosteroids or cyclosporine and many antineoplastic chemotherapeutics. Chronic and serious illness has also been associated with leukopenia, with infection the most significant adverse effect related to any leukopenia. Infection requiring hospitalization occurs in 10% to 60% of patients with cancer. The estimated cost of hospitalization for febrile neutropenia is $19,400, involving an additional 7 to 10 days of hospitalization. The incidence of leukopenia ranges from a small

risk to 100% of patients treated with certain antineoplastic regimens, with a higher incidence of febrile neutropenia in older adults, often requiring longer hospitalization (23).

Pathophysiology

The primary clinical consequence of leukopenia is infection. The greater the depletion of WBCs, the higher is the risk of life-threatening infection (24). Assessment of the severity or grade of leukopenia is a common practice to define this risk. Depletion of specific WBCs produces risk of infection with microbes normally neutralized by that cell. Neutropenia places patients at risk for bacterial infection, and for fungal infection when prolonged. Lymphopenia places patients at risk for infection with viral and opportunistic organisms and fungal disease as well (23).

Clinical Presentation

Many patients with leukopenia are asymptomatic until infection occurs. Vague constitutional symptoms such as fatigue or weakness are reported by some patients. Fever is considered the symptom of greatest importance, specificity because the lack of inflammatory cells prevents production of exudates, precluding usual indications of infection such as sputum production and pus formation (2). Although fever is considered the classic symptom, a subnormal temperature may occur with lymphopenia, serious sepsis, and gram-negative organisms (23). The presence of microbes infecting different parts of the body produces organ-specific signs and symptoms. Organ-specific signs and symptoms are noted in Table 14-5 (23).

Diagnosis

When the etiology of leukopenia is unknown, it may become necessary to perform a bone marrow aspirate and biopsy to determine if the source of leukopenia is inadequate stem cell precursors or bone marrow cell production. The presence of excessive immature cells, termed blasts, is a common indicator of acute leukemia, classified as lymphocytic or nonlymphocytic. Low neutrophil precursors without blasts may indicate chronic metabolic demands as seen in sepsis or medication toxicity. Low lymphocytic precursors are a common manifestation of HIV disease.

The usual method of diagnosing leukopenia is the serum WBC differential examination. Grading of neutropenia or lymphopenia by absolute counts is categorized as mild, moderate, and severe. Each level infers a specific risk for infection or the types of microbes likely to cause infection. On rare occasions, the source of leukopenia can be splenic sequestration that is most commonly detected with noncontrast CT scan. Follow-up assessment of all possible infectious sites with microbial cultures of blood and tissue may differentiate the type and location of infection.

TABLE 14–5 Organ-Specific Signs and Symptoms of Infection

Organ System	Infection
Neurological	Encephalitis
	Meningitis
Pulmonary	Bronchitis
	Pneumonitis
Cardiac	Endocarditis
	Myocarditis
	Pericarditis
Gastrointestinal	Colitis
	Enteritis
	Mucositis
	Pharyngitis
Genitourinary	Cystitis
	Nephritis
	Urethritis
Integumentary	Cellulitis

Management

Patients with leukopenia should be carefully assessed from head to toe for evidence of infection. Since inflammatory symptoms may be blunted due to lack of WBCs, careful evaluation of pain, erythema, or swelling should be evaluated further. Vital signs are monitored frequently for presence of hypothermia or hyperthermia, tachycardia, tachypnea, or hypotension with low diastolic blood pressure or wide pulse pressure. When a central venous catheter is available, a central venous pressure reading will be helpful for assessing the degree of vasodilation and response to fluid administration. Other signs and symptoms of altered tissue perfusion may be present in sepsis. Worrisome symptoms include oliguria and altered mental status (25).

When leukopenia is suspected or present, infection prevention measures should be implemented. The stringency and extensiveness of these measures are based on the severity of WBC deficit. For patients with mild depletion, they may be advised to avoid crowds and enhance hygiene measures. For patients with more severe WBC depletion, more caution and protective measures are advised. Some institutions that are unable to congregate high-risk patients may admit these patients to single-patient rooms, use single-use disposables, and implement additional visitor or transport limitations (26). Table 14-6 includes common infection prevention precautions for leukopenic patients (2).

Patients at risk for leukopenia may be prescribed prophylactic hematopoietic growth factors or antimicrobials. Hematopoietic growth factors are also termed colony-stimulating factors. They target the bone marrow precursor or stem cells, causing greater stem cell commitment to a particular cell line.

TABLE 14–6 Immunocompromise Precautions

Precaution	Evidence-Based Support
Have patient avoid public crowds, screen their visitors, and limit contact with pets and small children to avoid exposure to communicable diseases.	High Evidence
Hygiene should consist of bathing once a day and performing perineal care twice a day; linens should be changed each day; oral care should be performed 3 or 4 times per day.	High Evidence
Patient should wear a high particulate filter mask if being exposed to any construction.	High Evidence
Patients should wear a particulate filter mask and gloves while gardening. There should be no fresh flowers in water or soil in close contact with the patient.	High Evidence
Practice safe handling of foods by thoroughly cleaning and cooking before consumption. Avoid purchasing foods with possible contaminants, i.e., meats, eggs, seafood, and mayonnaise, if the preparation process is unknown. Fresh foods with no preservatives should be stored no longer than 2 to 3 days in the refrigerator. A "neutropenic diet" has not been proven to prevent infection (low evidence).	High Evidence except for neutropenic diet

Continued

TABLE 14-6 Immunocompromise Precautions—cont'd

Precaution	Evidence-Based Support
Intravenous (IV) tubing with blood and parenteral nutrition infusions should be changed daily. Stopcocks should not be used on IV lines to prevent a source of infection.	High Evidence
Rooms that are negative pressure or filtered with HEPA filters reduce the risk of a patient acquiring airborne fungal pathogens.	High Evidence
To avoid regrowth and resistance to microbes, administer therapeutic and prophylactic antimicrobials as prescribed. Monitor drug levels with peaks and troughs. Assess the patient for factors that may influence the absorption of a drug. Assess variables that would influence the drug level.	High Evidence
Consider making cohorted nursing assignments to avoid cross-care between high-risk patients and infected patients. Patients with leukopenia should be placed in a private room or cohorted with like patients.	High Evidence
Use strict hand washing and hand hygiene between each patient and between procedures. Encourage families and patients to practice hand hygiene before eating and after toileting by providing cleaning products in the hospital setting.	
All nondisposable multipurpose equipment should be thoroughly cleaned between each patient. If possible, provide each patient with single-use equipment and disposable supplies.	High Evidence
Immunization of patients should be considered due to the suppression of lymphocytes. Patients may receive the flu shot but not the nasal inoculation. Evaluate each patient's need for pneumococcal and meningitis vaccines. All members of the health care team should receive the influenza vaccination to prevent transmission to the patients.	High Evidence
Hematopoietic growth factors are to be administered in patients >65 years of age or those on chemotherapy agents likely to cause neutropenia in >20% of patients between 24 and 72 hours after the last chemotherapy treatment.	High Evidence
Patients that are returning home should be advised to keep their windows closed. Their living environment should be kept clean, avoiding food wastes left on the table and countertops.	Moderate Evidence
In the event of contact where moderate or high risk of respiratory infection is possible, the patient should wear a mask and change it at least every 30 minutes while in contact with that person.	Moderate Evidence
Instruct the patient to maintain good health. Stress the importance of rest, nutrition, and sleep. Blood glucose levels should be well controlled.	Moderate Evidence
Vascular access devices should be managed with sterile technique while the patient is in the hospital. Instruct the patient on institutional protocols for clean versus sterile management of their devices.	Moderate Evidence
Encourage deep breathing, coughing, and incentive spirometry to prevent atelectasis. Encourage ambulation as tolerated.	Moderate Evidence
Keep all open lesions covered with a sterile dressing. Change dressing for draining wounds per specific institutional guidelines.	Moderate Evidence
If possible, avoid rectal procedures, for example, rectal temperatures.	Moderate Evidence
Any procedure that is considered invasive must be performed using sterile technique.	Moderate Evidence

TABLE 14–6 Immunocompromise Precautions—cont'd

Precaution	Evidence-Based Support
If patient has an artificial airway, use an inline endotracheal/tracheal suction system with a flush to clean out the catheter after use.	Moderate Evidence
If patient is unable to take food by mouth, consider enteral feeding as opposed to parenteral feeding. Using the gastrointestinal tract, even if the feeding rate is small, will maintain the mucosal integrity. Enteral feeding also eliminates the need for a high-dextrose solution through an IV line.	Moderate Evidence
Encourage patients to drink only processed drinks or bottled water.	Low Evidence
For areas on the skin at high risk for infection development (e.g., skinfolds), consider using antimicrobial ointments and powders.	Low Evidence
Any oxygen therapy treatment should be changed when there are obvious signs of contamination or breaks in integrity.	Low Evidence
Administer IGIV if indicated by patient's immunoglobulin level (IgG level <300 mcg/dL).	Low Evidence

Granulocyte colony-stimulating factor and granulocyte-macrophage colony-stimulating factor are the available products used for stimulation of WBC production. The most common adverse effects of these agents are fever, bone pain, arthralgias, and myalgias. They are administered 24 to 72 hours after completion of antineoplastic therapies or routinely on a defined schedule with antiretroviral therapy (27). Prophylactic antimicrobials administered to patients with prolonged neutropenia or lymphopenia are targeted to the specific microorganisms that are usual infecting organisms. For neutropenia, this involves broad-spectrum antimicrobials directed at common gram-positive and gram-negative organisms. In lymphopenia, antimicrobials directed at *Pneumocystis carinii, Mycobacterium avium intracellulare,* or cytomegalovirus are used. Antimicrobials administered to prevent these infections are usually administered throughout the period of myelosuppression, and often at lower doses than when used for therapeutic treatment of infection (26).

When leukopenia is severe, prolonged, and in the presence of sepsis, granulocyte transfusions may be administered (26). Granulocytes are harvested from donors and separated from other blood components into a concentrated product of granulocytes bathed in plasma. The validation process and administration is similar to other blood components except the number of cells in the product are calculated and a precise infusion rate is recommended by the blood bank (23). Granulocyte transfusions are more likely to produce febrile and allergic reactions than other blood components, and consequently require premedication with acetaminophen and diphenhydramine with frequent monitoring during transfusion.

When leukopenia is permanent and not amenable to supportive strategies, HSCT may be considered as a potential treatment option for some patients. This involves the infusion and migration of donor stem cells from anther individual to the bone marrow of the patient and is plagued by potential serious complications of inadequate engraftment or rejection.

In some clinical conditions, leukopenia may not be avoidable, while in others it may be significantly minimized. Healthy living and absence of chronic illness are considered the optimal safeguards against leukopenia. Adequate nutrition and sleep are considered important for normal blood cell development and may reduce leukopenia in cases where chronic illness or metabolic demands have contributed to the disorder.

The development of neutropenia risk models to predict which patients will develop clinically significant neutropenia is an important area of current research in oncology where many of these patients are managed (23, 26). These risk assessment tools are administered at the beginning of treatment or when designing the therapy plan to identify patients who would benefit from prophylactic infection prevention. Risk models to further define individuals who are most likely to then develop serious infections are less well developed at this time. It is hoped that the future will bring more evidence-based knowledge of how to identify these highest-risk patients and best practices to prevent infection.

Clinical Nurse Specialist Competencies and Spheres of Influence
Clinical Expert/Direct Care and Consultation
The APRN serves as an essential bridge between specialty and general care. Patients who receive

marrow-suppressing therapies may encounter health care professionals in clinics, emergency departments, intensive care units, operating rooms, and diagnostic testing centers. Specialized infection prevention precautions directed against these patients at extreme risk for infection may be unfamiliar to professionals working in these general care areas.

Patients with neutropenia often receive growth factors for support of the WBC suppression related to chemotherapy. These medications are expensive and often only partly covered by patients' medication insurance coverage. The CNS is instrumental in providing information and referrals for patients who may require assistance to access reimbursement support for growth factors.

Coaching/Teaching/Mentoring

Nurses caring for patients with leukopenia often recognize the need for higher level of caution to prevent infection but may be unsure of their role in ensuring this practice by others. The CNS is an ideal mentor to assist staff in developing unit-based standards, routines, and mechanisms to ensure protection from infection. The CNS is also a key resource for staff that provide education and discharge planning for these patients' special needs. The CNS who is expert in management of these patients will design educational curricula for staff and patients that incorporate best practices and essential adult education principles.

Systems Leadership, Collaboration, and Research/Evidence-Based Practice

Patients with leukopenia are at high risk for infection and hospital practices may be inadequate to protect them from hospital-acquired infection. The CNS plays an important role as a leader in guiding staffing patterns, ensuring patient cohorting, and evaluating products that are optimal for care of these patients. It may involve evaluation of many supplies and equipment used in direct patients care to ensure they meet the highest infection prevention standards. Use of single-patient-use items is recommended for neutropenic patients, but the CNS may need to provide research-based documentation to encourage the institution to adopt these practices.

The CNS is an essential clinical expert who may advise or compose hospital policies and procedures to address the special needs of patients with leukopenia. National guidelines for venous access device management, isolation, and management of fever are available to assist in collecting quality improvement data and defining institutional standards. The CNS's expertise in systems management will aid in identifying opportunities for practice improvement such as emergency department wait time for neutropenic patients, reduction of wait time for antibiotic approval, or development

of specialized patient menus for patients with immune compromise.

THROMBOCYTOPENIA

Etiology

Thrombocytopenia is defined as a platelet count below 150,000; with a usual normal range of 150,000 to 450,000/mm^3, although some variability between laboratories is common. It is ascribed a severity classification according to the degree of deficit. Mild thrombocytopenia connotes only small increased risk of bleeding, but exponential bleeding risk occurs as the count drops lower than 20,000/mm^3 (2). Common causes of thrombocytopenia are bone marrow suppression, increased metabolic demands, chronic excessive alcohol use, massive tissue injury, autoimmune destruction, and large indwelling vascular devices (28). Other less common etiologies include an autoimmune disorder called HELLP syndrome of pregnancy, which involves *H*emolysis, *E*levated *L*iver enzymes, and *L*ow *P*latelet count (29); a serious adverse immunological platelet autolysis syndrome associated with heparin use called heparin-induced thrombocytopenia (HIT) (30); and thrombotic thrombocytopenia purpura (TTP), an uncommon disorder that may arise for undefined reasons (idiopathic) or may be related to immune processes such as pregnancy, viral infection, or lymphoid malignancies (31). Unique and specific risk factors for development of thrombocytopenia, including specific medications, are included in Table 14-7 (1, 2).

Pathophysiology

The absence of adequate platelets leads to incomplete development of platelet plugs in the presence of small vessel injury. Vessel injury leads to risk for bleeding into tissues. Any breaks in vascular integrity are normally immediately detected by the body, causing serotonin release and vasoconstriction to limit blood extravasation, followed by release of ADP that triggers platelet migration to the area and aggregation into a platelet plug to temporarily prevent bleeding. This platelet plug lasts 2 to 5 hours but is shortened or inadequate when thrombocytopenia is present. The clinical consequence of thrombocytopenia with inadequate platelet plugs is bleeding via mucous membranes or into subcutaneous tissue (1).

Clinical Presentation

Because the greatest effects of these platelet plugs are in the microvasculature, small vessel bleeding evidenced by petechiae and ecchymoses are classic manifestations of thrombocytopenia. Bleeding first appears where small vessels lie close to the body surface. Mucosal bleeding in the naso-oropharynx, urogenital system, gastrointestinal system, and skin or

TABLE 14-7 Etiologies of Thrombocytopenia

Mechanism	Examples
Destruction of platelets from immunological sources	Thrombotic thrombocytopenia purpura (TTP) Immune thrombocytopenia purpura (ITP) Heparin-induced thrombocytopenia (HIT) Mononucleosis Immunizations Viral Illnesses
Sources of blood loss	Gastrointestinal bleeding Hemoptysis Retroperitoneal bleed (e.g., blunt trauma) Vascular surgeries Hematuria Epistaxis
Bone marrow production of abnormal platelets	**Drugs:** hormones, allopurinol, antineoplastic chemotherapy (especially platinols), chloramphenicol, flucytosine, H2 blockers, alcohol, thiazide diuretics, linezolid **Conditions:** aplastic anemia, burns, catecholamine release, histoplasmosis, nutritional deficiencies, radiation exposure, liver transplant
Processes causing consumption of platelets	Damaged heart valves Blood transfusion Disseminated intravascular coagulation (DIC) Large tumors Sepsis Heat stroke Large-bore vascular catheters (e.g., balloon pump, dialysis catheter) Sulfonamides Trimethoprim-sulfamethoxazole
Sources of platelet function interference	**Drugs:** dextran, aminoglycosides, vitamin E, loop diuretics, NSAIDS, phenothiazines, salicylates, tricyclic antidepressants **Conditions:** diabetes, sarcoidosis, catecholamine release, hepatic cirrhosis, hyperthermia, hypothermia, uremia, thyrotoxicosis, systemic lupus erythematosus, scleroderma, malignant lymphomas

soft tissue is most common. When injury to major vessels occurs as a result of falls, phlebotomy, insertion of vascular access devices, or surgical procedures, major bleeding can occur. The severity of bleeding is directly related to both the platelet count and size of vascular injury. Diffuse organ bleeding can occur, producing complications such as intracranial hemorrhage, hemoptysis, cardiac tamponade, hepatomegaly, retroperitoneal hematoma, or hydronephrosis. Intraorgan bleeding is often subtle and manifests as fluid in the organ or organ dysfunction such as enlarged and tender organs,

oliguria, decreased bowel sounds, hypoxemia, or muffled heart sounds (32).

In thrombocytopenic disorders associated with immune destruction and simultaneous clotting such as HELLP syndrome or TTP, thrombotic complications such as venous thromboembolism (VTE) or pulmonary embolism may also be present despite a low platelet count (33). HIT is characterized by sudden decrease in platelets approximately 7 days after exposure. The thrombocytopenia in HIT is also associated with massive organ-dispersed clots composed of fibrin and platelets, giving the clot a white appearance, which led to the nickname for this disorder: white clot syndrome (30).

Diagnosis

The primary diagnostic tool in thrombocytopenia is the total platelet count. This test is part of the CBC and can be obtained quickly with 2 to 3 mL of blood. Some laboratories produce a blood smear and hand-count when the cell count is very low. On occasions, the actual platelet count may not be reflective of the degree of bleeding and a qualitative test of platelet function called the bleeding time may be performed. This requires a skin prick with a standardized instrument and timed blotting until the site stops bleeding. This usually is performed on the wrist or ear lobe. Normal bleeding time is less than 2 minutes, but patients may require more than 15 to 30 minutes to achieve hemostasis with severe problems of platelet quality. This test is presumed to be abnormal if the patient has actual thrombocytopenia. Immune thrombocytopenia may also be detected by the presence of platelet antibodies.

In patients with suspected HIT, a heparin antibody titer may be drawn. The presence of heparin antibodies indicates a platelet rejection phenomenon that involves platelet destruction with a propensity for clotting. TTP is diagnosed by platelet count, CBC and peripheral blood smear, and mucus membrane biopsy; bilirubin and urinalysis may be done to rule out differential diagnoses (2).

Management

Patients with thrombocytopenia require frequent vital signs and head-to-toe assessments for signs and symptoms of bleeding. Special attention to the qualities of excrement and testing for occult blood may also be helpful. Vital signs may be stable, but heart rate elevations are considered the most sensitive indicator of excessive bleeding. Immediate assessment for potential etiological factors allows for early implementation of corrective strategies such as discontinuation of medications, removal of large venous catheters, or fever control.

Thrombocytopenia may not be treated unless the patient is bleeding, requires an invasive procedure, is started on anticoagulation, or reaches a defined safe threshold. Hematologists suggest that for most patients without injury risk or high metabolic demands, a platelet count as low as $10,000/mm^3$ is safe without significant bleeding risk (34). If treatment is required, platelet transfusions are the usual best therapeutic option. The target platelet count may vary with individual risk factors for bleeding. Platelets for transfusion are usually obtained in small quantities during usual blood donation. Normally, each platelet product is termed a unit and is comprised of 30 to 60 mL. Each unit comes from a different donor. Platelets have more antigenic properties and commonly cause febrile and allergic reactions. It is desirable for patients who need to receive many platelet transfusions to receive pooled single-donor products that are the equivalent of 6 to 10 units of platelets. Large quantities of platelets from a single donor during a pheresis procedure require intentional planning for platelet harvesting. Each single unit of platelet should boost the patient's platelet count by 2,000 to $5,000/mm^3$, and pooled single-donor platelets usually produce a platelet count bump of $30,000/mm^3$ (2). No premedications for reactions are administered until the patient develops reactions, and then the premedication may be directed to the type of reaction, such as acetaminophen for febrile or diphenhydramine for allergic reactions. A condition termed alloimmunization may also occur in patients receiving frequent platelet transfusions, which is a direct rejection of the transfused platelets as foreign proteins. A major sign that patients are developing this complication is a failure to boost the platelet count after transfusion. A post-transfusion platelet count should be obtained 10 minutes to 1 hour after transfusion for best assessment of transfusion effectiveness. Platelet counts drawn later may not allow for differentiation between immune and nonimmune causes of platelet transfusion refractoriness (35).

Topical hemostatic agents may be used to halt mucosal bleeding. There are several available agents, and some are considered products, while others are pharmacological agents. While used for other coagulopathic disorders such as dessiminated intravascular coagulation (DIC), they are particularly useful with thrombocytopenia since most bleeding in this disorder is mucosal. A summary of topical hemostatics and their ideal indications is included in Table 14-8 (1).

In patients with chronic thrombocytopenia due to chemotherapy, a hematopoietic stem cell growth factor targeting platelets, oprelvekin (Neumega), may be administered to provide stimulation for platelet development. Neumega is a cytokine with similar consequences to naturally occurring thrombopoietin that acts by a different mechanism. This growth factor will be ineffective if the hematopoietic stem cell has been permanently damaged and is unable to generate new precursor cells. Romiplostim (N-plate) is a recombinant thrombopoietin that has recently been licensed for stimulation of platelet production in patients with ITP (36).

Immune thrombocytopenia may be treated with corticosteroids or immunosuppressive agents (33). This suppresses the mechanism of platelet destruction. The most concerning adverse effect of this treatment is the potential for infections to arise despite correction of the platelet count. Plasmapheresis has demonstrated efficacy in treating TTP, but not ITP (31). The theoretical reason for this is that antiplatelet antibodies are thought to be circulating in the plasma with TTP but die due to direct cytotoxicity of immune cells in ITP.

TABLE 14–8 Topical Hemostatics

Agent	Application Instructions	Indications
Absorbable gelatin sponge (Gelfoam™)		Puncture wounds such as vascular access sites or bone marrow aspiration sites
Negatol (Negatan™)		Saturated biodegradable clothlike product used for surgical wound or cervical bleeding
QuickClot™ Combat Gauze		
Microfibrillar collagen hemostat (Avitine™)		Adjunct to procedures or surgery, bleeding from wounds or soft tissue
Oxidized cellulose (Surgicel™)		Hemostatic powder applied to bleeding soft tissue, wounds, around vascular access devices, or for oral bleeding
Topical thrombin (Fibrindex™, Thrombinar™)		

On rare occasions, thrombocytopenia is prolonged and refractory to traditional treatments, necessitating HSCT. Infusion of donor bone marrow or peripherally harvested stem cells migrate to the recipient's bone marrow and replace dysfunctional stem cells.

Bleeding precautions to prevent unnecessary bleeding are implemented for patients with significant risk. There are few evidence-based interventions to guide clinicians, so many traditional interventions are used without a clear understanding of their benefit. Science and research do support use of prolonged pressure after venous access, fall risk prevention, and avoidance of excess pressure on the subcutaneous tissue such as with noninvasive blood pressure cuffs (34) is effective in controlling bleeding. Research also supports the continued use of normal tooth brushing and flossing unless bleeding occurs, although a common myth is that patients should alter their normal oral hygiene practices (34). Practical strategies commonly implemented include avoidance of traumatic muscular and subcutaneous interventions such as intramuscular injections, and invasive rectal devices. Automatic blood pressure devices exert very high pressures on initial readings, and so should be avoided when possible or dedicated to an individual patient and intermittently timed. Most of these devices adjust their reinflation pressure when set for routine checks. Most respiratory therapists will defer chest physiotherapy and use of nasal airways with platelet counts less than 50,000/mm³. Occupational and physical therapy professionals also implement restrictions for patients with low platelet counts. Head of bed elevation to reduce intracranial pressure and risk of spontaneous intracranial hemorrhage may be necessary for patients with very low platelet counts. Individual modifications such as use of stool softeners in patients with hemorrhoids or extra skin emollients for dry or fragile skin are often implemented (34).

Establishment of platelet levels for which transfusions are indicated is done to prevent bleeding. Patients who need to undergo an invasive procedure or surgery may have a goal of 50,000/mm³. This threshold is also considered standard for patients receiving therapeutic anticoagulation. When patients have a history of serious bleeding, the threshold may also be adjusted above the level where they experienced bleeding. This individualization of platelet goal necessitates effective communication among the health care team to avoid risk of bleeding.

Increased knowledge of safe platelet thresholds and evidence-based bleeding precautions has transformed recent management of thrombocytopenia. Future advances in stimulation of platelet growth are expected as the science of growth factor therapy continues to expand. Research with hemostatic agents that can replace the need for platelet transfusions is also a growing body of science.

Clinical Nurse Specialist Competencies and Spheres of Influence
Clinical Expert/Direct Care and Consultation

Patients with thrombocytopenia-related bleeding present with skin, mucous membrane, and soft tissue bleeding. The location and nature of this bleeding lends itself to management with alternative hemostatic agents. The CNS as an expert clinician will be aware of hemostatic alternatives such as topical thrombin, Avetine, Gelfoam, and Surgicel (see Table 14-8).

Patients with thrombocytopenia are likely to require a multiple of invasive procedures ranging from diagnostic tests, catheter insertions, and operative procedures. Each procedure has varying recommended platelet levels to be achieved, and the CNS will assist in planning transfusions to support these levels. Since platelet counts are essential thresholds required for specific patient care, it is especially important for the nurse to obtain accurate postplatelet counts and the CNS is actively involved in ensuring that postplatelet counts are drawn according to best practice. Administration of platelets is not as common as RBC transfusions so retaining knowledge is sometimes problematic. Platelet transfusions require special filters and administration procedures; the CNS provides vital assistance to ensure safe transfusion practices.

Coaching/Teaching/Mentoring

Patients with thrombocytopenia are likely to receive frequent platelet transfusions. Because there is a greater risk for transfusion reactions with platelets than with RBCs, the CNS will counsel staff and provide assistance in recognizing and managing febrile and allergic transfusion reactions. Staff and patient education regarding bleeding risk and precautions are often within the expected role of the acute care CNS. When unusual etiologies of thrombocytopenia such as ITP or heparin-associated thrombocytopenia are the cause, unusual and special antibody tests must be drawn. The CNS has the knowledge base and access to laboratory resources to assist nurses in properly obtaining these laboratory tests.

Systems Leadership, Collaboration, Research/Evidence-Based Practice

Patients with thrombocytopenia require specialized bleeding precautions and the CNS is likely to lead the institution's efforts in developing evidence-based guidelines to prevent bleeding. Since platelet transfusions are more likely to produce reactions, it is common for APRNs to collaborate with physicians and pharmacists to create rapid access to medications to treat transfusion reactions. This may involve standing orders or kits of medications to act quickly when reactions occur.

Platelet growth factors are indicated in only a few instances of thrombocytopenia. The special indications and administration procedures may warrant standard orders and patient education, which is often coordinated by the CNS overseeing care of this patient population.

DISSEMINATED INTRAVASCULAR COAGULATION

Etiology

Disseminated intravascular coagulation is well known by the acronym DIC. It is a disorder of inappropriate and excessive hypercoagulability that is associated with severe tissue injury and triggering of the clotting cascade. The most common causes of this secondary disorder are sepsis (37), burns (38), shock, and trauma (39); although any significant body insult may trigger the clotting cascade. It is a relatively infrequent disorder; however, it is highly morbid and carries a mortality rate of approximately 60% to 80% even when detected in its early stages (40).

Pathophysiology

At one time, DIC was thought to result from any trigger for excessive clotting. It is now known to be linked more frequently to tissue injury and the generation of tissue thromboplastin. Tissue thromboplastin causes activation of the extrinsic coagulation pathway, producing massive intravascular clotting that causes organ thromboses or infarction (41). The degree of microclotting relates to end-organ function, although a common later manifestation is that of bleeding due to multiple causes (41). The microvascular clots deplete the body's supply of platelets, and perfusion pressure against clotted vessels can lead to vessel rupture in the face of thrombocytopenia and inadequate initial components for the platelet plug (41, 42). Tissue ischemia, acidosis, and the anticoagulant effect of fibrin breakdown products add to the bleeding risk (41).

Clinical Presentation

Initial signs and symptoms of DIC usually correlate to the early thrombotic phase of the disease. Soft tissue clotting is evidenced by a classic acral cyanosis of the digits where a clear demarcation between perfused and thrombosed tissue appears to create "lines" across the fingers or toes. The distal portions begin with cyanosis and can progress to gangrenous tissue infarction. Other signs and symptoms of thromboses may include decreased bowel sounds, abdominal pain, oliguria, hypoxemia, changes in pupil sizes, or decreased level of consciousness, depending on the target organ effected (43).

As the disorder progresses to the hemorrhagic phase, bleeding becomes the predominant feature. Initial bleeding symptoms are similar to those experienced with thrombocytopenia, such as petechiae, ecchymoses, and bleeding via mucosal organs (e.g., oral cavity, uroendothelium, or gastrointestinal track) (43). Bleeding of larger vessels and into major organs such as the liver, lungs, and other body spaces such as the eye or brain is an indication of more severe coagulopathy. The most common cause of death for these patients is intracranial hemorrhage (41).

Diagnosis

The diagnosis of DIC is made by detection of clotting component depletion and excessive clot degradation. Since thromboses are the initial physiological alteration, thrombocytopenia and hypofibrinogenemia occur early (44). Validation of excessive clot breakdown is evidenced by increased fibrin degradation products

(FDPs) and D-dimer. FDPs are the breakdown products of clots and are elevated when there is a significant microvascular clotting. The d-dimer is a "d-fragment" of the clot breakdown that aids in differentiating DIC from abnormal fibrinogen (45). Diagnosis of DIC is made by a combination of risk factors, clinical symptoms, and classic diagnostic test findings, which also provide the basis for a grading system of severity (41). Other abnormal laboratory tests include decreased Hgb and hematocrit from blood loss, elevated bilirubin from RBC lysis products, acidosis, and abnormal coagulation tests. The presence of schistocytes on blood smear indicates fragmented RBCs in the circulating bloodstream (43).

Management

The most immediate observations for patients with DIC concern organ dysfunction that signifies thrombosis or hemorrhage. Each body system is assessed for signs of ischemia or bleeding that are addressed specifically. Assessment for significant blood loss such as orthostatic vital signs and central venous pressure is complemented with assessment for blood such as inspection of excrement or abdominal and limb girths. Careful physical assessment for petechiae, ecchymoses, hematomas, and bleeding around IV exit sites provides an indication of progression to the hemorrhagic phase of the disease.

Frequent laboratory assessments of CBC and coagulation studies provide ongoing information regarding adequacy of blood component therapy. The DIC panel includes partial thromboplastin time (PTT), prothrombin time (PT), fibrinogen level, FDPs, and D-dimer (43).

The most important immediate intervention in DIC is to correct the underlying etiology. DIC is a secondary disorder that is triggered by a primary event that causes excessive and inappropriate clotting stimulus. If the triggering event is not corrected, it is nearly impossible to reverse the pathophysiological process of DIC.

Supportive management of thrombus-induced organ ischemia with IV fluids, colloids, or replacement blood components is considered the mainstay of initial treatment. Some researchers have questioned whether administration of blood components acts to "feed the disease" rather than treat it, but it is generally accepted practice to replace lost components with transfusion of platelets, fresh-frozen plasma, cryoprecipitate, antithrombin III, and RBCs. Although specific blood component therapy may be administered with other hematological disorders, the most comprehensive product transfusion is administered with DIC and is described in Table 14-9 (43).

During the thrombotic phase of DIC, some patients respond to anticoagulation with unfractionated heparin. This therapy has documented efficacy in DIC associated with some malignancies and pregnancy but is considered controversial in other settings (43). The platelet count or fibrinogen level is used to titrate therapy. Platelet counts of less than 50,000/mm^3 are considered appropriate triggers to start heparin therapy unless there are other clinical reasons for thrombocytopenia such as sepsis, medication triggers, or large indwelling catheters. In patients with preexisting thrombocytopenia, a fibrinogen level less than 100 mg/dL is considered diagnostic of DIC and used as an indication to begin heparin therapy. Heparin doses are lower than used when treating venous thromboembolism and the normal laboratory parameters may not be the trigger for dose titration. Usual heparin doses are 200 to 800 units/hr, and symptoms or stabilization of

TABLE 14–9 Blood Component Therapy

Blood component	Indications/characteristics
Red blood cells	Contains red cells from one whole unit of blood plus a small amount of plasma and anticoagulant; leukocyte reduced; may be used for patients with symptomatic deficit in oxygen carry capacity and hemoglobin <6
Platelets	Obtained by apheresis from a donor; also contains 200–350 mL of plasma with citrate as the anticoagulant; indicated for patients with thrombocytopenic disorders
Fresh-frozen plasma	Plasma separated from a unit of whole blood; contains ABO antibodies; contains coagulation factors; indicated for patients with a documented deficiency of coagulation factor, correction of INR from anticoagulants, and coagulopathy due to massive transfusion
Cryoprecipitate	Treatment of patients with von Willebrand's and factor VII deficiency; protein derived from fresh plasma
Factor VII	Factor VII deficiency
Factor VIII	Factor VIII deficiency

platelet counts or fibrinogen levels are considered signs of effective therapy.

When bleeding associated with DIC is due to vascular rupture, interventional radiology may become involved to diagnose the exact location of bleeding. They may also provide interventions to halt excessive bleeding such as cautery, cryoablation, or vascular coils. When bleeding occurs into confined body areas such as the pericardial or pleural spaces, interventional radiology may be consulted to emergently drain the space or accurately place a drainage catheter.

The best method of DIC prevention is recognition of high-risk individuals, and aggressive treatment of possible causes. Patients with sepsis are at highest risk for DIC, and early goal-directed therapy with fluids and broad-spectrum antimicrobials is essential (41). Since this disorder is triggered by inflammation and tissue injury inherent among the high-risk groups, there may be limited opportunities to prevent this complication.

Knowledge of the pathophysiology and subsequent best treatments of DIC continues to evolve. With this new knowledge will be newer targeted and more effective therapies. Some fibrinolytic agents are in phase III trials and are expected to come to market in upcoming years. These agents are targeted to the pathophysiology, require less monitoring, and are safer for patients. Newer tests of fibrinolytic activity that detect DIC at an earlier phase are also in experimental phases of development. Studies of antithrombin III administration have shown considerable promise in stabilizing the coagulopathy associated with DIC (41). A newer agent used for treatment of DIC is activated factor VIIa (Novo Seven RT). It is currently available and approved for hemophilia and factor II deficiency and may be indicated for compassionate use with DIC (46).

Clinical Nurse Specialist Competencies and Spheres of Influence
Clinical Expert/Direct Care and Consultation
DIC is an unusual but potentially life-threatening complication of a variety of medical surgical disorders. Recognition of high-risk patients such as those experiencing infection, sepsis, shock, trauma, and complications of pregnancy provide a window of opportunity to prevent the most severe symptoms. The CNS is aware of these complications and risk factors and can alert members of the health care team to patients who should be more carefully monitored or tested for early alterations signifying DIC.

Patients with DIC require complex assessment and management of thrombosis and bleeding. Staff require assistance in anticipating and preventing organ failure or serious bleeding. Massive transfusion of multiple blood products predisposes patients to adverse effects such as fluid volume overload, hyperammonemia, hypocalcemia, acidosis, and hypothermia. The CNS will guide staff in designing a plan of care that incorporates blood warming, administration of coagulation factors, and calcium replacement as indicated.

Due to the complexity of care for these patients, a comprehensive assessment plan encompassing frequent vital signs and physical examination to detect occult bleeding is coordinated by the CNS.

Coaching/Teaching/Mentoring
The acute care CNS is available to staff to provide emotional and professional support when caring for these acutely ill patients with a tenuous prognosis. The acuity of these patients and high risk of mortality require commitment and skill of bedside nurses. Assessment for bleeding and thrombosis requires advanced assessment skills and diagnostic test interpretation that can be role modeled and taught by the acute care CNS. In nursing areas that routinely care for patients with sepsis, shock, burns, trauma, or high-risk obstetrics, the CNS may provide staff orientation or inservice education regarding specialized care of these patients. In clinical areas where these patients are rarely placed, the CNS can be instrumental in identifying these patients early in the disease process and facilitating their transfer to a higher level of care.

Systems Leadership, Collaboration, and Research/Evidence-Based Practice
Patients with DIC require clinical advisement from a variety of clinical specialty providers. The CNS will coordinate advice from hematology, blood bank medicine, interventional radiology, or intensivist consultations to ensure best care for patients. The CNS will also assist the health care team in coordinating invasive procedures such as central line insertion, wound care, or diagnostic procedures while ensuring timing of blood and coagulation factor infusion.

The diagnosis of DIC is still considered an acutely ill and highly morbid condition; however, it may present as a chronic disorder in patients with persistent tissue and vascular injury. Addressing the patients with chronic DIC through collaborative assessment and monitoring of laboratory indicators can contribute to improved outcomes for these patients. Development of a standard order set of laboratory tests, or "DIC panel," will encourage monitoring of at-risk patients.

ONCOLOGICAL DISORDERS: HEMATOLOGICAL CANCERS (Leukemia, Lymphoma, Multiple Myeloma)

Oncological disorders that may require acute and critical care management include the complex hematological disorders of leukemia, lymphoma, and multiple myeloma or oncological emergencies that arise due to tumor or antineoplastic therapy. Each disorder has unique clinical risk factors and specialty nursing care.

Hematological malignancies are a group of cancers that arise from the hematopoietic cells. The point of the maturation process in which the cell becomes malignant predicts the type of cancer that occurs. Each malignancy and its cell affected will predict the clinical findings and inform appropriate treatment. Each hematological malignancy is also associated with a precursor syndrome that precedes and predicts for the malignant disease. These are addressed with the pathophysiology of each disorder.

All hematological malignancies demonstrate an error in maturation of WBCs and their by-products. They are caused by common etiological triggers such as ionizing radiation, chemical or medicinal carcinogens, and viral pathogens. The universal potential catastrophe associated with all of these disorders is risk for infection due to dysfunctional WBCs. Some disorders present with reduced number or immature cells, while others present with high WBC counts. All hematological malignancies are diagnosed by evaluating the WBC involved through bone marrow, lymph node, and bloodstream evaluation. Because cytogenetics is now recognized as an important tool for predicting prognosis or responsiveness to specific therapies in all of these malignancies, flow cytometry complements other diagnostic procedures for all of these disorders. Unlike the defined mass of solid tumors, all hematological malignancies except early-stage Hodgkin's disease are considered diffuse and "metastatic" at the time of diagnosis. For this reason, primary treatment always includes systemic chemotherapy, even if localized treatment of tumor cell masses such as directed radiation therapy is used to reduce specific masses.

Clinical Nurse Specialist Competencies and Spheres of Influence
Clinical Expert/Direct Care and Consultation

The CNS in acute care is more likely to be consulted for assistance in patients with hematological malignancies than with solid tumor malignancies. These patients present with acute clinical problems and can become unstable quickly. One in 10 of these patients experiences critical illness during their course of therapy (47, 48). The most common causes of acute illness are infection, pulmonary disorders, bleeding, or oncological emergencies (48, 49). These patients develop frequent, refractory infections, often with unusual or resistant microbes. Patient management may involve unusual and complex therapies such as unusual antimicrobials, pheresis procedures, and platelet or WBC transfusions. There are many opportunities for CNS consultation in assisting staff to navigate the challenging clinical issues in this population of patients.

Coaching/Teaching/Mentoring

Specialty care of patients with hematological malignancies is a practice that lends itself to a primary care model of nursing practice in acute care. Patients experience prolonged hospitalizations and frequent clinic visits with intensive nursing assessment and interventions. When nursing staff see these patients on a regular basis, many clinical settings have found it helpful to develop a core group of nursing staff to provide care. The CNS serves as a key educator and mentor for nurses who provide this care.

Few nursing orientation programs address the special needs of patients with hematological malignancies since they are encountered infrequently in general practice. Despite this, nurses will still be expected to provide care on an emergent, limited basis. Educational programs that address these patients' special needs are available through professional organizations and can be coordinated by the CNS. While the diversity of chemotherapeutic agents is less variable with hematological malignancies than with other solid tumor malignancies, the CNS is directly involved in ensuring safe administration and personal safety precautions by staff administering the chemotherapy. Annual chemotherapy administration, monitoring and symptom management nursing competencies are considered standard of practice.

Systems Leadership, Collaboration, and Research/Evidence-Based Practice

The role of the CNS in care of patients with hematological malignancies often involves collaborative management with oncology specialists. The patients receive high-dose systemic chemotherapy and require significant symptom management that can involve pharmacists, physical therapists, respiratory therapists, interventional procedures, and medical consultants. Evidence-based symptom management resources are available from professional organizations for optimal symptom management of these patients.

The CNS may also need to evaluate available services in their practice area to ensure these patients will have readily available clinical care. These patients require 24-hour availability of respiratory therapy and transfusion medicine services, quick access to antibiotics, and frequent laboratory evaluations. Some oncological emergencies common in these patients require emergent radiation therapy that should be available in the institution or via rapid transfer. The CNS may need to create proposals for access to additional supplies, services, or staff training to accommodate these demands of care.

HEMATOLOGICAL CANCERS: LEUKEMIA

Etiology

Leukemia is a malignant transformation of the WBC occurring during the developmental phase within the bone marrow. Although comprising only 1% to 2% of all cancers, it is the most common cancer in young children. The average survival for these patients is widely variable and dependent on host risk factors and clinical characteristics related to the malignant cell line. Factors that influence prognosis include how early in the cell line the malignant clone emerged, association with genetic abnormalities, and the specific type of leukemia (50). In general, leukemia is considered advanced and widespread at the time of diagnosis. The first remission is usually the longest and, for some patients with high risk for recurrence, is an important time to pursue potentially curative therapies such as HSCT.

The presence of excessive immature malignant cells is termed acute leukemia, and overproduction of mature cells is classified as chronic leukemia. Within each category, leukemia is further subdivided as occurring in the lymphocyte cell line or the myelocyte cell line (50). Leukemia may occur in children or adults but is usually associated with a better prognosis in children. A summary of all the subtypes of leukemia and their common clinical features is included in Table 14-10 (50).

The most common causes of leukemia are exposure to carcinogenic medications or ionizing radiation. Secondary leukemia after receiving antineoplastic treatment for another cancer comprises a small percentage of patients. Secondary leukemia after treatment with immunosuppressives for autoimmune disease or solid organ transplant has an occurrence rate of hematological malignancies (leukemia or lymphoma) of less than 1% but is no less tragic when it occurs (50, 51). All secondary leukemias are considered high risk for morbidity with a poor prognosis from the onset of disease. Medications known to enhance risk for leukemia include antineoplastic agents, antivirals, antimalarials, corticosteroids, and immunosuppressives. Exposure to toxic chemicals such as pesticides and benzenes can also induce leukemia. Some types of leukemia have been linked to unique viruses such as human T-cell leukemia virus (HTLV-1, HTLV-2). There are also genetic mutations that have been associated with leukemia of all aged individuals. The importance of genetic mutations, called cytogenetics, in children has been long recognized and considered in the overall treatment plan. The implications of genetic abnormalities in adult leukemia have only recently been recognized and are now an essential component of diagnosis and planning treatment (52-54).

Pathophysiology

Leukemia is characterized by the malignant transformation of the WBC during its maturation within the bone marrow. The degree of immaturity and cells affected define the type of leukemia and some of its characteristic features. The cell that is malignant does not function normally, so antimicrobial phagocytosis, inflammation, and deactivation of foreign antigens are impaired. These patients are at high risk for infection due to inadequate immune recognition and microbe destruction mechanisms.

Acute leukemia involves cells early in the maturation process, so there are excessive numbers of large immature cells called blasts. These blasts crowd other cells in the bone marrow and spill over into the serum. Excess circulating blasts cause hyperviscosity with thromboses and organ failure, called leukostasis (48, 55, 56). Leukostasis is considered an oncological emergency. It is most likely to occur when the myelocyte cell line is affected, the total WBC count is greater than 100,000/mm^3, or the serum blast percentage is more than 15% of the total WBC (55, 56). Other considerations that increase risk of clinically significant leukostasis include the WBC rate of rise, the presence of dehydration, or vasoconstriction.

Chronic leukemias overproduce matures cell with less risk for thrombotic organ failure. Excess mature WBCs are also more functional, and serious infections are less likely to occur early in the disease. Patients with chronic leukemias may have less acute symptoms and be diagnosed less quickly. Some of the patients with chronic leukemia will convert to a blastic acute phase leukemia, while others produce a long-term chronic disease unlikely to contribute to death (57, 58).

A disorder termed myelodysplasic syndrome (MDS) is an abnormality of hematopoietic cell production with less than the defined percentage of blasts to constitute acute leukemia. Most patients with myelodysplasia will develop acute leukemia in the months to years after diagnosis of MDS. At one time these patients were considered as having "preleukemia," but definitive treatment was deferred until leukemic conversion. These patients present with a particularly refractory leukemia, and specific treatments are used to correct the bone marrow dysfunction before the onset of leukemia. These agents are still categorized as antineoplastics and patients are treated by oncologists, but they are not the same treatments used for leukemia (59, 60).

Clinical Presentation

Although the primary feature of leukemia is the malignant WBC, the presence of these malignant cells crowds the bone marrow, preventing normal production of all hematopoietic cells. The classic signs and symptoms are associated with anemia, thrombocytopenia, and leukopenia as described in previous sections of this chapter. Bone pain is common due to marrow overproduction and packing with cells. Constitutional symptoms such as fatigue, weakness, myalgias, and arthralgias are common for all patients. On occasion, leukemic cells accumulate into masses on or near the bones, termed leukemic infiltrates or chloromas. High

TABLE 14–10 Overview of Leukemia

Leukemia Subtype	FAB classification	Epidemiology	Clinical Features	Prognosis
Acute lymphocytic leukemia	L1	Common in children	Hepatomegaly, lymphadenopathy, CNS involvement, splenomegaly; age of onset usually 2–3 years	CNS involvement, infant with t(4;11), patient with t(9;22), t(1;19), high WBC count, age <1 or >10 yr, or a longer time to achieve remission is associated with poor prognosis
Chronic lymphocytic leukemia		Most common type of leukemia in adults with age of onset usually >60 yr may be familial	Prone to viral infections, may not require treatment for years if low risk	Low-risk patients die mostly of other causes; median survival is 4–6 yr; CLL patients with low risk usually die from complications within a few months of diagnosis
Acute myelocytic leukemia	M1	WBC infiltrate organs and causes CNS changes	High WBC count on presentation; splenomegaly, heptomegaly, and lymphadenopathy	Median survival 10–15 mo if remission is not achieved
Acute myelomonocytic leukemia	M2	Increase in WBCs that infiltrates other organs	High WBC count, gum hypertrophy, splenomegaly	65%–80% achieve remission with therapy, but if remission not achieved, survival is usually 10–15 mo
Acute progranulocytic leukemia	M3			
Acute monocytic leukemia	M5	Increase in WBC causing infiltration to other organs such as the spleen; often involves MLL gene	CNS involvement, hepatomegaly, lymphadenopathy	Remission rate 65%–80%, without remission median survival is 10–15 mo

WBC counts rather than leukopenia, especially in patients with immature cells called blasts, produce leukostasis. For unclear reasons, leukostasis most commonly affects the brain and lungs. Mental status changes, signs of stroke, or respiratory distress are considered emergent and may be rapidly progressive to life-threatening crises (55).

Each type of leukemia has clinical features unique to the cell type and acuity. They may be associated with effusions, gum infiltration, coagulopathy, or meningeal involvement. These specific clinical identifiers of leukemias are included in Table 14-10 (50). Acute leukemia notably presents with infection or bleeding. Since granulocytes live only hours, the depletion of effective WBCs is most immediately noticeable at the onset of disease. The life span of platelets is 7 to 10 days, so failure to replace platelets, leading to a bleeding tendency, is also early in the disease. Since RBCs live 80 to 120 days, it may be months until signs and symptoms of anemia are evident.

Patients with MDS present much like leukemia patients but without malignant transformation of the bone marrow. Because they are chronically myelosuppressed, they receive a large volume of blood products and prophylactic or therapeutic antimicrobials. Iron toxicity with hepatic dysfunction, skin discoloration, and gastrointestinal symptoms is common. Adverse effects of antimicrobials such as renal dysfunction, gastrointestinal upset, and superinfections also occur with these patients (60).

Chronic leukemia produces subtle and far less debilitating symptoms than acute leukemia or MDS. Patients may have slow healing wounds, gum bleeding, and many symptoms of chronic anemia. A number of these patients are able to continue normal activities of daily living while receiving treatment. Some have carried normal pregnancies to term, or underwent serious surgical procedures with little impact on their health.

Diagnosis

The most common screening test to demonstrate probable leukemia is the CBC. There may be decreased or elevated WBCs, and in acute leukemia, systemic blasts may be present. The bloodstream normally carries less than 5% blasts, but in acute, newly diagnosed, or recurrent leukemia, the blast percentage may be as high as 50% of the WBC. Indicators of leukemia dissemination in the liver and kidneys include elevated liver function tests and elevated serum creatinine (61).

The most definitive diagnostic test for confirmation of leukemia is bone marrow aspiration and biopsy. This test allows examination of the bone marrow precursor cells and can demonstrate the malignant cell changes. The bone marrow is also tested for cytopathology and molecular changes that assist in specific definition of the type of leukemia and the specific mutations. Cytogenetics is helpful in planning treatment and identifying prognostic factors (53, 62).

Management

The patient with leukemia is usually acutely ill and often admitted to the hospital immediately after diagnosis. Evaluation for significant infection or bleeding is the most important initial assessments. Patients may be unable to mount inflammatory responses due to dysfunctional WBCs and have few traditional signs and symptoms of infection. Fever and pain are the most reliable indicators of infection. Without functional WBCs, the risk of rapid progression of infection to sepsis is a serious concern. For this reason, temperatures of 38.0°C (100.4°F) are considered represent potential infection (63). If infection is suspected, broad-based bacterial, fungal, and sometimes viral cultures are performed to detect microbes, and broad-spectrum antimicrobials are started within 1 hour of fever (26). The localization of infection is essential for ensuring appropriate antimicrobial agents are prescribed. The nurse's full head-to-toe assessment including careful visualization of skinfolds, and orifices may provide clues to sources of infection and guide treatment decisions. Throughout treatment of leukemia, patients may receive antimicrobials, either as prophylaxis or as part of treatment for fever of unknown origin.

Patients with leukemia are administered systemic chemotherapy or targeted antineoplastic agents. Many of these medications have significant immediate and ongoing adverse effects. The nurse plans assessment and monitoring for these adverse effects so that optimal preventive strategies and timely treatments can be implemented. If the chemotherapy agent causes nausea and vomiting, a preventive antiemetic regimen is prescribed with additional medications for breakthrough symptoms. Other common clinical effects of antileukemia chemotherapy can be capillary leak syndrome with edema or effusions, mucositis, dysrhythmias, cardiomyopathy, diarrhea, peripheral neuropathies, skin eruptions, sleep-wake disturbances, or renal dysfunction (50).

Patients with leukemia require immediate systemic antineoplastic therapy to prevent disease-related organ failure or the adverse consequences of myelosuppression. These therapies often require frequent phlebotomy, multiple IV medications, parenteral nutrition, and blood transfusions. Most patients have long-term indwelling venous catheters inserted for the duration of treatment. Ideally, these should be placed prior to the start of therapy, as myelosuppression and infection risk worsen with targeted therapy and chemotherapy.

When administering targeted therapy or chemotherapy, special hazard precautions should be implemented to protect the nurse against exposure to carcinogens. Patients and families should also be taught protective measures to be implemented through 48 hours after the last therapy. Some of these patients will take daily therapy for months to years. If the agent is a vesicant, additional precautions to prevent extravasation are implemented.

Chemotherapeutic regimens differ with each subclassification of leukemia. Subtypes within the same cell line may receive similar treatment but cytogenetics and unique individual features often dictate different treatments (50). Each regimen is associated with an adverse effect profile that will dictate the supportive medications needed. Patients receiving daunorubicin or cyclophosphamide will need antiemetics, whereas patients receiving high-dose cytarabine may require diuretics. Oncological texts provide advice of greater detail to guide the acute care nurse (50).

Most patients with leukemia receiving antineoplastic therapy can anticipate prolonged and severe aplasia. This suppressed hematopoietic cell production may result in administration of prophylactic antimicrobials to prevent infection or chronic transfusions for anemia and thrombocytopenia. Because myelosuppression is so prolonged, the incidence of infection with unusual or resistant microbes necessitates administration of several and less common antimicrobials. Prophylaxis for gram-negative organisms and fungal infections with oral agents such as norfloxacin, polymyxin, nystatin, or an azole antifungal agent is common (64).

When leukemia patients present with high WBC counts, the viscosity of the blood places patients at high risk for thrombotic events. Immediate administration of chemotherapy agents may cause massive tumor cell lysis, and while this is the intended objective of therapy, the accumulation of toxic metabolic products in the serum can be life-threatening. Patients with high WBC counts, rapid rate of rise, or high percentage of blasts may have leukapheresis prior to starting chemotherapy (55, 65). Performed by hemapheresis professionals, the process of removing excess WBC and reinfusing plasma leads to reduction of WBCs without dehydration. In facilities without pheresis services, exchange transfusions may be performed instead. Most pheresis procedures will reduce the WBC count by 20,000 to 30,000 cells/mm³ per given treatment (55). With very high WBC counts, pheresis may be performed while also administering a rapid-acting antineoplastic such as hydroxyurea or cyclophosphamide, whereby removing cells while also beginning the cell destruction process.

Patients with leukemia who are at high risk for relapse may undergo HSCT after their first remission (66, 67). Replacement of the defective marrow with the stem cells of a donor serves to correct the defect. Successful long-term disease remission with HSCT in leukemia is widely variable and dependent on host risk factors as well as leukemia-specific prognostics. The most common complications of this therapy are failure to engraft or rejection phenomenon. Tumor relapse occurs as well, but the risk decreases after the initial 9 to 15 months post-transplant (68).

The best prevention of leukemia is avoidance and protection from carcinogens. Healthy living, masks for carcinogenic aerosols, and skin shielding against UV rays are all specific interventions used to protect against carcinogenic exposure. Autoimmune disorders treated long-term with immunosuppressants or corticosteroids also comprise a population of patients who need to be monitored for early changes in the bone marrow and, when possible, rotation of treatments to minimize exposure to these carcinogens.

Some patients receiving induction chemotherapy for newly diagnosed acute leukemia may remain hospitalized for 30 to 60 days, but an emerging trend is to identify patients at lower risk for severe infection and to manage their infections in an intensive ambulatory clinic with good caregiver support while at home or at nearby housing facilities. Considerations for individuals who may be candidates for this alternative care include those with knowledgeable caregivers, individuals housed close to the hospital/clinic, efficient triage and emergent antibiotics availability, patients with previous good performance status, or infections acquired outside the acute care setting (69). It is considered more risky when the infection is respiratory in origin, in patients with previous invasive fungal infection, or in patients after HSCT (69, 70).

The leukemia patient in many cases now is receiving oral targeted antineoplastic therapies. Specific genetic mutations have been identified and can be targeted with these oral agents. While optimal in providing patients more opportunities to continue normal activities of daily living, there are considerable educational challenges associated with these agents. Each of them requires specific instructions for ingestion with or without food or in conjunction with other medications. In addition, patients must be reliable with medication use. There are a number of these oral agents, and while highly effective, they may not be adequately covered by outpatient medication insurance and require costly copayments.

The specialty practice of HSCT has progressed in such proportions that it is no longer essential to have a matched bone marrow donor in order to offer this therapeutic option to patients with leukemia that is high risk for relapse. Nonmyeloablative transplant, also known as mini-transplant, allows donor marrow to be partially matched and donor leukocyte reinfusions can boost the engraftment of the donor marrow. This modality provides an avenue for transplant to patients who previously had too many or severe comorbidities or for whom no marrow match could be found. Development of more and highly efficacious immunosuppressant agents prevents rejection. It is anticipated that current toxicities and failure to engraft will become even less frequent as this technology continues to be perfected.

Clinical Nurse Specialist Competencies and Spheres of Influence
Clinical Expert/Direct Care and Consultation

Caring for patients with leukemia in the general medical-surgical, emergency, or intensive care setting may be unusual. Although concepts of managing myelosuppression are universal, other clinical problems experienced by these patients are unique and complex. Chemotherapy regimens for patients with acute leukemia are usually complex and involve an induction phase where all leukemia cells are eradicated, followed by a consolidation phase where additional chemotherapy administered to patients with a normalized bone marrow is aimed at preventing disease relapse. Some therapy plans vary in agent and administration patterns across several months, and others require chemotherapy for several years or administered intrathecally. The development of a treatment planning calendar, planning for timely hospital admissions, and coordination of ambulatory services are care issues ideally suited to the skills of the acute care CNS.

The practice of HSCT is a common therapeutic option for patients with leukemia. This involves unique and advanced knowledge of the processes of cell harvest, preparative regimens, stem cell infusion, and antirejection treatments. Complications of HSCT are inclusive of other oncological therapies, but there are also several unique to this specialty. The acute care CNS who works with these patients and advises staff and the health care team is familiar with preparative regimen toxicities such as engraftment syndrome, hepatic veno-occlusive disease, alveolar hemorrhage, hemolytic uremic syndrome, posterior reversible encephalopathy, and viral infections such as cytomegalovirus, respiratory syncytial virus, John Cunningham virus (JCV), or BK virus. Knowledge of risks, clinical findings, timing, and optimal management strategies allows the CNS to provide expert consultation in care of these patients.

Patients with leukemia have prolonged and extreme immunosuppression, making them vulnerable to common and unusual infections alike. Due to frequent antibiotic exposure, patients are often prescribed less common antimicrobials and agents reserved for patients with resistant infections. The administration of these atypical antibiotics and antifungals requires specialized nursing knowledge. Interpretation of culture results and antibiotic serum levels is a necessary skill for the acute care CNS caring for these patients.

Coaching/Teaching/Mentoring

The CNS assisting nurses who care for patients with leukemia will be instrumental is guiding safe administration of chemotherapy and special extravasation precautions for agents such as daunorubicin or vincristine. Chemotherapeutic agents commonly used to treat leukemia also may produce hypersensitivity reactions (L-asparaginase), neurotoxicity (cytarabine, vincristine), or cardiotoxicity (arsenic trioxide). Each agent administered has a specific adverse effect profile and nursing staff must provide patient education. The CNS will play an active role in assisting nurses to access specialized cancer nursing knowledge and patient education materials available.

New oral agents used to manage leukemia patients are especially important to emphasize as most are metabolized by the cytochrome 450 pathway and have many drug–drug or drug–food interactions that will affect efficacy and toxicity. Staff and patients must understand the importance of adherence to the treatment plan and special precautions needed to ensure their efficacy. The CNS may need to act as case manager and navigator for this patient population or provide significant advice and support for others providing this care.

Most patients receiving treatment for their leukemia must take prophylactic antimicrobials. It is important for the CNS to help staff understand the importance of verifying adherence with prophylactic antimicrobials. Patients must not be made to feel guilty if they are unable to tolerate the prescribed therapy but must know that without these agents the risk of serious infection is escalated. There are a variety of choices of prophylactic agents to select, and patients unable to tolerate one may be switched if they inform their caregivers. Since prophylactic antimicrobials are also oral and may be attained on ambulatory medication insurance, it is important to ensure that patients can afford and obtain these agents.

Due to the importance and longevity of antimicrobial therapy and the risks of hepatic or renal dysfunction, antimicrobial serum levels must be drawn. The CNS will be instrumental in advising staff the timing and information needed to ensure accurate serum levels are drawn and appropriate antimicrobial adjustments are made. Some agents require a before-and-after antimicrobial blood draw, some "post" blood samples are drawn in 30 minutes while others are drawn at 60 minutes, and all require accounting of the exact time of the immediate past dose and total doses for the past 24 hours.

Systems Leadership, Collaboration, and Research/Evidence-Based Practice

The acute care CNS involved in care of the leukemia patient is likely to be involved with multiple health care disciplines. These patients often present while acutely ill and may require intermediate or intensive care during the initial phases of their stabilization and first chemotherapy. They require central venous access yet need to remain as mobile as possible to reduce complications. Physical therapy and occupational therapy are consulted for their assistance with many patients. The potency and complexity of their therapy require the involvement of consultant physicians from intensive care, nephrology, gastroenterology, and infectious disease medicine. Since many of these therapies are inpatient and prolonged, patients will need support of social workers to address insurance coverage, home care needs, return to work, or disrupted family dynamics.

Ambulatory practice for patients with leukemia is a growing trend but requires significant coordination and patient education. Patient and caregiver education and policies for out of hospital care should be structured and precise. Accommodations for urgent care should be well-planned and documented. The acute care CNS leads the team in these efforts and implements quality monitoring to ensure safe patient care. Standards of care for these patients may differ significantly from other cancer patients at less risk for severe infection.

Due to the high risk for infection and critical illness experienced by these patients, close relationships with the intensive care unit and infectious disease departments is essential. The CNS is a core systems expert that is ideally suited to develop and maintain protocols for collaboration. It is estimated that more than 90% of patients with leukemia will develop infection, and while some are not difficult to manage, others are extremely challenging to diagnose and eradicate. Rapid availability of antimicrobial agents may hinge on antibiotic approval programs coordinated between infectious disease and pharmacy. The CNS must ensure these programs demonstrate antibiotic stewardship without compromising rapid intervention for patients. One in every 7 to 10 patients with leukemia will develop a critical illness during their disease trajectory. The most common reasons for critical illness are respiratory distress, sepsis, bleeding, hypotension, and oncological emergencies. The CNS will coordinate education and algorithms with intensivists, and rapid response teams to ensure these complications are managed appropriate to these patients' unique needs.

HEMATOLOGICAL CANCERS: LYMPHOMA

Etiology

Lymphomas are a group of malignancies of the WBC that arise from malignant transformation within the lymph node. Two major subtypes of lymphoma occur—Hodgkin disease (HD) and non-Hodgkin lymphoma (NHL). These cancers affect both adults and children, with a propensity for Hodgkin lymphoma in young adults younger than 35 years or in the fifth or sixth decade of life. NHL is a more diverse disease, with more than 20 different cytopathologies occurring in individuals of all ages. Like leukemia, the molecular genetics of NHL are important for treatment planning and prognostics (71).

Unlike leukemia, the incidence of lymphomas has been rising over the past decade, currently comprising 7% to 11% of all cancers, and is the fifth most common type of cancer (71). The major proposed reason for this increase is the number of patients with immunosuppression. These include patients surviving organ transplant, longer life expectancy for patients infected with HIV, and greater success with immunosuppressive agents used to treat autoimmune diseases. Risk factors for development of most lymphomas are genetic abnormalities, immunosuppression, and viral illness (72, 73). Patients with lymphoma have widely variable survival rates that depend on the subtype, cytogenetics, and etiological factors. Secondary lymphoma occurring after immune suppression or previous antineoplastic therapy is known to be more refractory to therapy than disease arising de novo without immune-related risk factors (73, 74).

The prognosis of lymphoma varies with histology and molecular features. Patients with most subtypes of HD have a better than 90% chance of 5-year survival, and 60% to 70% may be cured (71). NHL overall has a less promising prognosis; however, indolent lymphoma is associated with a chronic disease trajectory lasting 5 to 15 years after diagnosis. High-grade lymphomas are rapidly fatal if untreated and carry a 40% to 60% initial response rate but less than 20% survival at 5 years unless the patient receives an HSCT. Intermediate-grade lymphomas have moderate prognosis and disease course.

Pathophysiology

The lymphocyte is the only WBC that is affected in lymphoma; however the T-lymphocyte is more often the cause of HL and the B-lymphocyte is affected in approximately 85% of NHLs. Lymphocytes become malignant within different portions of the lymph node and are named by their cellular origin and microscopic appearance. The specific implications of each of the subtypes of both HD and NHL are well-described in oncology nursing references (71). These disorders are staged differently and managed with unique chemotherapeutic agents. NHL disease is generally considered the more severe and invasive of the two disorders and is systemic at the time of diagnosis. HD may present with disease in a single or two lymph node groups and be treated with local therapy such as radiation (75, 76).

HD arises from a specific cell mutation and classic T-lymphocyte cell appearance named the Reed-Sternberg cell. There are five subtypes of HD, the most common being nodular sclerosing. HD has a more indolent clinical course than NHL, and since it usually initially arises in a single lymph node group, is staged by the Ann Arbor staging system. This system considers how many lymph node groups are involved and whether disease is above or below the diaphragm, plus additional nonmyeloid sites.

HD is a malignancy that is usually moderately aggressive, although some types are more proliferative. Since it is characterized by a single cell type, it is likely to be responsive to systemic therapy. Patients with HD, even with multiple lymph node groups, may be highly responsive with long-term remission or cure (75). Since HD involves the T-lymphocyte, viral infections commonly destroyed by the T-lymphocyte are more problematic for these patients. During postchemotherapy immunosuppression, patients are given antiviral prophylaxis (77).

NHL is characterized by the malignant transformation of the lymphocyte within the lymph node. Types of lymphoma are named by the origin of the cell (e.g., mantle cell, follicular) within the lymph node and also by its growth rate or proliferative potential with consideration of molecular characteristics such as marker cells or receptor sites. These various types of lymphomas are then grouped by growth rate and prognostic implications into low, intermediate, or high grades. Low-grade lymphomas have a slow growth rate and may also be termed indolent lymphomas. These patients may have long-term, non–life-threatening disease, although there is a low cure potential with these lymphomas. High-grade lymphomas such as Burkitt's lymphoma have a high proliferation rate, and cells are less mature. This disease can be rapidly fatal if not treated immediately but is more responsive to systemic therapy. The clinical staging of NHL is very different than that with HD and considered advanced at diagnosis. The presence of disease in nonimmunological organs such as the abdomen, liver, and lungs is not uncommon. The high propensity for involvement of B-lymphocytes in NHL results in bacterial and fungal infections but less risk for viral illness (71).

Clinical Presentation

Lymphomas of every subtype consistently present with enlarged lymph nodes. NHL is noteworthy for both enlarged lymph nodes and lymphomatous masses producing complications similar to solid tumors. Layperson educators suggest that lymph nodes greater than 2 cm for longer than 2 weeks are considered a node suspicious for malignancy. Enlarged lymph nodes with infection and inflammation are painful and moveable, but malignant nodes are often painless and have irregular borders that are not moveable. Lymphomatous masses can interfere with organ function in any part of the body, and masses cause compression of lungs, bowel, ureters, or other organs.

Constitutional symptoms such as fatigue, fever, night sweats, and itching occur in some patients and are considered poor prognostic signs. The symptoms are termed "B" symptoms and may trigger the decision to provide more comprehensive therapy to avoid later disease relapse.

For unclear reasons, patients with lymphoma are prone to metabolic paraneoplastic syndromes. It is proposed this may be related to the level of inflammation associated with this disease, yet others believe it is related to hormonal characteristics of the tumors. Syndrome of inappropriate antidiuretic hormone is common in patients with advanced disease, and hypercalcemia occurs in a moderate number of patients. Lambert-Eaton neuropathy and DIC are less common and usually a reflection of more severe disease.

Diagnosis

The most definitive diagnostic tool for confirmation of lymphoma is a lymph node biopsy. Since malignancy is suspected, the node should not undergo needle or incisional biopsy as this induces a risk of tracking malignant cells through the subcutaneous tissue and provides an avenue for recurrence. If no enlarged lymph nodes are readily available for excisional biopsy, exploratory operative procedures are performed to obtain a good specimen.

Cytopathology physicians will examine the total lymph node and its cells to assess for malignant cells. Immunohistochemistry tests are performed to detect cell surface markers such as CD20 or CD22 that signify specific types of lymphoma and prognostic markers. Once a cytopathological diagnosis of lymphoma has been confirmed, other nonspecific diagnostic tests such as CT or positron emission tomography (PET) scans are used to assess extensiveness of disease or responsiveness to therapy. Most patients have repeated CT scans to monitor the status of their disease or evaluate for recurrence. The lactate dehydrogenase (LDH) serum value is considered an accurate surrogate marker for severity of disease and used to establish a baseline and monitor for response to treatment. Extensive NHL, particularly with high growth rates, will have LDH levels 5 to 10 times normal. Higher LDH levels are predictive for patients at risk to develop a complication of rapid cell lysis termed tumor lysis syndrome (TLS) (78). Other tests that may be abnormal in patients with lymphoma but are not diagnostic for the disease itself include alkaline phosphatase levels, serum WBC count, hypoalbuminemia, or C-reactive protein. Other diagnostic tests are monitored to detect organ dysfunction caused by mass compression and may include CBC, renal function studies, transaminases, or bilirubin (71).

Management

Patients with lymphomas have multiple clinical presentations based on the location of enlarged lymph nodes or lymphomatous masses, and disease is often widespread at diagnosis. Assessment of these patients should be comprehensive and include evaluation of all sites of known disease and all body systems. Since the risk of infection is high, assessment for infection or sepsis is also included in initial and ongoing assessments.

Once therapy has been initiated, careful observation and frequent laboratory tests are implemented to detect tumor lysis syndrome. While not all patients are at risk, approximately 10% of patients have some electrolyte abnormalities. Since TLS can also lead to renal failure, urine output should be maintained at approximately 2 mL/kg/hr. Slowing of urine output may warrant additional diagnostic tests and increased IV fluid infusion rates.

Patients with lymphoma may be treated in either inpatient or outpatient settings. At initial diagnosis, these patients may have significant tumor burden and risk for tumor lysis, requiring inpatient care. Most of the ongoing standard chemotherapy regimens are amenable to outpatient care. The treatment of lymphomas is usually targeted and chemotherapy except in early-stage HD can be provided as outpatient care. Many patients with high-grade lymphoma require emergent chemotherapy or urgent radiation in addition to immediately shrink tumor masses.

Chemotherapy is given as a planned regimen approximately every 3 weeks for 4 to 6 months. Unlike leukemia management, there is no induction followed by consolidation, but instead it is delivered as multiple cycles of the same chemotherapy plan. Patients who are optimal candidates for HSCT will receive fewer cycles, followed by transplantation and patients who are not eligible for transplantation receive more monthly chemotherapy cycles. The decision to progress to transplantation is based on the histology, molecular features, stage of disease at diagnosis, and risk for early disease relapse after treatment.

The role of invasive therapies such as surgery or management of malignant lymphomas is primarily limited to early-stage HD with limited lymph node involvement for diagnostic purposes in patients with NHL. Surgical procedures to obtain biopsy specimens for diagnosis is common when disease is limited to the chest or abdomen and no peripheral lymph nodes appear to be involved. Many palliative and supportive surgical procedures may be performed to provide ongoing care but are not considered treatments.

Clear measures to prevent lymphoma are related to minimizing risk factor exposures. Patients can actively prevent acquisition of human immunodeficiency virus (HIV) and thus prevent lymphoma, but other variables may be less avoidable. Individuals receiving immunosuppressant therapy or antineoplastic agents may have severe life-threatening diseases that require treatment with these agents and will be counseled on the risks and benefits of these agents when they are used in other conditions. Follow-up monitoring of these high-risk patients is also implemented to enhance early recognition of lymphadenopathy or lymphoma. It is

unclear with other viral illnesses such as Epstein-Barr virus (EBV), which patients will develop malignant responses to the presence of the virus and hence it is difficult to define preventive actions.

Knowledge of the pathobiology of lymphomas has greatly advanced over the past decade and targeted therapies have generated successful long-term remissions or second responses in patients who previously died of recurrent disease. It is conceivable that the implications of molecular markers and prognostic variables with more targeted therapies will continue to advance management of lymphoma. It is also expected that with more effective marker identification, preventive therapies or gene therapies may become more prevalent strategies to manage lymphoma.

Clinical Nurse Specialist Competencies and Spheres of Influence
Clinical Expert/Direct Care and Consultation

Patients with malignant lymphoma may present in medical surgical, ambulatory, and emergency settings with a wide variety of clinical symptoms. Patients often present to surgeons and medical-surgical settings with symptoms of pain, masses, and organ dysfunction that are not immediately recognizable as lymphadenopathy. The acute care CNS is involved in assisting staff with assessment and care planning for these patients. Common problems include fevers, night sweats, and symptoms of lymphadenopathy or lymphomatous mass–induced complications. Patients should be thoroughly assessed for dyspnea, gastrointestinal distress, biliary obstruction, mental status changes, electrolyte disturbances, and renal dysfunction. In patients with high-grade non-Hodgkin lymphomas, HD with large bulky tumors, patients with high LDH levels, abdominal disease, or hypoalbuminemia, careful observation for TLS is essential.

Patients with lymphoma have risks for a variety of oncological emergencies discussed within this chapter. The rapid tumor growth rate and tendency for mass rapid development of masses can lead to structural emergencies such as pleural effusions, pericardial effusions, ascites, tracheobronchial obstruction (TBO), or SVCS. The CNS is a key clinical expert for staff to consult for development of assessment and nursing care strategies.

Coaching/Teaching/Mentoring

Staff caring for patients with lymphoma should have advanced assessment and critical thinking skills. These patients are at risk for multisystem symptoms that can rapidly progress to life-threatening complications. The CNS is an expert clinician and educator who will be key in coordinating pertinent staff education, or multidisciplinary inservices for pharmacy, respiratory therapy, physical therapy, or laboratory clinicians involved in care of these patients. Specialized oncology nursing resources for care of these patients are readily available (71).

Patient education content for individuals with lymphoma is extensive and involves information about the disease, therapy options, supportive care, medications, diagnostic tests, and self-care. There are several complex treatments such as hematopoietic growth factors or targeted therapies that may require assessment of insurance coverage. Many of these patients need assistance at home or follow-up teaching for wound care or IV catheter care. Since therapies span several months, patients may need to discuss work leave and obtain disability information from the hospital. The CNS is likely to be involved in developing or guiding staff in providing this education. If patients are frequently seen in the clinical area, specialized information should be packaged and organized to provide information over time.

Systems Leadership, Collaboration, and Research/Evidence-Based Practice

Patients with malignant lymphoma will require consultation from many health professional and specialty services. The acute care CNS as coordinator of care is central to developing collaborative relationships with these specialists. Patients often receive multiple cycles of chemotherapy, require frequent phlebotomy specimens, and are at risk for infection, so semipermanent indwelling central venous catheters or ports are implanted for the duration of therapy. Home care plans for these devices may need to be designed and shared with local home care companies.

Collaboration with other departments for management of oncological emergencies is also an important aspect of care for these patients. Although not a primary treatment modality, emergency radiation treatment to rapidly shrink tumor masses compressing body organs or causing effusions may be necessary. If the CNS's hospital does not provide radiation services, advanced planning with other facilities that will provide this care is necessary. In cases of SVCS, TBO, and spinal cord compression (SCC), transfer may be advised to ensure the patient has rapid access to skilled surgical services or continuous dialysis if TLS occurs.

HEMATOLOGICAL CANCERS: MULTIPLE MYELOMA

Etiology

Multiple myeloma (MM) is a type of hematological cancer resulting from malignant transformation of B-cell destined plasma cells. The disease is characterized by secretion of a malignant clonal immunoglobulin, excessive production of cytokines, and bone metastases

in 95% to 100% of patients (79). Plasma cells are lymphocytes that secrete immunoglobulins that are protective in the inflammatory response and provide for immune competence. In MM, the malignant plasma cells produce excessive quantities of dysfunctional immunoglobulins, "myeloma proteins," inducing an immunoglobulinopathy. Any immunoglobulin (IgG, IgA, IgD, IgE) can be involved; however, IgM is most common. IgA is the largest protein molecule and produces the highest incidence of hyperviscosity and thrombotic events (80, 81).

MM is classified into four disease categories, according to plasma cell manifestation: (1) monoclonal gammopathy of undetermined significance (MGUS), (2) smoldering multiple myeloma (SMM), (3) indolent multiple myeloma (IMM), and (4) symptomatic multiple myeloma. The Durie and Salmon Staging System entails three stages, based on plasma cell proliferation. Stage I is characterized by low cell mass; Stage II, intermediate cell mass; and Stage III, high cell mass. The disease is further subclassified into Subclassification A, in which there is normal renal function, and Subclassification B, with abnormal renal function (82).

The incidence of MM is 4 in 100,000 people, representing 1% to 2% of all cancers and 20% of hematological malignancies. Approximately 14,500 new cases are diagnosed annually, with 10,500 deaths per year. A 29% survival rate at 2 years is predicted. The prognosis for MM is less promising than that for many other types of malignancies. The average life expectancy for people with MM is 31 to 39 months regardless of an existing "pre-myeloma" syndrome. There is reportedly a 5-year survival rate in 31% of cases, 10-year survival in 10%, and 20-year survival rate in 4% of cases. The survival statistics are largely unchanged since 1985 (82, 83).

Risk factors include older age (average age 66 years at diagnosis), with fewer than 11% under the age of 50. The malignancy is more common in African Americans and occurs in twice as many men than women. Forty-two percent of cases have a strong family history of hematological malignancy. Exposure to environmental toxins such as benzene, pesticides, herbicides, and ionizing radiation increases the risk for MM. Also, immune-modulating conditions such as chronic inflammatory disease and allergies may be a risk. The herpes virus is thought to enhance conversion from MGUS of undetermined significance to MM (84).

Pathophysiology

MM is a malignancy of the plasma cell, a derivative of B-lymphocytes, expressing abnormal cell surface glycoproteins, including CD38, CD56, CD138, and CD20. It is a genetic disorder, with deletion of chromosomes 13 and 17 (83). The pathophysiology involves excessive production of cytokines, namely interleukin (IL)-6 and plasma cell growth factor. Other cytokines involved include tumor necrosis factor α (TNF-α), IL-1, vascular endothelial growth factor, transforming growth factor β, and receptor activator of necrosis factor (NF)-κB (85). The interaction between malignant plasma cells, bone marrow stromal cells, and osteoclasts in the bone causes destructive bone lesions and stimulation of bone marrow angiogenesis.

Clinical Presentation

Bone pain is usually the first symptom of MM, occurring in approximately 58% of patients (79). The pain is usually in the back or chest; extremity pain is unusual. The pain is induced by movement and rarely occurs at night unless associated with position change. Bone pain stems from two pathophysiological processes. First are cytokine effects: IL-1 and IL-6 activate osteoclasts, which cause bone demineralization and loss of infrastructure. Second, myeloma proteins directly invade the bone, resulting in destruction of osteoblasts and dominance of osteoclasts. Bone demineralization causes hypercalcemia in approximately 13% of patients (86).

Plasmacytomas, large purple-colored, fixed, subcutaneous masses, are the sole presenting symptoms in approximately 5% of patients. They are usually located in the brain/leptomeninges, intramedullary in the thoracic paravertebra, the skull, the ribs, and the long bones. Plasmacytomas are also found in extramedullary tissue in the head and neck region, upper airways, digestive tract, bladder, and breast/testes (87).

Bone marrow suppression causes a decreased production of erythrocytes and leukocytes, leading to anemia and infection. The most common organisms include *Streptococcus pneumoniae*, gram-negative bacteria, and *Candida*. Inhibited antibody responses can also lead to infection with previously experienced infections such as herpes simplex and measles. The most frequent infections are pneumonia and urinary tract (79).

Renal dysfunction is common, with elevated blood urea nitrogen and creatinine and decreased creatinine clearance. Weight loss, lymphadenopathy, and hepatosplenomegaly are sometimes present. Skin changes occur, including unexplained pruritus (related to gammopathy), and thickened skin, especially on the palms of the hands and soles of the feet. Yellowish plaques appear along skin creases, proposed to be lipid-based deposits related to gammopathy and interference with lipid metabolism. Acral cyanosis may also occur. Patients sometimes complain of neuropathies, especially with osteosclerotic myeloma and a constellation of signs, including polyneuropathy, organomegaly, endocrinopathy, monoclonal gammopathy, and skin changes, called POEMS syndrome (88).

Hyperviscosity is caused by circulating large plasma cells and excess immunoglobulin. This leads to sluggish blood flow and increases the risk for thromboembolic events, including deep vein thrombosis, pulmonary embolism, stroke, and cardiac ischemia, predisposing to heart failure (80).

Diagnosis

Diagnostic testing includes general laboratory studies, testing specifically for MM, and imaging studies. Laboratory tests include serum electrolytes, especially for calcium levels; chemistry profile to evaluate albumin and renal and liver function; and CBC to identify anemia and infection. Also, coagulation studies and serum B12, folate, and ferritin levels should be determined. Serum and urine electrophoresis is done for monoclonal protein identification. Standard radiographs of the spine, pelvis, skull, humeri, and femurs are taken to evaluate bone lesions and fractures; MRI and bone scans cannot differentiate bone lesions from fractures. Bone mineral densometry is done to evaluate lytic lesions. Bone marrow aspiration is done and should include flow cytometrics and cytogenetics. A bone marrow specimen with plasma cells OR plasmacytoma AND at least one of the following confirms the diagnosis of MM: monoclonal protein in the serum, monoclonal protein in the urine, or presence of organ tissue impairment: increased *C*alcium, *R*enal insufficiency, *A*nemia, and *B*one lesions (CRAB) (85).

Management

Clinical treatment options include (1) an aggressive attempt for remission with high-dose chemotherapy, biological therapy (e.g., thalidomide), and HSCT; (2) treatment of refractory disease with special transplant techniques and/or multimodal therapy; and (3) palliative care to include pain management, bone disease management, and renal disease management. With the recent development of highly effective targeted therapies, patients are more likely to have a significant disease-free period and less likely to receive an HSCT in early disease.

Chemotherapy regimens include several drug combinations, such as melphalan and prednisone; cyclophosphamide and prednisone; vincristine, BCNU, cyclophosphamide, and melphalan; vincristine, Adriamycin, and dexamethasone (VAD); and cyclophosphamide and VAD (hyper-CVAD). Response to treatment and patient tolerance determine whether additional or different agents are needed. Newer targeted and chemotherapy agents such as bortezimib (Velcade), thalidomide, and lenalidomide have provided significant advancements in patient outcomes (89, 90).

HSCT often provides a prolonged disease-free state but does not significantly increase survival. However, high refractiveness of myeloma cells make transplant appealing. Some disadvantages to stem cell transplantation include a higher incidence of graft-versus-host disease than in other patients and a higher incidence of infectious deaths than in other patients with cancer. Some new variations showing promise include double transplant, allogeneic transplant followed by mini-transplant, and vaccine linked to transplant (91).

A new therapeutic agent is bortezomib (Velcade), which targets a core proteosome responsible for cell replication. Therapeutic actions include antiangiogenesis, enhancement of apoptosis, interference with cellular interferons, overriding resistant Bcl2 resistance, and is effective in hypoxic conditions. Adverse effects of the drug include paresthesias (circumoral, esophageal, other), gastrointestinal distress, and thrombocytopenia.

Bisphosphonates are used to prevent skeletal events and hypercalcemia. Zoledronic acid is commonly used and is effective through several mechanisms, through (1) reducing bone resorption by potently inhibiting osteoclast hyperactivity; (2) functional suppression of mature osteoclasts; (3) inhibition of osteoclast maturation; (4) inhibition of osteoclast recruitment to the site; (5) reduction in the production of cytokines (e.g., IL-1, IL-6); (6) inhibition of tumor cell invasion and adhesion to bone matrix; and (7) inhibition of osteoclasts and cytokines, which presumably slows growth of myeloma cells (92).

Clinical Nurse Specialist Competencies and Spheres of Influence
Clinical Expert Direct Care and Coaching/Teaching/Mentoring
Patients with MM require CNSs with expert knowledge of the disease process, treatment protocols, and risk for complications of both. Nurses play a key role in the management of patients with MM, and CNSs serve as important resources for frontline caregivers. Nursing care includes several important safety measures, including infection prevention and protection against pathological fractures. Assessment for neurological and cardiac symptoms due to hypercalcemia is important. Significant mental status changes can place patients at risk for aspiration. Nurses are instrumental in assessment for thromboembolic complications due to hyperviscosity and implementation of prophylactic treatment. Fluid balance requires vigilant attention due to renal insufficiency and cardiac involvement. Finally, nurses must address age-related complications and prevention strategies for elderly patients with MM (79).

Patients with MM are at high risk for hypercalcemia. The calculation of corrected calcium is not common knowledge for staff nurses and not always provided by laboratory reporting. Since serum calcium is only that which is bound to albumin, patients are more likely to have underestimated calcium levels with low albumin. The serum calcium and albumin are used by the CNS to calculate corrected calcium.

Systems Leadership, Collaboration, and Research/Evidence-Based Practice
Management of patients with MM requires collaboration between nursing, oncology, nephrology, cardiology, and infectious disease medicine, depending on the trajectory of the disease process and clinical presentation. Palliative and spiritual care services may be indicated. Fluid and electrolyte management is a priority due to renal and cardiac compromise and is often accomplished by protocol, with CNSs playing an instrumental role in development and implementation: medicine, laboratory, and pharmacy services provide input. Research in fall prevention and other safety concerns is very active; CNSs must maintain surveillance of the literature and develop and test clinical practice guidelines accordingly.

ONCOLOGICAL DISORDERS: ONCOLOGICAL EMERGENCIES

Oncological emergencies are a group of disorders that are primarily associated with the presence of malignancy. Some are present due to the disease itself, and others are unique complications that occur almost exclusively with antineoplastic therapies. The emergencies are generally classified into three different subheadings: structural complications, metabolic complications, or hematological complications. To some degree, these classifications also guide diagnostic test selection and best management strategies. This text lists them in alphabetical order.

Clinical Nurse Specialist Competencies and Spheres of Influence
Clinical Expert/Direct Care and Consultation
Patients at risk for oncological emergencies can be recognized prior to acute crisis. The CNS can use advanced knowledge of anatomy and physiology, pathophysiology, and advanced nursing knowledge to assist staff in identifying these high-risk patients and planning assessment to detect early symptoms of decompensation. Oncological emergencies often present similarly to other clinical medical-surgical problems but require very different management strategies.

Oncological emergencies present throughout the continuum of care for patients with cancer, but may warrant different interventions when present at initial diagnosis or as an indicator of progressive and refractory disease. Nursing and medical care will also vary according to the current goals of care. The CNS will provide nursing staff with assistance in critical thinking skills needed to differentiate these conflicting data. These patients' unusual treatments require the specialized knowledge that a CNS can offer.

Coaching/Teaching/Mentoring
With implementation of patient-centered assessment and clinical care, patients with oncologic emergencies can usually be managed in medical-surgical settings with minimal ICU care. The CNS is ideally matched to mentor and teach staff to care for these patients. Each

oncological emergency has established malignant associations and prognostic implications. Some units that care for oncological patients on an intermittent basis have periodic educational offerings on oncological emergencies to update and refresh staff knowledge and skills.

Systems Leadership, Collaboration, and Research/Evidence-Based Practice

Patients with certain oncological emergencies require radiation or blood component therapy that may not be available in every institution. The CNS must assess their institutional resources and staff capabilities. The development of practice standards, documentation tools, and services requires multidisciplinary collaboration. Additional medical-surgical supplies may need to be procured to support best practices for these patients. Some patient services may need to be contracted outside of the facility, and plans for patient transport or urgent referral may need to be developed.

HEMORRHAGIC CYSTITIS

Etiology

Hemorrhagic cystitis is described as mucosal irritation of the bladder (93). Many of the anti-neoplastic agents that act by cell-cycle nonspecific destruction of rapidly dividing cells can produce mucosal destruction in gastrointestinal and genitourinary systems. The alkylating agents such as cyclophosphamide, ifosphamide, or busulfan are the most likely to produce genitourinary-specific mucosal destruction (94). Antimetabolites such as methotrexate and pemetrexed, and radiotherapy to the pelvic region are also known for producing hemorrhagic cystitis, although newer techniques have reduced the incidence over the past decade (94). Recent literature has also implicated the important contribution of concomitant viral illnesses such as cytomegalovirus, BK virus, and John Cunningham virus as risk factors for this complication (95). Reduced incidence and severity of hemorrhagic cystitis are primarily attributed to enhanced scientific knowledge of medication dosing, pharmacokinetics, and clearance. Recognition of the need for concomitant hydration and development of toxicity protection with agents such as mesna and folinic acid have also enhanced patient outcomes. While this complication is not usually considered life-threatening, unusual cases of severe toxicity has produced long-term morbidity and need for cystectomy for some individuals.

Pathophysiology

When hemorrhagic cystitis is due to antineoplastic therapy, the proposed mechanism of injury is drug metabolite destruction of the rapidly dividing cells of the urogenital mucosa of the bladder and urethra. Destruction of the mucosal layer exposes the vascular endothelium to toxins in the urine and leads to bleeding vessels and hematuria. Viral organism–induced hemorrhagic cystitis does not have such a clear pathology and may in fact seldom cause this complication unless accompanied by another triggering agent.

Clinical Presentation

Universally, the key presenting symptom is occult or frank hematuria, although most patients report dysuria that precedes the presence of visible blood. When bleeding is significant and clots are retained in the bladder, patients commonly develop painful bladder spasms.

Diagnosis

The most common diagnostic examination for hemorrhagic cystitis is cystoscopy. This permits definitive diagnosis and evaluation of the extent of erosion. If specific lesions are the source of bleeding, immediate cautery may also be performed to abrogate acute bleeding. Although not diagnostic of the disorder, both serum and urinary hematocrit and hemoglobin may be measured to assess the amount of blood loss. High hematocrit and hemoglobin values of the urine reveal that most output is blood as opposed to urine or irrigation fluid.

Management

The two major clinical priorities for these patients are to maintain fluid flow from the bladder, without development of clot retention, and alleviation of pain. Most patients will be advised to increase fluid intake to 5 liters per day. Careful intake and output measurement is essential to ensure that urine output is adequate and hydronephrosis does not occur. Frequent vital signs to assess for blood-loss related orthostasis or hypotension may also be necessary.

Patients at risk for chemotherapy-related hemorrhagic cystitis are administered rescue agents aimed at reducing the toxic chemotherapy metabolites that pass through the bladder. Neutralization of the metabolite prevents erosion of the mucosa. Rescue agents are administered prior to the first dose of chemotherapy and continued for approximately 24 hours after the last dose of chemotherapy is completed. Methotrexate is rescued with IV folinic acid and cyclophosphamide and ifosphamide are rescued with mesna (94). Other specific agents and identified rescue agents are not available. There is considerable debate whether additional hydration or insertion of a Foley catheter provides additive protection, and these practices are based on clinician preference.

Patients who develop hemorrhagic cystitis are not candidates to receive protective agents after they have experienced this complication. The goal of therapy is then directed toward methods of enhancing hemostasis at the site(s) of bleeding without producing excessive intrabladder clotting. Agents that have been infused or instilled into the bladder for this purpose include prosta-cyclin E, alum, and formalin (96, 97).

Patients with hemorrhagic cystitis often have significant bladder spasms. While traditional pain medications may be necessary, the first line of therapy is antispasmodic or anticholinergic agents aimed to reduce bladder spasms. Common medications used for this purpose include dantrolene, pyridium, and anticholinergic agents such as oxybutynin chloride and tolterodine.

If urine flow is not adequate to prevent clot retention in the bladder, continuous bladder irrigation (CBI) is initiated. Free-flowing saline is infused through one lumen of the Foley catheter and returns through a drainage bag. Sometimes the flow rate is ordered, but more often the nurse adjusts the rate to achieve a light pink return. The greater amount of bleeding necessitates a brisker irrigation rate. It is very important for nurses to adjust the intake and output values to accommodate the fluid overfill in most irrigation containers that may range from 30 to 150 mL. Inadequate accounting of overfill will lead to overestimation of urine output.

When CBI and medication instillation are not successful at resolving hemorrhagic cystitis, hyperbaric oxygen or surgery may be considered. Hyperbaric oxygen is only available at specialized wound care centers. Inpatients will require daily transportation to the center for several weeks. Intraoperative cystoscopic medication instillation or cautery may be used as an initial strategy. Partial or complete cystectomy is considered as a last resort.

While not always preventable, some etiologies of therapy-related hemorrhagic cystitis may be minimized or avoided with use of appropriate protective agents. Mesna is used from the beginning to 24 hours after administration of cyclophosphamide and ifosfamide. Methotrexate is neutralized with infusion of folinic acid starting with chemotherapy and continuing until serum levels return to normal. Additional hydration to achieve a brisk urine output also ensures that the toxic metabolite responsive for mucosal erosion is exposed to the bladder for short periods of time. Nurses usually administer hydration with titration incrementally increased until a goal urine output of approximately 2 mL/kg/hr is achieved.

Additional neutralizing agents and new administration procedures of existing protective agents are currently under investigation. It is hoped that increasing knowledge of bladder protective agents will enable further reduction in the incidence of this painful and debilitating complication.

Clinical Nurse Specialist Competencies and Spheres of Influence
Clinical Expert/Direct Care and Consultation
Identification of patients at risk for hemorrhagic cystitis and proactively planning infusion of protective agents,

ensuring hydration, and monitoring are important components of the plan for care for these patients. The acute care CNS who is aware of therapies provided in the clinical areas they cover will be actively involved in this process, providing direct consultation to design preventive and proactive plans. Nurses who infrequently provide continuous bladder irrigation therapies or need to manually flush catheters will need assistance in these ordering supplies, practicing titration, and documenting care.

Staff should have reinforcement of the importance of accurate and frequent intake and output measurement measures to ensure sufficient urine output. If clots form in the bladder, obstruction of ureters and hydronephrosis can occur, producing postrenal failure.

Coaching/Teaching/Mentoring
Performing continuous bladder irrigation, particularly with irrigation additives such as alum or formalin, will be taught to bedside nurses. Fluid titration to create pink returns may require frequent adjustment in infusion rates. If retained fluid or clots are suspected, staff may require training in use of a bladder scanner that demonstrates fluid within the bladder. While the bladder scanner is an easy to use bedside device, it requires different settings for men and women after hysterectomy than for women with a uterus.

Systems Leadership, Collaboration, and Research/Evidence-Based Practice
Patients develop hemorrhagic cystitis infrequently, but it is a complication with tremendous implications for impaired quality of life. Proactive correct administration of protective agents is essential to minimize these potential adverse outcomes. The CNS and pharmacists will collaborate with prescribers to ensure the exact dose and timing of protective agents is defined in standard order sets or individual plans of care. The acute care CNS will also be actively involved in creation of documentation tools for irrigation fluids and returns.

HYPERCALCEMIA

Etiology
Hypercalcemia has historically been viewed as the most common metabolic oncological emergency, affecting up to 20% of patients with cancer. It is less common in today's oncological care because high-risk patients have been identified and effective preventive measures are available. When present, it usually signifies active malignant disease or refractory bone metastases. Hypercalcemia is defined as a corrected serum calcium greater than 11 mg/dL, although clinical symptoms are not usually present until the calcium is greater than 12 mg/dL, and life-threatening complications are not common until the calcium exceeds 15 mg/dL.

Accounting for more than two-thirds of malignancy-associated hypercalcemia is bone metastasis with demineralization. Cancers linked to a high incidence of hypercalcemia include breast, multiple myeloma, and small cell lung cancer (also pancreatic cancer and renal cell carcinoma). Renal dysfunction and dehydration are known to exacerbate this condition because of altered renal excretion of calcium.

Pathophysiology

Hypercalcemia is a direct reflection of levels of serum calcium that exceed the kidney's excretion capabilities. It occurs when the number of osteoclasts (bone demineralization cells) exceeds the osteoblasts (immature bone cells) needed to maintain normal bone structure. There are three distinct pathophysiological mechanisms causing imbalanced osteoclasts and osteoblasts and resulting hypercalcemia. The most common etiology is excess calcium caused by bone invasion with malignant cells. Other malignancy-associated hypercalcemia occurs due to malignant cell production of a parathormone-like substance. The third mechanism of hypercalcemia is production of excess inflammatory cytokines that trigger bone demineralization.

Clinical Presentation

Calcium is an electrolyte primarily necessary for neuromuscular and cardiac function and bone integrity. Excess calcium leads to overactivity of the calcium influx mechanisms responsible for neuromuscular activity. The severity of signs and symptoms of hypercalcemia often correlates with the corrected serum calcium level. The most common presenting symptoms include nausea, constipation, polyuria, and mental status changes. Most patients present with somnolence, combativeness, or confusion (98). Cardiac symptoms include bradycardia with a short PR interval, junctional rhythm, and heart block. Extremely high levels of calcium can lead to seizures, coma, or cardiac arrest.

Diagnosis

Calcium is present in its active ionized form and as an inactive electrolyte bound to albumin. The only calcium reflected in the normal serum value is that bound to albumin. In cases of hypoalbuminemia, the serum calcium may be underestimated if only the serum calcium is considered. For this reason, calcium levels must be corrected to accurately diagnose hypercalcemia. The formula for correction of serum calcium with hypoalbuminemia can be obtained by subtracting the patient's albumin from the low normal albumin value, multiplying this number by the correction factor of 0.8, and adding this to the reported serum calcium (99, 100). Serum ionized calcium levels are accurate, but because the normal value is 1.0 mEq/L (±0.02), it is a less sensitive indicator of hypercalcemia, but used more often for management of hypocalcemia. In addition to increased calcium levels, patients often also exhibit elevated alkaline phosphatase and immunoreactive parathyroid hormone (99, 100).

Management

Patients with hypercalcemia require an immediate baseline physical examination and identification of life-threatening complications such as seizures, aspiration risk, or life-threatening dysrhythmias. Patients with significant mental status changes and confusion or combativeness have major safety risks and may develop seizures. Seizure precautions include padded bedrails, additional activity limitations, and no oral temperatures. Hypoventilation and inability to protect the airway may require airway assistance with oxygen therapy, oral airway devices, or bilevel positive pressure ventilation.

At the time of admission with suspected or confirmed hypercalcemia, laboratory tests such as serum and urinary osmolarity, electrolyte panel, and alkaline phosphatase are performed. A 12-lead ECG is also obtained to search for evidence of bradycardia, heart block, or a shortened PR interval. Abnormalities in cardiac rhythm or severely elevated calcium levels warrant continuous cardiac, oxygen saturation, and apnea monitoring. The severity of hypercalcemia will also predict the risk of dehydration from profuse polyuria. An indwelling urinary catheter may be placed to ensure accurate urinary output measurement, and central venous pressures or orthostatic vital signs may be used to provide valuable information regarding fluid volume status.

The most immediate management of hypercalcemia is dilution of blood calcium levels with IV hydration. IV fluids with 0.9% normal saline is the preferred fluid because saline enhances renal excretion of calcium. Fluids are administered at 150 to 300 mL/hr to induce urine output in excess of 2 mL/kg/hr. This measure alone may be successful at lowering calcium, especially if the patient is also suffering from hypovolemia. In cases where the calcium continues to be elevated, enhancement of renal calcium excretion with pharmacological therapies is indicated. In severe emergent hypercalcemia, hemodialysis with a calcium-free dialysate can successfully lower blood calcium levels temporarily, but more permanent measures to halt bone resorption are necessary to prevent recurrence of this condition.

Initial enhancement of renal calcium excretion is usually achieved with diuretic agents that increase glomerular filtration rates. Loop diuretics are preferred as many of the thiazide diuretics actually cause calcium reabsorption. For patients whose hypercalcemia is related to production of tumor-induced parathormone-like substances, anticancer therapy is the most effective treatment.

Patients who do not respond to immediate fluid and diuretic therapies or whose tumor control is not adequate to control recurrence of hypercalcemia are treated with bisphosphonates. Currently available IV bisphosphonates are pamidronate and zolendronate. Patients who continue to have hypercalcemia despite these traditional therapies may be treated with more potent and side effect–producing therapies such as corticosteroids, calcitonin, or strontium-98. Pharmacological support of secondary effects of hypercalcemia may also be necessary. Recognizing that confusion is related to the correctable electrolyte abnormality, anxiolytics may still be needed to control patient behavior. Nausea is often alleviated with fluid replenishment. Constipation may require treatment and is best managed with motility agents since the major causes of constipation are slowed peristalsis and dehydration. Other medications that may be prescribed include anticonvulsants, vagolytics (e.g., atropine), or sympathomimetics.

Optimal prevention of hypercalcemia involves recognition of high-risk patients and implementation of hydration and exercise regimens. Patients who remain mobile enhance calcium reabsorption by bones, minimizing the serum calcium level. Hydration of approximately 2 liters per day will enhance the glomerular filtration rate and renal excretion of calcium.

Over recent years, the development of more rapid-acting and potent bisphosphonates has enabled many patients with bone metastases to be managed on an outpatient basis. Originally these agents were used only to treat hypercalcemia, but it is now recognized that patients with bone metastases should be proactively administered a bisphosphonate to reduce the risk of both hypercalcemia and pathological fractures. It is hoped that this prophylactic management will serve to reduce this complication to a rare occurrence. New diuretic agents in a pharmacological category called vaptens are in the last phases of clinical research and may be available in the near future to optimize diuresis of these patients.

Clinical Nurse Specialist Competencies and Spheres of Influence

Clinical Expert/Direct Care and Consultation

Patients at high risk for hypercalcemia should be pre-identified with vigilant assessment and interventions accessible prior to an acute decompensation of symptoms. Patient and caregiver education regarding preventive strategies and reportable signs and symptoms have been proven to reduce the incidence and morbidity of this complication. Patients are advised to drink at least 2 quarts of fluid per day, consume salty fluids (e.g., broths, sports drinks), or increase dietary salt. At the same time, patients are advised to maintain mobility, with the goal of walking at least 1 mile per day. When patients are unable to walk, active range-of-motion exercises are still beneficial to maintain bone integrity. Reportable

conditions include headaches, personality changes, confusion, irritableness, difficulty breathing, nausea, constipation, or frequent urination. Patients without live-in caregivers may require periodic visits from friends and family or home health aides taught to recognize mental status changes and impaired judgment of patients.

When patients present acutely symptomatic, the acute care CNS is an ideal consultant to identify the patient's most immediate problems and recommend monitoring. Patients may require interventions of rapid response teams or transfer to a higher level of care.

Coaching/Teaching/Mentoring

The acute care CNS plays an active role in both staff and patient education regarding hypercalcemia. Standard teaching plans for patients with this common oncological emergency should be readily available. A number of opportunities for informal staff education exist by assisting staff with proper assessment of orthostatic vital signs or measurement of central venous pressure. Administration of bisphosphonates may also present a learning opportunity. Pamidronate is not currently administered as defined by the package insert and therefore many drug handbooks. The package insert describes several different doses and states it is administered over 90 minutes to 24 hours. In reality, a full dose of 90 mg is safe to administer over 30 to 60 minutes.

Since mental status changes are an indicator of significant hypercalcemia, subtle decline in mental faculties should be noted and reported. One sensitive method of assessing mental status changes is with the Mini-Mental Status Exam (MMSE) because it assesses orientation, cognitive function, calculating skills, and reasoning abilities. Performance of the MMSE requires training and explanations that are within the expertise of the acute care CNS.

Systems Leadership, Collaboration, and Research/Evidence-Based Practice

Patients with hypercalcemia may present to neurological or cardiac units despite their primary diagnosis and etiology of symptoms being cancer related. The acute care CNS acts as a coordinator of care across several subspecialities involved in the care of this patient. The multi-system physical changes require synchronization of care and continuous reassessment. Since several medications may be prescribed, assessment of medication interactions is essential. Patients may have significant mental status suppression or respiratory muscle weakness to be at risk for aspiration with oral medications. This may require adjustment of the medication plan.

The varied pattern and chronic nature of hypercalcemia-related signs and symptoms warrant a number of consultations. In the acute phase, patients may need consultation from neurology, speech and swallow assessment, or cardiology services. These patients are ideal candidates for palliative care services due to their symptom profile and probable association with advanced disease. Early physical therapy consultation is considered an important standard of practice. Mobility is a tremendous deterrent for bone demineralization and hypercalcemia. Consultation with dieticians is also recommended when the patient and caregivers are considered near discharge. A home assessment for safety risks may also be recommended.

PLEURAL EFFUSIONS

Etiology

A pleural effusion is defined as excess accumulation of fluid in the space between the visceral and parietal pleura. A small amount of fluid is usually present, allowing for ease of lung expansion. Normally fluid is constantly recirculated throughout the thorax, allowing only 15 to 50 mL to remain. Venous congestion, pleural inflammation, capillary permeability, and lymphatic obstruction impair normal fluid dynamics, causing fluid accumulation (101). The outcomes are increased work of breathing, inadequate lung expansion, and hypoxemia.

Although many nonmalignant conditions (e.g., congestive heart failure, hypothyroidism, renal failure) may cause pleural effusion, malignant infiltration or lymphatic obstruction has the same consequences. Pleural effusions occurring due to volume overload, capillary permeability, or lymphatic obstruction are transudative and characterized by the presence of albumin (102, 103). Infections of the pleura or malignant cell infiltration cause inflammatory exudative effusions, distinguished by the presence of RBCs, WBCs, and LDH into the pleural fluid (103).

Up to 50% of patients with cancer experience pleural effusions during the course of their disease, particularly in cancers of the lung or breast (101, 104, 105). Other tumors that originate or metastasize to the chest or obstruct lymphatic flow such as malignant lymphoma, pancreatic cancer, and ovarian cancer are also associated with disabling pleural effusions. The presence of pleural effusion is associated with a poor prognosis, and an average life expectancy of 3 to 12 months after diagnosis (104, 106, 107). Predictors for better outcome include specific types of cancer and patients with higher performance status at diagnosis of effusion (107).

Pathophysiology

Excess pleural fluid between the visceral and parietal pleural impedes lung expansion by exerting a positive pressure within the space. Fluid accumulation within the pleural space applies pressure on the lung parenchyma, and alveoli collapse. The work of breathing is significantly increased as the patient attempts to fill alveoli.

Failure to expand alveoli leads to decreased gas exchange with hypoxemia and hypercarbia (101). Fluid accumulation is initially free-flowing and can track anywhere in the pleural space based on body position. Most lung collapse begins in the bases, and rises until larger and more rigid bronchioles force fluid along the lateral wall.

Clinical Presentation

The signs and symptoms of pleural effusion are directly related to the two major physiological changes: increased work of breathing and alveolar collapse. Excess pleural pressures decrease lung compliance, causing additional negative pressure to create chest expansion. Patients must exert greater muscular effort and often feel short of breath. The work of breathing may be so great, that patients are dyspneic, anxious, and unable to lie down. Visible use of accessory muscles to breathe, and unequal chest excursion on the affected side are common physical findings. When patients are in an upright position, the force of gravity pulls the fluid to the base of the pleural space, and breath sounds are diminished to the level of fluid. Symptoms that relate to this pathological process are diminished breath sounds, unequal chest excursion, tracheal shift away from the effusion, and signs of hypoxemia (e.g., dyspnea, anxiety, confusion, oliguria, decreased bowel sounds) (101, 105). The work of breathing also impairs the ability to eat, and weight loss is common. With progressive worsening of pleural effusion, patients may also have disrupted sleep with cognitive impairment, daytime sleepiness, and chest discomfort.

Diagnosis

After pleural fluid is confirmed by noninvasive methods such as radiography or CT scan, a cytological evaluation of pleural fluid is obtained for evaluation of etiology. Via thoracentesis, pleural fluid is extracted and sent for chemistry and cytology evaluation. Pleural fluid is categorized as transudative or exudative, which assists in determination of the etiology of the effusion. Cytological studies require at least 50 mL fluid to confirm the presence or absence of malignant cells. Despite a large amount of fluid, cytology is only accurate approximately one-third of the time, and several separate thoracentesis specimens may be required for confirmation (104, 108, 109). When fluid cytology is inconclusive, pleural biopsy may be helpful in diagnosis of malignant infiltration (110).

The first diagnostic test performed to validate the presence of pleural effusion is an upright chest radiograph. (104). When upright, gravitation pull causes the fluid to accumulate in the lower lung, causing a blunted diaphragmatic dome on radiography and decreased radiolucence where alveoli are collapsed. Fluid accumulation often produces a meniscus of decreased radiolucence and a thickened lateral pleural lining, indicating fluid tracking up the side. When alternative pleural diagnoses such as hemothorax, infection, or tumor infiltrates are possible, the CT scan may be more accurate.

Management

Patients presenting with pleural effusions have varying degrees of disability and clinical signs or symptoms. The nurse must assess the impact pleural effusions have on the patient's general health and vital functions. Monitoring respiratory rate, work of breathing, and oxygen saturation provides insight into the patient's ability to compensate for collapsed alveoli. With increasing effusion, the work of breathing becomes consuming, and air hunger is more evident. Signs and symptoms of hypoxemia are assessed and warrant intervention.

The most immediate interventions for patients with pleural effusion are aimed at optimization of comfort. Most patients will be severely dyspneic with physical activity and may require sitting upright to breathe. Oxygen therapy may provide some relief of dyspnea, even if hypoxemia is not evident. Although not an option in the hospital setting, patients describe relief of dyspnea with a fan directed at them. Providing a quiet and cool environment may also assist patients in feeling less anxious about breathing difficulties. Patients who require thoracentesis or chest catheter drainage may need analgesia or sedation for the procedure.

Definitive management of pleural effusion depends on the etiological mechanism, rapidity of symptom onset, and degree of respiratory compromise (101, 111). Since many patients with malignant pleural effusion have limited survival, the selection of an optimal treatment that enhances quality of life with minimal morbidity or recovery is a priority. When pleural effusions are small or have a nonmalignant cause, observation without definitive treatment may be indicated. Aggressive antineoplastic therapy may be indicated when a large tumor and significant pleural effusion are present.

If insertion of a chest catheter is the initial treatment, the nurse should observe carefully for complications associated with rapid pleural fluid removal. When the chest catheter is placed and large amounts of fluid drains rapidly, interstitial fluid shifts may cause hypotension. After fluid removal of more than 1,500 to 2,000 mL, reexpansion pulmonary edema has been reported. The collapsed alveoli reexpand but become fluid permeable due to inflammatory responses. Both of these complications are more prevalent in patients with large, long-standing effusions at the time of initial drainage (112).

Ambulatory patients who have evacuation of large pleural effusions should be observed for about 1 hour postprocedure for the onset of thee complications. Although unusual, pneumothorax or pleural hemorrhage may also occur during thoracentesis and can present with sudden and severe dyspnea, hypoxemia, unilateral jugular vein distention, new tracheal deviation, and marked reduction in chest excursion.

The discomfort of breathing associated with pleural effusions may induce painful dyspnea or chest discomfort. Opiate medications are often administered orally, intravenously, or by inhalation to reduce these sensations and provide relaxation. Although the primary pathophysiological mechanism is compressed alveoli, bronchodilators or corticosteroids may be administered in which to optimize airway dilation and air movement. In cases where catheter drainage is unsuccessful, intracavitary chemotherapy with cisplatin, interferon, or pemetrexed has been used with moderate success (104, 108, 111, 113).

When malignant cells are present in the pleural fluid, management may be determined by overall treatment goals. Repeated therapeutic thoracentesis is often the initial therapy while providing more definitive anticancer treatment (101, 104, 105, 111). Patients who require repeated thoracenteses develop pleural scarring and effusions may become loculated or difficult to access. The clinician performing thoracentesis may have to needle access a higher rib level and will be unable to completely drain the effusion. More definitive interventions should be used before these complications occur.

When the patient's life expectancy is longer, and pleural effusions do not resolve with anticancer therapy and intermittent thoracenteses, treatment includes methods to drain the pleura or eliminate the potential pleural space. The most patient friendly method achieving this today is with a long-term chest catheter drainage. Insertion of a soft tunneled catheter (e.g., Pleurex catheter) allows patients to have a means of draining excess fluid while continuing their activities of daily living (114-118). In operative settings, a variety of chest catheters are used for pleural drainage, including traditional chest tubes, Blake tubes, pigtail catheters, or tunneled catheters. Each is associated with unique nursing management strategies. If the drainage slows and patients become a good candidate for pleurodesis, they are admitted to the hospital for medical or surgical pleurodesis. Medical pleurodesis involves placement of a traditional chest catheter and instillation of a sclerosing agent. Pleurodesis, also called pleural sclerosing, involves intrapleural administration of a chemical (e.g., doxycycline, bleomycin) or a mechanical agent (e.g., talc slurry) to alter the pH of the pleural fluid and cause inflammatory adherence of the visceral and parietal pleura to each other (108, 111). These medications are not systemically absorbed, but instead have local irritating effects. Sclerosed pleura do not have the normal lubricating pleural fluid, and restrictive lung disease is the long-term consequence. Pleurodesis is successful only about 67% of the time, necessitating the availability of additional treatment options. Pleurectomy is a thoracic surgical procedure that removes the entire pleura. Pleurectomy is effective but can be difficult to perform when long-term inflammation and pleurodesis attempts cause a friable pleura that is not easily separated. Chronic, long-term pleuroperitoneal shunts or implanted access devices have been used for intermittent fluid removal, but catheters often become occluded with fibrin sheaths (105, 111).

While it may be impossible to eliminate all pleural effusions, there are some measures thought to reduce their severity and impact on quality of life. Patients with lymphatic disruption in the chest may be able to minimize fluid accumulation by maintaining a normal activity level. Ambulation serves to massage the lymph system in the chest and enhance fluid recirculation. Some clinicians have suggested that patients with pleural effusions be placed on fluid restrictions based on a belief that excess vascular volume leads to increased extravasation of fluid into the pleural space. These measures are not evidence-based and are likely to negatively influence patients' quality of life.

There are new laboratory methods of evaluating pleural fluid that are in developmental stages but are considered promising to improve the accuracy of diagnosis. DNA methylation studies of the pleural fluid or testing for tumor markers may provide more accurate and sensitive diagnostic measures. This could reduce the need for frequent diagnostic thoracenteses to achieve and confirmation of malignancy.

The use of semipermanent indwelling pleural catheters has become increasingly more popular due to their ease of insertion and use. Patients are able to independently drain their catheter when uncomfortable. It is anticipated that development of greater skill at providing rapid interventional radiology or bedside insertion of these catheters will lead to even higher use. There is some concern about the costs of ambulatory disposables incurred with these catheters, but many insurers recognize the savings in hospital and medical consultation fees.

Clinical Nurse Specialist Competencies and Spheres of Influence
Clinical Expert/Direct Care and Consultation
The CNS is actively involved in treatment planning discussion with prescribers and patients. It is often helpful for the CNS to provide additional information and follow-up reinforcement for patients and their loved ones to understand the gravity and prognostic implications of a new diagnosis of pleural effusion. The CNS can help patients understand the treatment options available and benefits or problems with each.

Patients with pleural effusion having traditional or newer innovative chest catheters will often be admitted to the acute care nursing unit with little advance notice. The CNS is ideally positioned to assist staff in understanding the nuances of each catheter and drainage system. In patients who receive a pleuropericardial window, there will be chest catheters in both the pleural and mediastinal spaces. Expected drainage and tube assessment and nursing care will be different with these two catheters; an air leak would not be normal with a mediastinal drain, although often present with a pleural catheter immediately after surgery. At times pigtail catheters or Blake tubes are used for this purpose, and may not be easily fitted to closed chest suction drainage apparatuses or require flushing that would not be normal with traditional chest catheters.

Nursing care with pleurodesis is unusual and at times counterintuitive. Prescribers may be the only professionals permitted to instill intrapleural pleurodesis agents but are not likely to appreciate the difficulty of accessing a chest catheter that does not have a normal IV-type connection. The CNS is actively involved in assisting the health care team to plan for instillation of the pleurodesis agent, flushing the agent into the space, clamping the tube, and replacing the tubing and drainage system.

Coaching/Teaching/Mentoring
Chest tube management is a highly technical and high-risk clinical procedure that may not be common for staff on some nursing units. Informal daily educational support may be supplemented with formal education or competency validation in practice setting where patients with pleural effusions are managed. Staff and patient education of long-term indwelling devices are also precise and device-specific and may require coordination by the CNS. Development or instructions to access public domain educational materials for care of these catheters is often managed by the CNS.

Systems Leadership, Collaboration, and Research/Evidence-Based Practice
The patient with pleural effusion requires frequent procedures and may be hospitalized for symptom management or procedural interventions. During these times of acute symptomatology, the acute care CNS is a key coordinator of their care. Surgical procedures such as pleuropericardial windows, pleuroperitoneal shunts, and various tubes in the pleural or mediastinal spaces should be well documented to ensure the nurses can plan appropriate care. The CNS works with surgeons or interventional radiology to optimize communication between disciplines.

Hospital protocols for management of chest tubes may be inadequate to address the special needs and variety of treatment measures used for these patients. The acute care CNS will be central to revising or amending these protocols to describe care for pigtail or tunneled pleural catheters, for administering pleurodesis agents or intrapleural analgesia and chemotherapy.

While evidence-based recommendations for management of pleural effusion are limited, there a few small studies regarding pleurodesis. Evidence states that only 60% to 70% of patients will have successful pleurodesis with chest tube instillation of any agent, while thoracoscopic pleurodesis with talc is successful approximately 90% of the time (115). Studies have shown conclusively that after instillation of pleurodesis there is no benefit in rotating the patient's position to ensure fluid distribution as has been traditionally done (115).

SPINAL CORD COMPRESSION

Etiology

Spinal cord compression (SCC) occurs when tumor cells or collapsed vertebrae invade in the epidural space and exert pressure on the spinal cord or its blood supply. Prolonged pressure not diagnosed and treated promptly will result in permanent nerve dysfunction with paralysis. The most common cause of SCC is bone metastasis with vertebral compression fracture and vertebral collapse (119). The incidence of epidural involvement with metastatic disease is poorly documented but present in about 5% of patients with metastatic disease at autopsy (120). Factors associated with effective local control and long-term survival after SCC include favorable histological diagnosis, no visceral metastases, and a long-course radiation therapy schedule (119, 120).

Pathophysiology

The three most common pathophysiological mechanisms to result in SCC are bony metastases causing vertebral collapse, interference with blood supply of the spinal cord, or tumors arising within the epidural space through vertebral or lymphatic spread (119-121). Spinal nerve root compression causes permanent neurological damage. Other disorders producing signs and symptoms of cord compression are paraneoplastic syndromes, radiation myelopathy, herpes zoster, pain from a pelvic or long bone metastasis, or cytotoxic drug effects (120). The tumors most likely to cause cord compression are those with a propensity for metastasis to the bone such as cancers of the breast, colon, kidney, lung, and prostate and lymphoma that develops into lymph node masses. The location of cancerous disease predicts the level of compression and subsequent symptoms.

Clinical Presentation

When a primary tumor slowly grows and invades into the epidural space, signs and symptoms usually develop slowly. Rapidly growing disease such as lymphoma and metastatic lesions produce more acute signs and symptoms. The earliest symptom of SCC is radicular back pain located centrally with or without radiation that can be aggravated by manual palpation, weight bearing, or other activities using back muscles. Sitting often relieves this pain (122, 123).

Once patients experience pain, other sensory changes such as paresthesias, numbness, or cold sensitivity occur (123, 124). Patients complain that leg or arm aching and heaviness and decreased sensation of pressure becomes more pronounced through the day and is worst at night or after prolonged activity. These are followed by weakness and ataxia (124). Some describe unsteadiness and inability to sense body position. Other patients lose the ability to sense light touch, pain, and temperature. Over time, weakness may progress to spasm, paralysis, and muscle atrophy.

The most frequent site of SCC is the thoracic region of the spinal cord, causing lower extremity paresis. Compression of the lower thoracic and lumbar spine causes neurogenic bladder with urinary retention and incontinence. Patients with this level of compression may also be unable to produce a Valsalva and lose the urge to defecate. Men on occasion lose the ability to have or maintain an erection. Metastases to the cauda equina occurring with tumors of the prostate, testicle, or sigmoid colon frequently produce impaired urethral, vaginal, and rectal sensations; bladder dysfunction; and decreased sensation in the lumbosacral dermatomes (124).

It is possible to determine the level of cord compression by the patient's report of pain location during straight leg raising, neck flexion, or vertebral percussion. The upper limit of the pain sensation is usually one or two vertebral bodies below the site of compression (124). Deep tendon reflexes can be brisk with cord compression and diminished with nerve root compression.

Diagnosis

A myelogram involving injection of dye into the spine with follow-up scanning to observe areas of blocked flow used to be a common diagnostic test to detect SCC but has been replaced with highly effective less invasive diagnostic tests. Rarely, surgical exploration with planned surgical correction may be used for diagnostic purposes.

A screening spinal radiograph is used for rapid initial evaluation of high-risk patients with probable SCC, as it will detect up to 80% of vertebral fractures (125). MRI is the diagnostic test of choice due to its high sensitivity for neurological tissues and would be preferred over radiographs if immediately available. MRI can clearly demonstrate all epidural metastases as well as complete or partial blockages of the spinal cord (126, 127). A CT scan may reveal spinal tumors, but these studies are less sensitive for diagnosing the presence and extent of cord compression. Lumbar puncture, which is used to obtain cerebrospinal fluid, reveals malignant cells in the presence of epidural disease but is considered a diagnostic tool to validate the etiology of SCC rather than diagnose the presence of SCC (126).

Management

Since pain is the most common clinical finding of SCC, pain assessment and management are key priorities of care. Pain assessment should include location, duration, character, intensity, aggravating factors, and alleviating factors. Manual palpation and assessment of pain with neck or knee flexion provide helpful information regarding the potential location of cord compression. Other associated sensory changes should also be documented.

Frequent assessment for sensory and motor neurological deficits is essential to detect progression of cord compression. Since sensory changes are the earliest to occur, evaluating patients' ability to detect pressure and pain in the lower extremities is the first level of assessment. Assessment of motor weakness of the lower extremities is assessed by asking the patient to display flexion and extension against resistance. If high thoracic or cervical compression is present, the upper extremities or breathing may also be affected. Patients with a weak shoulder shrug are at high risk to develop respiratory complications.

Factors considered in the selection of the best therapeutic option are the level of cord compression, the rate of neurological deterioration, and previous use of radiation therapy. (121). Immediate interventions are aimed at reducing inflammation as a contributor to cord compression, while providing spine stabilization. Patients should be on complete bedrest until the degree of cord compression is verified, as standing or walking with partial compression can lead to spinal injury with permanent paralysis.

If the tumor is determined to be radiosensitive, radiation therapy should be initiated as soon as the diagnosis of cord compression has been confirmed (122). Radiation fields include the entire area of blockage and two vertebral bodies above and below this area. More than 50% of patients with rapid neurological deterioration improve with radiation therapy; however, patients with autonomic dysfunction or paraplegia have a poor prognosis with any therapy (125, 128). A number of patients receive maximal tolerated radiation to the spinal cord, and there is recurrence despite therapy. These patients will then require surgical intervention or supportive therapy.

Bowel retraining and intermittent urinary catheterization may be necessary. Frequent turning, skin care, and range-of-motion exercises are essential to prevent complications. Surgical wounds are particularly susceptible to skin breakdown (with possible wound dehiscence) because of limited mobility and the effects of concomitant corticosteroid therapy (122).

Corticosteroids decrease inflammation and edema around the tumor and can improve neurological dysfunction. In patients with acute neurological symptoms, dexamethasone 10 mg is administered emergently as an initial dose prior to diagnostic procedures. dexamethasone 4 to 20 mg every 6 hours is continued during radiation therapy and then tapered (120, 121, 125, 128). Although steroid therapy is considered appropriate standard of care, it is not clear whether steroid therapy affects final patient outcome. If the tumor is chemosensitive, chemotherapy is administered concurrently or soon after completion of radiation therapy or surgery. Chemotherapy may also be effective in patients with multiple myeloma who have had previous radiation therapy (129). Systemic chemotherapy or hormonal therapy is most useful in certain types of tumors, such as lymphoma or prostatic cancer.

Immediate decompression of the spinal cord is achieved with laminectomy, with or without placement of stabilization rods in the nearby vertebral bodies (129, 130). The posterior approach is preferred but is often difficult because most metastases arise in the vertebral bodies anterior to the spinal cord (126, 129). The anterior approach is warranted for people with tumors that are believed to be resectable, making the clinical risks worth the aggressive surgical intervention (130). Postoperative radiation therapy is used to shrink residual tumor, relieve pain, and improve the patient's functional status. Surgery is usually contraindicated if there is a collapsed vertebral body or if there are several areas of cord compression. If there is no previous histological diagnosis of cancer or if infection or epidural hematoma must be ruled out, then laminectomy can be used for both diagnosis and treatment. If high cervical cord compression precludes surgery, a neurologist should stabilize the patient's neck in halo traction to prevent respiratory paralysis (129). If the patient continues to deteriorate neurologically despite high doses of steroids and radiation therapy, then emergency decompression may be necessary (130).

In some people, stabilization of the spine with vertebroplasty with or without kyphoplasty represents a less invasive and equally effective short-term resolution for acute cord compression and its associated pain (129, 131, 132). Injection of physiological cement (kyphoplasty) to re-expand collapsed vertebrae has been used to successfully prevention progression to SCC (132).

Although SCC often cannot be prevented, the time to significant bone metastases, and the severity of bone destruction can be ameliorated by administration of bisphosphonates to high-risk patients. The incidence of clinically significant SCC has greatly reduced since the routine use of bisphosphonates in patients with breast cancer and MM. Proactive recognition of patients at risk for SCC due to compression fractures can lead to early vertebroplasty and spine stabilization before SCC occurs.

Less invasive vertebral surgeries such as vertebroplasty and kyphoplasty are a useful strategy for early management of vertebral collapse. When used with early bone metastasis, SCC can be prevented. With highly sensitive and specific diagnostic tests, the implementation of these therapies is likely to increase in patients with bone metastasis.

Clinical Nurse Specialist Competencies and Spheres of Influence
Clinical Expert/Direct Care and Consultation

The patient with SCC presents with acute pain and sensory changes requiring immediate pain management and safety interventions. Unless nurses routinely care for patients with spine surgery or traumatic spinal cord injury, they may not be familiar with the immediate needs of these patients. The acute care CNS has expert neurological assessment skills that can be implemented and used as role modeling for staff providing follow-up care. Sensory, pressure, and pain assessment of lower extremities and strength assessment without and against resistance are not part of routine assessment skills but may be required for these patients. If the acute care facility does not provide radiation therapy services, it is highly likely these patients will be transferred to another facility.

Coaching/Teaching/Mentoring

The CNS is responsible for assessing and providing staff education and consultation. Since this is common in patients with cancer, the CNS may elect to provide staff education at orientation for these nurses. When infrequently encountered, education for staff on a case-by-case basis can be supplemented with fast facts sheets with the most important nursing priorities. Emphasis should be on identification of high-risk patients, that pain and sensory changes occur early, but that weakness or autonomic dysfunction potentially signals high risk for paralysis and warrants immediate mobility restrictions and diagnostic testing. Since SCC can cause autonomic dysfunction, staff are taught the importance of assessment for urinary retention or constipation. The use of a bladder scanner to evaluate the volume of urine in the bladder may require additional staff training. Staff should anticipate and deliver stat doses of high-dose rapid-acting steroids.

Since several different cancers can cause SCC and there are a variety of treatment options, patient education should be generic and nonspecific regarding selection of specific treatments or prognostic implications. There are a number of commercial products providing videos of the pathophysiology and methodology of vertebroplasty procedures targeted for understanding by lay personnel. Development of patient education materials and links to appropriate public materials are ideally suited to the expertise of the APN.

Systems Leadership, Collaboration, and Research/Evidence-Based Practice

The coordination of rapid diagnostic testing, expert neurological consultation, and immediate treatment is essential for optimal outcomes in patients with SCC. The CNS is in a key role to facilitate these efforts. Since SCC is a common complication for patients with certain types of cancer, the CNS can assist nursing staff to modify the standard assessment for patients in order to detect early signs and symptoms of SCC. Relationship building and education for radiology and MRI departments can result in rapid responses for diagnostic testing. In some circumstances, obtainment of an outpatient MRI can prevent an unnecessary admission by rapidly ruling out SCC in high-risk patients with back pain. Diagnostic algorithms to ensure that spine radiographs are used to perform initial screening can reduce the number of MRI procedures that will be required (121).

Standard nursing plans of care developed by the acute care CNS incorporate immediate and ongoing interventions that will assist in ensuring comprehensive management. The standard plan will include unique spinal neurological assessments, physical care to prevent injury, assessment of bladder volumes, and prevention of constipation. Incorporation of management of potential complications such as postradiation myelopathy and wound dehiscence with radiation to surgical sites ensures all caregivers are working from the same framework. Collaboration with physical therapists, surgeons, medical oncology, and radiation oncology in development of the plan of care also allows all caregivers to anticipate when their expertise will be required.

SUPERIOR VENA CAVAL COMPRESSION SYNDROME

Etiology

Obstruction of the SVC by external compression, tumor invasion, or intraluminal occlusion results in an oncological complication termed SVCS. Impediment of venous return to the right heart produces venous congestion with facial, chest, arm, and neck edema (133, 134). Severe obstruction has also been associated with pleural effusion, tracheal obstruction, and cerebral edema. This disorder is most common in patients with malignancies involving the central chest. More than 80% of all SVCS is related to bronchogenic cancer, and 10% to 15% of the remaining cases are attributed to breast cancer and lymphoma (133-137). All other malignancies and nonmalignant causes (e.g., infection, thrombus) comprise the remaining cases. Obstruction of the vessel lumen by a thrombus is most often related to indwelling central venous catheters and enhanced by the hypercoagulability of cancer (133-135, 138). Patients with a previous history of venous thromboembolism (VTE) and an SVC filter may develop SVCS if additional clots are trapped by the filter. All patients with a filter should be taught to monitor for early signs and symptoms of SVCS.

SVCS occurs in 3% to 5% of patients overall but is as high as 20% in patients with advanced cancers of the chest (134). It is generally considered a poor prognostic marker. If SVCS is an initial presenting symptom in the newly diagnosed patients with cancer, it is often highly responsive to therapy but recurs in 10% to 30% of patients (134). Therapy is usually emergent and involves collaboration among a number of specialized clinicians.

Pathophysiology

The SVC is a thin-walled, low-pressure vein located in the mediastinal cavity that drains blood from the head and neck and the upper thoracic cavity. The mediastinal bones include the sternum, ribs, and spine, and surround the SVC and other central vessels. This region also houses more than 20 lymph nodes. When a mass is present or lymph nodes are enlarged with tumor infiltration, the SVC is easily compressed and impedes venous return from the upper body. There are three distinct pathophysiological consequences that may occur independently or together. They include (1) external compression by a mass, (2) direct invasion with tumor, or (3) an intraluminal thrombus. Therapy is designed to match the specific pathological finding.

Clinical Presentation

The clinical presentation of SVCS depends on the rapidity of onset and severity of SVC compression. If the SVC is compressed gradually and collateral circulation develops, clinical findings of SVCS are more subtle (135, 137). Initial symptoms include periorbital and conjunctival edema, facial swelling, and Stokes' sign (tightness of the shirt collar) most prominent in the early morning (134). After the patient is mobile and upright for several hours the congestion abates and symptoms may lessen. The patient may also complain of visual disturbances and headache. Altered consciousness and focal neurological signs are uncommon and result from cerebral edema and impaired cardiac filling. Late and chronic signs and symptoms include distention of the veins of the thorax and upper extremities (137), dysphagia, dyspnea, cough, hoarseness, and tachypnea. All patients, including children, most commonly visit health care providers because of dyspnea (134, 136). Pleural effusions are present in approximately 60% of cases, compounding respiratory symptoms and providing a complex dimension for treatment planning (139). Most pleural effusions are transudative and related to obstruction of pleural and lymphatic outflow. Pericardial effusion may also be present independently or due to pulmonary hypertension associated with SVCS. Physical findings that uniquely support the diagnosis of SVCS include the upper body edema, blood pressure higher in the right arm.

Several complications may occur in patients with SVCS. Right-sided heart failure is the most common (133). Such heart failure is usually self-limiting and treated symptomatically with fluid restrictions and diuretics. Vessel rupture in SVCS occurs when a tumor invades the vena cava and is at greatest risk with SVCS when the tumor shrinks with treatment. The incidence of vessel rupture is highest in patients with esophageal and lung cancer; and peak incidence is 3 to 4 weeks after initiation of therapy (133). Warning signs of vessel rupture are acute and sudden dyspnea, hypoxia, cough, and hypotension.

Diagnosis

The risk profile and clinical findings often provide the strongest clues for the diagnosis of SVCS. Although not diagnostic, a chest radiograph is often performed as an initial screen for SVCS. This will show the proximity of masses or lymph nodes to the SVC. The spiral CT scan with contrast currently provides the most accurate information about tumor location and involvement of the vena cava and may be the only diagnostic test performed (140). If, however, biopsy or cytological tests are required to establish a cytopathological diagnosis of malignancy, biopsies may be required (135). Venography, angiography, and radionuclide scans are no longer necessary for validation of SVCS.

Management

Patients initially presenting with SVCS will have or be at risk for significant hypoxemia from venous congestion and impaired cardiac output. Maintenance of a patent airway is of the highest priority (133). Because many patients have severe dyspnea, they are unable to lie flat for their radiation therapy, and short-term airway intubation may be necessary. When the patient is in bed, the head should be at least in a semi-Fowler's position. Elevation of the arms on pillows helps alleviate swelling; however, elevation of the legs is not helpful because this increases fluid volume in the torso. For ambulatory patients, the nurse teaches the patient not to bend over and to avoid Valsalva maneuvers.

Supportive care is an essential part of the patient's plan of care. Patients with SVCS experience significant dyspnea and anxiety due to their condition and the body image changes that occur. Oxygenation should be maximized, although it may not be effective against the dyspnea induced by heart failure and edema. Body position, skin care, and rest aid in compensation for significant symptoms. Patients may require cardiac and respiratory monitoring for acute decompensation. Neurological symptoms are usually moderate and include non–life-threatening blurred vision or headache, but significant changes in mental status, one-sided sensory or motor deficits, unequal pupils, or altered speech may signal severe increased intracranial pressure or stroke. Prevention of constipation is important to avoid Valsalva maneuvers that may further increase intracranial pressure.

The primary treatment of choice for cancer-related SVCS is radiation therapy. Dosage depends on the size of the tumor and its radiosensitivity. Radiation therapy is initially given in high daily fractions (total dose of 30 to 50 rad) for 14 to 21 days, and symptom relief occurs in 7 to 14 days (134). Radiation therapy is palliative for SVCS in 70% of patients with lung cancer and for more than 95% of patients with lymphoma (136). Radiation of the mediastinal, hilar, and supraclavicular lymph nodes and any adjacent parenchymal lesions is appropriate in patients with locally advanced lung cancer. If the tumor is more chemosensitive, antineoplastic medications may be immediately initiated.

Patients who receive radiation therapy experience increased cough within 3 days of the start of therapy. During the initial 7 to 10 days, secretions are increased because of inflammation, but a dry irritation then develops, resulting in a dry, hacking cough with few secretions but possible bleeding (133).

While awaiting effective anticancer effects, patients are provided cardiopulmonary supportive care. The head of bed should remain elevated, and chest or upper extremity procedures and IV lines should be avoided. In general, fluids are restricted due to the known venous congestion; however; it is difficult to determine which patients may require and be able to tolerate diuretics to decrease venous return.

Chemotherapy may be the treatment of choice for SVCS in patients with disseminated disease, such as small cell anaplastic carcinoma or lymphoma. The agents used most often include high-dose regimens containing cyclophosphamide, cisplatin or carboplatin, bleomycin, etoposide, and doxorubicin (133, 136). The most common adverse effects of these agents include bone marrow suppression, cardiac toxicity, and renal dysfunction.

Treatment of SVCS caused by a thrombus around a central venous catheter may include thrombolytics (e.g., tissue plasminogen activator), fibrinolytics (e.g., activated protein C), or anticoagulants and possibly surgical removal of the catheter (141). In any case, chest and neck central venous catheter placements should be avoided until effective treatment has been delivered.

Clinicians may prescribe oxygen therapy, diuretics, steroids, and heparin, and their administration requires careful observation of patient response. If necessary, administration of corticosteroids for 3 to 7 days to decrease the edema associated with the disease and treatment is warranted (135). Anxiolytics are used judiciously while always assessing the adequacy of their airway.

In some circumstances, the placement of stents or vascular grafts in the SVC provides immediate symptomatic relief while patients receive definitive therapy (135, 142, 143). Patients are only considered for this therapy when skilled interventionalists are present, the patient's life-expectancy warrants a more permanent therapy, and their clinical status is stable enough to safely perform an operative procedure. It is unclear whether long-term anticoagulation is required for assured patency of these interventions. Caution must be taken and intensive observations are made to enhance early detection of bleeding as the tumor shrinks (144). In some patients with refractory disease or where additional radiation is contraindicated, stenting of the vena cava is a viable treatment option.

The best method of preventing SVCS is early recognition and intervention for chest tumors. New patients presenting with SVCS may not be prevented, but patient and family education of reportable signs and symptoms can reduce this complication in high-risk individuals. Prompt treatment for early symptoms can diminish the number of individuals who develop life-threatening SVCS. In some patients with known and refractory chest tumors near the SVC, prophylactic insertion of a venal caval stent can maintain vessel patency during treatment or to support other palliative care measures.

The development of new interventional radiology techniques will continue to allow growth of direct vessel maneuvers such as catheter directed thrombolytics, or vascular stents will enable high-risk patients to remain symptom-free for longer periods of time. As more effective antineoplastic regimens are developed, more patients with chest tumors will live longer, so it is possible that despite advances in treatment, the actual incidence of SVCS may increase in the near future. This possible trend reinforces the importance of having continuing discussions with patients about their cancer, realistic goals of treatment, and advanced care planning for metastatic and refractory disease.

Clinical Nurse Specialist Competencies and Spheres of Influence
Clinical Expert/Direct Care and Consultation

Patients with SVCS present with moderate to severe symptoms signaling disrupted cardiopulmonary function. The need for immediate recognition differentiating this syndrome from other similar disorders such as pneumonia, TBO, pulmonary embolism, stroke, or pericardial effusion may necessitate CNS consultation. The CNS will assist staff in implementing immediate interventions such as administration of corticosteroids and bronchodilators or oxygen therapy and head of bed elevation.

The CNS's expert knowledge of this disorder will guide staff to implement unique assessment strategies such as assessment of blood pressure in both arms since the right side is often higher or avoidance of upper extremity and chest vessels for venous catheter insertion. Patients should have oxygenation and vital signs assessed in various positions in order to determine alterations that are position-dependent due to pressure on central vessels. Some patients have severe enough chest pressure from existing tumor and venous congestion that they develop dysrhythmias when laid supine.

Patients who require emergent radiation therapy despite respiratory extremis requires creative use of anxiolytics and complementary relaxation therapy to facilitate radiation treatments in the supine position without severe respiratory distress. When these measures are unsuccessful, endotracheal intubation with mechanical ventilation and moderate sedation may be necessary to deliver treatment. Patients who do not tolerate supine position without hypotension, dysrhythmias, respiratory distress, or mental status changes may need to have radiation technique adjusted to be delivered in the prone position.

Coaching/Teaching/Mentoring

SVCS is more common in newly diagnosed patients with cancers of the chest. The acute care CNS should assess the patient case mix to determine the frequency with which this complication will be encountered. If the clinical setting does not provide radiation therapy services, it is highly likely these patients will be transferred to another facility.

When caring for patients with SVCS, the nurse will need to understand and anticipate the common adverse effects of chemotherapy or radiation therapy. The acute care CNS will guide staff in recognition and management of radiation effects such as cough, airway secretions, skin reactions, hoarseness, or sore throat. It may be difficult to differentiate radiation effects from infectious complications such as esophagitis or pneumonia.

Patients with SVCS who receive chemotherapy treatment require implementation of hazard precautions for 48 hours after administration. The specific chemotherapy regimen varies according to the primary cancer but will be high dose and systemic in order to achieve maximum destruction of tumor. Most of these therapies warrant pretreatment antiemetics and posttreatment hematopoietic growth factors. Chemotherapy competency assessments for staff are coordinated by the CNS when chemotherapy administration is performed by nursing staff.

Systems Leadership, Collaboration, and Research/Evidence-Based Practice

The care of patients with SVCS requires skills and input from a multitude of professionals. Patients with SVCS are often on the inpatient unit until the upper body and extremity edema has resolved. Patients often receive more than one treatment modality, combining radiation, chemotherapy, and anticoagulation therapy. They may also require invasive treatments by the interventional radiology service. Follow-up CT scans to assess thromboses, vascular compression, lymphadenopathy, and tumor size are usually performed after at least 4 to 6 weeks of therapy. Follow-up may be sooner if assessing the efficacy and evaluation of dose reduction of anticoagulation or thrombolytic treatment. The CNS will confer with multiple clinical experts to coordinate care for these patients. Rare but serious complications that can occur 3 to 8 weeks after initiation of radiation therapy are development of a tracheoesophageal fistula or vascular rupture. The proximity of tumor or malignant lymph nodes to the esophagus and major vessels places patients at risk for these complications when tumors shrink.

TRACHEOBRONCHIAL OBSTRUCTION

Etiology

TBO is defined as the compression of major conducting airways with tumor or enlarged lymph nodes. The mediastinal region contains more than 20 lymph nodes and is encased with bony structures such as the sternum. The growth of malignancy in the high chest or neck region predisposes patients to a tumor compression of one of the higher airways such as mainstem bronchi or trachea. It is estimated to occur in less than 1% of all cancer patients but as high as 20% of patients with bronchogenic cancers, or about 10% of patients with mediastinal lymphoma. Although lung cancer has the highest incidence of TBO, small cell lung patients are actually the highest risk group due to the common central location of their tumor but also to the rapid growth rate of this type of lung cancer (145). Adenocarcinomas may also grow centrally but are more likely to have slower onset of symptoms. Other cancers that have been associated with TBO include head/neck cancer, thyroid cancer, sarcoma, and melanoma. These patients usually present with acute life-threatening respiratory distress and require rapid assessment and invasive interventions. Nonmalignant disorders (e.g., amyloidosis, bronchomalacia) may also cause airway obstruction. Rare instances of leukemia infiltrates causing airway obstruction have also been reported (146).

Pathophysiology

Obstruction of the large bronchi or trachea with tumor results in respiratory distress and hypoxemia. The severity of symptoms depends on the rapidity of obstruction and degree of closure (145, 147). As the airway becomes occluded, both inspiration and expiration are impaired. The turbulent airflow produces bronchospasm with wheezes or stridor and both hypoxemia and hypercarbia. It is estimated that symptoms become noticeable at approximately 50% to 75% obstruction, but severe compromise usually indicates 90% to 95% obstruction. Although most symptoms are location dependent, it is less common to have obstruction of the trachea because of its greater rigidity and the presence of tracheal rings to maintain its position.

Clinical Presentation

Patients with TBO present with varying degrees of dyspnea depending on the amount and location of the obstruction and the rapidity of onset. Some patients with slowly developing tumors have compensated respiratory acidosis and minimal symptoms even with nearly complete obstruction. Other patients, especially those with lymphoma or small cell lung carcinoma, have rapidly growing tumors and severe symptoms even when the airway is less than 75% obstructed. Stridor is present in tracheal obstruction, and wheezing with unequal chest excursion is seen with bronchial obstruction (145). Some patients presenting with severe respiratory distress actually have only partial airway obstruction, but the resultant narrowed airway leads to concomitant atelectasis or trapped secretions with pneumonia that may be mistaken as more severe tumor obstruction (145).

Two severe complications that may occur are total airway occlusion and hemorrhage caused by tumor erosion into the nearby pulmonary vessels. Treatment of total obstruction is the same as that of partial obstruction when an improvement in symptoms can be reasonably expected as a result of therapy. Treatment of hemorrhage, when recognized before massive bleeding occurs, may involve embolization. If severe hemorrhage occurs, it is necessary to insert a dual-lumen endotracheal tube or single-sided intubation and occlude the bleeding lung while ventilating the good lung until surgical repair can be performed. Airway obstruction may also lead to erosion through the airway and accompanying pneumothorax. In these circumstances, supportive therapy such as chest tube insertion may be used but is rarely helpful.

Diagnosis

The first screening examination performed is usually a chest radiograph. Strong suspicion of tumor near the major ventilating airways is likely to be confirmed by CT angiography. These tests provide a three-dimensional view of the normal anatomical structures and level of malignant involvement. Bronchoscopy makes it easy to detect tracheal or bronchial obstruction and grade its severity. However, bronchoscopy does not always reveal whether the airways are compressed extrinsically or invaded with tumor (147). Bronchoscopy is always used in conjunction with spiral CT scans to provide a comprehensive description of the obstructive process that is used to guide therapy (148).

Management

Patients with TBO must be immediately assessed for severity of oxygen deprivation or carbon dioxide retention. Continuous cardiac rhythm and oxygen saturation monitoring are usually indicated. Arterial blood gases are the most accurate reflection of hypoxemia, hypercarbia, and the extent of compensation for airway obstruction. Arterial access is more invasive than venous phlebotomy, so frequent assessment may warrant insertion of an arterial line for monitoring blood pressure and obtaining arterial blood specimens.

Patients with narrowed airways are at even greater risk of mucus plug obstruction than those with other lung disorders. The inflammation and atelectasis lead to inflammation and production of sputum. Hydration, humidification, and assessment of sputum returns are important initial parameters to implement. This will reduce the risk of a mucus plug in an already narrow airway. Signs of mucus plugging include sudden increased respiratory distress, absence of secretions, unequal chest excursion, and pleuritic chest pain. If preventive measures are not adequate, nebulizer treatments with coughing, bronchodilators, and expectorant such as mucomyst or guaifenesin are administered to maintain airway patency. Changes in mental status are considered a cardinal emergency symptom. The most difficult aspect of this oncological emergency is that any definitive intervention minimally requires a CT scan and bronchoscopy to identify the exact location and severity of airway occlusion.

Clinically significant obstruction of the major airways always necessitates immediate treatment, although the therapeutic plan varies according to tumor-specific factors and therapeutic goals. Emergent treatment of airway occlusive-induced hypoxemia or hypercapnia may require nasal inhalation or heliox-based nebulizer treatments. A combination of oxygen and helium that is lighter than pure oxygen, heliox enhances movement of the air beyond the area of obstruction and provides palliative relief until more aggressive operative measures are possible (149). If airway obstruction is more oropharyngeal or high tracheal, an emergent tracheostomy may be performed.

If air movement is adequate, bronchodilators and corticosteroids are administered to enhance ventilation. If pneumonia is suspected, antimicrobial therapy is instituted (145). It may be difficult to differentiate which of the patient's symptoms are due to the obstructive mass in contrast to the exudates of infection. Patients with symptoms of mucus plugs may be administered increased hydration, mucomyst, or expectorants. Immediate chemotherapy may be implemented in patients with chemosensitive tumors, but other interventions may be required while awaiting tumor shrinkage.

Effective treatment for endobronchial tumors includes laser, cautery, photodynamic therapy, and endobronchial brachytherapy (150-153). These therapies for tumors invading the major airways are highly successful for prolonging life as well as improving its quality. Most procedures entail use of a rigid bronchoscope under anesthesia, and patients usually experience a rapid recovery with little more than a sore throat and annoying cough for a few days afterward. (152, 153). Endobronchial brachytherapy involves endotracheal intubation with precisely directed radiation therapy through an endobronchial catheter (154). In laser therapy, electrocautery, photodynamic therapy, and endobronchial brachytherapy, close observation for airway bleeding is necessary, and clinicians may prescribe cough suppressants or low-dose corticosteroids to reduce the incidence of bleeding (151, 152).

Airway opening with tracheal or bronchial stents may provide temporary symptomatic relief while definitive anticancer treatment is implemented for palliative relief of symptoms near the end of life (150, 152, 155-157). For insertion of an airway stent, a rigid bronchoscope and light anesthesia are necessary, and multiple bronchoscopic procedures to assess or adjust placement are required. The most common problem with stents, especially if placed before shrinking the tumor, is displacement because the airway naturally opens with the reduction of tumor. Displaced stents usually cause severe and sudden respiratory distress and require immediate interventional adjustment. In rare circumstances, or when stenting is not possible, patient positioning to shift the chest tumor off the major airway (e.g., prone positioning) may provide temporary symptomatic relief while cancer therapy is used to shrink the tumor (152, 155).

Realistic prevention of cancer-related airway obstruction lies primarily with public education regarding the signs and symptoms of malignancy. Many patients with TBO have newly diagnosed disease. In patients with known chest tumors, the occurrence of tracheobronchial disease is a part of the natural history of disease progression. Proactive conversations about best management should consider this expected symptom of progressive disease and whether it is best managed aggressively or palliatively.

Airway management for TBO has advanced tremendously in recent years with the advent of endobronchial interventions. The perfection of endobronchial brachytherapy and lasar will increase potential treatment efficacy for these patients. In even a few years, the development of more tissue-compatible stent materials have enabled more patients to receive this therapy, and this is expected to continue to develop. During this time of development, the ability to provide endobronchial therapies or placement of stent has only been available at major medical centers, but this is an expanding science that will likely reach more patients in the future. The recent knowledge that patients with reexpansion therapies have greater penetration by radiation and chemotherapy suggests that in the future, more patients should be offered these interventions prior to antineoplastic therapy.

The use of heliox therapy is also new to many medical-surgical units, but its efficacy in high airway obstruction and ease of use will probably lead to more widespread availability to future patients with airway obstruction.

Clinical Nurse Specialist Competencies and Spheres of Influence
Clinical Expert/Direct Care and Consultation
Patients with TBO are often acutely symptomatic and require rapid decisive life-support interventions such as oxygen or heliox, secretion management, and airway protection followed by diagnostic tests. It may be tempting to delay diagnostic testing in hopes of waiting for the patient to stabilize, but this is tactically incorrect. The more rapidly those diagnostic tests can be performed, the more quickly that differential diagnoses can be evaluated and evaluation for invasive treatment of airway obstruction can be implemented. The CNS who recognizes the classic risk factors and clinical presentation of these patients can facilitate these initial emergency interventions.

Although heliox is usually administered by respiratory therapy department personnel, a well-informed CNS will know that the heliox tank is large and space-consuming and should have its own flowmeter and face mask. Although a patient may be dependent on 100% oxygen and the heliox does not deliver this high of percentage (usually oxygen 75% to 80% with helium 20% to 25%), the lightweight helium may facilitate better delivery of the 80% oxygen it is mixed with and allow enhanced oxygen blood levels despite delivery of lower oxygen concentrations.

Coaching/Teaching/Mentoring
Patients with TBO comprise a small percentage of patients with cancer and come from a defined high-risk group of individuals. The CNS who is involved in complex patients, who are admitted to the medical-surgical unit, can identify these patients and the staff and patient education needs. Few professional resources and almost no patient education materials are pre-created and readily available and thus must be developed by the CNS or provided in consultation on a case-by-case basis. Patients with similar respiratory problems such as otolaryngology or asthma patients may provide a template for the CNS to use in creation of educational resources. At this time, invasive management of TBO may mean that many medical-surgical areas are primarily responsible for recognizing key symptoms and facilitating rapid transfer to a more comprehensive medical center.

Systems Leadership, Collaboration, and Research/Evidence-Based Practice
Patients with small cell lung cancer and malignant lymphoma are treated in many community and university medical centers. These patients are not only at highest risk for TBO, but also have rapidly proliferative tumors that may lead to a more acute onset of TBO. The CNS should assess the institutional capability to manage these patients and collaborate with interventional pulmonologists, thoracic surgeons, otolaryngologists, intensivists, radiology personnel, and respiratory therapists to ensure that all the necessary personnel, supportive equipment, and supplies are available for these patients when needed. A rapid call response tree should also be developed to ensure emergent airway management if necessary. If determined that these patients should be transferred to another facility, advance discussion of the collaborative care for these patients should be explored to ensure efficient hand-off when the patient is in crisis.

Patients with high airway obstruction should also be assessed in advance for a possible difficult airway. Patients with TBO and tumors in the neck are high risk for a difficult airway intubation if mechanical ventilator support is needed. Proactive assessment of the airway by anesthesia in advance of a crisis will allow all professionals to obtain special equipment that may be needed for airway protection.

Speech therapy is often involved with these patients to ensure they can safely swallow and protect their airway.

TUMOR LYSIS SYNDROME

Etiology

TLS is a metabolic syndrome caused by rapid cancer cell death and release of toxic metabolites in excess of which can be cleared by the kidneys. Clinically symptomatic disease occurs in only 2% to 4% of high-risk patients (158). Tumor lysis usually presents 1 to 5 days after initiation of therapy in patients with chemosensitive or radiosensitive tumors; however, it may onset as late at 7 days after therapy initiation (158, 159). Despite its name, there are also documented instances of TLS in rapidly proliferating disease such as acute leukemia or high-grade lymphoma even before treatment initiation (159). Patients who are at highest risk for TLS are those with bulky tumors having a high growth rate (e.g., acute leukemia or Burkitt's lymphoma) and those with highly radiosensitive or chemosensitive tumors such as small cell lung cancer and most malignant lymphomas (158-160). The amount of disease is often reflected in the severity of rise in the LDH or alkaline phosphatase. Patients with preexisting renal dysfunction may be at greatest risk owing to their difficulty in clearing the metabolic waste products fast enough to prevent clinical complications (159, 161). Dehydration also causes higher concentration of the lysis products and may enhance symptomatic disease. Other patients at high risk are those with Merkel's tumor, hepatoblastoma, and medulloblastoma (159).

Pathophysiology

Rapid cell death causes the release of intracellular contents (potassium, phosphorus, and nucleic acids) into the circulating serum. The normal filtration mechanisms in the kidneys should immediately detect the levels of metabolic waste products and attempt to excrete them. If production is more rapid than excretion or renal insufficiency is present, serum accumulation of electrolytes and uric acid will occur. The most common metabolic findings include hyperkalemia, hyperphosphatemia, and hyperuricemia (159). High phosphorus causes the kidneys to excrete calcium, causing hypocalcemia. Hyperuricemia causes deposition of uric acid crystals in the urinary tract and may lead to renal failure (158, 161, 162).

Clinical Presentation

Signs and symptoms of TLS are related to the specific electrolyte imbalances involved and renal dysfunction. Hyperkalemia, hyperphosphatemia, hypocalcemia, hyperuricemia, and acidosis may occur. Table 14-11 lists the typical clinical signs and symptoms associated with the metabolic abnormalities of TLS (159).

Diagnosis

The electrolyte panel is used to identify key abnormalities in patients at risk for tumor lysis syndrome. Elevated serum potassium, phosphate, uric acid, blood urea nitrogen, and creatinine, with low calcium, are

TABLE 14–11 Clinical Presentation of Tumor Lysis Syndrome

Laboratory Abnormality	Signs and Symptoms	Management
POTASSIUM >5.5 MEQ/L OR >25% INCREASE FROM BASELINE		
	• Increased bowel sounds • Abdominal cramping and diarrhea • Nausea • Muscle weakness, flaccidity • Fatigue • Paresthesias • Progressive ECG changes: First stage—peaked T waves, shortened PR interval, ST depression; second phase—widened QRS, prolonged PR interval, decreased amplitude of P wave; third phase—flattened QRS into ventricular fibrillation • Palpitations • Tachycardia—atrial, supraventricular, or ventricular • Increased premature beats (atrial, junctional, or ventricular)	• Kaexylate orally or by enema will bind with K+ ions and remove via loose stool • Sodium bicarbonate (1 mEq/kg) causes potassium ions to move into the cells • Calcium gluconate 1 amp (4.5 mEq) intravenous (this is not preferred choice if symptoms are mild or only ECG change is peaked T waves) • Dextrose 50% and Regular insulin 10 units intravenous • Force fluids, sodium based to enhance electrolyte excretion • Loop diuretics (e.g., furosemide) • Dialysis

TABLE 14-11 Clinical Presentation of Tumor Lysis Syndrome—cont'd

Laboratory Abnormality	Signs and Symptoms	Management
PHOSPHATE >8.0 MG/DL OR 25% INCREASE FROM BASELINE		
	• Renal dysfunction • Muscle weakness • Joint pain • Limited joint movement • Pruritus • Red eye or conjunctivitis • Mental status changes ranging from mild confusion to obtundation or seizures • Cataracts • Paresthesias • Prolonged QT segment of ECG • Leukopenia • Thrombocytopenia • Hypocalcemia	• Force fluids, sodium based to enhance electrolyte excretion • Phosphate binding agents (e.g., aluminum hydroxide) • Dialysis • Bone marrow growth factors
URIC ACID >8.0 MG/DL OR INCREASE FROM BASELINE		
	• Renal dysfunction evidenced by elevated creatinine • Oliguria, anuria • Hematuria • Enlarged and tender kidney with possible tubular obstruction	• Allopurinol • Rasburicase • Force fluids • Diuretics • Dialysis
CALCIUM <8.0 MG/DL OR 25% DECREASE FROM BASELINE		
	• Muscle contraction/tetany • Painful twitching/fasciculation of small muscle • Increased deep tendon reflexes • Abdominal cramping, diarrhea, increased bowel sounds • Irritable heart rhythms—tachycardia, atrial fibrillation/flutter, premature beats • Nausea	• Calcium replacement—ONLY after phosphorous has been reduced • Phosphorous reduction
ARTERIAL PH <7.25 MM HG		
	• Bradycardia, junctional rhythm, heart block • Hypotension • Cyanosis • Smooth muscle contraction-abdominal cramping, uterine cramping	• Increase blood volume with fluids, blood products, colloids • Maximize oxygenation of tissues with oxygen supplements if levels are deficient. • Support blood pressure with vasopressor agents (e.g., dopamine, norepinephrine) • Sodium bicarbonate 1 mEq/kg intravenous

reported. Acidosis may be present in patients with severely compromised renal function. The urinary uric acid/creatinine ratio is greater than 1. Renal ultrasonography is used to exclude ureteral obstruction (163).

Management

The focus of nursing care is on careful monitoring of fluid therapy, intake and output, and electrolyte balance. To measure urine output more accurately, insertion of a Foley catheter into the bladder is usually necessary. If oliguria or anuria develops, ureteral or urethral obstruction must be excluded prior to declaring the patient as having intrarenal failure due to TLS. The use of prophylactic allopurinol, aggressive hydration, and early intervention with continuous renal replacement therapy (CRRT) has reduced the incidence and severity of TLS (159).

Treatment involves recognition of high-risk patients and promoting prevention through aggressive hydration, as well as administration of phosphate-binding agents and allopurinol for at least 48 hours before beginning chemotherapy. It is necessary to avoid agents that block tubular reabsorption of uric acid (e.g., aspirin, radiographic contrast, probenecid, thiazide diuretics). The goal is to keep the serum uric acid level within normal limits. Electrolyte disturbances are specifically treated as needed (164, 158).

IV fluids are given to ensure a urine volume of more than 3 L/day. In the past, IV sodium bicarbonate (4 g initially, then 1 to 2 g every 4 hours) has been administered to alkalinize the urine and reduce uric acid crystallization in the kidney tubules. Clinicians are now less likely to initiate alkalinization if the phosphate is high because calcium-phosphate precipitation is equally likely to cause renal failure (160, 164).

Phosphate-binding agents such as aluminum hydroxide are given every 2 to 4 hours in an effort to keep phosphate levels below 4 mg/dL (159). Concomitant diuresis or medications such as kayexalate that enhance gastrointestinal excretion of potassium may effectively manage elevated serum potassium levels not prevented with hydration. Allopurinol, a xanthine oxidase inhibitor that blocks uric acid production, is administered in doses ranging from 300 to 900 mg/day. Because it is now available in an IV form given as 200 to 400 mg/m^2/day, rapid normalization of uric acid levels is an achievable objective (159). Its greatest limitation is that it cannot assist in breakdown or clearance of already existing uric acid (165). Rasburicase (Elitek), a new agent, acts like the natural enzyme urate oxidase to oxidize uric acid to allantoin for excretion (164, 165). Rasburicase is used cautiously in patients at risk for GPD deficiency because of increased risk for hemolytic anemia. Severe hypersensitivity reactions have also been reported and warrant careful observation during infusion. The uric acid serum blood levels drawn on patients receiving rasburicase must be placed in an iced blood tube and transported to the laboratory on ice to ensure accurate levels (164-167).

If diuresis does not occur within a few hours after the initiation of treatment, renal replacement therapy is needed. An initial hemodialysis treatment usually reduces the patient's uric acid levels by 50%, but most patients then receive several additional days of CRRT until electrolyte abnormalities and hyperuricemia resolve (158, 162). A low-calcium dialysate is used to prevent calcium phosphate precipitation. If peritoneal dialysis is used, albumin is added to the dialysate to increase uric acid protein binding and removal.

Optimal prevention of TLS is achieved with effective hydration and glomerular filtration that leads to a urinary output of at least 2 mL/kg/hr. Recognition of patients at high risk for tumor lysis based on their tumor type, tumor's growth rate, amount of tumor mass, and treatment sensitivity allows tailored fluid therapy and potential initiation of protective agents prior to beginning the anticancer therapy. For patients with high WBC counts and acute leukemia, leukapheresis may be performed to lower the WBC count prior to starting antineoplastic therapy, hence also reducing the risk for TLS.

Patients with pretreatment and acute therapy-related TLS fair much better today than a decade ago because early recognition allows timely pretreatment allopurinol and phosphate binding or leukapheresis to prevent severe TLS. Recent research has also provided evidence-supported best practice hydration strategies using normal saline solution rather than a bicarbonate-based solution.

Possibly the most significant recent advance in management of TLS has been development of an effective gentle continuous dialysis that permits constant fluid and metabolic toxin removal during the period of tumor lysis. The use of CRRT early during an episode of tumor lysis can prevent renal failure and life-threatening electrolyte disturbances. Future research defining best dialysate solutions, dialysis modality, blood flow rates, or types of filters are likely to define future best care for these patients. Just as a new medication has become available for management of hyperuricemia, it is likely that enhanced management of hyperkalemia will also become a research priority, allowing for less invasive management of many patients with TLS. Leukapheresis is still not universally employed in patients with high WBCs in leukemia because some clinicians do not believe there is adequate evidence that patient outcomes are altered with this expensive and labor-intensive therapy. Further research that includes quality of life measures as well as outcome measures is needed to assist in guiding this clinical practice.

Clinical Nurse Specialist Competencies and Spheres of Influence
Clinical Expert/Direct Care and Consultation

Patients with TLS may be asymptomatic until they are having an electrolyte crisis, reinforcing the importance of recognizing and proactive monitoring patients at high risk for this syndrome. The subtle signs or symptoms that precede dysrhythmias or mental status changes are noticeable for expert clinicians like the CNS who are closely monitoring patients with highly proliferative or rapidly growing tumors with known risk for TLS. Abdominal cramping, muscle cramping, nausea, increased bowel sounds, or diarrhea are symptoms that may indicate electrolyte abnormalities. Expert clinicians will ensure that appropriate prophylactic medications are prescribed as soon as possible prior to starting therapy and continued throughout the 7 to 10 days of tumor lysis. Uric acid–blocking agents have adverse effects such as bone marrow suppression, hemolysis, or rash, and phosphate-binding agents can cause gastrointestinal distress, providing a clinical picture similar to the disease itself. If rasburicase is being administered, it must be dosed according to uric acid levels, but special caution must be taken to send all uric acid levels in a previous refrigerated tube placed on ice in order for values to be accurate. False low values by not following these laboratory monitoring guidelines can cause dangerous underdosing of this medication.

Serum chemistry panel with addition of phosphate and magnesium are monitored at least every 12 hours and possibly as frequent as every 6 hours. When possible, other sources of electrolytes or acidosis risks such as banked blood, electrolyte drinks and foods, dark colas, and milk products are avoided during this high-risk time. It is important to replenish calcium cautiously because if calcium is administered when the phosphate is high, calcium-phosphate precipitants can exacerbate renal dysfunction.

Coaching/Teaching/Mentoring

Acute care CNSs should invest the most staff education in assisting nurses to recognize the patients who are at risk for TLS and assisting them in proactively discussing management of this complication with the multidisciplinary team. Nurses caring for patients with risk for TLS must be familiar with the acute management of life-threatening electrolyte disturbances, most common in this disorder being hyperkalemia and hypocalcemia. Immediately in patients with high count leukemia, or within 24 to 72 hours after initiation of effective treatment with other tumors with high growth rates, the rise for lysis electrolyte levels can span only a few hours. Once symptoms begin, little time may be available to institute more hydration, dialysis, or active counteractive measures. Nurses should proactively advocate for initiation of preventive measures such as hydration, phosphate binders, and uric acid inhibitors that should be instituted before or immediately with treatment.

Continuous dialysis is a complex therapy managed by bedside intensive care nurses and is often implemented on an emergent basis. Nurses caring for patients at risk for TLS should be competent at managing this therapy or be able to access nurses who are skilled within a 2-hour timeframe. This may necessitate emergency patient transfer or shared nursing resources. Since most of these dialysis pumps do not have a battery, the ability to transfer or transport this patient in the midst of severe tumor lysis is very risky.

Systems Leadership, Collaboration, and Research/Evidence-Based Practice

The rapid onset of acuity in patients with TLS requires significant proactive planning for care of these patients. The acute care CNS should consider these factors when faced with care of any patients with acute leukemia, high-grade lymphomas, small cell lung cancer, germ cell tumors (e.g., testicular cancer), or other defined highly proliferative cancers. It is appropriate for the CNS to coordinate multidisciplinary meetings with ambulatory care, oncology, intensivists, nephrologists, dialysis staff, critical care nurses, and laboratory services to ensure that prompt recognition and management of TLS is possible in the institution. If dialysis catheters are placed by interventional radiology services, they may also be involved in discussion of best practice. Due to severe acidosis, specialty high bicarbonate dialysate solutions may be required and are usually mixed by pharmacy personnel. It is advisable to stock dialysate in pharmacy or ensure rapid availability to guarantee a 1-hour bedside availability. Rapid availability of less than one hour for screening tests and less than 10 minutes for immediate test results should be available, but often requires discussion with laboratory personnel or a named unit laboratory set called "tumor lysis labs" to alert laboratory staff of the urgency of results. Intensive care unit staff may be very unfamiliar with this serious but unique complication of malignancy. It is similar to rhabdomyolysis and this can be used for comparison when discussing the clinical management of these patients. It is important for them to realize this acute complication is actually a clinical indicator of response to anticancer treatment and should be managed aggressively to ensure the best outcome for patients.

References

1. Shelton BK, Rome SI, Lewis SL. Nursing assessment: Hematological system. In Lewis SL, Heitkemper MM, Dirkson SR, et al, editors. Medical-Surgical Nursing: Assessment and Management of Clinical Problems. 7th ed. Philadelphia: Elsevier; 2007:665-683.

2. Shelton BK General Toxicity: Myelosuppression and secondary malignancies. In Gobel B, Triest-Robertson S, Vogel WH, editors. Advanced Oncology Certification Review and Resource Manual. Pittsburgh, PA: Oncology Nursing Society Press; 2009:405-442.

3. Smith RE Jr. The clinical and economic burden of anemia. Am J Manage Care 2010;16(suppl): S59-S66.

4. Hussein M, Haddad RY. Approach to anemia. Dis Mon 2010;56(8): 449-455.

5. Bayraktar UD, Bayraktar S. Treatment of iron deficiency anemia associated with gastrointestinal tract diseases, World J Gastroenterol 2010;1(22):2720-2725.

6. Salim-Ur-Rehman S, Huma N, et al. Efficacy of non-heme iron fortified diets: a review. Crit Rev Fod Sci Nutr 2010;50(5): 403-413.

7. Harder L, Boshkov L. The optimal hematocrit. Crit Care Clin 2010;26(2):335-354.

8. Fishbane S. The role of erythropoiesis-stimulating agents in the treatment of anemia. Am J Manage Care 2010;16(suppl): S67-S73.

9. Barbera L, Thomas G. Erythropoiesis stimulating agents, thrombosis and cancer. Radiother Oncol 2010;95(3):269-276.

10. Prittie JE. Controversies related to red blood cell transfusion in critically ill patients. J Vet Emerg Crit Care 2010;20(2):167-176.

11. Lippi G, Franchini M, Favaloro EJ. Thrombotic complications of erythropoiesis-stimulating agents. Semin Thromb Hemost 2010;36(5):537-549.

12. Mousa SA, Qari MH. Diagnosis and management of sickle cell disorders. Methods Mol Biol 2010;663:291-307.

13. Prabhakar H, Haywood C Jr, Molokie R. Sickle cell disease in the United States: looking back and forward at 100 years of progress in management and survival. Am J Hematol 2010;85:346-353.

14. Barabino GA, Platt MO, Kaul DK. Sickle cell biomechanics. Annu Rev Biomed Eng 2010;12:345-367.

15. Wright J, Ahmedzai SH. The management of painful crisis in sickle cell disease. Curr Opin Support Palliat Care 2010;4(2): 97-106.

16. Akinsheye I, Klings ES. Sickle cell anemia and vascular dysfunction: the nitric oxide connection. J Cell Physiol 2010; 224(3):620-625.

17. Vij R, Machado RF. Pulmonary complications of hemoglobinopathies. Chest 2010;138(4):973-983.

18. Ramakrishnan M, Moisi JC, Klugman KP, et al. Increased risk of invasive bacterial infections in African people with sickle cell disease: a systematic review and meta-analysis. Lancet Infect Dis 2010;10(5):329-337.

19. Verduzco LA, Nathan DG. Sickle cell disease and stroke. Blood 2009;114(25):5117-5125.

20. Thein SL, Menzel S, Lathrop M, et al. Control of fetal hemoglobin: new insights emerging from genomics and clinical implications. Hum Mol Genet 2009;18(R2): R216-R223.

21. Ataga KI. Novel therapies in sickle cell disease. Hematol Am Soc Hematol Educ Progr 2009;54-61.

22. Shelton BK. Oncological emergencies. In Morton PG, editor. Critical Care Nursing. Philadelphia: Elsevier; 2009:1248-1309.

23. Shelton BK. Infections, In Yarbro CH, Wujcik D, Gobel BH, editors. Cancer Nursing Principles and Practice. 7th ed. Boston, MA: Jones and Bartlett; 2011:713-744.

24. Friese C. Prevention of infection in patients with cancer. Semin Oncol Nurs 2007;23(3):174-183.

25. Dellinger RP, Levy MM, Carlet JM, et al. Surviving sepsis campaign: international guidelines for management of severe sepsis and septic shock. Crit Care Med 2008;36(1):296-327.

26. NCCN. Prevention and management of infections in patients with cancer, v2010.1. Retrieved December 2, 2010, from www.nccn.org

27. National Comprehensive Cancer Network (NCCN). National clinical practice guidelines in oncology. Myeloid growth factors. Retrieved August 17, 2011, from http://www.nccn.org/ professionals/physician_gls/f_guidelines.asp#supportive

28. DeLoughery TG. Thrombocytopenia and other hot topics. Am J Clin Oncol 2009;32(4 suppl) S13-S17.

29. Kirkpatrick CA. The HELLP syndrome. Acta Clin Belg 2010;65(2):91-97.

30. Otis SA, Zehnder JL. Heparin-induced thrombocytopenia: current status, and diagnostic challenges. Am J Hematol 2010;85(9):700-706.

31. Kiss JE. Thrombotic thrombocytopenia purpura: recognition and management. Int J Hematol 2010;91(1):36-45.

32. Eklund EA. Thrombocytopenia and cancer. Cancer Treat Res 2009;148:279-293.

33. Cines DB, Liebman H, Stasi R. Pathobiology of secondary immune thrombocytopenia, Semin Hematol 2009;22(2): S2-S14.

34. Damron BH, Brant JM, Belansky HB, et al. Putting evidence into practice: prevention and management of bleeding in patients with cancer. Clin J Oncol Nurs 2009;13(5):573-583.

35. University of Michigan. Five blood transfusion guidelines and utilization review. Retrieved December 2, 2010, from http://www.pathology.med.umich.edu/bloodbank/manual/ bbch_5/index.html

36. Molieux G, Newland A. Development of romiplostim for the treatment of patients with chronic immune thrombocytopenia purpura: from bench to bedside. Br J Haematol 2010;150(1): 9-20.

37. Levi M, Schultz M, van der Poll T. Disseminated intravascular coagulation in infectious disease. Semin Thromb Hemost 2010;36(4):367-377.

38. Lippi G, Ippolito L, Cervellin G. Disseminated intravascular coagulation in burn injury. Semin Thromb Hemost 2010;36(4): 429-436.

39. Lippi G, Cervellin G. Disseminated intravascular coagulation in trauma injuries. Semin Thromb Hemost 2010;36(4):378-387.

40. Levi M. Disseminated intravascular coagulation. Crit Care Med 2007;35(9):2191-2195.

41. Levi M, Toh CH, Thachil J, et al. Guidelines for the diagnosis and management of disseminated intravascular coagulation. Br Comm Stand Haematol 2009;145(1):24-33.

42. Kitchens CS. Thrombocytopenia and thrombosis in disseminated intravascular coagulation (DIC). Hematol Am Soc Hematol Educ Progr Book January, 2009, 240-246.

43. Shelton BK. Disseminated intravascular coagulation. In Chernecky CC, Murphy-Ende K, editors. Acute Care Oncology Nursing. 2nd ed. Philadelphia: Saunders; 2009:122-136.

44. Favaloro EJ. Laboratory testing in disseminated intravascular coagulation. Semin Thromb Hemost 2010;36(4):458-467.

45. Thachil J, Fitzmaurice DA, Toh CH. Appropriate use of D-dimer in hospital patients. Am J Med 2010;123(1):17-19.

46. NovoNordisk. NovoSevenRT. Retrieved from http://www. novosevenrt.com/hcp/index.html

Oncological Malignancies General

47. Shelton BK. Admission criteria and prognostication in patients with cancer admitted to the intensive care unit. Crit Care Clin 2010;26(1):1-20.

48. Carlson KS, De Sancho MT. Hematological issues in critically ill patients with cancer. Crit Care Clin 2010;26(1):107-132.

49. Hill QA. Intensify, resuscitate or palliatate: decision making in the critically ill patient with haematological malignancy. Blood Rev 2010;24(1):17-25.

50. Kurtin SE. Leukemia. In Yarbro CH, Wujcik D, Gobel BH, editors. Cancer Nursing Principles and Practice. 7th ed. Boston, MA: Jones and Bartlett; 2011:1369-1398.

51. Larson RA. Is secondary leukemia an independent prognostic factor in acute myeloid leukemia? Best Pract Res Haematol 2007;20(1):29-37.

52. Berheom A. Cytogenomics of cancers: from chromosome to sequence. Mol Oncol 2010;4(4):309-322.

53. Motyckova G, Stone RM. The role of molecular tests in acute myelogenous leukemia treatment decisions. Curr Hematol Malig Rep 2010;5(2):109-117.

54. Collins-Underwood JR, Mulligham CG. Genomic profiling of high-risk acute lymphoblastic leukemia. Leukemia 2010;24(10):1676-1685.

55. Marbello L, Ricci F, Nosari AM, et al. Outcome of hyperleukocytic adult acute myeloid leukemia: a single-center retrospective study and review of literature. Leuk Res 2008;32(8):1221-1227.

56. Montoya L. Managing hematological toxicities in the oncology patient. J Infus Nurs 2007;30(3):168-172.

57. Perotti D, Jamieson C, Goldman J, et al. Chronic myeloid leukemia: mechanisms of blastic transformation. J Clin Invest 2010;20(7):2254-2264.

58. Ostreicher P. What's blasting off in CML? ONS Connect 2007;22(8 suppl):71-72.

59. Goldberg SL, Chen E, Corral M, et al. Incidence and clinical consequences of myelodysplastic syndromes among United States Medicare beneficiaries. J Clin Oncol 2010;28(7):2847-2852.

60. Barzi A, Sekeres MA. Myelodysplastic syndromes: a practical approach to diagnosis and treatment. Cleve Clin J Med 2010;77(1):37-44.

61. Betz BL, Hess JL. Acute myeloid leukemia diagnosis in the 21st century. Arch Pathol Lab Med 2010;134(10):1427-1433.

62. Quintas-Cardama A, Kantarjian H, Cortes JE. Applying cytogenetic and molecular information in the clinic: implications for the treatment of chronic myeloid leukemia. Clin Lymphoma Myeloma Leuk 2010;10(suppl 1): S20-S26.

63. Bow EJ. Neutropenic fever syndromes in patients undergoing cytotoxic therapy for acute leukemia and myelodysplastic syndromes. Semin Hematol 2009;46(3):259-268.

64. Shelton BK. Evidence-based care for the neutropenic patient with leukemia. Semin Oncol Nursing 2003;19(2):133-141.

65. Blum W, Porcu P. Therapeutic apheresis in hyperleukocytosis and hyperviscosity syndrome. Semin Thromb Hemost 2007;33(4):350-354.

66. Wang J, Ouyang J, Zhou R, et al. Autologous hematopoietic stem cell transplantation for acute myeloid leukemia in first complete remission: a meta analysis of randomized trials. Acta Haematol 2010;124(2):61-71.

67. Hill BT, Copelan EA. Acute myeloid leukemia: when to transplant in first complete remission. Curr Hematol Malig Rep 2010;5(2):101-108.

68. Wayne AS, Baird K, Egeler RM. Hematopoietic stem cell transplantation for leukemia, Pediatr Clin North Am 2010; 57(1):1-25.

69. Carstensen M, Sorensen JB. Outpatient management of febrile neutropenia: time to revise the present treatment strategy. J Support Oncol 2008;6(5):199-208.

70. Friese C. Prevention of infection in patients with cancer. Semin Oncol Nurs 2007;23(3):174-183.

71. Manson SD, Porter C. Lymphoma. In Yarbro CH, Wujcik D, Gobel BH, editors. Cancer Nursing Principles and Practice. 7th ed. Boston, MA: Jones and Bartlett; 2011:1458-1512.

72. Schenk M, Purdue MP, Colt JS, et al. Occupational/industry and risk of non-Hodgkin's lymphoma in the United States. Occup Environ Med 2009;66(1):23-31.

73. Calzone KA, Lea DH, Masny A. Non-Hodgkin's lymphoma as an exemplar of the effects of genetics and genomics. J Nurs Scholarship 2006;38(4):335- 343.

74. Nagpal S, Glantz MJ, Recht L. Treatment and prevention of secondary CNS lymphoma. Semin Neurol 2010;30(3):263-272.

75. Armitage JO. Early-stage Hodgkin's lymphoma. N Engl J Med 2010;363(7):653-662.

76. Fortez-Vila J, Fraga M. Differential diagnosis of classic Hodgkin's lymphoma. Int J Surg Pathol 2010;18(3 suppl):124S-127S.

77. Mullen E, Zhong Y. Hodgkin lymphoma: an update. J Nurs Pract 2007;3(6):393-403.

78. Fortez-Vila J, Fraga M. Burkitt lymphoma and diffuse aggressive B-cell lymphoma. Int J Surg Pathol 2010;18(3 suppl):133S-135S.

79. Faiman B. Clinical updates and nursing considerations for patients with multiple myeloma. Clin J Oncol Nurs 2007;11(6):831-840.

80. Mullen E, Mendez N. Hyperviscosity syndrome in patients with multiple myeloma. Oncol Nurs Forum 2008;35(3):350-352.

81. Wiley KE. Multiple myeloma and treatment-related thromboembolism: oncology nurses' role in prevention, assessment, and diagnosis. Clin J Oncol Nurs 2007;11(6):847-851.

82. Engelhardt M, Kleber M, Udi J, et al. Consensus statement from European experts on the diagnosis, management, and treatment of multiple myeloma: from standard therapy to novel approaches. Leuk Lymphoma 2010;51(8):1424-1443.

83. Lonial S. Presentation and risk stratification: improving prognosis for patients with multiple myeloma. Cancer Treat Rev, 2010; 36(suppl):S12-S17.

84. Wadhera RK, Rajkumar SV. Prevalence of monoclonal gammopathy of undetermined significance: a systematic review. Mayo Clin Proc 2010;85(10):933-942.

85. Cleveland Clinic MedEd. Multiple myeloma. Retrieved December 2, 2010, from http://www.clevelandclinicmeded.com/medicalpubs/diseasemanagement/hematology

86. Berenson JR. Therapeutic options in the management of myeloma bone disease. Semin Oncol 2010;37(Suppl 1):S20-S29.

87. Nair B. Solitary extramedullary and bone plasmacytomas versus multiple myeloma with extramedullary manifestation. Oncology (Williston Park) 2010;24(9):836.

88. Mateos MV. Management of treatment-related adverse events in patients with multiple myeloma, Cancer Treat Rev 2010;36(suppl 2):S24-S32.

89. Zhou FL, Meng S, Zhang WG, et al. Peptide-based immunotherapy for multiple myeloma: current approaches. Vaccine 2010;28(37):5939-5946.

90. Chanan-Khan AA, Borrello I, et al. Development of target-specific treatments in multiple myeloma. Br J Haematol 2010;151(1):3-15.

91. Lokhorst H, Einsele H, Vesole D, et al. International Myeloma Working Group consensus statement regarding the current status of allogeneic stem-cell transplantation for multiple myeloma. J Clin Oncol 2010;28(29):4521-4530.

92. Lipton A. Bone continuum of cancer. Am J Clin Oncol 2010;33(3 suppl):S1-S7.

93. Moy B. Cystitis in patients with cancer. UpToDate online version 18.3; last updated January 27, 2009; accessed Dec 10, 2010.

94. Polovich M, Whitford JM, Olsen M, editors. Oncology Nursing Society Chemotherapy and Biotherapy Guidelines and Recommendations for Practice. 3rd ed. Pittsburgh: Oncology Nursing Press.

95. Federoff A. BK virus in hematopoietic stem cell transplantation recipients. Clin J Oncol Nurs 2008;12(6):895-900.

96. Sylvanus T. Prevention of hemorrhagic cystitis: the evidence says what? Oncol Nurs Forum 2007;34(2):574.

97. Bogris SL, Johal NS, Hussein I, et al. Is it safe to use aluminum in the treatment of pediatric hemorrhagic cystitis? A case discussion of aluminum intoxication and review of the literature. J Pediatr Oncol 2009;31(4):285-288.

98. Kacprowicz RF, Lloyd JD. Electrolyte complications of malignancy. Hematol Oncol Clin North Am 2010;24(3):553-565.

99. Ijaz A, Mehmood T, Qureshi AH, et al. Estimation of ionized calcium and total calcium and albumin corrected calcium for the diagnosis of hypercalcemia of malignancy. J Coll Phys Surg Pakistan 2006;16(1):49-52.

100. Shane E. Diagnostic approach to hypercalcemia. UpToDate online version 18.1, last updated January 13, 2010; accessed July 12, 2010.

101. Cope D. Pleural effusions: malignant. In Chernecky CC, Murphy-Ende K, editors. Acute Care Oncology Nursing. 2nd ed. St Louis: Saunders; 2009;435-441.

102. Porcel JM. Pearls and myths in pleural fluid analysis. Respiraology 2010. Epub ahead of print.

103. Korczynski P, Krenke R, Safianowska A, et al. Diagnostic utility of pleural fluid and serum markers in differentiation between malignant and non-malignant pleural effusions. Eur J Med Res 2009;14(suppl 4):128-133.

104. Heffner JE. Management of malignant pleural effusion. UpToDate online version 18.1, last updated January 26, 2010; accessed June 23, 2010.

105. Held-Warmkessel J, & Schieh L. Caring for the patient with malignant pleural effusion. Nursing 2008;38(1):43-48.

106. Barbetakis N, Asteriou C, Papadopoulou F, et al. Early and late morbidity and mortality and life expectancy following thoracoscopic talc insufflations for control of malignant pleural effusions: a review of 400 cases. J Cardiothorac Surg 2010;5:27.

107. Ozyurtkan MO, Balci AE, Cakmak M. Predictors of mortality within three months in the patients with malignant pleural effusion. Eur J Intern Med 2010;21(1):30-34.

108. Moore AJ, Parker AJ, Wiggins J. Malignant mesothelioma. Orphanet J Rare Dis 2008;3:34.

109. Abouzgheib W, Bartter T, Dagher H, et al. A prospective study of the volume of pleural fluid required for accurate diagnosis of malignant pleural effusion. Chest 2008;135:999-1001.

110. James P, Gupta R, Christopher DJ, et al. Evaluation of the diagnostic yield and safety of closed pleural biopsy in the diagnosis of pleural effusion. Indian J Tuberc 2010;57(1):19-24.

111. Doelken P. Management of refractory nonmalignant pleural effusions. UpToDate online version 18.1, last updated June 16, 2009; accessed July 7, 2010.

112. Adegboye VO, Falade A, Osinusi K, et al. Reexpansion pulmonary oedema as a complication of pleural drainage. Nigerian Postgrad Med J 2002;9(4):214-220.

113. Zhao WZ, Wang JK, Zhang XL. Clinical research on recombinant human Ad-p53 injection combined with cisplatin in treatment of malignant pleural effusion induced by lung cancer. Clin J Cancer 2009;28(1):1324-1327.

114. Walker SJ, Bryden G. Managing pleural effusions: nursing care of patients with a Teckhoff catheter. Clin J Oncol Nurs 2010;14(1):59-64.

115. Uzbeck MH, Almeida FA, Sarkiss MG, et al. Management of malignant pleural effusions. Adv Ther 2010;27(6):334-347.

116. Varela G, Jimenez MF, Novoa N. Portable chest drainage systems and outpatient chest tube management. Thorac Surg Clin 2010; 20(3):421-426.

117. Adeoye PO et al. Early experience with outpatient tube drainage for management of pleural collections. West Afr J Med 2009;28(6):364-367.

118. Thornton RH, Miller Z, Covey AM, et al. Tunneled pleural catheters for treatment of recurrent malignant pleural effusion following failed pleurodesis. J Vasc Interv Radiol 2010;21(5): 696-700.

119. Cole J, Patchell R. Metastatic epidural spinal cord compression. Lancet Neurol 2008;7(5):459-466.

120. Bartels RH, van der Linden YM, van der Graaf WT. Spinal extradural metastasis: review of current treatment options. CA Cancer J Clin 2008;58(4):245-259.

121. Coleman RE, Guise TA, Lipton A, et al. Advancing treatment for metastatic bone cancer: consensus recommendations from the Second Cambridge Conference. Clin Cancer Res 2008; 14(20):6387-6395.

122. Lowey SE: Spinal cord compression: an oncological emergency associated with metastatic cancer—evaluation and management for the home health clinician. Home Health Nurse 2006; 24(7):439-448.

123. Miaskowski C. Spinal cord compression. In Chernecky CC, Murphy-Ende K, editors. Acute Care Oncology Nursing. 2nd ed. St. Louis: Saunders; 2009:492-498.

124. Colen FN. Oncological emergencies: superior vena cava syndrome, tumor lysis syndrome, and spinal cord compression. J Emerg Nurs 2008;34(6):535-537.

125. Wilkinson AN, Viola R, Brindage MD. Managing skeletal-related events resulting from bone metastases. BMJ 2008;371:a2041.

126. Acharya S, Ratra GS. Posterior spinal cord compression: outcome and results. Spine 2006;31(7):E74-E78.

127. Sevaggi K, Abrahm J. Metastatic spinal cord compression: the hidden danger. Nat Clin Pract Oncol 2006;3(6).

128. Hitron A, Adams V. The pharmacological management of skeletal-related events from metastatic tumors. Orthopedics 2010;32(3):188-192.

129. Sun H, Nemecek AN. Optimal management of malignant epidural spinal cord compression. Hematol Oncol Clin North Am 2010;24(3):537-551.

130. Gerber DE, Grossman SA. Does decompressive surgery improve outcome in patients with metastatic epidural spinal-cord compression? Nat Clin Pract Neurol 2006;2(1):10-11.

131. Saliou G, el Kocheida M, Lehmann P, et al. Percutaneous vertebroplasty for pain management in malignant fractures of the spine with epidural involvement. Radiology 2010;254(3):882-890.

132. Gofeld M, Bhatia A, Burton AW. Vertebroplasty in the management of painful bony metastases. Curr Pain Headache Rep 2009;13(4):288-294.

133. Drews RE, Rabkin DJ. Malignancy-related superior vena cava syndrome. Up-to-Date Online 18.1, last updated March 23, 2009; retrieved June 30, 2010, from http://www.uptodate.com

134. Wan JF, Bezjak A. Superior vena cava syndrome. Emerg Med Clin N Am 2009;27:243-255.

135. Wilson LD, Detterbeck FC, Yahalom J. Clinical practice: superior vena cava syndrome with malignant causes. N Engl J Med 2007;356:18.

136. Nunnelee JD. Superior vena cava syndrome. J Vasc Nurs 2007; 25:2-5.

137. Bruno TF. Superior vena cava syndrome and telangiectasia in a man with lymphoma. CMAJ 2007;177(10):1177-1179.

138. Canon R, Shah M, Suydam E, et al. Early thrombosis of the superior vena cava in a patient with a central venous catheter and carcinoma of the ampulla of Vater. Am Surg 2008;74: 1195-1197.

139. Rice TW. Pleural effusion in SVCS: Prevalence, characteristics, and proposed pathophysiology. Curr Opin Pulmon Med 2007;13(4):324-327.

140. Plekker D, Ellis T, Irusen EM, et al. Clinical and radiological grading of superior vena cava obstruction. Respiration 2008;32:585-589.

141. Kostopoulou V, Tsiatas ML, Kelekis DA, et al. Endovascular stenting for the management of port-a-cath associated with superior vena cava syndrome. Emerg Radiol 2009;16: 143-146.

142. Uberoi R. Quality assurance guidelines for superior vena cava stenting in malignant disease. Cardiovasc Intervent Radiol 2006;29:319-322.

143. Morales JP, Sabharwal T, Man-Hurun S, et al. Alleviation of severe compressive symptoms in a patient with advanced lung carcinoma using tracheal and superior vena cava stents. J Palliat Care 2007;10:24-29.

144. Ploegmakers MJM, Rutten MJCM. Fatal pericardial tamponade after superior vena cava stenting. Cardiovasc Intervent Radiol 2008;32:585-589.

145. Theodore PR. Emergent management of malignancy-related acute airway obstruction. Emerg Med Clin N Am 2008;27: 310-312.

146. Singer J, Henry S. Upper airway obstruction as the presenting manifestation of leukemia. Pediatr Emerg Care 2008;24(5): 231-241.

147. Liberman M. Bronchoscopic evaluation of the trachea and dilatation of the trachea. Semin Thorac Cardiovasc Surg 2009;21(3):255-262.

148. Shin JH, Sing HY, Kim KR, et al. Radiological and clinical outcomes with special reference to tumor involvement pattern after stent placement for malignant bronchial obstructions. Acta Radiol 2009;50(9):1011-1018.

149. Feller-Kopman DJ, O'Donnell C. Physiology and clinical use of heliox, 2006. Up-to-Date Online 15.2; retrieved August 24, 2007, from http://www.uptodate.com

150. Beeson J. Palliation of tracheobronchial carcinoma: the role of cryosurgery. JPP 2007;17(7):332-339.

151. Ernst A, LoCicero J III. Photodynamic therapy of lung cancer. UpToDate online version 18.1, last updated January 22, 2010; accessed July 7, 2010.

152. Colt HG. Endobronchial electrocautery. UpToDate online version 18.1; last updated October 6, 2009; accessed July 7, 2010.

153. Collins AS, Garner M. Caring for lung cancer patients receiving photodynamic therapy. Crit Care Nurse 2007; 27(2):53-60.

154. Fortunato M, Felijo S, Almeida T, et al. Endoluminal high dose rate brachytherapy in the treatment of primary and recurrent bronchogenic tree malignancies. Rev Port Pneumol 2009; 15(2):151-164.

155. Furukawa K, Ishida J, Yamaguchi G, et al. The role of airway stent placement in the management of tracheobronchial stenosis caused by inoperable advanced lung cancer. Surg Today 2010;40:315-320.

156. Kim H, Shin JH, Song H, et al. Palliative treatment of inoperable malignant tracheobronchial obstruction: temporary stenting combined with radiation therapy and/or chemotherapy. AJR 2009;193:W38-W42.

157. Oki M, Saka H, Kitagawa C, et al. Double Y-stent placement for tracheobronchial stenosis. Respiration 2010;79:245-249.

Tumor Lysis Syndrome

158. Cairo MS, Coiffier B, Reiter A, et al; TLS Expert Panel. Recommendations for the evaluation of risk and prophylaxis of tumour lysis syndrome (TLS) in adults and children with malignant diseases: an expert TLS panel consensus. British Journal of Haematology, 2010;149(4):578-586.

159. Shelton BK. Tumor lysis syndrome. In Chernecky CC, Murphy-Ende K, editors. Acute Care Oncology Nursing. 2nd ed. Philadelphia: Saunders; 2009:545-559.

160. Tosi P, Barosi G, Lazzaro C, et al. Consensus conference on the management of tumor lysis syndrome. Haematologica 2008;93(12):1877-1885.

161. Tiu RY, Mountonakis SE, Dunbar AJ, et al. Tumor lysis syndrome. Semin Thromb Hematol 2007;33(4):397-404.

162. Choi KA, Lee JE, Kim YG, et al. Efficacy of continuous venovenous hemofiltration with chemotherapy in patients with Burkitt lymphoma and leukemia at high risk for tumor lysis syndrome. Ann Hematol 2009;88(7):639-645.

163. Ikeda AK, Sakamoto K, Krishnan K, et al. Tumor lysis syndrome. EMedicine http://emedicine.medscape.com/article/989050-overview. Last updated Sept 26, 2008.

164. Coiffer B, Altman A, Pui CH, et al. Guidelines for the management of pediatric and adult tumor lysis syndrome: an evidence-based review. J Clin Oncol 2008;26(16): 2767-2778.

165. Hochberg J, Cairo MS. Rasburicase: Future directions in tumor lysis management. Exp Opin Biol Ther 2008;8(10): 1595-1604.

166. Mayne N, Keady S, Thacker M: Rasburicase in the prevention and treatment of tumor lysis syndrome. Intens Crit Care Nurse 2008;24(1):59-62.

167. Campara M, Shord SS, Haaf CM. Single-dose rasburicase for tumour lysis syndrome in adults: weight-based approach. J Clin Pharm Ther 2009;34(2):207-213.

15

Immune Problems

Jan Foster, PhD, APRN, CNS, Tari Gilbert, MSN, FNP-BC, and Rebecca Long, MS, RN, CMSRN, ACNS-BC

INTRODUCTION

Immune problems represent a broad category of diverse conditions, some due to an accelerated acute hypersensitivity reaction, some to an exaggerated chronic autoimmune response, others the result of an immune deficient condition with susceptibility to various types of infection, and others the result of an abrupt cascade of inflammatory mediators. Immune problems faced by clinical nurse specialists (CNSs) in acute care may present as secondary problems for patients who are hospitalized for other illnesses or they may be the primary reason for hospitalization. Because of an abrupt presentation, seriousness in response, systemic complications, and potential for CNSs to make an impact, the acute hypersensitivity reactions to be addressed in this chapter include allergic response, three types of blood transfusion reaction, reaction to contrast media, and anaphylaxis. Due to the incidence and comorbidity of the diseases, systemic involvement, complexity in management, and economic impact, the chronic immune diseases discussed in this chapter include two autoimmune disorders: systemic lupus erythematosus (SLE) and rheumatoid arthritis (RA). Management of human immunodeficiency virus (HIV) and acquired immunodeficiency syndrome (AIDS) takes place predominately in the primary care setting versus acute care. However, opportunistic infections, sepsis, and organ dysfunction often necessitate hospitalization, and due to the complexity in care, require the expertise of CNSs and are therefore covered in this chapter. Sepsis/systemic inflammatory response syndrome (SIRS), one of the most rapidly developing, complex complications of infection and injury, requires prompt recognition and therapeutic intervention for success in achieving desirable clinical outcomes and minimizing resource consumption. There are many opportunities for CNSs to affect care for patients with sepsis/SIRS, many of which are included in this chapter.

BLOOD TRANSFUSION REACTION

Transfusion complications may be classified as either immunologic or nonimmunologic in origin. Nonimmunologic includes conditions such as volume overload; complications of massive transfusion, including hypothermia, hemodilutional effects, and pulmonary microemboli; and transfusion hemosiderosis (1). Most nonimmunologic reactions occur in people who require many or repeated transfusions. Immunologic reactions, on the other hand, can be a sudden event and occur without previous transfusion, depending on the type. There are several kinds of immunologic reactions; the most common include acute hemolytic transfusion reaction (AHTR), delayed hemolytic transfusion reaction, transfusion-related acute lung injury, febrile nonhemolytic transfusion reaction, and allergic reactions. Delayed hemolytic transfusion reactions are usually mild (and are often missed completely), with red cell destruction beginning approximately 2 to 10 days after the transfusion, with no specific therapy required. Febrile nonhemolytic reactions are also generally mild, with a chill, and occasionally headache and vomiting that last for several hours. Allergic reactions are common, most involving only hives and other skin reactions. Occasionally, however, the allergic reaction can include angioedema, bronchospasm, and develop into full-blown anaphylaxis. The most serious reactions are acute hemolytic reaction due to ABO incompatible transfusion and transfusion-related acute lung injury (TRALI), which carry very high mortality rates.

ACUTE (IMMEDIATE, INTRAVASCULAR) HEMOLYTIC TRANSFUSION REACTION

Etiology

Incidence of AHTR varies across sources, and interpretation is sometimes problematic. For example, one source reports the sum of both delayed and AHTRs, ranging from 1 in 1,400 to 1 in 6,400 transfusions (1). Combining the reaction types along with such disparate numbers makes it difficult to ascertain the number of AHTRs. Some experts estimate approximately 20 people die annually in the United States from AHTR, a seemingly modest number considering approximately 12 million units of red blood cells (RBCs) are transfused annually in the United States (1). The mortality of AHTR corresponds to the amount of RBCs transfused, with 44% reported in patients transfused with more than one liter of incompatible blood (1). Most reactions are caused by ABO blood group incompatibility. Most of these are due to mislabeling the recipient's pretransfusion sample at collection, failing to match the recipient with the blood product immediately before transfusion, and other clerical errors (1).

Pathophysiology

AHTR represents a type II hypersensitivy reaction and is a complement dependent reaction, involving IgG and IgM antibodies. The underlying mechanism involves the interaction between the antigen on the red cell surface and circulating antibody, development of immune complexes, activation of the complement cascade with release of C3a and C5a, and the coagulation system, with release of cytokines and factor XII, precipitating consumption of coagulation factors and production of bradykinin (1). Anti-A and anti-B antibodies (as in ABO blood type A and B) are able to bind with complement; the antigen–antibody complex triggers complement activation, which destroys the antigen on the cell surface of circulating donor or recipient RBCs, although destruction of donor cells is more common (2). Hemolysis can result from ABO/Rh incompatibility, plasma antibodies, or hemolyzed or fragile RBCs (e.g., by overwarming stored blood or contact with hypotonic IV solutions). Hemolysis is most common and most severe when incompatible donor RBCs are hemolyzed by antibodies in the recipient's plasma. Mediator release includes histamine, serotonin, and cytokines. This leads to systemic vasodilatation and may result in shock. During AHTR, hemolysis is intravascular, causing hemoglobinuria and possibly DIC. Hypoperfusion, vasoconstriction in the renal vascular bed, and renal tubular obstruction with microthrombi are factors contributing to acute renal failure associated with AHTR (1).

Clinical Presentation

The severity of AHTR depends on the degree of incompatibility, the amount of blood given, the rate of administration, and the integrity of the kidneys, liver, and heart. Transfusions of 100 mL or more of incompatible blood can result in permanent renal failure, shock, and death. The reaction usually develops within 1 hour of initiating the transfusion, but it may occur later during the transfusion or immediately following. Onset is usually abrupt. The patient may complain of discomfort and anxiety, nausea, and vomiting. Dyspnea, fever, chills, facial flushing, and severe pain may occur, especially in the lumbar area. Jaundice may follow acute hemolysis (2).

Diagnosis

If AHTR is suspected, the sample and patient identifications should be immediately rechecked. Diagnosis is confirmed by sampling urinary hemoglobin (Hgb), serum lactate dehydrogenase (LDH), bilirubin, and haptoglobin. Intravascular hemolysis produces free Hgb in the plasma and urine; haptoglobin levels are low, and bilirubin may be elevated (2).

Management

The transfusion should be stopped immediately and normal saline should be initiated through another line. The goal of initial therapy is to achieve and maintain adequate blood pressure and renal perfusion with intravenous 0.9% saline and furosemide and/or mannitol. Intravenous saline is given to maintain urine output of 100 mL/hr for 24 hours. The initial furosemide dose is 40 to 80 mg, with later doses adjusted to maintain urinary flow greater than 100 mL/hr during the first day of the reaction. Antihypertensive drugs should be administered with caution. Pressors that reduce renal blood flow such as epinephrine, norepinephrine, and dopamine are contraindicated. A nephrologist should be consulted as early as possible, particularly if no diuretic response occurs within 2 to 3 hours after initiating therapy, which may indicate acute tubular necrosis. Further fluid and diuretic therapy may be contraindicated, and early dialysis may be helpful. The coagulopathy may require management with anticoagulation; moderate dose heparin is sometimes used (1).

Delayed hemolytic transfusion reactions are usually not as dramatic as AHTR. In fact, patients may be asymptomatic or have only a slight fever, with severe symptoms occurring rarely. Occasionally, a patient who has been sensitized to an RBC antigen has low antibody levels and pretransfusion tests during blood typing and crossmatching are negative. After transfusion with RBCs bearing this antigen, a primary reaction may result (usually in 1 to 4 weeks) and trigger a delayed hemolytic transfusion reaction. Usually, only destruction of the transfused RBCs (with the antigen attached) occurs, resulting in a falling hematocrit and a slight rise in LDH and bilirubin. Delayed hemolytic transfusion reactions are usually mild, self-limited, and often unidentified, manifested by an unexplained drop in hemoglobin compared with the pretransfusion level. If the reaction is severe, treatment is the same as for acute reactions (1).

Clinical Nurse Specialist Competencies and Spheres of Influence
Clinical Expert/Direct Care and Consultation

AHTRs occur unexpectedly and may require critical care intervention. As a result, the CNS competencies of clinical expert and consultation in the patient/family and nurse spheres of influence are priorities at this time. The bedside nurse should be educated to call for the rapid response team when an AHTR is suspected or when patients exhibit classic signs and symptoms but the nurse is uncertain of the underlying problem. The CNS applies expert knowledge in quickly assessing surrounding events (transfusion or not) and recognizes a need for fluids, diuretics, and airway management. She or her uses her/his skills or consults with an appropriate practitioner for intravenous line insertion and endotracheal intubation if needed. The CNS facilitates patient transfer to a higher level of care if needed, through nursing and medical administrative channels.

TRANSFUSION-RELATED ACUTE LUNG INJURY

Etiology

TRALI is a serious complication of blood transfusion that often goes unnoticed because many times patients have other etiology for acute lung injury. It is the most common cause of transfusion related death in the United States, with incidence exceeding that of AHTR secondary to incompatibility and bacterial contamination of blood products (3). Incidence is reportedly 1 in 5,000 transfusions but may go unrecognized in many more, diagnosed as another type of pulmonary problem. There are four components that define TRALI: presentation within 6 hours of transfusion; hypoxemia demonstrated by a SpO_2 less than 90% or PaO_2/FiO_2 ratio less than 300 mm Hg on room air; new bilateral infiltrates consistent with edema on an anterior-posterior view chest radiograph; and absence of left atrial fluid overload (4).

Pathophysiology

TRALI is caused by a reaction to white blood cell (WBC) antibodies in donor plasma directed against an antigen on the recipient's leukocytes. Antibodies may be directed against HLA class I or class II antigens, or non-HLA neutrophil antigens (4). The antibodies activate neutrophils, causing plasma to leak into alveoli in the lungs creating pulmonary edema. It is postulated that agglutination of granulocytes combines with complement

activation in the pulmonary vessels, which causes endothelial injury and capillary leak (1). Donors more likely to harbor these WBC antibodies include women with past pregnancy and exposure to fetal blood and blood donors who have received a transfusion or organ transplant in the past (3).

Clinical Presentation

The individual presents with acute respiratory distress and hypoxemia (SpO_2 less than 90% or PaO_2/FiO_2 ratio less than 300 mm Hg) within 6 hours of a blood transfusion. Chest pain, cyanosis, chills, and fever may also be evident. Auscultation of the lungs reveals crackles. An assessment of cardiovascular function and fluid balance is negative for fluid volume overload and cardiogenic pulmonary edema. A summary of clinical manifestations with pathophysiology and treatment is in Table 15-1.

Diagnosis

Diagnosis is made on the basis of clinical presentation and history of blood transfusion, along with confirmatory findings on chest radiograph. Other sources of lung injury must be ruled out, including aspiration, pneumonia, toxin inhalation, lung contusion, and near drowning. The chest radiograph will show fluffy, white, bilateral infiltrates indicative of pulmonary edema. Arterial blood gases may be obtained, substantiating a hypoxemia and to rule out other acid-base imbalances, although hypoxemia can be determined noninvasively via pulse oximetry (3).

Management

The mainstay of management for TRALI is supportive care. As soon as TRALI is recognized, treatment should begin. This includes oxygen supplementation and possible intubation with mechanical ventilatory support, fluid restriction, and diuresis until the lungs clear. Hemodynamic monitoring to manage fluids may be indicated. When mechanical ventilation and hemodynamic monitoring are necessary, patients will need to be cared for in the intensive care unit (1).

Clinical Nurse Specialist Competencies and Spheres of Influence
Clinical Expert/Direct Care and Coaching/Teaching/Mentoring

Risk-reduction and prevention of TRALI are essential management strategies and mainly involve transfusion and blood donor services. A fundamental approach is to minimize the preparation of high-plasma volume components, which would in turn limit exposure of donor antibodies to recipient WBC antigens. High plasma-volume blood components include any plasma components such as fresh frozen plasma, cryoprecipitate, or platelets derived from whole blood, apheresis, or phlebotomy within 24 hours. CNSs may apply this knowledge when high plasma-volume blood products are administered and when the use of 24-hour processing recommendation

TABLE 15-1 Clinical Connections: Transfusion-Related Acute Lung Injury

Clinical Manifestations	Pathophysiology	Assessment Finding	Laboratory/ Diagnostic tests	Treatment
Acute respiratory distress	Neutrophil activation by antibodies in donor plasma against antigen on recipient's leukocytes with plasma leak into alveoli	SPo₂ <90% Pao₂/Fio₂ ratio <300 mm Hg within 6 hours of blood transfusion Crackles Chest pain Cyanosis	Chest x-ray shows fluffy, white bilateral infiltrates	*Oxygen *Ventilatory support *Fluid restriction *Diuretics
· Chills	Reaction of antibodies in donor plasma against recipient leukocytes			
Fever	Reaction of antibodies in donor plasma against recipient leukocytes	Temperature ≥10° F		*Acetaminophen

is unknown. Education for bedside clinicians about the risks of TRALI when these products are transfused is fundamental. Recognizing the signs and symptoms of TRALI is vital to timely intervention, and stabilizing the patient's pulmonary and hemodynamic status is critical to overall patient outcome. Blending the competencies of clinical expertise with teaching/mentoring to provide background education about TRALI along with educating caregivers abut "how to know it when they see it," and application of clinical expertise to assist with immediate stabilization of the patient are important roles for CNSs within the patient/family and nursing/other professionals spheres of influence.

ALLERGIC DISORDERS

Allergy and allergic reaction is the most common overall health-related disorder, and involves responses to a multitude of environmental, chemical, pharmaceutical, food, and other allergens. The immune system is designed to protect the organism from countless harmful environmental assaults, tumor cells, and invading microorganisms. The immediate host defense immune response involves interplay between immunoglobulin E (IgE), cytokine release, T- and B-lymphocytes, mast cells, macrophages, and basophils. This complex sequence of events serves to protect the individual from bacteria,

parasites, and other sources of infection. However, a heightened response can lead to potentially life threatening illnesses and devastating complications.

Because of the unexpected nature of allergic responses in hospitalized patients and differential diagnostic challenge, CNSs are often called on emergent consultation to assist with intervention and stabilization concurrently or even before a diagnostic evaluation is undertaken. Potentially serious allergic responses that CNSs should anticipate in acute care include contrast media reaction and anaphylaxis to food or medications.

Radiocontrast Media
Etiology

Many radiographic and fluoroscopic exams require the use of contrast agents because they are radiopaque and elucidate excellent views of soft tissue. Radiocontrast agents are either ionic or nonionic, with the latter causing fewer allergic-type responses and nephropathy and because of these advantages are used exclusively at some institutions. However, in those using ionic contrast agents, allergic reactions should be anticipated.

Unlike many anaphylactic reactions, the reaction to contrast media is not IgE mediated. Some immunologists have classified IgE-mediated reactions as anaphylactic in nature and those that are non–IgE mediated as anaphylactoid. However, anaphylactoid reactions are clinically indistinguishable from anaphylaxis and may in fact be more dangerous because the reaction does not require a second exposure. These reactions occur via direct stimulation of mast cells or via immune complexes that activate complement. The most common triggers are iodinated radiographic radiopaque dye, aspirin, other nonsteroidal anti-inflammatory drugs (NSAIDs), opioids, blood transfusion, immunoglobulin, and exercise (5).

One of the dangers of contrast media–induced response is that because it is not IgE mediated, a reaction can occur with first time exposure. On the other hand, it can occur with a repeated exposure with no past reactions. With no index of suspicion from experiencing a previous mild response, for example, a skin rash, a false sense of security with subsequent exposure may cause lag time in recognition of the problem when it does present.

Most reactions to radiocontrast are mild, with approximately 10% of those occurring with first exposure. If individuals have a severe reaction progressing to anaphylaxis, more than likely they will have a similar reaction with subsequent exposure. Intravenous administration is more likely to trigger a reaction than if taken orally. Risk factors for radiocontrast media allergic reaction include other food and drug allergies, previous allergic-type reactions, and asthma. Also, adults are more likely to demonstrate a reaction to radiocontrast than children, possibly the result of repeated exposure, hypersensitivity, or a combination of both factors (5).

Pathophysiology

The mechanism for radiocontrast media allergic reactions is not certain. However, it is thought to be a result of direct degranulation of mast cells and basophils. Histamine is released almost immediately upon activation of mast cells. This causes smooth muscle contraction in the airways, coronary arteries, and gastrointestinal tract. Vasodilatation and increased vascular permeability contribute to hypotension. There is also stimulation of sensory nerve endings, resulting in reflexive activation of vagal pathways and myocardial depression. Platelet activating factor is synthesized from mast cells and basophils, although the role in this process is unclear. This may cause disseminated intravascular dissemination. Adenosine is released from degranulation of mast cells, triggering bronchoconstriction and respiratory distress, along with vasodilatation and hypotension (5). Other inflammatory responses are triggered as a result of mediator activation. For example, mast cell and basophil release of kininogenase and kallikrein, respectively, may active the kinin system. Kallikrein activation of the complement system leads to release of fibrinogen. Chemotactic agents attract eosinophils, which potentiates the intensity and prolongs the reaction (5).

Clinical Presentation

The response to contrast agents may be mild or severe. Mild to moderate signs and symptoms include itching, flushing, nausea, vomiting, and chills. Severe reactions include anaphylactoid, laryngeal edema, bronchospasm, hypotension, tachycardia, bradycardia, cardiopulmonary arrest, seizures, and even death (Table 15-2).

Diagnosis

In the emergent situation, the diagnosis is based on clinical presentation and history of exposure to radiocontrast. Analysis of urine and blood samples taken following the reaction or stabilization of the patient may reveal histamine and beta-tryptase (5).

Management

Treatment begins with halting the procedure, gaining full view of the patient, and stopping the infusion. Diphenhydramine 25 to 50 mg intravenously should be given for mild to moderate reactions. Oxygen, intravenous epinephrine, and fluids are indicated for severe reactions, with application of Advanced Cardiac Life Support measures as indicated (5).

Clinical Nurse Specialist Competencies and Spheres of Influence
Collaboration

In order to prevent and/or anticipate potential reactions due to cross allergy, all patients undergoing diagnostic

TABLE 15–2 Clinical Connections: Radiocontrast Media Reaction

Clinical Manifestations	Pathophysiology	Assessment Finding	Treatment
Hypotension	Histamine release from mast cells causes vascular vasodilatation	MAP <65	Epinephrine Intravenous normal saline Glucagon to those receiving β-blockers
Tachycardia, palpitations	Compensatory mechanism for hypotension	Heart rate >99/min	Treat hypotension
Bradycardia	Release of adenosine from mast cells	Heart rate <60/min	Atropine

TABLE 15-2 Clinical Connections: Radiocontrast Media Reaction—cont'd

Clinical Manifestations	Pathophysiology	Assessment Finding	Treatment
Dyspnea, wheezing, cyanosis	Histamine release from mast causes smooth muscle contraction, laryngeal edema Adenosine release from mast cells causes bronchoconstriction	Poor air exchange, stridor, hypoxemia	Diphenhydramine Cimetidine Inhaled β-agonists such as albuterol Oxygen
Flushing, chills Nausea, vomiting	Vasodilatation Histamine release		Diphenhydramine

procedures with contrast agents should be carefully screened for past food and drug reactions and asthma. Communication among providers via documentation tools, patient identifying mechanisms, and electronic health records is critical to prevention of catastrophic events. CNSs may take responsibility for development of screening and documentation tools for capturing patient allergy history.

Coaching/Teaching/Mentoring

All radiographic and fluoroscopic technologists, technicians, and transportation aides should be educated in the risks of allergic response and patient monitoring skills for early detection of and intervention for a reaction. Emergency life-supporting drugs and equipment should be readily available, with a process in place for summoning help. CNSs may be influential in implementing an interdepartmental safety program for prevention and management of allergic responses.

Anaphylaxis
Etiology

Anaphylaxis is an acute, life-threatening, IgE-mediated allergic reaction that occurs in previously sensitized individuals when they are reexposed to the sensitizing antigen. Anaphylaxis represents a Type I immediate IgE antibody mediated allergic response. The most common causes of anaphylaxis include animal venom; foods such as nuts, seafood, and eggs; drugs such as beta-lactam antibiotics, insulin, and streptokinase; proteins such as tetanus antitoxin, and blood transfusions; and of particular importance to health care workers, latex. While less than 1% of the general population shows sensitivity to latex, the U.S. Occupational Safety and Health Administration (OSHA) estimates that 8% to 12% of health care workers are sensitized (6). Additionally, hospitalization for angioedema associated with use of angiotensin-converting enzyme inhibitors (ACEIs), which is a type I IgE-mediated response, has increased over the years during the same time hospitalization for nonangioedema allergic disorders has declined as these drugs are increasingly prescribed for cardiovascular disease (7).

Pathophysiology

During anaphylaxis the allergen binds to IgE antibodies, which are then attracted to the surface of mast cells and basophils, triggering the release of mediators. Histamine and leukotrienes are released from intracellular granules of mast cells, which are concentrated in skin, lungs, and gastrointestinal (GI) mucosa. Activation of both H1 and H2 receptors induce vasodilation within the vascular bed. H1 receptors stimulate release of nitric oxide from endothelial cells, which acts upon the blood vessels, whereas H2 receptors act directly on vascular smooth muscle. The histamine effects cause local vasodilation, increased capillary permeability and edema, surrounding arteriolar vasodilation mediated by neuronal reflex mechanisms, and stimulation of sensory nerves. Cardiac effects are largely mediated by H2 receptors, which increase the heart rate and force of contraction. However, stimulation of H1 receptors causes increased sinoatrial node depolarization, which increases heart rate (5). Systemic vasodilation also occurs, causing peripheral pooling of blood and hypotension, along with cerebral vasodilation, which induces headache. With increased capillary permeability, plasma and plasma proteins leak from the vascular space and can worsen circulatory shock (7).

Histamine (H1) causes smooth muscle contraction and bronchoconstriction in the airways, which causes wheezing and increased bronchial gland secretions. In the GI tract, stimulation of H1 receptors induces increased bowel motility and salivation. H1 receptor stimulation induces mild uterine contraction, with H2 stimulation causing uterine relaxation.

Clinical Presentation

Generally, patients present with involvement of the skin, upper or lower airways, cardiovascular system, or GI tract. One or more systems may be affected but do not necessarily progress to involvement of all systems. Each patient typically shows the same reaction to each subsequent exposure, so if an individual mounts a serious, multi-system response initially, subsequent reactions pose imminent danger.

Signs and symptoms range from mild to severe and include flushing, pruritus, urticaria, angioedema, sneezing, rhinorrhea, dyspnea, wheezing, cyanosis, nausea, diarrhea, abdominal cramps, palpitations, hypotension, tachycardia, dizziness, and syncope. Distributive shock can develop within minutes, and patients may experience seizures, become unresponsive, and die, even in the absence of respiratory or other symptoms. (See Table 15-3.)

Diagnosis

The working diagnosis is made based on clinical presentation and history of allergen exposure. As in mast cell degranulating reactions, IgE-mediated anaphylaxis may be tentatively diagnosed after the reaction by the presence of histamine and beta-trypsin levels in the blood and urine. Differential diagnoses include other acute events that involve hypotension, tachycardia, and respiratory distress. These include vasovagal syncope, acute myocardial infarction, cardiac dysrhythmia, and pulmonary embolism. Other chronic conditions that manifest more cutaneous and gastrointestinal signs than hemodynamic and/or respiratory distress include carcinoid syndrome, hereditary angioedema, and mastocytosis. Also, seizure disorder should be considered in the differential (5). Primary prevention and desensitization are indicated to avoid future reactions.

TABLE 15–3 Clinical Connections: Anaphylaxis

Clinical Manifestations	Pathophysiology	Assessment Finding	Treatment
Hypotension	Histamine release causes vascular permeability; vasodilatation	MAP <65	Epinephrine Intravenous normal saline Dopamine Glucagon to those receiving β-blockers
Tachycardia, palpitations	Compensatory mechanism for hypotension	Heart rate >99/min	Treat hypotension
Dyspnea, wheezing, cyanosis	Histamine release causes bronchoconstriction	Poor air exchange, stridor, hypoxemia	Oxygen Diphenhydramine Cimetidine Inhaled β-agonists such as albuterol Cricothyrotomy
Rhinorrhea, sneezing	Leukotriene release from mast cells and basophils		Diphenhydramine
Dizziness, syncope	Decreased cerebral perfusion		Epinephrine Intravenous normal saline
Flushing	Vasodilatation		
Pruritus, urticaria	IgE-mediated histamine release		Diphenhydramine
Angioedema	Vascular permeability from histamine release		Epinephrine
Nausea, diarrhea, abdominal cramps	Increased bowel motility secondary to histamine release		Diphenhydramine

Management

Epinephrine is the principal treatment for anaphylaxis and should be administered immediately. It can be given subcutaneously or for best absorption, intramuscularly into the lateral thigh. The usual dose is 0.3 to 0.5 mL of a 1:1000 solution in adults and repeated every 10 to 30 minutes. For patients with cardiovascular collapse or severe airway obstruction, epinephrine may be given intravenously in a single dose, 3 to 5 mL of a 1:10,000 solution over 5 minutes or by continuous infusion mixing 1 mg in 250 mL of 5% dextrose and water. The infusion should be initiated at 1 mcg per minute and increased to 4 mcg per minute as needed. Epinephrine may also be given by sublingual injection (0.5 mL of 1:1,000 solution) or through an endotracheal tube should intubation be necessary (3 to 5 mL of a 1:10,000 solution diluted to 10 mL with saline). Glucagon (1 mg bolus followed by 1 mg/hr continuous infusion) should be given to patients taking oral beta-blockers, which interfere with the effect of epinephrine.

Hypotension is treated with 1 to 2 liters of isotonic intravenous fluids. Intravenous epinephrine or dopamine is indicated for refractory hypotension. Oxygen and early endotracheal intubation is recommended for individuals who have stridor and wheezing unresponsive to epinephrine, as awaiting a response to epinephrine may allow upper airway edema to progress to the point of necessitating cricothyrotomy. Antihistamines such as diphenhydramine 50 to 100 mg and cimetidine 300 mg intravenously should be given every 6 hours until wheezing subsides. Inhaled beta-agonists such as albuterol 5 to 10 mg by continuous nebulization should be administered (8). Table 15-4 summarizes the treatment for anaphylaxis.

Clinical Nurse Specialist Competencies and Spheres of Influence
Systems Leadership

Implementation of a standardized, color-coded wrist identification band to alert all hospital personnel about potential for allergy is an important safety strategy that has been effective across many hospitals in the western United States. In 2006, the Colorado Hospital Association in collaboration with the Western Alliance for Patient Safety (WRAPS) published recommendations for a standardized color-coded system, following a near-miss situation in which a patient was almost resuscitated at a hospital because the patient's wristband color indicated Do Not Resuscitate in another facility but not in this hospital. The system they developed includes allergy and latex allergy as well as Do Not Resuscitate, Restricted Extremity, and Fall Risk. In addition to wristbands, the Alliance recommends the same color-coding for any placards, stickers, etc; to communicate patient allergy (Box 15-1) (9).

BOX 15–1	Standardized Color-Coded Allergy Wristbands
Allergy	Red
Latex Allergy	Green
DNR	Purple
Fall Risk	Yellow
Restricted Extremity	Pink

TABLE 15–4 Treatment for Anaphylaxis

	SQ/IM	IV Bolus	IV Continuous	SL Injection	ETT	Neb
Epinephrine	0.3-0.5 mL 1:1,000 every 10-30 minutes	3-5 mL 1: 10,000 over 5 minutes	1 mg/250 D5W 1-4 mcg/min	0.5 mL 1:1,000	3-5 mL 1:10,000 in 10 mL NS	
Glucagon for patients receiving beta-blockers		1 mg	1 mg/hr			
Diphenhydramine		50-100 mg every 6 hours				
Cimetidine		300 mg every 6 hours				
Albuterol						5-10 mg every 6 hours

AUTOIMMUNE DISORDERS

There are over 80 different types of autoimmune disorders, with many individuals afflicted with more than one type of disorder. Autoimmune disorders can be classified as systemic, effecting multiple tissues, organs, and functions, or localized with specific target organs such as the pancreas in diabetes mellitus or the nervous system in multiple sclerosis (Table 15-5) (10). Rheumatoid arthritis (RA) and systemic lupus erythematosus (SLE) are discussed in this chapter because of multisystem involvement with widespread organ dysfunction. As such, SLE is considered the prototype of autoimmune diseases. RA and SLE commonly coexist with other diseases and health care problems. For example, patients with RA often present in cardiac care and heart transplant units because of debilitating cardiovascular disease; have an increased risk for opportunistic infection even prior to transplant due to use of glucocorticoids for treatment; and have challenging blood glucose management. Patients with SLE commonly present in general medicine and renal transplant units due to end-stage renal disease. Complications due to anemia associated with chronic disease typify both disorders, with wound healing delays, fatigue, and immobility-associated problems such as impaired skin integrity and pneumonia.

RHEUMATOID ARTHRITIS

Etiology

RA is the most common systemic autoimmune disease in the United States, and affects 0.8% of the adult population worldwide. It is the most common inflammatory arthritis and the most destructive to joints. It is a progressively chronic, inflammatory, systemic debilitating disease that initially affects the synovial joints. It affects women more than men by a 2.5-to-3.1:1 ratio. There is no dominance of any ethnic group. Incidence increases with age, peaking between ages 40 to 60. With remissions and exacerbations, joint deformity increases over time, interfering with function as well as self-image and self-esteem. Although primarily affecting the joints, the cardiovascular, cerebrovascular, pulmonary, and renal systems are also affected. RA is associated with increased cardiovascular mortality, with a decrease in life expectancy of 10 to 15 years, compared with the general population (11). It is also a very debilitating disease, with 20% of individuals unable to work within two years of diagnosis, and within 10 years, almost 50% of patients are severely work-disabled. RA accounts for approximately 250,000 hospitalizations and 9 million physician visits annually, largely due to the systemic effects (12). Functional limitations and treatment of the disease often complicate the course of the hospital stay, necessitating multidisciplinary collaboration and leadership from CNSs.

Multiple phenomena including infection, autoimmunity, environmental, and hormonal factors have been linked to RA; however, no specific cause has been identified. A familial pattern is typical, and in monozygotic twins, there is a 30% concordance rate, suggesting a genetic origin (11). There is much evidence to indicate there is an association between several class II major histocompatibility complexes (MHCs) and the development and severity of RA. HLA-DR1 and DR4, gene products of MHC, cause a specific arthrogenic peptide presentation to CD4 T lymphocytes. Similar amino acid sequencing in the same position on the HLA-DR molecule is seen in individuals with RA and are absent in those without RA (11).

Pathophysiology

Two major theories of the pathophysiology of RA are currently in vogue. The first proposes that the pathogenesis is orchestrated by T-lymphocytes, which activate the inflammatory cascade in response to locally released antigens within the synovial joint and subsequently continue

TABLE 15–5 Autoimmune Disorders

Systemic Autoimmune Disorders	Localized Autoimmune Disorders
Rheumatoid Arthritis	Type 1 Diabetes Mellitus (pancreas islets)
Systemic Lupus Erythematosus	Hashimoto's thyroiditis, Graves' Disease (thyroid)
Scleroderma	Celiac disease, Crohn's Disease, Ulcerative Colitis (GI tract)
Sjögren's Syndrome	Multiple Sclerosis
Goodpasture's Syndrome	Addison's Disease (adrenal)
Wegener's Granulomatosis	Primary Biliary Cirrhosis, Sclerosing Cholangitis, Autoimmune Hepatitis (liver)
Polymyalgia Rheumatica	Temporal Arteritis/Giant Cell Arteritis (arteries of the head and neck)
Guillain-Barré Syndrome	

the chronic inflammatory process. The stimulating antigen may be an autoimmune substance. The second theory suggests that the T cell is key to initiation of the process; however, the chronic inflammation characterized by the disease is propagated by macrophages and fibroblasts independent of T-cell activity (13).

Joint destruction in RA begins with proliferation of macrophages and fibroblasts following an immune trigger. CD4 T cells, B cells, and monocytes migrate into the synovial interstitium in response to a chemotactic stimuli and interaction of cellular adhesion molecules or extracellular matrix molecules such as collagen and/or fibronectin. Macrophages migrate to the effected synovium in early disease; increased macrophage-derived lining cells are prominent along with vessel inflammation later in the disease. The T-cell theory holds that the chronic inflammation is due to T-cell activity perpetuating this cellular interaction. However, although the CD4 cells are prevalent in the synovial joints long after the initial response, they appear to be inactive. On the other hand, the macrophage model of chronic inflammation is based on the observation that cytokines produced by macrophages and fibroblasts, such as interleukin-1 (IL-1), interleukin-6 (IL-6), tumor necrosis factor (TNF), interleukin-8 (IL-8), and granulocyte-macrophage colony-stimulating factor (GM-CSF), are abundant in the joints and may perpetuate the inflammatory process. Rheumatologists continue to study the pathophysiologic process, largely in search of better treatment (13).

Plasma cells, produced by joint migratory B cells, produce antibodies known as rheumatoid factor (RF) that form antigen–antibody complexes; however, destructive arthritis can occur in the absence of RF. Macrophages and lymphocytes produce proinflammatory cytokines and chemokines, including TNF, GM-CSF, various interleukins, and interferon-γ in the synovium. Release of inflammatory mediators contributes to the systemic and joint manifestations of RA.

Joint destruction results from the action of several of the aforementioned mediators produced during the inflammatory process. Both cartilage and bone are affected. The synovial lining cells produce various materials, including collagenase and stromelysin, which contribute to cartilage destruction, and IL-1 and TNF-α, which stimulate the cartilaginous destructive process. Bone destruction occurs by osteoclast-mediated bone absorption and release of prostaglandins and proteases. Prostaglandin release potentiates the inflammatory response.

Besides destruction of cartilage and bone tissue, joint mobility and dysfunction results from synovial involvement. The synovium is normally very thin (1 to 3 mm thick). In RA, the synovium thickens and develops many villous folds, becoming a hyperplastic synovial tissue membrane, called a pannus. The pannus in turn releases inflammatory mediators, which further erode cartilage, subchondral bone, articular capsule, and ligaments. The pannus consists of granulated vascular tissue extending from the vascular bed into the joint and has increased angiogenesis properties. However, the newly formed vessels are unable to provide adequate blood supply to the highly proliferative joints, contributing to joint ischemia. Additionally, fibrin deposition and fibrosis cause increased intra-articular pressure, leading to further joint ischemia and necrosis. Besides the synovia of the joints, the pannus invades layers of the heart muscle, cardiac valves, pulmonary visceral pleura, sclera, spleen, larynx, and dura mater, accounting for many of the systemic effects of RA (14).

Extra-articular, systemic effects of the inflammatory processes associated with RA are found in the cardiovascular (CV), cerebrovascular, and pulmonary systems. Cutaneous lesions, ocular involvement, and other systemic manifestations may also be present. Early research suggests that kidney disease is highly prevalent in patients with RA, which must be taken into consideration for treatment, with dosing adjustments in medications to avoid exacerbating renal impairment (15).

The most common CV effect of RA is pericarditis and occurs in approximately 50% of individuals. Often patients with pericarditis present with a concomitant pleuritis. Patients are usually asymptomatic, however, and cardiac tamponade rarely develops. On occasion pericardiocentesis is necessary for symptom relief or differential diagnosis; pericardial fluid low in glucose and complement levels is a significant finding for ruling in RA (16).

RA is a known risk factor for coronary artery disease (CAD). Individuals with both RA and CAD have a reduced life expectancy of approximately 10 to 15 years, compared to those with neither disease (17). The chronic inflammatory process of RA including endothelial involvement and local vasodilation contribute to the atherosclerotic process, which effects coronary artery and other cardiovascular disease. The inflammatory mediators released within the joints enter the systemic circulation and contribute to atherogenesis in the coronary arteries. Elevated levels of C-reactive protein, a known mediator and procoagulant in the inflammatory response and major risk factor for CAD, has been demonstrated in patients who have been diagnosed with RA diagnosed less than 1 year (18). Individuals with RA are at increased risk for ischemic stroke, resulting from the same process associated with CAD (19).

The most common pulmonary manifestations of RA include bronchiectasis and pleural effusion. Interestingly, both conditions occur more in men, even though the incidence of RA is much higher in women. Bronchiectasis, characterized by dilation and destruction of larger bronchi caused by chronic infection and inflammation, is found in men with a long-running course of RA.

There is a chronic cough with production of copious, purulent sputum, sometimes fever, and dyspnea. Pleural effusions are more likely to be found in older men with rheumatoid nodules and severe arthritic deformities. Effusions may be transudative or exudative, be asymptomatic, or cause severe dyspnea and pleuritic chest pain (11).

Cutaneous lesions develop in approximately one-third of individuals with RA. Nodules most commonly develop in the olecronon bursa of the elbow, dorsum of the hand, Achilles tendon, and occiput of the head. Vasculitis may affect blood vessels of all sizes; however most commonly the small vessels in the hands are affected, causing microhemorrhages. This may lead to polyneuropathy, as well (11).

Ocular involvement includes a dry, gritty sensation in the eyes, a common complaint among individuals with RA. This may be an indication of Sjögren syndrome, which affects approximately 10% to 20% of those with RA. Sjögren syndrome results from a lymphocytic infiltration of the lacrimal glands, which interferes with tear production and loss of the protective covering of the superficial portion of the eyeball. Keratoconjunctivitis

may develop as a result. Irritation of the sclera from episcleritis is also a common ocular manifestation of RA (11).

Clinical Presentation

RA typically presents as a slow, insidious disease over several weeks to months, with the initial complaints consisting of pain in multiple joints, early morning stiffness, and fatigue later in the day. In approximately 15% of affected individuals, the onset is more sudden, over days to weeks, usually following an infection (11). Other complaints include anorexia, generalized weakness, and low-grade fever.

The joints most frequently affected are those with the greatest ratio of synovium to cartilage, including the wrists and the proximal interphalangeal and metacarpophalangeal joints. Other less commonly involved joints include the metatarsophalangeal joints, shoulders, elbows, hips, knees, and ankles. Rarely is the distal interphalangeal joint or the spine affected. Joints are usually tender and warm to touch but are not erythematous. Sometimes the epitrochlear, cervical, and axillary lymph nodes are enlarged. Muscles adjacent to involved joints sometimes atrophy (11). See Table 15-6 for a summary of articular and extra-articular manifestations of RA, with associated pathophysiology.

TABLE 15–6 Clinical Connections: Rheumatoid Arthritis

Clinical Manifestations	Pathophysiology	Assessment Finding	Laboratory/ Diagnostic tests	Treatment
Joint swelling (predominately metacarpophalangeal, proximal interphalangeal)	Synovial fluid accumulation, hypertrophy of the synovium, thickened joint capsule	Swelling, pain, stiffness of the metacar-pophalangeal, proximal interphalangeal joints in the hands		
Joint pain	Abundant supply of pain fibers within the joint capsule that are sensitive to stretching and distention	Pain in fingers and hands, especially after periods of inactivity		
Joint warmth	Synovial inflammation	Hands and fingers warm to touch		
Joint deformity	Muscle atrophy, imbalance in forces transmitted across the joints, tendon flaccidity	Mild flexion, nodular appearance of metacar-pophalangeal,		

TABLE 15–6 Clinical Connections: Rheumatoid Arthritis—cont'd

Clinical Manifestations	Pathophysiology	Assessment Finding	Laboratory/ Diagnostic tests	Treatment
	or shortness, tendon or liga-ment rupture, weakened joint capsule, cartilage destruction	proximal inter-phalangeal joints in the hands		
Skeletal muscle weakness	Muscle atrophy Steroid myopathy 2nd treatment	Atrophied mus-cles adjacent to affected joints, weak-ness and poor mobility	Biopsy shows atrophy of type II mus-cle fibers; sometimes myositis	
Constitutional signs/ symptoms	Inflammatory flare-up	Fever, diaphore-sis, anorexia, weight loss, lymphadenopa-thy, weakness, fatigue		
Ocular involvement	Lymphatic infiltra-tion of lacrimal glands and decreased tear production (Sjögren syndrome)	Dry eyes, gritty sensation	Schirmer test (filter paper under the eyelid) indicates low tear production Rose bengal staining shows dessicated corneal epithelium	Artificial tears at regular intervals
Cutaneous nodules	Necrotic collagen fibrils, noncolla-gen filaments, cellular debris, macrophages, granulation tissue	Nodular lesions surround ole-cranon bursa, Achilles tendon, occiput, dor-sum of hands	High titers of rheumatoid factor	
Pulmonary: Pleural effusion Interstitial disease	Inflammatory process Methotrexate toxicity	Usually asympto-matic; may cause respira-tory distress, hypoxemia	Pleural fluid is exudative with low glucose and complement levels Chest x-ray: reticular nodular pattern; pneumonitis	Thoracentesis Oxygen Glucocorticoids

Continued

TABLE 15–6 Clinical Connections: Rheumatoid Arthritis—cont'd

Clinical Manifestations	Pathophysiology	Assessment Finding	Laboratory/ Diagnostic tests	Treatment
Cardiac: Pericarditis Myocarditis Coronary artery disease	Inflammatory process Inflammatory mediators released from joints contribute to atherosclerotic process, endothelial involvement, and vasodilatation in the coronary arteries	Usually asymptomatic; may cause low cardiac output syndrome Consistent with acute coronary syndrome	Pericardial fluid is exudative with low glucose and complement levels Elevated C-reactive protein levels	Pericardiocentesis Cardioprotective medications; Appropriate treatment for acute coronary syndrome (see Chapter 9)
Renal: Amyloidosis Glomerular membrane alterations Decreased glomerular filtration rate Nephrotic syndrome Renal tubular acidosis	Systemic inflammatory response Drugs used for treatment (NSAIDS)		Histologic exam positive for amyloid deposits Urine may show proteinurea Reduced glomerular filtration rate	
Neurologic: Myelopathy Neuropathy	Arthritic involvement of the spine with nerve entrapment	Cervical spine joint subluxation or spondylolisthesis Neck pain, headache Neurologic deficit (paresthesia, weakness)	Positive radiographs	Surgical intervention for significant neurologic deficit
Gastrointestinal: Xerostomia Amyloidosis Elevated liver function tests Peptic ulcer disease	Decreased saliva production Chronic inflammatory process Drugs used for treatment (NSAIDS, glucocorticoids)	Dryness of the mouth Abdominal pain	Elevated ALT, AST Endoscopy positive for peptic ulcer	Artificial saliva, oral care Appropriate treatment for peptic ulcer disease (see Chapter 12)
Hematologic: Anemia Eosinophilia Thrombocytosis	Chronic disease/iron dysutilization Inflammatory process	Activity intolerance, fatigue, pallor, tachycardia Thromboembolic events	Decreased RBC, Hgb, Hct Elevated eosinophil count, platelet count	Iron supplement, nutrition counseling Prophylaxis for thromboembolic events

Diagnosis

Diagnosis of RA is largely a clinical diagnosis, which encompasses joint signs and symptoms, radiographic findings, and some laboratory tests. Any four criteria must be present to for a definitive diagnosis (Table 15-7) (20). Although a positive rheumatoid factor (RF) is one of the diagnostic criteria and is present in approximately 70% of patients with RA, it is positive in other diseases such as other connective tissue disorders, granulomatous diseases, chronic infections, and some cancers. Other laboratory findings may include positive anticyclic citrullinated peptide antibody (anti-CCP); elevated C-reactive protein, erythrocyte sedimentation rate, alkaline phosphatase, platelets, and leukocytes; and decreased hemoglobin and hematocrit. Synovial fluid contains elevated neutrophils (20).

Differential diagnoses include other connective soft tissue and joint diseases. Autoimmune rheumatic disorders include eosinophilic fasciitis, mixed connective tissue disease, polymyositis and dermatomyositis, relapsing polychondritis, Sjögrens syndrome, SLE, and systemic sclerosis. Additionally, sarcoidosis, various neoplasms, and viral polyarthritis should be ruled out. RF will be negative in the presence of most neoplasms. Hepatitis C and rubella should be considered when ruling out viral polyarthritis. Osteoarthritis is a consideration but rarely effects the wrists and metacarpophalangeal joints as in RA. Also, the thumb carpophalangeal joint is affected in osteoarthritis but not in RA. Gout as a differential diagnosis is ruled out with negative synovial fluid aspirate for urate crystals (20).

Management

Goals of treatment include preserving function and quality of life, minimizing pain, maintaining joint integrity, and prevention and control of systemic complications. Management includes three classes of medications, NSAIDs, glucocorticoids, and disease-modifying antirheumatic drugs (DMARDs), along with supportive adjunct therapy. (See Table 15-8 for a summary of

TABLE 15–7 Diagnostic Criteria for Rheumatoid Arthritis: Any Four Criteria Must be Present for a Diagnosis

Morning stiffness >1 hour
Arthritis of ≥3 joints
Hand joint involvement
Symmetrical arthritis
Rheumatoid nodules
Positive serum rheumatoid factor (RF)
Radiographic changes: hand and wrist showing
   typical changes and erosions

medications and recommended doses.) DMARDS should be initiated as soon as a definitive diagnosis is available, in order to slow disease progression. NSAIDS, salicylates, and cyclooxygenase-2 inhibitors are used to control pain and reduce swelling however, because they do not modify the disease, they should not be used alone. Prednisone 7.5 milligrams daily reduces symptoms and slows joint destruction (12, 21).

Various types of adjunct therapy have shown some benefit and include physical and occupational therapy, heat and cold applications, exercise, rest, acupuncture, splinting, journaling, meditation, and dietary supplements of herbals and essential fatty acids. Surgery for unacceptable pain and severe functional impairment should be considered (22).

Clinical Nurse Specialist Competencies and Spheres of Influence

The effective management of chronic illnesses such as RA requires timely, appropriate, and comprehensive clinical care to achieve optimal outcomes. An organized delivery system within the acute care environment with complementary community resources requires patients to engage in self-care management, which entails goal-setting and monitoring of one's own health status. The clinical nurse specialist competencies of patient teaching-coaching within the patient/family sphere of influence, and collaboration among various providers within the nurse and systems spheres come into play in the management of RA.

Coaching/Teaching/Mentoring

Patient and family/caregiver education focuses on the goals of therapy; medication dosing and administration schedules, effects and side effects; and adjunct therapies. Additionally, patients require education on the cardiovascular risks of RA, blood pressure management, signs and symptoms of acute myocardial infarction and stroke, and advisement on when to seek emergent health care. Due to the chronic and debilitating nature of RA, much support of the patient and caregiver is needed. Referral to community support groups has been a traditional mainstay of support and patient education. However, not all individuals are comfortable in group settings. Internet-based self-management programs is an option, with patients reporting improvement in health status variables such as pain, fatigue, activity, and disability as a result of education and support materials provided through electronic media (23).

Collaboration

An interdisciplinary, comprehensive educational program covering practice guidelines for the management of patients with RA has been shown to be successful in fostering interdisciplinary collaboration and patient self-management (24). This approach to learning allows each discipline firsthand knowledge of the scope of others' knowledge and practice, fosters trust, and facilitates communication.

Self-management entails mutual goal setting between patient and provider and integrates individual differences

TABLE 15–8 Treatment for Rheumatoid Arthritis: DMARDS

Abatacept	<60 kg: 500 mg; 60-100 kg: 750 milligrams; >100 kg 1,000 mg intravenously over 30 minutes at week zero, 2 weeks, 4 weeks, then every 4 weeks
Adalimumab	40 milligrams subcutaneously every 2 weeks
Anakinra	100-150 milligrams subcutaneously per day
Auranofin	6 milligrams orally per day
Azathioprine	50-150 milligrams orally per day
Cyclosporine	2.5 to 5 milligrams per kilogram orally per day
D-Penicillane	250-750 milligrams orally per day
Etanercept	25 milligrams subcutaneously twice per week
Hydroxychloroquine	200 to 400 milligrams orally per day
Infliximab	3 milligrams per kilogram intravenously at weeks zero, 2, and 6, then every 8 weeks
Leflunomide	100 milligrams orally per day for 3 days then 10 to 20 milligrams per day
Methotrexate	12 to 25 milligrams orally, subcutaneously, or intramuscularly per week
Minocycline	100 milligrams orally twice per day
Sulfasalazine	2 to 3 grams orally per day in divided doses

in presentation of RA, while using evidence-based practice guidelines. Patients are active decision-makers in their care and prioritize management behaviors accordingly. Communication among providers is foundational to self-management, patient-driven care. With rheumatologists, family practice physicians, cardiologists, physical therapists, and advanced practice nurses participating together in an educational program, using patient education specialists, team learning, and networking approaches, collaborative and complementary care facilitates self-management and fosters best outcomes for patients.

SYSTEMIC LUPUS ERYTHEMATOSUS

Etiology

SLE is an autoimmune, connective tissue disorder affecting multiple systems with a wide range of clinical presentations. It predominately affects women during childbearing age, with a peak onset of 15 to 40 years, and a ratio of women to men 9:1. For men, onset is later in life, usually age 60 to 70 years. The overall prevalence in the United States is 15 to 50 cases per 100,000, with an incidence of 1.8 to 7.6 cases per 100,000 per year. The incidence of SLE is 3 to 4 times higher in black females, and has more serious renal involvement and higher mortality rates than other groups. Asian, Hispanic, and women from certain North American Indian tribes have a greater risk for developing SLE than those from European ancestors (25).

SLE appears to result from the interplay of genetic, environmental, and hormonal factors. Disease prevalence among family members and twins emerged as the first evidence of a genetic basis of the disease. There is a 15- to 20-fold increase among siblings and a 24% concordance rate among identical twins versus 2% among fraternal twins. More recently, several genes on the long arm of chromosome 1, 1q23-24, have been isolated in many populations with SLE. Additionally, an allele of C-reactive protein associated with antinuclear antibody production, a key diagnostic marker for SLE, has been identified (26).

Empirical evidence clearly indicates the influence of environmental factors on expression of clinical manifestations of SLE. Sunlight exposure triggers appearance of the characteristic skin rash, and exacerbation of the disease following viral and bacterial infections has been observed. Some studies suggest exposure to environmental toxins such as silica and mercury among agricultural workers contributes to development of the disease (25, 26).

Although the evidence is mixed, the general consensus is that both endogenous and exogenous exposure to estrogens may increase the risk of developing SLE. The disease occurs during child-bearing years and eruptions are common during pregnancy, not only complicating maternal aspects of the pregnancy but compromising the health of the fetus and newborn as well.

Oral contraceptives and postmenopausal hormone replacement therapy have shown in some studies to increase the risk of developing SLE; though not conclusive, because of increased thromboembolic risk for patients with SLE, oral contraceptives are discouraged (26).

Pathophysiology

The pathophysiology of SLE is unclear, although recent cytogenetic research has elucidated several underlying mechanisms. A key pathophysiologic finding is the production of autoantibodies that mediate the disease process. Some autoantibodies are directed toward the cell surface of RBCs, platelets, neutrophils, and neuronal cells. Other autoantibodies are directed toward the DNA and RNA of cells, thus the term antinuclear antibodies (ANAs). Additionally, CD4 T cells, T-cell cytokines, T-cell co-stimulation and T-cell/B-cell interactions play a role in the disease process (26).

What triggers the autoantibody response is unclear, although apoptosis may offer some explanation. Autoantigens are released by apoptotic and necrotic cells; a defect in clearance of apoptotic cells may lead to anomalous uptake by tissue macrophages, followed by presentation of previously intracellular antigens to B and T cells. This in turn perpetuates the autoimmune process (27).

The pathophysiologic process affects multiple organs and plays out in many different ways among individuals with SLE. However, approximately 50% of all patients have clinically apparent renal involvement. Urinalysis abnormalities include hematuria, proteinuria, or casts, and functional impairment is indicated by decreased creatinine clearance. The World Health Organization has established a five-class histologic classification system for lupus nephritis, the criteria determined by renal biopsy, immunofluorescence, and electron microscopy. In class I, only urinalysis and creatinine clearance are abnormal, with normal biopsy results. In class II, mesangial deposits of immune complexes and hypercellularity are evident on biopsy. Class III shows focal, proliferative inflammatory lesions in less than 50% of the glomeruli, with capillary loop immune complex deposits. In Class IV, more than 50% of the glomeruli are involved, with diffuse glomerulonephritis and deposits of immune complexes. In class V, there is generalized thickening of the capillary loops, with deep deposits of immune complexes (28, 29).

SLE is associated with increased risk of cardiovascular (CV) disease. Pericarditis is the most common CV manifestation of SLE, followed by endocarditis and valve disease (26). Coronary artery disease (CAD) for patients with SLE is reportedly 50-folder higher than in people without SLE. CV disease is largely due to systemwide inflammation and an accelerated atherosclerotic process, provoked by inflammatory mediators and prothrombotic factors. Elevated levels of C-reactive protein, CD40 ligand, and sVCAM-1 have been detected in patients

with SLE. This may account for the inflammatory response by the pericardium and the endocardium, as well as increased atherosclerosis. Small artery elasticity, a measure of endothelial health and vessel wall stiffness, in conjunction with atherosclerosis, contributes to CAD, acute myocardial infarction, and sudden cardiac death (30). Antiphospholipid antibodies, which contribute to thrombosis, likely account for valve disease as well as contribute to coronary artery disease.

A variety of central nervous system effects of SLE are seen, some considered neuropsychiatric effects, and depending on the defining criteria applied occur in as many as 15% to 75% of individuals. Neurologic manifestations can be as mild as a headache and as severe as seizures, cognitive dysfunction, aseptic meningitis, movement disorders, coma, and death. Psychiatric disorders include depression and psychosis. Depression is reported in more than 50% of patients with SLE, and is significantly higher than in non–SLE-afflicted individuals. It is thought that lupus antibodies cross-react with DNA and N-methyl-D-aspartate (NMDA) receptors in SLE and account for depression; this is consistent with a mechanism of depression in non-SLE individuals. Depression in turn interferes with cognitive function. Fatigue is the most commonly reported symptom of SLE overall. There is evidence to suggest that higher levels of depression, fatigue, cognitive dysfunction, and even pain occur in individuals with SLE, are interrelated, and are due to global changes in the central nervous system as a result of the disease (31, 32).

Transischemic attacks and stroke are common, due in part to thomboembolic events and vessel occlusion owing to antiphospholipid antibodies. Other pathophysiologic processes include the action of antineuronal antibodies, increased IgG levels, oligoclonal bands in cerebrospinal fluid, elevated levels of antibodies to ribosomal P proteins, and activation of cytokines. All of these immune products target central nervous system tissue in a diffuse fashion, resulting in widespread effects (26).

The hematologic system, including all cell lines, is usually affected in SLE. Autoantibodies directed against erythroblasts induce an RBC aplasia anemia. However, most people have normocytic, normochromic anemia of chronic disease associated with active systemic inflammation. Leukopenia is present, both granulocytic and lymphocytic, owing to antilymphocytic antibodies. Mild thrombocytopenia is common and in a subset of patients, due to antiphospholipid antibodies. These individuals usually have more severe disease and experience arterial and venous thromboembolic events such as stroke, myocardial infarction, cardiac valve disease, pulmonary embolism, deep vein thrombosis, and autoimmune hemolytic anemia. In addition to antiphospholipid antibodies, they usually test positive for beta-2-glycoprotein I complex and cardiolipin as well. Beta-2-glycoprotein has an anticoagulant effect, which is blocked by the antiphosphospholipid antibodies, leading to thrombus formation (26).

Musculoskeletal involvement includes arthralgia and myalgia, with complaints of joint pain in over 90% of patients. Edema and pain is limited to the fingers and hands. Circulating inflammatory mediators account for the musculoskeletal effects of SLE. Skin involvement is common, with over 80% of patients manifesting rashes on the face and scalp. Most patients with cutaneous lesions have elevated antibodies to Ro/SS-A, a self-protein (26).

Clinical Presentation

Most patients present for initial diagnosis with complaints of fatigue, malaise, depression, sleep difficulties, joint pain, and fever; the facial "butterfly" rash may be present also, as this flares up during active disease, particularly following exposure to sunshine. Acutely ill, hospitalized patients, previously diagnosed or not, commonly present with thromboembolic events or complications of renal disease. Stroke, acute myocardial infarction, pulmonary embolism, ischemic bowel, renal artery infarction, acute arterial occlusion, and deep vein thrombosis may be reasons for admission (32). Additionally, complications of treatment such as hyperglycemia, infection, and fluid and electrolyte imbalances with resulting sequelae may be present, even if not the primary reason for hospitalization. When evaluating patients with any of these problems, advanced practice nurses should always be cognizant of the potential for SLE as a comorbidity. (See Table 15-9 for a summary of clinical manifestations, pathophysiology, diagnostic tests, and management of SLE.)

TABLE 15–9 Clinical Connections: Systemic Lupus Erythematosus

Clinical Manifestations	Pathophysiology	Assessment Finding	Laboratory/ Diagnostic tests	Treatment
Mucocutaneous: Rashes Photosensitivity Alopecia Vasculitis Raynaud's phenomenon Angioedema Mucosal ulcers Leg ulcers	Possible autoantibody binding to nuclear antigen on cell surfaces; occurs during active disease	Facial butterfly rash	Positive antinuclear-antibody tests	Antimalarial drugs (hydroxychloroquine) Dehydroepian-drosterone Topical fluorinated corticosteroids for alopecia and acute cutaneous lesions Avoidance of sun exposure; 30 SPF sunscreen Avoidance of irritating mouthwashes, i.e. alcohol, meticulous oral hygiene see Chapter 7 for leg ulcer care
Constitutional signs/symptoms	Active disease	Fever, anorexia, weight loss, fatigue	Elevated erythrocyte sedimentation rate, C-reactive protein	Rest Antipyretics NSAIDS Antimalarial drugs (hydroxychloroquine)

TABLE 15–9 Clinical Connections: Systemic Lupus Erythematosus—cont'd

Clinical Manifestations	Pathophysiology	Assessment Finding	Laboratory/ Diagnostic tests	Treatment
				Dehydroepian-drosterone Treatment of constitutional symptoms may benefit cutaneous and musculoskeletal findings
Musculoskeletal: Arthralgia Myalgia Avascular bone necrosis Osteopenia	Active disease Glucocorticoid myopathy and bone demineralization Myositis	Joint pain Symmetrical polyarthritis of metacarpopha-langeal, proximal interphalangeal joints Skeletal muscle weakness Destruction of hips	Elevated erythro-cyte sedimenta-tion rate, C-reactive protein Elevated CPK Electromyography Muscle biopsy	
Renal: Glomerular nephritis Hypertension	Deposition of immune complexes		Elevated serum creatinine Elevated creatinine clearance Urinalysis positive for RBCs, WBCs, casts, protein	
Pulmonary: Pleural effusion Pneumonitis Interstitial disease Hemorrhage Pulmonary hypertension	Active disease	Cough, hemoptysis, fever, dyspnea, hypoxemia, diminished breath sounds	Chest x-ray: Infiltrates Hemorrhage	Thoracentesis Oxygen Antipyretics
Cardiac: Pericarditis Myocarditis Coronary artery disease Hypertension Valve disease	Inflammatory process; contributes to atherosclerotic process, endothe-lial involvement, and vasodilatation in the coronary arteries Antiphospholipid antibodies	Tachycardia Hypertension Findings consistent with acute coro-nary syndrome Murmurs (usually associated with mitral valve)	Chest x-ray shows cardiomegaly Echocardiogram positive for pericardial fluid Lipid profiles may be elevated C-reactive protein levels may be elevated during active disease	Pericardiocentesis Cardioprotective medications; Appropriate treatment for acute coronary syndrome (see Chapter 9)

Continued

TABLE 15-9 Clinical Connections: Systemic Lupus Erythematosus—cont'd

Clinical Manifestations	Pathophysiology	Assessment Finding	Laboratory/ Diagnostic tests	Treatment
Gastrointestinal: Nausea/vomiting Peritonitis Pancreatitis Intestinal vasculitis Hepatomegaly Hepatitis	Glucocorticoids, aspirin, NSAIDS for treatment	Dryness of the mouth Abdominal pain	Elevated ALT, AST Liver biopsy may show inflammatory cells Endoscopy positive for peptic ulcer	Artificial saliva, oral care Appropriate treatment for peptic ulcer disease (see Chapter 12)
Hematologic: Anemia Thrombocytopenia Neutropenia Thrombosis/ emboli Bleeding diasthesis	Chronic disease/ iron dysutilization Autoantibodies binding to cell surface antigens	Activity intolerance, fatigue, pallor, tachycardia Thromboembolic events	Decreased RBC, Hgb, Hct, WBC platelet count	Iron supplement, nutrition counseling Prophylaxis for thromboembolic events
Neurologic: Headache/ migraines Stroke syndromes Seizures Movement disorders Neurocognitive disorders Psychosis, depression Aseptic meningitis Peripheral neuropathy	Antineuronal antibodies interfere with neuronal function	Can occur during active or quiescent periods of disease: Complaints of headache Seizure activity Focal weakness, paresthesias, slurred speech indicative of stroke Neurocognitive impairment Psychotic behaviors Poor sleep habits, anorexia, lack of initiative and other signs and symptoms of depression	Elevated serum IgG MRI may show cerebral vasculitis, stroke	Standard treatment specific to presenting neurologic disorder (See Chapter 8)

Diagnosis

Eleven criteria have been established by the American College of Rheumatology; only four of the eleven are required to make a diagnosis of SLE (32). (See Table 15-10 for a complete summary of diagnostic criteria.) Diagnosis of SLE begins with a complete history and physical exam, which then drives the diagnostic plan. Laboratory tests are the primary method of diagnosing SLE and should include a complete blood count (CBC) to evaluate anemia, leukopenia, and thrombocytopenia. A basic metabolic profile to evaluate renal function and electrolytes, and serum albumin, which may be reduced secondary to nephropathy, should be done. Urinalysis to evaluate protein, RBCs, WBCs, and casts is imperative, along with creatinine clearance for evaluation of renal function. Antibody screening for ANA, double-stranded

TABLE 15–10 Diagnostic Criteria for Systemic Lupus Erythematosus: Presence of Any Four Criteria Sufficient for Diagnosis

Criterion	Description
Malar rash	Fixed erythema over malar area
Discoid rash	Erythematous raised patches with keratotic scaling
Photosensitivity	Skin rash with recent sun exposure
Oral ulcers	In mouth or oropharynx, usually painless
Arthritis	In 2 or more peripheral joints
Serositis	Pleuritis or pericarditis
Renal involvement	Persistent proteinuria >0.5 grams per day
Neuropsychological disorder	Seizures, psychosis
Hematologic involvement	Hemolytic anemia plus elevated reticulocytes, or leukopenia (<4,000), or lymphopenia (<1500), or thrombocytopenia (<100,00)
Immunologic involvement	Positive LE, or anti-DNA titer, or anti-Sm, or false positive test for syphilis
Antinuclear antibody	Abnormal titer by immunoflorescnce

and single-stranded DNA, antiphospholipids, and anti-Ro/SS-A, along with complement levels, and C-reactive protein should be done. Elevated ANA and C-reactive protein are not specific to SLE and diagnosis should not be based on this alone; referral to a rheumatologist is appropriate with positive findings on baseline screening tests (26).

Imaging tests should be guided by the clinical presentation. Radiography, ventilation-perfusion scanning, and echocardiography are appropriate for patients presenting with pulmonary and/or cardiac signs and symptoms. Evaluation for stroke and acute myocardial infarction should include computed axial tomography, magnetic resonance imaging, and cardiac imaging studies, which should be determined by a neurologist and cardiologist, respectively.

Differential diagnoses for SLE include other connective or nonconnective tissue disorders, including RA if arthritic symptoms predominate. Mixed connective tissue disease can mimic SLE but also may involve features of systemic sclerosis, rheumatoid-like polyarthritis, and polymyositis or dermatomyositis. Certain infections such as bacterial endocarditis and histoplasmosis can imitate SLE and may develop as a result of therapy-induced immunosuppression. Other differential diagnoses may include sarcoidosis and paraneoplastic syndromes (26).

Management

Management of SLE includes supportive care and treatment of acute exacerbations of the disease. The overriding goals of therapy are to suppress disease manifestations, curtail complications of the disease, minimize toxicity of treatment, and optimize quality of life. Treatment is tailored toward patient presentation, which is typified by exacerbations that require intervention to achieve a steady state.

Traditional medical treatment has consisted of high-dose glucocorticoids and cytotoxic drugs. Newer treatment with monoclonal antibodies, immunoglobulins, and autologous stem-cell transplantation shows promising results.

High-dose glucocorticoids are indicated for patients with no prior treatment, those with lupus nephritis, central nervous system involvement, hemolytic anemia, immune thrombocytopenia, visceral vasculitis, lupus pneumonitis, serositis with complications, and severe systemic disease. Cytotoxic drugs are indicated for patients refractory to high-dose glucocorticoids or with severe complications of glucocorticoids (26).

High-dose glucocorticoid therapy consists of prednisone 1 mg per kilogram per day in divided doses, approximately 60 to 80 mg/day. Several weeks may be required to see results in improved renal function. After the creatinine has returned to normal and proteinuria decreased, the dosage should be reduced by approximately 10 mg every 2 weeks to a maintenance dose of 40 mg/day; thereafter, the lowest possible dose to maintain renal function is desired. During high-dose glucocorticoid therapy, patients should be vigilantly monitored for endocrine, fluid, and electrolyte complications; opportunistic infection; myopathy and avascular joint necrosis; glaucoma and cataracts; and psychological problems such as anxiety and absolute psychosis (26).

Cytotoxic drug therapy has traditionally included cyclophosphamide. The recommended dose is 0.5 to 1 g/m² body surface area intravenously over 60 minutes. Recommendations include five additional doses every month followed by a dose at 3-month intervals. The leukocyte count should be closely monitored and not exceed a nadir of 1,500 neutrophils per microliter. Renal protection with hydration is required, along with protection from opportunistic infection (26).

Rituximab is a newer drug for use with SLE. It is a murine monoclonal antibody directed toward CD20 antigens on B lymphocytes and their precursors. Achievement of and sustaining longer remission for patients resistant to other drug therapy have been observed in some patients. Intravenous immunoglobulins are useful in the treatment of patients with active lupus and concomitant infection in whom high-dose steroids and immune suppression would be risky. Various protocols using combinations of rituximab in conjunction with intravenous cyclophosphamide and methylprednisoline are in progress to evaluate B cell re-accumulation and disease exacerbation (27).

Clinical Nurse Specialist Competencies and Spheres of Influence
Consultation

Clearly, the CNS competency of consultation is an important strategy for ensuring quality outcomes in the management of patients hospitalized with SLE. The multisystem effects of both the chronic and acute manifestations of the disease need to be addressed. Frontline caregivers are likely (and appropriately) to focus on the acute complaint or diagnosis such as chest pain associated with acute myocardial infarction or electrolyte imbalance stemming from glucocorticoid treatment. Assistance with comprehensive

management of the patient to address other issues such as peptic ulcer (secondary to glucocorticoids or stress of acute illness) prophylaxis or monitoring and assessment for protection from opportunistic infection is a vital contribution of CNSs to the patients and nurses alike.

CNS consultation may occur through either a consultee-initiated or a CNS-initiated process. The CNS as consultant may participate indirectly by sharing clinical judgment and making recommendations on an as-needed basis when contacted by frontline caregivers. The attributes necessary for this approach include mutual trust, ongoing evidence of knowledge and expertise, and ready availability; the staff nurse must be able to rely on the CNS to respond when called upon and offer the requested assistance with managing the patient when complications of SLE arise, for example (33).

Clinical rounds is an example of CNS-initiated consultation. For success with this approach, the individual must possess good time management and organizational skills, self-confidence, resourcefulness, initiative, leadership, assertiveness, and good interpersonal skills (34). One must be an astute listener, appreciating subtleties and decoding information provided in order to uncover problems and issues that may only be apparent to a true expert. Box 15-2 illustrates an example of an instrument

---

BOX 15–2 CNS Rounds Documentation

Patient Identification Information
Date/Hospital Day#11-25-08/5

Admitting Diagnoses/CC	Fatigue, cough – pericarditis, pleuritis
Systems Review	
Chronic Disease/Problem	Rheumatoid arthritis × 4 years
Acute Disease/Problem	Hyperglycemia
Neurologic	
Behavior/Psych	
CV	Distant heart sounds; pericardial friction rub, pericarditis
Pulmonary	Distant breath sounds, cough subsiding, mild chest pain, pleuritis
Endocrine	Glucose 120-160 past 24 hours; E-lytes WNL
MS/Mobility	Poor activity tolerance with minimal ambulation
	Bilateral joint deformity in hands
Integumentary/Wounds	
GI/GU/Elimination	On PUD prophylaxis
Nutrition	Appetite improving, regular reduced fat diet
Hydration/Fluids	
Laboratory	Elevated C-reactive protein coming down, WBC 10.4 ^PMNs (coming down), decreased lymphs; platelets 160,000; Hgb 9.2 Hct 27.3 (stable).; BUN 21 Creat 1.8; Glucose 132
Pain	Pleuritic and joint pain controlled with NSAIDS
Family	Husband comes after work in evening; paraplegic S/P motorcycle collision 2 years ago
Social/Economic	
Precautions	Fall; immunosuppressive
Current Plan	Continue tapering IV steroids, rheumatologist will determine when to DC and initiate DMARDS
Recommendations	IV insulin protocol to get better control of blood glucose
Follow-up/	Will follow up with rheumatology re: endocrinology consult.
Consult/Education	Nsg resources re: patient's risk for CAD and assessment for ACS

that may be used for clinical rounds on the unit. The CNS should establish criteria for rounding, such as frequency, time, selection of patients and criteria if not all patients are included, personnel attendance, and format. Traditionally, the primary nurses or bedside caregivers provide a brief report on the patients in their care. The CNS then uses prompts as needed to elucidate potential or brewing problems, summarizes the plan, makes recommendations, and follows up with other professionals. An instrument such as this can be used for development of a quality, outcome, and administrative database as well as documentation of specific patient information and tracking of progress during the hospitalization. The form can be loaded onto a tablet personal computer (tablet PC) or personal digital assistant (PDA), and the patient data can easily be aggregated on a cumulative basis, providing data on length-of-stay, complications, and outcomes of interventions. Calculation of financial and human costs and other factors can then be determined and the CNS is able to demonstrate his or her worth to the organization.

Consultation, either consultee- or CNS-initiated, is one of the best opportunities for realizing the benefits of CNS practice. She or he can establish an environment of clinical inquiry, in which the status quo is always questioned, answers are sought in the literature versus tradition, and improved care is always the goal (34). This sets the stage for evidence-based practice, which is critical now with an emphasis on quality and safety and a reimbursement climate that places the financial burden of poor quality on hospitals. Conducting clinical rounds on a consistent basis allows for visibility of the CNS and provides an opportunity to influence practice with infusion of state-of-the-science interventions. Ongoing staff education and professional development through CNS role modeling and facilitation of learning are other benefits to clinical rounds, which strengthen the professional practice milieu and foster a culture of quality and excellence in care.

Clinical Expert/Direct Care

Clinical expertise is a prerequisite for effective consultation. Clinical expertise, or clinical judgment as termed by the American Association of Critical Care Nurses in the Synergy Model, involves analysis and synthesis of assessment data, formulation and prioritization of differential diagnoses, and establishing a plan to achieve desired outcomes for patients, nurses, and the organization (35). The CNS must appreciate not only the chronic nature of SLE but also significant features of the disease and treatment that trigger acute events and necessitate hospitalization. Various thromboembolic events, ramifications of electrolyte imbalance, and expectations of potential psychotic reactions, for example, are critical aspects of this chronic immune disease for which CNSs

must be knowledgeable. Through consultation for patients with SLE, patient complications are averted, and nurses learn chronic and acute aspects of the disease, along with current management and preventive approaches. The system enjoys benefits such as high patient satisfaction ratings and lower costs of care through shorter lengths of stay associated with prevention of infection and patient falls, for example.

Research/Evidence-Based Practice

Application of research is another important competency for CNSs. Proficiency in database searching is an important skill set for CNSs so that systematic reviews, practice guidelines, and other electronic resources can be accessed. During the past decade, major advances have been achieved in understanding the genetic and inflammatory processes involved in the development of SLE. This understanding, in turn, has led to new, more efficacious treatment, which previously was limited to symptom control. Because knowledge grows and practice changes so rapidly, CNSs must be able to use technology, access electronic sources, and critically appraise evidence for appropriate use in practice.

Safe and effective care of hospitalized patients with SLE depends on utilization of research and sound clinical judgment. CNS consultation is one avenue for implementation of other CNS competencies.

Coaching/Teaching/Mentoring

Case study examples are ideal methods of teaching, with prospective application of learned content. CNSs may use case examples in a nursing grand rounds milieu or in a classroom setting. Case Study 15-1 provides an example of a typical presentation of a patient with SLE. This approach stimulates interactiv e learning, a method nurses and other health care professionals generally find beneficial.

SEPSIS AND SYSTEMIC INFLAMMATORY RESPONSE SYNDROME

Systemic inflammatory response syndrome (SIRS) was first introduced in 1992 by a consensus of members of the American College of Chest Physicians and Society of Critical Care Medicine and is part of a group of definitions relative to systemic infection and organ dysfunction. Infection is the most common etiology of SIRS and thus is often referred to as sepsis or severe sepsis. However, SIRS is a complex process of immune responses and mediator activation triggered by insults other than infection, including pancreatitis, traumatic injury, and thermal injury, to name a few. All of the definitions of the consensus group are described in Table 15-11 (36).

CASE STUDY 15-1

CHIEF COMPLAINT: Pain and feeling tired, with difficulty sleeping.

HISTORY OF PRESENT ILLNESS: A 34-year-old African-American woman presents with complaints of worsening fatigue, headache, and feeling poorly "all over". She complains of pain and swelling in her knees and difficulty using the keyboard on her computer. She is wearing dark glasses when you approach her.

HISTORY & PHYSICAL EXAM

Generally, she appears ill and pale.

INTEGUMENTARY Warm dry skin, with splinter hemorrhages on the fingertips and scattered on her toes. A macular rash is apparent between the knuckles of 4 fingers on the right hand and 3 fingers on the left hand. Open lesions in her mouth, which she says she has not noticed.

NEUROLOGIC Alert and oriented ×3. PERRLA. DTRs 1+. Reports photophobia. Denies history of seizures.

MUSCULOSKELETA Arm and leg strength is 4/5, moves all extremities equally bilaterally. Right knee with moderate swelling.

PULMONARY Lungs clear to auscultation bilaterally with a pleural friction rub. No use of accessory muscles. Denies SOB.

CARDIOVASCULAR Heart sounds S_1 S_2 are regular, systolic murmur heard best 4th intercostal space, left sternal border. No gallops, heart sounds somewhat muffled.

GASTROINTESTINAL Abdomen is soft and nontender with active bowel sounds in all quadrants. No rebound tenderness. Reports intermittent generalized abdominal pain, poor appetite, unsure of weight loss. Unable to give history of changes in bowel elimination.

GENITOURINARY Reports no changes in urinary habits. Pelvic exam deferred at this time.

LABORATORY RBC 3.1, Hgb 9.5 Hct 28

WBC 4,000

Platelets 98,000

Urinalysis: specific gravity 1.022, WBCs 0, RBCs 0, bacteria 0, few casts, protein 3+,

ALT 95, AST 78

Alkaline phosphatase 55

Amylase 35

Albumin 3.0

BUN 24, Creatinine 2.4

Glucose 95

Electrolytes Na 137, K 4.2, Cl 96, Ca 10.4

QUESTIONS (See DavisPlus for answers)

1. What are the significant findings in the history and physical?

2. What are the differential diagnoses?

3. What additional diagnostic tests are indicated?

4. The rheumatoid factor is negative, ANA is positive, C-reactive protein 0.8, serum albumin 1.5, creatinine clearance 60 milliliters per minute. What is the working diagnosis?

5. What are the appropriate management strategies for this patient?

6. Are there other findings that you may expect to see with a diagnosis of SLE?

7. What genetic counseling is indicated, if any?

8. What management-related patient education is necessary for this patient?

9. What disease-related patient education is needed for this patient?

10. How does SLE differ from scleroderma?

TABLE 15–11 Definitions of SIRS, Sepsis, Severe Sepsis, and Septic Shock

Syndrome	Definition
SIRS	2 or more of the following: Temperature >38 C (100.4° F) or <36 C (96.8° F) Pulse >90 per minute Respiratory rate >20 per minute or Paco$_2$ <32 mm Hg White blood cell count >12,000/mm^3 or <4,000/mm^3 or >10% immature forms (bands)
Sepsis	SIRS due to suspected or confirmed infection
Severe sepsis	Sepsis associated with organ dysfunction, hypoperfusion or hypotension
Septic shock	Sepsis-induced hypotension despite fluid resuscitation + perfusion abnormalities

Etiology

The pathophysiology of SIRS/sepsis and end-organ dysfunction involves a complicated interplay of genetics, immunity and inflammatory mediators, procoagulation-anticoagulation imbalance, cellular metabolic derangements, endocrine dysfunction, and hypoxia. Of the 750,000 cases of sepsis/SIRS diagnosed in the United States annually, approximately 215,000 die (9.3% of all deaths). Hospital mortality ranges from 18% to 30%, with lengths of stay averaging 20 days, half of those in the intensive care unit. Estimated costs for the hospitalization exceed $16 billion, with many more dollars consumed during prolonged recovery phases.

Pathophysiology

Sepsis/SIRS results from the interaction between an infecting microorganism (when the etiology is infection) and host immune, inflammatory, coagulation, and cellular factors, culminating in tissue injury and multiorgan dysfunction (Table 15-12). Because the response to inflammation, injury, and infection varies among individuals, it is likely that genetics and genomics play an important role. Elevated levels of serum proinflammatory mediators are associated with early mortality from infection and have a genetic link. For example, high levels of TNF-α have been found in patients with septic shock and death from severe sepsis; through molecular biology, a gene that codes for TNF-α has been isolated. Specific genes have been identified for at least 10 other proinflammatory, anti-inflammatory, and procoagulant mediators (37).

Host defenses in sepsis encompass both innate and adaptive immune responses. The innate system responds initially to an insult through pattern-recognition receptors, which stimulates intracellular signaling, causing increased production of proinflammatory molecules such as TNF-α and IL-β and antiinflammatory cytokines. These activate neutrophils to kill microorganisms and injure endothelium via mediator release. Vascular permeability increases, edema forms, and nitric oxide release causes profound vasodilatation.

Adaptive immunity involves release of immunoglobulins from B lymphocytes that bind to microorganisms, facilitating presentation to natural killer lymphocytes and neutrophils for destruction. Immune suppression is thought to occur late during sepsis/SIRS and is associated with death due to secondary infection when the individual survives the initial septic episode.

TABLE 15–12 Mediators of Sepsis/SIRS

Pathway	Mediators
Pattern recognition receptors interact with molecules in microorganism	Superantigens TSST-1 Streptococcal exotoxins Lipopolysaccharide (endotoxins)
Innate immunity	Toll-like receptors (TLRs): TLR-2, TLR-4 Monocytes, macrophages Neutrophils
Adaptive immunity	B cells, plasma cells, immunoglobulins CD4+T cells (type 1 or 2 helper cells)
Immunosuppression or apoptosis	Lymphocyte apoptosis Intestinal epithelial cell apoptosis

Continued

TABLE 15–12 Mediators of Sepsis/SIRS—cont'd

Pathway	Mediators
Proinflammatory pathway	Tumor necrosis factor α (TNF-a)
	Interleukin-1 β
	Interleukin-6
	Prostaglandins, leukotrienes
	Bradykinin
	Platelet-activating factor
	Proteases
	Oxidants
	Nitric oxide
Antiinflammatory	Interleukin-10
	TNF-alpha receptors
Procoagulant pathway	Decreased protein C
	Decreased protein S
	Decreased antithrombin III
	Decreased tissue factor-pathway inhibitor
	Increased plasminogen-activator inhibitor-1
Cellular metabolism: abnormalities in carbohydrate, lipid, protein metabolism	Anaerobic metabolism
	Lactate production
	Mitochondrial dysfunction
Endocrine	Adrenal insufficiency
	Vasopressin deficiency
	Hyperglycemia
Hypoxia	Hypoxia-inducing factor 1a
	Vascular endothelial growth factor

Procoagulation factors increase, along with a decrease in anticoagulation factors in sepsis, leading to formation of disseminated microthrombi. Fibrinogen converts to fibrin, which becomes trapped in the microvasculature. Levels of protein C, protein S, antithrombin III, and tissue factor-pathway inhibitor, all important anticoagulant factors, are diminished in sepsis, which leads to excessive clotting. Ischemia from hypoperfusion and hypoxia from acute lung injury intensify the proinflammatory and procoagulation processes (38).

Carbohydrate, protein, and lipid metabolism is disrupted in sepsis/SIRS. Hyperglycemia occurs in essentially all patients with sepsis/SIRS and exaggerates many of the responses, including procoagulation; interferes with neutrophil function and phagocytosis; impairs wound healing; and predisposes to further infection. Insulin may have other beneficial properties during sepsis, providing the rationale for tight glycemic control to reduce the known harmful effects of hyperglycemia.

Adrenal insufficiency often occurs in sepsis/SIRS as a manifestation of the stress response. Mechanisms are not well understood, however, and are thought to be due to decreased production of and diminished receptors for corticotrophin-releasing hormone (CRH), adrenocorticotropin hormone (ACTH), and cortisol. Adrenal insufficiency is often manifested by low cortisol and vasopressin levels, resulting in persistent hypotension. Diminished glucocorticoid activity results in excessive production of proinflammatory mediators, thus a cycle of inflammation—adrenal insufficiency—and further inflammation is set into motion (38).

Inadequate cellular oxygen delivery due to reduced capillary blood flow and decreased cardiac output may contribute to anaerobic metabolism and lactate production. Mitochondrial dysfunction may contribute to poor oxygen extraction and utilization at the cellular level (39).

Clinical Presentation

The clinical presentation varies according to the source of sepsis/SIRS and point in the trajectory of the syndrome, early or late, although early recognition and treatment are critical to survival and fewer complications. Most individuals present with signs of systemic infection, including elevated temperature, tachycardia, tachypnea, hypotension, and change in mental status. The elderly, however, commonly present with mental status changes without fever. The same holds true for others who, due to an underlying immune defect, are unable to mount a febrile response. Abdominal pain, nausea, vomiting, and diarrhea are common in those with in intra-abdominal source of infection. Other cardiovascular system changes include low mean arterial pressure, mottled extremities, delayed capillary refill, low cardiac output, and low oxygen saturation. Respiratory signs include a PaO_2/FIO_2 ratio less than 300, hypoxemia and distress necessitating endotracheal intubation and mechanical ventilator support, and chest radiograph abnormalities owing to acute respiratory distress syndrome and/or pneumonia as the primary source of sepsis/SIRS. Renal indicators include oliguria and elevated creatinine. Hepatic dysfunction is manifested by elevated transaminases and bilirubin levels. Hypoperfusion may cause an intestinal ileus. Hematology system changes show abnormal coagulation, including elevated international normalized ratio (INR), elevated partial thromboplastin time (PTT), elevated D-dimer, thrombocytopenia, and DIC. Metabolic changes include acidosis, elevated lactate, elevated base deficit, and low serum pH (40). (See Table 15-13.)

Diagnosis

When sepsis/SIRS is suspected based on the clinical presentation and focused history and physical, diagnostic testing should begin immediately and in conjunction with initial resuscitation. Laboratory tests include serum lactate level, CBC with WBC count differential, renal and liver function tests, arterial blood gases, electrolytes, and coagulation studies to include PTT, prothrombin time, INR, and D-dimer. At least two blood cultures should be done before initiating antimicrobial therapy to identify the causative organism for sepsis. When vascular access devices are present, one sample should come from each catheter lumen and one drawn percutaneously. Imaging studies include chest and abdominal radiographs, CT scan, and magnetic resonance imaging if the patient is stable enough for transport and when an abscess, bowel perforation, or biliary tract infection is suspected. Bedside ultrasonography may be useful when patients are not stable enough for transport. Specific source identification and control should take place within the first 6 hours following presentation with evidence of sepsis/SIRS (40).

TABLE 15–13 Clinical Connections: Sepsis/SIRS

Clinical Manifestations	Pathophysiology	Assessment Finding	Laboratory/ Diagnostic Tests	Treatment
Hypotension	*Decrease in systemic vascular resistance *Vascular permeability causes loss of fluid from the vascular bed *Nitric oxide release causes vasodilatation *Adrenal insufficiency Adrenocorticotropic hormone deficiency	MAP <65		Intravenous fluids 500-1000 mL/30 minutes Norepinephrine or dopamine Packed red blood cells Hydrocortisone <300 mg/day Fludrocortisone 50 mcg/day
Tachycardia	Increase in cardiac output (initially)	Heart rate >90/min		
Tachypnea	Compensatory mechanism for tissue hypoxia and metabolic acidosis	Respiratory rate >20/min PCO2 <32 mm Hg	Arterial blood gases	
Change in mental status	Decreased cerebral perfusion; fever	Confusion, agitation		
Hyperglycemia	Epinephrine release		Serum glucose >110	Insulin intravenously bolus or continuous infusion

Continued

TABLE 15–13 Clinical Connections: Sepsis/SIRS—cont'd

Clinical Manifestations	Pathophysiology	Assessment Finding	Laboratory/ Diagnostic Tests	Treatment
Fever	Mediator release	Core temperature >38°×C (100.4°×F)	Blood cultures	Appropriate antimicrobials (after blood cultures drawn) Acetaminophen
Oliguria	Decreased renal perfusion	Urinary output <1 mL/kg/hr		Intravenous fluids 500-1000 mL/30 minutes
Abdominal distention	Ileus secondary to hypoperfusion	Distention, hypoactive or absent bowel sounds, abdominal pain, nausea, vomiting		Intravenous fluids 500-1000 mL/30 minutes Nasogastric tube insertion

Management

Many interventions are designed for critical care. However, the greatest improvements in outcomes for patients with sepsis/SIRS will come as a result of education, early recognition and intervention, and process improvements across acute and community-based care (41).

Treatment for sepsis/SIRS is organized according to early and later stages, with protocolized, goal-directed management of early severe sepsis as the key to best outcomes.

During the first 6 hours of severe sepsis/SIRS, in which tissue hypoperfusion is a characteristic feature, the goals of initial resuscitation are to restore perfusion with aggressive fluid administration to achieve a central venous pressure of 8 to 12 mm Hg, mean arterial pressure 65 mm Hg or greater, and urine output 0.5 mL/kg.hr or greater, and central or mixed venous oxygen saturation 70% or greater or 65%, respectively. Fluids can be either colloids or crystalloids, with a minimum of 1,000 mL of crystalloid or 3 to 500 mL of colloid over 30 minutes.

When fluid administration fails to achieve the targeted mean arterial pressure, vasopressors should be initiated. Norepinephrine or dopamine are the drugs of choice, followed by epinephrine if a mean arterial pressure of 65 mm Hg is not reached. Dobutamine is indicated if myocardial dysfunction becomes evident by elevated cardiac filling pressures and low cardiac output. After tissue hypoperfusion has been restored, RBC transfusion is recommended when hemoglobin falls to less than 7.0 g/dL in order to increase oxygen delivery.

Antimicrobial therapy should be initiated within one hour of recognition of severe sepsis. Choice of agent is made empirically, based on patient history, underlying disease process, clinical issues, susceptibility patterns in the hospital and community, and drug intolerance. Drugs used recently for an infection or prophylaxis should be avoided. Once the offending organism/s is/are identified, antimicrobial therapy should be customized immediately to reduce the problem of drug resistance and optimize positive outcomes through appropriate therapy.

Continuous monitoring of mean arterial pressure, central venous pressure, and oxygenation is necessary to evaluate the response to treatment. Initial resuscitation is feasible and should occur in any acute care setting. However, transfer to a critical care unit is necessary for ongoing, vigilant monitoring; more invasive methods of evaluation and treatment; and expert care by critical care practitioners during both early and later stages of sepsis/SIRS. Table 15-14 describes early, goal-directed therapy (42).

Management of sepsis/SIRS during the later stages consists largely of supportive care for organ dysfunction and assessment for resolution and recognition of complications. Assessment centers on adjustment of the antimicrobial regimen as culture reports become available. Sepsis source control continues, which includes measures such as drainage of abscesses and empyema, treatment of cholecystitis/cholangitis, relief of urinary obstruction, surgery for isolation and resection of infarcted bowel tissue, and surgical excision of necrotizing fasciitis and

TABLE 15-14 Management of Sepsis: Early, Goal-Directed Therapy (first 6 hours following recognition of severe sepsis/SIRS)

Goals	Therapeutic Interventions
Central venous pressure 8-12 mm Hg Mean arterial pressure ≥65 mm Hg Urine output ≥0.5 mL per kg per hour Central venous (superior vena cava) or mixed venous oxygen saturation ≥70%	Fluid administration 500-1000 mL crystalloids or 300-500 mL colloids over 30 minutes; repeat according to goals achieved or evidence of intravascular volume overload
	Vasopressors if mean arterial pressure not achieved with fluids: norepinephrine or dopamine
	Packed red blood cells if central venous pressure or mixed venous oxygen saturation not achieved with fluids
Proper diagnosis	At least two blood cultures: one percutaneously and one from each vascular access device
Antimicrobial therapy	Empiric antibiotic therapy within one hour of recognition of severe sepsis/SIRS

gas gangrene (41). Supportive care for organ dysfunction may include cardiovascular support with inotropes, pulmonary protective mechanical ventilation with low volumes and pressure relief, renal replacement therapy, and activated protein C in selected patients. Ongoing management by the critical care team focuses on detection, treatment, and support for newly arising complications such as secondary and/or hospital acquired infection, new-onset organ dysfunction such as hepatic or hematologic failure, DIC, and complications of antimicrobial therapy (41).

Clinical Nurse Specialist Competencies and Spheres of Influence

Sepsis/SIRS progresses very quickly, with high morbidity and mortality rates. Because of proven efficacy of early, goal-directed therapy, timely recognition for positive outcomes is critical. CNSs play a pivotal role in facilitating successful outcomes of sepsis/SIRS for patients and hospitals through application of several CNS competencies, including teaching/mentoring, implementation of evidence-based practice, consultation, and collaboration with numerous health care providers.

Coaching/Teaching/Mentoring

Both formal and informal teaching activities are instrumental in developing knowledgeable caregivers in recognizing a presentation of severe sepsis/SIRS in order to initiate early, goal-directed therapy. Although most teaching takes place in classrooms, most learning does not. One of the greatest assets of CNS practice to the hospital is the availability of expert nurses for informal

teaching of frontline caregivers to guide them through unplanned critical patient events, such as onset of severe sepsis/SIRS. Formal education that focuses on a core group of frontline providers as resource nurses is one approach. These individuals would in turn serve as local "sepsis/SIRS experts," with ongoing availability for assisting other unit nurses with interpretation of relevant clinical data and prompt action. Employing multiple strategies, including classroom sessions, poster boards displayed on the unit, and PowerPoint presentations distributed via email or placed on the institution's intranet increase opportunities for reaching many individuals and are available for continued review of content (43). Topics should include background and statistics of morbidity and mortality of sepsis/SIRS, along with examples of key research findings stressing the beneficial outcomes of early recognition and intervention, with the burden of responsibility for early detection falling largely on the shoulders of the bedside nurse, hence establishing the need-to-know. Recognition of clinical signs of severe sepsis/SIRS is critical content as most of these findings are generally discovered during basic nursing assessment; nurses must realize the potential meaning and urgent need for reporting and summoning medical intervention. Finally, the interventions described in Table 15-14 for early, goal-directed therapy must be stressed so that nurses can begin to assemble supplies and equipment for insertion of intravenous and urinary catheters and administration of fluids and antimicrobials. Nurses must also set into motion processes for transferring the patient to a higher level of care if the patient is not already in the appropriate unit.

A Sepsis Alert Program has been shown to be effective in reducing mortality rate, shortening hospital length of stay, and increasing the proportion of patients discharged to home versus long-term care facility (43). This program consisted of an interdisciplinary group who devised an educational program to increase recognition of sepsis/SIRS and multiple resources to streamline patient identification and implementation of a management plan. Additionally, a management protocol, treatment algorithm to be initiated in the emergency department, and standardized order set were developed as part of the program. This exemplifies the success that can be achieved by integrating several CNS competencies, namely implementation of research in practice, collaboration among primary caregivers, and implementation of a comprehensive education program.

Research/Evidence-Based Practice

Implementing research into practice for improved patient outcomes is a hallmark of CNS practice (44). Severe sepsis/SIRS is a well-researched topic, with much support for the components of early, goal-directed therapy. The CNS may choose one of several models to guide implementation of the severe sepsis guidelines, such as the Iowa Model of Evidence-Based Practice to Promote Quality Care (45), the Stetler Model (46), and ACE Star Model of Evidence (47) to name a few. All of the models require an appraisal of the literature and hierarchical leveling of the evidence, which has been well established and is published with the Surviving Sepsis Campaign Guidelines for Management of Severe Sepsis and Septic Shock (42). Thus, the CNS can then focus on the implementation phase of the selected model, along with baseline and post-implementation data collection of identified outcomes (i.e., decreased incidence of failure-to-rescue, earlier recognition of sepsis, timely administration of antibiotics, and decreased mortality rates).

Consultation

The CNS may need to teach nursing staff how and when to consult the CNS for assistance in managing complex patients such as those who develop severe sepsis/SIRS. A good place to begin is with educating the staff about the predisposing risk factors and subtle signs of early sepsis. CNSs should urge the bedside nurse to contact him/her when seeing these signs for the first time, in order to validate the assessment as well as facilitate rapid intervention and collaboration with the medical team. Once trusting relationships are established and staff realize the CNS is respectful and approachable, they will routinely initiate consultation for challenging patient situations. CNSs commonly participate on Rapid Response Teams (RRT) (48), which is a prime opportunity for staff nurse and CNS consultation. Recognizing when to appropriately access

the RRT is critical to success of the program and in averting undesirable patient outcomes, hence the CNS should provide in depth, up-front education on the presentation of early sepsis and triggers for calling the RRT.

Collaboration

Communication and collaboration among nurses, physicians, pharmacists, and laboratory personnel are fundamental to management of patients with sepsis/SIRS, and contributes to lower mortality rates (49). The bedside clinician is in the best position to recognize initial changes in vital signs and altered mental status. This information must ultimately be communicated to an appropriate physician such as a hospitalist or intensivist for critical care management. However, the CNS often mediates between the bedside clinician and physician to expedite initial fluid resuscitation and other patient stabilizing efforts, along with diagnostic testing and transportation to a higher level of care. Laboratory personnel must recognize the urgency in responding to requests for STAT cultures and prioritize workload accordingly. Likewise, pharmacy personnel must realize the expediency with which antimicrobials must be made available, either through stock drug inventories on the nursing units or rapid delivery upon request. Additionally, doctorally prepared pharmacists (PharmDs) are invaluable resources for prescribing recommendations in septic patients infected with drug resistant organisms, drug allergies, and knowledge of prevalent local organisms. Family members should not be forgotten during this critical time in which events happen quickly; they are typically frightened, have many questions, and need much support; often the CNS identifies and responds to these needs while other team members are active in stabilizing and transporting the patient. Team members working together collaboratively promote prompt intervention and heighten success in the management of patients with severe sepsis/SIRS.

HUMAN IMMUNODEFICIENCY VIRUS INFECTION

HIV and its sequelae have significantly altered the field of immunology since clinical cases were first described in 1981. AIDS was the nomenclature applied to the constellation of immunologic symptoms that includes uncommon infections and/or malignancies in previously healthy individuals and can progress to profound immune collapse and death. Discovery in 1983 of HIV, the virus responsible for AIDS, was an important landmark; once the pathogen was identified, the search for a cure, as well as prevention efforts, became more focused. Although a cure has remained elusive, universal precautions for prevention that became the norm in clinical settings during this time period remain in place today.

Of the two different types of HIV, HIV-1, and HIV-2, HIV-1 is more prevalent, more virulent, but also more responsive to antiretroviral (ARV) medication. HIV-2 is primarily confined to Western Africa. Within the HIV-1 type, there are multiple clades, or subtypes, that are distributed geographically; clade B is most common in the United States, Europe, Japan, and Australia. Disease trajectory, transmission potential, health management, and medication responsiveness do not vary significantly between the different clades. For the purpose of this chapter, we will confine our discussion to HIV-1.

In the United States, the CDC estimates that there are currently between 1 and 1.3 million HIV-1 infected individuals. Experts postulate that between 40,000 and 55,000 people become infected annually in the United States. Approximately one-quarter of infected persons do not know their status, a finding that led to the CDC's recommendation for universal HIV testing for all adolescents and adults. Transmission rates are 3.5 times higher in those unaware of their serostatus, a fact which underscores the important role of universal testing in prevention (50, 51).

Although the epidemic remains primarily identified with gay culture in the United States as in other resource-rich countries, those who are not gay-identified but are nonetheless men who have sex with men (MSM) are perhaps most at risk, due, in part to their detachment from the greater gay culture where prevention efforts are focused and normalized. Globally, at least half of all HIV-positive individuals are women, with their primary source of transmission being heterosexual sex. Parent to child transmission (PTCT) has dramatically decreased since the early days of the epidemic, through the use of ARVs; however, PTCT still occurs, particularly in the absence of prenatal care. In the United States, people of color and young adults 18 to 24 years old are disproportionately represented among HIV-positive individuals, especially the recently diagnosed.

Research studies related to HIV/AIDS have exploded in number over the last decades as the complexity and severity of the illness have provided many fertile study opportunities. The Division of Acquired Immunodeficiency Syndrome (DAIDS), an office under National Institute of Allergy and Infectious Diseases (NIAID) of the National Institutes of Health (NIH), was formed in 1986 to develop and implement the national research agenda to address the HIV/AIDS epidemic. Their efforts are directed in the areas of discovering the basics of HIV/AIDS, HIV medicines as prevention, finding an effective vaccine, topical microbicides, the next-generation of treatment, and behavioral interventions (52).

The Association of Nurses in AIDS Care (ANAC) describes their mission "to promote the individual and collective professional development of nurses involved in the delivery of health care to persons infected or affected by the Human Immunodeficiency virus (HIV) and to promote the health and welfare of infected persons". Their mission includes creating an effective network among nurses in AIDS Care and promoting social awareness concerning issues related to HIV/AIDS. ANAC strives to accomplish the above through research, providing a network of information exchange and advocating, and providing leadership. Inherent in their goals is a commitment to the prevention of HIV infection (53).

In 1989, the Guidelines for Prophylaxis against *Pneumocystis carinii* pneumonia for persons infected with the human immunodeficiency virus became the first HIV-related treatment guideline published by the U.S. Public Health Service, Centers for Disease Control and Prevention (CDC) (54). As of July 2009, over 31 clinical guidelines have been published by national and international government agencies and organizations related to the care and treatment of HIV/AIDS.

Although no specific figures are available regarding HIV/AIDS patients needing acute care, it is clear that hospitalizations as well as mortality for primary HIV/AIDS illness has decreased dramatically since the introduction of HAART therapy. Respiratory infection is the most common reason for admission; however, it is not unusual for patients to have comorbidities that necessitate acute care hospitalization and sometimes it is during these care episodes that a diagnosis of HIV or AIDS is discovered.

Patients with advanced immunosuppression may have prolonged survival, although usually with exacerbations and remissions complicated by therapy-related toxicity and medical and psychiatric comorbid conditions (55).

The HIV/AIDS epidemic contributed to the development and use of needle-free devices. With the passage of the Needlestick Safety and Prevention Act in 2000 by the United States, product design and availability of such systems have improved. However, the use of needle-free systems still varies in the United States.

Etiology

HIV transmission can occur with any introduction of infected body fluids into a susceptible host. While HIV virions are present in all body fluids, they are most prevalent in genital secretions, blood, and breast milk. The amount of virions present in other body fluids is not considered sufficient for transmission. Factors that facilitate sexual transmission include high levels of viremia, "high-risk" sexual behaviors such as unprotected intercourse, and co-infection with ulcerative genital disease in either partner.

Receptive sexual partners are most vulnerable to acquiring infection, but transmission can occur from any sexual activity with body fluid present. Nonconsensual sex is a strong risk factor, whether historical or recent. Other risk behaviors include needle-sharing, which can occur with injection drug use or tattooing, and vertical PTCT during childbirth or breastfeeding. Our understanding of all factors that lead to HIV transmission is incomplete. Fuller understanding of transmission is an important area of research, as new infections rates have remained stagnant in the United States and even increased in some groups, particularly among MSM, 18- to 24-year-olds, and people of color.

Pathophysiology

The ability of HIV to proliferate, despite the presence of innate, adapted, and intrinsic immunity, is responsible for the current pandemic state of the disease. HIV is able to utilize cellular pathways while either neutralizing or effectively hiding from other components of the immune system (56).

Upon transmission, HIV enters the target cell, which is a specialized WBC known as a CD4 cell (sometimes commonly called a T cell), without creating initial damage. The entry process itself appears to trigger a cascade of signals which results in viral replication (56). Following entry, subsequent binding results in conformational changes of the CD4 and ultimately in fusion between the virion and CD4 receptor cell. During fusion, the viral core is injected into the cellular cytoplasm of the CD4 cell and the viral genome is converted into DNA via the reverse transcriptase enzyme of the virus. This enzyme is quite prone to error and lacks proofreading ability, thus resulting in frequent formations of distinct viral variants.

Another viral enzyme, integrase, combines with host factors to insert the viral genome into the host's DNA. Finally, CD4 cells become a veritable virus factory, as mature, infectious virions are produced with the aid of the viral enzyme protease. The incorporation of host DNA into mature virions is a vital factor in HIV's ability to elude host immune response. By completion of this step, infectious virions resemble the cells in which they were produced, thereby not stimulating host response (57).

After transmission, viral replication initially takes place in regional lymph organs. From there, infected CD4 cells and virions migrate systemically, via the blood stream, and result in profound infection. When measured shortly after transmission, initial HIV viral levels in the plasma are dramatically high, often recorded as millions of virions in each milliliter of blood, but as the immune system is activated and begins to exert some level of immune control, viral proliferation decreases to a more steady state, ultimately finding a set point, or range within which the viral level remains for months to years (58).

Clinical Presentation

The first 72 hours after exposure to HIV offers a small window in which transmission can be averted through the use of post-exposure prophylaxis (PEP), which involves treatment with highly active antiretroviral therapy (HAART). The closer to the time of HIV exposure that PEP is initiated, the more effective it will be to prevent infection. During the first 72 hours, if unchecked, the virus replicates at the site of entry and infiltrates the surrounding lymph nodes. By day seven post-transmission, HIV infection becomes systemic, affecting all lymph tissue compartments. Within 10 days, most CD4 cells are infected with HIV; the majority of them are depleted between days 10 and 21 (57). CD4 depletion is most profound in the gut-associated lymphoid tissue (GALT), which is the largest lymph organ in the body (59, 60).

Individuals who are newly infected with HIV often experience symptoms from their high viremic state. Severity of symptoms ranges from none to life-threatening, with most people describing their symptoms as ". . . the worse flu I've ever had." Approximately two-thirds of those newly infected experience some degree of symptoms (56). People frequently seek testing at this point, although traditional HIV tests can take weeks to months to convert to seropositivity.

Symptoms that may bring newly infected people into acute care include fever, rash, gastrointestinal symptoms, headache, pharyngitis with or without ulcers, myalgia, arthralgia, and lymphadenopathy. Table 15-15 shows the signs and symptoms most commonly associated with

TABLE 15–15 Signs and Symptoms Associated With Having Acute HIV Infection

Sign or Symptom	Approximate Prevalence (%)[a]
Fever	>70
Lymphadenopathy	35-70
Sore throat	40-70
Rash	20-70
Joint pain	30-60
Diarrhea	25-50
Anorexia or weight loss	15-70
Night sweats	50
Myalgia	40-70
Malaise or fatigue	>70
Headache	30-40
Vomiting	10-30
Too sick to work	60
Hospitalized	10-20
Oral or genital ulcer disease	10-20

From Zatola and Pilcher (2007): Diagnosis and management of acute HIV infection. Infectious Disease Clinics of North America; 21(1). Kidlington, Oxford, OXS 1GB, UK, with permission).

acute HIV infection (59). Severity of symptoms is often predictive of prognosis.

Diagnosis

Evaluation of suspected acute HIV infection should include a complete history and physical examination and laboratory testing. Specific HIV testing should include two HIV tests for confirmation; among the options are rapid HIV antibody (Ab) tests, Western blot, Ab enzyme immunoassay (EIA), indirect fluorescent AB (IFA), p24 antigen (Ag), and/or an HIV RNA. In the presence of an indeterminate or positive HIV test, the results of a less sensitive Ab test, often called a "detuned," can support the diagnosis of acute or early HIV infection.

Further laboratory testing should include CD4 count, CBC, chemistry panel, and assessment for the presence of other infectious diseases, such as sexually transmitted infections (STIs) and hepatitis A, B, and C. If diagnosed, a phenotype and/or genotype of the virus should be ordered, to determine the presence of any transmitted viral mutations. Laboratory findings often include leukopenia, CD4 lymphopenia, thrombocytopenia, and elevated liver function tests. Co-infection with other STIs is also not uncommon. Physical findings include diffuse lymphadenopathy; fever to 40°C; pharyngitis; rash; oral, anal, or vaginal ulcerations; meningeal signs; and oral or vaginal thrush (58).

All people who present to the hospital with severe flulike symptoms, especially if they have a history of behaviors that are considered high risk, should be screened for HIV. Acute HIV should also be on the differential diagnosis of any person diagnosed with aseptic meningitis.

Management

Once a diagnosis has been made, management of acute HIV-1 includes supportive care, use of antibiotics as needed, and consideration of HAART. Viral replication is the target of HIV-1 therapies, with the overarching goals of HAART being nonreplication of the virus and improved immunologic status. HAART initiated during the acute phase of HIV takes advantage of an important window of opportunity to alter the course of the disease. If prescribed during acute or early HIV infection, HAART can improve the clinical outcomes and seroconversion symptoms of the acutely infected individual and may offer long-term benefits. These include limiting latent HIV reservoirs, limiting HIV diversification that can arise during early exponential replication, protection of host immune response, and reduction in immune activation in the patient. Long-term benefits are manifested in lower rates of opportunistic infections (OIs), greater and more specific CD4 cell recovery, and less progression to AIDS in patients who received HAART during the acute stages of HIV (61, 62).

The decision to initiate HAART shortly after HIV transmission must include consideration of the potential for transmitted viral mutations. In one cohort of acutely infected individuals, 10% were infected with viral mutations (63). Some mutations were benign; however, some were treatment-limiting. One single mutation, K103N, can confer resistance to an entire class of ARVs, the non-nucleotide reverse transcriptase inhibitors (NNRTIs). Phenotype and/or genotype tests, drawn as soon as HIV is suspected, may take up to 4 weeks for results; therefore, early HAART should not include the NNRTI class of medications until lack of the K103N mutation is proved.

Currently there are five classes of ARVs, each targeting a different stage of viral replication. The first ARV class developed, the nucleoside/nucleotide reverse transcriptase inhibitors (NRTIs), inhibit the reverse transcriptase enzyme necessary for the first step of viral replication. A combination of two or even three NRTIs is not strong enough to halt viral replication, although they form an important backbone of therapy. At least one other class of ARVs must be added to prescribe full HAART. NNRTIs also inhibit the same enzyme, but are generally more effective at viral suppression than NRTIs and have a longer half-life. Their addition to two NRTIs would create a sufficient HAART regimen (64, 65).

Protease inhibitors (PIs) inhibit the enzyme protease. This was the second class of ARVs developed and the use of PIs, in combination with NRTIs, changed the trajectory of the disease. HAART, commonly known as the "AIDS cocktail" because of the necessity to combine at least two different classes of medication, became possible with the introduction of PIs and changed HIV from an almost universally fatal disease to a chronic one.

The other two classes of ARVs, integrase inhibitors (IIs) and entry inhibitors (EIs), are generally reserved for later stages of AIDS, although studies are under way to determine their role in acute HIV treatment. IIs target the enzyme integrase, which helps HIV incorporate in host DNA. EIs halt either the initial fusion of the HIV virion onto the CD4 cell or entry of viral genome into the target cell.

Treatment considerations involve choosing the strongest, most effective HAART regimen with the least side effects. As mentioned earlier, NNRTIs should be avoided until phenotype and/or genotype results are available. If NNRTIs were prescribed to an individual with resistant virus, results could be incomplete viral suppression, which, in turn, could lead to further viral mutations.

ACQUIRED IMMUNODEFICIENCY SYNDROME (AIDS): HIV/AIDS PROGRESSION

In the current HAART milieu, HIV-positive individuals have experienced a significant decrease in AIDS-related morbidity and mortality compared with the nascent days of the epidemic. Early diagnosis, consistent health maintenance and access to HAART have led to longer life expectancy and a dramatic decrease in complications which can lead to hospitalization. Health issues that present with normal aging are similar between infected and uninfected persons, although those who are HIV-positive experience an accelerated aging process compared with uninfected individuals, the reasons for which remain elusive (66).

A wide array of health issues may bring the HIV-positive individual into acute care. HIV/AIDS may be the presenting diagnosis with hospitalization or may be an incidental diagnosis. Although a critical factor in a patient's medical history, HIV has assumed a more chronic role in health management. This section will focus on AIDS progression, opportunistic infections (OIs), co-infections, and other HIV considerations.

Etiology

Infection with the HIV virus is necessary for the development of AIDS, although other factors are often cited as increasing the risk of AIDS diagnosis. Poverty, limited access to health care, gender inequities (especially when associated with inability to negotiate sexual safety), stigma, racism, internalized homophobia, lack of social support, depression, and substance abuse have all been noted as potential co-factors for AIDS (67). Progression to AIDS is not inevitable for HIV-positive individuals, especially if patients are able to engage in their health care consistently and from an early stage in their illness.

Pathophysiology

Acute and early HIV infection pathophysiology, as discussed earlier, results in tremendous changes in one's immune system. Many HIV-positive patients are not diagnosed in this stage, however, and their immunologic changes are effectively silent. Primary HIV, generally considered the first 6 months post-transmission, is followed for most people by a prolonged period of asymptomatic disease, which typically lasts between 2 and 10 years. Post-transmission, after the virus has established itself systemically and is present in multiple latent reservoirs, the immune system remains in a state of chronic activation. Regardless of the presence or absence of overt symptoms, CD4 depletion continues as HIV replication persists in untreated HIV (67).

Symptomatic HIV infection usually occurs between 2 and 10 years post-transmission. Gradual decline in CD4 counts signals loss of immune control and is often an indicator for HAART initiation. Symptomatic HIV can occur at any CD4 level, but is most often associated with CD4 counts ranging from 200 to 500 cells/mm³. Symptoms accompanying CD4 depletion may include fatigue, fever, weight loss, and frequent infections; patients often initiate HAART during this stage (65).

Advanced HIV disease, or AIDS, is defined by the CDC as a CD4 count less than 200 cells/mm³ and/or the presence of an OI, HIV-related malignancy, or wasting syndrome. Without treatment, progression to AIDS is inevitable for most HIV-positive individuals (68). One subgroup of HIV-positive people, known as long-term non-progressors (LTNPs), does not follow the normal trajectory from transmission to AIDS. This small subgroup, also known as "elite controllers," have a unique ability to control the replication of HIV without medications. Even with complete viral control, however, some loss of CD4 cells occurs. LTNPs can also be affected by the introduction of another viral strain which could override the immunologic control previously achieved. Other than the possible exception of LTNPs, HIV-positive individuals will require HAART at some point in their disease trajectory, to prevent AIDS.

Clinical Presentation

Advanced AIDS is much less common in the HAART era, particularly in resource-rich settings. Introduction of effective therapy halts viral replication, decreases the rate of CD4 depletion, preserves immune response and prevents the development of devastating infections that are associated with the profound immune collapse of AIDS. Some patients, however, present to the hospital with a disease or diseases that result from full immune suppression; their HIV and AIDS diagnoses may occur simultaneously within the acute care setting. These individuals may have never previously tested for HIV or, despite having tested positive years earlier, have either not accessed health care or have chosen not to pursue traditional medication therapies.

Aids-Defining Conditions

Late-stage AIDS is associated with multiple complications. OIs and malignancies are foremost among severe late stage sequelae. OIs are infections, often relatively commonplace and controllable with an intact immune system, which can be physically devastating in the absence of immune control. A full list of OIs is found in the CDC's AIDS-defining conditions (Table 15-16) and includes cytomegalovirus (CMV), toxoplasmosis, cryptococcal meningitis (CM), and progressive multifocal leukoencephalopathy (PML). Patients who present in an immunocompromised state but have not developed an OI should receive prophylactic treatment to prevent the development of an OI (68-70).

Specific medication that should be prescribed for OI prevention and the different CD4 levels that require prophylaxis are listed in Table 15-17. Beyond prevention of an OI, treatment for OIs includes appropriate antibiotic, antifungal, and/or antiviral medication and careful consideration of HAART initiation. Delay of HAART is associated with HIV progression; however, treatment initiation in the setting of immunologic compromise can lead to a paradoxical worsening of the presenting infection

TABLE 15–16 AIDS-Defining Conditions

AIDS-Defining Conditions

- Bacterial infections, multiple or recurrent
- Candidiasis of bronchi, trachea, or lungs
- Candidiasis of esophagus
- Cervical cancer, invasive
- Coccidiocomycosis, disseminated or extrapulmonary
- Cryptococcosis, extrapulmonary
- Cryptosporidiosis, chronic (>1 month duration)
- Cytomegalovirus (other than liver, spleen, or nodes), onset at age >1 month
- Cytomegalovirus retinitis (with loss of vision)
- Encephalopathy, HIV-related
- Herpes simplex: chronic ulcer (>1 month duration) or bronchitis, pneumonitis, or esophagitis (onset at age >1 month)
- Histoplasmosis, disseminated or extrapulmonary
- Isosporiasis, chronic intestinal (>1 month duration)
- Kaposi sarcoma
- Lymphoid interstitial pneumonia or pulmonary lymphoid hyperplasia complex
- Lymphoma, Burkitt (or equivalent term)
- Lymphoma, immunoblastic (or equivalent term)
- Lymphoma, primary, of brain
- *Mycobacterium avium* complex or *Mycobacterium kansasii,* disseminated or extrapulmonary
- *Mycobacterium tuberculosis* of any site, pulmonary, disseminated or extrapulmonary
- *Mycobacterium,* other species or unidentified species, disseminated or extrapulmonary
- *Pneumocystis jirovecii (previously carinii)* pneumonia
- Pneumonia, recurrent
- Progressive multifocal leukoencephalopathy
- *Salmonella* septicemia, recurrent
- Toxoplasmosis of brain, onset at age >1 month
- Wasting syndrome attributed to HIV

TABLE 15–17 CD4 Levels and Appropriate Medications for OI prevention

CD4 Level	Preventive Regimen	Alternative Regimen	Disease Prevention
<200 cells/mm^3	TMP/Sulfa	• Dapsone plus Pyrimethamine and Leucovirin • Aerosolized Pentamidine	*Pneumocystis carinii* (now known as *Pneumocystis jirovecii*) pneumonia
<100 cells/mm^3	TMP/Sulfa	• Dapsone plus Pyrimethamine • Atovaquone	*Toxoplasma gondii*
<50 cells/ mm^3	Azithromycin *or* Clarithromycin	• Rifabutin	*Mycobacterium avium* complex
Any CD4 level	Vaccinations		HBV, HAV, influenza, VZV, and *streptococcus pneumonia*

known as immune reconstitution inflammatory syndrome (IRIS). Either worsening of a current infection or reactivation of a past infection can occur with IRIS, which generally develops within 8 weeks of HAART initiation. Patients whose CD4 counts were less than 50 cells/mm when starting HAART are most at risk for development of IRIS (68, 70).

IRIS management depends on the specific infection, but often includes continuation of both OI therapy and HAART. Since inflammation is the underlying pathology, treatment with either corticosteroids or NSAIDs may relieve symptoms. Corticosteroids are particularly useful in life-threatening complications of IRIS such as tracheal compression or ARDS (70).

Malignancies which are AIDS-defining include lymphomas, invasive cervical cancer, and Kaposi sarcoma. As previously noted, the presence of any of these OIs or malignancies is considered an AIDS-defining event by the CDC. AIDS-related malignancies are best treated by a multidisciplinary team in a facility that has extensive experience with their management. Therapies depend on the specific diagnosis, but may include localized treatment, chemotherapy, radiation therapy, or surgical excision, as well as HAART initiation or optimization (71). As in the case of OIs, introduction of HAART may result in IRIS, which also requires intensive medical oversight.

Co-Infections

Although not considered AIDS-defining, co-infections are relatively common and may increase HIV complications. The most common co-infections, tuberculosis (TB), hepatitis C (HCV) and hepatitis B (HBV) are discussed below.

TB is a frequent co-infection with HIV, particularly in resource-limited settings. Guidelines for TB treatment are not based on HIV seropositivity, although intermittent TB regimens may not be recommended for HIV-positive individuals. Likewise, HAART guidelines are not changed by TB status; a patient who needs to initiate HAART should not await completion of TB therapy to do so. IRIS, as described above, is a potential complication with treatment. In the case of IRIS associated with TB, a 4-week course of prednisone for mild to moderate TB-related IRIS can lead to reduction in hospitalizations and greater improvement of symptoms (70).

HCV is another important co-infection with HIV. Due, in part, to shared epidemiologic risk factors, between 30% and 50% of HIV infected people are co-infected with HCV. The importance of HCV in HIV care was highlighted with the finding in the post-HAART era that once HIV was controlled with HAART, liver disease became the leading cause of mortality among HIV-positive persons. HCV was the most prevalent co-factor in these deaths (72-74). Co-infection can hasten progression to end-stage liver disease (ESLD) and necessitates careful management of both infections.

A multidisciplinary team, including infectious disease experts, hepatologists, advanced practice nurses, and social workers should manage HCV treatment for HIV/HCV co-infected individuals.

Pegylated interferon in combination with weight-based ribavirin for 48 to 72 weeks is the current HCV treatment of choice for patients with compensated liver disease. Sustained virologic response (SVR) or eradication of HCV is the goal of this therapy and, while less common with co-infected patients than those infected with HCV alone, this goal is attainable. Patients with decompensated liver disease or ESLD should be referred for liver transplant evaluation (74). Careful oversight of HAART must be maintained, as many ARVs undergo hepatic metabolization and may interact with anti-HCV therapies.

Hepatitis B (HBV) co-infection is also prevalent in certain parts of the world. Although less prevalent in resource-rich areas, co-infection with HBV and HIV requires special consideration, particularly regarding medications. Several ARVs also have HBV suppressive qualities and must be carefully managed, to avoid either HIV- or HBV-resistant mutations arising from incorrect use and/or dosage. A recent study indicates good efficacy, in relation to viral suppression of both viruses, of tenofovir-containing regimens for those co-infected with HIV and HBV (73).

Diagnosis

Universal HIV testing became a CDC mandate in 2006, with the goal that HIV testing become incorporated into routine health care (52). At least 25% of people who are HIV-positive do not know their serostatus, which increases the risk of continued transmission. In some settings, opt-out HIV testing is performed on all hospitalized patients, in order to both normalize and destigmatize the testing process (75). Positive results may be incidental to the acute episode, or they may help to guide management decisions.

Case Report.

A 49-year-old Caucasian male is admitted to the hospital with "back pain." Tested for HIV as a part of the CDC's universal mandate, the patient is found to have a preliminary positive HIV result. He denied risk factors for HIV, but acknowledged no previous testing. His work-up for back pain revealed diffuse abdominal lymphadenopathy and an abdominal mass. Armed with this finding and his HIV test results, the team ordered confirmatory HIV testing (repeat Ab and IFA, as well as RNA and CD4 tests) and an abdominal MRI and biopsy. HIV infection was confirmed, and he was found to have abdominal lymphoma. Appropriate treatment for both disease entities was instituted.

The above case study illustrates the importance of universal testing, even in persons considered to be low risk. Diagnosis of HIV in an individual with late-stage AIDS may be confounded by the possibility of a negative HIV Ab test due to attenuated immune response. In a patient with a high index of suspicion for HIV, HIV RNA testing may be necessary.

Management

HIV-positive persons are often faced with a multitude of issues. HIV affects one's physical status, as well as psychosocial, emotional, and spiritual well-being. An interprofessional approach is most effective in partnering with patients for their optimal care. Although nurses affect each patient's life regardless of the diagnosis, in the case of HIV nursing, a strong association exists between patient/provider relationships and patient engagement and satisfaction, as well as quality and access to care and adherence to medications.

Support, education, and treatment are all important components of HIV management. Patient education must include prevention information, to help prevent further transmission and protect the HIV-positive individual from becoming either superinfected with a different strain of HIV or co-infected with another pathogen. While many people are aware of how HIV is transmitted, a lack of understanding persists in how HIV is not transmitted. Many overestimate transmission potential through casual contact, which can result in isolating or stigmatizing behaviors (76). Nursing advocacy and education can help ameliorate these issues.

HAART, as previously noted, is necessary at some point in HIV's trajectory to halt viral replication and enhance immune response. Optimal timing of treatment initiation and choice of initial ARVs remains subjective, and many factors must be taken into consideration. Presence of other comorbidities, such as cardiovascular, hepatic or renal disease, a history of diabetes mellitus and/or hyperlipidemia, presence of co-infections, reproductive status, and concomitant medications should all be assessed (65).

Current WHO and International AIDS Society (IAS) guidelines are being revised to reflect recent findings that earlier treatment results in improved morbidity and mortality rates and may be associated with fewer side effects.

These findings are preliminary, but may result in changes in treatment initiation guidelines. Table 15-18 reflects current guidelines and new findings (65).

Current recommendations suggest a combination of 2 nucleoside/nucleotide reverse transcriptase inhibitors (NRTIs) and either a non-nucleoside reverse transcriptase inhibitor (NNRTI) or a boosted protease inhibitor (PI) regimen to be optimal for initial therapy. No current studies have established the superiority of either NNRTI-based or PI-based regimens, and these can be safely switched once viral suppression has occurred (65). A NRTI backbone with either an EI or II is not generally used for initial therapies, although studies are currently ongoing to determine the efficacy and tolerability of such regimens for the treatment-naïve population.

Patient monitoring of treatment response includes HIV RNA testing, with the goal being an undetectable viral load (currently less than 50 copies/mL), and CD4 counts to ascertain immune response. A metabolic panel and CBC will allow assessment of potential toxicities. Adherence is of particular concern with HAART. Studies have shown that less than 95% adherence is associated with treatment failure and can result in viral mutations, which may be treatment-limiting.

Special Populations
Pregnancy

Universal HIV testing is recommended as a routine part of prenatal care for all pregnant women in the United States. HIV screening should be performed with standard prenatal testing and, if indicated, repeated in the third trimester. Indications for repeat testing include geographical areas with high rates of HIV among pregnant women, and a patient history of high risk behaviors and/or any symptoms which may indicate early infection (52).

Expectant mothers who are HIV-positive must be monitored by an obstetrician who is well-versed in HIV care. If the patient was on HAART prior to pregnancy, she should normally continue HAART throughout her pregnancy, although specific ARVs may need to be altered. Efavirenz (EFV), an NNRTI, should be avoided

TABLE 15–18 Guidelines Related to Treatment Initiation of HAART

Clinical Presentation	CD4 Count	HIV RNA	Treatment
Symptomatic	Any	Any	Initiate HAART
Asymptomatic	<200 cells/mm³	Any	Initiate HAART, OI prophylaxis
Asymptomatic	201-350 cells/mm³	Any	Recommend HAART
Asymptomatic	>350 cells/mm³	>100,000 copies/mL	Consider HAART
Asymptomatic	>350 cells/mm³	<100,000 copies/mL	Discuss HAART

for its teratogenicity, and two NRTIs, stavudine (d4T) or didanosine (ddI), should also be avoided, if possible, to reduce the risk of lactic acidosis. If d4T and ddI cannot be avoided, lactate levels must be monitored throughout the pregnancy. OI prophylaxis, if necessary, must be carefully monitored, and folic acid supplements should be encouraged (77).

Treatment-naïve women who do not meet the guidelines for HAART initiation should be prescribed short-term antiretroviral therapy (START) in their second trimester, for prevention of parent-to-child transmission (PTCT). Their START regimen should not include EFV, d4T, or ddI, as noted above, and may be discontinued after delivery, ideally when the mother's viral load is undetectable. Discontinuation of START should take into consideration the half-life of each separate ARV component, to avoid a less-than fully suppressive regimen and the potential of subsequent viral mutations (77).

Elective vaginal delivery is a reasonable option for HIV-positive women who have an undetectable HIV RNA. A cesarean section should be scheduled for mothers with a detectable viral load with any complications. Post-exposure prophylaxis (PEP) is indicated for the infant in the case of detectable maternal viremia. PEP should also be offered if maternal HIV diagnosis occurs simultaneously with or just following delivery. If an expectant mother presents in labor, an HIV screen should be obtained and PEP offered, if indicated (77).

Post-delivery, breastfeeding should be avoided if possible. Mothers in resource-limited settings may not have formula feeding as an option for their neonates; however, in the settings in which many CNSs practice in the United States, this should not be an issue. Another important postnatal concern is maternal contraception. Contraceptive issues must take into account potential interactions between hormonal therapies and HAART. For the infant, post-delivery HAART should be continued for the first 4 weeks of life, and HIV DNA Ab testing should be performed serially for the first 3 months of the infant's life (77).

Psychiatric Issues

Psychiatric concerns play a very important role in HIV. Any psychiatric diagnosis can increase the risk of HIV acquisition; comorbid HIV and psychiatric diagnoses can also worsen either condition. Psychiatric complications with HIV are generally divided into three categories: cognitive impairment, affective disorders, and psychotic disorders.

Cognitive changes in HIV can range from mild impairment to severe dementia. Subtle neurocognitive changes can be appreciated even in early HIV, but profound dysfunction is most noted in late-stage AIDS. HAART has significantly decreased the rates of HIV-associated dementia, but the central nervous system (CNS) remains vulnerable to HIV infection. Many ARVs have limited penetration of the blood-brain barrier, allowing localized viral replication to persist (78).

Affective disorders are disproportionately found in the HIV-positive population. Depression is reported in 15% to 40% of all HIV persons. This diagnosis increases HIV transmission, both independently and by increasing the risk of substance use, which leads to further increased HIV risk. In those already infected with HIV, depression impairs immune response and frequently leads to nonadherence with medications (72). Stigma, social isolation, discrimination, and substance abuse are all potential precursors for depression and can also exacerbate the depression that may arise from the diagnosis of HIV (76, 78). Antidepressants, support groups, and counseling are all possible therapies for HIV-related depression.

Another affective disorder, manic syndrome, is noted in about 8% of HIV-positive individuals. Diagnosis of mania is challenging; whether it is a separate diagnosis or related to AIDS-dementia can be difficult to ascertain. Traditional treatment with mood-stabilizers has not proven effective, and antipsychotics appear to be a better choice of medications in treatment for mania within the HIV-positive population (78).

Between 0.5% and 20% of HIV-infected people experience psychoses. As with other psychiatric disorders, a preexisting diagnosis of psychotic disorder can increase risk of HIV transmission. A psychotic disorder may also be difficult to delineate from HIV-associated cognitive impairment, although psychosis is distinguishable from HIV encephalopathy (78).

Finally, substance use confounds the psychiatric picture of HIV-positive individuals. Prevalence of use is high in patients with either HIV or psychiatric diagnoses. Up to 75% of HIV-infected persons report illicit drug use. Drug use increases transmission risks; it has also been hypothesized that drug use hastens HIV progression (72, 78). Additionally, some patients self-medicate with alcohol or drugs to ameliorate psychiatric or HIV symptoms. A thorough psychiatric history, including substance use, is warranted on all HIV-positive patients.

Incidental HIV

As HIV has moved from a terminal to more chronic disease, HIV-positive persons are living longer and experiencing the effects of normal, although accelerated, aging processes. Patients may be hospitalized with diagnoses unrelated to HIV as the general population and their HIV history, although pertinent, may be incidental to their hospitalization. A critical point to remember is that, if the hospitalized HIV-positive patient is taking HAART, they must continue their therapy as previously ordered unless there is contraindication to doing so. Even brief interruptions in HAART may result in treatment-limiting viral mutations that arise from incomplete suppression of HIV replication. Some ARVs are available in liquid form, for those unable to swallow pills.

If HAART suspension is indicated, care must be taken to ensure correct discontinuation. The half-life of ARVs varies and at no point should there be presence of one ARV without a full complement of suppressive medication. Guidance by HIV specialists and/or pharmacists is critical to avoid later complications.

An interprofessional approach is most effective in working with HIV-positive patients. As HIV is a rapidly evolving field, the presence of an HIV specialist is critical for HIV care. Advanced practice nurses add both nursing and collaborative perspectives, and provide the patient and their family with care and support. Consultation with additional specialties, as indicated, will ensure optimal outcome for HIV-positive patients in acute care settings.

Clinical Nurse Specialist Competencies and Spheres of Influence

Most acute care CNS's will at some point be coordinating the care for HIV/AIDS patients and will need to facilitate quality care via the nursing staff and in the system in which he/she practices. Thus, the various CNS competencies are generally interchangeable due to the close association between these complex illnesses.

Clinical Expert/Direct Care and Coaching/Teaching/Mentoring

Assisting the staff nurses in providing current evidence-based care is a key role of the acute care CNS. Role-modeling a warm, nonjudgmental approach that nurtures patient participation, connection, and validation is most effective in HIV care (79). CNS's are uniquely qualified to offer these attributes and to partner with patients for best outcomes.

If HIV is a new diagnosis for the patient, assisting the patient care team to understand the psychological implications for the patient will be relevant. Although there is much patient education that pertains to a new diagnosis of HIV, an absolutely essential concept for the patient and family is to have an accurate concept of mode of transmission. Patient teaching related to HAART therapy, if initiated, is paramount prior to discharge, as patients must understand their regimens and commit to the importance of adherence, lest they risk development of resistant virus. A strong patient/provider relationship also reaps benefits in improved adherence (79). CNSs can play an important role in ensuring the patient is "plugged in" to appropriate follow-up care and support and that patient and significant others understand the benefits of such follow-up.

Supportive care includes adequate hydration, nutrition, and treatment of co-infections, all which the CNS can impact by their clinical availability via bedside rounds and participation in interprofessional care conferences. Generally, hospitalizations for acute HIV infections are brief. Discharge planning must include referral to appropriate providers who are well versed in HIV care.

Promotion of specialty certification to staff nurses in order to enhance patient safety is a valuable way in which the CNS can contribute. Role or specialty certification may be relevant, dependent upon the area of practice and/or coverage. The HIV/AIDS Nursing Certification Board offers an ACRN (AIDS Certified Registered Nurse) to RN's who meet eligibility criteria (80).

Consultation

CNS's may serve as experts to guide protocols of care. Assessing staff nurse's knowledge related to HIV/AIDS and identifying opportunities for staff development demonstrates the consultant role. The CNS can also facilitate product evaluations related to medical therapy and pharmaceuticals used in the care of HIV/AIDS patients. Working closely with the interprofessional team to keep a close eye on any interruption in HAART medications for various diagnostics or comorbidities which would alter the medication regimen is critical. "Partial menus" of HAART therapy can lead to virus mutation. Due to the nature of HIV, consultation with medical sub-specialties such as infectious disease will be important in order to establish an appropriate pharmacologic regimen based on current illness.

Systems Leadership

Safety principles include reviewing the mode of transmission for staff exposures and reassuring of the extremely low risk of transmission, unless an adverse event occurred. Ordinary precautions which are taken for any body substance are appropriate for the care of HIV-infected patients. The CNS can facilitate communication of the procedure for any exposures and the reasons for immediate action in pursuing possible treatment for such exposure. Blood-borne exposures contain the highest risk of exposure to nurses. Facilitation of needleless systems, if not in use, is an important system wide focus of the CNS.

Universal HIV testing of all patients in the hospital is now proposed by a variety of government and professional organizations as one solution to aid in earlier diagnosis. Benefits would include actual cost-savings by offering earlier treatment which may result in fewer complications. It is also suggested that by offering testing to every hospitalized patient regardless of risk factors, stigmatization would decrease. Certainly, the CNS has a valuable role in assisting with adoption of such a policy. The CNS could assist in the education of various disciplines and in the systemwide implementation of universal testing.

Collaboration

Collaboration with other disciplines is essential in the care of the HIV patient. Patients with HIV require a multitude of services and often benefit from a case management approach. Social work, pharmacy, chaplaincy, dietary, and rehabilitation services are just some of the disciplines that are often involved in patients diagnosed with HIV. CNSs who serve as case managers would offer invaluable care toward managing these complex patients. If dedicated case managers are not present within the patient's system of care, then referrals to ensure that the patient has appropriate assessment of needs and follow-up care, including a holistic approach, are essential. Support groups exist for both patient and significant others.

Research/Evidence-Based Practice

Staying abreast and communicating best care practices in the field of HIV/AIDS care is important. As guidelines and clinical research become available, awareness and communication of such standards related to nursing care is an important role for the CNS. Facilitation of any research protocols within the acute care environment provides opportunities for the CNS to educate staff nurses on the elements of research and to participate in the process. Conducting a "journal club" focusing on HIV/AIDS nursing is an excellent method of facilitating application of evidence-based nursing.

Ethical Decision-Making/Moral Agency/Advocacy

The CNS is in a unique role to impact policy at the bedside and in the greater health care arena. Advocating for the HIV/AIDS patient by supporting them in initiation of advance directives is important. Keeping a keen eye and ear to the patient's situation may provide unique opportunities for the CNS to intervene on their behalf and facilitate both inpatient and community referrals.

As CNS's recognize their greater role related to health care policy, participation in political arenas to impact policy and regulations which contribute to patient safety and outcomes is essential. Supporting the proposed universal testing measures via membership in a professional organization which promotes this change would be one way of advocating for patients with HIV/AIDS. Liddicoat notes that targeted testing on the basis of risk behaviors fails to identify a substantial number of persons who are HIV infected (81). See Table 15-19 for CDC published recommendations in 2006 which include HIV testing in all health-care settings (82).

As CNs are educators, a visit with their government representatives to help them analyze the above change would open lines of communication and provide one more opportunity for nursing to be a necessary voice in making such national and international policy decisions.

As Lewis states, "the goal of practice for CNS's in HIV/AIDS is high-quality health care, that is, care that has a significant and measureable effect on patient outcomes, cost-effectiveness, and nursing care practices. CNSs can achieve these goals through the integration of research and education, manipulation of organizational factors, contributions toward social policy, and political actions for change (83)."

TABLE 15–19 CDC Recommendations for HIV Testing in Health care Settings

- HIV screening is recommended for patients in all health care settings after the patient is notified that testing will be performed unless the patient declines (opt-out screening).
- Persons at high risk for HIV infection should be screened for HIV at least annually.
- Separate written consent for HIV testing should not be required; general consent for medical care should be considered sufficient to encompass consent for HIV testing.
- Prevention counseling should not be required with HIV diagnostic testing or as part of HIV screening programs in health care settings

References

1. Galel SA, Malone JM, Viele MK. Transfusion medicine. In Greer JP, Foerster J, Lukens JN, et al, editors. Wintrobe's Clinical Hematology. 11th edition. Philadelphia: Lippincott Williams & Wilkins; 2004:831-882.

2. Monahan FD, Neighbors M, Sands JK, et al. Phipp's Medical-Surgical Nursing: Health and Illness Perspectives. 8th edition. St. Louis, MO: Mosby; 2007:2427-2431.

3. Transfusion-Related Acute Lung Injury. Retrieved September 24, 2008, from http://www.aabb.org/Content/About_Blood/Facts_About_Blood_and_Blood_Banking/fabloodtrali.htm

4. Kleinman S, Gajic O, Nunes E. Promoting recognition and prevention of transfusion-related acute lung injury. Crit Care Nurse 2007;27(4):49-53.

5. Lieberman LL. Anaphylaxis and Anaphylactoid reactions. In Adkinson FF, Yuninger JW, Busse WW, et al, editors. Middleton's Allergy Principles & Practice. 6th edition. St Louis, MO: Mosby; 2003:1497-1522.

6. Toraason M, Sussman G, Biagini R, et al. Latex allergy in the workplace. Toxicol Sci 2000;58 (1):5-14.

7. Lin RY, Shah SN. Increasing hospitalizations due to angioedema in the United States. Ann Allergy Asthma Immunol 2008;101(2): 185-192.

8. Anaphylaxis. Retrieved August 18, 2011 from http://www.merckmanuals.com/professional/sec14/ch176/ch176c.html?qt=anaphylaxis&alt=sh#v996084

9. Colorado Hospital Association. Colorado Wristband Standardization Project, 2006. Retrieved August 18, 2011 from http://www.cha.com/index.php?option=com_content&task=view&id=939&Itemid=179

10. Rich RR, Fleisher TA, Shearer WT, et al, editors. Preface. In Clinical Immunology. 2nd edition. London: Mosby; 2001:1.

11. Lipsky P, Kavanaugh A. Rheumatoid arthritis. In Rich RR, Fleisher TA, Shearer WT, et al, editors. Clinical Immunology. 2nd edition. London: Mosby; 2001:61.1-20.

12. Rindfleisch JA, Muller D. Diagnosis and management of rheumatoid arthritis. Am Fam Phys 2005;72(6). Retrieved October 23, 2008. http://www.hopkins-arthritis.org/arthritis-info/rheumatoid-arthritis/rheum_clin_path.html

13. Bathon JM. Rheumatoid arthritis pathophysiology. Retrieved October 23, 2008, from http://www.hopkins-arthritis.org/arthritis-info/rheumatoid-arthritis/rheum_clin_path.html

14. Firestein GS. Etiology and pathogenesis of rheumatoid arthritis. In Ruddy S, Harris ED, Sledge CB, et al, editors. Kelley's Textbook of Rheumatology. 7th edition. Philadelphia: WB Saunders; 2005:996-1042.

15. Karie S, Gandjbakhch F, Janus N, et al. Kidney management in RA patients: prevalence and implication on RA-related drugs management: the MATRIX study. Rheumatology 2008;47:350-354.

16. Harris ED. Clinical features of rheumatoid arthritis. In Ruddy S, Harris ED, Sledge CB, et al, editors. Kelley's Textbook of Rheumatology. 7th edition. Philadelphia: WB Saunders; 2005:1043-1078.

17. Ciftci O, Yilmaz S, Topcu S, et al. Impaired microvascular function and increased intima-media thickness in rheumatoid arthritis. Atherosclerosis 2007;198(2):332-337.

18. Hannawi S, Haluska B, Marwick TH, et al. Atherosclerotic disease is increased in recent-onset rheumatoid arthritis: a critical role for inflammation. Arthritis Res Ther 2007;9(6):116-124.

19. Symmons D. Ischemic stroke: Another feature of accelerated atherosclerosis in rheumatoid factor? Arthritis Rheum 2008;59(8):1051-1053.

20. Saraux A, Betrthelot M, Cales G, et al. Ability of the American College of Rheumatology 1987 criteria to predict rheumatoid arthritis in patients with early arthritis and classification of these patients two years later. Arthritis Rheum 2001;44:2485-2491.

21. Barr C. A nursing guide to infusion therapy with abatacept for the treatment of rheumatoid arthritis. J Infus Nurs 2007;30(2):96-104.

22. American College of Rheumatology Subcommittee on Rheumatoid Arthritis Guidelines. Guidelines for the management of rheumatoid arthritis: 2002 update. Arthritis Rheum 2002;46:328-346.

23. Lorig KR, Ritter PL, Laurent DD, et al. The Internet-based self-management program: a one-year randomized trial for patients with arthritis or fibromyalgia. Arthritis Rheum 2008;59(7):1009-1017.

24. Lineker SC, Bell MJ, Boyle J, et al. Implementing clinical practice guidelines in primary care. Med Teach 2008;Sept 29:1-8.

25. Porter BO, Jones SG, Winland-Brown JE. Hematology and immune problems. In Dunphy LM, Winland-Brown JE, Porter BO, et al, editors. Primary Care: The Art and Science of Advanced Practice Nursing. 2nd edition. Philadelphia: FA Davis; 2007:848-952.

26. Kotzin BL, West SG. Systemic lupus erythematosus. In Rich RR, Fleisher TA, Shearer WT, et al, eds. Clinical Immunology. 2nd edition. London: Mosby; 2001:60.1-24.

27. D'Cruz DP, Khamashta MA, Hughes GR. Systemic lupus erythematosus. Lancet 2007;369(9561):587-597.

28. Munoz LE, Gaipl US, Franz S, et al. SLE: A disease of clearance deficiency? Rheumatology 2005;44:1101-1107.

29. Kotzin BL, Achenbach GA, West SG. Renal involvement in systemic lupus erythematosus. In Schriner RW, Gottschalk CW, editors. Diseases of the Kidney. 6th edition. Boston: Little Brown; 1997:1781.

30. Lee AB, Godfrey T, Rowley KG, et al. Traditional risk factor assessment does not capture the extent of cardiovascular risk in systemic lupus erythematosus. Intern Med J 2006;36:237-243.

31. Kozora E, Ellison M, West S. Depression, fatigue, and pain in systemic lupus erythematosus (SLE): relationship to the American College of Rheumatology SLE Neuropsychological Battery. Arthritis Rheum 2006;55(4):628-645.

32. Merck Company. Retrieved November 19, 2008, from http://www.merck.com/mmpe/sec04/ch032/ch032g.html#sec04-ch032-ch032g-213

33. Beitz JM. The clinical nurse specialist consultant role: issues and pragmatics. In Zuzelo PR, editor. The Clinical Nurse Specialist Handbook. Boston: Jones & Bartlett; 2007:199-225.

34. Schulman C. Clinical inquiry. In McKinley M, editor. Acute and Critical Care Clinical Nurse Specialists: Synergy for Best Practices. St Louis, MO: Saunders; 2007:77-90.

35. Kaplow R. Synergy model guiding the practice of the CNS in acute and critical care. In McKinley M, editor. Acute and Critical Care Clinical Nurse Specialists: Synergy for Best Practices. St Louis, MO: Saunders; 2007:29-47.

36. Bone RC, Balk RA, Cerra FB, et al. Definitions for sepsis and organ failure and guidelines for the use of innovative therapies in sepsis. The ACCP/SCCM Consensus Conference Committee. American College of Chest Physicians/Society of Critical Care Medicine. Chest 1992;101(6):1644-1655.

37. Winkelman C. Inflammation and genomics in the critical care unit. Crit Care Nursing Clin N Am 2008;20(2):213-221.

38. Hotchkiss RS, Karl IE. The pathophysiology and treatment of sepsis. N Engl J Med 2003;348(2):138-150.

39. Marik PE. Mechanisms and clinical consequences of critical illness associated adrenal insufficiency. Curr Opin Crit Care 2007;13(4):363-369.

40. O'Brian JM, Ali NA, Aberegg SK, et al. Sepsis. Am J Med 2007;120:1012-1022.

41. Russell JA. Management of sepsis. N Engl J Med 2006;355:1699-1713.

42. Dellinger RP, Levy MM, Carlett JM, et al. Surviving sepsis campaign: international guidelines for management of severe sepsis and septic shock: 2008. Crit Care Med 2008;36(1):296-327.

43. Zubrow MD, Sweeney TA, Fulda GJ, et al. Improving care of the sepsis patient. Jt Comm J Qual Patient Saf 2008;34(4):187-191.

44. National Association of Clinical Nurse Specialists. Statement on Clinical Nurse Specialist Practice and Education, 2004. Harrisburg, PA: Author.

45. Titler MG, Kleiber C, Steelman VJ, et al. Iowa model of evidence-based practice to promote quality care. Crit Care Nurs Clin North Am 2001;13(4):497-509.

46. Stetler CB. Updating the Stetler model of research utilization to facilitate evidence-based practice. Nursing Outlook 2001;49:272-279.

47. Stevens KR. ACE Star Model of EBP: Knowledge Transformation. Academic Center for Evidence-based Practice, 2004. The University of Texas Health Science Center at San Antonio.

48. Institute for Health Improvement. Retrieved April 2, 2009, from www.ihi.org.

49. Knaus WA, Draper EA, Wagner DP, et al. An evaluation of outcome from intensive care in major medical centers. Ann Intern Med 1986;104:410-418.

50. Branson B. Current epidemiology and revised recommendations for HIV testing in health-care settings. J Med Virol 2007;79:S6-S10.

51. Branson B, Handsfield HH, Lampe MA, et al. Revised recommendations for HIV testing of adults, adolescents, and pregnant women in health care settings. MMWR 2006;55:1-17.

52. National Institutes of Health, NIAID. Retrieved June 29, 2009, from http://www.3.niaid,nih,gov/about/otganization/daids/DAIDSOverview.htm

53. Nurses in AIDS care. Retrieved July 24, 2009, from http://www.nursesinaidscare.org/

54. Guidelines for prophylaxis against *Pneumocystis carinii* pneumonia for persons infected with human immunodeficiency virus. MMWR 1989;38:1-9.

55. Morris A, Creasman J, Turner J, et al: Intensive care of human immunodeficiency virus infected patients during the era of highly active antiretroviral therapy. Resp and Crit Care Med 2006;34(suppl):S245-S250.

56. Simon V, Ho DD, Abdool Karim Q. HIV/AIDS epidemiology, pathogenesis, prevention and treatment. Lancet 2009;5:489-504.

57. Fiebig EW, Rawal BD, Garrett PE, et al. Dynamics of HIV viremia and antibody seroconversion in plasma donors: implications for diagnosis and staging of primary HIV infection. AIDS 2003;17:1871-1879.

58. Zetola N., Pilcher CD. Diagnosis and management of acute HIV infection. Inf Dis Clin N Am 2007;21:19-48.

59. Brenchley J M, Price DA, Schacker TW, et al. Microbial translocation is a cause of systemic immune activation in chronic HIV infection. Nat Med 2006;12:1365-1371.

60. Douek D, Brenchley JM, Price DA, International AIDS Society–USA, et al. HIV disease progression: immune activation, microbes, and a leaky gut. Top HIV Med 2007;15(4):114-117.

61. Kassutto S, Johnston MN, etal. Longitudinal analysis of clinical markers following antiretroviral therapy initiated during acute or early HIV type 1 infection. Clin Infect Dis 2006;42(7):1024-1032.

62. Kinloch-DeLoes SH, Hoen B, et al. A controlled trial of zidovudine in primary human immunodeficiency virus infection. N Engl J Med1995;333(7):408-413.

63. Little SJ, Holte S, Routy JP, et al. Antiretroviral-drug resistance among patients recently infected with HIV. N Engl J Med 2002;347(6):385-394.

64. Hammer SM, SM Schechter M, et al .Treatment for adult HIV infection: 2006 recommendations of the International AIDS Society: USA panel. JAMA 2006;296(7):827-843.

65. Deeks SG, Phillips AN. HIV infection, antiretroviral treatment, ageing, and non-AIDS related morbidity. BMJ 2009;338:a3172.

66. Barroso JA, et al. Metasynthesis of qualitative research on living with HIV infection. Qual Health Res 2007;10:340-353.

67. Ray G. Pathophysiology: Human immunodeficiency virus and its life cycle. In Guberski TADG, editor. Clinical Challenges in HIV/AIDS: A Practice Handbook for Nurse Practitioners and Physician Assistants. Cranbury, NJ: NP Communications; 2006.

68. Centers for Disease Control and Prevention. AIDS defining conditions. Retrieved May 17, 2009, from http://www.cdc.gov/mmwr/preview/mmwrhtml/rr5710a2.htm

69. Kaplan J, Masur S, Holmes KK. Guidelines for preventing opportunistic infections among HIV-positive persons. MMWR 2002;51:1-46.

70. Murdoch D, Venter WDF, Van Rie A, et al. Immune reconstitution inflammatory syndrome (IRIS): review of common infectious manifestations and treatment options. AIDS Res Ther 2007;4(9).

71. Bower M, Collins S, Cottrill C, et al; on behalf of the AIDS Malignancy Subcommittee. British HIV Association guidelines for HIV-associated malignancies for 2008. HIV Med 2009; 336-388.

72. Currier JS, Havlir DV. Complications of HIV disease and antiretroviral therapy. Top HIV Med 2009;17(2):57-67.

73. Salmon-Ceron D, Lewden C, Morlat P, et al; Mortality Study Group 2000. Liver disease as a major cause of death among HIV infected patients: role of hepatitis C and B viruses and alcohol. J Hepatol 2005;42(6):799-805.

74. Strader D, Wright T, Thomas DL, et al. Diagnosis, management and treatment of hepatitis C. Hepatology 2004;39(4):1147-1171.

75. Santangelo J. Routine HIV testing: The opt-out program at UCSD. Paper presented at the University of California at San Diego Nursing Research Conference, 2009.

76. Centers for Disease Control (CDC). HIV-related knowledge and stigma. HIV-related knowledge and stigma—United States, 2000. MMWR 2000;49:1062-1064.

77. de Ruiter A, Anderson J, Chakrborty R, et al. British HIV Association and Children's HIV Association guidelines for the management of HIV infection in pregnant women. HIV Med 2008;9:452-502.

78. Koutsilieri E, Sopper S, ter Meulen V, et al. Psychiatric complications in human immunodeficiency virus infection. J Neurovirol 2002;8(suppl 2):129-133.

79. Mallinson RK, Coleman S. The provider role in client engagement in HIV care. AIDS Patient Care STDS 2007;21(S1):S77-S84.

80. HIV/AIDS Nursing Certification Board. ACRN. Retrieved August 18, 2011 from http://www.hancb.org/.

81. Liddicoat RV, Horton NJ, Urban R, et al. Assessing missed opportunities for HIV testing in medical settings. J Gen Intern Med 2004;19:349-356.

82. CDC. Revised Recommendations for HIV testing of adults, adolescents, and pregnant women in health-care settings. MMWR 2006;55(RR14):1-17.

83. Lewis Y. Clinical nurse specialist practice: Addressing populations with HIV/AIDS. Clin Nurse Spec 2002;16:306-311.

CHAPTER 16

Genitourinary and Gynecologic Problems

Kate Moore, DNP, RN, CCRN, CEN, ACNP-BC, ANP-BC, GNP-BC, and Sharon E. Lock, PhD, ARNP, FNP-BC

INTRODUCTION

Male genitourinary and female gynecologic problems in the acute care setting can present numerous challenges for the clinical nurse specialist. Many of these health problems can lead to catastrophic outcomes, including infertility or even death if not diagnosed early and treated appropriately. This chapter will review common and some less common but risky male genitourinary and female gynecologic problems encountered in the acute care setting.

Male genitourinary problems addressed in this chapter are acute urinary retention, testicular torsion, priapism, Fournier's gangrene, and paraphimosis. These acute problems generally present as the result of an underlying chronic problem left undiagnosed. In the acute presentation, acute urinary retention, testicular torsion, priapism, Fournier's gangrene, and paraphimosis are medical emergencies and must be treated as such.

Gynecologic problems such as ectopic pregnancy, ruptured ovarian cyst, and spontaneous abortion can become life threatening if not diagnosed early and managed appropriately. Pelvic inflammatory disease (PID) can lead to infertility. Adnexal torsion can lead to loss of an ovary. Vaginal bleeding is a complication of many gynecologic problems. These gynecologic problems will be discussed in this chapter as well as toxic shock syndrome (TSS) and the use of hormone replacement therapy (HRT). Urinary incontinence, although not specific to women, will also be addressed here. Urinary tract infection is covered in Chapter 13, Renal Problems.

This chapter will provide information about the etiology, pathophysiology, risk factors, clinical presentation, diagnosis, and management of these conditions. In addition, the CNS competencies and spheres of influence will be examined.

MALE GENITOURINARY PROBLEMS

Acute Urinary Retention Etiology

Acute urinary retention is the sudden and often painful inability to void despite having a full bladder (1). The causes of urinary retention vary and may be categorized as obstructive, infectious and inflammatory, pharmacologic, neurologic, or other (2-4). In studies of men aged 40 to 83 years, the overall incidence of acute urinary retention was 4.5 to 6.8 per 1,000 men per year. The incidence increases with age. A man aged 70 or greater has a 10% chance of experiencing urinary retention, and a man aged 80 or greater has a 30% chance (5, 6).

Obstructive

Obstructive urinary retention may be intrinsic (prostatic enlargement, bladder stones, urethral stricture) or extrinsic (gastrointestinal mass compressing the bladder neck obstructing the outlet). The most common cause is benign prostatic hyperplasia (BPH) (1, 3). Other causes include prostate cancer, phimosis, paraphimosis, urethral strictures, stones, fecal impaction, and gastrointestinal or retroperitoneal masses, foreign bodies, and external-constricting devices applied to the penis (7).

Infectious and Inflammatory

The most common cause of infectious acute urinary retention is acute prostatitis. The causative organism is generally gram-negative, such as *Escherichia coli* and *Proteus*. As a result of the infection, the prostate becomes acutely inflamed, which leads to urinary retention (1). Urethritis from a urinary tract infection or sexually transmitted infection (STI) can cause urethral edema, resulting in urinary retention.

Pharmacologic

Medications with anticholinergic properties (e.g., tricyclic antidepressants) or sympathomimetic drugs (e.g., oral decongestants) can cause urinary retention. Other drugs that may lead to acute urinary retention include antiarrhythmics, antihypertensives, and nonsteroidal anti-inflammatory drugs (NSAIDs) (3, 8).

Neurologic

Functions of the bladder and urinary tract depend on complex interactions between the brain, the autonomic nervous system, and the somatic nerves. *Neurogenic* or *neuropathic bladder* is defined as any defective functioning of the bladder caused by impaired innervations (9). Acute urinary retention caused by neurogenic bladder may be the result of stroke, diabetic peripheral neuropathy, multiple sclerosis, disk herniation, spinal trauma, and cord compression (10-13).

Other Causes

Two other causes of acute urinary retention in men are postoperative complications and trauma. Postoperative urinary retention may be due to pain, traumatic instrumentation, bladder overdistention, and pharmacologic agents. Surgical procedures most likely to be followed by acute urinary retention include rectal surgery and hip arthroplasty (14).

Traumatic injury to the urethra, penis, or bladder may cause acute urinary retention. Pelvic fracture or traumatic instrumentation may lead to bladder rupture and urethral disruption (5).

Pathophysiology

The pathophysiology of acute urinary retention is a direct reflection of the physiology of urination. The bladder stores urine then empties as a result of the complex integration of musculoskeletal, neurologic, and psychological functions. As a person's bladder begins to fill, impulses are conducted to cause the sensation of fullness in the bladder, triggering the urge to void. Additional impulses relax the sphincters, causing emptying of urine from the bladder (3).

Clinical Presentation

Urinary retention is the inability to void despite a distended bladder. As the obstruction increases, the urinary stream decreases in strength and flow despite forceful and prolonged muscle contraction (15, 16). A patient presenting with acute urinary retention is generally ambulatory, restless, and in a good deal of discomfort. Deep suprapubic palpitation will exacerbate their discomfort (16).

Diagnosis

As with most disorders, a careful history is essential to diagnosis of acute urinary retention. In collecting the past medical history and history of present illness, the clinician should first focus on the genitourinary system to include questions about frequency, urgency, dysuria,

hematuria, fever, chills, low back pain, or rash. It is also important to establish if there has been any recent trauma or procedure that might account for the urinary retention. For example, recent catheterization or an injury to the genital area may account for urinary retention. In taking the genitourinary history, ensure a thorough gastrointestinal history is taken as well to include bowel habits and perirectal pain. A sexual history is also important and should include sexual habits to include rectal intercourse and any rectal or urethral foreign bodies that might be present. Since there is the potential for neurologic causes, a careful neurologic history should be included. A complete medication history is also critical.

In addition to the focused examination of the genitourinary system, the clinician should include a full detailed examination including vital signs. Fever, tachycardia, or hypotension may indicate infection or even sepsis. Tachycardia associated with the discomfort of urinary retention should resolve once the bladder fullness has been relieved. The physical examination should include a rectal examination to include palpation of the prostate, evaluation for fecal impaction, rectal tone, perineal sensation, and masses. The abdominal examination should be thorough, with particular attention to bladder percussion. The external genitalia should also be carefully examined for phimosis, paraphimosis, meatal stenosis, foreign bodies, tumors, or rashes. A thorough neurologic examination should focus on strength, sensation, reflexes, and muscle tone, with particular attention to the lower extremities. A neurologic etiology should be suspected when other sources have been ruled out, especially in the younger population.

Diagnostic testing, especially in the acute care setting, may be limited to a urinalysis and possible urine culture. In the acute setting, a urinalysis will provide the necessary information to either move forward with a diagnosis or provide the clues necessary to proceed with other diagnostics. Optimally, the urine culture should be obtained before initiating antibiotic treatment. The placement of a Foley catheter may be not only diagnostic but also therapeutic. If there is suspicion of infection, a complete blood count should be obtained and a chemistry panel should be done to assess renal function and electrolyte status. Radiographic studies may include a film of the kidney, ureters, and bladder; an ultrasound of the abdomen and or pelvis; and possibly computed tomography (CT) of the abdomen. With suspicion of trauma or masses, lumbar spine films may be helpful. Beyond these diagnostics, referral to urology for further diagnostics would be recommended.

Management

The immediate decompression of the bladder is both diagnostic and therapeutic for the patient presenting with acute urinary retention (7, 17, 18). The placement of a transuretheral catheter is the primary method for bladder decompression. A 14- to 18-French Foley catheter should be easily placed and provide immediate relief. In the event of difficulty passing a 14- to 18-French Foley catheter, a firm angular Coudé catheter should be attempted. If attempts to pass these catheters are unsuccessful, a urologist should be consulted.

Clinical Nurse Specialist Competencies and Spheres of Influence
Clinical Expert/Direct Care, Consultation, and Collaboration

Acute urinary retention has the potential to be a medical emergency and the patient generally presents with severe discomfort. The CNS competencies of direct care, consultation, and collaboration are priorities at this time. Direct care is provided by assessing, diagnosing, and assisting with the management of the patient with urinary retention. The CNS will consult and collaborate with the patient and nursing and medical staff in an effort to treat the patient's problem, and reassure the family to ensure the best care and treatment.

Testicular Torsion Etiology

Testicular torsion is a medical and urologic emergency that can lead to permanent ischemic injury of the involved testis (19, 20). The incidence rate of testicular torsion in men less than 25 years old is 1 in 4,000. Of men presenting with testicular torsion, Cummings et al. reported nearly 61% were younger than 25 years old (21). The etiology of torsion is based on age and anatomy. The two ages most closely associated with testicular torsion are the neonatal period and near puberty, around 13 years of age (22).

The two types of testicular torsion are intravaginal, the more common type, and extravaginal, usually only seen in the prenatal or neonatal period. Intravaginal testicular torsion is an anatomical anomaly of a narrow attachment of the tunica vaginalis from the spermatic cord to the testes secondary to high insertion of the tunica on the spermatic cord (23). Intravaginal testicular torsion is commonly seen in adolescents and elderly males and commonly occurs during sleep. Torsion may also occur secondary to trauma.

Pathophysiology

Testicular torsion is the rotation of the testicular vascular pedicle, which results in testicular ischemia and ultimately infarction if not addressed immediately. The extent of ischemia and infarction depends on the duration and degree of the torsion (23).

Clinical Presentation

Patients generally present with acute and excruciating hemiscrotal pain. On palpation, the involved testes may be so exquisitely tender that clinical examination may be impossible. The affected testis generally tends to be retracted, higher in the scrotum and unilateral to the left. There may also be a complaint of abdominal pain, and nausea and vomiting are generally present. In the later stages, the patient may exhibit a low-grade fever. Patients usually deny urinary problems (24).

Diagnosis

A male presenting with acute scrotal swelling and pain should be considered to have torsion unless the history, examination, or imaging suggests otherwise. Other acute causes of acute scrotal pain include strangulated hernias, orchitis, epididymitis, and torsions of the testicular appendages (23).

Diagnostic tests to confirm testicular torsion include Doppler ultrasound of the testes, magnetic resonance imaging (MRI), radionuclide scintigraphy, and infrared thermography. Doppler ultrasound is the diagnostic of choice when testicular torsion is high on the list of differential diagnoses (25, 26).

Management

Testicular torsion is a urologic emergency and should be referred immediately. Providing intravenous access and appropriate analgesia are the most immediate primary management techniques. The urologist may elect to attempt manual detorsion, but the acute scrotum generally requires urgent surgical intervention (27).

Clinical Nurse Specialist Competencies and Spheres of Influence
Collaboration

The primary competency to be exhibited by the CNS when encountering patients with testicular torsion is collaboration. This condition is a urologic emergency and requires immediate consultation with a urologist to salvage the testicle. The CNS may be instrumental in mobilizing the surgical services.

Priapism Etiology

Priapism is defined as a prolonged and persistent penile erection unassociated with sexual interest or stimulation. It is a true disorder of erection physiology, associated with risks for structural damage of the penis and erectile dysfunction. Priapsim is relatively rare, with an incidence of between 0.5 and 1 case per 100,000 person-years (28). There are specific segments of the male population at risk. Individuals undergoing pharmacologic therapy for erectile dysfunction have been identified as a group at risk for priapism. Populations with sickle cell disease have demonstrated lifetime probabilities of developing priapism of 29% to 42% (29). Other causes of priapism under consideration include neurogenic, drug-induced, and idiopathic forms (30).

Pathophysiology

Persistent engorgement of the corpora cavernosa of the penis results in priapism. Venous stasis and decreased venous outflow in the penis are the primary features. This pathophysiologic presentation supports the findings of priapism in sickle cell disease, hematologic dyscrasias, hemodialysis, heparin-induced platelet aggregation, and local primary or metastatic neoplasia (31, 32).

Clinical Presentation

Priapism generally presents as a penile erection not associated with sexual interest or stimulation. The erection may last a few hours or longer and will eventually resolve, although there may be permanent damage to the penis as a result of ischemia (33).

Diagnosis

The goal of diagnosis is to determine if the presentation is ischemic, a urologic emergency, or nonischemic. The initial diagnostic work-up includes history and physical examination to include onset, presence of pain, duration of priapism, causative factors, information about prior episodes, prior successful treatment, and a thorough evaluation of all medications and past medical history. Pain is typically considered to be the differentiating factor of ischemic priapism. If the patient with priapism presents with pain, the priapism should be considered a urologic emergency and referred.

Further evaluation may include laboratory testing to include a complete blood count and drug screening. Radiologic evaluation may be made with color duplex ultrasonography. Additional diagnostics may be obtained through the penile diagnostic of aspirated blood from the corpus cavernosum (31).

Management

Ischemic priapism is a urologic emergency and should be referred immediately to a urologist. The initial management of nonischemic priapism should be observation because spontaneous resolution occurs in up to 62% of reported cases. However, nonischemic priapism that does not resolve spontaneously should be referred to a urologist (33).

Clinical Nurse Specialist Competencies and Spheres of Influence
Clinical Expert/Direct Care, Consultation, and Collaboration

Priapism can be an embarrassing situation for patients and accompanying significant others. The CNS may be consulted to assist the bedside clinician with patient history taking and physical examination for a sensitive problem. This condition is a urologic emergency and requires immediate consultation to a urologist to ensure integrity of the penile and surrounding tissue.

Fournier's Gangrene Etiology

Fournier's gangrene is a rare urologic emergency characterized by progressive necrotizing infection of the external genitalia or perineum. The incidence of Fournier's gangrene is 1.6 per 100,000 males. The mortality rate ranges from 20% to 40%, with some studies placing the fatality rate as high as 88% (34, 35). It is an extremely life-threatening form of necrotizing fasciitis of the perineum and genital area. The cause of Fournier's gangrene is generally perineal, perianal or genital trauma to include anal fissures, colonic perforations, lacerations, abrasions, blunt force trauma, traumatic catheterization, or frostbite (36, 37).

Pathophysiology

There is generally more than one causative organism cultured from the wound in Fournier's gangrene. Those found include both anaerobic and aerobic bacteria such as *Escherichia coli*, *Pseudomonas*, *Streptococcus*, and *Bacteroides*. Regardless of the causative organism, the pathophysiology is the same: anaerobic and aerobic microbes working in synergy to cause thrombi formation within the blood vessels and ultimate tissue destruction and death. Necrosis develops along the planes of the fascia and can progress as rapidly as 2 to 3 cm/hr (37, 38).

Clinical Presentation

The onset of Fournier's gangrene is insidious and the initial complaints range from general malaise to abdominal or scrotal discomfort. The patient rapidly progresses to overt sepsis. The hallmark finding on examination is crepitus caused by gas-forming organisms. This condition left untreated will progress to sepsis, multiple organ failure, and death (37).

Diagnosis

Diagnosis is based on history and physical examination. A complete blood count, metabolic panel, and wound cultures may prove helpful as well as arterial blood gases. This patient will rapidly deteriorate into sepsis and even septic shock (37).

Management

Fournier's gangrene is managed surgically by urology and plastic surgery with extensive debridement. Broad-spectrum antibiotics should be administered as soon as possible to cover gram-positive, gram-negative, aerobic, and anaerobic bacteria (38).

Clinical Nurse Specialist Competencies and Spheres of Influence
Clinical Expert/Direct Care, and Collaboration

The primary competencies to be exhibited by the CNS in Fournier's gangrene are direct care and collaboration. The CNS must be able to recognize this condition and appreciate the progression to sepsis if not emergently treated. This condition requires immediate consultation with a urologist to avert the devastation of sepsis, septic shock, and organ failure. The patient will need assessment and monitoring in the intensive care unit even when hemodynamically stable due to the risk of rapid progression to septic shock.

Paraphimosis Etiology

Paraphimosis, a urologic emergency, occurs in uncircumcised men when the retracted foreskin becomes entrapped behind the glans penis (39, 40). Risk factors for paraphimosis include forceful retraction of the foreskin; failure to replace the foreskin after bathing, voiding, or after catheterization; vigorous sexual activity; and chronic balanoposthitis.

Pathophysiology

The foreskin becomes trapped proximal to the glans and forms a constricting band that impairs the flow of blood and lymph to and from the glans and foreskin. The result is vascular engorgement. Treated appropriately and immediately, it is not a serious condition. Left untreated, paraphimosis can lead to necrosis, and in the worst case scenario, amputation of the penis (39, 40).

Clinical Presentation

On examination, the glans appears enlarged and congested, bound by a tight and generally edematous foreskin. The foreskin is retracted and cannot be replaced. Patients presenting with paraphimosis are generally quite anxious.

Diagnosis

The diagnosis is made by clinical presentation. A history of preceding events will aid in identification of patient or caregiver learning needs in order to prevent future episodes of paraphimosis.

Management

Reduction is the preferred treatment and can generally be performed by a urologist. In the event reduction cannot be performed or is unsuccessful, the condition may require a puncture technique or incision (40). The tourniquet effect of the foreskin is released when the tissue is punctured or incised and allows for resumption of perfusion.

Clinical Nurse Specialist Competencies and Spheres of Influence
Clinical Expert/Direct Care, Collaboration, and Coaching/Teaching/Mentoring

The primary competencies required of the CNS in addressing paraphimosis are direct care in order to promptly recognize the condition and collaboration with other providers. This condition requires intervention by a urologist and may become a urologic emergency if immediate resolution is not achieved. Additionally, coaching/teaching/mentoring may be indicated to provide education in proper hygiene, especially if the patient is newly dependent on others for self-care needs and the caregiver lacks knowledge of correct bathing technique. The caregiver will need instruction in retracting the foreskin, cleansing, and drying the tissue, with emphasis on replacing the foreskin.

GYNECOLOGIC PROBLEMS

The gynecologic problems discussed in this chapter can lead to infertility or even death if not managed appropriately and in a timely manner. In the acute care setting the CNS is an integral member of the health care team in providing care to women with gynecologic problems. In this chapter the following gynecologic problems will be discussed: ectopic pregnancy, ruptured ovarian cyst, vaginal bleeding, spontaneous abortion, TSS, PID, and adnexal torsion. The use of HRT in the acute care setting will also be discussed.

Ectopic Pregnancy Etiology

The most common cause of ectopic pregnancy is salpingitis, an inflammation of the fallopian tube. Inflammation can decrease the diameter of the lumen of the fallopian tube, making it difficult for the fertilized ovum to travel through the tube and implant in the uterus. If the fertilized ovum does not complete its travel through the fallopian tube within 7 days, implantation will occur in the fallopian tube or outside the uterine cavity. Another cause of ectopic pregnancy is altered ciliary motility in the fallopian tube, which is caused by hormonal imbalances or tobacco abuse. Other etiology include pelvic masses, which can alter the structure of the tubes, and surgeries, which can cause tubal adhesions (41).

Pathophysiology

Implantation of the blastocyst anywhere other than the uterine cavity is considered an ectopic pregnancy (42). About 2 in 100 pregnancies are ectopic and over 95% of those are implanted in the fallopian tubes. Implantation can also occur in the abdomen, cervix, ovary, or uterine cornua (43).

Risk Factors

Risk factors for ectopic pregnancy include prior tubal surgery, previous ectopic pregnancy, previous salpingitis, previous STIs, PID, smoking, and tubal adhesions caused by infection, appendicitis, or endometriosis (44). In addition, assisted reproductive procedures such as gamete intrafallopian transfer (GIFT) and in vitro fertilization (IVF) are risk factors (45). About half of women diagnosed with ectopic pregnancy have no risk factors (41, 43).

Clinical Presentation

The cardinal symptoms of ectopic pregnancy are amenorrhea, abdominal pain, and vaginal bleeding (41). However, not every woman will present with all three symptoms (44). The majority of women (56% to 100%) will present with abdominal pain, 62% to 84% will present with amenorrhea, and 55% to 84% will present with vaginal bleeding (41). Signs and symptoms of ectopic pregnancy are presented in Table 16-1. A woman with a

TABLE 16–1 Signs and Symptoms of Ectopic Pregnancy

Diagnosis	Signs and Symptoms
Ruptured ectopic regnancy	Severe abdominal pain
	Abdominal distention
	Abdominal guarding and rebound tenderness
	Ipsilateral shoulder pain
	Tachycardia
	Hypotension
	Possible cervical motion tenderness
	Possible enlarged uterus
	May not have palpable mass
Probable ectopic pregnancy	Lower abdominal pain
	Vaginal bleeding
	Possible amenorrhea
	Possible abdominal, adnexal, and cervical motion tenderness
Possible ectopic pregnancy	Lower abdominal pain
	Vaginal spotting or bleeding
	Amenorrhea or abnormal LMP
	Possible adnexal mass
	Uterus may be enlarged or normal size

ruptured ectopic pregnancy may present with severe abdominal pain as well as tachycardia and hypotension and ipsilateral shoulder pain. On exam, her abdomen may be distended with guarding and rebound tenderness. She might have cervical motion tenderness and an enlarged uterus but may not have a palpable adnexal mass. Any woman of reproductive age who complains of abdominal pain should be given a pregnancy test (46).

Women with a *probable ectopic pregnancy* may present with lower abdominal pain and vaginal bleeding with or without amenorrhea. The abdomen may be tender with adnexal or cervical motion tenderness (46).

Women with a *possible ectopic pregnancy* may present with lower abdominal pain and vaginal spotting or bleeding. Women usually have amenorrhea or an abnormal last menstrual period (LMP). On exam, the patient may have an adnexal mass. The uterus may be normal size or slightly enlarged and the ultrasound shows a thickened endometrial stripe (46).

Diagnosis

The differential diagnosis of ectopic pregnancy includes gynecologic and nongynecologic problems. Gynecologic problems included in the differential are threatened or incomplete abortion, ruptured ovarian cyst, PID, adnexal torsion, and degenerating leiomyoma. Nongynecologic problems included in the differential are acute appendicitis, pyelonephritis, and pancreatitis. Transvaginal ultrasound and testing of serum quantitative beta-human chorionic gonadotropin (β-hCG) are the two primary

methods of diagnosis of ectopic pregnancy (44). As the fertilized egg begins to divide, it will produce β-hCG even before implantation. In the first trimester, serum β-hCG titers increase exponentially, doubling every 2 days with the maximum at 8 to 10 weeks (47). Current testing is so sensitive that β-hCG can be detected in serum 8 days after ovulation. Urine pregnancy tests will detect β-hCG as low as 25 mIU/mL and will detect a pregnancy 11 days after ovulation (47). An intrauterine pregnancy is usually seen on ultrasound when the serum β-hCG is 1,500 to 2,000 mIU/mL. If serum β-hCG titers are plateauing or decreasing or increasing abnormally, the pregnancy is abnormal (44). A serum progesterone level greater than 20 ng/mL indicates a normal intrauterine pregnancy. A level below 5 ng/mL suggests an abnormal pregnancy. However, serum progesterone levels are not good for diagnosing ectopic pregnancy because of the length of time needed to obtain results (almost 24 hours) and usually the results fall between 5 and 25 ng/mL (43, 44).

Transvaginal ultrasound is the standard for diagnosing ectopic pregnancy. Intrauterine pregnancy can be seen on ultrasound after 5 weeks of amenorrhea (or 3 weeks after conception). If an intrauterine gestational sac is not seen when the β-hCG is between 1,500 and 2,000 mIU/mL, there is a probable ectopic pregnancy. Multifetal pregnancies can produce more β-hCG without visible sacs (43, 44).

Ultrasound has decreased the need for culdocentesis, but this procedure may still be done to determine the need for surgery. On vaginal exam, a needle in is inserted through the vaginal fornix into the posterior cul-de-sac.

If nonclotting blood is found, the patient probably has an ectopic pregnancy (46).

Management
Surgical Management
If the woman is unstable hemodynamically, a laparotomy should be performed to gain rapid access to the bleeding site. If the patient is hemodynamically stable, a laporoscopy is preferred due to fewer days of hospitalization, decreased postoperative pain, and faster recovery. If the fallopian tube has been damaged and if less than 6 cm of functional tube remains, the entire fallopian tube should be removed (salpingectomy). Removal of a portion of the tube (partial salpingectomy) is only done if the ectopic pregnancy is implanted in the ampullary portion of the tube (44).

Salpingotomy and salpingostomy are also surgical options. Both surgeries involve making an incision in the fallopian tube at the site of the ectopic and removing the pregnancy. In salpingotomy, the incision is closed and in salpingostomy, the incision is left open. This type of surgery runs the risk of leaving residual trophoblastic tissue. Repeat β-hCG titers should be done 3 to 7 days postoperatively to confirm that no hormone-producing cells remain.

Medical Management
If ectopic pregnancy is diagnosed early, ambulatory medical management with methotrexate (MTX) is an option. Methotrexate is a folic acid antagonist that is toxic to replicating tissues. Medical management is an option for women who meet the following criteria: (1) hemodynamically stable, (2) no severe or persistent abdominal pain, (3) woman's commitment to follow-up until ectopic pregnancy is resolved, and (4) normal liver and renal function tests at before treatment (48).

Absolute contraindications for medical management with MTX include intrauterine pregnancy, immunodeficiency, moderate to severe anemia, leukopenia or thrombocytopenia, sensitivity to MTX, active pulmonary or peptic ulcer disease, clinically important hepatic or renal dysfunction, and breastfeeding (48). Relative contraindications include embryonic cardiac activity detected by transvaginal ultrasound, initial hCG greater than 5,000 mIU/mL, ectopic pregnancy greater than 4 cm in size, refusal to accept blood transfusion, and inability to provide follow-up (48).

Before administering the first dose of MTX, a complete blood count, liver function tests, serum creatinine, blood type, and Rh are obtained. A chest radiograph should be performed on women who have a history of pulmonary disease due to the risk of interstitial pneumonitis (48). Single- and multiple-dose MTX regimens are commonly used. The single 50 mg/m^2 dose is given intramuscularly. For the multiple-dose regimen, MTX is dosed at 1.0 mg/kg and is given intramuscularly and followed with a leucovorin rescue injection of 0.1 mg/kg.

Serial β-hCG measurements should be obtained until the level is less than 5 mIU/mL. If the woman is Rh negative, RhoGAM should be administered (43, 48).

Clinical Nurse Specialist Competencies and Spheres of Influence
Consultation and Collaboration
The CNS should collaborate with the nursing and medical staff to ensure that preliminary laboratory and diagnostic tests have been performed prior to surgery or administration of MTX. Nursing staff will need to be knowledgeable about the dosage, route of administration, side effects and drug interactions of MTX. Patients who are Rh negative should be administered Rh(D) immune globulin (RhoGAM) (42, 48).

Coaching/Teaching/Mentoring
When the patient is receiving MTX, she should be instructed on the mechanism of action and possible side effects. MTX will make the patient photosensitive, so she should be told to avoid the sun. She should be instructed of the possible common side effects of MTX such as, stomatitis and conjunctivitis as well as rare side effects such as pleuritis, gastritis, dermatitis, alopecia, enteritis, increased liver enzymes, and bone marrow suppression. Since MTX is a folate antagonist, the patient should be instructed to discontinue folic acid supplements until treatment with MTX has ended. She should be instructed to immediately report severe abdominal pain, which may indicate impending or actual rupture. The patient should be instructed to return in 1 week for follow-up and testing of β-hCG. In addition, she will need to return for weekly testing until β-hCG is less than 5 mIU/mL (41). Contraception should be prescribed and the woman instructed to avoid pregnancy for at least 3 months, giving the tissue in the fallopian tube time to heal (46).

Ruptured Ovarian Cyst Etiology
Ovarian cysts are more common the first year after initiation of ovulation (49). In the premenopausal woman, the ovary undergoes a hormonal cycle each month leading to development of the follicles, emergence of a dominant follicle, ovulation, and the formation of the corpus luteum. Cystic enlargement of any of these structures is common and is considered functional rather than malignant. Follicular cysts are fluid filled and are a result of a follicle that has not ovulated or does not regress after ovulation. Corpus luteum cysts may arise from prolonged secretion of progesterone, are usually larger than follicular cysts, and are more likely to cause symptoms.

Pathophysiology
Two to 4 days after ovulation, the ovary becomes very vascular and blood fills the cyst cavity. The cyst may either reabsorb the blood or rupture if there is a large amount of bleeding (41).

Clinical Presentation

Women usually complain of dull, unilateral lower abdominal and pelvic pain. On pelvic exam, the ovary may be enlarged and tender. The pain of a bleeding corpus luteum is similar to the pain of a ruptured ectopic pregnancy (50). The patient may also have gastrointestinal symptoms such as nausea, vomiting, or diarrhea (41).

Diagnosis

A serum β-hCG should be performed to rule out an ectopic pregnancy. Transvaginal ultrasound may establish the diagnosis of ovarian cyst (41, 50). If the patient is having acute pain, CT without contrast is recommended to determine if bleeding is active or if a hemoperitoneum has developed (41, 50)

Management

Follicular cysts usually are not symptomatic and do not require treatment. Unruptured corpus luteum cysts are managed conservatively with continued observation and repeat ultrasound in 4 to 6 weeks. In addition, oral contraception may be prescribed to stop further ovulation (41). However, there is evidence to show that oral contraceptives may not be beneficial in preventing the development of functional ovarian cysts (51). The patient who is managed conservatively should be cautioned that sexual intercourse, exercise, or trauma may rupture the cyst. The patient should be instructed to return with the onset of severe lower abdominal or pelvic pain, which could indicate that the cyst has ruptured. If the cyst has ruptured and the patient is hemodynamically unstable, she should receive adequate volume and blood replacement. If the bleeding from a ruptured cyst is confirmed, then emergency laparotomy is performed, the cyst is removed and hemostasis achieved. In the event a diagnosis is uncertain, a laparoscopy is indicated (51).

Clinical Nurse Specialist Competencies and Spheres of Influence
Collaboration and Consultation

For a patient who is hemodynamically unstable, the CNS will collaborate with the nursing and medical staff to ensure that emergency procedures are performed in a timely manner. The CNS may be consulted for assistance with stabilizing the patient and executing the chain of command to facilitate preparation of the patient for emergency surgery.

Coaching/Teaching/Mentoring

For the patient who is hemodynamically stable and will be conservatively managed, the CNS will assist the nursing staff in teaching the patient about the etiology of ovarian cysts and what would signal a potential rupture of the ovarian cyst. In addition, the CNS would assist in instructing the patient that sexual intercourse, exercise and trauma could lead to rupture of the cyst.

Vaginal Bleeding Etiology

Gynecologic hemorrhage may be caused by hormonal problems, structural problems, neoplasms, or other problems. Hormonal problems include anovulation and irregular ovulation. Structural problems include polyps, fibroids, arteriovenous malformations, and neoplasms, such as endometrial cancer. Other problems that can cause vaginal bleeding include but are not limited to endometritis (52).

Pathophysiology

In anovulatory cycles, an excess amount of estrogen is secreted by the granulose-theca cell complex, but progesterone is not secreted. Estrogen causes stimulation and thickening of the endometrium. Without the secretion of progesterone, the endometrial tissue is randomly broken down, which leads to irregular, excessive bleeding. Irregular ovulation during perimenopause and menopause can also lead to excess estrogen stimulation and thickening of the endometrium (52). In adolescence, the hypothalamic-pituitary system may fail to respond to the positive feedback of estrogen causing anovulatory uterine bleeding. Postmenarcheal anovulatory bleeding is usually caused by the ovaries' declining function (53).

Vaginal bleeding caused by leiomyomas (fibroids) depends on the location in the uterus. Submucosal leiomyomas protrude into the uterus and have a poorly developed endometrium over the surface of the leiomyoma, leading to chronic inflammation and bleeding (52). Endometrial polyps are caused by overgrowth of endometrial tissue and can lead to irregular vaginal bleeding due to vascular fragility and erosions (52). Arteriovenous malformations are rare and can be caused either congenitally or by uterine trauma or after early pregnancy loss. Bleeding associated with endometrial cancer is caused by necrosis of malignant tissue (52).

Risk Factors

Anovulatory cycles are particularly common during adolescence and the premenopausal period, but can also occur anytime during the reproductive years. Thyroid disorders can cause anovulatory cycles. Sexual abuse, trauma, pregnancy, coagulation disorders, PID, endometriosis, and malignancy are also risk factors. Risk factors for developing leiomyomas include advancing age, ethnicity, nulliparity, and family history. Based on current research, statistics show that African American women are two to three times more likely to develop fibroids than are Caucasian women (54).

Clinical Presentation

Patients will present with complaints of regular or irregular bleeding, which can vary from spotting to heavy. Uterine bleeding greater than 7 days at regular intervals is referred to as menorrhagia. Uterine bleeding that occurs at irregular intervals is referred to as metrorrhagia. Menometrorrhagia refers to heavy irregular uterine bleeding. Patients may also present with anemia, due to blood loss (53).

Diagnosis

Since it is difficult to accurately determine the amount of blood loss, laboratory tests should be drawn to determine if the patient is anemic or has another condition that might cause the bleeding. Laboratory tests include complete blood count with platelets, coagulation studies, liver function tests, thyroid-stimulating hormone, and a pregnancy test. A pelvic exam with Papanicolaou (Pap) smear and cultures for gonorrhea and *Chlamydia* should be obtained. Endometrial biopsy also should be performed to rule out malignancy. If the endometrial biopsy results show insufficient tissue, a dilation and curettage should be performed. A transvaginal ultrasound should be performed to evaluate the endometrial lining for polyps and the myometrium for leiomyomas (fibroids). If an intrauterine device (IUD) is present, it should be removed and sent for culture of gonorrhea and *Chlamydia* (41, 53).

Management

Treatment is based on the cause of uterine bleeding. If bleeding is due to a hormonal problem, cyclic estrogen and progesterone may be prescribed. For moderate menometrorrhagia, 1.25 mg of conjugated estrogen may be given every day for 25 days and progesterone 10 mg is added for the last 10 days. Another option is to give oral contraceptives or insert a levonorgestrel-releasing IUD. Endometrial ablation may be necessary if the patient does not respond to medical therapy. Patients with leiomyomas and menorrhagia should be referred to a gynecologist for evaluation. Women who are postmenopausal with vaginal bleeding should always be referred to a gynecologist for endometrial biopsy. If medical therapy and endometrial ablation do not resolve the bleeding, a vaginal hysterectomy may be necessary (53, 55).

Clinical Nurse Specialist Competencies and Spheres of Influence
Clinical Expert/Direct Care and Consultation

The CNS should work with the nursing staff to ensure that blood loss is monitored. If hemorrhage is severe, perineal pads may need to be weighed to determine a more accurate blood loss (1 g = 1 mL). The staff may need assistance with measurement of vital signs, volume, and blood replacement. Patients discharged home on cyclic estrogen and progesterone will need to be educated on how to correctly take the medication.

Spontaneous Abortion Etiology

Spontaneous abortion (also known as miscarriage) is defined as a pregnancy that spontaneously ends before the fetus has reached viability at about 23 weeks' gestation (56).

The World Health Organization defines *spontaneous abortion* as "the loss of a clinical pregnancy that occurs before 20 completed weeks of gestational age (18 weeks post fertilization) or, if gestational age is unknown, the loss of an embryo/fetus of less than 400 grams" (57). Up to 20% of recognized pregnancies under 20 weeks' gestation end in spontaneous abortion, and 80% of these occur in the first 12 weeks of gestation (42). In the first trimester, the fetus usually dies before expulsion (42). About 50% to 60% of spontaneously aborted embryos and fetuses had chromosomal abnormalities (42). Invasive uterine procedures such as amniocentesis or chorionic villi sampling increase the incidence of spontaneous abortion. Maternal uterine abnormalities can interfere with implantation, causing spontaneous abortion. Acute maternal infection such as rubella or toxoplasmosis can cause abortion.

Pathophysiology

During a spontaneous abortion, hemorrhage into the deciduas basalis usually occurs followed by necrosis of tissue. If this happens early in the pregnancy, the fertilized ovum detaches, which stimulates uterine contractions and expulsion of the fertilized ovum. In later-term abortions, the retained fetus may become macerated.

Risk Factors

Advanced maternal age is the greatest risk factor in healthy women due to the increased incidence of fetal aneuploidy (56). By age 35 years, 20% of pregnancies will end in spontaneous abortion; 40%, by age 40; and 80%, by age 45 (42). The rate of spontaneous abortion increases with each subsequent abortion (56). Women who smoke are at increased risk for spontaneous abortion (56) possibly due to vasoconstriction, which reduces uterine and placental blood flow (42). In addition, moderate to high consumption of alcohol is associated with an increased risk of spontaneous abortion (56).

Clinical Presentation, Diagnosis, and Management

Spontaneous abortion is categorized as threatened, inevitable, complete or incomplete, missed, and recurrent (Table 16-2). *Threatened abortion* is "presumed" when bleeding is observed through a closed cervical os during the first half of pregnancy (42). About half of these pregnancies will end in spontaneous abortion; however, the risk of abortion decreases if fetal cardiac activity is documented. Even women who have a threatened abortion and do not abort are at increased risk for preterm delivery, low birth weight, and perinatal death. Ectopic pregnancy also should be considered in the differential diagnosis for threatened abortion. Although women with threatened abortions are often put on bed rest, it does not change the outcome (42). Transvaginal ultrasound, serial serum quantitative hCG levels, and serum progesterone

TABLE 16-2 Categories of Spontaneous Abortion

Category	Definition
Threatened abortion	Bleeding observed through closed cervical os during first half of pregnancy
Inevitable abortion	Gross rupture of membranes with leaking amniotic fluid and cervical dilation
Complete abortion	Expulsion of the fetus and placenta after which the internal cervical os closes
Incomplete abortion	Internal cervical os remains open with fetus and placenta either in utero or partially extruding from the os
Missed abortion	Dead products of conception are retained in the uterus for days or weeks
Recurrent abortion	Three or more consecutive spontaneous abortions

levels alone or in combination may help determine if the fetus is alive and its location.

Inevitable abortion occurs when there is gross ruptured membranes with leaking amniotic fluid and cervical dilation, suggesting almost certain abortion (42). Uterine contractions usually begin soon after rupture of membranes, resulting in abortion or infection develops. The woman should be put on bed rest and observed. If after 48 hours amniotic fluid stops leaking and there is no bleeding, pain, or fever, the woman may resume her usual activities except for vaginal penetration. If bleeding, pain, or fever is present after rupture of membranes, abortion should be considered inevitable and the uterus emptied of the products of conception.

Complete abortion occurs with expulsion of the fetus and placenta, after which the internal cervical os closes (42). After complete abortion, the woman should be monitored for bleeding and infection. With an *incomplete abortion,* the internal os remains open with the fetus and placenta either in utero or partially extruding from the os (42). A cervical dilation and curettage may be required with an incomplete abortion. Afterward, the woman should be monitored for bleeding and infection.

In a *missed abortion*, dead products of conception are retained in the uterus for days or weeks (42). There may or may not be vaginal bleeding. The uterus stops growing and eventually decreases in size. Most missed abortions will be expulsed spontaneously, but some will have to undergo dilation and curettage. If there is prolonged retention of the dead products of conception, coagulation problems can result.

Recurrent abortion refers to three or more consecutive spontaneous abortions (42). Usually recurrent abortions are due to chance, but parental cytogenetic analysis can identify genetic problems with the fetus and may identify couples at risk for subsequent pregnancies with genetic problems (58). Testing for immunologic factors such as antiphospholipid antibodies may also be helpful in identifying the cause of recurrent abortion (58). Women with recurrent abortion due to antiphospholipid antibodies may be treated with low-dose aspirin and unfractionated heparin (58).

Clinical Nurse Specialist Competencies and Spheres of Influence
Clinical Expert/Direct Care and Consultation
After a spontaneous abortion, the level of parental grief varies and is unique for each individual (59, 60). The CNS will need to be prepared to consult with the nursing staff about how to approach the family and strategies for grief counseling. The meaning and significance of the loss should be evaluated before intervening with the family. The mother and father should be encouraged to express their feelings to each other. A support group or bereavement counseling may be recommended (60).

Toxic Shock Syndrome Etiology
TSS emerged in 1978 primarily among menstruating women 12 to 24 years old. In 1980, the Centers for Disease Control and Prevention (CDC) established national surveillance to determine the magnitude and trends of the disease (61). In 1980, several case-control studies indicated that women who used tampons were more likely to develop TSS. The CDC study found that women who used tampons continuously were at higher risk (62). In addition, studies have shown that women with TSS used tampons with very high absorbency (61). In 1982, the U.S. Food and Drug Administration (FDA) required manufacturers to lower the absorbency of tampons and to advise women to use the lowest absorbency needed. Since tampons with very high absorbency were taken off the market, the incidence of TSS has decreased dramatically to 6 to 7 per 100,000 menstruating women annually (61, 63).

Pathophysiology
TSS is caused by preformed toxins produced by the aerobic gram-positive cocci, *Staphylococcus aureus*. These toxins release large amounts of cytokines, which cause systemic vascular resistance and nonhydrostatic leaking of fluid from the intravascular space to the interstitial space, which causes hypotension (64). Highly absorbent tampons may obstruct the vagina, causing retrograde menstruation leading to peritoneal absorption of bacteria.

Oxygen trapped in interfibrous spaces of the tampon may lead to increased numbers of aerobic bacteria (61).

Risk Factors

Women who use tampons with super absorbency are at increased risk for TSS. In addition, the longer a tampon is left in place, the higher is the risk for the development of TSS (61).

Clinical Presentation

The CDC case definition of TSS was awkward revised in 1982 (65) and includes temperature greater than or equal to 38.9°C (102°F), diffuse macular rash, hypotension, desquamation (especially palms and soles of feet) 1 to 2 weeks after onset on illness, and involvement of three or more organs. Gastrointestinal symptoms can include vomiting and diarrhea. Muscular symptoms can include severe myalgia or creatinine phosphokinase level at least twice the upper limit of normal. Vaginal, oropharyngeal, or conjunctival mucous membranes may be hyperemic. Renal signs can include elevated blood urea nitrogen or creatinine or urinary sediment with pyuria. Liver function tests may be elevated. Central nervous system symptoms include disorientation or alteration in consciousness without focal neurologic signs when fever and hypotension are absent (65).

Diagnosis

The diagnosis of TSS is based on the clinical presentation and the CDC case definition. In addition, a vaginal exam should be performed, and if a tampon is present, it should be removed. A vaginal culture for *S. aureus* should be obtained. Other laboratory tests include a complete blood count with differential, electrolytes, and liver and renal function tests. Cultures from blood, throat, and cerebrospinal fluid will assist in the diagnosis (61).

Management

Fluid and electrolyte replacement should be done initially to maintain adequate vascular perfusion. Dopamine at 2 to 5 mcg /min may be needed to control hypotension. Central venous or pulmonary wedge pressure and urinary output should be monitored. Mechanical ventilation may be necessary if acute respiratory syndrome develops. In addition, hemodialysis may be needed if renal failure develops. Corticosteroids may decrease fever and the severity of illness. A β-lacatamase–resistant antibiotic such as nafcillin or oxacillin (2 g IV every 4 hours) should be given. If the patient is allergic to penicillin, vancomycin can be given instead. Until gram-negative sepsis is ruled out, an aminoglycoside should be given cautiously because of altered renal function (61).

Clinical Nurse Specialist Competencies and Spheres of Influence
Clinical Expert/Direct Care, Consultation, and /Teaching/Coaching/Mentoring

If the patient is unstable, the CNS may need to assist the medical and nursing staff in fluid and electrolyte resuscitation and monitoring of the patient. In addition, the CNS should work with the nursing staff in developing teaching strategies for prevention of menstrual TSS. Patient education includes instructing the patient to use a tampon with the lowest absorbency possible and to change tampons at least every 4 to 6 hours.

Pelvic Inflammatory Disease Etiology

PID is a community-acquired infection caused by a sexually transmitted organism that causes an acute infection of a woman's upper genital tract (i.e., uterus, fallopian tubes, and ovaries). In 2007, the estimated number of visits to physicians' offices for PID was 146,000 (66). Hospitalizations for PID have declined steadily over the past 20 years but have remained constant since 2000 at around 60,000 to 70,000 admissions per year (67).

Pathophysiology

The endocervical canal serves as a barrier to protect the usually sterile upper genital tract from pathogenic organisms in the vagina. If this barrier is disrupted, pathogenic organisms can ascend into the upper genital tract infecting the endometrium and fallopian tubes. About 75% of cases of PID occur within 7 days of menses when the quality of cervical mucus facilitates the ascension of bacterial organisms in the vagina (68). Almost 44% of cases of PID are caused by *N. gonorrheae,* about 10% of cases are caused by *Chlamydia,* and about 12% of cases are caused by both *N. gonorrheae* and *Chlamydia.* Other organisms that cause PID are microflora associated with bacterial vaginosis and aneorobes such as *Prevotella, Bacterioides*, and *Peptostreptococcus* (68, 69).

Risk Factors

Risk factors include multiple partners, the clinical status of the partner, young age, previous PID, and race. Studies have shown that the incidence of PID is increased by 3 to 20 times in women with multiple sex partners (68, 69). Adolescents may be more at risk for PID due to the immature cervix, which has a greater proportion of columnar epithelium on the ectocervix than that of older women, which provides a larger surface area for bacterial infection (68, 69). Adolescents are also more likely to be exposed to STIs due to engaging in unprotected sexual intercourse and multiple partners (69).

Clinical Presentation

Women with PID will usually present with lower abdominal pain, usually bilateral with duration of 2 weeks or less. Women may complain of pain shortly after menses. On physical exam, about half of women will have a fever. There is diffuse abdominal tenderness, especially in the lower quadrants. On pelvic exam, a purulent endocervical discharge and/or cervical motion or adnexal tenderness strongly suggests PID. Case Study 16-1 provides an example of a typical presentation of a patient with PID.

CASE STUDY 16-1 | Pelvic Inflammatory Disease (PID)

CHIEF COMPLAINT: Lower abdominal pain

A 17-year-old white girl complains of lower abdominal pain for 1 week. She rates the pain 9 of a possible 10. She has been sexually active for 3 years and has had 4 partners. She and her current partner have been together for 3 months, and they last had sexual intercourse 2 weeks ago. She takes birth control pills but does not always use condoms.

HISTORY & PHYSICAL EXAM

GENERAL: Temperature is 101.4°F, pulse is 90, respirations are 20, and blood pressure is 126/70. The patient is lying on the exam table in the fetal position and is crying.

GASTROINTESTINAL: Some nausea, vomiting, but no diarrhea or constipation. Positive bowel sounds in all four quadrants. Abdominal is diffusely tender. No masses. No organomegaly.

GENITOURINARY: Gravida 0. Last menstrual period (LMP) 6 days ago. Menses every 28 days, 5 days duration. No history of sexually transmitted infection. On pelvic exam there is purulent endocervical discharge and cervical motion tenderness.

INITIAL LABORATORY STUDIES

Urine hCG negative
Vaginal microscopy: Numerous WBCs
RBC 3.4 Hgb 12.0 Hct: 40
WBC 12,000
ESR 30

QUESTIONS

1. What are the differential diagnoses?

2. What additional diagnostic tests are indicated?

3. Based on the history and physical exam, what is the working diagnosis?

4. Should this patient be hospitalized or treated as an outpatient and why?

5. What medication regimen should be used to treat this patient and for how long?

6. What patient education is needed for this patient?

Diagnosis

The diagnosis of PID is usually based on clinical findings. In women presenting with abdominal pain, the minimum criteria for diagnosis of PID are cervical motion tenderness or uterine tenderness or adnexal tenderness (70). Supportive criteria for diagnosis includes oral temperature greater than 101°F, mucopurulent cervical or vaginal discharge, abundant white blood cells on microscopy of vaginal secretions, elevated erythrocyte sedimentation rate, elevated C-reactive protein, and laboratory documentation of cervical infection with *N. gonorrheae* or *Chlamydia* (70).

Management

Women with mild or moderate PID can be treated successfully on an outpatient basis. Empiric therapy is recommended for women who meet the minimum criteria for diagnosis of PID and are at risk. Antibiotic therapy should provide coverage for *N. gonorrheae*, *Chlamydia*, and anaerobes (70). The CDC recommends a single dose of ceftriaxone 250 mg intramuscularly *plus* doxycycline 100 mg orally twice a day for 14 days *with or without metronidazole* 500 mg orally twice a day for 14 days (71). A single dose of cefoxitin 2 g intramuscularly with a single dose of probenecid 1 g orally may be substituted for ceftriaxone (Table 16-3). Other third-generation parenteral cephalosporins (e.g., ceftizoxime or cefotaxime) may also be substituted for the single-dose ceftriaxone or cefoxitin. Women treated on an outpatient basis should follow-up in 3 days after initiation of treatment to evaluate clinical improvement. If the woman has not demonstrated substantial clinical improvement after 72 hours of outpatient therapy (e.g., normal temperature, decrease in abdominal tenderness, and decrease in uterine, adnexal and cervical motion tenderness), the woman should be hospitalized and parenteral therapy begun.

The CDC recommends the following criteria for hospitalization: (1) cannot exclude a surgical emergency (e.g., appendicitis), (2) patient is pregnant, (3) does not respond clinically to antibiotics, (4) is not able to follow or tolerate an outpatient regimen, (5) is severely ill with nausea and vomiting and fever, and (6) has a tubo-ovarian abscess (70).

The CDC recommends two parenteral regimens for the inpatient treatment of PID (Table 16-3) (70). Parenteral Regimen A uses cefotetan 2 g IV every 12 hours or cefoxitin 2 g IV every 6 hours plus doxycycline 100 mg orally or IV every 12 hours. Since doxycycline is painful when administered intravenously, it should be given orally when possible. The intravenous regimen can be discontinued 24 hours after the patient improves clinically and doxycycline 100 mg twice a day can be given for 14 more days. If the patient has a tubo-ovarian abscess, many providers use clindamycin or metronidazole with doxycycline for more effective anaerobic coverage.

Parenteral Regimen B uses clindamycin 900 mg IV every 8 hours plus gentamicin loading dose IV or IM (2 mg/kg of body weight), followed by a maintenance dose (1.5 mg/kg) every 8 hours. Single daily dosing may be substituted. Intravenous therapy can be discontinued 24 hours after the patient improves clinically and oral therapy can begin with doxycycline 100 mg orally twice a day or clindamycin 450 mg orally four times a day for 14 days. If the patient has a tubo-ovarian abscess, many providers will use clindamycin for continued therapy, rather than doxycycline for better anaerobic coverage. If the patient does not respond to parenteral therapy a diagnostic laparoscopy may be needed to look for alternative diagnoses (70).

Clinical Nurse Specialist Competencies and Spheres of Influence
Coaching/Teaching/Mentoring
The patient treated on an outpatient basis should be instructed on how to correctly take medication and to

TABLE 16–3 Recommendations for Outpatient and Inpatient Pharmacotherapy for PID

Outpatient Therapy

Single dose of ceftriaxone 250 mg IM (may substitute a single dose of cefoxitin 2 g IM and a single dose of probenecid 1 g orally)
PLUS
Doxycycline 100 mg orally twice a day for 14 days
WITH or WITHOUT
Metronidazole 500 mg orally twice a day for 14 days

Inpatient Therapy

Parenteral Regimen A
Cefotetan 2 g IV every 12 hours
OR
Cefoxitin 2 g IV every 6 hours
PLUS
Doxycycline 100 mg orally or IV every 12 hours
IV therapy may be discontinued after 24 hours if patient improves, then continue doxycycline for 14 more days.
Parenteral Regimen B
Clindamycin 900 mg IV every 8 hours
PLUS
Loading dose of gentamicin IV or IM (2 mg/kg of body weight) followed by a maintenance dose (1.5 mg/kg) every 8 hours.
IV therapy may be discontinued after 24 hours if patient improves and oral therapy can begin with doxycycline 100 mg orally twice a day for 14 days OR clindamycin 450 mg orally four times a day for 14 days.

Centers for Disease Control and Prevention. Sexually transmitted diseases treatment guidelines, 2010. MMWR Morb Mortal Wkly Rep 2010;59(RR-12):1-114.

take the full course. She should also be instructed to return to the clinic in 72 hours for follow-up. Male sex partners should be tested for STIs if they have had sexual contact with the patient in the 60 days before the patient began having symptoms. The partner should be treated if the test is positive for an STI (70). In addition, the patient should be instructed on prevention of STIs.

Adnexal Torsion Etiology

Ovarian or adnexal torsion occurs when an enlarged ovary causes increased force on the supporting ligaments, which causes the ovary to twist upon itself. Fallopian tubes can also be involved. Ovarian torsion is almost always associated with ovarian tumors such as functional cysts or benign neoplasms (72).

Pathophysiology

In a partial torsion, there is enough arterial pressure to allow blood flow to the adnexa. However, as the torsion worsens, venous blood is unable to return, arterial blood flow is reduced and is then unable to oxygenate the ovary and surrounding tissue leading to necrosis. Lymphatic drainage is also blocked, which causes edema (72). Patients having in vitro fertilization are at greatest risk for adnexal torsion due to hyperstimulation of ovarian follicles (41, 72). In addition, pregnancy may cause torsion as the uterus becomes enlarged and pushes the ovaries anteriorly (41).

Clinical Presentation

Patients may present with acute, intermittent, and unilateral abdominal pain. Pain can be made worse with change of position. About 70% of patients will have gastrointestinal complaints such as nausea and vomiting. On exam, a tender, unilateral adnexal mass can be palpated about 70% of the time. A fever may develop if necrosis occurs (41, 72).

Diagnosis

A pregnancy test should be performed to rule out ectopic pregnancy. Cultures for *N. gonorrheae* and *Chlamydia* should be performed to rule out PID. A pelvic ultrasound with color Doppler can suggest adnexal torsion, but it does not provide a definitive diagnosis. An abdominal CT may be performed to rule out appendicitis (41). A definitive diagnosis is made in surgery (41, 72).

Management

Surgical reduction is the treatment for ovarian torsion. Recently, more conservative surgery, performing a gentle untwisting of the ovary and tacking the ovary to the pelvic sidewall has been successful rather than removing the tube and ovary. If there has been severe vascular damage, tube and ovary are removed (41).

Clinical Nurse Specialist Competencies and Spheres of Influence
Clinical Expert/Direct Care

The CNS should assist the medical and nursing staff in the diagnosis and management of the patient with adnexal torsion. If adnexal torsion is suspected, the patient will need to be quickly prepared for diagnostic tests and surgery. The CNS may be instrumental in facilitating timely and safe passage through the diagnostic process and transport to surgery.

Hormone Replacement Therapy

HRT historically has been prescribed to allay the symptoms of menopause, including the vascular response that triggers "hot flashes," skin and vaginal dryness, depression, and osteoporosis, as well as for presumed protection against cardiovascular disease. However, as a result of the Women's Health Initiative (WHI) study conducted in the 1990s to the 2000s, HRT is no longer first-line treatment for menopause. In this study, one group of women who had undergone hysterectomy received estrogen alone compared with placebo, and a second group of women without hysterectomy received estrogen plus progestin compared with placebo. In the estrogen plus progestin group, there was an increase in heart disease, thromboembolic disease, stroke, and breast cancer and, as a result, the study was aborted. In the estrogen-alone-hysterectomy group, there was a decrease in coronary artery calcium buildup, suggesting some promise for cardioprotection for women following hysterectomy. More research is required before making recommendations for estrogen therapy for prevention of cardiovascular disease, however. Because of the complexities of estrogen therapy, HRT is recommended only for moderate to severe menopausal symptoms in the lowest possible dose. One outcome of the study, because of the striking differences in results among the groups, was acceptance of new nomenclature for hormone therapy: estrogen therapy alone is referred to as ET and estrogen plus progestin as EPT (73).

Despite findings from the WHI, many women who initiated HRT prior to release of this study are unwilling to endure the symptoms of menopause by discontinuing therapy. Clinicians should be mindful of the risk of comorbidity in women taking HRT who present for other health conditions. Because of a higher risk for venous thromboembolism (VTE) (74), some experts recommend that prior to surgery, all women older than 40 years old who are taking hormone replacements should receive perioperative VTE prophylaxis, especially if they will be immobile for a period of time (75). Prophylaxis can include graduated compression stockings, pneumatic compression, low-dose unfractionated heparin, or low-molecular-weight heparin. In addition, some women may decide to discontinue hormone therapy four weeks before surgery if they anticipate prolonged immobility, but there is no research to support that practice. Once the patient is ambulatory, she may resume hormone therapy (75).

Clinical Nurse Specialist Competencies and Spheres of Influence
Coaching/Teaching/Mentoring and Collaboration

Patients require education on the risks of cardiovascular disease, thromboembolic events, and stroke when taking oral estrogens. CNSs should provide counseling on the synergistic effects of HRT and tobacco smoking and risk for VTE and initiate referral for smoking cessation programs. Patients should be advised to guard against dehydration, especially in warm climates, air travel, and outdoor sports. Weight loss counseling should be addressed. Hospitalized patients should be educated about the risk for VTE related to immobility. Patients need education and advisement on when to seek emergent health care in the event of a thromboembolic event.

For any hospitalized woman undergoing surgery, the CNS ensures that screening for hormone therapy has been documented in the medical record. Like herbals and other complementary therapy, many patients do not consider hormones to be medications; careful questioning is sometimes required to elicit this information. The CNS collaborates with the surgical team for decisions about VTE prophylaxis.

URINARY INCONTINENCE IN MEN AND WOMEN

Etiology

Approximately 17 million people in the United State experience urinary incontinence. More than one-third of hospitalized adults have urinary incontinence, which creates problems for patients and caregivers, consumes enormous resources in nursing time and hygiene supplies, and leads to numerous complications. Etiology for urinary incontinence includes patient, environmental, and iatrogenic factors. Patient conditions consist of neurologic deficits such as stroke, dementia, delirium, and spinal cord or brain injury; gynecologic anatomical deviations; diabetes mellitus; and immobility. Older adults may experience urinary incontinence due to poor hydration and nutrition and constipation or fecal impaction. Hospitalized patients may have difficulty ambulating to the bathroom, especially with intravenous catheters, monitoring equipment, and other attachments. Side effects of medications, especially cardiac drugs and diuretics, are iatrogenic causes of urinary incontinence (76).

Pathophysiology

There are five types of urinary incontinence. Stress incontinence occurs from conditions that cause increased intra-abdominal pressure. Examples include pregnancy, tumor, ascites, obesity, and distended bowel secondary to constipation. Urge incontinence results from an overdistended bladder that creates an extreme urgent need to void. Mixed urinary incontinence has elements of stress and urge incontinence. Overflow incontinence occurs with loss of urine when the bladder is overdistended and may result from a poorly functioning bladder detrusor muscle or obstruction of urinary outflow. Finally, functional incontinence comes from nongenitourinary problems such as cognitive or physical limitations that interfere with independent toileting; this type often afflicts older adults (76).

Clinical Presentation

Depending on the type and origin, patients may volunteer they are experiencing urinary incontinence. In patients with cognitive impairment, however, nurses must conduct a thorough assessment and may need to obtain a history from other family members. Compromised skin integrity and evaluation for urinary related dermatitis should be included.

Diagnosis

Urinary incontinence is diagnosed largely through clinical presentation and history. Several screening instruments to identify and determine the type of urinary incontinence are available. Examples include the Urinary Distress Inventory-6 (UDI-6) and the Incontinence Impact Questionnaire-7 (IIQ-7) (76). Urodynamic tests may be indicated to evaluate urine flow, retention, and obstruction in complex situations or when the diagnosis is unclear after the history and physical exam; urodynamic testing is not recommended for routine evaluation of urinary incontinence, however. Abdominal radiographs will show excessive stool throughout the bowel when constipation and fecal impaction cause urinary incontinence. Additional testing to rule out any underlying pathology may be indicated, which should be done by specialists.

Management

Management of urinary incontinence depends on the type, etiology, and gender of the patient. For women, lifestyle changes such as weight loss and scheduled voiding regimen may help prevent stress incontinence. Physical therapy and Kegal exercises are aimed at strengthening pelvic floor muscles that may help with stress, urge, and mixed incontinence. Bladder training and timed voiding are effective in patients with cognitive or functional impairment. Complicated cases should be referred to a specialist, who may offer options such as placement of vaginal cones, electrical or magnetic stimulation, or a variety of surgical modifications of the genitourinary tract (77).

For men, management of urinary incontinence may include lifestyle modifications, pelvic floor muscle training, and scheduled voiding. When basic approaches are ineffective, referral to a specialist may be necessary. Treatment options may include additional testing such as urodynamics to identify underlying pathology, electrical stimulation, pharmacologic agents such as alpha-blockers or 5-alpha-reductase inhibitors, or surgery for anatomical modification (78).

For both men and women admitted to the hospital, especially elder adults, identification and treatment of the underlying causes is the initial step in management. Effective prehospital strategies should be continued. Indwelling catheters should be avoided. All patients should have fluid intake and output measured to gauge level of hydration. Skin assessment and prevention strategies such as cleansing and use of barrier products should be initiated to prevent dermatitis, maceration, and breakdown. The environment should be safe for ambulation to the bathroom. For stress incontinence, pelvic floor muscle exercises and assistance with toileting are recommended. For urge incontinence in the cognitive intact individual, bladder training is indicated, along with pharmacologic therapy. For overflow incontinence, adequate time for bladder emptying should be provided. Patients may need bedside ultrasonography to determine postvoid residual urine amounts, and instruction in double voiding with Crede's maneuver to facilitate complete bladder emptying. People with functional incontinence may benefit from cuing to void, with strict scheduling (79).

Pharmacologic therapy may include a variety of medications, but most are not recommended for first-line treatment. The patient's type of urinary incontinence, comorbidities, and other medications should be considered when selecting medications. A list of medications for possible use is available in Guidelines on Urinary Incontinence US Department of Health and Human Services Agency for Healt care Research and Quality (80).

Clinical Nurse Specialist Competencies and Spheres of Influence
Clinical Expert/Direct Care
CNSs apply clinical expertise in recognizing when patients present with risk factors for urinary incontinence. The CNS completes a thorough history for identification and, for hospitalized patients, ensures that prehospital management strategies are followed whenever possible. For cognitively and functionally impaired individuals in particular, the CNS conducts a thorough skin assessment and prescribes appropriate therapy for treatment and prevention of incontinence dermatitis and skin breakdown. The CNS recognizes when referral to a specialist is indicated.

Consultation, Systems Leadership, Coaching/Teaching/Mentoring, and Research/Evidence-Based Practice
The CNS assists in identifying the type of urinary incontinence and helps to establish an appropriate plan of care. Urinary incontinence–associated dermatitis can be severe; he or she may be consulted for assistance with managing these challenging skin problems. The CNS may be instrumental in leading systemwide initiatives such as a bladder training programs, implementation of incontinence screening tools, and translation of evidence-based practice guidelines for prevention of urinary incontinence. Limited use of indwelling catheters has been a vast undertaking in some facilities; persistence and vigilance by CNS leaders, who are committed to quality, cost-effective care with fewer catheter-related infections, and prevention of urinary incontinence, are necessary for success. CNSs bring resources such as practice guidelines and research-based clinical protocols to frontline clinicians for use in managing patients with urinary incontinence.

References

1. Rosenstein D, McAninch JW. Urologic emergencies. Med Clin North Am 2004;88(2):495-518.

2. Ellerkmann RM, McBride A, Management of obstructive voiding dysfunction. Drugs Today (Barc) 2003;39(7):513-540.

3. Curtis LA, Dolan TS, Cespedes RD. Acute urinary retention and urinary incontinence. Emerg Med Clin North Am 2001;19(3):591-619.

4. Choong S, Emberton M. Acute urinary retention. BJU Int 2000; 85(2):186-201.

5. Meigs JB, et al. Incidence rates and risk factors for acute urinary retention. The Health Professionals Followup Study. J Urol 1999; 162(2):376-382.

6. Jacobsen SJ, et al. Natural history of prostatism: risk factors for acute urinary retention. J Urol 1997;158(2):481-487.

7. Fuselier HA Jr. Etiology and management of acute urinary retention. Compre Ther 1993;19(1):31-36.

8. Verhamme KM, et al. Nonsteroidal anti-inflammatory drugs and increased risk of acute urinary retention. Arch Intern Med 2005;165(13):1547-1551.

9. Fowler CJ, O'Malley KJ. Investigation and management of neurogenic bladder dysfunction. J Neurol Neurosurg Psychiatry 2003;74(suppl 4):iv27-iv31.

10. Kong KH, Young S. Incidence and outcome of poststroke urinary retention: a prospective study. Arch Phys Med Rehabil 2000; 81(11):1464-1467.

11. Sasaki K, Yoshimura N, Chancellor MB. Implications of diabetes mellitus in urology. Urol Clin North Am 2003;30(1):1-12.

12. Barbalias GA, Nikiforidis G, Liatsikos EN. Vesicourethral dysfunction associated with multiple sclerosis: clinical and urodynamic perspectives. J Urol 1998;160(1):106-111.

13. Tintinalli JE. Acute urinary retention as a presenting sign of spinal cord compression. Ann Emerg Med 1986;15(10):1235-1237.

14. Ruhl M. Postoperative voiding criteria for ambulatory surgery patients. AORN J 2009;89(5):871-874.

15. Dalton JE, editor. Basic Clinical Urology. Philadelphia: JB Lippincott; 1983.

16. Fontanarosa PB, Roush WR. Acute urinary retention. Emerg Med Clin North Am 1988;6(3):419-437.

17. Fontanarosa PB. Radiologic contrast-induced renal failure. Emerg Med Clin North Am 1988;6(3):601-616.

18. Pickard R, Emberton M, Neal DE. The management of men with acute urinary retention. National Prostatectomy Audit Steering Group. Br J Urol 1998;81(5):712-720.

19. Nussbaum Blask AR, et al. Color Doppler sonography and scintigraphy of the testis: a prospective, comparative analysis in children with acute scrotal pain. Pediatr Emerg Care 2002;18(2):67-71.

20. McAndrew HF, et al. The incidence and investigation of acute scrotal problems in children. Pediatr Surg Int 2002;18(5-6):435-437.

21. Cummings JM, et al. Adult testicular torsion. J Urol 2002;167(5):2109-2110.

22. Gunther P, et al. Acute testicular torsion in children: the role of sonography in the diagnostic workup. Eur Radiol 2006;16(11):2527-2532.

23. Kapoor S. Testicular torsion: a race against time. Int J Clin Pract 2008;62(5):821-827.

24. Lavallee ME, Cash J. Testicular torsion: evaluation and management. Curr Sports Med Rep 2005;4(2):102-104.

25. DeMauro CA, Horrow MM. Diagnosis: incomplete testicular torsion progressing to complete torsion. Ultrasound Q 2008;24(2):121-123.

26. Kapasi Z, Halliday S. Best evidence topic report. Ultrasound in the diagnosis of testicular torsion. Emerg Med J 2005;22(8):559-560.

27. Cole FL, Vogler R. The acute, nontraumatic scrotum: assessment, diagnosis, and management. J Am Acad Nurse Pract 2004;16(2):50-56.

28. Eland IA, et al. Incidence of priapism in the general population. Urology 2001;57(5):970-972.

29. Adeyoju AB, et al. Priapism in sickle-cell disease; incidence, risk factors and complications: an international multicentre study. BJU Int 2002;90(9):898-902.

30. Burnett AL, Bivalacqua TJ. Priapism: current principles and practice. Urol Clin North Am 2007;34(4):631-642, viii.

31. Burnett AL. Pathophysiology of priapism: dysregulatory erection physiology thesis. J Urol 2003;170(1):26-34.

32. Levine JF, et al. Recurrent prolonged erections and priapism as a sequela of priapism: pathophysiology and management. J Urol 1991;145(4):764-767.

33. Montague DK, et al. American Urological Association guideline on the management of priapism. J Urol 2003;170(4 Pt 1):1318-1324.

34. Stone HH, Martin JD Jr. Synergistic necrotizing cellulitis. Ann Surg 1972;175(5):702-711.

35. Sorensen MD, et al. Fournier's gangrene: population based epidemiology and outcomes. J Urol 2009;181(5):2120-2126.

36. Hammer CC, Santucci RA. Genitourinary emergencies: how to appropriately manage GU injuries & illnesses. JEMS 2005;30(3):120-122, 124, 126-128 passim; quiz 136.

37. Bradway C, Rodgers J. Evaluation and management of genitourinary emergencies. Nurse Pract 2009;34(5):36-43; quiz 43-44.

38. Thwaini A, et al. Fournier's gangrene and its emergency management. Postgrad Med J 2006;82(970):516-519.

39. Paynter M. Paraphimosis. Emerg Nurse 2006;14(4):18-19.

40. Little B, White M. Treatment options for paraphimosis. Int J Clin Pract 2005;59(5):591-593.

41. McWilliams GDE, Hill MJ, Dietrich CS. Gynecologic emergencies. Surg Clin North Am 2008;88(2):265-283.

42. Cunningham FG, et al. Williams Obstetrics. 22nd edition. New York: McGraw-Hill; 2005.

43. American College of Obstetrics & Gynecology, ACOG practice bulletin: Medical management of ectopic pregnancy. Obstet Gynecol 2008;111(6):1479-1485.

44. Nama V, Manyonda I. Tubal ectopic pregnancy: diagnosis and management. Arch Gynecol Obstet 2009;279:443-453.

45. Chandrasekhar C. Ectopic pregnancy: a pictorial review. Clin Imaging 2008;32(6):468-473.

46. Nelson AL, DeUgarte CM, Gambone JC. Ectopic pregnancy. In Hacker NF, Gambone JC, Hobel CJ, editors. Essentials of Obstetrics and Gynecology. Philadelphia: Saunders; 2009. p. 325-333.

47. Chung K, Allen R. The use of serial human chorionic gonadotropin levels to establish a viable or a nonviable pregnancy. Semin Reprod Med 2008;26(05):383-390.

48. The Practice Committee of the American Society for Reproductive Medicine [ASRM Practice Committee]. Medical treatment of ectopic pregnancy. Fertil Steril 2008;90(suppl 3):S206-S212.

49. Song AH, Advincula AP. Adolescent chronic pelvic pain. J Pediatr Adolesc Gynecol 2005;18(6):371-377.

50. Podczaski ES, Kramer PR. Gynecologic considerations for the general surgeon. In Ashley SW, et al, editors. ACS Surgery: Principles and Practice. Philadelphia: B.C. Decker; 2009.

51. Grimes DA, et al. Oral contraceptives for functional ovarian cysts. Cochrane Database Syst Rev 2009(2).

52. McFarlin BL. Ultrasound assessment of the endometrium for irregular vaginal bleeding. J Midwif Womens Health 2006;51(6):440-449.

53. Moore JG, Gambone JC. Dysfunction uterine bleeding. In Hacker NF, Gambone JC, Hobel CJ, editors. Essentials of obstetrics and Gynecology. Philadelphia: Saunders; 2009:409-412.

54. Moore JG, Nelson AL. Congenital anomalies and benign conditions of the uterine corpus and cervix. In Hacker NF, Gambone JC, Hobel CJ, editors. Essentials of Obstetrics and Gynecology. Philadelphia: Saunders; 2009:268-276.

55. Colin CM, Shushan A. Complications of menstruation: abnormal uterine bleeding. In DeCherney AH, et al, editors. Current Diagnosis and Treatment Obstetrics and Gynecology. New York: McGraw-Hill; 2007.

56. Brown S. Miscarriage and its associations. Semin Reprod Med 2008;26(05):391-400.

57. Zegers-Hochschild F, et al. The International Committee for Monitoring Assisted Reproductive Technology (ICMART and the World Health Organization (WHO) revised glossary on ART terminology 2009. Hum Reprod 2009;24(11):2683-2687.

58. Stephenson M, Kutteh W. Evaluation and management of recurrent early pregnancy loss. Clin Obstet Gynecol 2007;50(1):132-145.

59. Brier N. Grief following miscarriage: a comprehensive review of the literature. J Womens Health 2008;17(3):451-464.

60. Hutti MH. Social and professional support needs of families after perinatal loss. JOGNN 2005;34(5):630-638.

61. Ainbinder SW, Ramin SM, DeCherney AH. Sexually transmitted diseases and pelvic infections. In DeCherney AH, et al, editors. Current Diagnosis and Treatment Obstetrics and Gynecology. New York: McGraw-Hill; 2007.

62. Centers for Disease Control and Prevention (CDC). Historical perspectives reduced incidence of menstrual toxic-shock syndrome: United States, 1980-1990. MMWR Morb Mortal Wkly Rep 1990;39(25):421-423.

63. Hajjeh RA, et al. Toxic shock syndrome in the United States: surveillance update, 1979-1996. Emerg Infect Dis 1999;5(6):807-810.

64. Lappin, E., Ferguson, A. Gram-positive toxic shock syndromes. The Lanst Infectious Diseases, 2009;9(5):281-290 doi:10.1016/S1473-3099(09)70066-0.

65. Reingold AL, et al. Toxic shock syndrome surveillance in the United States, 1980 to 1981. Ann Intern Med 1982;96 (6 Pt 2):875-880.

66. CDC. Sexually transmitted disease surveillance 2007. Atlanta, GA: US Department of Health and Human Services; 2008.

67. CDC. Sexually transmitted disease surveillance 2007. Available from: http://www.cdc.gov/std/stats07/Surv2007FINAL.pdf

68. Lareau SM, Beigi RH. Pelvic inflammatory disease and tubo-ovarian abscess. Infect Dis Clin North Am 2008;22:693-708.

69. Gray-Swain MR, Peipert JF. Pelvic inflammatory disease in adolescents. Curr Opin Obstet Gynecol 2006;18:503-510.

70. CDC. Sexually transmitted diseases treatment guidelines, 2010. MMWR Morb Mortal Wkly Rep 2010;**59**(RR-12):1-114.

71. CDC. Update to CDC's sexually transmitted diseases treatment guidelines: 2006:—fluoroquinolones no longer recommended for treatment of gonococcal infections. MMWR Morb Mortal Wkly Rep 2007;56(14):332-336.

72. Stevens E, Gilbert-Cohen J. Surgical considerations in early pregnancy: ectopic pregnancy and ovarian torsion. Perinat Neonat Nursing 2006;21(1):22-29.

73. National Institutes of Health. Women's Health Initiative. Estrogen therapy and coronary artery calcification. Retrieved April 29, 2011 from http://www.nhlbi.nih.gov/whi/estro_alone.htm

74. Canonico M, et al. Hormone replacement therapy and risk of venous thromboembolism in postmenopausal women: systematic review and meta-analysis. Br Med J 2008;336:1227-1231.

75. Speroff L. Should hormone therapy stop before surgery? Geriatrics 2008;63(8):29-30.

76. Dowling-Castronovo A. urinary incontinence nursing standard of practice protocol: urinary incontinence (UI) in older adults admitted to acute care. Hartford for Geriatric Nursing. Consult GerRn.org. http://consultgerirn.org/topics/urinary_incontinence/want_to_know_more#item_2

77. US Department of Health and Human Services Agency for Healthcare Research and Quality. Incontinence in women. In Guidelines on urinary incontinence. (2) 2010 addendum to 2009 urinary incontinence guidelines. Retrieved May 2, 2011 from www.guideline.gov

78. US Department of Health and Human Services Agency for Healthcare Research and Quality. Incontinence in men. In Guidelines on urinary incontinence. Retrieved May 2, 2011 from www.guideline.gov

79. US Department of Health and Human Services Agency for Healthcare Research and Quality. Urinary incontinence (UI) in older adults admitted to acute care. In: Evidence-based geriatric nursing protocols for best practice. Retrieved May 2, 2011 from www.guideline.gov

80. US Department of Health and Human Services Agency for Healthcare Research and Quality. Pharmacotherapy. In Guidelines on urinary incontinence. (2) 2010 addendum to 2009 urinary incontinence guidelines. Retrieved May 2, 2011 from www.guideline.gov

CHAPTER 17

Musculoskeletal Problems

Jan Powers, PhD, RN, CCNS, CCRN, CNRN, FCCM,
and Diana Jones, MSN, RN, ACNS-BC

INTRODUCTION

Common types of musculoskeletal problems include traumatic injuries, osteoarthritis (OA), amputations. Some of these are the results of traumatic injuries, or they may be the result of the aging process. Along with these conditions, there are also devastating complications that may occur such as compartment syndrome, venous thromboembolism (VTE), fat embolism and pulmonary embolism. Regardless of the cause, musculoskeletal injuries can be devastating to the individual, resulting in changes in functional status and ongoing functional issues. These conditions present challenges to bedside caregivers as well as the Clinical Nurse Specialist (CNS). The CNS evaluates the individual patient as well as the orthopedic patient population as a whole and determines process requirements from a system perspective to best meet orthopedic patients' needs (1).

OSTEOARTHRITIS AND JOINT REPLACEMENT SURGERY

There are two types of arthritis, rheumatoid arthritis and osteoarthritis. Together they represent two of the most prevalent chronic health problems and most common causes of disability (2). OA, a degenerative joint disease characterized by the breakdown of joint cartilage, is the most common form of arthritis, affecting over 27 million Americans, most over the age of 45 (3). Approximately 40% of people with arthritis have employment limitations due to physical disabilities (3). By the year 2030, it is projected that 25% of the U.S. population (nearly 67 million people) will have OA (4). This will be an increasing burden on the health care system. Health care providers in all types of settings will continue to see the number of arthritis-related illnesses increase with the aging population. It is estimated that over 70% of people aged 70 years or older have radiographic evidence of OA. Arthritis and related conditions cost the U.S. economy

nearly $128 billion per year in medical care and indirect expenses, including lost wages and productivity (5).

Etiology

The causes of OA are uncertain. There are certain risk factors that may contribute to the development of idiopathic (primary) or secondary disease. Risk factors for primary OA include aging, female gender, and genetics. (6). Over time, as joints are continually subjected to movement and friction, cartilage breaks down, causing irritation and potentially bone to bone contact. This leads to joint pain and swelling, and causes disability. For those with a total loss of cartilage there is increasing pain and limitation to joint movement. There is an increased incidence of OA in aging women. This may be related to estrogen reduction with menopause. Finally, there is evidence to suggest that OA may be hereditary in nature, due to the disease presence in multiple members of the same family (6). Researchers have also found that the daughters of women who have osteoarthritic knees have significant increase in cartilage breakdown, making them more susceptible to the disease. Development of a genetic test for OA is in progress (7).

Modifiable risk factors for OA include but are not limited to obesity, overuse of joints, and repeated trauma. These factors contribute to secondary OA, which is associated with another disease or condition. Obesity contributes to development of OA by increasing the mechanical stress on the cartilage. Even modest weight loss can reduce symptoms of OA by easing the strain on weight-bearing joints such as the hips and knees. If a person undergoes joint replacement surgery for OA in a weight-bearing joint, weight reduction can significantly improve their ability to rehabilitate afterward as well as decrease the risk of perioperative complications. Because injured joints are more vulnerable to OA, repeated trauma to joint tissues such as ligaments, bones, and cartilage leads to early OA. There are numerous occupations such as nursing, packaging/shipping/delivery workers, and certain factory workers, whose jobs demand repetitive motion, which pose a higher risk for work-related injuries. Athletes who participate in strenuous exercise with quick stopping and pivoting while playing sports such as soccer, football, and basketball have an increased risk for developing OA in the knees (8).

OA is not curable, but lifestyle modifications can improve function and reduce pain. Eating a healthy diet to maintain a weight that reduces stress on joints, avoiding extreme sports that may cause injury, and taking precautions on the job when repetitive motion is required by following workplace safe practices and guidelines contribute to better quality of life.

Pathophysiology

OA is the most common of the noninflammatory type of degenerative joint disease. Both forms of OA, primary and secondary, have the same general characteristics: articular cartilage erosion, sclerosis (thickening) of the bone underneath the cartilage, and the formation of osteophytes (bone spurs).

Normally, when a synovial joint is at rest, cartilage absorbs synovial fluid; when the joint is in motion, this fluid flushes out. This continual flushing occurs repeatedly during the course of a day. Over time, the protective barriers begin to erode. A person's body weight is not evenly distributed and rests largely on the knees, which are typically the first to become affected by OA. Persons with OA will likely present with complaints of stiffness and occasional pain, which becomes progressively worse.

Enzymatic destruction of the articular cartilage begins in the matrix, with destruction of proteoglycans and collagen fibers. The cartilage matrix is made up of proteoglycans, glycosaminoglycans (carbohydrates that contain amino sugars), chondrocytes, and collagen (a fibrous structural protein). Normally, all four elements—collagen, proteoglycans, chondrocytes, and water—work together to ensure smooth, pain-free movement.

Enzymes are released to break down the large molecules of these components into diffusable fragments, which are then taken up by the chondrocytes and digested by the cell's own lysosomal enzymes. Scientists are not certain where or how these enzymes are formed. One theory is that some may lie dormant in the matrix or in the cartilage itself. Another explanation may be that the enzymes originate in the synovial membrane, blood plasma, or leukocytes and migrate into the synovial cavity. Further speculation is that activation of these enzymes may be the result of injury, dietary allergies, inflammation, or other conditions that trigger an excessive release of enzymes in the joint. Whatever the reason, these enzymes are fundamental to both the health and destruction of bone.

Any change in the structure of proteoglycans disrupts the pumping action that regulates the movement of synovial fluid into and out of cartilage. Without this regulatory action, the cartilage accumulates excessive fluid and becomes less able to withstand the stresses of weight bearing. The synovium has many nerve endings and pain receptors, which sends pain messages to the brain. In response, the brain signals the synovium to produce more fluid. This results in a flooding of the area, which causes more pain and swelling. The synovium itself may also swell and exude a pus-like material.

As the disease progresses, the cartilage begins to soften and crack, resulting in longitudinal fissures (fibrillation). In advanced cases, bone spurs (osteophytes), abnormal bone hardening (eburnation), and fluid-filled pockets in the bone (subchondral cysts) can form. Pressure builds in the cysts until its contents are forced into the synovial cavity, breaking through the articular cartilage on the way. As the articular cartilage erodes, cartilage-coated osteophytes may grow outward from the underlying bone. These spurlike bony projections enlarge until small pieces, called "joint mice," break off into the synovial cavity. These fragments can cause irritation, resulting in an accumulation of unwanted fluid (joint effusion) and the cycle begins again.

As the cartilage degenerates, more stress is placed on the joint, which speeds up the destruction of even more cartilage. The bones then become damaged, and the afflicted joint may become deformed. The bones thicken or change shape, narrowing the space within a joint. Bone spurs twist the joint contours, making it difficult for the bones to move. Presentation of a healthy knee joint compared to an arthritic joint is found in Figure 17-1

Clinical Presentation

A typical presentation of a person with OA is limited movement and joint pain. In the early stages of OA one may be unaware of the disease, as it tends to progress insidiously. One may notice pain following physical activity during work or while exercising initially. Next, the individual is unable to perform tasks that were achievable in the past. There may be deep aching of the joints, with pain becoming more persistent.

One may begin to experience joint stiffness, particularly first thing in the morning when getting out of bed or after being in the same position for a long period of time. An indication that the disease has progressed is when there is noticeable pain that becomes more predominant following times of prolonged rest. Joint deformity is another visual cue. Visible bony overgrowths may appear on the hands (Heberden's nodes) or on the toes (Bouchard's nodes).

Diagnosis

Obtaining a history and performing a physical examination will be most useful in gaining pertinent subjective and objective information from the patient. There is not a specific laboratory test to diagnose OA. A diagnosis will

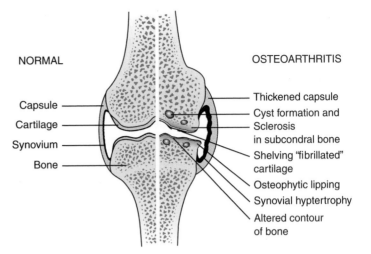

NORMAL

OSTEOARTHRITIS

Capsule

Cartilage

Synovium

Bone

Thickened capsule

Cyst formation and
Sclerosis
in subcondral bone

Shelving "fibrillated"
cartilage

Osteophytic lipping

Synovial hyptertrophy

Altered contour
of bone

FIGURE 17–1: Osteoarthritis.

be based on the combination of a patient's medical history, physical exam, radiographs, and possibly a sampling of synovial fluid from an affected joint. Tables 17-1 and 17-2 summarize the laboratory and other tests.

Radiographs are not very useful to detect early OA because the films do not show significant changes in cartilage, which is where the earliest abnormalities occur. The findings may not correlate with what the patient describes in the history. Magnetic resonance imaging (MRI) can reveal early changes in cartilage, but it is rarely needed for the diagnosis. However, MRI is more sensitive than a radiograph in identifying progressive joint destruction.

Management

The CNS plays a collaborative role with a host of other disciplines to care for people with OA. A multidisciplinary approach will achieve the most appropriate and optimal outcome for the patient. The following list of professionals may assume direct care or act as a consultant during the course of OA treatment. Primary care physicians often determine the initial diagnosis and may treat patients with OA before they are referred to other specialists in the health care system. Rheumatologists provide specialized ongoing treatment of OA over the course of the disease. Orthopedists are consulted for advisement on surgical options for joint repair or replacement. Physical therapists can effectively work with patients to improve joint function. Occupational therapists provide patient education on ways to protect joints, minimize pain, perform activities of daily living, and conserve energy. Dietitians provide patient education in ways to use proper nutrition to improve health and maintain a healthy weight. Patient educators and

TABLE 17-1 Laboratory Tests

Test	Description
Rheumatoid factor (RF)	A blood sample determines the diagnosis of rheumatoid arthritis.
Cyclic citrullinated peptide antibody (CCP)	The test differentiates rheumatoid arthritis from other forms of arthritis. A CCP is ordered if the RF result is negative.
Erythrocyte sedimentation rate (ESR)	Indicates presence of inflammation. ESR will be elevated in rheumatoid arthritis but not in osteoarthritis.
C-reactive protein (CRP)	A test used to differentiate osteoarthritis and rheumatoid arthritis. An increased level of CRP occurs in rheumatoid arthritis but not in osteoarthritis.
Complete blood count (CBC)	To evaluate red and white blood cells. To monitor the side effects of some osteoarthritis treatments.
Comprehensive metabolic panel (CMP)	To evaluate and monitor function of the kidney and liver for side effects of some medications used for treatment.
Synovial fluid analysis	Fluid sample is obtained from a joint by inserting a needle in the space between bone and joint. Changes in the fluid indicate presence of disease.

TABLE 17-2 Nonlaboratory Tests

Test	Description
Radiograph	Can identify cartilage and narrowing of the joint space but will not show significant changes early in the disease. This study is useful to rule out injury and to offer a baseline reference from the time treatment begins.
Magnetic resonance imaging (MRI)	Provides accurate information of the joint structure, bones, and soft tissue. The test is an adjunct to the medical history and physical examination and following a radiograph. The test is supportive to the medial history and physical examination and following a radiograph.

nurses assist patients in understanding their overall condition, implementation of treatment plans, and lifestyle modifications. Physiatrists (rehabilitation specialists) may provide specialty care to assist patients with optimizing physical potential. Licensed acupuncture therapists provide complementary therapy options for pain reduction and improved physical functioning. Psychologists are sometimes consulted to help patients cope with difficulties in the home and workplace resulting from OA. Social workers often assist patients with the social challenges caused by disability, unemployment, financial hardships, home health care, and other needs resulting from the limitations of OA. Advanced practice nurses may work independently or collaboratively with physicians in the management of the disease.

The approach to treatment focuses on reducing pain, improving mobility, and slowing the progression of the disease. The therapeutic plan may include pharmacologic, nonpharmacologic, or both approaches.

Nonpharmacologic

Exercise can improve psychological well-being, which can greatly impact pain management and quality of life. Individuals with OA may want to avoid exercise due to the concern that pain may occur. Conservative exercises of low impact can actually improve mobility and increase strength. Walking, swimming, and water-based exercise programs are considered low impact and are generally well tolerated. Of course, exercises will vary by individual case depending on the severity of symptoms and location of discomfort. In addition to low-impact exercises, one can also participate in weight training activities that will help strengthen muscle around joints. Simply avoiding exercise reduces muscle strength, mobility, and overall energy and increases joint stiffness. An exercise regimen also facilitates weight loss. Prior to starting an exercise program it is critical for the patient with OA to have a discussion with a health care provider about which types of exercise routines fit best with their current health condition.

Physical Therapy

A licensed physical therapist (PT) can assess the need to use special equipment as necessary. A therapist may determine that the patient with OA could benefit from the use of devices such as a cane, crutches, walker, neck collar, or elastic knee support to protect joints from overuse. Using a device such as a cane or walker helps to redistribute the weight so there is less difficulty with weight-bearing joints.

In addition to a PT consult patients may benefit from occupational therapy (OT) consultation, for the patient who exhibits difficulty with activities of daily living. The OT may be able to recommend activities that minimize pain and conserve energy and help the patient incorporate activities into their lifestyle.

In addition to the therapist recommending assistive devices, they may also perform specific therapies that can reduce OA pain. The joints of the person with OA are very sensitive. Massage will assist with blood flow and provide warmth to the joints. The technique mimics more of a light stroke and kneading opposed to deep massage. The therapist will need to adjust the amount of touch based on the subjective information provided by the patient. Heat or cold (or a combination of the two) can be useful for joint pain. Heat can be applied in a number of different ways—with warm towels, hot packs, or a warm bath or shower—to increase blood flow and ease pain and stiffness. In some cases, cold packs (bags of ice or frozen vegetables wrapped in a towel), can relieve pain or numb the sore area (9). Techniques for heat and cold therapy are recommended based on treatment goals at a particular time. When nonpharmacologic treatment modalities fail to control pain, leading to reduced mobility and participation in activities of daily living, it may be necessary to discuss pharmacologic options to complement current interventions.

Pharmacologic

Medication is used to supplement the interventions of physical activity and exercise. Using one intervention will not promote progression of wellness. It is imperative that medications are used to reduce symptoms and thus allow more normal daily activities. A nonopiate analgesic such as acetaminophen may be all that is needed for mild to moderate pain. This may be safe for people who are unable to take NSAIDs due to allergies, kidney or peptic ulcer disease, or bleeding risk. Because of its low cost, effectiveness and safety, acetaminophen is recommended as a first-line option against OA pain. Some people require the addition of a mild opiate. Finally, some people use NSAIDs in addition to acetaminophen for added pain relief. Commonly used analgesics are presented in Table 17-3.

Nonsteroidal Anti-inflammatory Drugs

NSAIDs fall into two basic categories: traditional NSAIDs and Cox-2 inhibitors. All NSAIDs work by blocking prostaglandins—hormone-like substances that contribute to pain, inflammation, fever, and muscle cramps.

Traditional NSAIDs

The original category of NSAIDs includes aspirin and is still preferred by many patients and providers. Even non-prescription versions of NSAIDs carry a risk of side effects, including stomach upset and gastrointestinal bleeding, especially in people over 60 years of age. Receiving a prescription for an NSAID prompts diligence in taking the medication exactly as prescribed and necessitates a conversation with a health care provider or pharmacist if any problems occur. Listings of medications are given in Table 17-4 and 17-5.

NSAIDs work well to relieve pain, decrease fever, and reduce swelling and inflammation caused by an injury or

TABLE 17–3 Analgesics

Drug	Brand	Dosage	Precautions	Side Effects
Acetaminophen	Anacin (aspirin free), Exedrin, Panadol, Tylenol, Tylenol Arthritis	Range from 325 mg to 1,000 mg every 4–6 hr as needed. Warning: not to exceed 4,000 mg/day. For the use of Tylenol Arthritis: 1,300 mg every 8 hours as needed; no more than 3,900 mg in 24 hr.	Not to be used in combination with any other product containing acetaminophen. This medication is not to be used for more than 10 days for pain, unless directed by a provider.	Taken as directed, this medication is usually not associated with side effects.
Acetaminophen with codeine	Phenaphen with Codeine, Tylenol with Codeine #3	15–60 mg codeine every 4 hr as needed (150–600 mg acetaminophen)	High doses of this drug can cause respiratory depression. It is not recommended to take more of this drug than is prescribed.	Constipation, nausea/vomiting, dizziness, light-headedness, sedation, and shortness of breath.
Hydrocodone with acetaminophen	Dolacet, Hydrocet, Lorcet, Lortab, Vicodin	2.5–10 mg hydrocodone every 4 to 6 hours as needed. Note: The acetaminophen portion of these medications will vary.	Driving or operating machinery is not recommended until able to understand how the body reacts to the drug. It is not recommended to take more of this medication than prescribed as the side effects will increase.	Constipation, dizziness or the feeling of being lightheaded, mood changes, nausea/vomiting, sedation, shortness of breath, and urinary retention

Continued

TABLE 17–3 Analgesics—cont'd

Drug	Brand	Dosage	Precautions	Side Effects
			Tolerance to this medication will increase as higher dosages are taken. Abrupt discontinuation of this medication should only be done under the advisement of a provider.	
Morphine sulfate	Avinza, Oramorph SR	Avinza: Single dose of 30 mg/day Oramorph SR: 30–100 mg every 12 hr	Driving or operating machinery is not recommended until able to understand how the body reacts to the drug. This medication is to be swallowed whole. It is not to be chewed or crushed. Can be taken with or without food. It is recommended to take the medication at the same time each day. Abrupt discontinuation of this medication should only be done under the advisement of a provider.	Constipation, drowsiness, nausea
Oxycodone	OxyContin, Roxicodone, OxyFAST, OxyIR (liquid)	OxyContin: 10 mg every 12 hr Roxicodone, OxyFAST, OxyIR (liquid): 5 mg every 6 hr as needed	Note: if this medication is released too rapidly it can become a potentially fatal dose. The medication can be mixed with liquid or soft foods such as pudding or applesauce. Never chew this medication.	Constipation, dizziness, drowsiness, dry mouth, headache, increased sweating, itching of the skin, nausea/vomiting, shortness of breath, weakness

TABLE 17–3 Analgesics—cont'd

Drug	Brand	Dosage	Precautions	Side Effects
Oxycodone with acetaminophen	Percocet, Endocet	5 mg oxycodone every 6 hr as needed. Depending on whether taking the medication in pill or capsule form the portion of acetaminophen will vary.	Note: if this medication is released too rapidly it can become a potentially fatal dose. The medication can be mixed with liquid or soft foods such as pudding or applesauce. Never chew this medication.	Constipation, dizziness, drowsiness, dry mouth, headache, increased sweating, itching of the skin, nausea/ vomiting, short- ness of breath, weakness
Tramadol with acetaminophen	Ultracet	75 mg tramadol every 4–6 hours as needed for up to 5 days (no more than 600 mg/day)	Driving or operating machinery is not recommended until able to under- stand how the body reacts to the drug. Abrupt discontinuation of this medication should only be done under the advisement of a provider. It is not recommended to take with medica- tions that contain acetaminophen.	Constipation diarrhea, dizziness, drowsiness, increased sweating, loss of appetite, nausea
Tramadol	Ultram, Ultram-ER	50–100 mg every 4–6 hours as needed	Driving or operating machinery is not recommended until able to understand how the body reacts to the drug. Abrupt discontinuation of this medication should only be done under the advise- ment of a physician.	Constipation diar- rhea, dizziness, drowsiness, increased sweating, loss of appetite, nausea

disease (10). There are side effects that are commonly associated with the use of NSAIDs. Most frequently the experience is mild, causing upset stomach and possible heartburn. More alarming are development of gastric ulcers and skin rashes. Taking NSAIDS with food helps prevent some of the problems. NSAIDs are contraindi- cated in patients with ulcers or a history of gastrointestinal (GI) bleeding. Restrictions should also be placed on NSAID use for patients who drink more than three alcoholic drinks a day as these agents can increase the risk of GI bleeding. Other conditions for which NSAIDs are contraindicated or should be used with caution are high blood pressure and kidney, liver, or heart disease (10).

TABLE 17–4 No Prescription Needed (Not a Complete List)

Generic Name	Brand Name
Ibuprofen	Advil, Motrin
Naproxen sodium	Aleve
Aspirin	Bayer, Bufferin

TABLE 17–5 Prescription Nonsteroidal Anti-inflammatory Drugs (Not a Complete List)

Generic Name	Brand Name
Celecoxib	Celebrex
Ibuprofen	Motrin
Ketoprofen	
Naproxen sodium	Anaprox
Piroxicam	Feldene
Sulindac	Clinoril

COX-2 inhibitors

Like traditional NSAIDs, COX-2 inhibitors help reduce pain and inflammation but are designed to be safer for the stomach. Studies have shown COX-2 inhibitors cause less GI bleeding compared to traditional NSAIDs; however, COX-2s have not been used as long as other NSAIDs (10).

Opiates

Opiates are often used in conjunction with NSAIDs for relief of pain with orthopedic injuries. Because opiates offer no reduction in inflammation and edema formation, a major source of pain with acute injury, they should not be prescribed independently of NSAIDs and offer the best analgesic effect when the two drugs are used together. A listing of the most common opiates is found in Table 17-6.

Beyond taking prescription or over-the-counter medications there are other pharmacologic interventions that have been suggested. Patients with persistent pain may benefit from corticosteroid injection. However, relief only lasts for a short time. Many people use over-the-counter remedies such as glucosamine and chondroitin sulfate. Capsaicin (Zostrix) skin cream may also help relieve pain. A warm, stinging sensation may be felt when the cream is first applied. This sensation goes away after a few days of use. Pain relief usually begins within 1 to 2 weeks.

TABLE 17–6 Opiates Recommended for Orthopedic Injuries

Generic Name	Brand Name
Codeine	
Hydrocodone	Vicodin
Oxycodone	OxyContin, Roxicodone
Tramadol	Ultram

Procedures

If OA interferes with everyday life and the symptoms do not improve with pharmacologic or nonpharmacologic interventions, joint replacement surgery is an option. Joint replacement is usually successful, almost always improving motion and function and dramatically decreasing pain. Therefore, joint replacement should be considered when pain is unmanageable and function becomes limited. Because the artificial joint does not last for a lifetime, the procedure is often delayed as long as possible in young people so the need for repeated replacements can be minimized (11). While joint replacement surgery certainly has its place in the management of arthritic diseases, it should be considered the final option after all other medical options have been exhausted. The joints that are most often replaced are those of the knee and hip. Possible options for procedural intervention are outlined in Table 17-7.

Clinical Nurse Specialist Competencies and Spheres of Influence
Collaboration

Treating arthritis often requires a multidisciplinary or team approach. Many types of health professionals care for people with arthritis. The CNS in an acute care setting

TABLE 17-7 Procedures

Arthroscopy	Surgery to trim torn and damaged cartilage
Osteotomy	A procedure to change the alignment of a bone to relieve stress on the bone or joint
Arthrodesis	Surgical procedure performed on arthritic joints. This procedure is done when it is necessary to perform a joint fusion.
Arthroplasty	Total or partial replacement of a damaged joint with an artificial joint

offers the opportunity to orchestrate and coordinate plans of care through collaboration and communication. The efforts of the CNS will focus on ensuring appropriate consults have been made to include physical therapy for mobility needs that go beyond the autonomous scope of nursing practice and social work to inquire about any financial setbacks due to disability and to raise concern of home care needs. The CNS can further identify the need to consult with a dietician to promote eating habits that will improve health and achieve and maintain a healthy weight. It is most important to remember that the patient is also a part of the team and that their suggestions are as valuable as any other member of the team. Improved clinical outcomes are more likely to be achieved when patients are encouraged to participate in his or her plan of care.

OSTEOPOROSIS

Osteoporosis is the thinning of bone tissue and loss of bone density over time. It is a life-long metabolic bone disease that causes bones to be fragile and increases the risk of fractures to the hip, spine, and wrist. It is a silent disease with no signs or symptoms until a fracture occurs. The exact etiology of this disease is not known, it may be iatrogenic or secondary to other disorders. Predisposing factors include menopause, long-term corticosteroid use, prolonged immobilization, and nutritional deficiency.

Etiology

In the United States today, an estimated 10 million people over the age of 50 years have osteoporosis and nearly 34 million have low bone mass that puts them at increased risk for developing the disease. Four of five people who have osteoporosis are women, but about 2 million men in the United States also have the disease and 14 million more have low bone mass that puts them at risk for it. One in two women and as many as one in four men over age 50 will have an osteoporosis-related fracture in their lifetime (11).

A major cause of osteoporosis is less than optimal bone growth during childhood and adolescence, resulting in failure to reach optimal peak bone mass. Thus, peak bone mass attained early in life is one of the most important factors affecting the risk of osteoporosis in later years. People who start out with greater reserves of bone (higher peak bone mass) are less likely to develop osteoporosis when bone loss occurs as a result of aging, menopause, or other factors. Other causes of osteoporosis are bone loss due to a greater than expected rate of bone resorption, a decreased rate of bone formation, or both (12). Nutritional factors include low dietary intake of calcium and vitamin D.

Pathophysiology

In osteoporosis, the rate of bone loss (i.e., resorption) exceeds bone formation, resulting in a decrease in total bone mass. Bones affected by osteoporosis lose calcium and phosphate salts, resulting in porous brittle bones that are susceptible to fractures (11).

Clinical Presentation

A fracture is often the first complaint that brings the patient with osteoporosis in contact with a primary care provider. Many times the disease process goes undetected until a fracture occurs. Other signs may include diminished height, rounded shoulders, and the visually noticeable dowagers hump. Symptoms may include back or neck pain as well.

Diagnosis

Before performing any tests, the primary care provider will complete a physical examination and record information about medical history and lifestyle. The collection of information will center on risk factors, family history, medication history, and dietary intake, particularly the amount of calcium and vitamin D. For females, there will be an interest in learning the menstruation history as well.

Once the physical examination is complete, diagnostic studies such as computed tomography (CT) scan or various radiographs that detect skeletal problems will be warranted. A standard radiograph does not reveal osteoporotic changes until about 30% of bone mineral density (BMD) is lost (7).

A BMD test is the best way to determine bone health. This test can identify osteoporosis, determine risk for fractures, and measure response to osteoporosis treatment. The most widely recognized BMD test is a dual-energy radiograph absorptiometry, or DXA test. The BMD test involves much less exposure to radiation than plain films. It measures bone density at the hip and spine.

The DXA test is the gold standard for diagnosis of osteoporosis; results are reported as a T score, which is the difference between the patient's BMD and that of a young adult of the same gender (7). When a T-score appears as a negative number (such as −1, −2, or −2.5), it indicates low bone mass. The greater the negative number, the greater is the risk of fracture (9). Although no bone density test is 100% accurate, this type of test is the single most important predictor of a fracture in the future. Diagnosis may include serum and urine markers of bone remodeling. Osteocalcin is synthesized by the osteoblasts and is increased in conditions of rapid bone turnover. Urinary alkaline phosphatase is a marker of bone resorption. Markers do not indicate BMD and are not an indicator of fracture risk (7). Blood and urine tests will detect the amount of calcium, vitamin D, and thyroid hormone in the body. The most common blood tests are outlined in Table 17-8.

The most common urine tests are the 24-hour urine collection to measure calcium metabolism, which is a test to measure the rate of bone resorption. In addition to the history and physical, the provider will note

TABLE 17-8 Common Blood Tests

serum calcium levels
serum vitamin D levels
Thyroid function
Parathyroid hormone levels
Estradiol levels to measure estrogen (in women)
Follicle-stimulating hormone (FSH) test to establish menopause status
Testosterone levels (in men)
Osteocalcin levels to measure bone formation

medical problems and medications being taking that can contribute to bone loss, including glucocorticoids, such as cortisone. It is also important for the care provider to measure height for changes and posture to note any curvature of the spine from vertebral fractures. Any complaint of back pain warrants a radiograph to detect any fractures of the spine.

Management

In order to understand how to prevent further health-related problems associated with osteoporosis, it is crucial to understand modifiable and nonmodifiable risk factors. Table 17-9 shows risk factors that are nonmodifiable as well as those related to lifestyle.

A comprehensive program that consists of a well-balanced diet rich in calcium and vitamin D, physical activity, and a healthy lifestyle will aid in moderating the modifiable risk factors. Lifestyle changes including smoking cessation, avoiding excessive alcohol use, and

TABLE 17-9 Risk Factors

Nonmodifiable Risk Factors	Risk Factors Related to Lifestyle
Gender (increased risk for women)	Inadequate calcium intake
A thin, small frame	Nutritional disorders (anorexia nervosa)
Family history of osteoporosis	Lack of weight-bearing exercise
Menopause before age 45	Smoking
Over age 50.	Alcohol consumption
Use of certain medications for a long time, such as hormones	

recognizing that some prescription medications and chronic diseases can cause bone loss.

Medications should not be relied on entirely as the only treatment for osteoporosis. Practices such as exercise, particularly weight-bearing physical activity, strengthen bones and improves balance. The more active and fit that patients are, the less likely they will be to fall and fracture bones. Good nutrition is also important, healthy eating habits will ensure that the intake of calcium and vitamin D are adequate. Being underweight or losing significant weight unintentionally is associated with poorer bone health and a higher risk of fracture—even when taking a bisphosphonate. Using tobacco products speeds up bone loss, so stopping will improve health and reduce the risk. Alcohol consumption should be limited to one drink a day or less, on influence for optimal health. The CNS can positively impact tobacco cessation and excessive alcohol use by making referrals to outpatient agencies that assist with quitting tactics through individualized coaching.

Pharmacologic

Many medications have been associated with the development of osteoporosis. A list of medications commonly associated with osteoporosis can be found in Table 17-10. Management of the patient with osteoporosis includes maintaining the lowest possible doses of these medications and increasing vigilance of bone density assessment.

Bisphosphonates are the cornerstone of pharmacologic therapy. Fosamax, along with its generic equivalent alendronate, is a commonly prescribed bisphosphonate that has been on the market for more than 10 years. These medications tend to be well tolerated, for the most part, by the women who take them. A listing of these medications is located in Table 17-11.

Bisphosphonates slow bone resorption. These drugs effectively preserve or maintain bone density during menopause—and decrease the risk of fractures.

TABLE 17-10 Medications Associated With Osteoporosis

Anticoagulants (heparin)
Anticonvulsants
Cyclosporine A and tacrolimus
Cancer chemotherapy drugs
Glucocorticoids (and adrenocorticotropic hormone [ACTH])
Gonadotropin-releasing hormone agonists
Lithium
Methotrexate
Parenteral nutrition
Thyroxine

TABLE 17-11 Bisphosphonates

Generic Name	Brand Name
Alendronate	Fosamax
Risedronate	Actonel
Ibandronate	Boniva
Zoledronic acid	Reclast

Hormones, such as estrogen, and some hormone-like medications approved for preventing and treating osteoporosis, such as raloxifene (Evista), also play a role in osteoporosis treatment. Fewer women take these medications for osteoporosis treatment because the bisphosphonates are so effective, especially if there is no other reason to choose hormonal therapy, such as breast cancer prevention.

Due to the increased risk of fractures associated with osteoporosis, it is important to avoid falls for patients with OA. The patient's environment should be assessed for factors that may contribute to fall risk.

Clinical Nurse Specialist Competencies and Spheres of Influence
Coaching/Teaching/Mentoring

The CNS will assist the nurse and patient with education; emphasis will be centered around patient education to ensure promotion of a healthy lifestyle. It is imperative for the CNS to perform an environmental assessment to identify factors or items that would place the patient at increased risk for falls, such as loose rugs, items in the pathway of walking, and lack of bath mats in the shower or tub.

TRAUMATIC INJURIES

Fractures, Dislocations, Sprains, and Strains
Etiology

Orthopedic injuries are a common concomitant injury occurring with other traumatic injuries. The incidence of orthopedic injuries associated with motor vehicle crashes (MVCs) and motorcycle crashes (MCCs), sports-related injuries, and falls is very high. Approximately 85% of multiple trauma patients have one or more skeletal injuries. Females older than 85 years have the highest rate of pelvic fractures. Of all traumatic injuries, the most common is lower extremity, representing 47% of orthopaedic injuries and 35% involve the upper extremity. The most severe injuries are pelvic fractures and traumatic amputations, which often result in hemodynamic instability (12).

There are many types of injuries that may occur as a result of trauma. These include dislocation, subluxation, sprains/strains, fractures, and amputations. Each of these will be discussed briefly, including pathophysiology and treatment. Patients may experience one of these as isolated injuries or may also have multiple injuries simultaneously (i.e., fracture and dislocation of the lower extremity). Complications associated with orthopaedic trauma include compartment syndrome, venous thromboembolism (VTE), infection, and osteomyelitis. Spinal fractures are also a common type of orthopaedic injury related to trauma but are not within the scope of this chapter. Evaluation, diagnosis, and treatment of orthopedic injuries in trauma patients should follow appropriate evaluation of airway, breathing, circulation, and neurologic status. In order to appropriately diagnose injuries, one must first determine relevant history, mechanism of injury, location, and amount of time since original injury. Initial history and physical exam, patient level of functioning, radiographs, and laboratory results are important to reflect an accurate picture of type of injury (13).

Initial assessment of any traumatic orthopedic injury includes inspection, palpation, and diagnostic studies. Initial inspection should include the position of the patient, position of extremities, bleeding/estimated blood loss, any obvious deformities, presence of open or closed fractures, extremity color, ecchymosis, muscle spasm, and swelling. Palpation includes pulse, capillary refill, range of motion (passive or active), sensation, pain, interruption in bone integrity, crepitus, and temperature. It is important to assess the zone of injury, including the area affected by traumatic forces. Damage to soft tissue structures is often greater than what it initially appears. It is important to be highly suspicious of not only the injured area but areas above and below the injury. Diagnostic studies include plain film radiographs including joints above and below, CT, angiography, CT myelography, and possibly MRI.

Dislocations

A dislocation occurs in a joint when the articulating surfaces come out of anatomic position. Joints most commonly dislocated include shoulder, elbow, wrist, hip, knee, and ankle.

Dislocations, as with other traumatic conditions, can result from a variety of mechanisms. Blunt injuries and falls commonly result in dislocations, specifically of the upper extremity. These injuries commonly occur from sports injuries or falling on outstretched arms.

The glenohumoral joint of the shoulder is the most commonly dislocated joint in the body (14). Posterior shoulder dislocation is an infrequent event, with a reported incidence of only 1% to 4% of all shoulder dislocations. These may often be misdiagnosed, which results in significant delays in treatment and the potential for resulting disability (14). Early recognition requires a high level of suspicion and a careful patient history and physical examination, confirmed with appropriate radiographs. Dislocation at the elbow or wrist may accompany an upper extremity traumatic injury and can lead to significant long-term morbidity if left undiagnosed and untreated. These associated injuries are frequently subtle and consequently missed on initial emergency department presentation.

Hip dislocations commonly occur after MVCs and should be considered an orthopaedic emergency. Posterior dislocations are the most common, occurring in 90% to 95% of patients with hip dislocation (15). These require immediate reduction within 12 hours. Typically, closed reduction is adequate and can be performed immediately. However, for unstable dislocations and with associated fractures, open reduction and internal fixation (ORIF) will be required.

Complications associated with hip dislocations are recurrent dislocation, avascular necrosis, and post-traumatic arthritis. Hip dislocations are typically diagnosed based on physical assessment with one limb shorter than the other, external rotation of the limb, and complaint of pain. Diagnosis is further delineated based on radiologic exam. Patients with hip dislocations are at risk for sciatic and femoral nerve injuries as well as vessel injuries. Diligent nursing assessment of neurovascular and perfusion status is imperative.

Initial assessment for dislocations as well as other orthopedic injuries involves assessment of the 6 Ps: Pain, Pallor, Parasthesia, Poikilothermia, Paralysis, and Pulselessness. Neurovascular compromise may occur as bones are displaced and may impinge on neurovascular structures. A thorough assessment needs to be completed and timely interventions implemented in order to decrease associated morbidity.

Management
Initial treatment requires immobilization of the dislocated joint above and below the affected joint. It is extremely important to treat pain appropriately; this is especially important at the time of closed reduction.

Most common treatment for dislocations involves closed reduction under moderate sedation. Once reduction is obtained, it is maintained with an immobilization device. Failure of closed reduction or chronic dislocations may necessitate surgery.

Subluxation is an incomplete or partial dislocation of a joint. With a subluxation, the adjacent bones are out of alignment with one another. A subluxation may cause a pinched nerve and pain.

Sprains and Strains
A sprain is a tear in a ligament surrounding a joint. Common areas for sprains involve the ankle, knee, elbow, or wrist.

A strain is an overstretching injury to muscles or tendons. The most common strains occur in the hamstring, groin, and back muscles.

One of the most common diagnoses made in the injured upper extremity is wrist sprain. The wrist is a complex structure with multiple bones and joints with which there are a numerous combinations of positions and motions (14). Wrist sprains should only be entertained after careful physical and radiographic examinations have ruled out fracture and dislocation in this region.

Management
Initial treatment for sprains or strains involves RICE: Rest, Ice, Compression, and Elevation. The application of Ice must be applied cautiously to avoid additional injuries from the application of cold. Ice should be applied for 20 minutes at a time and 20 minutes off. Avoid direct application of the ice on the skin; a cloth layer should be placed between the ice and the skin.

Fractures
There are many specific types of fractures; it is beyond the scope of this chapter to capture every type of fracture. A more general overview of all fractures will be provided and then further delineated as upper extremity, lower extremity, and pelvic fractures. Variations in treatment for closed versus open fractures will also be discussed.

Common types of fractures include comminuted, spiral, impacted, transverse undisplaced, and oblique. Comminuted fractures are fractures with more than two fragments noted. Spiral fractures have a torsional component. Impacted fractures are typically very stable, one where fractured ends are compressed together. Transverse fractures run perpendicular to the bone. An oblique fracture has no torsional or twisting component present, but usually runs across the bone at an angle of 45 to 60 degrees (16) (Figure 17-2).

Closed Fractures Versus Open Fractures
Closed fractures occur with the skin remaining intact. Open fractures involve an open wound and can be further classified according to the extent of skin and soft tissue damage. Complicated fractures are associated with other types of injuries as well, including muscular, neurovascular, and ligamentous damage (Table 17-12).

Clinical Presentation
There are many mechanisms of injury associated with fractures. These include crushing force or a direct blow, sudden twisting motion (common in those with osteoporosis), forceful muscle contraction, and even neoplasm or malignancy. Direct forces cause a fracture that will usually result in a transverse, oblique, or comminuted fracture. Indirect forces may also cause a fracture by transmitting energy to the fracture site; a common example of this would be a stress fracture or a rotational injury resulting in a spiral fracture (16).

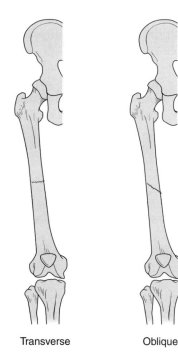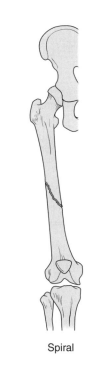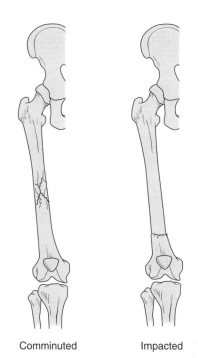

| Transverse | Oblique | Spiral | Comminuted | Impacted |

FIGURE 17-2: Types of fractures.

TABLE 17-12 Classifications of Open Fractures

Type I	Wound less than 1 cm Moderately clean, minimal contamination Simple fracture Minimal soft tissue damage
Type II	Wound greater than 1 cm Moderate contamination Fracture—moderate communition/crush injury Moderate soft tissue damage
Type III	High degree of contamination Fracture—severe communition and instability Extensive soft tissue damage Traumatic amputation
Type IIIa	Soft tissue coverage of fracture is adequate Fracture—segmental of severely comminuted
Type IIIb	Extensive injury to or loss of soft tissue, and exposure of bone Massive contamination Fracture—severe communition
Type IIIc	Any open fracture associated with arterial injury that must be repaired regardless of degree of soft tissue injury

Diagnosis

Diagnosis of fractures is based on clinical assessment as well as definitive radiologic testing. Clinical features include general appearance, pain, deformity, angulation, shortening, rotation, swelling, ecchymosis, inability to bear weight, decreased range of motion, or pain and crepitus on motion. Integrity of injured skin (soft tissue damage, avulsions, or bleeding) should also be assessed. Abnormal vascular or neurologic exam, lacerations, or other soft tissue injury necessitate further evaluation and intervention. Other assessment parameters include mechanism and history of injury. Primary assessment measures can be summarized by using the "six Ps." Other important features to assess are temperature and decreased capillary refill.

Radiographic exams are typically required to appropriately diagnose any musculoskeletal injury. The most common exams used are the anteroposterior (AP) and lateral views of injured site and joints above and below the injury. Fractures at joints also require oblique films. Fractures in areas that are difficult to visualize on a plain film may also require a CT scan for accurate diagnosis. MRI is more helpful for visualization of soft tissue, ligament, and tendon injuries.

Concurrent injuries often occur with orthopedic injuries. The most common injuries associated with fractures are neurovascular injuries. Vascular injuries occur in arteries in the region of the fracture or dislocation. Pulses may be absent due to spasm or compression of the artery. This will cause ischemia distal to the fracture if not corrected urgently. Neurologic injuries occur with fractures where there is a high density of nerves. This type of complication is more common with dislocations: posterior hip dislocation, knee dislocation, elbow fracture or dislocation, and supracondylar and shaft fractures of the humerus and shoulder dislocation.

Others injuries include multiple fractures of various bones depending on the type of injury. A fractured calcaneous from falls or jumps is commonly associated with other lower extremity fractures. Bilateral wrist fractures or thoracolumbar spine fracture are concomitant injuries with falls as well. Patellar fractures due to dashboard impact are commonly associated with femur and posterior hip fracture as well as possible popliteal artery damage. Femur and pelvic fractures lead to hypovolemia due to blood sequestration. It is important for the health care professional to be aware of common concomitant injuries and evaluate for these during the initial physical exam.

Management

Following a thorough assessment and physical exam, fracture management is based on type of fracture. All fractures will require definitive reduction and/or stabilization depending on type and location of fracture. When splinting fractures, it is important to splint the joint above and below the fracture site. Avoid excessive movement of fractured bone fragments in order to decrease the risk for fat emboli. It is important to perform a neurovascular assessment before and after splinting. Various types of splints are available for stabilization of the fractured extremity. These include rigid, soft-air, Hare, Sager, and Thomas. Management of fractures is based upon the principle of RICE.

The fundamental principles for treatment of open fractures have remained unchanged for years. These principles include urgent and appropriate wound debridement, timely administration of intravenous antibiotics, skeletal stabilization to facilitate wound management, and early appropriate soft tissue coverage (17). Initial treatment of open fractures involves removal of any gross debris and application of a sterile dressing followed by reduction and splinting of the affected area. Treatment should then include tetanus injection followed by operative treatment within 8 hours and intravenous antibiotics. Operative treatment may include multiple incision and drainage (I&D) procedures before hardware placement. In addition to closed versus open, other considerations with fractures include stability, mechanism of injury, and joint injuries. Unstable fractures tend to displace after reduction whereas stable fractures do not.

Common complications of open fractures include infection, delayed union, and nonunion of the fracture. The rates of deep infection have been declining with improvements in recognition of importance of surgical debridement and improved techniques of fracture stabilization and soft tissue closure (18). Studies have shown the efficacy of timely wound management and use of antibiotics in reducing infection rates (19).

In general, patients will benefit from early stabilization and total care of their musculoskeletal injuries after appropriate initial resuscitation (20). It is important to determine adequate resuscitation markers and collaborate with general trauma surgeons regarding planning the timing of definitive orthopedic repairs. It is imperative to judiciously time the repair of orthopedic injuries in the multisystem trauma patient with other life-threatening injuries (i.e., increased intracranial pressure, respiratory insufficiency, and hypotension).

Pelvic Fractures

Pelvic ring fractures are common with high velocity trauma; the majority of these do not require surgical repair (21). The most common type of pelvic fracture is lateral compression fracture. This type of injury may also be associated with head, thorax, and abdominal injuries. Typically with this injury, the sacroiliac (SI) joints or iliac wing is compressed, and the femoral head disrupts the pubic rami and can extend into the acetabulum. There are fewer long-term problems associated with this type of injury. Another type of pelvic fracture is anteroposterior compression, or open book fracture—external rotation. This type of fracture causes the symphysis pubis to spring open and there is a rupture of the anterior SI and sacrospinous ligaments. This is the most morbid type of pelvic fracture due to bleeding and may have high transfusion needs. Other pelvic fractures may result in unilateral or bilateral both anterior and posterior rings disruption. These injuries may be unstable, with bone and soft tissue disruption. It takes great force to produce this type of fracture. Vessel and nerve injury may also accompany this type of injury due to disruption of the SI joint.

Acetabular fractures typically occur from injury to femur/femoral head in high impact fall or motor vehicle accidents. The location of the fracture depends on angle of injury (e.g., anterior force leads to fracture of posterior acetabulum). Diagnosis of these types of fractures is based on AP pelvis with Judet views (obliques), but may also require a CT scan.

With any pelvic fracture, concomitant spinal fractures and spinal cord injury must also be ruled out. This is due to the force necessary to fracture the pelvis and the close proximity to the spinal column.

Management

In severe pelvic injuries, bone instability can be associated with severe hemodynamic instability and can lead to life-threatening hemorrhage (13). The mortality rate for high-energy pelvic fractures is 10% to 20%, this increases to 50% in the presence of hemodynamic instability (22, 23). A patient with a mechanically unstable posterior pelvic ring and hemodynamic instability (systolic blood pressure less than 90 mm Hg) in a patient who is inconsistently responsive or unresponsive to fluid resuscitation, early pelvic stabilization should be part of the resuscitation effort (24). Clinical series have shown that early, aggressive resuscitation of the patient has resulted in decreased mortality in patients with significant pelvic ring injuries (25). Emergent management of pelvic fractures includes the use of external stabilizing devices for initial management. More definitive management of pelvic fractures may include the use of external fixators or internal fixation (symphyseal or open plating, percutaneous or iliosacral screws).

After external stabilization, arteriography and embolization may be necessary to locate the source of bleeding. Direct exploration may be necessary if unable to locate the source of bleeding with angiography.

There is a 16% incidence of urologic injuries associated with pelvic fractures. These are most commonly urethral or bladder ruptures and tears. Urethral injury is a relatively common sequelae of complex anterior ring injuries in males. Blood at the urethral meatus is highly suspicious of a urethral injury, and a retrograde urethrogram is recommended before attempting to insert a Foley catheter (26). The nurse must suspect urethral injury with blood at the urethral meatus and notify the physician immediately and should not attempt insertion of a Foley catheter. The patient should be closely examined for occult injuries associated with pelvic fractures such as a perineal wound or vaginal vault wound. Patients with blood in the vaginal vault requires a manual vaginal examination (13).

A delayed risk following pelvic fractures is infection from Foley catheters and suprapubic tubes, as well as from any hardware placed on anterior pelvic ring fractures or external fixators. With posterior pelvic fractures there is also the risk of sacral plexus/sciatic nerve injury.

Management of acetabular fracture requires open reduction and internal fixation (ORIF). Surgery may be delayed 3 to 5 days after injury to reduce bleeding. Complications commonly associated with acetabular fracture include post-traumatic arthritis. This is a result of incongruity of displaced surfaces of the femoral head and posterior wall fractures. Another less common complication is heterotopic ossification (HO), which results from abnormal formation of bone in soft tissue.

Lower Extremity Fractures

Lower extremity fractures include femur and tibia/fibula fractures. Femur fractures typically occur with high-energy injuries and are often accompanied by hematomas from disrupted blood supply. Open femur fractures require immediate surgical intervention with ORIF as well as external fixation if grossly contaminated.

Supracondylar femur fracture of the distal femur and femoral neck fractures frequently occur in the elderly (from a low-energy fall) who have multiple comorbidities and osteoporosis. There is a 10% mortality associated with these injuries in the elderly when treatment includes internal fixation; this increases to 60% for those patients treated with bedrest. Within 1 month of injury, death occurs in 21% of women and 37% of men over the age of 84 years (27). Even though these injuries are more common in the elderly, they may also occur in the young as a result of a high-energy injury. Treatment of femur fractures requires surgical stabilization within hours of injury. Commonly this consists of intramedullary nailing or rod placement. It is imperative to assess for concomitant vascular injuries associated with femur fractures. Early ORIF decreases complications and facilitates early rehabilitation.

Patellar fractures typically result from a direct blow to the front of the knee. It is important to assess for knee ligament, femur fracture, and posterior hip dislocation. Patellar fractures are nonoperative injuries for minimally displaced or nondisplaced fractures. However, operative repair is preferred if displacement or extensor mechanism is disrupted. Complications associated with patellar fractures include post-traumatic arthritis; nonunion may also occur but is rare.

When a tibial plateau fracture is present, it is important to also assess ligaments for stability due to twisting injury or fall. Stabilization, reduction, and early mobilization are goals. Internal or external fixation is used for stabilization. Nonoperative treatment includes casts, bracing, and non–weight bearing. Complications include post-traumatic arthritis and wound infection.

Tibial shaft fracture management is typically nonoperative with long leg cast for four weeks or patellar bending cast. External fixation may be used if there is concern about viability of soft tissue; vascular repair may be indicated. When operative management is required, this consists of intramedullary nailing.

COMPLICATIONS OF FRACTURES

Nonunion, delayed union, malunion, infection, and osteomyelitis are all potential complications of fractures. Soft tissue loss and bone defects need vigilant assessment. Observation for other complications of fractures include arterial injury, compartment syndrome, fat embolism syndrome, VTE, and blood loss. VTE includes both deep venous thrombosis (DVT) and pulmonary embolism (PE). These will be discussed in detail later in the chapter.

Most fractures heal within 8 to 12 weeks. Failure of bone to heal normally after a fracture is seen more commonly with inadequate fixation, with comminuted fractures and in older patients. Avascular necrosis may also occur; this is seen as death of the bone due to collapse or infarcted bone. This is more commonly seen with hip fracture, hip dislocation, and femur fracture.

Management

Initial fracture management includes a thorough physical examination along with initial immobilization followed by more definitive stabilization. Initial immobilization includes stabilizing the joint above and below the fracture site with splints, bandages, or traction. Stabilization includes initial reduction and realignment, which may include open or closed methods. The purpose of splinting extremities is to avoid excessive movement of fractured bone fragments. It is important to perform a thorough neurovascular assessment before and after splinting.

Rehabilitation after fractures is of the utmost importance. Early operative fixation allows earlier mobility. It is important to obtain physical and occupational therapy consults to facilitate recovery. Most pelvic and acetabular fractures require non–weight bearing for a period of time depending on extent of injury and surgical procedure; this may be as long as 8 to 12 weeks. Acetabular fractures usually have a flexion restriction of 60 to 70 degrees. Mobility restrictions will be ordered by the orthopedic surgeon based on type of injury, type of fixation, and other comorbid conditions.

Casts. Casts are a mainstay of treatment for fractures and are an effective method of stabilization. More definitive stabilization may involve the use of pins, wires, screws, or other hardware. If casts are used for stabilization, it is important for the nurse to pad any bony areas and assess skin for breakdown. Monitor neurovascular status above and below the cast: capillary refill, color, temperature, presence of edema, sensation, movement, and pain. Elevate the extremity above the heart level. Teach patient to never place any foreign objects in the cast.

Traction. Orthopedic traction involves placing tension on a limb, bone, or muscle group. Traction may be used to reduce the fracture, maintain alignment, or decrease muscle spasm. Traction typically reduces pain by preventing motion of bone fragments. Various types of traction may be used including noninvasive devices such as Buck's traction and traction-hair splints or invasive skeletal traction. Invasive or skeletal traction involves the use of metal pins inserted into bone.

When traction is used, the physician will order weights to be applied to the traction apparatus. Prereduction and postreduction radiographs should be completed. The nurse should always check that the ordered weights are in place and in alignment. Do not lift weights when moving the patient in bed. If weighs must be removed, the traction must be maintained on the extremity to prevent displacement of bony surfaces.

Nursing care of patients in traction includes ongoing assessment and monitoring of neurovascular status, skin assessment, and monitoring for any pressure areas. Pressure relief is a must for patients in traction to prevent skin breakdown from immobility. Common areas of skin breakdown are the occiput, sacrum, and heels, with the heels being most vulnerable. Pin care with traction or external fixators should be conducted each shift and when necessary. Care includes cleaning sites, preferably with chlorhexidine; no ointments/creams should be applied to the site, site should be wrapped with gauze, and increased drainage and signs of infection should be reported.

Clinical Nurse Specialist Competencies and Spheres of Influence
Clinical Expert/Direct Care and Coaching/Teaching/Mentoring

The CNS needs to provide consultation with bedside caregivers to ensure all patient needs are being met and preventive and safety measures are appropriately implemented. Following initial resuscitation and treatment for the traumatic injury, prevention of complications is a priority in care. The nurse must be diligent in assessment and administer fluids aggressively while monitoring hemodynamic status. The CNS role models diligent initial assessment for urologic injury and ongoing assessment for signs of infection.

The CNS teaches the importance of pressure relief for prevention of skin breakdown, with attention to the occiput, sacrum, and heels and assessment of pressure areas under casts, splints, and traction. Education on proper use and care of traction weights and pin care to nurses and family caregivers should be included.

Assessment of environmental factors, physical limitation, and psychosocial situations that may affect patient safety is also important.

Collaboration and Consultation

Communication of the plan of care among all interdisciplinary providers is critical to ensure progression of functional mobility and prevention of complications. The CNS may take responsibility for coordination of interdisciplinary care and ensure that all care providers are moving toward the same discharge goals for the patient. The CNS needs to consult with appropriate rehabilitation services and home care agencies.

Amputation
Etiology

Amputations can occur as a result of a traumatic injury, as a planned event following an extremity injury, or as surgery to manage complications of peripheral vascular disease and diabetes mellitus. Amputation after an injury is generally completed only after all efforts to salvage the limb have been exhausted. Traumatic amputations are classified according to the degree of soft tissue, nerve, and vascular injury. Various types of amputations can occur. A guillotine amputation has well-defined wound edges and localized damage to soft tissues, nerves, and vessels. A crush amputation has more soft tissue damage, especially to the arterial intima. An avulsion amputation is caused by the forceful stretching and tearing away of tissue.

Management

Advances in microsurgery techniques to reattach amputated parts have made it a priority to correctly care for the part until determination can be made regarding feasibility of surgical reattachment.

Direct contact with iced solutions is contraindicated as it causes more damage to the tissue cells, decreasing the probability that reattachment will be successful. Dry ice should never be used. The body part should be loosely wrapped in gauze, placed in a plastic bag, and then placed in a ice-and-water solution. Crush or avulsion injuries have a low reattachment success rate therefore the procedure is usually not attempted. However, the amputated part should be cared for correctly until that decision has been made.

The decision whether to amputate or reconstruct a severely injured leg remains the subject of extensive debate in the orthopedic trauma literature. Scoring algorithms are available, which can provide some direction to the surgeon; however, subjectivity is inherent in the algorithms. Soft tissue injury severity has the greatest impact on decision making regarding limb salvage versus amputation (28). It may also be an immediate decision or a delayed decision after initial attempts to salvage the injured limb. The type of amputation depends on the extent of injury as well as underlying medical conditions or diseases. Attempts at revascularization and limb salvage are the first priorities before amputations. Closed amputation creates a weight-bearing residual limb. Disarticulation involves an amputation through a joint.

Clinical Nurse Specialist Competencies and Spheres of Influence
Clinical Expert/Direct Care and Coaching/ Teaching/Mentoring

Application of the direct care competency includes monitoring for and prevention of complications, including correct application of compression dressings, alignment of the residual limb, and assessment for infection. Patient and family teaching focuses on care of the residual limb and prosthesis and promotion of functional recovery and mobility training. Consultation with appropriate rehabilitation services for prosthesis training and mobility should occur early on in the postoperative recovery period for best clinical outcomes and prevention of complications. Education and management of phantom limb sensation and pain is a priority in the short- and long-term recovery phases. Alternative techniques such as mirror therapy have been shown to be effective for treatment of phantom limb pain.

Compartment Syndrome
Etiology

Compartment syndrome is an uncommon but serious condition that can occur after musculoskeletal trauma and orthopaedic surgery (Figure 17-3). Compartment syndrome may occur after fractures, crush injuries, circumferential burns, and arterial injuries. It develops when there is increased pressure within a a muscle compartment bound by dense fascial sheaths. The exact incidence of compartment syndrome is unknown (14). Three quarters of cases are associated with fractures, with tibia fracture having the highest incidence (29).

Compartments in the arm and lower leg are most vulnerable to this syndrome but can also occur in the hand, foot, thigh, shoulder, back, and buttocks. Early diagnosis and treatment is crucial to prevent the devastating complications of this condition (14).

Pathophysiology

Compartment syndrome is caused by increased tissue pressure inside an osseofacial compartment resulting in ischemia (13). The circulation and function of muscle within a closed fascial space are compromised by the increasing pressure within that space. The increased pressure within a confined space causes neurovascular compromise, tissue damage, impaired function, and if no

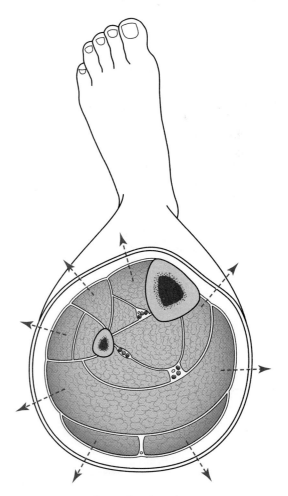

FIGURE 17–3: Compartment syndrome.

intervention, soft tissue necrosis requiring surgical debridement and even amputation.

Clinical Presentation

The most striking clinical features that manifest compartment syndrome are increasing numbness and parasthesias in nerves that traverse the involved compartment. Parasthesia or burning pain is an early sign due to nerve sensitivity. Common assessment findings include increasing pain that is exacerbated with range of motion and pain out of proportion to physical findings. The physical exam will reveal an increase in tissue pressure or firmness of the involved extremity. If compartment syndrome is not recognized and intervened upon early, it can result in loss of limb. Neurovascular assessment should be done using the six Ps.

Besides trauma and orthopedic surgery, compartment syndrome can also result from treatments that restrict compartment size. These include casts, splints, dressings, closure of fascial defects, and fracture reduction. Other less common factors include intracompartmental infusions, muscle edema, massive intravenous infusions, rhabdomyolysis, sepsis, and muscle hypertrophy from exertion.

Diagnosis

Diagnosis is dependent on history and physical exam. Definitive diagnosis is made based on compartment pressures, which are measured with a needle placed in the fascial compartment connected to a transducer. There are also commercial devices manufactured for the purpose of measuring compartment pressures (Figure 17-4).

Compartment pressures less than 30 mm Hg are considered normal. Pressures greater than 30 mm Hg typically result in pain and parasthesia.

Management

Nonsurgical interventions for compartment syndrome include early identification of high-risk patients, relief of constriction, and elevation to heart level. Do not elevate extremity above heart level or apply ice, these interventions may further compromise blood flow and cause more ischemia. Surgical intervention for elevated compartment syndrome is fasciotomy. This is typically performed for compartment pressures of 30 to 60 mm Hg. Prompt notification of the surgeon for physical findings of compartment syndrome is imperative. Fasciotomy will prevent muscle necrosis if performed immediately.

Postfasciotomy care includes loose dressings, elevation of extremity, debridement, and monitoring for reoccurrence of symptoms. Fasciotomy dressing and closure with dynamic wound closure in conjunction with Wound VAC™ (KCI) may also be beneficial in facilitating wound healing and closure (30).

Assess for complications of infection and loss of viable tissue and muscle. It is also important to monitor for myoglobinuria renal failure, which could indicate rhabdomyolysis. Treatment for myoglobinuria includes administration of large volumes of fluid, alkalinization of urine, and maintainance of high urine output (75 to 100 mL/hr).

Clinical Nurse Specialist Competencies and Spheres of Influence
Clinical Expert/Direct Care and Consultation

Compartment syndrome occurs as a complication of fractures and other musculoskeletal disorders. Early detection is imperative to prevent adverse sequelae from occurring. CNSs oversee and teach front-line nursing personnel diligent assessment, evaluation, and anticipation of this potential complication of orthopedic injury and joint replacement surgery. Timely consultation with the orthopedic, vascular, or neurosurgeon can be paramount to limb preservation.

Other Complications of Musculoskeletal Injuries

The most common and concerning complication with musculoskeletal injuries is VTE. These conditions

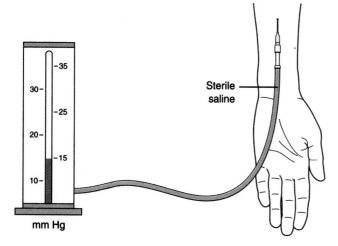

FIGURE 17-4: Compartment pressure measuring device.

include fat emboli, DVT, and pulmonary embolism. These conditions are summarized in Table 17-13.

Fat Embolism Syndrome

Fat embolism syndrome (FES) is seen more with unstabilized long bone fractures (femur fractures). Fat embolism occurs in almost all patients with pelvic and femur fractures but is often asymptomatic (16). Fat is released from fractured marrow and/or vasculature and migrates to pulmonary capillaries. This syndrome occurs when intramedullary fat is released into the venous circulation resulting in emboli to lungs, brain, and skin. This typically occurs 12 to 72 hours after injury to long bones. Symptoms of FES include sudden onset of shortness of breath from arterial hypoxemia. Other symptoms include restlessness, confusion, disorientation, tachycardia, and petechiae on chest, axilla, neck, and conjunctiva. The classic triad of FES includes pulmonary distress, mental status changes, and petechial rash that develops within 72 hours after injury.

Diagnostics include positive fat in urine and a chest radiograph demonstrating an acute respiratory distress syndrome (ARDS) pattern. Treatment in the intensive care unit is mostly supportive with early fracture stabilization, oxygen administration, and heparin administration.

Venous Thromboembolism

The most common type of VTE with orthopedic injuries is DVT, which is a major problem in patients with orthopedic trauma. Incidence without prophylaxis is reportedly 61 of 100 patients with pelvic fracture, 59 of 74 patients with femur fracture, and 66 of 86 patients with tibia fracture (31). Most authors recommend some form of prophylaxis for DVT patients with major fractures (32).

Clinical findings of DVT are typically unilateral and include pain made worse by walking, swelling, erythema, and warmth of the affected leg above or below the knee. Fever, skin discoloration, venous distention and lower extremity cyanosis may also be present. Homan sign and Moses sign occur infrequently and are often nonspecific. Risk factors for DVT may be absent; the clinical diagnosis is correct only 50% of the time, so diagnostic testing is mandatory whenever DVT is suspected.

Diagnosis

Venous Doppler ultrasound is used for detecting disruption in velocity of blood flow due to thrombus occlusion.

This can be performed at the bedside and is noninvasive. It is recommended to perform the exam on both extremities even when only unilateral involvement is suspected.

Venogram is the gold standard for diagnosis of DVT. However, this requires an invasive procedure that is associated with increased risk of complications.

The DVT prophylaxis is imperative for any musculoskeletal injury and many other medical conditions. The most effective prophylactic treatment is pharmacologic therapy. Pharmacologic prophylaxis includes heparin,

TABLE 17–13 Traumatic Complications

Clinical Problem	Symptoms	Laboratory/ Diagnostic Tests	Treatment
Fat emboli	Sudden onset of shortness of breath, restlessness, confusion, disorientation, tachycardia, petechiae on chest, axilla, neck, and conjunctiva	Positive fat in urine Chest radiograph demonstrating an acute respiratory distress syndrome (ARDS) pattern	Early fracture stabilization Treatment in intensive care unit is mostly supportive with oxygen and heparin administration
Deep venous thrombosis	Pain in limb made worse by standing or walking. Pain better with rest and elevation Swelling of lower extremity Heaviness or aching of lower extremities Unilateral swelling, erythema, and warmth of the affected leg above or below the knee Fever Skin discoloration Venous distention	*Venous Doppler ultrasound* Bedside Noninvasive Do bilateral lower extremities *Venogram* Gold standard Invasive Increased risk of complications	Prophylaxis: Mechanical: Use in patients at high risk of bleeding Thromboembolic deterrent stockings (TEDS) Sequential compression devices

Continued

TABLE 17–13 Traumatic Complications—cont'd

Clinical Problem	Symptoms	Laboratory/ Diagnostic Tests	Treatment
	Homan sign and Moses sign occur infrequently and are often nonspecific (should not be relied on for definitive diagnosis)		Pharmacologic: Low molecular weight heparin (LMWH), unfractionated heparin (UFH), or fondaparinux
Pulmonary embolism	Dyspnea Tachypnea Crackles Accentuated S_2 Tachycardia Fever Diaphoresis S_3 or S_4 gallop Apprehension Cough Hemoptysis Hypoxemia Pleuritic rub Hypotension Tricuspid insufficiency Right heart failure Syncope	Spiral CT Pulmonary angiogram Ventilation/Perfusion (V/Q) scan nonspecific Pulmonary angiogram	Oxygen: Usually 100% non-rebreathing (NRB) mask Assess need for intubation Requires intensive care unit admission Establish venous access Consider PA catheter Consider thrombolytic treatment Initiate anticoagulant therapy if no contraindications (LMWH, UFH, or fondaparinux) Heparin IV bolus, then continuous infusion most widely used Pain management

low molecular weight heparin (LMWH), unfractionated heparin (UFH), or fondaparinux. Enoxaparin, a LMWH, should not be used if acute renal failure is present due to reduced excretion, which results in increased anticoagulation effect. Mechanical devices such as TED hose and sequential compression devices are not as effective and are only indicated with patients who have high bleeding risks.

Pulmonary Embolus

One of the most life-threatening complications associated with traumatic fractures is pulmonary embolism (PE). Signs of PE include tachypnea, crackles, accentuated S_2, tachycardia, fever, diaphoresis, S_3 or S_4 gallop, and thrombophlebitis. A patient with PE will present with symptoms of hypoxemia, pleuritic rub, hypotension, tricuspid insufficiency, and right heart failure. Symptoms of PE include unexplained dyspnea, pleuritic chest pain,

apprehension, cough, hemoptysis, diaphoresis, nonpleuritic chest pain, and syncope.

Typical PE presentation in the intensive care unit setting is worsening hypoxemia or hypocapnia in spontaneously ventilating patient or worsening hypoxemia and hypercapnia in a sedated patient on controlled mechanical ventilation. Unexplained fever and sudden increase in pulmonary artery of central venous pressures may also indicate a PE.

Management

Management of PE involves intensive care unit admission, administering supplemental oxygen (usually 100% nonrebreather mask), consideration of thrombolytic therapy treatment, along with the assessment for the possible need for intubation. Additional management includes establishment of venous access, consideration of pulmonary artery catheter need, and initiation of anticoagulant therapy if no contraindications. Pain management should also be considered.

Any patient with confirmed PE should be assessed for possible treatment of thrombolytic therapy The current initial treatment for PE is anticoagulant therapy with LMWH, UFH, or fondaparinux for at least 5 days. Heparin, most commonly delivered as an intravenous bolus followed by continuous infusion, is the most widely used regimen. Long-term therapy would then include a transition to treatment with warfarin.

Infection

Infection is a complication that may be seen with all musculoskeletal injuries. Wound infections, pin site infections with traction or osteomyelitis may occur. Open wounds may be contaminated due to the conditions in which the traumatic injury occurs. Gross wound contamination is common with segmental fracture, soil contamination, and farm and lawnmower injuries or close range shotgun wounds. The infection may be caused from the traumatic injury or infection from other tissues via the bloodstream. Manifestations of osteomyelitis include localized acute bone pain, edema, redness, and warm to touch, fever, and purulent drainage from skin abscess. Diagnostic tests will demonstrate a CBC with elevated white cell count, erythrocyte sedimentation rate (ESR) will be elevated, with positive blood and wound cultures. Definitive diagnosis is made via radiograph verification. Treatment for osteomyelitis includes administration of intravenous antibiotics and surgical aspiration and/or removal of dead bone and surrounding tissue Other infections that may be associated with orthopedic trauma and injuries are soft tissue infections. These typically consist of cellulitis and necrotizing infections. Necrotizing infections consist of necrotizing fasciitis and clostridial myonecrosis (gas gangrene).

Clinical Nurse Specialist Competencies and Spheres of Influence [Header like "Treatment" Key competencies for effective care of patients with musculoskeletal problems and orthopedic injuries have been addressed throughout this chapter. In addition, the requisite competencies for wound infection and sepsis are described in chapter 7 and 15; for DVT, PF and neurovascular compromise in chapter 9; and for compartment syndrome in chapter 12.

References

1. National Association of Clinical Nurse Specialists. Statement on Clinical Nurse Specialist Practice and Education. 2nd edition. Pittsburgh, PA: National Association of Clinical Nurse Specialists; 2004.

2. Centers for Disease Control and Prevention. Prevalence of disabilities and associated health conditions among adults: United States, 1999. MMWR Morb Mortal Wkly Rep 2001;50:120-125.

3. Helmick C, Felson D, Gabriel S, et al. Estimates of the prevalence of arthritis and other rheumatic conditions in the United States. Arthritis Rheum 2008;58(1):15-25.

4. Centers for Disease Control and Prevention. Prevalence of Doctor-Diagnosed Arthritis and Arthritis-Attributable Activity Limitation: United States, 2007—2009 MMWR Morb Mortal Wkly Rep 2006;55(40):1089-1092. Retrieved August 25, 2011 from http://www.cdc.gov/mmwr/preview/mmwrhtml/mm5939a1.htm

5. MMWR Centers for Disease Control and Prevention. National and State Medical Expenditures and Lost Earnings Attributable to Arthritis and Other Rheumatic Conditions—United States, 2003. Morb Mortal Wkly Rep 2007;56(01):4-7. Retrieved August 25, 2011 from http://www.cdc.gov/mmwr/preview/mmwrhtml/mm5601a2.htm

6. Lewis S, Heitkemper M, Dirksen S, et al. Medical Surgical Nursing Assessment and Management of Clinical Problems. 7th edition. St Louis, MO: Mosby; 2007.

7. National Institutes of Health, United States Department of Health and Human Services. National Institute of Arthritis and Musculoskeletal and Skin Diseases. Osteoarthritis. Retrieved August 25, 2011from http://www.niams.nih.gov/Health_Info/Osteoarthritis/default.asp

8. Bartz R, Laudicina L. Osteoarthritis after sports knee injuries. In Lewis S, Heitkemper M, Dirksen S, et al, editors. Medical Surgical Nursing Assessment and Management of Clinical Problems. 7th edition. St Louis, MO: Mosby; 2007

9. WebMD. Pain Management Health Center. Retrieved August 25, 2011 ffrom www.webmd.com/pain-management/nonsteroidal-anti-inflammatory-drugs-nsaids#tv8532

10. Gotzsche PC. Non-steroidal anti-inflammatory drugs. Retrieved from http://www.clinicalevidence.com

11. The Merck Manual Home Health Handbook for Patients and Caregivers. Osteoarthritis. Retrieved August 25, 2011from http://www.merckmanuals.com/home/sec05/ch063/ch063a.html

12. Perron AD, Brady WJ. Evaluation and management of the high risk orthopaedic emergency. Emerg Med Clin North Am 2003; 21:159-204.

13. Olson SA, Rhorer AS. Orthopaedic trauma for the general orthopaedist. Clin Orthop Relat Res 2005;433:30-37.

14. Perron AD, Brady WJ, Keats TE. Orthopedic pitfalls in the ED: acute compartment syndrome. Am J Emerg Med 2001;19(5):413-416.

15. Rudman N, McIlmail D. Emergency department evaluation and treatment of hip and thigh injuries. Emerg Med Clin North Am 2000;18(1):29.

16. Simon R, Sherman S, Koeningsknecht S. Complications in Emergency Orthopedics. 5th edition. New York: McGraw-Hill; 2001.

17. Gustilo RB, Merkow RL, Temleman D. The management of open fractures. J Bone Joint Surg 1990;72A:299-304.

18. Olson SA, Finkemeier CF, Moehring HD. Open fractures. In Bucholz F, Heckman JD, editors. Fractrures in Adults. 5th edition. Philadelphia: Lippincott Williams & Wilkins; 2001:285-317.

19. Ostermann PA, Henry SL, Seligson D. Timing of wound closure in severe compound fractures. Orthopedics 1994;17:397-399.

20. Pape HC, Giannoudis P, Krettek C. The timing of fracture treatment in polytrauma patients: relevance of damage control orthopaedic surgery. Am J Surg 2002;183:622-629.

21. Tile M. Pelvic ring fractures: should they be fixed? J Bone Joint Surg Br 1988;70:1-12.

22. Caviglia HA, Osorio PQ, Comando D. Classification and diagnosis of intracapsular fractures of the proximal femur. Clin Orthop Relat Res 2002;399:17.

23. DeLaMora SN, Gilbert M. Introduction of intracapsular hip fractures: anatomy and pathologic features. Clin Ortoped Relat Res 2002;399:9.

24. American College of Surgeons, Committee on Trauma. Advanced Life Support. 5th edition. Chicago, IL: American College of Surgeons; 1993.

25. Routt ML Jr, Simonian PT, Ballmer F.. A rational approach to pelvic trauma: resuscitation and early definitive stabilization. Clin Orthop 1995;318:61-74.

26. Lee J, Abrahamson BS, Harringon TG, et al. Urologic complications of diastasis of the pubic symphysis: a trauma case report and review of the world literature. J Trauma 2000;48:133-136.

27. Barnes R, Brown JT, Garden RS, et al. Subcapital fractures of the femur: a prospective review. J Bone Joint Surg Br 1976;58(1):2.

28. Swiontkowski MF, MacKenzie EJ, Bosse MJ, et al. Factors influencing the decision to amputate or reconstruct after high-energy lower extremity trauma. J Trauma Inj Infect Crit Care 2002;52(4):641-649.

29. Blick SS, Brumback RJ, Poka A, et al. Compartment syndrome in open tibial fractures. J. Bone Joint Surg Am 1986;68:1348-1353.

30. Singh N, Bluman E, Starnes B, et al. Dynamic wound closure for decompressive leg fasciotomy wounds. *Am Surg* 2008;74:217-220.

31. Geerts WH, Jay RM, et al. A prospective study of venous thromboembolism after major trauma. N Engl J Med 1994;331:1601-1606.

32. Irwin RS. Antithrombotic and thrombolytic therapy: American College of Chest Physicians evidence-based clinical practice guidelines (8th edition). Chest 2008;133(6):67S- 968S.

INDEX

Page numbers in italics indicate figures or tables.